CHILD ABUSE AND NEGLECT
Diagnosis, Treatment, and Evidence

CHILD ABUSE AND NEGLECT
Diagnosis, Treatment, and Evidence

CAROLE JENNY, MD, MBA, EDITOR

Professor of Pediatrics
Warren Alpert Medical School of Brown University;
Director, *ChildSafe* Child Protection Program
Hasbro Children's Hospital
Providence, Rhode Island

Associate Editors:

DEBORAH E. LOWEN, MD
Associate Professor
Director
Child Abuse Pediatrics Program
Department of Pediatrics
Vanderbilt University School of Medicine
Nashville, Tennessee

MARY CLYDE PIERCE, MD
Associate Professor of Pediatrics
Northwestern University Feinberg School of Medicine
Department of Pediatrics
Division of Emergency Medicine
Children's Memorial Hospital
Chicago, Illinois

NANCY D. KELLOGG, MD, FAAP
Professor of Pediatrics
Chief
Division of Child Abuse
University of Texas Health Science Center at San Antonio
San Antonio, Texas

LORI D. FRASIER, MD, FAAP
Professor of Pediatrics (Clinical)
Department of Pediatrics
University of Utah School of Medicine;
Medical Director
Center for Safe and Healthy Families
Primary Children's Medical Center
Salt Lake City, Utah

LISA AMAYA-JACKSON, MD, MPH
Associate Professor of Child and Adolescent Psychiatry
Department of Psychiatry
Duke University School of Medicine
Associate Director
National Center for Child Traumatic Stress
Durham, North Carolina

JUDITH A. COHEN, MD
Professor of Psychiatry
Drexel University School of Medicine
Medical Director
Center for Traumatic Stress in Children
    and Adolescents, Psychiatry
Allegheny General Hospital
Adjunct Assistant Professor
Child Advocacy Center
Department of Pediatrics
Children's Hospital of Pittsburgh
Pittsburgh, Pennsylvania

ANTOINETTE L. LASKEY, MD, MPH, FAAP
Assistant Professor of Pediatrics
Indiana University
Riley Hospital for Children
Indianapolis, Indiana

CHRISTINE E. BARRON, MD, FAAP
Assistant Professor of Pediatrics (Clinical)
The Warren Alpert Medical School of Brown University;
Clinical Director, The Child Protection Program
Hasbro Children's Hospital
Providence, Rhode Island

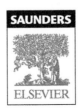

SAUNDERS

ELSEVIER

3251 Riverport Lane
St. Louis, Missouri 63043

CHILD ABUSE AND NEGLECT:
DIAGNOSIS, TREATMENT, AND EVIDENCE

ISBN: 978-1-4160-6393-3

Notices

Knowledge and best practice in this field are constantly changing. As new research and experience broaden our understanding, changes in research methods, professional practices, or medical treatment may become necessary.

Practitioners and researchers must always rely on their own experience and knowledge in evaluating and using any information, methods, compounds, or experiments described herein. In using such information or methods, they should be mindful of their own safety and the safety of others, including parties for whom they have a professional responsibility.

With respect to any drug or pharmaceutical products identified, readers are advised to check the most current information provided (i) on procedures featured or (ii) by the manufacturer of each product to be administered, to verify the recommended dose or formula, the method and duration of administration, and contraindications. It is the responsibility of practitioners, relying on their own experience and knowledge of their patients, to make diagnoses, to determine dosages and the best treatment for each individual patient, and to take all appropriate safety precautions.

To the fullest extent of the law, neither the Publisher nor the authors, contributors, or editors assume any liability for any injury and/or damage to persons or property as a matter of products liability, negligence or otherwise, or from any use or operation of any methods, products, instructions, or ideas contained in the material herein.

Library of Congress Cataloging-in-Publication Data

Child abuse and neglect : diagnosis, treatment, and evidence / [edited by] Carole Jenny.—1st ed.
      p. ; cm.
   Includes bibliographical references.
   ISBN 978-1-4160-6393-3
   1. Abused children.   I. Jenny, Carole.
   [DNLM: 1. Child Abuse–diagnosis.   2. Child Abuse–therapy.   3. Forensic Medicine.
WA 325 C5355 2010]
RJ507.A29C55 2010
618.92'858223–dc22

2010010118

Acquisitions Editor: Judith Fletcher
Associate Developmental Editor: Lora Sickora
Publishing Services Manager: Anne Altepeter
Project Manager/Senior Project Manager: Sukanthi Sukumar/Cheryl A. Abbott
Design Direction: Ellen Zanolle

To Thomas A. Roesler, MD, *husband extraordinaire!*

CONTRIBUTORS

Michelle Amaya, MD, MPH
Associate Professor of Pediatrics
Medical University of South Carolina
Charleston, South Carolina

Lisa Amaya-Jackson, MD, MPH
Associate Professor of Child and Adolescent Psychiatry
Department of Psychiatry
Duke University School of Medicine
Associate Director
National Center for Child Traumatic Stress
Durham, North Carolina

James Anderst, MD, MSCI
Assistant Professor
Department of Pediatrics
University of Missouri at Kansas City
Section Chief
Section on Child Abuse and Neglect
Children's Mercy Hospital and Clinics
Kansas City, Missouri

Kavita M. Babu, MD
Associate Professor
Division of Medical Toxicology
Department of Emergency Medicine
The Warren Alpert Medical School of Brown University
Rhode Island Hospital
Providence, Rhode Island

Christine E. Barron, MD
Assistant Professor of Pediatrics (Clinical)
Department of Pediatrics
The Warren Alpert Medical School of Brown University
Clinical Director
The Child Protection Program
Director
Fellowship Program in Child Abuse Pediatrics
Division of Child Protection
Hasbro Children's Hospital
Providence, Rhode Island

Jan Bays, MD
Child Abuse Examiner
Child Abuse Response and Evaluation Services (CARES) NW
Legacy Emanuel Children's Hospital
Portland, Oregon

Berkeley L. Bennett, MD, MS
Assistant Professor of Clinical Pediatrics
Division of Emergency Medicine
Cincinnati Children's Hospital Medical Center
Cincinnati, Ohio

Susan Bennett, MB, ChB, FRCP
Professor of Pediatrics and Psychiatry
University of Ottawa
Director
Child and Youth Protection Program
Children's Hospital of Eastern Ontario
Ottawa, Canada

Rachel P. Berger, MD, MPH
Assistant Professor of Pediatrics
University of Pittsburgh
Child Advocacy Center
Children's Hospital of Pittsburgh
University of Pittsburgh Medical Center
Pittsburgh, Pennsylvania

Gina Bertocci, PhD, PE
Professor
Department of Mechanical Engineering
Endowed Chair of Biomechanics
University of Louisville
Louisville, Kentucky

Maureen M. Black, PhD
John A. Scholl, MD, and Mary Louise Scholl, MD, Professor, Pediatrics
University of Maryland School of Medicine
Baltimore, Maryland

Robert W. Block, MD, FAAP
Daniel C. Plunket Chair
Department of Pediatrics
University of Oklahoma–Tulsa
Tulsa, Oklahoma

Stephen C. Boos, MD, FAAP
Assistant Professor
Department of Pediatrics
Tuft's University Medical School
Medical Director
Family Advocacy Center and Child Protection Team
Baystate Medical Center
Springfield Medical Center
Springfield, Massachusetts

Daniel D. Broughton, MD
Professor of Pediatrics and Adolescent Medicine
Department of Pediatric and Adolescent Medicine
Mayo Clinic
Rochester, Minnesota

Roger W. Byard, MD
Marks Chair of Pathology
Discipline of Pathology
The University of Adelaide
Senior Forensic Pathologist
Forensic Sciences SA
Adelaide, Australia

Kristine A. Campbell, MD, MSc
Assistant Professor
Department of Pediatrics
University of Utah
Center for Safe and Healthy Families
Primary Children's Medical Center
Salt Lake City, Utah

David L. Chadwick, MD
Director Emeritus
Chadwick Center for Children and Families
Rady Children's Hospital San Diego
San Diego, California

Kimberle C. Chapin, MD
Associate Professor
Department of Pathology and Laboratory Medicine
The Warren Albert Medical School of Brown University
Director of Microbiology
Lifespan Academic Medical Centers
Providence, Rhode Island

Brittany Coats, PhD
Assistant Professor
Department of Mechanical Engineering
Department of Pediatrics
University of Utah
Salt Lake City, Utah

Judith A. Cohen, MD
Professor
Department of Psychiatry
Drexel University College of Medicine
Medical Director
Center for Traumatic Stress in Children
   and Adolescents, Psychiatry
Allegheny General Hospital
Adjunct Assistant Professor
Child Advocacy Center
Pediatrics, Children's Hospital of Pittsburgh
Pittsburgh, Pennsylvania

David L. Corwin, MD
Professor and Chief
Child Protection and Family Health Division
Department of Pediatrics
University of Utah School of Medicine
Medical Director
Primary Children's Center for Safe and Healthy Families
Primary Children's Medical Center
Salt Lake City, Utah

Theresa M. Covington, MPH
Executive Director
National Center for Child Death Review
Michigan Public Health Institute
Washington, DC

Joseph C. Crozier, MD, PhD
Fellow
Division of Child and Adolescent Psychiatry
Duke University Hospital
Durham, North Carolina

Melissa L. Currie, MD
Director
Division of Forensic Medicine
Assistant Professor
Department of Pediatrics
University of Louisville School of Medicine
Louisville, Kentucky

Michael D. De Bellis, MD, MPH
Professor of Psychiatry and Behavioral Sciences
Psychiatry and Behavioral Sciences
Duke University Medical Center
Durham, North Carolina

Allan R. De Jong, MD
Clinical Professor
Department of Pediatrics
Jefferson Medical College of Thomas Jefferson University
Philadelphia, Pennsylvania;
Director
Children and Risk Evaluation (CARE) Program
Department of Pediatrics
Nemours-Alfred I. duPont Hospital for Children
Wilmington, Delaware;
Medical Director
Children's Advocacy Center of Delaware
Wilmington, Dover, and Georgetown, Delaware

Katherine P. Deye, MD
Child Abuse Pediatrician
Freddie Mac Foundation Child and Adolescent
   Protection Center
Children's National Medical Center
Washington, DC

Mark S. Dias, MD, FAAP
Professor of Neurosurgery and Pediatrics
Department of Neurosurgery
Penn State University College of Medicine
Vice Chair of Clinical Neurosurgery and Director
   of Pediatric Neurosurgery
Penn State Milton S. Hershey Medical Center
Hershey, Pennsylvania

Howard Dubowitz, MD, MS
Professor of Pediatrics
Chief
Division of Child Protection
University of Maryland School of Medicine
Baltimore, Maryland

Thomas L. Dwyer, MA
Director
Office of Foster Care and Adoption Services
Department of Children and Families,
    State of Connecticut
Hartford, Connecticut
Director of Child Welfare Services (Retired)
Department of Children, Youth, and Families
    State of Rhode Island
Providence, Rhode Island

Peter T. Evangelista, MD
Assistant Professor of Diagnostic Imaging
The Warren Alpert Medical School of Brown University
Director of Musculoskeletal Radiology
Department of Diagnostic Imaging
Rhode Island and Hasbro Children's Hospitals
Providence, Rhode Island

Linda Ewing-Cobbs, PhD
Director
Dan L. Duncan Children's Neurodevelopmental Clinic
Professor of Pediatrics and Psychiaty and Behavioral Sciences
Children's Learning Institute
The University of Texas Health Science Center at Houston
Houston, Texas

Russell A. Faust, PhD, MD, FAAP
Assistant Professor
Oral Biology
Ohio State University
Columbus, Ohio
Otolaryngologist
Neurosciences Institute and Craniofacial Institute
Ascension Health Michigan
Providence Park Hospital
Novi, Ohio

Kenneth Feldman, MD
Clinical Professor of Pediatrics
Department of Pediatrics
General Pediatric Division
University of Washington School of Medicine
Medical Director, Children's Protection Program
Seattle Children's Hospital
Seattle, Washington

Martin A. Finkel, DO
Professor of Pediatrics
Medical Director
Child Abuse Research Education and Service (CARES) Institute
University of Medicine and Dentistry of New Jersey
School of Osteopathic Medicine
Stratford, New Jersey

Emalee G. Flaherty, MD
Associate Professor
Department of Pediatrics
Northwestern University Feinberg School of Medicine
Medical Director
Protective Service Team
Department of Pediatrics
Children's Memorial Hospital
Chicago, Illinois

Kristine Fortin, MD, MPH
Teaching Fellow
Department of Pediatrics
The Warren Alpert Medical School of Brown University
Fellow
Child Abuse Pediatrics
Hasbro Children's Hospital
Providence, Rhode Island

Lori D. Frasier, MD, FAAP
Professor of Pediatrics (Clinical)
Department of Pediatrics
University of Utah School of Medicine
Medical Director
Medical Assessment Team
Center for Safe and Healthy Families
Primary Children's Medical Center
Salt Lake City, Utah

Nathan W. Galbreath, PhD, MFS
Licensed Clinical Psychologist
Forensic Science Specialist
Professorial Lecturer in Forensic Sciences
Department of Forensic Sciences
The George Washington University
Washington, DC

Rebecca Girardet, MD
Associate Professor and CARE Center Medical Director
Department of Pediatrics
The University of Texas–Houston Medical School
Pediatrician
Children's Memorial Hermann Hospital–Houston
Medical Director
The Forensic Assessment Center Network
Houston, Texas

Amy P. Goldberg, MD
Assistant Professor
Department of Pediatrics
The Warren Alpert Medical School of Brown University
Attending Physician
Department of Pediatrics
Child Protection Program
Hasbro Children's Hospital
Providence, Rhode Island

Arne H. Graff, MD
Associate Professor of Pediatrics
Department of Pediatrics
University of North Dakota School of Medicine
Grand Forks, North Dakota
Staff Consultant
Department of Pediatrics
Altru Health Systems
Grand Forks, North Dakota
Medical Director
Department of Pediatrics
Child and Adolescent Maltreatment Services
Fargo, North Dakota

Christopher S. Greeley, MD
Associate Professor
Department of Pediatrics
University of Texas Health Sciences Center at Houston
Children's Memorial Hermann Hospital
Houston, Texas

Elisabeth Guenther, MD, MPH
Associate Professor
Department of Pediatrics
Division of Pediatric Emergency Medicine
University of Utah School of Medicine
Attending Physician
Department of Pediatric Emergency Medicine
Primary Children's Medical Center
Salt Lake City, Utah

Nancy S. Harper, MD
Assistant Professor of Pediatrics
Department of Pediatrics
Texas A&M
College Station
Medical Director
CARE Team, Driscoll Children's Hospital
Corpus Christi, Texas

Tara L. Harris, MD
Assistant Professor of Clinical Pediatrics
Indiana University School of Medicine
Riley Hospital for Children
Indianapolis, Indiana

Rhea M. Haugseth, DMD
Private Practice
Post Oak Pediatric Dentistry
Marietta, Georgia

Sandra M. Herr, MD
Associate Professor of Pediatrics
Division of Pediatric Emergency Medicine
University of Louisville
Medical Director
Pediatric Emergency Medicine
Kosair Children's Hospital
Louisville, Kentucky

Stephen R. Hooper, PhD
Professor
Department of Psychiatry and Pediatrics
University of North Carolina School of Medicine
Associate Director
Center for Development and Learning
The University of North Carolina School of Medicine
Chapel Hill, North Carolina

Mark J. Hudson, MD
Child Abuse Pediatrician
Midwest Children's Resource Center
Children's Hospital and Clinics of Minnesota, St. Paul
Adjunct Instructor
Pediatrics, University of Minnesota
Minneapolis, Minnesota

Tammy Piazza Hurley, BA
Manager
Child Abuse and Neglect, Community and Specialty Pediatrics
American Academy of Pediatrics
Elk Grove Village, Illinois

Kent P. Hymel, MD
Professor of Pediatrics
Dartmouth Medical School
Hanover, New Hampshire
Medical Director, Child Advocacy and Protection Program
The Children's Hospital at Dartmouth–Hitchcock
    Medical Center
Lebanon, New Hampshire

Reena Isaac, MD
Assistant Professor of Pediatrics
Baylor College of Medicine
Attending Physician
Child Protection Section of Emergency Medicine Service
Texas Children's Hospital
Houston, Texas

Allison M. Jackson, MD, MPH
Associate Professor of Pediatrics
Department of Pediatrics
George Washington University School of Medicine
    and Health Sciences
Division Director
Freddie Mac Foundation Child and Adolescent
    Protection Center
Children's National Medical Center
Washington, DC

Brian M. Jackson, MD
Pediatric Resident
Department of Pediatrics
University of Colorado School of Medicine
The Children's Hospital
Aurora, Colorado

Carole Jenny, MD, MBA
Professor of Pediatrics
The Warren Alpert Medical School of Brown University
Director, *ChildSafe* Child Protection Program
Hasbro Children's Hospital
Providence, Rhode Island

Kim Kaczor, MS
Clinical Research Coordinator
Department of Pediatrics
Division of Emergency Medicine
Children's Memorial Hospital
Chicago, Illinois

Rich Kaplan, MD
Associate Professor
Department of Pediatrics
University of Minnesota
Minneapolis, Minnesota
Director, Center for Safe and Healthy Children
University of Minnesota
Clinician, Child Abuse Pediatric Group
Children's Hospital and Clinics of Minnesota
Minneapolis, Minnesota

Heather T. Keenan, MDCM, PhD
Associate Professor
Division of Critical Care
Department of Pediatrics
University of Utah
Salt Lake City, Utah

Brooks R. Keeshin, MD
Resident
Department of Pediatrics
Adult and Child Psychiatry
University of Utah School of Medicine
Salt Lake City, Utah

Nancy D. Kellogg, MD, FAAP
Professor of Pediatrics
Chief, Division of Child Abuse
University of Texas Health Science Center at San Antonio
San Antonio, Texas

John P. Kenney, DDS, MS, D-ABFO
Attending Physician
Department of Surgery/Division of Dentistry
Lutheran General Hospital and Children's Hospital
Park Ridge, Illinois
Deputy Coroner
DuPage County, Illinois Coroner's Office
Wheaton, Illinois

Kevin P. Kent, MD
Fellow in Medical Toxicology
Department of Emergency Medicine
University of Massachusetts
Worcester, Massachusetts

Barbara L. Knox, MD, FAAP
Assistant Professor
Department of Pediatrics
University of Wisconsin School of Medicine and Public Health
Medical Director
American Family Children's Hospital Child Protection Program
Madison, Wisconsin

David J. Kolko, PhD, ABPP
Professor of Psychiatry, Psychology, and Pediatrics
University of Pittsburgh School of Medicine;
Director
Special Services Unit
Western Psychiatric Institute and Clinic
Pittsburgh, Pennsylvania

Rachel P. Kolko, BA
Graduate Program in Clinical Psychology
Department of Psychology
Washington University
St. Louis, Missouri

Vesna Martich Kriss, MD
Educational Director
Kosair Children's Hospital
Department of Radiology
Professor
Department of Radiology and Pediatrics
University of Louisville School of Medicine
Louisville, Kentucky

Henry F. Krous, MD
Clinical Professor of Pathology and Pediatrics
University of California
San Diego College of Medicine–La Jolla
Director of Research
Department of Pathology
Rady Children's Hospital
Director
San Diego SIDS/SUDC Research Project
San Diego, California

Antoinette L. Laskey, MD, MPH, FAAP
Assistant Professor of Pediatrics
Department of Pediatrics
Indiana University
Riley Hospital for Children
Indianapolis, Indiana

Alex V. Levin, MD, MHSc, FAAP, FAAO, FRCSC
Professor
Department of Ophthalmology
Jefferson Medical College of Thomas Jefferson University
Chief
Pediatric Ophthalmology and Ocular Genetics
Wills Eye Institute
Philadelphia, Pennsylvania

Carolyn J. Levitt, MD
Professor
Department of Pediatrics
University of Minnesota
Minneapolis, Minnesota
Director
The Midwest Children's Resource Center
Children's Hospitals and Clinics of Minnesota
St. Paul and Minneapolis, Minnesota

Alicia F. Lieberman, PhD
Irving B. Harris Endowed Chair in Infant Mental Health
Department of Psychiatry
University of California–San Francisco
Director
Child Trauma Research Project
San Francisco General Hospital
San Francisco, California

Deborah E. Lowen, MD
Associate Professor
Director
Child Abuse Pediatrics Program
Department of Pediatrics
Vanderbilt University School of Medicine
Nashville, Tennessee

Kathi L. Makoroff, MD
Assistant Professor of Pediatrics
Department of Pediatrics
University of Cincinnati College of Medicine
Fellowship Director
Child Abuse Pediatrics
Mayerson Center for Safe and Healthy Children
Cincinnati Children's Hospital Medical Center
Cincinnati, Ohio

Susan Margulies, PhD
Professor
Department of Bioengineering
University of Pennsylvania
Philadelphia, Pennsylvania

Shelly D. Martin, MD
Assistant Professor of Pediatrics
Uniformed Services University of the Health Sciences
Child Abuse Physician
Walter Reed National Military Medical Center
Washington, DC

Kenneth McCann, MD, FAAP
Clinical Director
Regional Child Protection Center
Blank Children's Hospital
Des Moines, Iowa

Kathleen M. McCarten, MD, FACR
Associate Professor of Diagnostic Imaging
    and Pediatrics (Clinical)
The Warren Alpert Medical School of Brown University
Staff Radiologist
Diagnostic Imaging
Hasbro Children's Hospital
Rhode Island Hospital;
Staff Radiologist
Diagnostic Imaging
Women and Infants Hospital
Providence, Rhode Island

Megan L. McGraw, MD
Assistant Professor of Clinical Pediatrics
Department of Pediatrics
The Ohio State University College of Medicine
Assistant Professor of Clinical Pediatrics
Center for Child and Family Advocacy
Nationwide Children's Hospital
Columbus, Ohio

Sarah E. Oberlander, PhD
Post-Doctoral Fellow
Department of Pediatrics
University of Maryland School of Medicine
Baltimore, Maryland

Vincent J. Palusci, MD, MS
Professor of Pediatrics
Department of Pediatrics
New York University School of Medicine
Chair
Child Protection Committee
New York University Langone Center
Research Director
Frances L. Loeb Child Protection and Development Center
Bellevue Hospital Center
New York, New York

Karyn M. Patno, MD
Clinical Assistant Professor
Department of Pediatrics
University of Vermont Medical School
Consulting Physician in Child Abuse Pediatrics
Department of Pediatrics
Fletcher Allen Health Care
Burlington, Vermont
Staff Pediatrician
Department of Pediatrics
Northeastern Vermont Regional Hospital
St. Johnsbury, Vermont

Mary Clyde Pierce, MD
Associate Professor of Pediatrics
Northwestern University Feinberg School of Medicine
Pediatrics (Division of Emergency Medicine)
Children's Memorial Hospital
Chicago, Illinois

Mary R. Prasad, PhD
Assistant Professor of Pediatrics
Department of Pediatrics
The University of Texas Health Science Center at Houston
Houston, Texas

Kimberly A. Randell, MD, MSc
Attending Physician
Department of Pediatrics
Division of Emergency Medicine
Children's Mercy Hospital
Assistant Professor of Pediatrics
University of Missouri–Kansas City School of Medicine
Kansas City, Missouri

Lawrence R. Ricci, MD, FAAP
Associate Clinical Professor of Pediatrics
University of Vermont College of Medicine
Attending Pediatrician
Barbara Bush Children's Hospital
Co-Director
Spurwink Child Abuse Program
Portland, Maine

Thomas A. Roesler, MD
Associate Professor
Division of Child and Family Psychiatry
The Warren Alpert Medical School of Brown University
Co-Director
Hasbro Children's Partial Hospital Program
Hasbro Children's Hospital
Providence, Rhode Island

Lucy B. Rorke-Adams, MD
Clinical Professor of Pathology, Neurology, and Pediatrics
University of Pennsylvania School of Medicine
Senior Neuropathologist
Department of Clinical Laboratories and Anatomical Pathology
The Children's Hospital of Philadelphia
Consultant Forensic Neuropathologist
Office of the Medical Examiner
Philadelphia, Pennsylvania

Desmond K. Runyan, MD, DrPH
Professor
Social Medicine
The University of North Carolina
Attending Physician
Department of Pediatrics
North Carolina Children's Hospitals
Chapel Hill, North Carolina

Mark V. Sapp, MD
Instructor
Department of Pediatrics
Harvard Medical School
Complex Care Services
Children's Hospital Boston
Boston, Massachusetts

Patricia G. Schnitzer, PhD
Assistant Professor
Sinclair School of Nursing
University of Missouri
Columbia, Missouri

Philip V. Scribano, DO, MSCE
Chief
Division of Child and Family Advocacy
Associate Professor
Department of Pediatrics
The Ohio State University College of Medicine
Medical Director
Center for Child and Family Advocacy
Nationwide Children's Hospital
Columbus, Ohio

Rizwan Z. Shah, MD
Clinical Associate Professor
Pediatrics
University of Iowa
Carver College of Medicine
Iowa City, Iowa
Medical Director
Regional Child Protection Center
Blank Children's Hospital
Des Moines, Iowa

Meghan Shanahan, MPH
Doctoral Candidate
Maternal and Child Health
University of North Carolina Gillings School
    of Global Public Health
Chapel Hill, North Carolina

Andrew P. Sirotnak, MD, FAAP
Professor
Department of Pediatrics
University of Colorado School of Medicine
Director
Kempe Child Protection Team
The Children's Hospital
Aurora, Colorado

Katherine R. Snyder, MD, MPH
Fellow in Child Abuse Pediatrics
Department of Pediatrics
The Warren Alpert Medical School of Brown University
Teaching Fellow
Hasbro Children's Hospital
Providence, Rhode Island

Suzanne P. Starling, MD
Professor of Pediatrics
Eastern Virginia Medical School
Medical Director
Child Abuse Program
Children's Hospital of the King's Daughters
Norfolk, Virginia

Deborah Stewart, MD, FAAP
Section Chief and Medical Director
Department of Pediatrics
CAARE Diagnostic and Treatment Center
University of California–Davis Children's Hospital
Sacramento, California

Tanya F. Stockhammer, PhD
StrongMinds Child and Adolescent Psychology Specialists
Louisville, Kentucky

Rita Swan, PhD
President
Children's Healthcare is a Legal Duty
Sioux City, Iowa

Alice D. Swenson, MD
Assistant Professor
Department of Pediatrics
Medical College of Wisconsin
Staff Pediatrician
Child Advocacy and Protection Services Program
Children's Hospital of Wisconsin
Milwaukee, Wisconsin

Jonathan D. Thackeray, MD
Assistant Professor
Clinical Pediatrics
Department of Pediatrics
Center for Child and Family Advocacy
Nationwide Children's Hospital
Columbus, Ohio

Glenn A. Tung, MD, FACR
Professor of Diagnostic Imaging
The Warren Alpert Medical School of Brown University
Director
Division of Diagnostic Imaging
Rhode Island Hospital
Providence, Rhode Island

Patricia Van Horn, JD, PhD
Associate Clinical Professor
Psychiatry
University of California—San Francisco
Adjunct Professor
School of Law
University of San Francisco
San Francisco, California

Elizabeth E. Van Voorhees, PhD
Assistant Professor
Department of Psychiatry and Behavioral Sciences
Duke University Medical Center
Assistant Professor
Mental Illness Research, Education, and Clinical Center
Veterans Affairs Medical Center
Durham, North Carolina

Nichole G. Wallace, MD
Clinical Assistant Professor
Pediatrics
University of Oklahoma College of Medicine
Tulsa, Oklahoma

Adam J. Zolotor, MD, MPH
Assistant Professor
Department of Family Medicine
University of North Carolina at Chapel Hill
Chapel Hill, North Carolina

This book addresses a very difficult topic—child abuse and neglect. Almost every photograph and case study in the book represents a real-life tragedy—a child who needlessly suffered or died. Although recording and reporting their stories is necessary to educate health professionals and others, we continue to be reminded of the extraordinary amount of human suffering contained within the book's covers.

In 2009 the first cadre of board-certified child abuse pediatricians was recognized by the American Board of Pediatrics. This group of pediatricians has worked for many years to develop the subspecialty, dedicating their careers to the diagnosis, treatment, and prevention of child maltreatment. Knowledge in this field has exploded over the past 47 years since C. Henry Kempe published his landmark paper on "The Battered Child Syndrome." Although several excellent textbooks on medical aspects of child abuse are available, we believe this comprehensive volume will contribute significantly as a resource of evidence-based knowledge for the new subspecialty.

Child abuse and neglect were not thought of as "medical" problems until the 1960s. Since that time, an enormous amount of clinical research has led to a more sophisticated knowledge of the intersection between medicine and child maltreatment. The National Library of Medicine added the subject heading, "Child Abuse," to its catalog in 1963. That year, 12 articles were categorized as pertaining to child abuse. Currently approximately 600 articles are cataloged under the heading "Child Abuse" each year.

The National Association of Children's Hospitals and Related Institutions has recognized the importance of child maltreatment in pediatric medicine. In 2006 the organization published guidelines for children's hospitals' child protection teams, advising that every children's hospital should house a formal program to diagnose and treat child abuse.

The extraordinary effect that child maltreatment has over the lifespan has been overwhelmingly demonstrated. For example, the Adverse Childhood Experiences study done at the University of California–San Diego showed that childhood events such as experiencing physical abuse, sexual abuse, psychological abuse, and neglect increase the chances of an adult developing a wide variety of illnesses, including heart and lung disease, obesity, liver disease, and depression.

Adverse childhood events also were associated with disability and early death.

At this point, child maltreatment is as much a *medical* problem as it is a *social* problem. The active participation of health professionals in identifying, treating, and preventing child abuse and neglect has become imperative. Thus, this book was conceived to provide a complete overview of the crossroads of medicine and child maltreatment.

The book is divided into eight sections. The first section discusses the epidemiology of child abuse and neglect. The second section concentrates on interviewing children and families. The third section addresses sexual abuse, followed by a section on sexually transmitted diseases. Physical child abuse is covered in Section V. Section VI, containing 10 chapters, specifically addresses aspects of abusive head trauma. Section VII covers psychological aspects of child maltreatment, including diagnosis, treatments, and outcomes. The final section is a collection of 16 "special topics" that did not fit into any other category but nevertheless are important to address, such as child death review, failure to thrive, prevention of abuse and neglect, and medical child abuse.

Although the book was written as a *medical* text, there is much in this volume that will be helpful to other professionals who work with abused and neglected children, including attorneys, social workers, mental health professionals, law enforcement officers, and social service administrators. Our aim with this book is to create a "one-stop shopping" source of information on all aspects of child maltreatment. One noticeable omission is our lack of information on legal aspects of child protection. Fortunately, there are several outstanding texts and periodicals in existence that cover this topic extensively.

When possible, we strived to put the information in each chapter into context by commenting on the strength of the medical evidence and pointing out areas for which future research should be directed. Although controversy persists around many topics in child protection, the book demonstrates that there is extensive literature based on research and practice that is available to professionals in the field. We have attempted to put information from the best of this literature into a single volume.

Carole Jenny MD, MBA

This book represents the combined efforts of a magnificent team of editors and authors. The most important contributors were the eight associate editors—Deborah Lowen, Mary Clyde Pierce, Nancy Kellogg, Lisa Amaya-Jackson, Judith Cohen, Lori Frasier, Antoinette Laskey, and Christine Barron. Each took on one section of the book and worked with the authors to produce carefully researched and edited chapters. Their work has made this book complete and thorough. I cannot help but mention that this book is a post-feminist milestone. Although I did not set out to produce a book with an all-female editorial staff, I am proud that our editorial group of strong, intelligent women worked together so well!

I appreciate the patience and encouragement of our editor at Elsevier, Collen McGonigal. Working with her was a pleasure, and her efforts to make this a successful project are appreciated. Also deserving kudos is my secretary, Laurie Sawyer, who made sure chapters and correspondence went out in a timely fashion.

The authors of the 70 chapters also deserve an immense "thank you" for their efforts. They represent a geographically diverse collection of experts from 34 states and the District of Columbia, as well as Canada and Australia. I sought out people who are actively engaged in the field of child abuse pediatrics and related disciplines. To the person, they were cooperative, enthusiastic, and productive. I relied heavily on my current and past fellows from fellowship programs I have directed in Washington, Colorado, and Rhode Island. I am very proud of the contributions they have made to the book and to the profession.

Finally, this book would never have been completed without the encouragement and support of my family, including daughters Laura Roesler and Amelia Burke; granddaughter Nyssa Ann Burke; and husband, Tom Roesler. They were very patient with me when I spent evenings and weekends at the office working on this project.

Carole Jenny

CONTENTS

I Epidemiology of Child Maltreatment   1
Antoinette L. Laskey, MD, MPH, FAAP

1 Epidemiological Issues in Child Maltreatment Research, Surveillance, and Reporting   3
Antoinette L. Laskey, MD, MPH, FAAP

2 Epidemiology of Physical Abuse   10
Adam J. Zolotor, MD, MPH, and Meghan Shanahan, MPH

3 Epidemiology of Sexual Abuse   16
Vincent J. Palusci, MD, MS

4 Epidemiology of Intimate Partner Violence   23
Jonathan D. Thackeray, MD, and Kimberly A. Randell, MD, MSc

5 Epidemiology of Child Neglect   28
Howard Dubowitz, MD, MS

6 Epidemiology of Abusive Head Trauma   35
Heather T. Keenan, MDCM, PhD

II Interviewing   39
Nancy D. Kellogg, MD

7 Interviewing Children and Adolescents About Suspected Abuse   41
Nancy D. Kellogg, MD

8 Interviewing Caregivers of Suspected Child Abuse Victims   51
Katherine R. Snyder, MD, MPH, Melissa L. Currie, MD, and Tanya F. Stockhammer, PhD

III Sexual Abuse of Children   61
Nancy D. Kellogg, MD, FAAP

9 Physical Examination of the Child When Sexual Abuse Is Suspected   63
Reena Isaac, MD

10 Normal and Developmental Variations in the Anogenital Examination of Children   69
Nichole G. Wallace, MD, and Michelle Amaya, MD, MPH

11 Physical Findings in Children and Adolescents Experiencing Sexual Abuse or Assault   82
Deborah Stewart, MD, FAAP

12 Medical Conditions with Genital/Anal Findings That Can Be Confused with Sexual Abuse   93
Mark J. Hudson, MD, Alice D. Swenson, MD, Rich Kaplan, MD, and Carolyn J. Levitt, MD

13 The Forensic Evidence Kit   106
James Anderst, MD, MSCI

14 Tests Used to Analyze Forensic Evidence in Cases of Child Sexual Abuse and Assault   112
Allan R. De Jong, MD

15 Drug-Facilitated Sexual Assault   118
Nancy S. Harper, MD

16 Adolescent Sexual Assault and Statutory Rape   127
Martin A. Finkel, DO, and Mark V. Sapp, MD

17 Female Genital Mutilation/Cutting   134
Susan Bennett, MB, ChB, FRCP

18 Internet Child Sexual Exploitation   142
Daniel D. Broughton, MD

19 Evaluating Images in Child Pornography   147
Shelly D. Martin, MD

20 Child Molesters   152
Nathan W. Galbreath, PhD, MFS

IV   Sexually Transmitted Infections in Children—Epidemiology, Diagnosis, and Treatment   167
Lori D. Frasier, MD, FAAP

21   Nonsexually Transmitted Infections of the Genitalia and Anus of Prepubertal Children   169
Andrew P. Sirotnak, MD, FAAP

22   Bacterial Sexually Transmitted Infections in Children   174
Rebecca Girardet, MD

23   Viral and Parasitic Sexually Transmitted Infections in Children   179
Arne H. Graff, MD, and Laurie D. Frasier, MD, FAAP

24   HIV and AIDS in Child and Adolescent Victims of Sexual Abuse and Assault   186
Amy P. Goldberg, MD

25   Laboratory Methods for Diagnosing Sexually Transmitted Infections in Children and Adolescents   193
Kimberle C. Chapin, MD

V   Physical Abuse of Children   207
Mary Clyde Pierce, MD

26   Documenting the Medical History in Cases of Possible Physical Child Abuse   209
Allison M. Jackson, MD, MPH, and Brian M. Jackson, MD

27   Photodocumentation in Child Abuse Cases   215
Lawrence R. Ricci, MD, FAAP

28   Abusive Burns   222
Barbara L. Knox, MD, FAAP, and Suzanne P. Starling, MD

29   Bruises and Skin Lesions   239
Tara L. Harris, MD, and Emalee G. Flaherty, MD

30   Skin Conditions Confused with Child Abuse   252
Kathi L. Makoroff, MD, and Megan L. McGraw, MD

31   Bone Health and Development   260
Berkeley L. Bennett, MD, MS, and Mary Clyde Pierce, MD

32   Abusive Fractures   275
Kim Kaczor, MS, and Mary Clyde Pierce, MD

33   Imaging of Skeletal Trauma in Abused Children   296
Vesna Martich Kriss, MD

34   The Role of Cross-Sectional Imaging in Evaluating Pediatric Skeletal Trauma   308
Peter T. Evangelista, MD, and Kathleen M. McCarten, MD, FACR

35   Long Bone Fracture Biomechanics   317
Gina Bertocci, PhD, PE

36   Abdominal and Chest Injuries in Abused Children   326
Sandra M. Herr, MD

37   Ear, Nose, and Throat Injuries in Abused Children   332
Philip V. Scribano, DO, MSCE, and Russell A. Faust, PhD, MD, FAAP

38   Sudden Infant Death Syndrome or Asphyxia?   337
Henry F. Krous, MD, and Roger W. Byard, MD

VI   Abusive Head Trauma   347
Deborah E. Lowen, MD

39   Abusive Head Trauma   349
Kent P. Hymel, MD, and Katherine P. Deye, MD

40   Biomechanics of Head Trauma in Infants and Young Children   359
Susan Margulies, PhD, and Brittany Coats, PhD

41   The Case for Shaking   364
Mark S. Dias, MD, FAAP

42   Imaging of Abusive Head Trauma   373
Glenn A. Tung, MD, FACR

43   Neck and Spinal Cord Injuries in Child Abuse   392
Stephen C. Boos, MD, FAAP, and Kenneth Feldman, MD

44   Eye Injuries in Child Abuse   402
Alex V. Levin, MD, MHSc, FAAP, FAAO, FRCSC

45   Neuropathology of Abusive Head Trauma   413
Lucy B. Rorke-Adams, MD

46   Biochemical Markers of Head Trauma in Children   429
Rachel P. Berger, MD, MPH

47 Conditions Confused with Head
   Trauma   441
   Christopher S. Greeley, MD

48 Outcome of Abusive Head Trauma   451
   Linda Ewing-Cobbs, PhD, and Mary R. Prasad, PhD

VII Psychological Aspects of Child
   Maltreatment   459
   Lisa Amaya-Jackson, MD, MPH, and
   Judith A. Cohen, MD

49 Psychological Impact and Treatment of Sexual
   Abuse of Children   461
   Brooks R. Keeshin, MD, and David L. Corwin, MD

50 Psychological Impact and Treatment of
   Physical Abuse of Children   476
   David J. Kolko, PhD, ABPP, and Rachel P. Kolko, BA

51 Psychological Impact and Treatment of
   Neglect of Children   490
   Maureen M. Black, PhD, and Sarah E. Oberlander, PhD

52 Psychological Impact on and Treatment of
   Children Who Witness Domestic
   Violence   501
   Patricia Van Horn, JD, PhD, and
   Alicia F. Lieberman, PhD

53 Effects of Abuse and Neglect on Brain
   Development   516
   Joseph C. Crozier, MD, PhD,
   Elizabeth E. Van Voorhees, PhD,
   Stephen R. Hooper, PhD, and
   Michael D. De Bellis, MD, MPH

VIII Special Topics   527
   Christine E. Barron, MD, and
   Carole Jenny, MD, MBA

54 Substance Abuse and Child Abuse   529
   Rizwan Z. Shah, MD, and Kenneth McCann, MD, FAAP

55 Definitions and Categorization of
   Child Neglect   539
   Christine E. Barron, MD, and
   Carole Jenny, MD, MBA

56 Dental Neglect   544
   Rhea M. Haugseth, DMD

57 Failure to Thrive   547
   Deborah E. Lowen, MD

58 Detecting Drugs in Infants and
   Children   563
   Kevin P. Kent, MD, and Kavita M. Babu, MD

59 Injuries Resulting from Falls   570
   David L. Chadwick, MD, Gina Bertocci, PhD, PE,
   and Elisabeth Guenther, MD, MPH

60 Forensic Dentistry   579
   John P. Kenney, DDS, MS, D-ABFO

61 Medical Child Abuse   586
   Thomas A. Roesler, MD

62 Child Death Review   592
   Patricia G. Schnitzer, PhD, and
   Theresa M. Covington, MPH

63 Religion and Child Neglect   599
   Rita Swan, PhD

64 The Prevention of Child Abuse and
   Neglect   605
   Karyn M. Patno, MD

65 Caring for Foster Children   610
   Kristine Fortin, MD, MPH

66 The Response of Professional and Other
   Nonprofit Organizations to Child
   Maltreatment   615
   Robert W. Block, MD, FAAP, and
   Tammy Piazza Hurley, BA

67 International Issues in Child
   Maltreatment   620
   Desmond K. Runyan, MD, DrPH, and
   Adam J. Zolotor, MD, MPH

68 The Essentials of an Effective Child Welfare
   System   628
   Thomas L. Dwyer, MA

69 The Costs of Child Maltreatment   634
   Kristine A. Campbell, MD, MSc

70 Caring for the Caretakers   641
   Jan Bays, MD

CHILD ABUSE AND NEGLECT
Diagnosis, Treatment, and Evidence

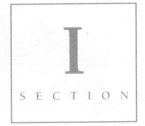

EPIDEMIOLOGY OF CHILD MALTREATMENT

Antoinette L. Laskey, MD, MPH

EPIDEMIOLOGICAL ISSUES IN CHILD MALTREATMENT RESEARCH, SURVEILLANCE, AND REPORTING

Antoinette L. Laskey, MD, MPH

INTRODUCTION

The science of medicine requires knowledge of more than just the effects of a disease process on the individual. A grasp of the epidemiology of a disease is necessary for clinicians to achieve a more complete understanding of the afflictions of their patients. In empirical samples, an *n* of 1 may not prove to be a valid data point. This is where the science of epidemiology steps in. This chapter covers the basics of epidemiology and issues that often challenge researchers in the area of family violence. The chapters that follow in this section will then more fully explore what is known about the epidemiology of family violence.

Defined by Merriam-Webster as "A branch of medical science that deals with the incidence, distribution, and control of disease in a population," or, "The sum of the factors controlling the presence or absence of a disease or pathogen," epidemiology can aid the clinician with a more complete understanding of a person's disease, and answers many different types of questions about diseases. (See Table 1-1.) The epidemiology of a disease covers a broad range of information that can be helpful in determining who is at risk for a given condition. When epidemiological data are gathered or interpreted incorrectly, those data can be misleading to clinicians. It is important to remember that a risk factor for a condition is different than a risk factor for an outcome. For example, high blood pressure is a risk factor for heart disease; low blood pressure during a heart attack is a risk factor for an adverse outcome.

For clinicians who care for victims of family violence, it is useful to know which families are at most risk and what factors are most amenable to intervention and prevention. Given that it is often difficult or impossible to obtain the history from an impartial witness when presented with injuries in a child that may be the result of abuse, we often use other factors to determine the need for further action. Some of these factors are determined by our knowledge of the literature; others are based on our anecdotal experience over our careers.

TERMINOLOGY

Research has shown that the medical literature is steadily becoming more complicated and even out of reach for some medical readers.[1] With a rapidly expanding body of increasingly difficult medical literature, it is essential that the fundamentals of epidemiology be understood. A command of the terminology used in epidemiology is crucial to an understanding of the medical literature.

The common epidemiological terms *incidence* and *prevalence* have worked their way into the general vernacular, perhaps without an understanding of their meanings. *Incidence* is the proportion of a group without a condition that will go on to develop the condition in a specific period of time. For example, the incidence of abusive head trauma would be the number of new cases in a year among the population at risk for abusive head trauma. *Prevalence* is defined as the proportion of a group who has the condition either at one point in time or during a period of time. For example, the prevalence of sexual abuse among women is said to be 25% or higher but most abuse would not have occurred in the past year.

It should be obvious that the method of data collection will strongly influence the determination of the incidence or prevalence of a disease. When physicians rely on their own personal experience to informally assess the prevalence of a disease, their anecdotal experience will be based on the peculiarities of their practices. It follows, then, that clinicians will be influenced to be alert to a given condition based on their perception of the prevalence of the disease in their population. For example, if a clinician tells a colleague, "I don't screen for domestic violence in my patient population because it doesn't occur often in my area," the clinician's perception of the prevalence of domestic violence (DV) among his patients influences his clinical decision not to screen for DV. This results in circularity of reasoning: there is little risk of DV in my patient population, so I do not need to screen for DV. I do not screen for DV in my patient population, so I do not identify DV. For this reason, clinicians must be especially aware of the hazards of relying on their anecdotal experiences. They should also carefully read the methodology sections of the research they rely on to determine the measured prevalence or incidence of a disease.

Accuracy and reliability in diagnosing conditions is a concern for all clinicians. If a patient's signs and symptoms are misdiagnosed as a condition attributable to abuse or neglect, there are adverse consequences to the family and the child, such as further unnecessary diagnostic testing or a child protective services investigation of the family. On the other hand, if a child is abused or neglected and their presenting condition is erroneously identified as being attributable to something else, then the child is underdiagnosed and

Table 1-1	Clinical Questions Answered By Understanding Epidemiology of Abuse and Neglect	
Issue	**Question**	
Abnormality	Is this child abused or neglected?	
Diagnosis	How accurate are the tests used to diagnose abuse or neglect?	
Frequency	How often are children abused or neglected?	
Risk	What are the risk factors for abuse or neglect?	
Prognosis	What are the outcomes and consequences for abuse or neglect?	
Treatment	How does treating (or diagnosing) child abuse or neglect change the course of the condition?	
Prevention	Does an intervention prevent abuse or neglect? Does early detection and intervention change the course?	
Cause	What leads to abuse or neglect? Or what are the mechanisms of the injuries?	
Cost	How much does it cost to care for abused or neglected children? How much does it cost to miss a case of severe physical abuse?	

Adapted from Fletcher RH, Fletcher SW, Wagner EH: *Clinical epidemiology: the essentials,* ed 3, Williams & Wilkins, Baltimore, 1996.[15]

	Disease present	Disease absent
Test positive	TRUE POSITIVE	FALSE POSITIVE
Test negative	FALSE NEGATIVE	TRUE NEGATIVE

FIGURE 1-1 Diagnostic outcomes in medical decision making.

the necessary cascade of events that should take place to assess and protect the child (and potentially other siblings in the home) does not take place, leaving the child in a potentially dangerous environment.

There are four possible outcomes that result when a diagnosis of abuse or neglect is considered: (1) The patient is correctly identified as abused or neglected, a *true positive* diagnosis; (2) the patient is correctly identified as *not* abused or neglected, a *true negative* diagnosis; (3) the patient is *not* abused or neglected, but is diagnosed as having been so, a *false positive* diagnosis; and, (4) the patient *is* abused or neglected and is not identified as having been so, a *false negative* diagnosis (Figure 1-1). To determine the accuracy of the diagnosis, one must know what the "gold standard" is. In other words, what is the most accurate way of knowing whether a given patient has a given disease at a given point in time? For many diseases, the gold standard is an autopsy. Since most patients will not have an autopsy to confirm a diagnosis, we are forced to rely on other tests to arrive at a diagnosis. We then weigh our results against what the results could be if we were able to perform the gold standard study.

Sensitivity and specificity are measures of diagnostic accuracy. The *sensitivity* of a test is defined as its ability to accurately identify the true positives. Increasing the sensitivity likely also results in generating more false positives as an unintended consequence. Very sensitive tests, therefore, are most helpful when the results are negative. Ruling out a condition with a sensitive test can assure the clinician (and the family) that the condition in question most likely does not exist. However, there will be patients who will test positive with sensitive tests that do not actually have the condition. These patients will possibly require further intervention or, in the case of suspected child abuse, further investigation. The *specificity* of a test is defined as its ability to accurately classify true negatives as persons *without* the disease in question. If a patient is screened with a highly specific test and the results are positive, it can be stated with certainty that the patient does indeed have the condition (i.e., it is unlikely that the positive test results could be attributed to another condition). Specific tests are more useful when the test is positive, as the condition has been ruled in by the positive results.

Balancing the specificity and the sensitivity of a test is challenging. A test with low sensitivity could miss true positives and result in a child left in a potentially abusive situation, whereas tests with low specificity can result in false positives, which may subject a family to intrusive investigations and a child to unnecessary testing. When the testing is being performed for a disease or condition where the consequences for missing the diagnosis are severe, it is important to choose the most sensitive test, sacrificing specificity if necessary.

By definition, the specificity and sensitivity of a given test in a given patient require information as to whether the patient truly has or does not have the condition. Because this information is not known when the clinician actually orders the test, it becomes necessary to understand the predictive value of the test for this patient. Two types of probability are used to describe the predictive value of a test: the positive predictive value (PPV) and the negative predictive value (NPV). The positive predictive value of a test is the likelihood that a patient has the condition when the test results indicate that they have the condition. The negative predictive value of a test is the likelihood that patient does *not* have the condition when the test results indicate that they do *not* have the condition.

The predictive value of a test is different than the test sensitivity and specificity. Sensitivity and specificity are characteristics of the test; the predictive value is a characteristic of the test *and* the prevalence of the disease in the patients being tested. Consider the situation where a condition has a very low prevalence in a given population; for example, HIV infections in U.S. children. In such a situation, if a test is highly sensitive and the results are positive, it is still most likely to be a false positive. If a highly sensitive test for HIV is performed in a child following a sexual assault, the pretest probability (the prevalence) is low. Therefore, the predictive value (or the posttest probability) of a positive HIV test remains low in this population. If the results are positive, there is a good chance it will be a false positive and will therefore require further testing.

In another example, consider the negative predictive value of the skeletal survey for rib fractures in the potentially abused infant. If an infant presents with a head injury, multiple bruises and a limb fracture and then receives a skeletal survey, the pretest probability is high that other fractures such as rib fractures will be found. Rib fractures are prevalent in abused infants. If no fractures are identified on the skeletal survey, it is quite possible this is a false negative result, despite x-rays being a sensitive test for rib fractures. For this reason, the negative predictive value of this study to correctly identify rib fractures is low and further testing is necessary to confirm the absence of this type of fracture if other data or history prompts concerns about physical abuse.

Clinicians must understand the prevalence of a condition in their patient population to accurately determine the predictive value of a test. As previously discussed, the prevalence of a condition can be difficult to accurately assess in clinicians' personal patient populations. Prevalence of abuse can be estimated by starting with the population prevalence and then considering risk factors such as persistent crying, demographics factors such as young maternal age, and the specific details of a clinical situation. By relying upon published epidemiological studies, clinicians can hone their skill at estimating the pretest probability of a given condition and therefore better assess the posttest probability when the results are received.

Still, the medical literature must be viewed through a cautious lens. Often, literature will describe risk factors associated with a given condition. Quantifying the effect of a risk factor on the likelihood of a condition can be done in different statistical fashions. One term is attributable risk (AR). The AR is the incidence of a condition in patients with a specific risk factor minus the incidence of the condition in patients without that risk factor. AR estimates should be reserved for situations in which the factors might be considered causal and not simply as confounders. For example, smoking is a causal risk factor associated with lung cancers but male gender is not thought to be causal and is a marker for increased rates of smoking (a confounder).

The relative risk (RR), also known as the risk ratio, describes the risk (probability) of developing a condition when a risk factor is present versus the risk of developing the same condition without the risk factor. One might ask, "What is the relative risk for an infant being fatally abused if there is an unrelated male caregiver in the home?" To answer this question, one would need to know the probability of an infant being fatally abused with and without an unrelated male caregiver. Relative risks are the statistic most often encountered in cohort studies (i.e., longitudinal studies of a defined group of individuals).

Odds ratios (OR) are distinct from RR, but are sometimes used interchangeably when the disease or outcome being looked at is rare. ORs are used in retrospective studies and case-control studies as measures of effect describing the strength of a relationship. They describe the ratio of the odds of having the exposure if you have the disease compared with the odds of having been exposed if you don't have the disease or outcome. If an OR is greater than 1, the first group has a higher odds of the condition relative to the second group; if the OR is less than 1, the first group has a

lower odds of the condition relative to the second group. It is apparent that the OR would be more appropriate in a case-control study or a retrospective study when you consider the fact that the condition (e.g., some type of abuse) is already present in the sample and the researcher is interested in knowing how often a risk factor is present in the group that is abused versus the group that is not. To use RR, the condition is not yet present, the risk factor is, and the researcher is watching to see which subjects develop the condition.

There are situations where a public health policy makes sense, even if it addresses a risk factor which is relatively weak, if that risk factor affects many people in a community. A risk factor with a small relative risk, but which is widely prevalent may play a larger role in the development of a condition than a risk factor that has a high relative risk but is rare in the population. The statistical measure that describes this impact is the population attributable risk (PAR). Public health initiatives related to lead abatement in urban population centers, for example, are targeting a known population attributable risk. In the field of child abuse research, the work on social capital as a modifiable risk factor is an example of attempting to address a PAR. By increasing the social capital in a neighborhood, the risk of abuse for the children in the neighborhood can be reduced more broadly than by attempting to address the risk factors in an individual home. Therefore, while the relative risk is smaller to the individual children in the neighborhood, the widely prevalent risk of decreased social capital will affect more children placing them at increased risk of being abused. This is the so called "prevention paradox.[2]"

EPIDEMIOLOGICAL STUDIES IN CHILD ABUSE

Countless studies address risk factors, prevalence, and incidence of child abuse and neglect in the extant body of medical literature. A few of these studies are widely referenced as sources for our understanding of the epidemiology of child abuse and neglect. The National Child Abuse and Neglect Data System (NCANDS)[3] and the National Incidence Studies (NIS)[4] are two of the most commonly cited studies. These studies both address rates of various forms of child abuse, but gather information in very different ways. Data collected in the NCANDS are compiled by child protection agencies across the United States. With an enormous data set consisting of millions of data points, numerous questions can be addressed but there are limitations that must be considered. Children represented in the NCANDS are only those who came to the attention of local authorities. It is unknown how many others are abused or neglected but aren't identified in this sample. Although many epidemiological questions can be answered by examining the case details and risk factors of children who are reported for suspicions of abuse or neglect, the sample is inherently biased, and these biases can influence our understanding of the problem.

The NIS is a survey that occurs about every 10 years as a form of active surveillance. The goal of this study is to more accurately identify the number of child abuse and neglect cases that occur in a community but that may not come to the attention of child protection authorities. By using community sentinels (i.e., trained observers to report abuse), cases can be identified at a broader population level. With probability sampling techniques, the NIS attempts to demonstrate the impact of abuse nationally through a more affordable research methodology than would be possible if the entire population were studied.

Direct sampling of the population is another methodology used to assess the rate or prevalence of abuse. Examples of this methodology include the CarolinaSAFE study,[5] the National Gallup Poll,[6] and the Juvenile Victimization Questionnaire.[7] In these types of studies, families are contacted and questioned about specific acts of child maltreatment. In some studies parents are questioned, and in others the children are questioned. Interestingly, despite the obvious concern that a parent would be reluctant to report acts of violence against, or inappropriate contact with, their children, these studies have repeatedly found this not to be the case.

Although the studies discussed above are essential tools for researchers, clinicians, and policy makers, there are numerous inherent challenges that researchers and epidemiologists face when designing studies on child abuse and neglect. All of the studies mentioned have some limitations.

PROBLEMS IN CONDUCTING RESEARCH IN CHILD ABUSE AND NEGLECT

Data Collection Issues

Studies can collect data in a number of ways: actively or passively, using primary data sources or official reports, anonymously, or through face-to-face interviews. The NCANDS study[3] is an example of passive data collection using official reports. Because this sample includes only cases that are brought to the attention of authorities, undoubtedly, the prevalence of child abuse is underestimated. Another methodological problem with this dataset is that individual states reporting data do not use uniform definitions. Because the determination of whether to substantiate a case of child abuse or neglect is made by the agency investigating the allegation, there is inherently a subjective component. Criteria to substantiate cases (i.e., meeting the legal burden of proof in a given state) can change over time and be subject to secular or legal trends.

Just as the variations in state legal definitions and the subjective nature of the substantiation of allegations affect the reported prevalence of abuse in studies such as the NCANDS, the reported prevalence and incidence of abuse in other types of research are directly impacted by the researchers' definitions. Circularity is an issue that can pose a particular problem in child abuse research. If a researcher defines a case of abusive head trauma (AHT) as a child who has (1) sustained a traumatic brain injury, (2) has a child protection team consult, and (3) this consult determines that the child is a victim of AHT, there is an inherent circularity that the reader must acknowledge when interpreting the findings of the study. Concluding that intracranial hemorrhage is a sign of abusive head trauma when the clinical

team only suspected abusive head trauma because of the presence of intracranial hemorrhage is an example of circular reasoning. Early research on child abuse often contained circular reasoning that made it difficult for the results to be taken at face value. That does not mean these studies are without value; it does mean that the field must strive to achieve more stringent (i.e., less circular) case definition criteria when conducting research. Numerous studies of AHT are now using elaborate protocols for case definitions to avoid previous issues with circularity.[8,9]

Data sources can introduce bias into a study. For example, random digit dial surveys rely on subjects answering survey questions honestly and as accurately as possible. In the CarolinaSAFE study,[5] 1435 households were called in North Carolina and South Carolina and questioned about the disciplinary practices, and potentially abusive practices, used by adults in the household against a randomly selected child under 18 years of age. Although this methodology allows a unique perspective on possible abuse, especially abuse that may never come to the attention of authorities or community sentinels, it is subject to both recall bias and desirability bias.

Researchers conducting this type of research often will use a time frame they want the subject to use when answering questions: "In the last 6 months, how often did you hit your child somewhere other than on the bottom?" This type of question is subject to a recall bias. For rare events, the recall may be accurate. If a parent rarely ever uses physical discipline, the one time it was used in the last 6 months might have been for an especially egregious infraction on the part of the child and the event will stand out in the mind of the parent. If parents routinely use physical discipline and whip their children with belts for every perceived wrong, it may be difficult to accurately recollect the number of times. However, in a case such as this, the upper level choice (e.g., more than 10 times) may adequately encompass the extent of the events.

Desirability bias is the bias introduced when the subject knows what the answer "should be," or what the researcher would like the answer to be. Most people recognize the social taboos associated with shaking a baby as a form of "discipline" and it would be expected that the parents would not self-report this behavior to avoid being perceived as a "bad parent." Although it cannot be determined if some parents chose not to report this behavior because of desirability bias, the fact remains that some parents in the CarolinaSAFE study[5] did report this alarming behavior. Desirability bias also plays a role when screening for violence of any type in a clinical setting. When a mother is asked if she experiences violence in the home, there are numerous reasons for her to withhold the truth if she is indeed a victim of interpersonal violence, including not wanting to appear to be a victim, fear of her abuser, or fear that the physician will report her to child protective services.

Some biases are introduced when subjects are enrolled into a study. A *selection bias* is a bias that can occur when subjects are chosen for a study in a way that reduces the likelihood that they are a representative sample of the larger population. For example, a researcher is interested in prevalence of retinal hemorrhages among all children less than 6 months of age who come to the emergency department (ED) for any reason. If the researcher's protocol requires that the potential subject must have both parents present to be enrolled in the study, a significant percentage will not be able to be enrolled. Are the patients who arrive at the ED with only one parent significantly different than those that arrive with two parents? Does this introduce a possible bias in the design? Another example is the situation where an institutional review board (IRB) requires that a researcher include language in the informed consent document that states, "If retinal hemorrhages are identified in your child, there is a chance this finding could be related to inflicted trauma, also known as child abuse. If this is the case, we are required by law to report our concerns to child protective services." Would this statement influence the likelihood that a family would consent to the study? It could be that parents who knew their child had sustained inflicted trauma would decline participation because they would be likely identified and reported if hemorrhages were found. On the other hand, it could be the parents did not abuse their child but might be afraid that hemorrhages would be identified (a false positive) and they would be reported and subjected to an unwarranted investigation, so they choose not to participate. Either or both of these situations would influence the researcher's ability to accurately determine how often retinal hemorrhages are present in infants seeking care in an ED.

Ecological fallacies occur when a characteristic of a group is attributed to an individual person, implying a causal association with an outcome. For example, if there was a high rate of neglect in a particular census tract, an ecological fallacy would be to suggest that an individual living in that census tract is highly likely to neglect a child. Living in the census tract does not mean one will be neglectful, but there are likely some characteristics of the population in the area that increases the occurrence of neglect. Stereotypes are an example of an ecological fallacy that can negatively influence the ability of a clinician or researcher to accurately diagnose or classify abuse or neglect. Although lower socioeconomic status (SES) is a known risk factor associated with many forms of abuse or neglect, not all poor families abuse their children. However, rates of abuse may be high in areas with high concentrations of low SES families. Failing to consider this association (i.e., a higher concentration of low SES families is associated with a higher rate of abuse in the population) could result in drawing incorrect conclusions about residents of these areas.

Researchers who recognize the potential pitfalls that ecological fallacies pose can address them through wise methodology. A stratified sampling strategy allows the researcher to control for variables by maintaining homogenous subsets of the sample. For example, early research on child abuse suggested that certain types of abuse were more common among minority populations. By generalizing in this fashion, the research fails to take into account that there are other features shared among members of a minority population besides their race or ethnicity. It is not uncommon that SES is correlated with minority status. If the research were conducted to control for the SES of the various racial groups, it might be that SES was a stronger determinant of risk of abuse than was race. This in fact is the case.

In the late 1970s, professionals dealing with child abuse and neglect attempted to describe the ubiquitous nature of child maltreatment. It was stated that abuse affects all religions, races, communities, and economic levels. This led researcher Leroy Pelton to address the so-called *Myth of Classlessness*.[10] Dr. Pelton demonstrated a real increased rate of abuse and neglect among lower SES groups. It has been suggested that cognitive biases can lead to differences in recognition and reporting of abuse and this explains the higher rates among poorer populations. However, this would not explain the apparent dose-effect of poverty on the rates of abuse. Data cited clearly show that rates of abuse increase as SES decreases. Dr. Pelton explained that when public awareness increased about child abuse and reporting, there was not a concomitant increase in the rate of reports on higher SES families. "We have no grounds for proclaiming that if middle-class and upper-class households were more open to public scrutiny, we would find proportionately as many abuse and neglect cases among them. Undiscovered evidence is no evidence at all.[10]" Although it is important to recognize that rates of abuse among the poor are higher, it does not suggest that being poor causes parents to harm or neglect children in their care. The myth of classlessness serves to minimize the unique stresses that poverty places on families and the more dangerous environments that children are exposed to when raised in poverty. This minimization results in a diversion from what could be a focused risk reduction effort, the reduction of the number of children living in poverty.

Ethical Issues

There are significant ethical considerations in research on child abuse and neglect. One overarching issue facing researchers is mandated reporting of suspected child maltreatment, which is required by law in all 50 U.S. states. Many potential subjects are aware of this law and might be reluctant to disclose information that could result in abuse being reported to the authorities. This could result in measurement bias, a bias directly related to the desirability bias.

With the rise of IRBs governing research, there has arisen an issue unique to child abuse research—should prospective subjects be warned of the possibility of a report being made if abuse or neglect is suspected? With no consensus existing and no standard approach to this issue, some IRBs require researchers to warn potential subjects (or, as is often the case in child abuse research, the proxy signing the consent), while other IRBs remain silent on the issue, assuming that mandated reporting is a known factor that exists regardless of the research being conducted. It is arguable even that reporting suspected abuse or neglect is not a risk to the patient, and rather, it could bring benefit by protecting the child from further harm. Further, it should be noted that the principle of informed consent being given by a proxy (in the case of children, often a parent) is founded on the concept of the subject's best interest. In the case of a parent as an abuser, there is an inherent conflict of interest that could preclude that parent from offering informed consent when the "risk" of reporting is disclosed. Although currently no answers have been reached by the research and bioethical community, this very topic is being actively addressed internationally to arrive at some approach that can balance the rights of the child (and family) and the need for quality research on child abuse and neglect.

DIFFICULTIES IDENTIFYING CHILD ABUSE AND NEGLECT

Both researchers and clinicians are faced with the issue of accurately identifying cases of abuse or neglect. Just as researchers must be cognizant of biases that adversely affect their studies, clinicians should also be aware of biases that adversely affect their ability to diagnose abuse or neglect accurately. These biases are referred to as cognitive biases or cognitive errors. Errors in the correct diagnosis of abuse can directly lead to inaccuracies in the reported epidemiology of abuse. Take, for example, the NCANDS data. Official reports of abuse are often based on the diagnosis of abuse by a medical professional. If medical professionals are systematically misdiagnosing (either over- or under-diagnosing) abuse, the official reported numbers will not be accurate, leading to a skewed understanding of the prevalence of abuse. Several types of cognitive bias are particularly relevant to the recognition of child maltreatment. For example, selection bias can influence whether a sample accurately reflects the underlying population. When selection bias affects a clinician in a clinical encounter, it can influence who is evaluated for a given condition. If a clinician feels that a family is a "nice family" and is therefore at low risk for abusing their children, injuries in their children will not be evaluated in the same way they would be if the child were from a "bad family." This selection bias will tend to create a self-fulfilling prophecy. If clinicians only search for abuse in "bad families," they will find examples in troubled families because they are looking for it. By failing to consider abuse in "nice families," they will fail to identify abuse and will feel justified in their continued practice of relying on their subjective sense of "good" versus "bad" families.

Confirmation bias can also appear in a clinician's evaluation for abuse. When abuse is in the differential diagnosis, we ask questions and order tests to strengthen our certainty of the diagnosis. We will tend to incorporate positive findings that support our theory and disregard information that does not fit into our cognitive framework for abuse. Similarly, when the patient with injuries that could be due to abuse is seen through the filter of a "good family," we will be subject to a measurement bias and will look for alternate explanations for the injury and disregard information that would lead us to believe that a "good family" could have harmed their child.

The concept of anchoring is important in a discussion of cognitive biases. With anchoring, we attach great significance to a piece of information and build from there. This focus can derail a clinical evaluation and result in overdiagnosing or underdiagnosing of abuse. As an example, consider a mother presenting to the ED with her 18-month-old child who is limping and refusing to bear weight on her leg. The mother reports this has been going on for 3 days and has progressed to the point where the child wants to be carried everywhere. The mother is young, unemployed, and has two other children under the age of 5 years at home. She appears tired and disheveled. While waiting for the physician, the nurse overhears the mother yelling at someone on her cell phone and using very explicit language. The physician examining the child is told about the overheard phone call before the examination. When examining the patient, the physician feels the mother is rude and abrupt with him. Given the social information up to this point, the physician believes this patient has a high likelihood of an abusive injury. Anchoring on these facts and the clinician's subjective assessment of the mother's appearance and behavior, he begins to question her specifically about discipline, other caregivers, and previous reports to child protective services. As the exchange escalates, the mother becomes extremely frustrated and attempts to explain that the child has been sick recently and has had low grade fevers. Because this information does not fit in with a diagnosis of abuse, the physician does not incorporate it into the overall clinical picture. He interprets her increasing hostility as a sign that she has harmed her child, again adding weight to his cognitive anchor. He now will make clinical and diagnostic decisions based on where he has arrived as a result of his anchor: an evaluation for child abuse. Consider the alternative scenario: a mother comes in with the same child but is neatly dressed and calm. She is young but married and employed. Her husband is at home with her other two small children. When the physician arrives to examine the child, he is struck by how articulately the mother describes the child's symptoms and clinical course. He begins to develop a diagnostic strategy to determine whether this is toxic synovitis. Both of these cognitive anchors drive the interactions and influence the diagnosis. What if the first child had toxic synovitis, but was incorrectly labeled as abused and the second child was abused and incorrectly labeled as toxic synovitis? Cognitive anchors must be consciously recognized to be sure one does not miss important diagnostic information.

Implicit biases or stereotypes are another example of potential cognitive pitfalls. It is clear that a patient's race plays a significant role in the type and quality of medical care received. The first three rounds of the NIS have failed to show a difference in the rate of abuse by race.[11] Despite this lack of evidence, researchers have shown that minority children, particularly African-American children, are more likely to be medically evaluated for the possibility of abusive injuries and are more likely to be reported to CPS, regardless of whether their injuries are likely accidental or inflicted.[12] A recent study clearly demonstrated that in children with identical injuries, minority children were significantly more likely to be reported to CPS than their white counterparts.[13] There is evidence that abusive head trauma will be missed more frequently in white children.[14] It is unknown whether minority children have greater errors of "overdiagnosis," but a detection bias is strongly suggested by the work of Lane et al.[13] Clinicians need to center their judgments about the presence or absence of child abuse on risk factors other than race since race has no known contribution to the *a priori* risk.

STRENGTH OF THE EVIDENCE

With the field of literature rapidly expanding, we are developing an increasing understanding of the public health impact of child abuse and neglect. We also are recognizing the need to accurately define and measure child maltreatment to identify how to prevent it. As researchers and clinicians become increasingly aware of cognitive pitfalls, we become better able to address them, strengthening our work along the way. It would be wrong to "throw the baby out with the bath water" and walk away from earlier studies because of the flaws we now recognize. The early literature is the foundation on which to build sound hypotheses that we can then test in a more rigorous fashion. Research, like the clinical diagnostic process, is an iterative process.

FUTURE DIRECTIONS

As we hone our abilities to effectively measure abuse and neglect, we will need to continue to sample diverse populations, both nationally and internationally, to more fully understand who is at risk and how we can modify that risk. We also need to begin to explore how to teach clinicians to be "better thinkers." We all rely on cognitive shortcuts without realizing it. Problems arise when we do not assess what we as a field know and apply that to what we as individual clinicians do in our clinical practice.

References

1. Hellems MA, Gurka MJ, Hayden GF: Statistical literacy for readers of pediatrics: a moving target. *Pediatrics* 2007;119:1083, 2007.
2. Rose G: Sick individuals and sick populations. *Int J Epidemiol* 1985;14:32-38.
3. Administration for Children and Families, U.S. Department of Health and Human Services: *The NCANDS survey instrument* (website): http://www.acf.hhs.gov/programs/cb/systems/ncands/survey.htm. Accessed December 26, 2008.
4. Child Welfare Information Gateway, Children's Bureau, Administration for Children and Families, U.S. Department of Health and Human Services: *The national incidence study* (website): http://www.childwelfare.gov/systemwide/statistics/nis.cfm. Accessed December 26, 2008.
5. Theodore AD, Chang JJ, Runyan DK, et al: Epidemiologic features of the physical and sexual maltreatment of children in the Carolinas. *Pediatrics* 2005;115:e331-e337.
6. Gallup G, Gallup GH Jr: *The Gallup poll. Public opinion 1995*. SR Books, Lanham, Md, 1995, pp 183-185.
7. Finkelhor D, Hamby SL, Ormrod R, et al: The juvenile victimization questionnaire: reliability, validity, and national norms. *Child Abuse Negl* 2005;29:383-412.
8. Hymel KP, Makoroff KL, Laskey AL, et al: Mechanisms, clinical presentations, injuries, and outcomes from inflicted versus noninflicted head trauma during infancy: results of a prospective, multicentered, comparative study. *Pediatrics* 2007;119:922-929.
9. Keenan HT, Runyan DK, Marshall SW, et al: A population-based study of inflicted traumatic brain injury in young children. *JAMA* 2003;290:621-626.
10. Pelton LH: Child abuse and neglect: the myth of classlessness. *Am J Orthopsychiatry* 1978;608-617.
11. Sedlak AJ, Broadhurst DD: *Executive summary of the third national incidence study of child abuse and neglect*, National Clearinghouse on Child Abuse and Neglect Information, Administration for Children and Families (website): http://basis.caliber.com/cwig/ws/library/docs/gateway/Record;jsessionid=8C16A14A68BA6E48D6D5D4B2AF1F50C3?w=+NATIVE%28%27IPDET+PH+IS+%27%27nis-3%27%27%27%29&upp=0&rpp=-10&order=+NATIVE%28%27year%2Fdescend%27%29&r=1&m=6&. Accessed December 26, 2008.
12. Lau AS, McCabe KM, Yeh M, et al: Race/ethnicity and rates of self-reported maltreatment among high-risk youth in public sectors of care. *Child Maltreat* 2003;8:183-194.
13. Lane WG, Rubin DM, Monteith R, et al: Racial differences in the evaluation of pediatric fractures for physical abuse. *JAMA* 2002;288:1603-1609.
14. Jenny C, Hymel KP, Ritzen A, et al: Analysis of missed cases of abusive head trauma. *JAMA* 1999;281:621-626.
15. Fletcher RH, Fletcher SW, Wagner EH: *Clinical epidemiology: the essentials*, ed 3, Williams & Wilkins, Baltimore, 1996.

EPIDEMIOLOGY OF PHYSICAL ABUSE

Adam J. Zolotor, MD, MPH, and Meghan Shanahan, MPH

INTRODUCTION

The measurement of the incidence or prevalence of physical abuse is methodologically challenging. The most important challenge is that in many acts of violence, only two people know about the act, the victim and the perpetrator. Estimates of the rate of physical abuse vary depending on methodology used. There are numerous ways to collect incidence data, namely active and passive surveillance, and population-based surveys. There are two major datasets that employ these methods, The National Child Abuse and Neglect Data System (NCANDS), and the National Incidence Study (NIS). This chapter describes these data systems and the incidence and prevalence of physical abuse, and also discusses risk factors for physical abuse and the epidemiology of specific types of abuse.

SCOPE OF THE PROBLEM

Surveillance refers to ongoing data collection, analysis, and dissemination.[1] Surveillance data describe the scope of physical abuse, the populations at-risk, and the risk factors for abuse. Active surveillance involves identifying cases through numerous data sources, including Child Protective Services (CPS), medical records, and law enforcement records. The cases are followed up through interviews with the parents/guardians of the child, the authorities, and if appropriate, the child. Passive surveillance involves extracting data from sources not designed to collect data about child maltreatment, but that contain those data. For example, death certificates and medical records include information regarding physical abuse. In passive surveillance, this information is extracted and recorded, but not followed up on through interviews or further investigations.[1]

Population surveys of physical abuse use probability samples to ascertain the incidence of abusive parenting behavior.[2] These are frequently conducted through anonymous telephone surveys. Most medical, legal, and social services definitions of abuse include physical harm, which is impossible to determine from telephone surveys. The behaviors identified as physically abusive often include beating, burning, kicking, shaking, or hitting a child with an object other than on the buttocks. A recent population-based study determined that physical abuse occurs at a rate of 43 cases per 1000 children in North Carolina and South Carolina.[3] A national study determined that 49 per 1000 children experience physical abuse.[4]

The National Child Abuse and Neglect Data System (NCANDS) is an example of passive surveillance. It was established by the National Center on Child Abuse and Neglect as result of the Child Abuse Prevention Act (CAPTA).[5] NCANDS data are collected annually from child protective service agencies and contain case level and aggregate data from all states.[6] The data include the number of reports of alleged abuse, dispositions on investigations, data on victims and perpetrators of substantiated and indicated cases, and on children who are the subject of reports.[6] According to NCANDS, in 2006 an estimated 905,000 children were maltreated nationally, for a rate of 12.1 abuse and neglect victims per 1000 children under the age of 18. Additionally, 142,041 children were physically abused (1.9/1000). Physical abuse was the second most common form of maltreatment; neglect was the most common.[6] NCANDS data has shown a 48% decline in rates of physical abuse with similar declines in sexual abuse and almost no change in neglect from 1990 to 2006.[7] It will be an important mark of success for child abuse prevention if other methodologies can validate this progress.

The National Incidence Study (NIS) is a congressionally mandated active surveillance system that takes place approximately every 10 years.[8] The goal of the NIS is to go beyond the cases of maltreatment that come to the attention of CPS and determine a more accurate estimate of the incidence of child maltreatment nationally. The NIS methodology assumes that the number of children who are known to CPS is only a portion of the true prevalence of maltreatment. This survey uses both CPS data and data collected from community sentinels to determine the number of children who are being maltreated nationally. The sentinels are members of the community who come in regular contact with children. Sentinels are selected for their involvement with specific agencies, such as public schools, hospitals, voluntary social service agencies, and police departments.[8,9] The NIS uses a national probability sample to ensure that the data collected and reported can be generalized. According to the third NIS, 1.5 million children are victims of abuse and neglect annually.[9] An estimated 381,700 children are physically abused annually for a rate of 5.7 children per 1000.[9] These data reflect the rate under the "harm standard," where children are actually harmed from abuse or neglect. When considering risk of harm (endangerment standard), rates of abuse and neglect are much higher.

The differences in the results from these studies highlight the importance of considering methodology when interpret-

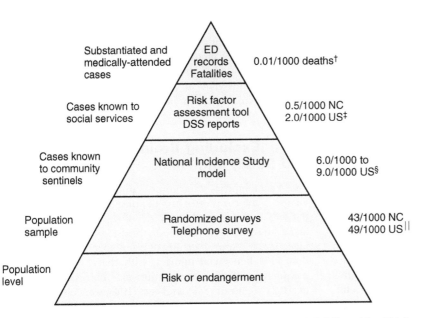

FIGURE 2-1 Child abuse surveillance pyramid.

† Rate based on 30 child abuse homicides reported in 2003 by the NC Office of the Chief Medical Examiner and census estimate of mid year population <18
‡ Substantiated reports to social services for physical abuse in 2006, NC and US estimates[52]
§ Physical abuse as reported by sentinels 1993, lower estimate for harm standard, upper estimate for endangerment or risk of harm standard[46]
‖ Estimates based on 2002 self-reported survey of parents reporting shaking a child <2, beating, burning, or kicking a child, or hitting a child with an object somewhere other than the buttocks[50] and a 1995 survey of US parents.[47]

ing the prevalence of physical abuse. NCANDS consistently reports fewer cases than the NIS.[52,46] It is clear that in only using CPS reports, the NCANDS data represent a smaller proportion of abused children. Anonymous population-based surveys consistently report higher rates of physical abuse.[6,9] The number of physical abuse cases known to CPS or community sentinels, and captured in the NCANDS and NIS studies, represent a small portion of children who actually experience physical abuse. Figure 2-1 demonstrates the range of rates depending on method of surveillance, with death certificates at the apex and surveillance of risk factors at the base considering the largest segment of the population.

Numerous risk factors have been identified for physical abuse. While many studies do not distinguish between types of maltreatment, this chapter will only include literature that has examined the specific risk factors for physical abuse. Risk factors at the child, caregiver, family, and community level will be discussed.

RISK FACTORS FOR PHYSICAL ABUSE

Child Characteristics

Age of child: Physical abuse is more common among older children than younger children.[6,8] The NIS-3 found that the rate of physical abuse among children ages 12 to 14 years was significantly higher than the incidence among children ages 0 to 2 years.[9] This may be due to a lack of identification among the younger children.[9] Children ages 0 to 2 years may have less exposure to people in the community than older children and be less likely identified as abused by community sentinels. NCANDS also reports a higher percentage

of physical abuse cases among older children, but is subject to the same biases as NIS. The association with age has been inconsistent with population-based surveys.[10]

Sex of child: Sex is an inconsistent risk factor for physical abuse.[6,8,9] One study determined that male children were more likely to be physically abused.[11] However, another recent study found that girls were at slightly higher risk for physical abuse.[10]

Race: The victim's race is sometimes found to be a risk factor for physical abuse.[6,10,11] NCANDS data revealed different rates of physical abuse by race; 14.6% of physical abuse victims were Asian, 12.9% were African-American, and 9.8% were white.[6] Other studies such as the NIS-3 have not found racial differences in rates of physical abuse.[9] Certain races may be more likely to come to the attention of CPS than others, which would bias the NCANDS results.

Caregiver Characteristics

Age of mother: Mothers younger than 26 years are more likely to physically abuse their children than older mothers.[12] A longitudinal study of 644 families determined that younger mothers were 2.37 times as likely to physically abuse their children.[13]

Mental health of mother: Children who have caregivers with depression[14,15] or substance abuse[11,15] are more at risk of being physically abused. Additionally, general maternal sociopathy has also been identified as a risk factor for physical abuse.[13]

Marital status: Caregiver marital status has also been found to be associated with physical abuse.[9,13,16] Children who live with only one parent are more likely to experience physical abuse than children who live with both parents.[9,13,16] Additionally, the NIS-3 determined that children who live with only their fathers are at a marginally higher risk of being physically abused than children who live with only their mothers.[9]

Family Characteristics

Poverty: Poverty has been found to be a significant predictor of experiencing physical abuse.[9,13,14,16] In the NIS, as income increases, the rate of physical abuse decreases through all income categories.[9]

Number in household: The number of individuals in the household has been found to be a risk factor for physical abuse. One study demonstrated that abused children lived in larger households (average 4.1 members) than children who were not abused (average 3.6 members).[11,15] Another study determined that children who live with four or five children are more likely to be physically abused than children who live in smaller or larger households.[11]

Domestic violence: Most studies examining the relationship between domestic violence and child abuse have shown that children who live in families where there is domestic violence are at an increased risk of experiencing physical abuse.[17-21] However, one report using a population-based survey found little relationship between domestic violence and physical abuse, but very strong relationships with other forms of child maltreatment.[22] Another study demonstrated that poor marital quality was associated with physical abuse.[13] Parental conflict and domestic violence might also be associated with physical abuse.

Corporal punishment: Parents who spank have been shown to be more likely to be physically abusive.[23] Two studies have shown that most physically abusive acts are either a result of escalated discipline or in response to a specific child misbehavior.[24,25] One study using cross-sectional data demonstrated that the risk of physical abuse increases with increasing frequency of spanking and the use of an object (e.g., belt or switch) on the buttocks.[10]

Neighborhood Characteristics

Children who live in impoverished neighborhoods are more likely to be physically abused than children who do not live in poor areas.[16,18] One study showed that decreasing neighborhood cohesion was associated with increasing rates of all types of maltreatment.[26] A more recent study examined the relationship of social capital to subtypes of abuse. Decreases in social capital were shown to be associated with neglect and psychological abuse but there was no observed association between social capital and physical abuse.[27] It has also been determined that the percentage of female headed households in a neighborhood and the concentration of alcohol vendors is positively associated with rates of physical abuse.[18]

PHYSICAL ABUSE EPIDEMIOLOGY BY INJURY TYPE OR BODY SECTION

Epidemiology can be used to better understand types of injury either by body location, organ system, or injury type. This can inform clinicians about the presentation of various types of injuries, about how commonly such injuries occur because of abuse versus other mechanisms, and about clinical and demographic risk factors for abuse. Some studies use diagnostic test terminology to characterize the relationship of a finding or injury type to abuse. This section reviews lessons from epidemiological studies specific to abuse injuries.

Head (Excluding Brain and Skull) and Neck

Face: Facial injuries are common among child physical abuse victims. One case series of 390 abused children seen as outpatients demonstrated that 59% of these children had orofacial injuries, most commonly bruising or abrasions of the face (95%).[28] A similar study of hospitalized children showed that 41% had facial injuries, with the cheek as the most common site (30% of facial injuries).[29] The eyes (25%), forehead (22%), nose (13%), and ears (10%) were also commonly involved. Injuries to the face involve lacerations, burns, and welts.[28-30] Most of the children with facial injuries in these case series were under 5 years.[28,29] In both large cohort studies, the perpetrator was most often male—usually the father of the child or the mother's boyfriend.[28,29]

Oropharynx: The mouth is a less frequent but important site of trauma from physical abuse. In some of the same studies cited above and in other retrospective cohort studies, the oropharynx was involved as a site of trauma in 1% to 11% of cases of physical abuse.[28-31] Tooth fractures, avulsions, labial lacerations, frenulum lacerations, mucosal injury, palatal injury, and fracture of the mandible or maxilla have all been reported.[29,31]

Injury of the labial frenulum has received somewhat more attention as an injury suggestive of abuse. A systematic review found 19 studies meeting inclusion criteria.[32] These included 30 cases of labial frenulum laceration. Most children suffered fatal abuse (27/30) and most were less than 5 years old (22/30). They identified two cases of frenulum laceration resulting from intubation, complicating the study of frenulum injury. Of the 30 cases, only two had an identified mechanism (direct blow to the face). It has been suggested that forced feeding or pulling of the lips may cause frenulum injury, but there were no documented cases in this review. The most serious limitation to this literature is the absence of cross-sectional or case-control data to understand the specificity or predictive value for frenulum injury and abuse.[32]

Neck: Skin injury to the neck, mostly bruising and abrasions, were included in several studies of facial trauma. In one cohort study, bruising of the neck was identified in 12% and abrasion in 7% of physical abuse victims. One study found that of children hospitalized for abuse, 6% are found to have neck injuries.[29] A series of pediatric cervical spine injuries at a trauma center found 3 of 103 injuries were due to abuse.[34] Abuse injuries were all classified as spinal cord injury without radiographic abnormality (SCIWORA), underscoring the challenge of diagnosing cervical spine injuries in abuse victims. All three of these patients were infants, two suffered head injuries, and the third massive injuries of the chest, abdomen, and bones.

The epidemiology of abusive head trauma is discussed in Chapter 6.

Visceral Injuries

Several case series have demonstrated a wide range of abdominal injuries from child abuse, including liver laceration, splenic laceration, renal contusion, and hollow viscus injury.[35-37] Several retrospective cohort studies have examined all admissions to large hospitals for children with abdominal injuries. The rates of abuse among these series range from 11% to 19%.[35,37,38] Children with inflicted abdominal injuries are more likely to have higher injury severity scores. Additionally they are more likely to have hollow viscus injury and extraabdominal injuries (such as bruises and rib fractures).[37] Of all children coming to an emergency department with injuries, abdominal injury from abuse is extremely uncommon (<1%); however, of all abdominal injuries seen in the emergency department, 4% were classified as abuse.[39]

Skeletal Injury

Estimates of fractures in physically abused children vary widely by setting (11%-31%).[40-42] One study found that unsuspected fractures were identified by skeletal survey in 26% of children admitted to a children's hospital for physical abuse.[43] Unsuspected fractures were most common in children with suspected fractures and head injuries, but uncommon in children admitted with burns. Most unsuspected fractures were found in children less than 1 year (80%).

Rib fractures: Rib fractures are a common skeletal manifestation of abuse. Most abusive rib fractures occur in children less than 2 years old.[42] One cohort study included only infants and found 82% of 39 infants with rib fractures were caused by abuse. Of the remaining seven cases not due to abuse, three were clearly due to unintentional injuries (one motor vehicle, one fall down stairs, and one crush injury), one to birth trauma, and three to bone fragility.[44] A second study included 78 children with a total of 336 rib fractures.[45] Sixty-two children were aged 3 years or younger and 82% were determined to have inflicted rib fractures by the child abuse team. The remaining 11 children (nonabused group) had postoperative rib fractures (5), skeletal dysplasias (3), osteoporosis of prematurity (2), or been in a motor vehicle crash (1). The positive predictive value of a rib fracture for abuse in children less than 3 years old is 95%, and if clinical and historical information are used to exclude children with other causes, the positive predictive value is 100%.

Many children with suspected abuse will undergo cardiopulmonary resuscitation (CPR) prior to first radiographic study. This raises the question of chest compressions as a potential cause of the rib fracture. A recent systematic review of rib fractures caused by CPR reviewed 427 studies, but only six met inclusion criteria. Of the 923 children who underwent CPR, only three had rib fractures, all anterior. Rib fractures from CPR are rare and only anterior fractures have been associated with CPR.[46] A recent study, however, did identify subtle rib fractures at autopsy in 11% of resuscitated infants after the parietal pleura was stripped from the ribs.[47] The fractures were anterior and lateral in location rather than posterior, and most were not visible before the pleura was removed.

Limb fractures: Among all children, femur fractures are rarely due to abuse. However, several studies have demonstrated that femur fractures among young children, especially preambulatory children, are more likely due to abuse. One study identified 139 children less than 4 years old with femur fractures.[48] The overall rate of fractures due to abuse was 9% with an average age of 1.1 years in the abuse group and 2.3 years in the unintentional injury group. Children who are not yet walking were more likely to be victims of abuse. A case-control study of fractures from abuse and unintentional injuries found that 93% of abuse injuries were in children aged less than 1 year.[49] This study found no differentiating characteristics either in fracture type or radiographic appearance. A study of a referral center's trauma registry found that abusive injuries accounted for 67% of lower extremity fractures for children under 18 months old compared with 1% for children 18 months or older.[50] Of children hospitalized with an abusive lower extremity fracture, 68% had femur fractures and 56% had tibia fractures. A study of a national administrative database found that 15% of all femur fractures in children under 2 years were coded as caused by abuse and almost no abusive fractures were reported among older children.[51] It is clear from these studies that abuse should be considered as a potential cause of long bone fractures in young children, especially those who are nonambulatory.

Fractures outside of the axial skeleton and lower extremities can be due to abuse, but such injuries have been the subject of less research. In a national U.S. study of a probability sample from administrative data, 1053 children were hospitalized for abuse with 1794 fractures.[52] The axial skeleton was the site of 50% of these fractures (59% skull, 37% rib, 3% vertebrae, 1% pelvis). Only 14% of fractures were to the upper extremity (45% humerus, 34% radius/ulna, 17% scapula/clavicle, 4% carpal/metacarpal). The lower extremity fractures accounted for 18% of these injuries (59% femur, 37% tibia/ fibula/ankle, 2% tarsal/metatarsal).[52]

Skin Injury

Bruises: Skin injury is one of the most common presentations for physical abuse, with bruises by far the most common injury. However, bruises are an extremely common injury in all children. A large prospective study of children seen for nontrauma reasons found that 76.6% had recent skin injuries, mostly bruises, and 17% had five or more injuries.[53] Epidemiological studies have been invaluable in characterizing normal versus abnormal bruising. Large case series of abused children, nonabused children, and case-control studies have been used to characterize normal and potentially abusive bruising.[33]

Nonabused children rarely have bruises before starting to transition to independent mobility (<1%).[54] The most common sites for nonabusive bruises are over the legs, bony prominences, and the head for infants and toddlers.[53-55] Child abuse victims commonly have bruises (28%-98%).[33] Bruises due to abuse tend to be greater in number, to be present with older injuries (i.e., scar or healing abrasion), and to be defensive in location (outer arm). Abusive bruises can carry the imprint of an implement such as a cord.[33] Bruises that are high in number (studies suggest 10-15), unusual in location or pattern, or occurring in young children not yet walking should be considered for abuse or bleeding disorder.[33,53,54]

Burns: Most epidemiological studies of burns compare cases of inflicted pediatric burns with unintentional burns. In series of hospitalized pediatric burn patients, the rates of abuse and/or neglect range from 4% to 16%.[56-60] These studies often combine abuse and neglect. A burn registry has recently allowed epidemiological study of nearly all serious pediatric burns in the United States.[61] This study found that 6% of children aged 12 years or younger admitted to burn units were suspected victims of abuse. The use of registries comes at the cost of detail, and the assessment of abuse is less clear and perhaps less standardized than a single center's approach.

Inflicted burns are most often due to liquid scald (78% of inflicted burns versus 59% of unintentional burns).[61] Abusive burns tend to be larger, involve younger children, have higher risk of mortality, and longer hospital stays.[60,61] They tend to be deeper and more often require grafting.[56,61] They more often involve both hands or both feet.[58] Social stress is a prominent risk factor in these injuries. Victims of abusive burns are more often from unstable families,[58,59] from single parent families,[56,57,59] live in poverty,[57,59] and have had prior involvement with protective services.[56]

FUTURE RESEARCH

Understanding the epidemiology of child physical abuse requires a combination of active and passive surveillance and population-based surveys. Passive surveillance allows for the systematic collection of large amounts of administrative data on an ongoing basis, but such systems only capture cases that present to care. Emergency department passive surveillance, a new approach to studying injury epidemiology, and hospital discharge data, similarly will only capture children who present to care and where the cause of injury is correctly identified and recorded. These systems can be helpful for studying severity and trends. Increasing collaboration in trauma registries and burn registries provide similar insight. A promising approach for understanding risk and abuse epidemiology is the combination of data by linking identifiers. This is occurring in some states, but concerns for privacy and interagency silos can hinder these productive efforts.

Active surveillance is more expensive and less practical. It allows for more complete case ascertainment of children in a variety of systems of care. This approach has been used to study children seen by many types of professionals in the National Incidence Studies[9] and specifically to study head trauma epidemiology,[62] and will be useful, especially in multicenter and national surveillance, to better understand the epidemiology of child physical abuse. Prospective studies of orthopedic and burn injuries would help clarify the epidemiology of these types of abuse as well.

References

1. World Health Organization: *Injury prevention and control: a guide to developing a multisectoral plan of action, surveillance and research* (website): http://www.emro.who.int/dsaf/dsa730.pdf. Accessed December 27, 2008.
2. Butchart A, Harvey AP, Mian M, et al: *Preventing child maltreatment: a guide to taking action and generating evidence*, World Health Organization (website): http://whqlibdoc.who.int/publications/2006/9241594365_eng.pdf. Accessed December 27, 2008.
3. Theodore AD, Chang JJ, Runyan DK, et al: Epidemiologic features of the physical and sexual maltreatment of children in the Carolinas. *Pediatrics* 2005;15:e331-e337.
4. Straus MA, Hamby SL, Finkelhor D, et al: Identification of child maltreatment with the Parent-Child Conflict Tactics Scales: development and psychometric data for a national sample of American parents. *Child Abuse Negl* 1998;22:249-270.
5. National Data Archive on Child Abuse and Neglect: *National child abuse and neglect data system (NCANDS) detailed case data component, 1998-1999* (website): http://www.ndacan.cornell.edu/NDACAN/Datasets/UserGuidePDFs/NCANDS_MultiYear_Guide.pdf. Accessed December 27, 2008.
6. U.S. Department of Health and Human Services, Administration for Children and Families: *Child maltreatment 2006* (website): http://www.acf.hhs.gov/programs/cb/pubs/cm06/cm06.pdf. Accessed December 27, 2008.
7. Finkelhor D, Jones L: *Updated trends in child maltreatment, 2006,* Berkman Center for Internet & Society (website): http://cyber.law.harvard.edu/sites/cyber.law.harvard.edu/files/Trends%20in%20Child%20Maltreatment.pdf. Accessed December 27, 2008.
8. Sedlak AJ: *A history of the national incidence study of child abuse and neglect.* Westat, Rockville, Md, 2001.
9. Sedlak AJ, Broadhurst DD: *Third national incidence study of child abuse and neglect.* National Clearinghouse on Child Abuse and Neglect Information, Washington, DC, 1996.
10. Zolotor AJ, Theodore AD, Chang JJ, et al: Speak softly—and forget the stick. Corporal punishment and child physical abuse. *Am J Prev Med* 2008;35:364-369.
11. Wolfner GD, Gelles RJ: A profile of violence toward children: a national study. *Child Abuse Negl* 1993;17:197-212.
12. Jones ED, McCurdy K: The links between types of maltreatment and demographic characteristics of children. *Child Abuse Negl* 1992;16:201-215.
13. Brown J, Cohen P, Johnson JG, et al: A longitudinal analysis of risk factors for child maltreatment: findings of a 17-year prospective study of officially recorded and self-reported child abuse and neglect. *Child Abuse Negl* 1998;22:1065-1078.
14. Cadzow SP, Armstrong KL, Fraser JA: Stressed parents with infants: reassessing physical abuse risk factors. *Child Abuse Negl* 1999;23:845-853.
15. Chaffin M, Kelleher K, Hollenberg J: Onset of physical abuse and neglect: psychiatric, substance abuse, and social risk factors from prospective community data. *Child Abuse Negl* 1996;20:191-203.
16. Coulton CJ, Korbin JE, Su M: Neighborhoods and child maltreatment: a multi-level study. *Child Abuse Negl* 1999;23:1019-1040.
17. Coohey C, Braun N: Toward an integrated framework for understanding child physical abuse. *Child Abuse Negl* 1997;21:1081-1094.
18. Freisthler B, Midanik LT, Gruenewald PJ: Alcohol outlets and child physical abuse and neglect: applying routine activities theory to the study of child maltreatment. *J Stud Alcohol* 2004;65:586-592.
19. McGuigan WM, Pratt CC: The predictive impact of domestic violence on three types of child maltreatment. *Child Abuse Negl* 2001;25:869-883.
20. Rumm PD, Cummings P, Krauss MR, et al: Identified spouse abuse as a risk factor for child abuse. *Child Abuse Negl* 2000;24:1375-1381.
21. Tajima EA: The relative importance of wife abuse as a risk factor for violence against children. *Child Abuse Negl* 2000;24:1383-1398.
22. Zolotor AJ, Theodore AD, Coyne-Beasley T, et al: Intimate partner violence and child maltreatment: overlapping risk. *Brief Treat Crisis Interv* 2007;7:305-321.
23. Gershoff ET: Corporal punishment by parents and associated child behaviors and experiences: a meta-analytic and theoretical review. *Psychol Bull* 2002;128:539-579.
24. Gil DG: *Violence against children.* Harvard University Press, Cambridge, Mass, 1973.
25. Kadushin A, Martin JA: *Child abuse: an interactional event.* Columbia University Press, New York, 1981.
26. Vinson T, Baldry E: *The spatial clustering of child maltreatment: are micro-social environments involved?* Australian Institute of Criminology, Canberra, Australia (website): http://aic.gov.au/documents/0/F/%7B0F2149F2-6563-4874-8C05-83541EF11743%7Dti119.pdf. Accessed February 15, 2010.
27. Zolotor AJ, Runyan DK: Social capital, family violence, and neglect. *Pediatrics* 2006;117:e1124-e1131.

28. Cairns AM, Mok JY, Welbury RR: Injuries to the head, face, mouth and neck in physically abused children in a community setting. *Int J Paediatr Dent* 2005;15:310-318.

29. Naidoo S: A profile of the oro-facial injuries in child physical abuse at a children's hospital. *Child Abuse Negl* 2000;24:521-534.

30. Jessee SA: Physical manifestations of child abuse to the head, face and mouth: a hospital survey. *ASDC J Dent Child* 1995;62:245-249.

31. da Fonseca MA, Feigal RJ, ten Bensel RW: Dental aspects of 1248 cases of child maltreatment on file at a major county hospital. *Pediatr Dent* 1992;14:152-157.

32. Maguire S, Hunter B, Hunter L, et al: Diagnosing abuse: a systematic review of torn frenum and other intra-oral injuries. *Arch Dis Child* 2007;92:1113-1117.

33. Maguire S, Mann MK, Sibert J, et al: Are there patterns of bruising in childhood which are diagnostic or suggestive of abuse? A systematic review. *Arch Dis Child* 2005;90:182-186.

34. Brown RL, Brunn MA, Garcia VF: Cervical spine injuries in children: a review of 103 patients treated consecutively at a level 1 pediatric trauma center. *J Pediatr Surg* 2001;36:1107-1014.

35. Canty TG Sr, Canty TG Jr, Brown C: Injuries of the gastrointestinal tract from blunt trauma in children: a 12-year experience at a designated pediatric trauma center. *J Trauma* 1999;46:234-240.

36. Ng CS, Hall CM, Shaw DG: The range of visceral manifestations of non-accidental injury. *Arch Dis Child* 1997;77:167-174.

37. Wood J, Rubin DM, Nance ML, et al: Distinguishing inflicted versus accidental abdominal injuries in young children. *J Trauma* 2005;59:1203-1208.

38. Ledbetter DJ, Hatch EI Jr, Feldman KW, et al: Diagnostic and surgical implications of child abuse. *Arch Surg* 1988;123:1101-1105.

39. Yamamoto LG, Wiebe RA, Matthews WJ Jr: A one-year prospective ED cohort of pediatric trauma. *Pediatr Emerg Care* 1991;7:267-274.

40. Galleno H, Oppenheim WL: The battered child syndrome revisited. *Clin Orthop Relat Res* 1982;4:1-7.

41. Herndon WA: Child abuse in a military population. *J Pediatr Orthop* 1983;3:73-76.

42. Merten DF, Radkowski MA, Leonidas JC: The abused child: a radiological reappraisal. *Radiology* 1983;146:377-381.

43. Belfer RA, Klein BL, Orr L: Use of the skeletal survey in the evaluation of child maltreatment. *Am J Emerg Med* 2001;19:122-124.

44. Bulloch B, Schubert CJ, Brophy PD, et al: Cause and clinical characteristics of rib fractures in infants. *Pediatrics* 2000;105:E48.

45. Barsness KA, Cha ES, Bensard DD, et al: The positive predictive value of rib fractures as an indicator of nonaccidental trauma in children. *J Trauma* 2003;54:1107-1110.

46. Maguire S, Mann M, John N, et al: Does cardiopulmonary resuscitation cause rib fractures in children? A systematic review. *Child Abuse Negl* 2006;30:739-751.

47. Dolinak D: Rib fractures in infants due to cardiopulmonary resuscitations efforts. *Am J Forensic Med Pathol* 2007;28:107-110.

48. Schwend RM, Werth C, Johnston A: Femur shaft fractures in toddlers and young children: rarely from child abuse. *J Pediatr Orthop* 2000;20:475-481.

49. Rex C, Kay PR: Features of femoral fractures in nonaccidental injury. *J Pediatr Orthop* 2000;20:411-413.

50. Coffey C, Haley K, Hayes J, et al: The risk of child abuse in infants and toddlers with lower extremity injuries. *J Pediatr Surg* 2005;40:120-123.

51. Loder RT, O'Donnell PW, Feinberg JR: Epidemiology and mechanisms of femur fractures in children. *J Pediatr Orthop* 2006;26:561-566.

52. Loder RT, Feinberg JR: Orthopaedic injuries in children with nonaccidental trauma: demographics and incidence from the 2000 kids' inpatient database. *J Pediatr Orthop* 2007;27(4):421-426.

53. Labbé J, Caouette G: Recent skin injuries in normal children. *Pediatrics* 2001;108:271-276.

54. Sugar NF, Taylor JA, Feldman KW: Bruises in infants and toddlers: those who don't cruise rarely bruise. Puget Sound Pediatric Research Network. *Arch Pediatr Adolesc Med* 1999;153:399-403.

55. Carpenter RF: The prevalence and distribution of bruising in babies. *Arch Dis Child* 1999;80:363-366.

56. Andronicus M, Oates RK, Peat J, et al: Non-accidental burns in children. *Burns* 1998;24:552-558.

57. Bennett B, Gamelli R: Profile of an abused burned child. *J Burn Care Rehabil* 1998;19:88-94.

58. Hight DW, Bakalar HR, Lloyd JR: Inflicted burns in children. Recognition and treatment. *JAMA* 1979;242:517-520.

59. Hummel RP 3rd, Greenhalgh DG, Barthel PP, et al: Outcome and socioeconomic aspects of suspected child abuse scald burns. *J Burn Care Rehabil* 1993;14:121-126.

60. Purdue GF, Hunt JL, Prescott PR: Child abuse by burning—an index of suspicion. *J Trauma* 1988;28:221-224.

61. Thombs BD: Patient and injury characteristics, mortality risk, and length of stay related to child abuse by burning: evidence from a national sample of 15,802 pediatric admissions. *Ann Surg* 2008;247:519-523.

62. Keenan HT, Runyan DK, Marshall SW, et al: A population-based study of inflicted traumatic brain injury in young children. *JAMA* 2003;290:621-626.

3

EPIDEMIOLOGY OF SEXUAL ABUSE

Vincent J. Palusci, MD, MS

HISTORY

As with other forms of child maltreatment, child sexual abuse (CSA) has likely occurred since the dawn of human history. But unlike physical abuse, neglect and psychological maltreatment, CSA has been shrouded by the cloak of social taboo surrounding sexual contact with children and human sexuality in general. This made determining the true number of CSA cases difficult, leading physicians and other scientists to believe it was an uncommon problem. In the 1970s in the United States, reports of CSA grew dramatically as the social changes associated with the women's movement revealed the plight of sexually victimized children. Early counts of CSA rose dramatically from a few thousand, to 44,700 annually in 1979.[1] CSA now consistently comprises 10% to 15% of child maltreatment (CM) reports in the United States and Canada.[2,3] Similar patterns have been noted in other countries, with initial reports of CSA being low or "nonexistent" in number, and more recently increasing case identification and reporting associated with social acceptance and improved professional response. Despite improved identification and reporting, a large proportion of CSA cases are thought to remain hidden from public view or investigation while real numbers appear to be declining in the United States.

TERMINOLOGY

A variety of sources reports aspects of the incidence and prevalence of child sexual victimization. Unfortunately, varying definitions of the type of sexual contact (direct or indirect, penetrative or nonpenetrative, harm or endangerment) and what constitutes a "child" can make assessment problematic.[4] *Rape*, which is often reported by law enforcement and criminal justice systems, has been generally defined as forceful, penetrative contact, and is further specified in state penal codes. *Sexual assault* refers to a broader collection of acts, including fondling and other nonpenetrating acts, and also is further refined in state penal codes. Other terms imply the relationship of the offender to the victim. *Incest* refers to sexual contact between family members, which is sometimes limited to immediate family but in other contexts can extend to fifth degree relationships (second cousin, once removed). *Sexual exploitation* generally refers to acts without sexual contact, such as having children pose for sexually explicit photographic or video images, having them witness sexual acts, or by adults exposing themselves to children inappropriately for the sexual gratification of the adult. Thus

a broad definition of *child sexual abuse* has been taken as the "... involvement of dependent, developmentally immature children and adolescents in sexual activities that they do not fully comprehend, to which they are unable to give informed consent, or that violate the social taboos of family roles.[5]" This has been modified for practical application to "... an act of commission, including intrusion or penetration, molestation with genital contact, or other forms of sexual acts in which children are used to provide sexual gratification for the perpetrator. This type of abuse also includes acts such as sexual exploitation and child pornography.[6]"

Case Finding

David Finkelhor[7] has noted that "because sexual abuse is usually a hidden offense, there are no statistics on how many cases actually occur each year. Official statistics include only the cases that are disclosed to child protection agencies or to law enforcement." There are several ways, however, that CSA can be identified. Cases are most often reported by witnesses or disclosed by the child. These reports are transmitted to law enforcement and child welfare agencies (child protective services [CPS] in the United States) as "suspected cases" until an investigation identifies credible evidence to make a determination that the child is a victim and/or that a crime has occurred. To identify more cases, screening has been proposed to find victims in the general pediatric population.[8] Screening procedures have been devised which use information from the parents, characteristics of the child, interview or physical examination findings, and other case factors. However, while some case characteristics have been found to be more predictive of CSA determination, there is no single "test" that identifies a child as a CSA victim.[9,10] That determination usually requires a finding by an investigatory agency, and the variability of these findings leads to variations in case findings in official statistics.

Incidence

Incidence refers to the number of CSA cases that occur each year, whereas prevalence is defined as the number of people who, at a given time, have been the victim of at least one act of CSA during their lifetime. These two approaches, measuring different aspects of the occurrence of CSA, come from different types of analyses and often appear to reach different conclusions about the extent of the problem. One can sometimes estimate the population prevalence of a condition from annual incidence statistics.

There are three principle sources of data on the incidence of CSA in the United States. Traditional criminal justice agencies collect information about a variety of crimes in the United States, including violent crimes such as homicide and rape, and property crimes. The U.S. Bureau of Justice reports that while violent crime decreased 26.3% from 1996 to 2005, the rate increased 1.3% from 2004 to 2005.[11] Although the National Crime Victimization Survey estimated there were 197,000 incidents of forcible rape and 110,000 other incidents of sexual assault of victims ages 12 and older in the United States, only one third were estimated to have been reported to law enforcement agencies in 1996. In the Federal Bureau of Investigation's Uniform Crime Reports in 12 U.S. states during 1991-1996, two thirds of the 60,991 sexual assault victims were less than 18 years of age.[11] Juvenile victims accounted for 75% or more of incidents of fondling, sodomy, and forcible assault with an object, but only 46% of rapes. Most offenders were male (96%) and older than 18 years (76.8%), but only 34% were family members, suggesting that only a relatively small proportion of the cases in this dataset are true CSA cases as defined by child protective services agencies and collected in the National Child Abuse and Neglect Data System.

The National Child Abuse and Neglect Data System (NCANDS) contains aggregate and case-level data on child abuse reports received by state agencies in the United States.[2] Data were first collected in the late 1980s from a small number of states, but there are now more than 45 states and territories providing information annually about the outcomes of child abuse reports, types of maltreatment, child and family factors, and services being provided. National estimates of the overall numbers of CM victims (substantiated or indicated reports) and victims identified with the major types of CM (physical abuse, sexual abuse, neglect, medical neglect, and psychological maltreatment) are provided in Figure 3-1. In NCANDS, the number of CM victims rose, fell, and then stabilized at approximately 900,000 annually since the year 2000, with rises in neglect and declines in physical abuse. The number of CSA victims, while rising during the late 1980s, actually declined during much of the 1990s and early into the twenty-first century. Cases declined from a peak of 144,760 cases in 1991 to 79,640 in 2006. CSA incidence rates also declined from 2.2 per 1000 children in 1990 to 1.1 per 1000 in 2006 (Figure 3-2).

National incidence surveys are an additional source of information. The Canadian Incidence Study (CIS) reported that 11% of confirmed CM reports were for sexual abuse, affecting 0.93 children per 1000 in 1998.[3] In the United States, the National Incidence Studies of child abuse and neglect (NIS) have provided separate, periodic estimates of a growing number of sentinel professionals in a representative group of U.S. counties to determine the actual number of CM victims.[12] In 1993, NIS-3 sampled more than 5600 professionals in 842 agencies serving 42 counties to identify children in any or all of the agencies under two standards: The harm standard (relatively stringent in that it generally requires that an act or omission result in demonstrable harm to be classified as abuse or neglect) and the endangerment standard (which allows children who were not yet harmed by maltreatment to be counted if the CM was confirmed by CPS or identified as endangerment by professionals outside

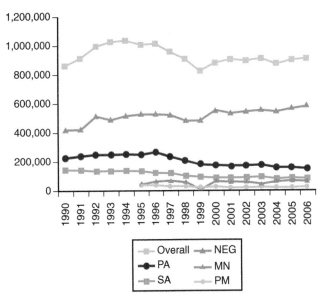

FIGURE 3-1 U.S. Child Maltreatment Victims, from the National Child Abuse and Neglect Data System. *PA*, Physical abuse; *SA*, Sexual abuse; *NEG*, Neglect; *MN*, Medical neglect; *PM*, Psychologic maltreatment. *(From U.S. Department of Health and Human Services: Child Maltreatment 1990-2006: Reports from the states to the national child abuse and neglect data system. U.S. Government Printing Office, Washington, DC, 1992-2008.)*

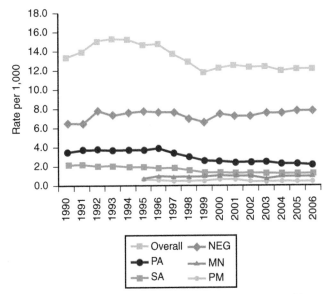

FIGURE 3-2 U.S. Child Maltreatment Victims, Rate per 1,000. *PA*, Physical abuse; *SA*, Sexual abuse; *NEG*, Neglect; *MN*, Medical neglect; *PM*, Psychologic maltreatment. *(From U.S. Department of Health and Human Services: Child Maltreatment 1990-2006: Reports from the states to the national child abuse and neglect data system. U.S. Government Printing Office, Washington, DC, 1992-2008.)*

CPS, either by their parents or other adults). It was found that there was a two thirds increase in the overall number of CM victims since the previous study (NIS-2) in 1986. Sexual abuse nearly doubled during this time period, rising to an estimated 217,700 cases under the "harm standard" and 338,900 cases under the "endangerment standard" in

1993. Differences in these estimates from those reported by NCANDS are thought to be explained by: (1) The fact that NCANDS reports victims that have been investigated and determined to include CSA and do not include unsubstantiated or unfounded cases; (2) NIS includes cases identified by community professionals at schools and hospitals, but which have not been reported to CPS; (3) NIS includes cases under the "endangerment standard," which do not meet CPS criteria for CSA case finding: and, (4) some cases are never revealed during the child's lifetime. In one analysis, the true number of CSA cases was thought to be closer to NIS estimates.[13] NIS-4 was conducted in 2006 and results are expected in 2009.

Prevalence

There are many studies which report the prevalence of CSA. Prospective designs may be more accurate than official CPS reports, but many prevalence studies are retrospective surveys in special populations at increased risk for CSA, suggesting potential biases might overestimate the true prevalence.[14,15] Early small studies reported prevalence rates as low as 3% for males and 12% for females, but with increasing social recognition and acceptance and improved survey techniques, rates of 25% or higher have been consistently identified. Prevalence studies have historically varied greatly in their definition of CSA and in their methods,[7] but they also likely include cases that have not been reported in prospective incidence studies, creating an apparent disparity in the numbers of cases. It is estimated, for example, that less than one third of all CSA cases are reflected in current incidence figures, mostly because cases are not disclosed to authorities. Thus prevalence studies can offer an opportunity to "capture" more cases than are officially reported.

In the selected sample of studies presented (Table 3-1), rates range from 1% in a population-based study in North and South Carolina to over 66% among pregnant adolescents in Washington.[16-29] These studies have been completed over a wide span of years (1988 through 2002) and have wide variations in the self-reported rates of CSA based on locality, sampling technique (convenience vs. population), victim gender, age, type of sexual contact (CSA vs. rape vs. unwanted sexual contact), condition of interest (medical vs. psychological), or criminal justice status (incarceration). Women with pregnancy and men with sexually transmitted infections (consequences of sexual activity) had higher lifetime prevalence of CSA. University students, incarcerated men, and those with injection drug use also had greater rates. This does not mean that these populations are more likely to be abused; rather, it implies that a history of CSA, when obtained by retrospective self-report, is more likely to be found in groups with certain medical, psychological, and social problems.

In contrast, meta-analyses and studies with national samples offer potentially more accurate CSA estimates for the general population (Table 3-2).[3,30-36] For example, the National Family Violence Survey in 1985 reported that 27% of adult women and 16% of adult men reported sexual contact or sexual abuse during childhood, but their relationship to the offender (a key element of CSA) was not specified.[30] Others later reported rates from as low as 4.5% to as high as 37%, varying by location and methodology.[3] A meta-analysis[32] of 59 studies from 1974-1995 noted that there were wide variations in definitions but that, in aggregate, college students reported rates of 16% for CSA with "close" family members and 35% for total CSA with "close" and "wider" family. These rates were 33% higher than the national studies used for comparison, but wide ranges of results were obtained depending on the sexual acts included in their definition.

International studies offer a window into other cultures and their social acceptance and reporting of CSA (Table 3-3).[37-46] Early reports from professionals in countries associated with the United Kingdom noted lower rates (3 per 1000), while later reports have rates similar to those in the United States The Canadian Incidence Study mentioned previously also showed similar rates. Reports from Asia, while limited, show smaller (but increasing) numbers. Other than CIS, these studies have not included national samples and should not be interpreted as representing true population prevalence estimates, especially when done with special populations.

WHY CSA IS DECLINING

Despite the variability, it does appear that overall CSA numbers and rates in the United States are declining (Figures 3-1 and 3-2). A variety of explanations have been offered.[47-49] In a survey of CPS state administrators in 43 U.S. states, Jones et al[47] note a 39% decline in annual incidence based on NCANDS data during 1992-1999. Increased evidentiary requirements, increased caseworker caution because of new legal rights for caregivers, and increasing limitations on the types of cases that are accepted to be investigated are given as potential causes, and the potential effects of prevention programs, increased prosecution, and public awareness campaigns. Some of these potential causes have also been associated with CSA declines outside of the United States.[50] Finkelhor and Jones[49] note that CSA substantiation by CPS declined 49% in the United States from 1990 to 2004, as did other family violence and crimes against children. Using four data sources (NCANDS, state CPS data, the National Crime Victimization Survey conducted by the U.S. Census, and the Minnesota student survey), Finkelhor[48] noted that data provided by CPS agencies offered little evidence that the decline was a result of the investigation decisions by CPS. Evidence was mixed that a social "backlash" had affected reporting. Finkelhor concluded that a significant proportion of the decline could reflect a real decrease in the incidence of CSA. While initial reports of this decline were met with skepticism, these declines in official reports paralleled declines in self-reports during the same period. And while physical abuse reports also declined, reports of neglect and other CM did not. While a general decline in crime has likely contributed to a decline in CSA, so too has a pattern of improved social conditions, economic prosperity, and prevention programs during the 1990s. Even more likely, "new agents of social control" and significantly increased rates of incarceration of offenders have played a pivotal role. Changing social norms and practices, psychopharmacology, and treatment for families may have also contributed to the decline. Unfortunately, the relative contributions of these factors to the decline have not been fully elucidated, and economic downturns and

Table 3-1	Selected CSA Prevalence Studies and Risk Factors in Special Populations			
Study	**Year Done**	**Population**	**Prevalence**	**Risk Factors***
Russell et al[16]	1978	930 adult women, San Francisco	38% (before age 18 yr)	
Boyer et al[17]	1988-1990	535 pregnant adolescents, Washington	66.2%	
Holmes[18]	1992	95 HIV- positive adult men	20%	
Ompad et al[19]	1997-1999	2143 injection drug users, 18-30 yr, five U.S. cities	14.3% (before age 18 yr)	Younger age injection drug use
Littleton et al[20]	1999-2000	1428 women, family planning clinics, 18-40 yr, Texas	19% (forced sex)	European women
Aspelmeier et al[21]	2000-2001	324 university undergraduates, females	37.7%	Protective: Attachment security in peer and parents relations
Van Gerko et al[22]	2000-2002	299 adult women with eating disorder	28.8%	
Harlow et al[23]	2000-2003	125 women with vulvodynia	18.4% (11.2% controls)	More vulvodynia with CSA
Trent et al[24]	2000	1698, 19-20 yr, Baltimore	16%	Female > male
Whetten et al[25]	2001-2003	611 HIV- positive adults, Deep South, U.S.	⅓ lifetime prevalence; 25% before age 13 yr	Females, nonheterosexual men; Alcoholic, depressed parents, DV
Johnson et al[26]	2001	100 men, county jail, Texas	59% (before puberty)	90% female perpetrators
Edwards et al[27]	2002	8667 adults, California	21.6%	
Theodore et al[28]	2002	1435, North and South Carolina	10.5/1,000 (1.05%)	Female (10×), adolescents
Senn et al[29]	2005	871 adults, STD Clinic, Rochester, NY, U.S.	51%	Minority race, less than high school education

*Odds or risk ratio.
STD, Sexually transmitted disease.

changes in other conditions and programs may portend a rebound in CSA.

Recurrence

CM recurrence has been studied to measure program effectiveness and to identify risk factors in cases which can be addressed to prevent further harm. A wide range of recurrence rates are reported (1%-66%) based on the type of maltreatment and whether re-reports or substantiated reports are used. Several studies have identified program, child, family, and services factors which affect subsequent maltreatment.[51-54] In general, factors that increase the likelihood that children will be reabused include younger aged children, children with more severe maltreatment, disabled children, white race, multiple CM types, multiple prior CM victimization, families with emotional problems, family abuse alcohol, and families with other violence histories.

Data regarding CSA recurrence are limited. In a longitudinal survey of 1467 sexually victimized children in 2002-2003, 39% were revictimized by the second year, with the odds of recurrence at 6.9, higher than property crime, assault, or other maltreatment.[54] My own analysis of NCANDS data for 2000-2004 has identified a CM resubstantiation rate of 10% within 2 years of the first confirmed CSA report, with over one third of the new confirmed reports being CSA. Factors associated with an increased risk of CSA recurrence were family housing problems or other family violence; the only services associated with decreased recurrence were counseling, mental health, and juvenile court petition.

Risk and Protective Factors

In addition to incidence and prevalence, epidemiological studies can also identify risk and protective factors, which

Table 3-2 Selected CSA Prevalence Studies with National Samples

Study	Year Done	Population	Prevalence	Risk Factors*
Finkelhor et al[30]	1985	2626 adults, U.S.	27% women, 16% men	Unhappy homes, single parents, West, inadequate sex education
Briere et al[31]		1442 adults, national sample, U.S.	23.3%	Females
Rind et al[32]	Meta-analysis	13,704 males, 21,999 females; college students	17% (3%-37%) females; 27% (8%-71%) males	Family environment factors
Adams et al[33]	1990-1992	4264, age 15-54 yr, U.S., national sample	7.4%	Female > male
Vogeltanz et al[34]	1991	1099 women, national sample, U.S.	21%-32%	Parental drinking, paternal rejection, single parents
Hussey et al[35]	2001-2002	15,197, national sample, U.S.	4.5%	Females (1.2), nonwhite race (1.4-2.0), parent education <high school (1.5), income <$15,000 (1.83), South (1.36)
Finkelhor et al[36]	2002-2003	2030 children, ages 2-17 yr, national sample, U.S.	8.2% (any sexual victimization)	Females, teens; poverty and other victimization (rape)

*Odds or risk ratio.

Table 3-3 Selected International CSA Prevalence Studies

Study	Year Done	Population	Prevalence	Risk Factors*
Mrazek et al[37]	1977-1978	1599 professionals, London, UK	3 per 1000	Female > male, family disturbances
May-Chahal et al[38]	1998-1999	2869, age 18-24 yr, UK	19%; 10% contact, 6% noncontact	Females, middle class
Dunne et al[39]	2000	1784, self-report, age 18-59 yr, Australia	32%	Females (2×), older women
Luo et al[40]	1999-2000	1994, China, adult reports	4.2%	Male > female, highest in age 20-29 yr
Senior et al[41]	1991-1992	10,641 adult women, SW England, UK	18.2% (early age)	Protective: white, high social support
Chen et al[42]	2002-2003	2300 students, 4 schools, survey, China	13.6%	Females (1.6)
Trocmé et al (CIS)[3]	2003	14,200 sample, Canada	National estimate: 17,321 (2.67/1000)	
Jirapramukpitak et al[43]	2005	202, age 16-25 yr, Bangkok, Thailand	5.8% (sexual penetration)	
Fanslow et al[44]	2005	2855 women, age 18-64 yr, 2 regions, New Zealand	23.5%/28.2%	Maori > European, rural > urban
Gladstone et al[45]	2004	125 depressed adult women, Australia	27.2%	More physical and other CM
McCrann et al[46]	2006	487, university students, Tanzania	27.7%	Poverty, superstition

*Odds or risk ratio.

can be addressed to reduce occurrence of CSA (see Tables 3-1 to 3-3). Females and certain race, origin, and age groups appear consistently to have elevated risk for CSA,[2,3,29,55] but these are not case characteristics that are easily modified (e.g., we would not want to reduce the number of girls to reduce CSA). Some factors, such as poverty[35,55] and single parent households,[30,34] are very difficult to address, and in many poor families with a single parent head of the household, no CSA occurs. We are then left with several factors such as alcohol use,[34] domestic violence,[25] less than high school education,[29] and mental illness,[25] which, if they could be reduced or prevented, could reduce the incidence (and therefore the lifetime prevalence) of CSA. And while up to half of sexually or physically abused adolescents have been found to be "resilient" or resistant to the effects of these adverse experiences,[56] further reductions could occur by increasing protective factors such as attachment security and social supports.[21,41,57] Few studies address the role of society in increasing the propensity for CSA, but some work has suggested we can identify particular neighborhoods for targeted prevention.[58] Interestingly, a lack of CSA education was found to be a risk factor for CSA in one study; this clearly could be addressed by currently available programs.[30,59] Unfortunately, most epidemiological studies fail to provide the proportion of CSA in the population that could be prevented by reducing a particular risk factor (the population attributable risk fraction, or PAR_f) or the specific type of intervention that could be used.

STRENGTH OF THE EVIDENCE AND DIRECTIONS FOR FUTURE RESEARCH

While several improvements have been suggested,[60] the National Child Abuse and Neglect Data System now includes report information from most U.S. states and territories, and the National Incidence Studies have identified numbers of CSA cases and risk factors supported by other independent research. However, current research has not identified the relative contribution of risk and protective factors to the occurrence or recurrence of CSA, and some of the factors identified vary among the populations studied. Other than in Canada, the full extent of CSA in other countries is just beginning to be understood. By increasing the size and representativeness of future incidence and prevalence samples, we will come to better understand the true proportion of our population affected by CSA.

References

1. Finkelhor D: Sexual abuse as a social problem. *In*: Finkelhor D (ed): *Child Sexual Abuse: New Theory and Research*. Free Press, New York, 1984, pp 1-22.
2. U.S. Department of Health and Human Services: *Child maltreatment 1990-2006: reports from the states to the national child abuse and neglect data system*. U.S. Government Printing Office, Washington, DC, 1992-2008.
3. Trocmé NM, Fallon B, MacLaurin B, et al: *Canadian incidence study of reported child abuse and neglect-2003: major findings*. Minister of Public Works and Government Services Canada, Ottawa, 2005.
4. Waterman J, Lusk R: Scope of the problem. *In*: MacFarlane K, Waterman J, Conerly S, et al (eds): *Sexual Abuse of Young Children: Evaluation and Treatment*. Guilford Press, New York, 1986, pp 3-12.
5. Rosenberg DA, Gary N: Sexual abuse of children. *In*: Briere J, Berliner L, Bulkley JA, et al (eds): *The APSAC Handbook on Child Maltreatment*. Sage, Thousand Oaks, Calif, 1996, pp 66-81.
6. English DJ: The extent and consequences of child maltreatment. *Future Child* 1998;8:39-53.
7. Finkelhor D: Current information on the scope and nature of child sexual abuse. *Future Child* 1994;4:31-53.
8. Palusci VJ, Palusci JV: Screening tools for child sexual abuse. *J Pediatr (Rio J)* 2006;82:409-410.
9. Palusci VJ, Cox EO, Cyrus TA, et al: Medical assessment and legal outcome in child sexual abuse. *Arch Pediatr Adolesc Med* 1999;153:388-392.
10. Palusci VJ, Cox EO, Shatz EM, et al: Urgent medical assessment after child sexual abuse. *Child Abuse Negl* 2006;30:367-380.
11. Snyder HN: *Sexual assault of young children as reported to law enforcement: victim, incident and offender characteristics*. U.S. Department of Justice, Bureau of Justice Statistics, Washington, DC, 2000.
12. Sedlak AJ, Broadhurst DD: *The third national incidence study of child abuse and neglect (NIS-3)*. U.S. Department of Health and Human Services, Washington, DC, 1996.
13. Runyan DK, Cox CE, Dubowitz H, et al: Describing maltreatment: do child protective service reports and research definitions agree? *Child Abuse Negl* 2005;29:461-477.
14. Shaffer A, Huston L, Egeland B: Identification of child maltreatment using prospective and self-report methodologies: a comparison of maltreatment incidence and relation to later psychopathology. *Child Abuse Negl* 2008;32:682-692.
15. Everson MD, Smith JB, Hussey JM, et al: Concordance between adolescent reports of childhood abuse and child protective service determinations in an at-risk sample of young adolescents. *Child Maltreat* 2008;13:14-26.
16. Russell DEH: The incidence and prevalence of intrafamilial sexual abuse of female children. *Child Abuse Negl* 1983;7:133-146.
17. Boyer D, Fine D: Sexual abuse as a factor in adolescent pregnancy and maltreatment. *Fam Plan Perspect* 1992;24:4-19.
18. Holmes WC: Association with a history of child sexual abuse and subsequent adolescent psychoactive substance abuse disorder in a sample of HIV seropositive men. *J Adolesc Health* 1997;20:414-419.
19. Ompad DC, Ikeda RM, Shah N, et al: Childhood sexual abuse and age at initiation of injection drug use. *Am J Public Health* 2005;95:703-709.
20. Littleton H, Breitkopf CR, Berenson A: Sexual and physical abuse history and adult sexual risk behaviors: relationships among women and potential mediators. *Child Abuse Negl* 2007;31:757-768.
21. Aspelmeier JE, Elliott, AN, Smith CH: Childhood sexual abuse, attachment, and trauma symptoms in college females: the moderating role of attachment. *Child Abuse Negl* 2007;31:549-566.
22. Van Gerko K, Hughes ML, Hamill M, et al: Reported childhood sexual abuse and eating-disorder cognitions and behaviors. *Child Abuse Negl* 2005;29:375-382.
23. Harlow BL, Stewart EG: Adult-onset vulvodynia in relation to childhood violence victimization. *Am J Epidemiol* 2005;161:871-880.
24. Trent M, Clum G, Roche KM: Sexual victimization and reproductive health outcomes in urban youth. *Ambul Pediatr* 2007;74:313-316.
25. Whetten K, Leserman J, Lowe K, et al: Prevalence of sexual abuse and physical trauma in an HIV-positive sample from the deep South. *Am J Public Health* 2006;96:1028-1030.
26. Johnson RJ, Ross MW, Taylor WC, et al: Prevalence of childhood sexual abuse among incarcerated males in county jail. *Child Abuse Negl* 2006;30:75-86.
27. Edwards VJ, Holden GW, Felitti VJ, et al: Relationship between multiple forms of childhood maltreatment and adult mental health in community respondents: results from the adverse childhood experiences study. *Am J Psychiatry* 2003;160:1453-1460.
28. Theodore AD, Chang JJ, Runyan DK, et al: Epidemiologic features of the physical and sexual maltreatment of children in the Carolinas. *Pediatrics* 2005;115:e331-e337.
29. Senn TE, Carey MP, Vanable PA, et al: Childhood sexual abuse and sexual risk behavior among men and women attending a sexually transmitted disease clinic. *J Consult Clin Psychol* 2006;74:720-731.
30. Finkelhor D, Hoteling G, Lewis IA, et al: Sexual abuse in a national survey of adult men and women: prevalence, characteristics and risk factors. *Child Abuse Negl* 1990;14:19-28.
31. Briere J, Elliott DM: Prevalence and psychological sequelae of self-reported childhood physical and sexual abuse in a general population sample of men and women. *Child Abuse Negl* 2003;27:1205-1222.

32. Rind B, Tromovitch P, Bauserman R: A meta-analytic evaluation of assumed properties of child sexual abuse using college samples. *Psychol Bull* 1998;124:22-53.

33. Adams RE, Burkowski WM: Relationships with mothers and peers moderate the association between childhood sexual abuse and anxiety disorders. *Child Abuse Negl* 2007;31:645-656.

34. Vogeltanz ND, Wilsnack SC, Harris TR, et al: Prevalence and risk factors for childhood sexual abuse in women: national survey findings. *Child Abuse Negl* 1999;23:579-592.

35. Hussey JM, Chang JJ, Kotch JB: Child maltreatment in the United States: prevalence, risk factors and adolescent health consequences. *Pediatrics* 2006;118:933-942.

36. Finkelhor D, Ormrod R, Turner H, et al: The victimization of children and youth: a comprehensive, national survey. *Child Maltreat* 2005;10:5-25.

37. Mrazek PJ, Lynch MA, Bentovin A: Sexual abuse of children in the United Kingdom. *Child Abuse Negl* 1983;7:147-153.

38. May-Chahal C, Cawson P: Measuring child maltreatment in the United Kingdom: a study of the prevalence of child abuse and neglect. *Child Abuse Negl* 2005;29:969-984.

39. Dunne MP, Purdie DM, Cook MD, et al: Is child sexual abuse declining? Evidence from a population-based survey of men and women in Australia. *Child Abuse Negl* 2003;27:141-152.

40. Luo Y, Parish WL, Laumann EO: A population-based study of childhood sexual contact in China: prevalence and long-term consequences. *Child Abuse Negl* 2008;32:721-731.

41. Senior R, Barnes J, Emberson JR, et al: Early experiences and the relationship to maternal eating disorder symptoms, both lifetime and during pregnancy. *Br J Psychiatry* 2005;187:268-273.

42. Chen J, Dunne MP, Han P: Child sexual abuse in China: a study of adolescents in four provinces. *Child Abuse Negl* 2004;28:1171-1186.

43. Jirapramukpitak T, Prince M, Harpham T: The experience of abuse and mental health in the young Thai population. *Soc Psychiatry Psychiatr Epidemiol* 2005;40:955-963.

44. Fanslow JL, Robinson EM, Crengle S, et al: Prevalence of child sexual abuse reported by a cross-sectional sample of New Zealand women. *Child Abuse Negl* 2007;31:935-945.

45. Gladstone GL, Parker GB, Mitchell PB, et al: Implications of childhood trauma for depressed women: an analysis of pathways from childhood sexual abuse to deliberate self-harm and revictimization. *Am J Psychiatry* 2004;161:1417-1425.

46. McCrann D, Lalor K, Katabaro JK: Childhood sexual abuse among university students in Tanzania. *Child Abuse Negl* 2006;30:1343-1351.

47. Jones LM, Finkelhor D, Kopiec K: Why is sexual abuse declining? A survey of state child protection administrators. *Child Abuse Negl* 2001;25:1139-1158.

48. Finkelhor D, Jones LM: Explanations for the decline in child sexual abuse cases. *Juvenile Justice Bulletin*, Office of Juvenile Justice and Delinquency Prevention, U.S. Dept. of Justice, Washington, DC, January, 2004 (website): http://www.ncjrs.gov/PDFfiles1/ojjdp/199290.PDF. Accessed February 15, 2010.

49. Finkelhor D, Jones L: Why have child maltreatment and child victimization declined? *J Soc Issues* 2006;62:685-716.

50. Jones LM, Finkelhor D: Putting together evidence on declining trends in sexual abuse: a complex puzzle. *Child Abuse Negl* 2003;27:133-135.

51. Fluke JD, Hollinshead DM: *Child maltreatment recurrence*. U.S. Department of Health and Human Services, Washington, DC, 2003.

52. Palusci VJ, Smith EG, Paneth N: Predicting and responding to physical abuse in young children using NCANDS. *Child Youth Serv Rev* 2005;27:667-682.

53. Fluke JD, Shusterman GR, Hollinshead DM, et al: Longitudinal analysis of repeated child abuse reporting and victimization: multistate analysis of associated factors. *Child Maltreat* 2008;12:76-88.

54. Finkelhor D, Ormrod RK, Turner HA: Re-victimization patterns in a national longitudinal sample of children and youth. *Child Abuse Negl* 2007;31:479-502.

55. Finkelhor D: Victims. *In*: Finkelhor D (ed): *Child Sexual Abuse: New Theory and Research*. Free Press, New York, 1984, pp 23-32.

56. DuMont KA, Widom, CS, Czaja SJ: Predictors of resilience in abuse and neglected children grown-up: the role of individual and neighborhood characteristics. *Child Abuse Negl* 2007;31:255-274.

57. Jonzon E, Lindblad F: Risk factors and protective factors in relation to subjective health among adult female victims of child sexual abuse. *Child Abuse Negl* 2006;30:127-143.

58. Tadoum RK, Smolij K, Lyn MA, et al: Predicting childhood sexual or physical abuse: a logistic regression geo-mapping approach to prevention. *AMIA Annu Symp Proc* 2005:1130.

59. Finkelhor D: Prevention of sexual abuse through educational programs directed toward children. *Pediatrics* 2007;120:640-645.

60. Finkelhor D, Wells M: Improving national data systems about juvenile victimization. *Child Abuse Negl* 2003;27:77-102.

4

EPIDEMIOLOGY OF INTIMATE PARTNER VIOLENCE

Jonathan D. Thackeray, MD, and Kimberly A. Randell, MD, MSc

INTRODUCTION

At its most basic level, intimate partner violence (IPV) involves the exertion of power and control by one person over another. IPV is pervasive in our society and no culture, ethnicity, or race should be considered immune. As practitioners, it is important to recognize the magnitude of the problem, to understand the complex social dynamics involved in these violent relationships, and most importantly, to appreciate the profound and long-lasting effects IPV can have on a person's physical, emotional, and behavioral health.

DEFINITIONS

The study of IPV has, in many ways, suffered from the inability of investigators to agree on the use of consistent terminology. Although often used interchangeably, the term "intimate partner violence" is distinct from other, more inclusive terms such as "family violence" or "domestic violence," which may encompass additional forms of violence, including child abuse and elder abuse. The term "intimate partner violence" should also be distinguished from the term "violence against women," which includes not only IPV, but sexual violence by unknown perpetrators and other forms of violence against women as well. Additionally, research has shown a lack of consistency in what people consider acts of "violence" and who represents an "intimate partner." Much of the early research in the field, for example, focused primarily on physical acts of aggression against women, without consideration of other forms of violence.[1]

For the purposes of this chapter, we define IPV using the definition adopted by the World Health Organization: "Any behavior within an intimate relationship that causes physical, psychological or sexual harm to those in the relationship.[2]" This definition is consistent with the Centers for Disease Control and Prevention (CDC), which defines IPV as "a pattern of coercive behaviors that may include repeated battering and injury, psychological abuse, sexual assault, progressive social isolation, deprivation and intimidation.[3]" What the definitions from these two organizations share is the recognition that IPV encompasses many forms of maltreatment, including physical abuse, sexual abuse, emotional abuse and neglect. Perhaps no organization has illustrated this concept better than the Domestic Abuse Intervention Project with the "Power and Control Wheel" (Figure 4-1). Although the figure is specific to abusive behaviors by men against women, "intimate partners" are defined by the CDC as current, divorced, or separated spouses (including common-law), and current or former dating or nonmarital partners, irrespective of gender, history of sexual involvement, or cohabitation status.[3]

SCOPE OF THE ISSUE

Given the variability in the published research, the true incidence and prevalence of IPV is difficult to determine. As a result, there are likely mixed conclusions as to the scope of the problem, and many believe that published statistics either underestimate or overexaggerate the issue. What is clear, however, is that IPV is a global health crisis. A review of 48 population-based surveys from around the world found that between 10% and 69% of women report being physically assaulted by an intimate partner at some point in their lives.[2] When considering additional and more common forms of IPV, such as intimidation, controlling behaviors, and humiliation, it is believed one in three women worldwide will be abused in her lifetime.[4] In the United States, it is estimated that 1.5 million women are physically or sexually assaulted by an intimate partner each year.[5] Many of these women are assaulted more than once, raising estimates to nearly 5 million assaults each year. It is important to recognize that patterns of dating violence begin early in life. Approximately 1 in 5 female high school students report being physically and/or sexually abused by a dating partner.[6]

RISK FACTORS

The risk factors leading to perpetration of and victimization by IPV are best thought of in a socioecological model that considers individual, relational, community, and societal concerns. Individually, perhaps one of the strongest risk factors for becoming a perpetrator of IPV is a history of family violence during childhood. This includes not only the child who suffers abuse, but also the child who is exposed to violence between his/her parents. Other recognized risk factors for an individual include mental health issues (specifically depression) and substance abuse. Women of lower socioeconomic status are disproportionately affected by IPV. Within relationships, risk factors for IPV include conflict, instability, or discord within the relationship, often centering around economic or job stress, or the stressors associated with pregnancy and childbirth. Communities are often poorly equipped to respond to IPV as a public health issue and may in part contribute to the issue by "refusing to take a stand" against the violence. Likewise, societies that devalue

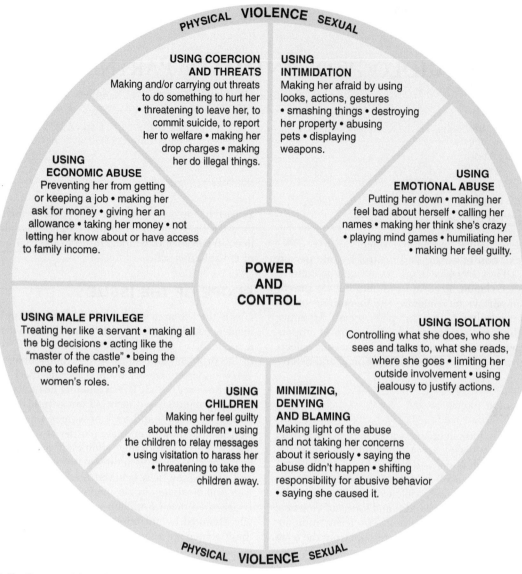

FIGURE 4-1 The Power and Control Wheel of the Domestic Abuse Intervention Project in Duluth, Minn., www.duluth-model.org.

the independence of women and promote violence as a means of resolving disputes likely foster an environment where IPV can thrive.

SOCIAL CONSIDERATIONS

With respect to how a woman views her abusive relationship, it has been proposed that there are several cognitive stages of change through which she may pass, ranging at one end from failure to even recognize IPV as a problem to the other where she has ended a relationship and is avoiding further abuse.[7] Because of this spectrum of response, caring for women who are in abusive relationships is a dynamic process and may be frustrating for a health care provider. For those women that do recognize abusive behavior as a problem, the decision to seek help is difficult and is compounded by numerous personal, systemic, and societal barriers. To effectively help women involved in these relationships, we must begin to understand the principal social dynamics of IPV, including the common barriers preventing

victims and providers from addressing IPV and the motivating factors for a woman to disclose IPV and seek help.

Barriers to Seeking Help

Before deciding to leave an abusive relationship, a woman must recognize that her relationship is a problem. Based on a childhood exposure to violence, or experience in past violent relationships, women may believe that a normal relationship is characterized by abusive behavior. Some also downplay the abuse as a problem unless one is injured severely enough to require medical attention.[8]

Even after recognizing the abuse as a problem, women often continue in the relationship. The decision to leave is confounded by conflicting emotional states. While recognizing the need to leave, many women continue to feel love for the perpetrator. Remembering the "good times" of the relationship, they hope for change and protect the perpetrator.[8-11] Additionally, low self-esteem, guilt, shame, and self-blame, all of which are often fostered by the perpetrator, prevent women from accessing help.[11-14] Fear of perpetrator reprisal against efforts to leave is an immense barrier.[8]

Practical concerns also impede leaving an abusive relationship. Many women are without jobs or access to household accounts and are therefore financially dependent upon their abuser.[8,9,11] There is the potential to lose the home and current lifestyle. Social isolation is a common weapon of abuse. Women may be separated emotionally or geographically from friends and family and they often do not know who to turn to for help.[9,15]

Women with children cite several unique barriers to accessing help, including the need to keep the family together and have the children know their father, not disrupting their children's lives, and fear of child protective services involvement and possible resultant loss of custody.[8-10,12,13]

In addition to the personal reasons cited above, women face societal and cultural barriers as well. Many women perceive a lack of community openness and support in discussing IPV.[8] They feel there is a stigma associated with shelter living.[12] Religious communities, families, and friends may invalidate the victim's disclosure by blaming her or refusing to believe her.[10,12] Cultural norms may condone IPV. Immigrant women face a unique set of barriers. In addition to the typical isolation of an abusive relationship, they must overcome language and cultural barriers as well. Concern about consequences related to immigration status also hinder disclosure.[9]

Finally, women may perceive barriers within the very systems intended to provide help. In regard to the criminal justice system, women are prevented from accessing help by the belief that, ultimately, the legal system is not helpful. Women cite the delay between a call to the police and their arrival, a bureaucratic system that is difficult to navigate, uncertain outcome, lack of support for victims, and the presence of a "good ol' boys" network as reasons for anticipating a lack of efficacy and therefore underutilization of the resources the criminal justice system offers.[13,15] With respect to health care resources, women cite the lack of health care providers' (HCP) understanding of the complexity of IPV, the lack of HCP knowledge of appropriate referral resources, lack of efficacy, fear that a disclosure of IPV will lead to a police or CPS report, cost of medical care, lack of knowledge that HCP can address IPV, and failure of the HCP to directly ask women about IPV.[11,13-15]

As evidenced by the discussion above, the barriers to leaving an abusive relationship are numerous and provide multiple areas where access to care can be improved.

Motivators for IPV Victims to Seek Help

Simply understanding and removing the barriers to IPV help-seeking is often not enough to convince a woman to leave an abusive relationship. Like many public health issues, before someone can access help, he or she must be willing and motivated to do so. Although not as well studied, the motivators for IPV help-seeking are no less important than the barriers to IPV help-seeking. In fact they may be interrelated and addressing the motivators may decrease certain barriers.

Many women cite increasing knowledge as a motivator for leaving an abusive relationship. This knowledge encompasses multiple domains: dynamics and definitions of IPV, availability and types of resources, and self-awareness.[8] Additionally, reaching an emotional or physical breaking point often triggers help-seeking.[8] For women with children, the many consequences of IPV for their children may be powerful motivators. These consequences include endangered physical safety, short and long-term effects of children's witnessing IPV on their emotional well-being, and CPS involvement with potential loss of custody.[8] A final motivator for leaving the abusive relationship is outside intervention. Interveners take many forms: legal professionals, friends, family, health care providers, and neighbors. One study suggests that the majority of women in shelter homes did not seek out information on resources on their own, but acted on information and suggestions provided by outside individuals.[16]

Understanding the motivators for help-seeking discussed previously allows directed interventions with the goal of increasing both disclosure and action.

Provider Barriers

Not only do women face barriers in discussing IPV, but there are well-documented barriers preventing health care providers from addressing the issue as well. Despite the overwhelming evidence to the contrary, many providers fail to recognize that IPV is an issue in their patient population.[17] Even when IPV is suspected, a provider may contextualize the issue as "nonmedical" and therefore be reluctant to directly question a patient.[18] The belief that direct questioning regarding IPV is somehow offensive or angering remains prevalent,[19] despite a wealth of research that demonstrates the majority of women are comfortable with being screened for IPV.[11,20-22] Some providers feel that patients would willingly volunteer a history of abuse if present, while others simply forget to ask.[23] Other common barriers that providers experience include limited time to conduct IPV assessments,[24-26] lack of formal training in evaluation and referral for IPV,[26-28] and concern with an inability to provide resources to those who disclose IPV.[19,26,29]

EFFECT OF INTIMATE PARTNER VIOLENCE ON CHILDREN

Children represent a special population at risk from IPV, both as victims of abuse and as witnesses to it. Rates of IPV are increased among households with children, and it is estimated that 3.3 to 15.5 million children are exposed to IPV in the United States each year.[30,31] Over the last several years, research has focused on the negative impact that IPV may have on a child's physical, emotional, and behavioral health. Recognizing the potential negative health outcomes for children, the American Academy of Pediatrics deemed the abuse of women a "pediatric issue" and recommended IPV screening for all female caregivers at well-child visits and the development of intervention plans for caregivers with positive screens.[32]

While estimates of the co-occurrence vary depending on study methodology, IPV is clearly associated with psychological, physical, sexual child maltreatment, and neglect. A large review found a median co-occurrence of 40% among battered women and abused children.[33] Community samples show co-occurrence rates of 5.6% to 55%.[34-36] A longitudinal study of at-risk families demonstrated an increased risk for physical and psychological abuse and neglect that persisted up to 5 years of age after IPV exposure in the first 6 months of life.[37] Evidence suggests that the combination of IPV exposure and child maltreatment has synergistic negative effects.[38,39]

Children also are at risk for physical harm as bystanders. A retrospective review showed that children of all ages are inadvertently injured during episodes of IPV.[40] Forty percent of the patients in this review had injuries requiring medical treatment. Young children were disproportionately represented among these patients and were more likely to incur head and facial injuries. It is likely that more children are accidentally injured during IPV episodes than health care providers recognize, as many may not come in for medical care and those that do may not disclose the true mechanism of injury for fear of reprisal.

Children of all ages, from infancy to adolescence, are affected by IPV exposure. Children exposed to IPV are at risk for internalizing and externalizing behavior problems, decreased cognitive performance, and suicide.[41-47] Internalizing problems include depression, anxiety, and social withdrawal. Externalizing problems include aggression, hyperactivity, and defiance of authority. Both internalizing and externalizing behaviors may negatively affect peer relationships, parent-child bonds, and school performance.

Additionally, childhood IPV exposure is a marker for other risk exposures. In the Adverse Childhood Experiences (ACE) study, 95% of respondents with histories of childhood IPV exposure experienced at least one additional adverse experience, including parental separation/divorce, household substance abuse, mental illness, and criminal activity.[36] These children are more likely to be exposed to other types of community violence as well. Increasing numbers of adverse exposures are associated with increasing negative outcomes.[38,47-49]

It is important to recognize that the negative effects of IPV exposure are not limited to childhood and can have serious health implications for the adult. Evidence links such exposure, alone and in combination with other adverse childhood experiences, with increased incidence of smoking, alcoholism, severe obesity, and diseases such as diabetes, ischemic heart disease, and depressive disorders.[38,48,49]

The degree to which each child is affected by IPV exposure depends upon a number of mediating factors: mother-child attachment, parenting styles, maternal depression, socioeconomic status, shelter status, child's temperament, and age at time of exposure.[41-43,50] However, children exposed to IPV are clearly at risk for both current and future problems in multiple areas. Identification of children exposed to IPV allows targeted interventions for at-risk children and the potential to ameliorate negative outcomes.

STRENGTH OF THE MEDICAL EVIDENCE

Intimate partner violence is inherently a difficult issue to study in that there is no gold standard test to measure its prevalence. With rare exceptions, the detection of IPV is the result of a complex dynamic between provider and patient, and ultimately the provider relies on the patient to disclose that IPV is present. True prevalence and incidence of the condition is therefore difficult to estimate. Further complicating the issue have been variations in study populations and a general inability of researchers to consistently define who constitutes an intimate partner and what constitutes a violent or abusive act. For all these reasons, the validity of conclusions that can be drawn from the research is, at the very least, subject to scrutiny. Only recently has the Centers for Disease Control published recommendations designed to promote consistency in the use of terminology and data collection related to intimate partner violence.[4] In the coming years, researchers will be challenged to incorporate consistent study methodologies to improve the value of the data collected.

DIRECTIONS FOR FUTURE RESEARCH

There remain many unexplored territories for IPV research. Despite a large body of work looking at how and when providers should best assess for IPV, there is almost no research that demonstrates improved outcomes when doing so. Could there potentially be harm caused by asking a woman about IPV? What can be done for those women who disclose IPV and for their children? These questions remain largely unanswered.

Despite ample research, which has traditionally focused on the subset of IPV that is violence perpetrated by males against females, there is a relative paucity of studies examining violence perpetrated by females against males or the dynamics of violence in gay, lesbian, bisexual, or transgender relationships. Targeted studies looking at these specific populations will be necessary in the coming years. Finally, it is becoming increasingly obvious that IPV is not just an issue that affects adult relationships, but also is pervasive in the adolescent population as well. Patterns of dating violence behavior often begin early and further work is needed to help pediatric/adolescent practitioners identify and address this issue with their patients and families.

References

1. Straus MA, Gelles RJ, Steinmetz SK: *Behind closed doors: violence in the American family*. Sage, Newbury Park, Calif, 1980.
2. Krug EG, Dahlberg LL, Mercy JA, et al *(eds): World report on violence and health*. World Health Organization, Geneva, 2002.
3. Saltzman LE, Fanslow JL, McMahon PM, et al: Intimate partner violence surveillance: uniform definitions and recommended data elements, Version 1.0, National Center for Injury Prevention and Control, Centers for Disease Control and Prevention (website): http://www.cdc.gov/ncipc/pub-res/ipv_surveillance/Intimate%20Partner%20Violence.pdf. Accessed January 28, 2009.
4. Heise L, Ellsberg M, Gottemoeller M: Ending violence against women. *Popul Rep L* 1999; 11 (website): Available at http://info.k4health.org/pr/l11edsum.shtml. Accessed February 15, 2010.
5. Tjaden P, Thoennes N: *Full report of the prevalence, incidence, and consequences of intimate partner violence: findings from the national violence against women survey*. National Institute of Justice, Washington, DC, 2000.
6. Silverman JG, Raj A, Mucci L, et al: Dating violence against adolescent girls and associated substance use, unhealthy weight control, sexual risk behavior, pregnancy, and suicidality. *JAMA* 2001;286:572-579.
7. Burke JG, Denison JA, Gielen AC, et al: Ending intimate partner violence: an application of the transtheoretical model. *Am J Health Behav* 2004;28:122-133.

8. Petersen R, Moracco KE, Goldstein KM: Moving beyond disclosure: women's perspectives on barriers and motivators to seeking assistance for intimate partner violence. *Women Health* 2004;40:63-76.

9. Fugate M, Landis L, Riordan K, et al: Barriers to domestic violence help seeking: implications for intervention. *Violence Against Women* 2005;11:290-310.

10. Lutenbacher M, Cohen A, Mitzel J: Do we really help? Perspectives of abused women. *Public Health Nurs* 2003;20:56-64.

11. Rodriguez MA, Quiroga SS, Bauer HM: Breaking the silence. Battered women's perspectives on medical care. *Arch Fam Med* 1996;5:153-158.

12. Feder GS, Hutson M, Ramsay, et al: Women exposed to intimate partner violence: expectations and experiences when they encounter healthcare professionals: a meta-analysis of qualitative studies. *Arch Intern Med* 2006;166:22-37.

13. Petersen R, Moracco KE, Goldstein KM, et al: Women's perspectives on intimate partner violence services: the hope in Pandora's box. *J Am Med Womens Assoc* 2003;58:185-190.

14. Wester W, Wong SLF, Lagro-Janssen ALM: What do abused women expect from their family physicians? A qualitative study among women in shelter homes. *Women Health* 2007;45:105-119.

15. Logan JK, Stevenson E, Evans L, et al: Rural and urban women's perspectives of barriers to health, mental health and criminal justice services: Implications for victim services. *Violence Vict* 2004;19:37-62.

16. Randell KA, Bledsoe L, Shroff P, et al: Motivators for intimate partner violence help seeking: implications for intervention in the pediatric emergency department. Unpublished data.

17. Sugg NK, Thompson RS, Thompson DC, et al: Domestic violence and primary care: attitudes, practices, and beliefs. *Arch Fam Med* 1999;8:301-306.

18. Tilden VP: Response of the health care delivery system to battered women. *Issues Ment Health Nurs* 1989;10:309-320.

19. Lapidus G, Beaulieu Cooke M, Gelven E, et al: A statewide survey of domestic violence screening behaviors among pediatricians and family physicians. *Arch Pediatr Adolesc Med* 2002;156:332-336.

20. Bacchus L, Mezey G, Bewley S: Women's perceptions and experiences of routine enquiry for domestic violence in a maternity service. *Br J Obstet Gynaecol* 2002;109:9-16.

21. Burge SK, Schneider FD, Ivy L, et al: Patients' advice to physicians about intervening in family conflict. *Ann Fam Med* 2005;3:248-254.

22. Friedman LS, Samet JH, Roberts MS, et al: Inquiry about victimization experiences. A survey of patient preferences and physician practices. *Arch Intern Med* 1992;152:1186-1190.

23. Elliott L, Nerney M, Jones T, et al: Barriers to screening for domestic violence. *J Gen Intern Med* 2002;17:112-116.

24. Davies J, Harris M, Roberts G, et al: Community health workers' response to violence against women. *Austr N Z J Ment Health Nurs* 1996;5:20-31.

25. McGrath ME, Bettacchi A, Duffy SJ, et al: Violence against women: provider barriers to intervention in emergency departments. *Acad Emerg Med* 1997;4:297-300.

26. Sugg NK, Inui T: Primary care physicians' response to domestic violence: opening Pandora's box. *JAMA* 1992;267:65-68.

27. Parsons LH, Zaccaro D, Wells B, et al: Methods of and attitudes toward screening obstetrics and gynecology patients for domestic violence. *Am J Obstet Gynecol* 1995;173:381-386.

28. Wright RJ, Wright RO, Isaac NE: Response to battered mothers in the pediatric emergency department: a call for an interdisciplinary approach to family violence. *Pediatrics* 1997;99:186-192.

29. Molliconi SA, Runyan C: Detecting domestic violence: a pilot study of family practitioners. *N C Med J* 1996;57:136-138.

30. Edleson JL: Children's witnessing of adult domestic violence. *J Interpers Violence* 1999;14:839-870.

31. McDonald R, Jouriles EN, Ramisetty-Mikler S, et al: Estimating the number of American children living in partner-violent families. *J Fam Psychol* 2006;20:137-142.

32. Committee on Child Abuse and Neglect: The role of the pediatrician in recognizing and intervening on behalf of abused children. *Pediatrics* 1998;101:1091-1092.

33. Appel AE, Holden GW: Co-occurrence of spouse and physical child abuse: a review and appraisal. *J Fam Psychol* 1998;12:578-599.

34. Zolotor AJ, Theodore AD, Coyne-Beasley T, et al: Intimate partner violence and child maltreatment: overlapping risk. *Brief Treat Crisis Interv* 2007;7:305-321.

35. Slep AM, O'Leary SG: Parent and partner violence in families with young children: rates, patterns and connections. *J Consult Clin Psychol* 2005;73:435-444.

36. Dong M, Anda RF, Felitti VJ, et al: The interrelatedness of multiple forms of childhood abuse, neglect and household dysfunction. *Child Abuse Negl* 2004;28:771-784.

37. McGuigan WM, Pratt CC: The effect of domestic violence on three types of child maltreatment. *Child Abuse Negl* 2001;25:869-883.

38. Felitti VJ, Anda RF, Nordenberg D, et al: Relationship of childhood abuse and household dysfunction to many of the leading causes of death in adults: the adverse childhood experiences study. *Am J Prev Med* 1998;14:245-258.

39. Antle BF, Barbee AP, Sullin D, et al: The relationship between domestic violence and child neglect. *Brief Treat Crisis Interv* 2007;7:364-382.

40. Christian CW, Scribano P, Seidl T, et al: Pediatric injury resulting from family violence. *Pediatrics* 1997;99:e8.

41. Hazen AL, Connelly CD, Kelleher KJ, et al: Female caregivers' experience with intimate partner violence and behavior problems in children investigated as victims of maltreatment. *Pediatrics* 2006;117:99-109.

42. Levendosky AA, Leahy KL, Bogat GA, et al: Domestic violence, maternal parenting, maternal mental health and infant externalizing behavior. *J Fam Psychol* 2006;20:544-552.

43. Fantuzzo JW, DePaola LM, Lambert L, et al: Effects of interparental violence on the psychological adjustment and competencies of young children. *J Consult Clin Psychol* 1991;59:258-265.

44. Huth-Bocks AC, Levendosky AA, Semel MA: The direct and indirect effects of domestic violence on young children's intellectual functioning. *J Fam Violence* 2001;16:269-290.

45. McDonald R, Jouriles EN, Rosenfield D, et al: Violence toward a family member, angry adult conflict, and child adjustment difficulties: relations in families with 1-to-3-year-old children. *J Fam Psychol* 2007;21:176-184.

46. Thompson, R, Briggs E, English DJ, et al: Suicidal ideation among 8-year-olds who are maltreated and at risk: findings from the LONGSCAN studies. *Child Maltreat* 2005;10:26-36.

47. Baliff-Spanvill B, Clayton CJ, Hendrix SB: Witness and nonwitness children's violent and peaceful behavior in different types of simulated conflict with peers. *Am J Orthopsychiatry* 2007;77:206-215.

48. Anda RF, Croft JB, Felitti VJ, et al: Adverse childhood experiences and smoking during adolescence and adulthood. *JAMA* 1999;282:1652-1658.

49. Dube SR, Anda RF, Felitti VJ, et al: Childhood abuse, household dysfunction and risk of attempted suicide throughout the life span: findings from the adverse childhood experiences study. *JAMA* 2001;286:3089-3096.

50. Levendosky AA, Huth-Bocks AC, Shapiro DL, et al: Impact of domestic violence on maternal-child relationship and preschool-age children's functioning. *J Fam Psychol* 2003;17:275-287.

5

EPIDEMIOLOGY OF CHILD NEGLECT

Howard Dubowitz, MD, MS

INTRODUCTION

Neglect is the most frequently identified form of child maltreatment, accounting for approximately two thirds of reports to child protective services.[1] This chapter covers a few key aspects concerning the epidemiology of child neglect: definitional issues, its incidence, and what is known about contributors to neglect. Related issues such as medical neglect as a result of not receiving health care for religious reasons and dental neglect are addressed in separate chapters.

DEFINITIONAL ISSUES

How Much Care is Adequate? Neglect and a Continuum of Care

The adequacy of care a child receives exists on a continuum from optimal to grossly inadequate, without natural cut points. A crude categorization of situations as "neglect" or "no neglect" is often simplistic. Seldom is a need met perfectly or not at all; cut-points are usually quite arbitrary. It is difficult to determine at what point inadequate household sanitation, for example, is associated with harmful outcomes. And, with relatively few extreme situations, the gray zone is large. Even a relatively concrete area such as establishing the daily requirement for key nutrients is not straightforward, and, it is difficult to measure the extent to which these are met.

Examples of adequate health care include: Reasonable efforts made for minor problems (e.g., cleaning a cut), professional care obtained for moderate to severe problems (e.g., trouble breathing), child receives adequate treatment to optimize outcome and limit complications (i.e., adequate adherence to treatment regimen), child receives recommended preventive health care (e.g., immunizations), and professional care meets accepted health care standards (i.e., appropriate treatment). The last example illustrates how deficits in care are not always due to parents. In keeping with the quality of care being on a continuum, it may be useful to categorize care, for example, as "excellent" (infant seat always used), "moderate" (infant seat usually used), or "inadequate" (seat seldom used).

The Quest for an Evidence-Based Definition

Ideally, a definition of neglect would be based on empirical data demonstrating the actual or probable harm associated with certain circumstances (e.g., not receiving adequate emotional support). Although evidence-based definitions are a good goal, they are difficult to achieve for most types of neglect.

Children's health, safety, and development occur within a complex ecology with many and interacting influences, making it difficult to study the impact of a single risk factor, such as inadequate emotional support. The context of children's experiences also influences the possible impact of a given circumstance; a mature 9-year-old, for example, may do well alone at home for a few hours, whereas an unsupervised child with a fire-setting problem is a scary proposition. In some areas, it is probably not necessary to have evidence documenting harm (e.g., hunger, homelessness, abandonment). It is very clear that these conditions impair children's safety, health, and development.

In practice, we need to apply the best available knowledge, albeit often less than we would like, to clarify whether a certain circumstance or pattern of experiences jeopardizes a child's wellbeing. Situations where the likelihood of harm is equivocal are best *not* considered to be neglect, although that should not preclude efforts to improve care. Research may help elucidate whether such circumstances should warrant concern.

Actual *vs.* Potential Harm

Most state legal definitions of neglect include circumstances of potential harm in addition to actual harm. However, approximately one third of states restrict their practice to circumstances involving actual harm.[2] Potential harm is of special concern because the impact of neglect may be apparent only years later. In addition, the goal of prevention may be served by addressing neglect even if no harm is yet apparent. However, it is often difficult to predict the likelihood and nature of future harm. In some instances, epidemiological data are useful. For example, we can estimate the increased risk of a serious head injury from a fall off a bicycle when not wearing a helmet compared with being protected.[3] In contrast, predicting the likelihood of harm when an 8-year-old is left home alone for a few hours is difficult. Such circumstances may come to light only if actual harm ensues. Even when we can estimate risks, opinions may vary as to how seriously to weigh a risk. In addition to the likelihood of harm, the nature of the potential harm should be considered. Even a high likelihood of minor harm (e.g., bruising from a short fall) might be acceptable. Life is not risk free. Indeed, children's development requires taking risks (e.g., learning to walk and falling). In contrast, even a low likelihood of severe harm (e.g., drowning) is unacceptable.

Further Refining the Definition of Neglect: A Heterogeneous Phenomenon

The different types of neglect children may experience represent a wide range of circumstances. In addition to characterizing different types of neglect—physical, emotional, supervisory, educational, etc.[4] —it is useful to describe other aspects of neglect: the severity, the duration (or chronicity), number of incidents (frequency), intentionality, and the context in which neglect occurs.

Severity is viewed in terms of the likelihood and seriousness of harm. Simply put, severe neglect occurs when the unmet need is associated with serious harm, actual or potential. And, the greater the likelihood of such harm, the more severe is the neglect.

Several researchers have pursued different strategies to rate the severity of neglect.[5-9] These approaches have limited clinical usefulness.

Chronicity, a pattern of needs not being met over time, is important albeit challenging to assess. One study[10] found that chronicity of maltreatment was related to child outcomes. Some experiences of neglect are usually only worrisome when they occur repeatedly (e.g., poor hygiene). The challenge to assessing chronicity is clear; caregivers seldom disclose socially undesirable information. Older children, however, may be helpful. A crude proxy of chronicity is the duration of child protective services (CPS) involvement, or the time between the first and most recent reports. The problem is clear. A CPS report reflects only when problems were identified; it is highly speculative to assume what transpired before and between reports.

Frequency is similarly difficult to assess. Caregivers or older children may disclose the information. The number of CPS reports again offers a crude proxy.

Intentionality is a question that arises regarding neglect—implicitly or explicitly. Intentionality may not apply to most neglectful situations. The Merriam-Webster dictionary defines *intentional* as "done by *intention* or design." In most cases, parents do not intend to neglect their children's needs. Rather, problems impair their ability to adequately meet these needs. Even the most egregious cases, such as those where parents appear to willfully deny their children food, probably involve significant parental psychopathology; labeling such instances "intentional" may be simplistic. In clinical practice, as we strive to strengthen families, viewing their shortcomings as intentional may be counterproductive, especially if it fosters a negative stance toward parents.

Finally, as a practical matter, it is very difficult to assess intentionality.

Cultural context is relevant to defining neglect. For example, in many cultures, young children help care for younger siblings. This is both a necessity and considered important in learning to be responsible. Others may view the practice as unreasonably burdensome for the child caregiver and too risky an arrangement. There is no easy resolution to such differences, and there can be dilemmas concerning new immigrants to the United States. Clearly, the risks here might be very different from those in the country of origin. We need to recognize the importance of cultural context and how it influences child rearing practices and the meaning and consequences of experiences for children. It is, however, also important to recognize that just because a certain practice is normative within a culture does not preclude possible harm.[11] One needs to be careful to avoid glibly accepting all culturally accepted practices; some may be clearly harmful and should not be sanctioned. At the same time, good practice should always involve understanding the culture and engaging the family respectfully.

Poverty is strongly linked with child neglect. For example, in the Third National Incidence Study (NIS-3), neglect was 44 more times likely to be identified in families earning less than $15,000 a year compared with those earning over $30,000.[4] There are also ample data demonstrating that poverty per se jeopardizes children's health, development, and safety.[12] Poverty can thus be construed as a form of societal neglect, particularly in a country with enormous resources. The child welfare system, however, focuses narrowly on parental or caregiver omissions in care (i.e., fault); 11 states and Washington, D.C., laws explicitly exclude circumstances attributable to poverty in their neglect definitions.

THE INCIDENCE OF CHILD NEGLECT

In 2006, 64% of the 905,000 substantiated CPS reports were for neglect, 2.2% for medical neglect, 16% for physical abuse, 8.8% for sexual abuse, and 6.6% for psychological maltreatment.[1] This translates to a rate of 8 per 1000 children identified as neglected, a rate that has been fairly steady since the early 1990s.[13] Medical personnel made 12% of all reports.

Child abuse and neglect, however, are often not observed, detected, or reported to CPS,[4] making it difficult to estimate their true incidence. A different approach was used in the NIS-3 conducted in 1993 in 42 counties representative of the United States.[4] Community professionals, including pediatricians, were trained as "sentinels" to document instances meeting study definitions of child maltreatment, regardless of whether they were reported to CPS. The definitions included both potential and actual harm. It was not possible, however, to include laypersons as sentinels, the source of almost half of CPS reports.

Neglect was identified in 14.6 per 1000 children, compared to rates of 4.9 and 2.1 for physical and sexual abuse. Seven forms of physical neglect were examined, including: (1) refusal of health care; (2) delay in health care; (3) abandonment; (4) expulsion of a child from the home; (5) other custody issues, such as repeatedly leaving a child with others for days or weeks; (6) inadequate supervision; and (7) other physical neglect, including inadequate nutrition, clothing, or hygiene. Delay in health care was defined as "failure to seek timely and appropriate medical care for a serious health problem, which any reasonable layman would have recognized as needing professional medical attention."

Seven forms of emotional neglect were examined, including: (1) Inadequate nurturance/affection; (2) chronic/extreme spouse abuse; (3) permitted drug/alcohol abuse (if the parent had been informed of the problem and had not attempted to intervene): (4) permitted other maladaptive behavior, such as chronic delinquency; (5) refusal of psychological care: (6) delay in psychological care; and (7) other emotional neglect, such as chronically applying inappropriate expectations of a child.

Educational neglect included three forms: (1) Permitted chronic truancy (if the parent had been informed of the problem and had not tried to intervene); (2) failure to enroll/other truancy, such as causing a child to miss at least 1 month of school; and (3) inattention to special educational needs. The special educational need criterion was defined as "refusal to allow or failure to obtain recommended remedial educational services, or neglect in obtaining or following through with treatment for a child's diagnosed learning disorder or other special education need without reasonable cause."

There are data from a variety of other sources that include concerns of societal neglect—circumstances where children's needs are not adequately met largely because of gaps in services and inadequate policies and programs. For example, children's mental health needs are often not met.[14] One study of youth between ages 9 and 17 years found that only 38% to 44% of children meeting stringent criteria for a psychiatric diagnosis in the prior 6 months had had a mental health contact in the previous year.[15] Neglected dental care is widespread. For example, a study of preschoolers found that 49% of 4-year-olds had cavities, and fewer than 10% were fully treated.[16] Another study found that 8.6% of kindergarteners needed urgent dental care.[17] Neglected health care is not rare, and if access to health care and health insurance is a basic need in the United States today, 8.7 million (11.7%) children experienced this form of neglect in 2006.[18]

Finally, in 2006, it is estimated that 74% of fatalities due to child maltreatment involved neglect, including 1.9% involving medical neglect.[19] Most of these were due to lapses in supervision contributing to deaths by drowning or in fires.

CONTRIBUTORS TO NEGLECT

Belsky[20] provided a theoretical framework for understanding the cause of child maltreatment, including neglect. There is no single cause of child neglect. Developmental-ecological theory posits that multiple and interacting factors at the individual (parent and child), familial, community, and societal levels contribute to child maltreatment. For example, although maternal depression is often associated with child neglect, it does not necessarily lead to neglect. However, the likelihood of neglect increases when maternal depression occurs together with other risks, such as poverty and little social support.

Individual Level

Parental Characteristics

Maternal problems in emotional health, intellectual abilities, and substance abuse have been associated with neglect. Emotional disturbances, particularly depression, have been a major finding among mothers of neglected children.[21-23] Mothers of neglected children have been described as more bored, depressed, restless, lonely, and less satisfied with life than mothers of nonneglected children,[23] and more hostile, impulsive, stressed, and less socialized than mothers of either abused or nonmaltreated children.[24] Intellectual impairment, including mental retardation and a lack of education, have also been associated with neglect.[23,25-27]

Maternal drug use during pregnancy has become a pervasive problem. Results from a national survey in 2002 and 2003[28] found that 4.3% of pregnant women (age 15-44 years) reported illicit drug use in the past month, compared to 10.4% among nonpregnant women in the same age range. Most illicit drugs pose risks to the fetus and child, and increasing evidence points to long-term problems.[29-32]

The compromised caregiving abilities of drug-abusing parents are a major concern. Parental substance abuse has been associated with child neglect[33-35] and increased rates of maltreatment recidivism.[36] Chaffin et al[37] reported that approximately half of the maltreating parents in their sample had a history of substance abuse, and this was associated with a threefold increase in child neglect. In addition, the potential harm to children of exposure to parental use of alcohol and other drugs has been amply documented.[38-41]

There has been relatively little research on fathers and neglect. One study reported that while a father's absence alone was not associated with neglect, fathers or father figures who had been involved for a shorter period of time, who felt less efficacious in their parenting, and who were less involved in household tasks were more likely to have neglected children.[42] There is also considerable research showing how children benefit from their relationships with their fathers. For example, one study found that father presence was associated with better cognitive development and greater perceived competence and social acceptance by the children. Children who described greater father support had a stronger sense of competence and social competence, and fewer depressive symptoms.[43] When a child lacks a positive relationship with his or her father, this can be seen as a form of, or contributor, to neglect.

Child Characteristics

Theories of child development and child maltreatment emphasize the importance of considering children's characteristics that may contribute to neglect and abuse.[44] For example, parents of children who are temperamentally difficult report more stress in providing care than parents of easygoing children. Situations that lead to parental stress may contribute to child maltreatment.[38]

Several studies have found low birth weight or prematurity to be significant risk factors for abuse and neglect.[45,46] Because these babies usually receive close pediatric follow-up and other interventions, it is possible that the increased reported maltreatment reflects greater surveillance. In addition, medical neglect might be expected to occur more often among children who require extensive health care;[47] their increased needs naturally place them at risk for their needs not being met.

Other studies have found increased rates of abuse and neglect among children with chronic disabilities. Diamond and Jaudes[48] found cerebral palsy to be a risk factor for neglect. Increased neglect, but not abuse, also was found among a group of disabled children who had been hospitalized.[49] Conversely, Benedict et al[50] found no increase in maltreatment among 500 moderately to profoundly retarded children, 82% of whom also had cerebral palsy. A more recent study found that children with mental health problems were at higher risk for maltreatment, but not those with developmental disabilities.[51]

Family Level

Problems in parent-child relationships have been found among families of neglected children. Research on dyadic interactions indicates less mutual engagement by both mother and child[52] and disturbances in attachment between mother and infant.[53,54] Compared to parents of abused and nonmaltreated children, parents of neglected children had the most negative interactions with their children.[55] Bousha and Twentyman[56] found that mothers of neglected children interacted least with their children compared with mothers of abused and nonmaltreated children.

Although mothers of neglected children may have unrealistic expectations of their young children compared with matched controls,[57] a lack of knowledge concerning child developmental milestones (e.g., when should an infant be able to sit unsupported) has not been clearly associated with neglect.[58] However, deficient parental problem-solving skills, poor parenting skills, and inadequate knowledge of children's developmental needs have been associated with neglect.[59-60]

In his work with neglected children, Kadushin[25] described chaotic families with impulsive mothers, who repeatedly demonstrated poor planning and judgment, coupled with either father absence (often abandonment or incarceration) or negative mother-father relationships. Neglect has been associated with social isolation.[24,61] Single parenthood without support from a spouse, family, or friends poses a risk for neglect. In one study, mothers of neglected children perceived themselves as isolated and as living in unfriendly neighborhoods.[62] Their neighbors saw them as deviant and avoided social contact with them. Mothers of neglected children may have less help with child care and fewer enjoyable social contacts compared with those where neglect was not a concern.[60] Another study found that maltreating parents showed lower levels of community integration, participation in community social activities, and use of formal and informal organizations than did parents providing adequate care.[63]

Giovannoni and Billingsley[64] described a pattern of estrangement from kin among mothers of neglected children that included a lack of supportive relationships. Seagull[65] asked whether social isolation is a contributory factor to neglect or a symptom of underlying dysfunction. In either case, social isolation appears to be strongly associated with child maltreatment, and particularly with neglect.

Stress also has been strongly associated with child maltreatment. In one study, the highest level of stress, reflecting concerns about unemployment, illness, eviction, and arrest was noted among families of neglected children compared with abusive and control families.[66] Lapp[67] found stress was frequent among parents reported to CPS for neglect, particularly regarding family, financial, and health problems.

Crittenden[68] described how distortions in information processing can lead to neglect. She described three types of neglect associated with deficits in cognitive processing, affective processing, or both: (1) disorganized, (2) emotionally neglecting, and (3) depressed. The first type, "disorganized," is characterized by families who respond impulsively and emotionally. The family operates in a crisis mode and appears chaotic and disorganized. Children may be caught in the midst of this crisis, and their needs are not met. The second type, "emotionally neglecting," includes families who are minimally attentive to their child's emotional needs. Parents may handle the demands of daily living (e.g., ensure food and clothing), but ignore how the child feels. The third type, "depressed," is the classic presentation of neglect. Parents are depressed and therefore unable to process either cognitive or affective information. Children may be left to fend for themselves emotionally and physically.

Community/Neighborhood Level

The community context and its resources, or social capital, influence parent-child relationships and are strongly associated with child maltreatment.[69] A community with much social capital, such as family-centered activities, quality and affordable child care, and a good transportation system, enhances the ability of families to nurture and protect their children. Informal support networks, safety, and recreational facilities also support healthy family functioning. Garbarino and Crouter[69] described the feedback process whereby neighbors may monitor each other's behavior, recognize difficulties, and intervene. This feedback can be supportive, diminish social isolation, and help families obtain services.

A comparison of neighborhoods with low and high rates for child maltreatment showed that families with the most needs tended to cluster in areas, often those with the least social services.[70] In addition to the role of personal histories, the authors attribute the formation of high-risk neighborhoods to political and economic forces. Families in a high-risk environment are less able to give and share and may be mistrustful of neighborly exchanges. In this way, a family's problems may be compounded rather than ameliorated by the neighborhood context, if dominated by other needy families. Garbarino and Crouter[69] found that parents' negative perceptions of the quality of life in the neighborhood were related to increased child maltreatment. In summary, communities can serve as valuable sources of support to families, or they may add to the stresses that families are experiencing.

Societal Level

Many factors at the broader societal level compromise the abilities of families to care adequately for their children. In addition, these societal or institutional problems can be directly neglectful of children. "More than a dozen blue-ribbon commissions and task forces over the past decade have warned of the inadequacy of America's educational system and urged reform."[36] Only 70% of youth complete high school.[37] In a national study, 70% of children with learning disabilities received special education services according to their parents; fewer than 20% of children receive needed mental health care.[38]

Poverty is defined as living in families with incomes below the federal poverty line ($21,200 for a family of four in 2008). Poverty appears to be strongly associated with neglect,[4,24,70] "...these families are the poorest of the poor."[64] The harmful effects of poverty on the health and development of children are pervasive.[38] In addition to its influence on family functioning, poverty directly threatens and harms children's health, development, and safety.[12,39-42] Children in poor families lag behind children in wealthier families in health insurance and in academic performance.[39] For many children, living in poverty means exposure to environmental hazards (e.g., lead, violence), hunger, few recreational opportunities, and inferior health and health care. According to the *National Center for Children in Poverty*, 20% of children under age 6 in America live in poverty, a rate two to three times higher than that of other major industrial nations. Of all the risk factors known to impair the health and well-being of children, poverty is clearly very important. It should be noted, however, that most low-income families are not neglectful of their children. Conversely, neglect is hardly limited to poor families.

The child welfare system,[40] the very system intended to assist children in need of care and protection, is another example of societal neglect. "If the nation had deliberately designed a system that would frustrate the professionals who staff it, anger the public who finance it, and abandon the children who depend on it, it could not have done a better job than the present child welfare system."[36] Inadequately financed, with staff who are generally undertrained and overwhelmed, and with poorly coordinated services, CPS are often unable to fulfill their mandate of protecting children.

Professional Level

As mentioned earlier, professionals may contribute to neglect in different ways. Problematic communication with parents not understanding their child's condition or treatment plan is pervasive.[71] Pediatricians sometimes do not comply with recommended procedures and treatments, thereby compromising children's health.[72] Pediatricians may fail to identify children's medical or psychosocial needs, perhaps contributing to their neglect.

PROTECTIVE FACTORS

The influence of risk factors can be buffered by protective factors. These may be internal characteristics (e.g., parental sense of competence) or external (e.g., social support). The concept of "social capital" has been applied to families' social relationships and connections to their communities (i.e., their social support network). Social capital appears to be related to children's development.[73] There is longstanding support for the protective effect of a strong social network.[74-76] Higher levels of social support are, for example,

associated with lower rates of physical neglect, and increased use of nonphysical disciplinary methods.[73,76]

Another potential protective factor is a parent's sense of competence regarding their parenting; it may offset the challenges of child rearing and help prevent neglect.[42] Neglect was less likely in families when fathers felt more competent in their parenting compared to those who felt less so. Perceived competence has been linked to positive parenting behaviors, such as responsiveness, stimulation, and nonpunitive caregiving.[42]

CONCLUSION

A clear definition of child neglect helps to guide pediatric practice. It is evident that neglect is a pervasive problem. It is also clear that its cause is complex, often involving multiple and interacting contributors. In addition, the presence of protective factors needs to be assessed; they are critical to strengths-based approaches. Addressing neglect requires careful attention to its cause and context, tailoring responses to the specific needs of children and families. Priorities for future research include developing and evaluating strategies to prevent and address child neglect.

References

1. Gaudiosi JA: *Child maltreatment 2006*, U.S. Department of Health and Human Services, Administration for Children and Families (website): http://www.acf.hhs.gov/programs/cb/pubs/cm06/cm06.pdf. Accessed December 27, 2008.
2. Zuravin SJ: Issues pertinent to defining child neglect. *In*: Morton TD, Salovitz B (eds): *The CPS Response to Child Neglect: An Administrator's Guide to Theory, Policy, Program Design and Case Practice.* National Resource Center on Child Maltreatment, Duluth, Ga, 2001, pp 37-59. http://www.nrccps.org/PDF/CPSResponsetoChildNeglect.pdf. Accessed on January 30, 2009.
3. Wesson D, Spence L, Hu X, et al: Trends in bicycling-related head injuries in children after implementation of a community-based bike helmet campaign. *J Pediatr Surg* 2000;35:688-689.
4. Sedlak AJ, Mettenburg J, Basena M, et al: *Fourth national incidence study of child abuse ande neglect (NIS-4): report to Congress.* U.S. Department of Heath and Human Services, Administration for Children and Families, Washington, DC, 2010.
5. Magura S, Moses B: *Outcome measures for child welfare services: theory and applications.* Child Welfare League of America, Washington, DC, 1986.
6. Barnett D, Manly JT, Cicchetti D: Defining child maltreatment: the interface between policy and research. *In*: Cicchetti D, Toth SL (eds): *Child Abuse, Child Development, and Social Policy.* Ablex Publishing, New York, 1993, pp 7-73.
7. Litrownik AJ, Lau A, English D, et al: Measuring the severity of child maltreatment. *Child Abuse Negl* 2005;29:461-477.
8. Dubowitz H, Pitts SC, Litrownik AJ, et al: Defining child neglect based on child protective services datra. *Child Abuse Negl* 2005;29(5):461-477.
9. McGee RA, Wolf D, Yuen SA, et al: The measurement of maltreatment: a comparison of approaches. *Child Abuse Negl* 1995;19(2):233-249.
10. English DJ, Graham JC, Litrownik AJ, et al: Defining maltreatment chronicity: are there differences in child outcomes? *Child Abuse Negl* 2005;29:575-595.
11. Korbin JE, Spilsbury JC: Cultural competence and child neglect. *In*: Dubowitz H (ed): *Neglected Children: Research, Practice, and Policy.* Sage, Thousand Oaks, Calif, 1999, pp 69-88.
12. Parker S, Greer S, Zuckerman B: Double jeopardy: the impact of poverty on early child development. *Pediatr Clin North Am* 1998;35:1227-1240.
13. Gaudiosi JA: *Child maltreatment—2004*, US Department of Health and Human Services, Administration on Children, Youth and Families (website): http://www.acf.hhs.gov/programs/cb/pubs/cm04/index.htm. Accessed January 30, 2009.

14. Jones LM, Finkelhor D, Holter S: Child maltreatment trends in the 1990s: why does neglect differ from sexual and physical abuse? *Child Maltreat* 2006;11:107-120.

15. U.S. Department of Health and Human Services: *Mental health: a report of the Surgeon General-executive summary* (website): http://www.surgeongeneral.gov/library/mentalhealth/pdfs/ExSummary-Final.pdf. Accessed January 30, 2009.

16. Leaf P, Alegria M, Cohen P, et al: Mental health service use in the community and schools: results from the four-community MACA study. *J Am Acad Child Adolesc Psychiatry* 1996;35:889-897.

17. Tang J, Altman D, Robertson D, et al: Dental caries: prevalence and treatment levels in Arizona preschool children. *Public Health Rep* 1997;112:319-331.

18. Chung LH, Shain SG, Stephen SM, et al: Oral health status of San Francisco public school kindergarteners 2000-2005. *J Public Health Dent* 2006;66:235-241. www.covertheuninsured.org. Accessed February 26, 2010.

19. Child Welfare Information Gateway: Child abuse and neglect fatalities: statistics and interventions (website): http://www.childwelfare.gov/pubs/factsheets/fatality.cfm#children. Accessed September 19, 2008.

20. Belsky J: Child maltreatment: an ecological integration. *Am Psychol* 1980;35:320-335.

21. Polansky N, Chalmers MA, Buttenwieser EW, et al: *Damaged parents: an anatomy of child neglect.* University of Chicago Press, Chicago, 1981.

22. Wolock I, Horowitz H: Child maltreatment and maternal deprivation among AFDC recipient families. *Soc Serv Rev* 1979;53:175-194.

23. Zuravin S: Child abuse, child neglect and maternal depression: is there a connection? *In: Child Neglect Monograph: Proceedings from a Symposium.* National Center on Child Abuse and Neglect, Washington, DC, 1988.

24. Friedrich WN, Tyler JA, Clark JA: Personality and psychophysiological variables: in abusive, neglectful, and low-income control mothers. *J Nerv Ment Dis* 1985;173:449-460.

25. Kadushin A: Neglect in families. *In:* Nunnally EW, Chilman CS, Cox FM (eds): *Mental Illness, Delinquency, Addictions, and Neglect.* Sage, Newbury Park, Calif, 1988.

26. Martin MJ, Walters J: Familial correlates of selected types of child abuse and neglect. *J Marriage Fam* 1982;44:267-276.

27. Ory N, Earp J: Child maltreatment and the use of social services. *Public Health Rep* 1981;96:238-245.

28. National Survey on Drug Use and Health: *The NSDUH report. Substance use during pregnancy: 2002 and 2003*, update, Substance Abuse and Mental Health Services Administration (website): http://www.oas.samhsa.gov/2k5/pregnancy/pregnancy.pdf. Accessed January 30, 2009.

29. Accornero VH, Morrow CE, Bandstra ES, et al: Behavioral outcome of preschoolers exposed prenatally to cocaine: role of maternal behavioral health. *J Pediatr Psychol* 2002;27:259-269.

30. Hurt H, Brodsky NL, Roth H, et al: School performance of children with gestational cocaine exposure. *Neurotoxicol Teratol* 2005;27:203-211.

31. Trezza V, Cuomo V, Vandershhuren LJ: Cannabis and the developing brain: insights from behavior. *Eur J Pharmacol* 2008;585(2-3):441-452.

32. Accornero VH, Amado AJ, Morrow CE, et al: Impact of prenatal cocaine exposure on attention and response inhibition as assessed by continuous performance tests. *J Dev Behav Pediatr* 2007;28:195-205.

33. Ondersma SJ: Predictors of neglect within low socioeconomic status families: the importance of substance abuse. *Am J Orthopsychiatry* 2002;72:383-391.

34. Wekerle C, Wall AM, Leung E, et al: Cumulative stress and substantiated maltreatment: the importance of caregiver vulnerability and adult partner violence. *Child Abuse Negl* 2007;31:427-443.

35. Harrington D, Dubowitz H, Black M, et al: Maternal substance use and neglectful parenting: relationships with children's development. *J Clin Child Psychol* 1995;24:258-263.

36. Connell CM, Bergeron N, Katz KH, et al: Re-referral to child protective services: The influence of child, family, and case characteristics on risk status. *Child Abuse Negl* 2007;31:573-588.

37. Chaffin M, Kelleher K, Hollenberg J: Onset of physical abuse and neglect. *Child Abuse Negl* 1996;20:191-200.

38. Besinger BA, Garland AF, Litrownik AJ, et al: Caregiver substance abuse among maltreated children placed in out-of-home care. *Child Welfare* 1999;78:221-239.

39. Chasnoff IL, Lowder LA: Prenatal alcohol and drug use and risk for child maltreatment: A timely approach to intervention. *In:* Dubowitz H (ed.): *Neglected Children: Research, Practice and Policy.* Sage Publications, Thousand Oaks, CA, 1999.

40. Marcenko MO, Kemp SP, Larson NC: Childhood experiences of abuse, later substance use, and parenting outcomes among low-income mothers. *Am J Orthopsychiatry* 2000;70:316-336.

41. Tronick EZ, Frank DA, Cabral H, et al: Late dose response effects of prenatal cocaine exposure on newborn neurobehavioral performance. *Pediatrics* 1996;98:76-83.

42. Dubowitz H, Black MM, Kerr M, et al: Fathers and child neglect. *Arch Pediatr Adolesc Med* 2000;154:135-141.

43. Dubowitz H, Black MM, Cox CE, et al: Father involvement and children's functioning at age 6 Years: a multisite study. *Child Maltreat* 2001;6:300-309.

44. Benedict M, White RB: Selected perinatal factors and child abuse. *Am J Public Health* 1985;75:780-781.

45. Herrenkohl EC, Herrenkohl RC: Some antecedents and developmental consequences of child maltreatment. *In:* Rizley R, Cicchetti D (eds): *Developmental Perspectives on Child Maltreatment.* Jossey-Bass, San Francisco, 1981.

46. Jaudes PK, Diamond LJ: Neglect of chronically ill children. *Am J Dis Child* 1986;140:655-658.

47. Diamond LJ, Jaudes PK: Child abuse and the cerebral palsied patient. *Dev Med Child Neurol* 1983;25:169-174.

48. Glaser D, Bentovim A: Abuse and risk to handicapped and chronically ill children. *Child Abuse Negl* 1979;3:565-575.

49. Benedict MI, White RB, Wulff LM, et al: Reported maltreatment in children with multiple disabilities. *Child Abuse Negl* 1990;14:207-217.

50. Jaudes PK, Mackey-Bilaver L: Do chronic conditions increase young children's risk of being maltreated? *Child Abuse Negl* 2008;32:671-681.

51. Dietrich KN, Starr RH, Weisfeld GE: Infant maltreatment: caretaker-infant interaction and developmental consequences at different levels of parenting failure. *Pediatrics* 1983;72:532-540.

52. Crittenden PM: Maltreated infants: vulnerability and resilience. *J Child Psychol Psychiatry* 1985;26:85-96.

53. Egeland B, Brunquell D: An at-risk approach to the study of child abuse and neglect. *J Am Acad Child Adolesc Psychiatry* 1979;18:219-235.

54. Burgess R, Conger R: Family interaction in abusive, neglectful, and normal families. *Child Dev* 1978;49:1163-1173.

55. Bousha DM, Twentyman CT: Mother-child interactional style in abuse, neglect, and control groups: naturalistic observations in the home. *J Abnorm Psychol* 1984;93:106-114.

56. Azar S, Robinson DR, Hekimian E, et al: Unrealistic expectations and problem solving ability in maltreating and comparison mothers. *J Consult Clin Psychol* 1984;52:687-691.

57. Twentyman C, Plotkin R: Unrealistic expectations of parents who maltreat their children: an educational deficit that pertains to child development. *J Clin Psychol* 1982;38:497-503.

58. Herrenkohl R, Herrenkohl E, Egolf B: Circumstances surrounding the occurrence of child maltreatment. *J Consult Clin Psychol* 1983;51:424-431.

59. Jones JM, McNeely RL: Mothers who neglect and those who do not: a comparative study. *Soc Casework* 1980;61:559-567.

60. Polansky NA, Ammons PW, Gaudin JM Jr: Loneliness and isolation in child neglect. *Soc Casework* 1985;66:38-47.

61. Polansky NA, Gaudin JM Jr, Ammons PW, et al: The psychological ecology of the neglectful mother. *Child Abuse Negl* 1985;9:265-275.

62. Gracia E, Musitu G: Social isolation from communities and child maltreatment: a cross-cultural comparison. *Child Abuse Negl* 2003;27:153-168.

63. Giovannoni JM, Billingsley A: Child neglect among the poor: a study of parental adequacy in families of three ethnic groups. *Child Welfare* 1970;84:196-214.

64. Seagull E: Social support and child maltreatment: a review of the evidence. *Child Abuse Negl* 1987;11:41-52.

65. Gaines R, Sangrund A, Green AH, et al: Etiological factors in child maltreatment: a multivariate study of abusing, neglecting, and normal mothers. *J Abnorm Psychol* 1978;87:531-540.

66. Lapp J: A profile of officially reported child neglect. *In:* Trainer CNI (ed): *The Dilemma of Child Neglect: Identification and Treatment.* The American Humane Association, Denver, 1983.

67. Crittenden PM: Child neglect: causes and contributors. *In:* Dubowitz H (ed): *Neglected Children: Research, Practice and Policy.* Sage, Thousand Oaks, Calif, 1999, pp 47-68.

68. Garbarino J, Crouter A: Defining the community context of parent-child relations. *Child Dev* 1978;49:604-616.

69. Garbarino J, Sherman D: High-risk neighborhoods and high-risk families: the human ecology of child maltreatment. *Child Dev* 1980;51: 188-198.

70. National Commission on Children: *Beyond rhetoric: a new American agenda for children and families.* National Commission on Children, Washington, DC, 1991.

71. Child Welfare Information Gateway: *How the Child Welfare System Works* (website). Available at http://www.childwelfare.gov/pubs/factsheet/cpsworks.cfm. Accessed January 30, 2009.

72. National Advisory Board on Child Abuse and Neglect: Creating Caring Communities: Blueprint for Effective Federal Policy on Child Abuse and Neglect. U.S. Department of Health and Human Services, Washington, DC, 1991.

73. Lyons SJ, Henly JR, Schuerman JR: Informal support in maltreating families: its effect on parenting practices. *Child Youth Serv Rev* 2005; 27:21-38.

74. Cohen S, Hoberman HM: Positive events and social supports as buffers of life change stress. *J Appl Soc Psychol* 1983;13:99-125.

75. McCurdy K: The influence of support and stress on maternal attitudes. *Child Abuse Negl* 2005;29:251-268.

76. Coleman PK, Karraker KH: Self-efficacy and parenting quality: findings and future applications. *Dev Rev* 1998;18:47-85.

77. Cohen S, Wills TA: Stress, social support, and the buffering hypothesis. *Psychol Bull* 1985;98:310-357.

6

EPIDEMIOLOGY OF ABUSIVE HEAD TRAUMA

Heather T. Keenan, MDCM, PhD

INTRODUCTION

The epidemiology of abusive head trauma (AHT) has been difficult to elucidate. Problems quantifying the number of children with this form of physical child abuse have included nonstandard research definitions, inconsistent nomenclature, disagreement about the mechanism of injury, and difficulty with case ascertainment.[1] Some of these challenges have been addressed in the past decade through consensus panels seeking to define cases and standardize nomenclature.[2] This chapter will use the nomenclature "abusive head trauma" (AHT), which recognizes that this subset of all closed head injury includes multiple mechanisms of injury (Figure 6-1).

Abusive head trauma was described first by Dr. John Caffey in 1946.[3] Dr. Caffey reported a case series of six infants with whiplash-shaken infant syndrome, all of whom had subdural hematomas and characteristic bone fractures. In 1962, a seminal paper by C. Henry Kempe[4] brought the battered child syndrome to public attention, including AHT. Shaking was proposed as a mechanism for the injuries seen in these infants by a British pediatric neurosurgeon, Dr. Norman Guthkelch.[5] "Shaken baby syndrome" was more formally described by Caffey in 1972 as a syndrome of intracranial and intraocular bleeding with no external signs of injury caused by vigorous shaking of infants.[6] Caffey questioned whether some of the developmental delays, cerebral palsy, and epilepsy diagnosed in children could be attributed to unrecognized brain damage caused by shaking. This question remains relevant in both developed and developing countries 35 years later.

Quantification of AHT is hampered by difficulties in ascertainment, including misclassification.[7] Studies reporting incidence have used different populations, including patients presenting to pediatric or subspecialty care, children admitted to intensive care units, victims of fatal abuse seen by medical examiners, and large administrative datasets.[8-11] Each of these data sources has areas of potential bias (Table 6-1). Ascertainment bias occurs when subpopulations of children are not included within the data set. For example, children with "subclinical" injury may not reach medical attention. Zolotar et al performed an anonymous phone survey of mothers with children under 2 years of age from a stratified random sample of birth certificates in North Carolina.[12] Preliminary results show that approximately 1% of parents with a child less than 2 years of age reported shaking their children. Mothers (0.7%) and mothers' partners (0.6%) shook children at similar rates. Thus shaking and possibly AHT occur more frequently within the population than is suggested by cases diagnosed in a medical setting. The rate of 1% reported by Zolotar would suggest that shaking is 54 times the rate of severe AHT prospectively observed in an earlier study in the same state.[9,12]

Additional evidence for unrecognized injury is provided by studies documenting old brain injuries in as many as 30% to 45% of children who are diagnosed with AHT.[13-15] Misclassification may lead to bias that can occur if a child is incorrectly diagnosed either when medical attention is sought or at postmortem. A retrospective review of 51 children with no neurological symptoms who were screened for AHT because of other injuries (rib fracture, healing fractures, or facial injury), revealed that 37% (95% CI: 24%-51%) also had a head injury. The status of the unscreened children having a similar finding is unknown.[16] A case series of children with confirmed AHT showed that 31% of the children had seen a clinician for symptoms of head trauma before a definitive diagnosis and the diagnosis had been initially missed.[14]

Deaths due to maltreatment are frequently not classified as homicides.[17] In a three-state study of death due to maltreatment, underascertainment of child maltreatment fatalities was found in all three states by both child welfare agencies and in death certificate data. The combination of the two data sets correctly identified 90% of fatalities due to maltreatment.[18] Thus both underascertainment and misclassification may falsely reduce the incidence in studies of AHT.

POPULATION-BASED INCIDENCE STUDIES OF ABUSIVE HEAD TRAUMA

There have been several population-based studies of the incidence of abusive head trauma.[8,10,11,19] Incidence is defined as the number of new cases diagnosed in a predetermined population over a specific amount of time, and is usually expressed in number of cases per unit of time. These incidence studies have all used different populations and slightly different definitions. Remarkably, the incidence estimates have been similar, which may reflect the fact that only the most severe cases are recognized. The prevalence of children in the population suffering from abusive head trauma is unknown.

Closed head injury

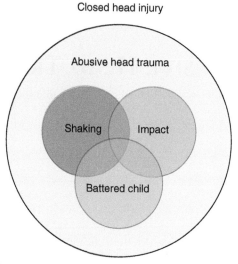

FIGURE 6-1 Abusive head trauma is a subset of closed head injury and can be caused by several mechanisms.

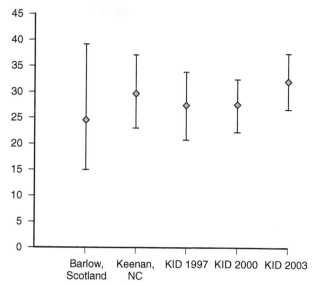

FIGURE 6-2 Incidence of abusive head trauma in infants per 100,000 person-years with 95% confidence intervals.

Table 6-1	Sources of Bias in Incidence Studies of Abusive Head Trauma

Ascertainment Bias

Subclinical injury
Prehospital deaths
ICU population only (severe injury)
Restricted age group

Misclassification

Misdiagnosis in hospital (not AHT)
Misdiagnosis on death certificate
Abusive head trauma vs. non-abusive head trauma

The first prospective, population-based, incidence study of AHT was performed by Barlow and Minns.[11] This study identified 19 cases of AHT over an 18-month period. The authors collected data from all hospital pediatric departments, pediatric intensive care units, neurosurgical units, and death records in Scotland. The calculated incidence of AHT was 24.6 per 100,000 infants per year (95% CI: 14.9, 38.5). The median age in this population was 2.2 months, with no child over 1 year of age. The main limitation of this study was its relatively small population base.

The first prospective population-based U.S. study of AHT was performed in North Carolina over a 2-year period.[9] The study collected cases of children with head trauma who were less than 2 years of age from all nine pediatric intensive care units in the state. The authors also reviewed the charts of all deaths among children under 2 years of age. Additionally, the three out-of-state hospitals likely to accept referrals for North Carolina residents were surveyed. Whether the case was abusive or non-abusive head trauma was decided by the treating medical personnel at each hospital, but was reviewed by the investigators. A

jury mechanism was developed to make decisions for cases that did not have a clear determination. Because of the larger population base, this study was able to provide more precise estimates than the Scottish study: 29.7/100,000 person-years (95% CI: 22.9, 36.7) in children less than 1 year of age; and 3.8/100,000 person-years (95% CI: 1.3, 6.4) for children during the second year of life.

The case fatality rate in this study was 22.5%. The median age at injury was 5.9 months. The median injury age was older in the North Carolina study than in the study of Barlow and Minns; however, this discrepancy is most likely due to the larger population base of the North Carolina study, which allowed case findings in children older than 1 year of age. The key limitation of the North Carolina study was its focus on severely injured children. Excluding children not admitted to an intensive care unit would tend to underestimate the incidence of AHT.

Ellingson[8] et al used the Kids' Inpatient Database (KID) for the years 1997, 2000, and 2003 in an effort to find a passive surveillance technique that could be used to monitor national trends in incidence rates of AHT. The KID dataset is part of the Healthcare Cost and Utilization Project (HCUP) collected by the U.S. Agency for Healthcare Research and Quality (AHRQ). The database contains an 80% sample of all non–birth-related discharges of children from all hospitals in participating states, which can be weighted to provide national estimates of disease. Using International Classification of Disease 9th Clinical Modification (ICD-9-CM) diagnosis codes to define cases in children less than 1 year of age, the authors calculated the national incidence estimate for KID 2000 at 27.5/100,000 person-years (95% CI: 22.6, 32.3).[19] This incidence rate is remarkably similar to that of infants in the North Carolina study conducted in 2000 and 2001, and the Scottish study (Figure 6-2). Limitations of the KID include exclusion of prehospital deaths, and the inability to verify each case. However, use of an existing surveillance mechanism is vastly less expensive than prospective case ascertainment. A 2008

U.S. Centers for Disease Control and Prevention panel is currently working on guidelines for the use of ICD-9-CM and ICD-10 codes to standardize ascertainment of AHT in hospital discharge datasets for research.[21]

In addition to the above studies of AHT, two population-based studies of subdural hemorrhage in young children have been conducted. A 3-year retrospective study of subdural hemorrhage in South Wales and southeast England found an incidence of subdural hemorrhage in children less than 2 years of age (n=33) of 21.0/100,000 person-years (95% CI: 7.5, 34.3) among infants, 82% of which were confirmed or suggestive of abuse.[22] The second such study, conducted in New Zealand, using both prospective enrollment by having health care providers send in notification cards and retrospective study of death certificates, found an incidence of 14.7 to 19.6 cases per 100,000 person-years in 2000-2002.[23] This study found a strikingly higher incidence in the Maori (native) population than in the general population.

POPULATION AT RISK

Societal Risk Factors

Injury occurs most often among socially disadvantaged families.[24] AHT appears to follow this pattern as well. Economic information regarding victim's families in the Lothian region of Scotland placed them in the lowest two quintiles of social deprivation based on the Scottish Index of Multiple Deprivation.[10] In the United States, the KID data captures insurance status, a proxy for income, which showed that nearly 70% of children identified with AHT used public insurance.[8]

Children may be more likely to experience abuse during times of societal and family stress. Social disruption in the form of military deployment increases maltreatment risk.[25,26] In dynamic models of risks, child maltreatment (abuse and neglect) in the first year of life was related both to parental stress, as measured by life event scores, and social support. Kotch et al[27] found a significant interaction between stress and social support in a cohort of families considered at risk for child maltreatment. In this model, the effect of family stress on increased child maltreatment reports was modified by the level of social support, with less social support predicting increased child maltreatment among stressed families. Abusive head trauma may fit this model as well. An example of a societal stressor that increased the rate of AHT is a natural disaster. The incidence of AHT increased approximately five times in the first 6 months after a hurricane in regions that experienced severe flooding compared with unaffected regions in an ecological study of AHT in North Carolina.[18] Additionally, children of military families, who may have decreased social support because of frequent moves, might be at higher risk for AHT.[27]

Family Characteristics

Children from all types of families are at risk for AHT; however, some family *characteristics* have been associated with increased risk of a child being a victim of AHT. Family characteristics of children with AHT differed from those of the general population in the North Carolina study.[9] In a model adjusted for multiple covariates including maternal education and marital status, AHT risk was associated with young maternal age, families with a multiple gestation, and minority families. When compared with a population of children with other types of brain injury, the association of AHT with maternal age remained, but there was no association with race. This suggests that race and ethnicity may be confounded by socioeconomic status, which was not measured in this study.

Adult Characteristics

Men and women self-report the shaking of young children at the same rate.[12,29] However, more men than women are identified as perpetrators in hospitalized cases.[9,30,31] Males make up more than 60% of perpetrators in cases of AHT, including fathers, mother's boyfriend, and stepfathers. Mothers account for approximately 15% of cases, and baby sitters account for about 11%. The reason for the disparity in self-report versus hospitalized cases of AHT might be due to the average relative strength of men and women with similar child handling behaviors.

Child Characteristics

The two child factors most consistently associated with AHT are male sex and young age. The North Carolina study estimated that boys are twice as likely as girls to be victims of AHT (adjusted odds 2.0; 95% CI: 1.1, 3.9).[9] Data from the KID confirmed these findings: approximately 64% of injured children were male.[8] Young child age is also a risk factor, with median age at injury reported from 2.2 months to 5.9 months.[8,9,11,30] Other child factors that may be associated with AHT include prematurity, multiple birth, and developmental delay.[9,32] However, these characteristics are relatively infrequent in the population and have not been confirmed in large data sets.

CRYING AS A POTENTIAL TRIGGER

Crying has been proposed as a trigger for AHT. This proposition comes from two sources of evidence: crying is often named as a trigger by those who admit to having injured a child,[33] and the peak incidence of normal infant crying occurs at around 5 to 6 weeks of age, just preceding the peak time of AHT injury.[34,35] A study using data from California hospital discharges using the ICD-9-CM code of 995.55 (Shaken Baby Syndrome) for children under 18 months of age found the peak age for admittance to a hospital with the relevant code to be between 10 and 13 weeks. Thus the peak period of crying precedes the time of injury.[34] Additionally, an Estonian study also correlated age of injury with crying as a stated trigger and found that peak crying coincided with or preceded the AHT.[32] While no causal relationship has been shown between crying and AHT, it is plausible that normal infant crying is a trigger for abuse in the context of an already stressed family or a family with low social support.

SUMMARY

Much progress has been made toward establishing the unique epidemiological features of AHT. This progress has been realized because of improved definitions, prospective population-based studies, and large data base studies. The strength of the evidence for the incidence of serious AHT is now strong, having been replicated in multiple populations. Quantifying the problem and understanding the societal, family, and child characteristics associated with AHT defines the population that would be most likely to benefit from primary prevention. The next challenge is to establish accurate and inexpensive ongoing surveillance for AHT.[36] Ongoing surveillance will allow for tracking of trends in incidence over time from which to measure the success of future prevention programs.

References

1. Runyan DK: The challenges of assessing the incidence of inflicted traumatic brain injury: a world perspective. *Am J Prev Med* 2008; 34:S112-S115.
2. Reece R, Nicholson C (eds): *Inflicted childhood neurotrauma*. American Academy of Pediatrics, Elk Grove Village, Ill, 2003.
3. Caffey J: Multiple fractures of long bones in infants suffering from chronic subdural hematoma. *AJR Am J Roentgenol* 1946;56:163-173.
4. Kempe CH, Silverman FN, Steele BF, et al: The battered-child syndrome. *JAMA* 1962;181:17-24.
5. Guthkelch AN: Infantile subdural haematoma and its relationship to whiplash injuries. *Br Med J* 1971;2:430-431.
6. Caffey J: On the theory and practice of shaking infants. Its potential residual effects of permanent brain damage and mental retardation. *Am J Dis Child* 1972;124:161-169.
7. Reece RM: What are we trying to measure? The problems of case ascertainment. *Am J Prev Med* 2008;34:S116-S119.
8. Ellingson KD, Leventhal JM, Weiss HB: Using hospital discharge data to track inflicted traumatic brain injury. *Am J Prev Med* 2008;34: S157-S162.
9. Keenan HT, Runyan DK, Marshall SW, et al: A population-based study of inflicted traumatic brain injury in young children. *JAMA* 2003;290:621-626.
10. Minns RA, Jones PA, Mok JY: Incidence and demography of nonaccidental head injury in southeast Scotland from a national database. *Am J Prev Med* 2008;34:S126-S133.
11. Barlow KM, Minns RA: Annual incidence of shaken impact syndrome in young children. *Lancet* 2000;356:1571-1572.
12. Zolotar A, Runyan D, Foster E, et al: *Reported shaking of children under two in North Carolina*. Pediatric Academic Society Meeting, Honolulu, 2008.
13. Ewing-Cobbs L, Kramer L, Prasad M, et al: Neuroimaging, physical, and developmental findings after inflicted and noninflicted traumatic brain injury in young children. *Pediatrics* 1998;102:300-307.
14. Jenny C, Hymel KP, Ritzen A, et al: Analysis of missed cases of abusive head trauma. *JAMA* 1999;281:621-626.
15. Keenan HT, Runyan DK, Marshall SW, et al: A population-based comparison of clinical and outcome characteristics of young children
with serious inflicted and noninflicted traumatic brain injury. *Pediatrics* 2004;114:633-639.
16. Rubin DM, Christian CW, Bilaniuk LT, et al: Occult head injury in high-risk abused children. *Pediatrics* 2003;111:1382-1386.
17. Herman-Giddens ME, Brown G, Verbiest S, et al: Underascertainment of child abuse mortality in the United States. *JAMA* 1999; 282:463-467.
18. Schnitzer PG, Covington TM, Wirtz SJ, et al: Public health surveillance of fatal child maltreatment: analysis of 3 state programs. *Am J Public Health* 2008;98:296-303.
19. Keenan HT, Marshall SW, Nocera MA, et al: Increased incidence of inflicted traumatic brain injury in children after a natural disaster. *Am J Prev Med* 2004;26:189-193.
20. National Center for Health Statistics: *International Classification of Diseases, ninth revision, clinical modification* (website): http://www.cdc.gov/nchs/icd9.htm#RTF. Accessed January 31, 2009.
21. Centers for Disease Control and Prevention: Workshop on abusive head trauma coding. Atlanta, March, 2008.
22. Jayawant S, Rawlinson A, Gibbon F, et al: Subdural haemorrhages in infants: population based study. *BMJ* 1998;317:1558-1561.
23. Kelly P, Farrant B: Shaken baby syndrome in New Zealand, 2000-2002. *J Paediatr Child Health* 2008;44:99-107.
24. Hippisley-Cox J, Groom L, Kendrick D, et al: Cross sectional survey of socioeconomic variations in severity and mechanism of childhood injuries in Trent 1992-1997. *BMJ* 2002;324:1132.
25. Gibbs DA, Martin SL, Kupper LL, et al: Child maltreatment in enlisted soldiers' families during combat-related deployments. *JAMA* 2007;298:528-535.
26. Rentz ED, Marshall SW, Loomis D, et al: Effect of deployment on the occurrence of child maltreatment in military and nonmilitary families. *Am J Epidemiol* 2007;165:1199-1206.
27. Kotch JB, Browne DC, Ringwalt CL, et al: Risk of child abuse or neglect in a cohort of low-income children. *Child Abuse Negl* 1995; 19:1115-1130.
28. Gessner RR, Runyan DK: The shaken infant: a military connection? *Arch Pediatr Adolesc Med* 1995;149:467-469.
29. Theodore AD, Chang JJ, Runyan DK, et al: Epidemiologic features of the physical and sexual maltreatment of children in the Carolinas. *Pediatrics* 2005;115:e331-e337.
30. King WJ, MacKay M, Sirnick A: Shaken baby syndrome in Canada: clinical characteristics and outcomes of hospital cases. *CMAJ* 2003; 168:155-159.
31. Starling SP, Holden JR, Jenny C: Abusive head trauma: the relationship of perpetrators to their victims. *Pediatrics* 1995;95:259-262.
32. Talvik I, Alexander RC, Talvik T: Shaken baby syndrome and a baby's cry. *Acta Paediatr* 2008;97:782-785.
33. Lee C, Barr RG, Catherine N, et al: Age-related incidence of publicly reported shaken baby syndrome cases: is crying a trigger for shaking? *J Dev Behav Pediatr* 2007;28:288-293.
34. Barr RG, Trent RB, Cross J: Age-related incidence curve of hospitalized shaken baby syndrome cases: convergent evidence for crying as a trigger to shaking. *Child Abuse Negl* 2006;30:7-16.
35. Brazelton TB: Crying in infancy. *Pediatrics* 1962;29:579-588.
36. Runyan DK, Berger RP, Barr RG: Defining an ideal system to establish the incidence of inflicted traumatic brain injury: summary of the consensus conference. *Am J Prev Med* 2008;34:S163-S168.

INTERVIEWING

Nancy D. Kellogg, MD

7

INTERVIEWING CHILDREN AND ADOLESCENTS ABOUT SUSPECTED ABUSE

Nancy D. Kellogg, MD

INTRODUCTION

Interviewing children and adolescents who are suspected victims of abuse requires knowledge of child development, including language acquisition, factors that influence the likelihood and type of disclosure, and appropriate questioning techniques. In addition, because a number of individuals might conduct interviews, collaboration and cooperation is needed to ensure that interviews are not unnecessarily redundant. Communities vary in interview approaches and protocols. While some permit or encourage gathering a medical history, others prefer limited interviews by medical professionals. Rationales for limiting additional interviews, such as physician interviews, include assertions that multiple interviews are traumatic for children, and interview inconsistencies are more likely and less defensible in court. However, because abused children commonly make partial or incremental disclosures initially, "Forensic evaluations that consist of a single interview may result in incomplete disclosure and less accurate determinations, especially in cases where medical or other external data are lacking or inconclusive.[1]"

Children interviewed by more than one person sometimes provide different or conflicting information. These differences do not necessarily diminish the credibility of the child. A number of factors can result in inconsistent histories provided by children to different interviewers. Table 7-1 summarizes these factors by characteristics of the interview, child characteristics, abuse-related factors, and family factors.

Disciplines involved in interviewing children can be investigative, diagnostic, or therapeutic. The role of investigative interviewers is to gather information to assess the likelihood of abuse to establish a safety plan for the child and/or initiate a criminal investigation. The purpose of the medical interview is to establish a diagnosis and treatment plan; the treatment plan might include another diagnostic assessment by a mental health professional and counseling or crisis intervention. An interview conducted for therapeutic purposes focuses on the sequelae and effects of abuse to establish an appropriate mental health treatment plan. While the purpose of each interview differs, there is often significant overlap in the type of information gathered from the child.

FORENSIC (INVESTIGATIVE) INTERVIEWS

In recent years, the focus of the criminal and civil justice systems on the forensic interview process has increased substantially, particularly for child sexual abuse investigations. In some states, child protective services are required by law to audiotape or videotape the investigative interviews conducted with children. In general, videotape has been preferred to audiotape so that the child's facial expressions, body language, and demeanor are recorded along with their words. Ideally, the forensic interview is conducted in a neutral, child-friendly environment such as a children's advocacy center where all professionals that require investigative information can watch and listen to the interview from a nearby observation room. This process prevents unnecessary multiple interviews while ensuring that the information needs of all the agencies involved are met.

Forensic interviewers are required to undergo specialized training. This individual may be a child protective services worker, a law enforcement professional, or an employee of a children's advocacy center. Regardless of who conducts the interview, other investigative and sometimes prosecutorial professionals involved in the case are usually present in the observation room (and are usually seated behind a one-way mirror) during the interview. While children younger than 12 years old are usually videotaped or recorded, protocols and mandates vary when children are 12 years and older. Older children can provide written statements, verbal statements that are transcribed and signed, or can be videotaped.

Videotaped forensic interviews of children are frequently used as evidence in grand jury proceedings, and these interviews also can assist investigators during questioning of alleged perpetrators. In some circumstances, the videotape is introduced during civil and/or criminal court proceedings, although the availability of a videotaped interview does not preclude a child from being required to testify during the trial.

Investigative protocols have been developed to guide interviewers in "best practices." One of these protocols, developed by the National Institute of Child Health and Human Development (NICHD) has been widely used for more than 10 years for investigative interviews of children

Table 7-1 **Factors that Can Alter Information Disclosed By Children and Adolescents**

Interviewer Characteristics

Gender
Experience
Types of questions asked
  Appropriate to child's development
  Nonleading
  Not suggestive
Knowledge of abuse dynamics and family factors
Knowledge of child language skills

Child Characteristics

Gender
Age
Memory of abusive events, including traumatic amnesia
Degree of guilt and self-blame for abuse
Protectiveness of abuser
Perceived degree of belief by nonabusive parent
Comfort level with interviewer
Relationship with adults and authority figures
Accommodation to abuse/acceptance of severe corporal
  punishment as "norm"

Abuse-Related Factors

Threats by abuser
Continued presence or absence of abuser
Intimate partner violence in the child's home
Disruption of family integrity
Victim knowledge of (or concern for) other victims

Family Factors

Parental degree of belief in the child
Family disruption after disclosure
  Anguish
  Retaliation against child or abuser
  Disbelief
Child placement out of home after disclosure

who are suspected victims of either physical or sexual abuse. This protocol provides guidelines for consecutive phases of the interview: The introductory phase where ground rules and expectations are established; a rapport-building phase that includes the child's description of a neutral event; and a substantive phase consisting of open-ended questions followed by focused or clarifying questions about the abuse.[2] A study that evaluated the effectiveness of the NICHD protocol found that "open-ended invitations" yielded more details from children than focused questions and nonprotocol interviews, but the total number of details elicited did not differ significantly among these various approaches.[3]

Investigative interviews may occur before or following the medical examination, depending on the circumstances of the specific case, including whether the child has already made a disclosure and where the child first presents with statements or symptoms of abuse. The history taken by a medical professional sometimes provides additional information the child might not have disclosed to the forensic interviewer,

and might represent important corroborative evidence regarding the validity of the child's history. From one jurisdiction to another, procedures vary in the types of professionals that interview children, and whether the forensic interviews precede, follow, or are a part of medical examinations. Regardless of the agreed-upon local protocols and procedures, the overarching goal common to all disciplines is to protect the child and preserve important information throughout the investigative process.

IMPORTANCE OF THE MEDICAL HISTORY

As with any medical assessment, a patient's history, including physical and behavioral symptoms, descriptions of events that may have affected medical and mental health, and social, family, and past medical and surgical histories, are fundamental to the diagnosis and treatment of the patient. Such information should be gathered from the parent and child when possible. A primary difference from general pediatric/clinical practice is the need to interview the child and parent separately when abuse is suspected to minimize influences on the child's history. Some children and adolescents may withhold hurtful, intimate details of abuse in the presence of their parents if they fear disapproval, distress, or disbelief.

The role of the child's medical history in the diagnosis of abuse often varies by the type of abuse. For example, the diagnosis of sexual abuse is primarily based on the child's history, and frequently there are no additional findings on physical examination. Examples of other medical diagnoses that are made based primarily on patient history are migraine headaches, seizures, and depression. In these cases, the idiosyncratic, experiential details provided by the patient establish the diagnosis. The diagnosis of physical abuse depends on the compatibility of the history (timing, mechanism of injury, symptoms of child, motor capabilities of child) with the characteristics of the child's injury(s). Unlike other medical diagnoses, the child's history is often discrepant from the parent's history, particularly when the parent is the abuser. Alternatively, the child may provide a vague or evasive history regarding their injury (or injuries) if they are trying to protect the abuser or they fear the consequences of disclosing abuse.[4]

Neglect in a medical setting usually involves preverbal children and observable compromises in the child's health or safety, attributable to some extent to inadequate parental care. In cases of neglect, the parent might deny, minimize, or claim ignorance about the child's condition. The diagnosis of neglect in young children and infants often depends upon an assessment of the parent's understanding of the child's medical condition and the extent to which the severity of the condition is attributable to parental causes. The medical history often focuses on the parent's ability and willingness to assume appropriate responsibility for ensuring that the basic needs of their child are met.

Of the types of evidence and information that can be collected during the medical assessment for suspected abuse, the history is usually the most important evidence. In most cases of child sexual abuse or assault, other types of evidence—semen/sperm, anogenital or bodily injuries, and sexually transmitted diseases—will not be present. Not all clinicians have the training or the luxury of time to conduct extensive interviews of children, but that should not preclude the clinician obtaining a medical history from the patient and/or family, sufficient for the performance of the medical evaluation.

Advantages to clinician interviews include:

- It helps establish rapport with the child, facilitating child relaxation and cooperation during the examination.
- Children generally see the physician as someone who helps them. This perception may facilitate disclosure of additional information not obtained by child protective services or law enforcement officers, whose role may be unknown or threatening to the child.
- A normal examination, taken in isolation from historical facts, can sometimes be misconstrued by the legal and lay community as meaning "nothing happened," thus the inclusion of the clinician's interview findings might improve the overall accuracy and effectiveness of the presentation of the medical assessment in court proceedings.

Disadvantages of extensive clinician interviews include time and inconvenience. Difficult interviews can take up to 1 hour. Most clinicians in private practice or in an emergency room setting are rarely able to set aside that much time on short notice. In addition, child abuse may provoke anger and even denial in some professionals. The medicolegal implications of diagnosing child abuse and the possibility of testimony and adversarial interactions in court are added disadvantages for some clinicians.

Decisions regarding how much and what type of information to gather from suspected victims of child abuse are clearly dependent upon each physician's personal preferences, availability of time, and access to other resources of assistance.

LEGAL CONSIDERATIONS

There are specific circumstances under which a medical professional may testify about the medical history gathered from the child in abuse evaluations, including:

1. Outcry witness. If the professional is the first person over the age of 18 years that the child has disclosed abuse to, then that person is the "outcry witness" and may testify as to what the child told him or her.
2. Hearsay exception: medical diagnosis and treatment. If the medical professional is asking the child for information important for medical diagnosis and treatment, then the medical professional may testify as to what the child told him or her and the medical records are sometimes admitted into evidence and can be reviewed by the judge or jury.
3. Hearsay exception: excited utterance. If the child suddenly discloses new information to a person because of the unique nature of the circumstances (i.e., disclosing sexual abuse during a genital examination or while testing for genital infections), the child's statements to the professional can be presented during testimony.

FACTORS THAT IMPACT PATTERNS OF DISCLOSURE

It is common for children to not disclose their abuse. In one study of more than 26,000 children investigated for abuse, disclosure rate for cases of sexual abuse was 71% and for cases of physical abuse was 61%.[2] However, retrospective studies of adults who were sexually abused as children indicate that only 30% to 40% recall ever disclosing their abuse as a child.[5] Adult survivors of child sexual abuse do report periods of time when the abuse is forgotten, and then independently recalled.[6] Other reasons for nondisclosure include denial, reticence, and lack of conceptual understanding of the abuse.[7] In one study,[7] the self-reports of 10 children were compared with the videotapes of their sexual abuse by one perpetrator. The videotapes of 102 incidents of sexual abuse involving these children (mean age 5.6 years) were compared with their statements, which were taken 3 to 23 months after the last incident of abuse (mean age 6.9 years). Every incident of sexual abuse that each child described was corroborated by video. However, three children did not disclose abuse and denials were correlated with a greater number of abusive incidents. Even with the use of confrontational interview techniques, leading questions, and accusatory suggestions, the abused children in this study denied or minimized their experiences. Two children in this study indicated they tried to actively forget the abuse, and another was described as having "childhood amnesia." As with many clinical situations, when the child indicates they "don't remember" the abuse, it is difficult to determine whether the memory is truly not accessible or whether the child is offering a deterrent because they do not want to talk about the traumatic event.

When disclosure does occur, it is often delayed, with up to 75% of sexually abused children waiting at least 1 year before telling someone about their abuse.[1] A national survey study of 288 women who experienced child sexual abuse revealed that 28% never disclosed and 47% waited more than 5 years to disclose.[8] Another survey study[9] found a 2.3 year average delay in child sexual abuse disclosures; median time to disclosure was 6 months, indicating a wide range of reported disclosure intervals. Reasons for nondisclosure and delay in disclosure are multifactorial, and include the child's fear of consequences, interpretation of the abuse, and attribution of blame. These factors additionally are modulated by the child's gender and age, the relationship between the child and abuser, threats made by the abuser, and the child's perception of support for their disclosure.

A number of studies have examined the effects of gender and age on children's disclosure of abuse. Boys are generally more reluctant to disclose abuse, especially sexual abuse, than girls, but gender differences are not consistent and vary by type of abuse as well.[2,10,11] Boys are thought to have higher levels of shame and embarrassment due to fears of being stigmatized as victims or homosexuals.[11-13] In addition, boys sexually abused by older women sometimes mistakenly view the abuse as desirable and minimize or deny their experience.[14] Perpetrators often prey upon gender-specific vulnerabilities in children by suggesting that the abusive experiences are enjoyable and a privilege for the child.

Numerous studies have indicated a relationship between victim age and disclosure. Younger victims are generally less likely to disclose.[8,13,15] This tendency holds for physical and sexual abuse,[2] although one study found that older children delayed disclosures longer than younger children because they understood and feared the consequences.[12] Low rates of disclosure in very young children can occur because interview protocols do not prompt the abuse statement or memory in a young child. Unfounded suspicions may be disproportionately higher in this age group compared with older children. Alternatively, younger children might be more easily coerced and deceived into silence by their abusers, especially because they are more likely to think they are responsible for, or have somehow caused, their own abuse.[16] Alternatively, they may be more susceptible to perpetrator tactics for maintaining secrecy.[15]

Developmental considerations, such as children's relationships with family and peers, also impact their tendencies to disclose. For example, preschool and school-age children tend to become strongly attached to their mother and father, and the preservation of the family's happiness and stability is a high priority. Once they reach adolescence, peer approval and intimacy may supersede close parental bonds, so that disclosure of parental abuse might be more likely; this developmental shift might explain why some disclosures occur during arguments between adolescents and their parents, and why older adolescents (ages 14-17) are more likely to tell peers about sexual abuse while younger children are more likely to tell adults.[15]

Certainly, older children and adolescents are cognizant of the consequences of disclosure of abuse and often fear consequences for themselves, the perpetrator, and other family members.[12,15] Their fears often stem directly from the threats of the abuser. Such threats may include breaking up the family, placement in foster care, punishment, and being responsible for the abuser's incarceration. Children victimized by family members living in the same house are more likely to be affected by these threats, supporting the finding that victims of parents or parental figures are more likely to delay or withhold disclosure, especially when the abuse is sexual.[2] Hershkovitz et al[2] found that victims of sexual abuse were more likely than victims of physical abuse to disclose and surmised that this difference was primarily attributable to the predominance of family member perpetrators of physical abuse when compared with sexual abuse. Children are explicitly entrusted with the integrity of the family when they are told their disclosure could destroy everything. Nondisclosure and longer delays in disclosure are more likely when the abuser is a family member rather than a nonfamily member.[2,12] Socioeconomic and cultural factors can also influence disclosure; among some Mexican-American cultures the girl's *quincenara*, a celebration of impending womanhood on her fifteenth birthday, is provided only if the girl is chaste and a virgin. Girls in families that place high values on virginity and chastity until marriage are often reluctant to disclose abuse and risk the anticipated disappointment of their families.[14] Isolation and lack of community security as seen in populations affected by discrimination, migration and poverty, are potential deterrents to disclose abuse.[14,17] Another study[15] found that sexually abused children that never lived with both parents were less likely to disclose their abuse, and those that lived with family members that abused drugs were more likely to disclose promptly. While the latter finding appears counterintuitive, the author proposed that

abused children in dysfunctional families may have stronger peer bonds, facilitating disclosure to their friends.

Children are also protective of their abusers, which affects the tendency and type of disclosure they are willing to provide. In a study of 47 children[18] whose sexual abuse was corroborated by perpetrator confession, 14% indicated they had been in love with the perpetrator and to some degree enjoyed the abuse experiences. One third of these children voluntarily returned to the abuser or took the initiative in sexual activities. As might be anticipated, those children who were attracted to or protective of their abusers had a longer delay in disclosure (mean 40 months) compared with victims who were not attracted to their abuser (mean 8 months). Even when children are not attracted to their abuser, they may still value the nonabusive components of their relationship and be reluctant to jeopardize the loss of that component by disclosing.

Abusers who reside in the home and who are demonstrably violent with others can effectively silence their child and adult victims with threats of harm should they disclose abuse.[19] Children with families characterized by intimate partner abuse, substance abuse, and ineffective parent-child bonding are less likely to perceive support for their disclosures and therefore less likely to disclose. Abusive corporal punishment of children often occurs in homes where intimate partner abuse occurs, but is often discovered when injuries are visible, not when the child discloses. In contrast to sexual abuse, victims of physical abuse tend to accommodate this practice, interpreting it as discipline rather than abuse. In general, children are more likely to disclose if they perceive their parents are supportive rather than skeptical of their disclosure; one study[20] found that 63% of children with supportive parents disclosed sexual abuse during their initial interview compared with only 17% of children whose caretakers were skeptical. In another study of 41 adult survivors of child sexual abuse, most of the victims who disclosed to their mother perceived a hostile or indifferent reaction.[4] While it is unknown whether the parents in these circumstances were actually supportive or believing of the children, it is the children's perception of support that ultimately influences their tendency to disclose.

Custody issues present unique challenges when abuse allegations arise. The number of sexual abuse reports arising from families involved in custody disputes do not differ significantly from those reported in families without custody disputes.[21] Children and adolescents do sometimes make false allegations of abuse. In a study of 576 child sexual abuse cases, 1.4% involved false allegations.[22] In another review of 551 child sexual abuse cases, there were 14 (2.5%) false reports; eight were false allegations by the child, 3 were false reports made in collusion with a parent, and 3 involved confusion or misinterpretation by the child.[23] It is important for the clinician to conduct unbiased and complete assessments of any child with a clear outcry of abuse, keeping in mind that while situations might be exaggerated or fabricated in particularly contentious child custody cases, separation of a child from their abuser can also prompt disclosure of valid abuse.

Given the various factors impacting the likelihood and timing of abuse disclosure by the child, it is not surprising that children may make partial (also referred to as "incremental") disclosures or full disclosures of abuse, and may recant part or all of their history depending on the responses following disclosure. Recantation rates for child sexual abuse range from 4% to 22%.[1,24-26] In one study,[26] 92% of the cases involving recantation of child sexual abuse were reaffirmed over a period of time. The clinician might interview the child early in the investigation before consequences of disclosure have occurred, or might interview the child later in the investigation, after investigators and family members have responded to the child's outcry. If the child perceives the responses as supportive, the medical history is more likely to reflect a full disclosure. Other times, the child victim can become alarmed by the response of their parent and become reluctant to provide further details. The clinician should have a sense of the factors that impact the child's history. If the child recants or appears to provide a partial history, the clinician should document observations that support retraction and conduct an examination that addresses suspected types of abuse, even if the child is recanting or minimizing their initial statement. For example, the medical examination of an 8-year-old child who recants a statement of vaginal-penile contact by her stepfather and whose mother chooses to believe the child is lying should include testing for sexually transmitted infections.

CLINICAL APPROACH TO THE MEDICAL HISTORY

Because the information gathered can be forensically significant and children experience considerable anxiety in discussing their abuse, the clinician's medical history encompasses several priorities, including the need to ask questions in a developmentally appropriate and forensically sound manner, and the provision of a neutral but appropriately supportive setting that optimizes the child's ability to share information about sensitive topics. As the interview progresses, the clinician sometimes needs to adjust his or her approach as the child's developmental capabilities and barriers to disclosure become more evident. These skills require knowledge of child development and appropriate interview approaches.

Language Acquisition and Development in Children (Table 7-2)

Clinicians should be well informed on how to interview children and adolescents of various ages and stages of development. In general, preschool children often are not capable of consistently understanding and appropriately responding to the kinds of questions asked during a medical history for suspected abuse. While they do respond well to directive yes/no questions such as, "Did anyone touch your private parts?" or "Has anyone ever hit you in the face?," their responses are difficult to verify. Younger children under the age of 6 years tend to provide less information spontaneously but do retain accurate memories.[27] However, they are more susceptible to highly leading and suggestive questions[28] than children older than 6 years, so it is particularly important to ask nonsuggestive questions such as, "How did you get that bruise?" rather than "Who hurt you there?" Young children have shorter attention spans, so medical histories should be

generally no longer than 20 minutes. In general, children are able to understand and respond appropriately to questions between the ages of 4 and 5 years.

School-age children have longer attention spans and are readily "interviewable" and often uncontrived in their responses. A more comprehensive medical history, including questions about their feelings, sleeping difficulties, and school functioning can be included. Adolescents also are able to provide detailed medical histories, but clarifications and verification of terms might still be needed.

Important Principles in Interviewing Children

By the nature of their profession, pediatricians have experience gaining the trust of their patients, and children understand that pediatricians are concerned about safety and health. It is appropriate to begin interviews of children who are suspected victims of abuse by reminding them that it is part of your job to take care of children's health and safety, and to "... find out how I can best help you and help your family keep you safe and healthy." This introduction explains the rationale for subsequent discussions of "uncomfortable, confusing, or threatening" events that occur in a child's life. Principles of respect, honesty, concern, and trust should be reinforced consistently with each child.

Each professional should give frequent and explicit permission to the child to talk about any uncomfortable or threatening experiences. Sometimes abuse victims disclose simply because someone asks. Many children do not disclose because they are fearful of their abuser, of not being believed, of getting in trouble, or of the effects on other family members.[29] When a child discloses abuse, acknowledgment of these fears is one way to show understanding and support for the child. Helpful questions include: "Does anything worry you?" "Some children worry about what people will think or do after they tell." "You're not in trouble here." "Thank you for talking to me about this." All of these are examples of statements that may facilitate disclosure in abused children who are reluctant to tell.

It is critically important that professionals not prompt or provide details for children when asking screening questions for abuse. The goal of screening questions is to obtain sufficient information to make a report and define the terms of the report. If the child has a physical finding or injury suspicious for abuse, ask the child to simply tell you "how this happened," or "everything about how these bruises happened." If the explanation is inconsistent with the pattern, age, or severity of the injury, the clinician should be honest with the child: "It's confusing to me how you would get two black eyes from falling down only one time. Sometimes children get bruises in other ways and they might feel scared to talk about it. I'm here to help. Is there anything else you can tell me about these bruises?" If the child does not disclose abuse but the physical examination findings are suspicious for abuse, a report to child protective services or the local law enforcement agency in accordance with state laws should be made.

Information the child shares should be made available only to the necessary individuals (child protective services, police, supervisors), and should be shared with respect and

Table 7-2	Language and Development of Children and Adolescents

Preschool Children (Ages 3-5)

Might be able to state:
  First name, age, and family members
  Who hurt or touched them
  Where they were hurt or touched
  Where they were when they were hurt or touched
  Whether event occurred "one time" or "more than one time"
  May give graphic, age-appropriate descriptions of body parts
Usually cannot state:
  Colors, or names for all body parts
  How many times event(s) occurred
  Reliably sequence events or tell you when an event occurred
Challenges specific to this age group:
  Language skills are widely variable and achieved at rapid rates
  Attention span is short, so interviews should be completed within 20 minutes
  Focused on the "here and now"; yesterday is "a long time ago"
  Demonstrative gestures are frequent and sometimes more detailed than verbal accounts
  Are reluctant to say "I don't know" or "I don't understand your question"
Able to recognize type of question (yes/no, "who" questions, etc.) and will sometimes try to "guess" the answer accordingly; for
  this reason, "yes/no" questions should be avoided
  Speech is often unintelligible

School-Age Children (Ages 6-11)

Will be able to state everything that preschool children can plus:
  Full name, ages, and members of family
  Colors, names for all body parts
  More details regarding type of abusive contact (bruising, bleeding, pain, etc.)
  Idiosyncratic details: what abuse felt like (conversations, smells, taste, etc.)
  Relative frequency of abusive events (daily, weekly, monthly, etc.)
  Age abuse began and ended
  Physical and behavioral symptoms
Might not be able to state/understand:
  Exact dates or abusive events in the correct sequence, if chronic
  Precise time frames for physical and behavioral symptoms
Abstract concepts such as (such as "what is truth?"), relations of time, speed, size, duration
Challenges specific to this age group:
Family responses and degree of belief are most important and can modify willingness to talk
  May not understand why they are *not* to blame for the abuse or family reactions

Adolescents (Ages 12-17)

Will be able to state everything that school-age children can plus:
  More idiosyncratic/experiential details
  Usually understand relations of time, speed, size, duration
Might not understand abstract concepts consistently
Challenges specific to this age group:
  Will sometimes provide excessive/extraneous details
Are generally unaware of adverse consequences of abuse (such as STIs) and might sensationalize information ("I may never get
  pregnant")
  Embarrassment more common and can compromise willingness to talk
  Still very concrete, so terms such as "spank" and "rape" still need to be clarified
Very focused on peer approval and whether or not they are "normal" (physically and otherwise)
  Concern about parental repercussions can compromise history about sexual activity

sensitivity to the child's needs. There should be no "shop talk" among professionals in the presence of children. The medical history is best gathered with the child or adolescent fully clothed; in cases of physical abuse, further questions can be asked during the course of the examination if additional injuries are uncovered.

Approach to the Interview

The clinician's initial approach will depend on whether the child has already disclosed abuse. If abuse is suspected because of physical, behavioral, or emotional symptoms but no abuse has been disclosed, the clinician should question the child in a careful, nonleading, nonsuggestive manner. If the child has already disclosed abuse, questions must still be carefully phrased, but the interview can be based in part on information already presented.

The medical interview of suspected abuse victims can take from 5 minutes (when they "do not want to talk about it") to 2 hours, depending on the extent of information gathered and the cooperation and verbal abilities of the child. In general, the clinician should gather the history out of the presence of the parent, but might wish to have another staff person such as a social worker or nurse present as a "neutral" witness. Because such histories can be prolonged and it is preferable to document the child's words, the clinician should take notes during the interview. If older children prefer, they can write their own answers. Some clinicians prefer to audiotape their history and have it transcribed into the medical record. Anatomically detailed dolls should only be used by trained individuals.

Children are often worried about the examination, and providing information about the examination procedures at the onset of the interview can alleviate anxiety and facilitate information gathering. The child should be allowed to describe in his or her own words "what happened" with little interruption, except to clarify terms. The clinician should clarify such statements as "… he touched me," or "… he hit me" by asking the following: (1) "Who is *he*?" (2) "Where did he touch (hit) you?" and (3) "What did he hit (touch) you with?" Questions should not be leading, where the answers are suggested in the question, such as "Somebody broke your arm, didn't they?" They also should not suggest an answer because components of the answer are projected by the questioner ("Did mommy hurt your arm?"). In general, it is recommended that questions begin with "what," "who," "where," "when," or "how," not "did" or "why."

During the interview, positive reinforcement should be provided cautiously and not just after statements of abuse. Neutral body language and maintenance of eye contact demonstrate the clinician is listening and hearing what the child says. Determining the time frame and frequency of abusive episodes are important for diagnosis and treatment. While it may be important to determine if anything "went inside" (when referring to vaginal-digital or vaginal-penile contact), children and adolescents might not be able to accurately distinguish partial (or vulvar) versus completed (or vaginal) penetration. Experiential and corroborative details that the child volunteers should be documented: visual/olfactory/taste characteristics of ejaculate; urge to defecate during or after sodomy; pornographic pictures or movies taken of a child in cases of sexual abuse; physically abused children's descriptions of the object used to hit them, threats, or conversations during the abusive events.

If a child stops while describing an incident of abuse, providing general support is appropriate ("I know this is hard for you but you are doing a good job," not, "I know when your daddy touched your privates you must have felt upset. I don't blame you."), followed by repetition of what was last said by the child so they are encouraged to continue. Clinicians may wish to employ reflective listening, a method of response that entails capturing the content or emotion of what a child says, and restating it to expand a frame of reference, reduce confusion, clarify emotions, develop neutral feedback, or simply to give the child more time to elaborate

their statement.[30] For example, if a child says, "I don't know how I feel about what happened," the clinician may reply, "It must be confusing to think about what your uncle did." Clinicians may offer the option of writing or whispering "what happened"; other props, such as dolls, puppets, or telephones, are useful in the hands of skilled interviewers but can also be distracting or suggestive to younger children.

Children will sometimes say they still love their abuser, or their nonbelieving mother. It is important for the clinician to acknowledge those feelings ("I know you love your mom") and clarify situations that may be confusing to the child ("While you live with your aunt, your mom will get help with learning how to keep you and your sister safe"). It is also appropriate for clinicians to acknowledge and clarify feelings of guilt expressed by the child. ("Other children I've talked with have also said they felt like what happened was their fault but the adult is responsible for what happened, not you.")

COMPONENTS OF THE MEDICAL HISTORY

Table 7-3 summarizes the components of the medical history in cases of suspected abuse.

Information About Abusive Events

Although the type of information (abuser identification, type of abusive contact, timing of contact) medical professionals rely on for diagnosis is similar for physical and sexual abuse, details gathered when sexual abuse is suspected differ from details gathered when other types of abuse are suspected. The type of sexual contact and timing of the most recent sexual contact will assist in the interpretation of examination findings and will determine whether emergent forensic evidence collection is indicated. Children and adolescents presenting within 48 to 72 hours of sexual abuse involving genital, anal, or oral contact, an evaluation for forensic evidence collection is often indicated. The medical history can provide important information about the need to collect other forensic materials such as assailant debris and hairs (pubic and head) that may be found on the child's body or clothing and linens from the scene of the event.

Information about the type of sexual contact will determine which examination procedures and tests are most appropriate. If there is a history of the perpetrator's genitals contacting the child's body, then testing for sexually transmitted infections (STIs) should be considered. With repeated genital contact, risk of STIs, including AIDS, increases. Condom use by the assailant reduces, but does not eliminate, the risks of pregnancy and diseases. The use of lubrication can reduce the likelihood of anal or genital trauma. The child, police, or caretakers might describe characteristics of the perpetrator that increase the risk of AIDS, such as known positive serology for HIV, stranger, gang member, intravenous drug user, and multiple sexual partners. When any of these characteristics are identified during the medical history, the clinician should discuss HIV testing with the child and family, enabling them to make an informed decision about whether to undergo testing, and possible prophylactic treatment in some circumstances (see Chapter 24).

Table 7-3 Medical History for Suspected Abuse

History of Event(s)

Frequency and most recent incident
Type(s) of sexual and/or physical contact or injury
Condom use
Perpetrator identity/risk factors for STIs, HIV (stranger, gang member, substance abuser, etc.)
Bodily injuries; attack/defense injuries

Physical/Emotional/Psychological Symptoms

Pain/tenderness over body surfaces
Bite marks (recent/healed)
Genital symptoms (pain/bleeding, dysuria, discharge, abdominal pain)
Recent drug/alcohol use; memory lapses, mental status changes
Symptoms of shock, depression, suicide
Sexualized, aggressive behaviors
Sleep disturbances, school dysfunction, weight/appetite changes

Gynecological History (Adolescents)

Prior gynecological evaluations/conditions/infections/pregnancy
Sexual history (timing and type[s] of previous sexual contact, contraceptive use, gender of partners)
Last menstrual period, including regularity of cycles, normal flow patterns

Family Background

Degree of support/belief in the child
Prior abuse in family members
Family violence
Parental and child coping
Changes in family structure/function since disclosure of abuse
Concerns for child: virginity/"damaged goods," AIDS, STDs, pregnancy, delinquency/runaway, depression

Safety Issues

Does the child fear repercussions at home because they have disclosed abuse?
Is the child actively suicidal?
Does the child feel safe going home?

Children and adolescents that present for medical evaluations after an acute sexual assault should be questioned and examined carefully for other nongenital injuries. Injuries can result from the assailant's blows, grabbing, restraining, or gagging, or from the defensive efforts of the victim. Assault injuries most frequently involve the face and neck and are inflicted to silence the victim. Slap marks, grab marks, and contusions from blows by a fist or object may be seen on the face, neck, head, and extremities. Areas where patients indicate they have been bitten or licked can yield important forensic information and should be swabbed and photographed in accordance with protocols.

Victims sometimes report tenderness over body surfaces after an acute sexual or physical assault. Victims of chronic sexual abuse often have genital concerns or complaints that have no identifiable pathological etiology. Children should be asked if they have had any pain, bleeding, or discharge. After examination, if appropriate, it is important to reassure children that they are normal. Genital symptoms that can indicate trauma or pathology, including bleeding, pain, dysuria, urinary tract infections, vaginal discharge, and abdominal pain. Recent drug/alcohol use or mental status changes suggest the need for drug testing or alcohol blood levels. In some states, criminal charges are affected by the victim's level of intoxication (and hence, inability to consent). Some victims require emergent or long-term treatment for substance abuse. The presence of illicit substances in child or adolescent victims of physical or sexual abuse should prompt careful questioning about prostitution and exploitation for pornography.

The initial approach to the interview of a child who is a suspected victim of physical abuse is similar to the approach for a suspected victim of sexual abuse. ("Can you tell me what you know or understand about why you are here to see me today?") In physical abuse cases, it is important to establish where the injuries are, when they occurred, and how they occurred. Descriptions of pain and disability will assist in assessing the need for further testing (such as radiographs) or follow-up examinations. Understanding the context and chronicity of the abuse, and the triggers that led to the child's injury can assist the physician in assessing whether the child is in ongoing danger. For example, injuries inflicted for minor, expected incidents (such as breaking a toy) and humiliation of a child in public might indicate greater risk of harm to the child in other, more provocative or less public situations. Physical abuse victims often provide limited information about the extent and severity of their injuries. It is not unusual for the physician to uncover additional acute and healed injuries during a child's examination that were not discussed or disclosed during the medical history. As injuries are revealed, the clinician should ask, "I see a long scar on your lower back here. What can you tell me about how this happened? Do you know when?" As with interviews of children who are suspected victims of sexual abuse, the clinician should be careful to clarify terms used by the victims. For example, many children say they are "spanked," but when asked to clarify, many will indicated that a spanking is when they are hit with a belt or another object.

Victims can have acute emotional shock, depression, and suicidal ideation. The clinician should ask victims of abuse directly about suicidal thoughts regardless of whether they have overt symptoms of depression. ("Have you ever felt so bad that you thought about killing or hurting yourself?" If the answer is yes, the clinician should establish the most recent suicidal thoughts/action and consider an immediate referral to a mental health professional. The clinician should be cautious in prescribing anxiolytic or antidepressant drugs, and should refer to a child psychiatrist whenever possible.

Other behavioral responses to abuse include aggressive behaviors, sleep disturbances, school dysfunction, weight changes, and delinquent behaviors (see chapters 49 and 50).

Gynecological History

Information regarding prior gynecological evaluations will assist the clinician and support staff in preparing the adolescent for an examination. Prior infections, pregnancies, and gynecological conditions should be noted. A menstrual history, including menarcheal age, last menstrual period, use of pads and/or tampons, and regularity of menstrual periods assist in determining the need for pregnancy testing. In addition, adolescents that have had prior gynecological examinations or who use tampons may tolerate certain examination procedures more readily. It is not unusual for physically abused adolescents to have also been sexually abused or sexually active and in need of a gynecological assessment.

A sexual history should include the gender and number of partners, type(s) of sexual contact (including anal and oral contact), and frequency of barrier contraceptive use so the type and optimal timing of testing can be determined. For example, venereal warts have a latency phase of 2 weeks to 2 years, averaging 2 months, so an examination might be indicated 2 months after the most recent sexual assault or contact. Information about the last menstrual period will determine risk and best timing for pregnancy testing.

Family History and Responses to Abuse Disclosure

Sometimes the child might reveal that the nonabusive caretaker does not believe them or is ambivalent about whether abuse has occurred. When there is compelling evidence of abuse, either in the child's history or in medical findings, the clinician should report any perceived lack of support or belief in the child to child protective services. Prior abuse history of the child or family should be noted. History of intimate adult partner abuse in the home of the child is particularly important as the risk of further violent outbursts and the risk of homicide increases when a battered adult leaves the batterer. In one study,[29] more than half of sexually abused children and adolescents reported adult intimate partner violence in their homes. When the abuse of the child by a batterer is revealed, this can be the first time the battered partner attempts to leave the batterer. This presents considerable risk to the adults and children in the home.

The child's coping depends on how the nonabusive adult reacts to the disclosure of abuse. Children perceive adults' distress as threatening, often affecting their willingness to talk about the abuse. Such concerns should be identified and addressed. The clinician should also ask children what concerns they have about the medical consequences of the abuse, including disfigurement, diseases, pregnancy, virginity, and alterations in body appearance or function. By providing answers and reassurance, clinicians can directly enhance the healing process.

Safety Issues

Adolescents assaulted by other adolescents also face fears related to family responses. Victims of "date rape" might fear physical punishment by parents for "letting that happen." Clinicians should ask teens if they feel safe going home and whether they have ever run away or thought about it.

Other Information

Some information is not frequently volunteered unless the clinician asks about it. Appropriate questions include:

- "Has anyone ever done anything like this to you before?"
- "Do you know if he (perpetrator) did this to anyone else?" (Some children have witnessed other children being victimized.)
- In sexual abuse cases, "Did he make you do anything to him?"
- "Did he take (or show) any pictures or movies of you (or other people) without your clothes on?"
- "What did he say about telling?"
- "What did he say would happen if you told?"

For many children and families, experiences with investigative agencies and professionals are intrusive, inconvenient, and/or time consuming despite best intentions. One 5-year-old girl said that when the police came to her house, "I thought they came to arrest me." Similarly, children expect physicians to give shots, or they may even think the physician has the power to take them away from their families. Clinicians should provide clear instructions on what will be done with the information given to them by a child ("I will write up a report which goes to the police, child protective services, and the district attorney's office") and what can be expected from medical staff ("You don't need to see me again unless any new problems come up; I will call you if any of the tests for infections come back positive"). It is important to note that if the physician determines that releasing any information to the parent of the child could endanger the child, the Federal HIPAA law (Health Information Portability and Accountability Act) provides exceptions to the release of verbal or written information under these circumstances. It is preferable, under these circumstances, to refer the parent to child protective services or law enforcement for more information on the medical assessment findings.

When releasing information to the parent of an adolescent, clinicians must respect the adolescent's right to confidential health care when discussing medical issues related to sexual activity with peers. As state child abuse reporting laws vary, the clinician should familiarize himself or herself with the definitions of sexual abuse as defined by statute and provisions for mandatory reporting of sexual activity that involves adolescents.

During closure after the interview and examination, the clinician should review the following:

- Explain findings and provide an interpretation (unless this could endanger the child, as discussed above). For example, child victims of sexual abuse should understand their examination is "normal" or their injuries are healing; a drawing may help the child and family understand that the hymen is "still there." Although children and especially teenagers rarely voice this concern, many are worried that their bodies may be "different."
- Answer any questions—spoken or unspoken—you think the child or parent might have. An exception would be sharing information with a parent of a child

who has been abused when there is a possibility that the parent is the abuser or is protective of the abuser.

- Give the family your name and contact information.
- Understand that further disclosures of abuse are not uncommon and may necessitate further evaluation in the future.

Abused children often depend on the clinician's honesty to maintain trust. Out of eagerness to assist such children, professionals sometimes predict or promise things that cannot be guaranteed. This may jeopardize the child's trust. *Do not* promise:

- That the child will never be abused again
- That their mother or caretaker will believe them or protect them
- That the abuser will be put in jail or arrested.

Do promise:

- To keep the child informed as to what you do, including examination procedures and the information that you share with others
- To answer any questions the child may have
- To be available for the child.

References

1. Elliott DM, Briere J: Forensic sexual abuse evaluations of older children: disclosures and symptomatology. *Behav Sci Law* 1994;12:261-277.
2. Hershkowitz I, Horowitz D, Lamb ME: Trends in children's disclosure of abuse in Israel: a national study. *Child Abuse Negl* 2005;29:1203-1214.
3. Orbach Y, Hershkowitz I, Lamb ME, et al: Assessing the value of structured protocols for forensic interviews of alleged child abuse victims. *Child Abuse Negl* 2000;24:733-752.
4. Somer E, Szwarcberg S: Variables in delayed disclosure of childhood sexual abuse. *Am J Orthopsychiatry* 2001;71:332-341.
5. London K, Bruck M, Ceci SJ, et al: Disclosure of child sexual abuse: what does the research tell us about the ways that children tell? *Psychol Public Policy Law* 2005;11:194-226.
6. Wilsnack SC, Wonderlich SA, Krisjanson AF, et al: Self-reports of forgetting and remembering childhood sexual abuse in a nationally representative sample of U.S. women. *Child Abuse Negl* 2002;26:139-147.
7. Sjoberg RL, Lindblad F: Limited disclosure of sexual abuse in children whose experiences were documented by videotape. *Am J Psychiatry* 2002;159:312-314.
8. Smith DW, Letourneau EJ, Saunders BE, et al: Delay in disclosure of childhood rape: results from a national survey. *Child Abuse Negl* 2000;24:273-287.
9. Kellogg ND, Huston RL: Unwanted sexual experiences in adolescents: patterns of disclosure. *Clin Pediatr* 1995;34:306-312.
10. Ghetti S, Goodman GS: Resisting distortion? *Psychologist* 2001;14:592-595.
11. Gries LT, Goh DS, Cavanaugh J: Factors associated with disclosure during child sexual abuse assessment. *J Child Sex Abus* 1996;5:1-20.
12. Goodman-Brown TB, Edelstein RS, Goodman GS, et al: Why children tell: a model of children's disclosure of sexual abuse. *Child Abuse Negl* 2003;27:525-540.
13. Keary K, Fitzpatrick C: Children's disclosure of sexual abuse during formal investigation. *Child Abuse Negl* 1994;18:543-548.
14. Alaggia R: Cultural and religious influences in maternal response to intrafamilial child sexual abuse: charting new territory for research and treatment. *J Child Sex Abus* 2001;10:41-61.
15. Kogan SM: Disclosing unwanted sexual experiences: results from a national sample of adolescent women. *Child Abuse Negl* 2004;28:147-165.
16. Hazzard A, Celano M, Gould J, et al: Predicting symptomatology and self-blame among child sex abuse victims. *Child Abuse Negl* 1995;19:707-714.
17. Fontes LA: Disclosures of sexual abuse by Puerto Rican children: oppression and cultural barriers. *J Child Sex Abus* 1993;2:21-35.
18. Sjoberg RL, Lindblad F: Delayed disclosure and disrupted communication during forensic investigation of child sexual abuse: a study of 47 corroborated cases. *Acta Paediatr* 2002;91:1391-1396.
19. Jaffe P, Geffner R: Child custody disputes and domestic violence: critical issues in mental health, social service, and legal professionals. *In:* Holden G, Geffner R, Jouriles E (eds): *Children Exposed to Marital Violence: Theory, Research, and Applied Issues.* American Psychological Association, Washington, DC, 1998, pp 371-408.
20. Lawson L, Chaffin M: False negatives in sexual abuse disclosure interviews: incidence and influence of caretaker's belief in abuse cases of accidental abuse discovery by diagnosis of STD. *J Interpers Violence* 1992;9:107-117.
21. Rieser M: Recantation in child sexual abuse cases. *Child Welfare* 1991;70:611-621.
22. Jones D, McGraw E, Melbourne E: Reliable and fictitious accounts of sexual abuse to children. *J Interpers Violence* 1987;2:27-46.
23. Oates RK, Jones D, Denson D, et al: Erroneous concerns about child sexual abuse. *Child Abuse Negl* 2000;24:149-157.
24. Bradley AR, Wood JM: How do children tell? The disclosure process in child sexual abuse. *Child Abuse Negl* 1996;20:881-891.
25. Faller KC, Henry J: Child sexual abuse: a case study in community collaboration. *Child Abuse Negl* 2000;24:1215-1225.
26. Sorenson T, Snow B: How children tell: the process of disclosure in child sexual abuse. *Child Welfare* 1991;70:3-15.
27. Oates K: Can we believe what children tell us? *J Paediatr Child Health* 2007;43:843-847.
28. Shrimpton S, Oates RK, Hayes S: Children's memory of events: effects of stress, age, time delay and place of interview. *Appl Cogn Psychol* 1998;12:133-143.
29. Kellogg ND, Menard SW: Violence among family members of children and adolescents evaluated for sexual abuse. *Child Abuse Negl* 2003;27:1367-1376.
30. Spaulding W: *Interviewing child victims of sexual exploitation.* National Center for Missing and Exploited Children, Washington, DC, 1987. http://eric.ed.gov/ERICDocs/data/ericdocs2sql/content_storage_01/0000019b/80/1e/bc/c8.pdf. Accessed February 6, 2009.

8

INTERVIEWING CAREGIVERS OF SUSPECTED CHILD ABUSE VICTIMS

Katherine R. Snyder, MD, MPH, Melissa L. Currie, MD, and Tanya F. Stockhammer, PhD

One of the most difficult aspects of dealing with cases of possible child maltreatment involves communicating with the caregivers of the child. Common questions that medical providers ask themselves when dealing with potential child abuse cases are, "Am I talking with a perpetrator?" "How do I take this history without getting angry?" "I'm not sure this is abuse—what do I do now?" "How do I ask these questions without making this parent angry or defensive?" Further complicating the issue are questions about the medical provider's role in the interviewing process. What questions do medical providers need to ask? What questions are best left for police and child protection investigators? More has been written about the interview of children in suspected abuse cases than about interviewing caregivers. The purpose of this chapter is to attempt to answer the above questions and to provide some practical tips and suggestions for communicating with caregivers in suspected maltreatment cases. Figure 8-1 illustrates an approach to the child maltreatment caregiver interview and summarizes the information in this chapter.

The volume of research about the assessment and diagnosis of child maltreatment has increased dramatically over the past 4 decades. However, there remains little research or guidance about best practices for the medical provider who interviews caregivers. Consequently, the information in this chapter is more practical and experience-based, although supportive research is cited when available.

THE PEDIATRIC HISTORY BEFORE CONCERN FOR MALTREATMENT

The first stage of the caregiver interview occurs before the medical provider has become concerned about the possibility of child maltreatment. During this time, the provider is obtaining a routine history during a well checkup or illness visit. Most important during this stage is asking the right screening questions that optimize the likelihood of recognizing maltreatment when it has occurred. It is rare to have "child abuse" as the chief complaint.[1] More common presenting complaints are "fussiness," "vomiting," "fell off couch," "starting to wet the bed at night," or "no concerns— here for school physical," among others. These routine patient encounters are sometimes the only opportunity to recognize the warning signs of child maltreatment. The first

and most important key to recognition is to keep child maltreatment (including physical abuse, sexual abuse, and neglect) in the differential diagnosis for every patient and every visit. As the common maxim goes, "You see what you look for, and you look for what you know."

Recognizing Red Flags During the History and Examination

When a nonverbal patient has an obvious injury, regardless of whether the injury is the reason for the visit, medical providers need to obtain enough detail to determine if the history is concerning for maltreatment and to document the explanation in case it changes or is later questioned.[2] It is most helpful to do this matter-of-factly. The tone for this type of questioning can vary based on the setting, the reason for the visit, and the depth of the relationship between the provider and the caregiver. For example, at times, a routine, "What happened here?" is the most direct and appropriate way to systematically assess skin findings. In other situations, particularly if the caregiver is defensive, a less formal tone can help with rapport. In this way, medical providers can gather basic information about the injury. They can quickly find out how, where, and when the injury occurred, and who the child was with at the time.

Oftentimes, the information is clearly consistent with the injury. It is particularly reassuring when caregivers report that other adults witnessed the injury. Sometimes, however, red flags begin to appear (Table 8-1). The history may not be consistent with the developmental ability of the child (an 8-month-old who turned on the hot water), the injuries may be too severe or too numerous to be explained by the history (bilateral depressed skull fractures after a roll off a couch onto carpeted flooring), or there may be no history of trauma offered ("I don't know … he just woke up one morning not using that arm.")[2] Sometimes a patient does not have a visible injury but with a chief complaint (will not stop crying), history (an apparent life-threatening event), pattern of behavior (precocious sexual behavior), or physical finding (limp) that can be consistent with occult injury or abuse.[1,2,9,10] Although some behaviors may not be independently diagnostic of maltreatment, such symptoms should heighten awareness of that possibility and prompt further questioning and evaluation.

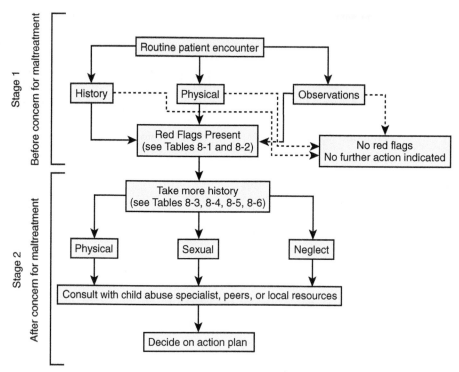

Stage 1 — Before concern for maltreatment

Stage 2 — After concern for maltreatment

FIGURE 8-1 Schema for Approach to Interview and Assessment.

Important Interactional Cues and Behavioral Observations

In addition to the history and physical examination, medical providers must also pay attention to the interaction, or lack thereof, between the caregiver and the child. Table 8-2 lists some common behavioral cues that can be indicators of abuse or neglect. Observation and documentation of these subtle findings is important supporting information if a case is being formally investigated.

Separation of Caregiver from the Child for the Interview

Interviewing the caregiver out of the child's presence is necessary if the child is verbal, the subject matter seems inappropriate for the child to hear, or if the caregiver merely appears to be uncomfortable discussing the issue in front of the child. It is also preferable for the child and caretaker to be interviewed separately to prevent any real or perceived coercion or leading of the verbal child.[8,14,15] If separation from the caregiver appears to be difficult for the child, then an alternative is to bring another adult into the room to attempt to distract the child while the history is being obtained. For example, after the history and physical for an adolescent or preadolescent, the provider could say, "Mrs. Jones, Sally is getting old enough now that I'd like to have a minute or two to speak with her privately. It gives her a chance to ask me any questions that she might be embarrassed to ask in front of you, and it helps start to prepare her for that day (too soon!) when she'll be grown up and coming to the doctor on her own."

For every well check, and as often as possible during illness visits, verbal children should be asked privately, "Do you feel safe at home?" This is a key screening question not only for child maltreatment, but also for identifying other issues such as domestic violence, a dangerous neighborhood, an out-of-control sibling, or a chaotic home environment.[16-18]

Beware of Bias

While much has been written about risk factors associated with child abuse, the absence of *risk factors* does not imply the absence of *risk*.[11] Similarly, the presence of risk factors does not necessarily mean that abuse has occurred.[11,19] Child maltreatment does not discriminate among socioeconomic level, education level, geography, or ethnicity. Research has shown that the most likely cases of abusive head injury to be missed by medical professionals involve Caucasian, middle-class, intact families,[1] a profile that also describes most medical professionals in America. It is natural to have opinions and biases. The clinician that is unaware of these biases may have misconceptions and provide less-than-optimal care for patients.[1,11,19-21] Therefore, medical providers must be self-aware and unwavering in their commitment to objectively evaluate every child and every family, regardless of where the family lives, what language they speak, or how many years of education they have.

THE DETAILED INTERVIEW ONCE THERE IS CONCERN FOR ABUSE

After the general history, the second stage of the interview occurs after the provider has developed concern for abuse (Figure 8-1). During this stage, questions are asked that help determine the likelihood of abuse. The assessment for child maltreatment is similar to any other clinical assessment in

Table 8-1	"Red Flags" that Can Indicate the Possibility of Child Maltreatment During Routine Patient Encounters[2-8]

Current History

History not consistent with developmental ability of the child

History not consistent with the injury type, severity, or number

History is vague or changes with time or different caregiver account

Absence of history for trauma in a child with injury

Child is described at clumsy

Delay in seeking medical care

History of multiple previous injuries/emergency department visits

Age inappropriate or intrusive/coercive sexual behaviors

Significant personality changes or changes in sleeping/eating habits

Symptoms

Infants with bruising

Infants with vomiting without diarrhea

Infants with unexplained fussiness

Depression

Behavioral issues

Past Medical History

Prematurity or prolonged NICU stay

Chronic medical conditions

Developmental delay

Special needs

Infant whose caregivers describe child as "easily bruised" or any previous bruising in an infant

Social History

History of child protective services involvement

Criminal history in family

Drug or alcohol abuse

One or both parents had previous children removed from their care

Nonrelated adult male in the household

Recent move, especially if vague explanation for move

Caregiver was victimized as a child

Domestic violence, past or current

Lack of social support network

Physical Examination

Infants

Any bruising

Full or bulging fontanelle

Rapidly increasing head circumference

Failure to thrive

Developmental delay

Any Age Child

Bruises in relatively protected areas such as ears, neck, flank, genitals, or buttocks

Patterned injury (handprints, submersion burns, contact burns, bite marks, loop marks)

Multiple healed injuries

Weight loss

Poor hygiene

Table 8-2	Observational and Nonverbal Cues that Help Identify Children at Risk[11-13]

Caregiver does not appear to appreciate the severity of child's condition

Caregiver does not attempt to comfort child

Child does not seek comfort from the caregiver

Caregiver speaks harshly to child

Caregiver has unrealistic developmental expectations of child

Child appears fearful of caregiver

Caregiver blames child for injuries or illness

Caregiver seems annoyed that child is requiring medical care

Caregiver treats one child in the room differently than others

There is tension between adult caregivers in the room

that questions are asked and the physical examination is performed to establish a differential diagnosis. The following section addresses the process of gathering information sensitively from caregivers once child maltreatment is being seriously considered.

First Things First

Once child maltreatment has become a distinct possibility, it is often overwhelming for medical providers to decide how to proceed.[21-24] Several factors should be considered to determine the next steps in the process. For example, is a potential perpetrator present, and if so, how is the safety of the child ensured while the workup proceeds? Does the medical provider ask more questions now, or send the child elsewhere for further evaluation? For many providers, it is necessary to step out of the room to gather thoughts and consider options. This is often an appropriate time to briefly consult with peers, supervisors, or local child protection experts. Some medical disciplines have published guidelines to address the specific role of the medical provider in forensic matters,[22,25] but the subtleties of these interactions remain challenging for the majority of providers.

Table 8-3 summarizes the major themes that need to be addressed during patient encounters once it is concerning that the patient might also be a victim. By systematically and deliberately addressing all of these themes, medical providers can feel confident that they have appropriately fulfilled their role in the assessment of suspected child maltreatment.

Rapport

While some patients may have clear-cut abuse, usually the evidence will be less clear and information from the caregiver will be essential to make an appropriate assessment of the case. Additionally, it might be unclear or unknown if the person who has brought the child for medical care is the abuser, a witness to the abuse, or is unaware or uninvolved. Sometimes it is impossible to determine this during the interview. An effective rapport with the child's caretaker is essential to gathering information that can clarify specifics of an

Table 8-3	Checklist of Major Themes to Be Addressed by the Medical Provider During an Abuse/Neglect Patient Encounter[2,14]

✓ Is the patient physiologically stable, and if not, what steps need to be taken immediately?

✓ Is the patient and hospital/office staff safe now? (If not, contact security or law enforcement.)

✓ If this patient may have been abused, then what studies can help confirm or refute that diagnosis?
  • What studies can help identify or rule out mimics of abuse?
  • What studies are needed to assess for occult injuries or associated medical issues (sexually transmitted infection)?

✓ If available, has the local child abuse medical team been consulted?

✓ Can this assessment be completed here, or does the patient require transfer?
  • If so, what is the safest method of transportation?

✓ Do any of the injuries require treatment?

✓ Is there medical or photographic evidence that needs collection or documentation?

✓ Have the necessary questions been asked of the caregivers to fully assess the injury (including timing, plausibility of mechanism, and alternative explanations)?

✓ If the child is old enough, has mental health been assessed and appropriate referrals been made?

✓ Have the necessary investigators (child protection series, law enforcement) been notified?
  • If not, when and by whom should the necessary investigators be notified?
  • If so, do the investigators understand the medical findings and their implications?

✓ Is there reason to be concerned for the patient's safety after discharge?
  • If so, has this been communicated to investigators and has an appropriate protection plan been developed?

✓ Are there siblings or other children in the same environment that need assessment or protection?
  • If so, has this been communicated to investigators?

✓ Are medical providers being as kind and supportive to the patient and caregivers as possible?

✓ Has the entire encounter been documented as thoroughly as possible?

abusive event or situation. Medical providers are often in the unique position of being the first nonperpetrator to recognize that maltreatment has occurred.[24,26] This provides an opportunity to record spontaneous responses to questions before the interview becomes rehearsed, altered, or guarded.

Often the most difficult aspect of developing this rapport involves overcoming feelings of anger or suspicion toward the caregivers or the situation in general. It is helpful to remember that the caregiver coming with the child is not necessarily the perpetrator and might be completely unaware of the true history. No harm is ever done when a medical provider is kind to a potential perpetrator. In fact, building rapport can allow the opportunity to obtain crucial detail about an event.[26] Irreparable harm is done, however, when nonperpetrators feel judged or criminalized by medical providers.

The degree of rapport that can be built or maintained is dependent on many factors. The length of the relationship between the medical provider and the family, the setting in which the encounter occurs, and the severity or urgency of the presenting complaint all play a role. Inevitably, regardless of the setting or the relationship between the medical provider and the family, cases of suspected child maltreatment are time-consuming and usually unexpected. Whenever possible, arrangements should be made as soon as possible to allow the medical provider to spend the necessary time to appropriately evaluate and care for the patient. This might involve rescheduling later patients, calling in assistance, or notifying office staff that there will be a significant delay for subsequent patient visits. If the provider is in a situation where there is a child abuse medical consultation service, this service can also be a resource to help obtain a complete and timely history and workup.[2,27]

Separation of Caregivers from One Another for the Interview

Separation of caregivers from one another during the interview is often impossible in the medical setting if rapport is to be maintained. In many cases, this technique is best reserved for law enforcement or child protection investigators, or at times, child abuse medical specialists. However, if it is practical or easily achievable (for example, one caregiver accompanies the child to radiology while the other stays to talk with the medical provider), this is always preferred for obtaining a spontaneous history. This is also the only acceptable way to screen for domestic violence. Screening questions about feeling safe at home or physical violence in the home should not be asked in front of a potentially abusive partner or caregiver.[28]

Key Details to Ask

Several key areas are important to address in the medical interview with caregivers. Table 8-4 summarizes the areas that should be covered during the history in most abuse or neglect cases. This information serves the purpose of establishing a timeline of events and list of people involved with the child. If the person providing the history is the perpetrator, gathering this information allows for clear documentation of the initial timeline and details provided, should those details change later.[2,24,26] Subsequent sections of this chapter provide questions that relate more specifically to the characteristics of the injury or maltreatment.

Specific Questions for Physical Abuse

Kellogg et al[2] have suggested guidelines for interviewing caregivers in cases of suspected physical child abuse. In the medical setting, whether inpatient or outpatient, such an interview will most often occur following a concerning history, physical, or radiological finding. Gathering the necessary detail around the injury event, or lack thereof, allows providers to better assess the plausibility of the explanation. Further, by attending to the details of the explanation, medical providers can identify inconsistencies. Table 8-5 describes questions that are important for specific physical abuse scenarios.

Table 8-4	General Information for Caregiver Interviews: the Key Areas[2,3,28,29]

What was the timeline of onset of events and symptoms? Who did what, when, where, and how?

Obtain a thorough past medical, family, and social history.

Ask about prior injuries or accidents in patient or siblings.

Ask about prior hospitalizations in patient or siblings.

Determine the child's developmental history and current developmental level.

Ask about physical and mental health history of parents.

Ask about parents' history of drug and alcohol use.

Ask about parents' criminal and child protection services history.

What medications are in the home?

Obtain pregnancy/adoption history, including miscarriages, planned/unplanned pregnancies, and fertility treatments.

Is there a family history of unexpected child deaths?

What is the composition of the family and household?

Are there pets in the home, and supervision of children when pets are present?

Are there other siblings who do not live in the home? What are their ages and what are the reasons for their absence?

Do the patient and caretakers feel safe in the home? What are the threats making them feel unsafe?*

Is there a history of domestic violence in the home?*

Discuss recent moves and relocations and reasons for the moves.

Does the child have other caregivers (babysitters, relatives, family friends)? When and where do they care for the child?

What methods are used by the caregivers for disciplining the child?

*Questions marked with * should not be asked in front of the caregiver/partner who might be a perpetrator.

Interview Questions Specific to Sexual Abuse

There are times in the primary care or emergency department setting when there has been no disclosure of sexual abuse, but presenting symptoms or physical examination findings have raised the possibility (see Table 8-1). In this instance, it is often helpful to start with the chief complaint when interviewing the caregiver (Table 8-6). When there has been a disclosure, questioning of nonabusive caregivers can focus on whether those caregivers believe abuse has occurred, their ability to protect the child, and assessment of any physical, emotional, and behavioral symptoms the child is experiencing because of the abuse. Often, these questions are best asked in a dedicated child advocacy center with a multidisciplinary team to address the spectrum of sequelae from the abuse. The child, if verbal, is likely to need a formal forensic interview (in addition to a medical history). (See Chapter 7.)

Interviewing About Suspected Child Neglect

An evaluation for neglect often requires several interviews with several caregivers over time. Consequently, building rapport with the family is a crucial component of the neglect assessment. One exception to this is the serious accidental, but preventable, injury to a child due to lack of supervision.[37] Often, however, what initially appears to be overt neglect is actually the consequence of some barrier that can be remedied outside of the child protection system. Interviews of caregivers in suspected neglect cases should focus on identifying barriers that have contributed to the situation, such as lack of transportation or telephone, caregiver misunderstanding of the illness, cultural differences in approach to illness, or poverty-related lack of resources. Once barriers are identified, the medical provider can document the discussion and any attempts to assist the caregiver in overcoming those barriers. For example, if a caregiver chronically misses the child's appointments due to lack of transportation, the medical provider can document that transportation was arranged through an insurer for subsequent visits. This accomplishes two important goals. First, effective intervention will allow the child to receive timely medical care. Second, if the caregiver continues to miss appointments, documentation of the efforts made by the medical provider, or other local resources, to assist the family provides valuable evidence for further assessment of medical neglect. This sort of documentation is critical evidence in the event child protection services ultimately become involved in the case.

While the majority of neglect cases that will be addressed by medical providers involve medical neglect, the same principles apply to evaluating other forms of neglect, such as physical neglect, failure to thrive, supervisional neglect, accidental ingestions, or delay in seeking care. The basic approach is to build rapport, gather information, identify barriers, use resources to overcome the barriers, and document all aspects of evaluation and treatment.[5,38] One important caveat to this approach involves neglect that could be immediately life-threatening for the patient. In that situation, immediate notification of child protective services is indicated to ensure the safety of the child.

When and How to Inform Caregivers About Concern for Maltreatment

Informing caregivers that the child may have an injury that is concerning for maltreatment, or that investigators are being notified, is often the most difficult part of the patient encounter. Medical providers often ask when it is appropriate to tell caregivers that child protection and/or law enforcement will be involved. There is also consternation surrounding how much detail to give caregivers about any occult injuries that have been identified and their possible mechanisms. Withholding such information can often present a true ethical dilemma for medical professionals, involving issues of trust, patient autonomy, and justice.[22,24] It is helpful to consider the patient's safety and well-being as the primary, guiding concern when trying to decide how to proceed in these cases. While in the ideal situation, it is usually best to be as honest as possible with caregivers, there are some situations that require a less forthright approach. For example, in the outpatient setting, when a child is being sent home with the caregiver because the evidence for abuse or neglect is vague, or the ability of local child protection to respond immediately is limited, it is usually best to not

Table 8-5 Details to Obtain During Caregiver Interview in Cases of Suspected Physical Abuse[2,30-35]

General Questions

Ask when the child was last known to be well, alert, smiling, and normal.
Obtain a detailed timeline from the time the child became symptomatic, including the child's behavior, activity, and appetite.
Obtain a detailed history of onset and progression of any symptoms.
Ask who has children for the child since before symptoms began.
Ask about any other known trauma (accident or otherwise).
If appropriate, ask the child directly about what happened.
If a history of an injury event is offered, obtain details about the mechanism of the injury event.

Questions About Falls

Did anyone see the child fall? If so, how did the child fall?
What was the child's position before the fall and after landing?
What was the nature of the impacted surface?
How far did the child fall?
Did the child cry right away, seem alert, lose consciousness, vomit, or have seizures?
If stairs were involved, how many steps were there? What were the dimensions of the stairs? Was there a stair railing present?
    What are the stairs and railing made of (wood, concrete, carpet, etc.)?
Did anyone fall with or on the child?
Did the child strike an object during the fall?
Did the child fall onto an object?

Questions About Head Injuries

Was there a history of birth trauma, prolonged labor, vacuum extractions, or forceps used?
What were the child's Apgar scores at birth?
Ask about family history of neurological diseases, seizure disorders, or developmental delays.
Obtain past growth parameters, including head circumferences.
Is there a past history of vomiting without diarrhea, unexplained fussiness, or altered consciousness?

Questions About Burns

What clothing (if any) was the child wearing?
If tap water was the source of the burn, what type of faucet/handle was involved?
Is the water from the faucet known to be particularly hot?

Questions About Long Bone Fractures

Was there an audible "pop" or "crack" at the time of injury?
Can you feel a popping, cracking, or creaking in the child's extremity?
When did the child last move/use the extremity normally?
Has child cried with certain activities, such as diaper changes or placement in the car seat?
Is there a history of birth trauma or difficult delivery?
Is there a family history of bone disease, frequent fractures, early hearing loss, or poor dentition?

Questions About Injuries Involving Bruising or Bleeding

Does the patient have a history of unusual bruising or bleeding?
After birth, was there unusual bleeding from the umbilicus or circumcision?
Is there a family history of easy bruising or bleeding disorders?
Is there a history of maternal postpartum hemorrhage, menorrhagia, or blood transfusions?

inform the caregiver that a report is being made. This allows child protection professionals the opportunity to observe an unaltered environment during their assessment and to minimize the likelihood that the child could be coerced or evidence destroyed while the caregivers await contact with child protection services. Obviously, if there is concern that the child is at imminent risk, it is not acceptable to send them home with a caregiver. In these instances, the child must be transferred to a secure facility that can provide assessment and protection while child protection professionals become involved. For example, the child can be sent to the local

emergency department by ambulance while child protection and/or law enforcement are being notified. It is often helpful to speak directly with community investigators and ask their thoughts on whether to share certain information with the caregiver.[2] Often, community investigators prefer not to give caregivers the opportunity to rehearse or alter histories to match an injury or mechanism. Medical providers must take all of these issues into account when deciding when and how much to tell caregivers about their concerns. It is important to note that HIPAA regulations permit the medical provider to withhold information from a legal guardian if there is a

Table 8-6	Details to Obtain During Caregiver Interview in Cases of Suspected Sexual Abuse[36]

Ask if there has been a disclosure of abuse by the child.

If so, ask to whom the disclosure was made. Using verbatim quotes, what did the child say?

Was the child's disclosure spontaneous, or was it in response to comments or questions from the caregiver? If so, what specifically did the caregiver say or ask?

How did the person to whom the child disclosed respond?

If the child (or caregiver) uses lingo/slang, clarify the terms used in the family for body parts or sexual acts.

How is the child doing now?

When was the last known contact with the alleged perpetrator (if known)?

Obtain details about the alleged perpetrator (name, age, medical history, sexually transmitted disease risks, address, perpetrator's knowledge of the child's disclosure, perpetrator's risk of violence against the family or child, other children the alleged perpetrator might have access to, etc.).

Has the child had any behavior changes? If so, describe.

Ascertain child's exposure to sexualized media or situations.

Is the caregiver's concern about abuse related to a physical sign or symptom? If so, what?

Is there anyone who makes you or your child feel unsafe or threatened?

perceived risk of harm to the child. If there is a suspicion of abuse and the perpetrator is unknown, it is reasonable for a clinician to withhold information about the likelihood of abuse until an investigation is conducted. Clinicians can refer parents to child protection for further information if they request it, or the clinician can call child protection and ask if the parent can receive the information. For the authors of this chapter, it has been helpful to remain in the role of a supportive medical provider, and in so doing, provide anticipatory guidance about the upcoming process. Of note, this should only be done if the child's safety is secure and both medical provider and investigative teams feel comfortable with the approach. For example, after the complete history has been taken, examination completed, and any appropriate testing ordered, the provider might say, "Ms. Jackson, I've asked you a lot of questions about Johnny and his injury, and I appreciate your patience with all of this. You are already aware that his leg is broken. The challenge we're now facing is that when we see fractures like this in children of Johnny's age, we have to be concerned about the possibility that someone might have caused this injury to him. *(Don't pause here…keep talking.)* Because of this, we are obligated to notify child protective services, and one of their representatives will be coming here to speak with you. *(Again, don't pause, keep talking.)* Part of my job is to help support you and Johnny through this process, so let me tell you a little about what will happen from here. A social worker will be coming to ask you a lot of questions similar to the ones I've already asked. It will be up to that person and his supervisor to determine what will happen next with Johnny. My job is to explain the medical findings to them and to you, and to answer any questions you have. I know this is difficult to

hear, but I want to do whatever I can to help your family through this process. Do you have any questions for me?"

In this way, the medical provider has both delivered some difficult information to the caregiver while clarifying his or her own role in the process. Further, the provider has assured the caregiver that she remains available to answer questions and provide support, and has not indicated in any way that the caregiver is suspected of doing anything wrong. The physician has also provided anticipatory guidance about the investigative process, which provides a buffer between the "bad news" and the moment when the caregiver responds to the information.

When caregivers ask about specific mechanisms of injury, it is usually best to give them as little detail as possible.[26] For example, if a child has a transverse, displaced femur fracture, but no history, the caregiver might ask, "What causes this kind of injury?" The medical provider can respond, "Actually, there are lots of different things that can cause it." When in doubt, it is always reasonable to explain that, "The answer is unclear at this time."

CONTEXTUAL ISSUES/SPECIAL CIRCUMSTANCES

When the Caregiver Is Also a Victim

In addition to whether the presenting caregiver is a perpetrator, other caregiver factors also impact the interview process and should be considered. Caregivers might also be current or past victims of violence, including sexual abuse. Such factors can adversely impact the quality of information they provide and their behaviors surrounding the questions asked.[39] For example, if caregivers have been sexually abused, they may overinterpret symptoms that to them indicate sexual abuse in their children. If a parent is simultaneously being victimized, she might attempt to cover for the perpetrator out of fear or loyalty.

Caregiver Substance Use/Abuse or Mental Illness

Parental substance use/abuse may also confound an interview.[39] If a parent is clearly intoxicated, the veracity of the information they are able to provide is questionable.[40] In addition, lack of supervision during an episode where the parent is intoxicated could lead to an accidental injury and/or poor reporting about the events surrounding an injury. Mental illness in the caregiver can pose similar complications.[39]

Cultural Factors

Language and cultural factors should be considered during the interview. The interview must be conducted in a language in which the parent has a reasonable degree of fluency to maximize the accuracy of the information. If the interview is done using an interpreter or translator, the interpreter's name and credentials should be documented. Caregiver attitudes on discipline and sexuality can directly impact both their perception of the situation and their ability to build rapport during the interview.[39] Information about these factors should be obtained in a sensitive and nonjudgmental manner.

Medical Child Abuse

When medical child abuse is suspected, a multidisciplinary approach is generally recommended. All available resources, including a child abuse pediatric specialist, should be used to decide how the team will proceed before any interviews with the caregivers (see Chapter 61).

THE IMPORTANCE OF DOCUMENTATION

Clear and complete documentation is critical in the assessment of potential child abuse and neglect. If a statement by a caregiver (or patient) is particularly noteworthy, it is helpful to document the statement as close to verbatim as possible, using quotation marks when appropriate.[2] It is also acceptable to document a caregiver's behavior during the interview if it seems pertinent. For example, when a child is brought to the emergency department with an injury, it would be important to document if the caregiver is stumbling about, slurring words, or smells of alcohol. It is much more helpful to document, "Father tripping over stools in an examination room, bumping into hospital personnel, singing, and smells of alcohol," rather than, "Father appears intoxicated," or, "Father behaving inappropriately in emergency room." The first example provides much more objective detail without the associated subjective interpretation of the behavior.

STRENGTH OF MEDICAL EVIDENCE

The interview of caregivers in cases of child maltreatment is a clinical skill that is learned over time. It is also an area of child maltreatment assessment that has not been extensively researched. Different geographical regions, cultures, and investigative protocols may influence the preferred approach to this difficult topic.

SUGGESTED DIRECTIONS FOR FUTURE RESEARCH

As child abuse pediatrics specialists develop best practice protocols, templates for interviewing caregivers will continue to aid in obtaining optimal information. Objective, rigorous study of different interview techniques and approaches will be necessary to achieve consistent, optimal outcomes from these interviews. Multidisciplinary collaborative research with community investigators would provide the ideal approach to this topic.

References

1. Jenny C, Hymel K, Ritzen A, et al: Analysis of missed cases of abusive head trauma. *JAMA* 1999;281:621-626.
2. Kellogg ND, Committee on Child Abuse and Neglect: Evaluation of suspected child physical abuse. *Pediatrics* 2007;119:1232-1241.
3. Stiffman M, Schnitzer PG, Adam P: Household composition and risk of fatal child maltreatment. *Pediatrics* 2002;109:615-621.
4. Sugar NF, Taylor JA, Feldman KW, et al: Bruises in infants and toddlers—those who don't cruise rarely bruise. *Arch Pediatr Adolesc Med* 1999;153:399-403.
5. Block RW, Krebs NF, Committee on Child Abuse and Neglect, et al: Failure to thrive as a manifestation of child neglect. *Pediatrics* 2005;116:1234-1237.
6. Arbogast KB, Margulies SS, Christian CW: Initial neurologic presentation in young children sustaining inflicted and unintentional fatal head injuries. *Pediatrics* 2005;116:180-184.
7. Hymel KP, Makoroff KL, Laskey AL, et al: Mechanisms, clinical presentations, injuries, and outcomes from inflicted versus noninflicted head trauma during infancy: results of a prospective, multicentered, comparative study. *Pediatrics* 2007;119:922-929.
8. American Academy of Pediatrics Committee on Child Abuse and Neglect: Shaken baby syndrome: rotational cranial injuries-technical report. *Pediatrics* 2001;108:206-210.
9. Pitetti RD, Maffei F, Chang K, et al: Prevalence of retinal hemorrhages and child abuse in children presenting with an apparent life-threatening event. *Pediatrics* 2002;110:557-562.
10. Samuels MP, Poets CF, Noyes JP, et al: Diagnosis and management after life threatening events in infants and young children who received cardiopulmonary resuscitation. *Br Med J* 1993;306:489-492.
11. Wolfe DA: Child-abusive parents: an empirical review and analysis. *Psychol Bull* 1985;97:462-482.
12. Twentyman CT, Plotkin RC: Unrealistic expectations of parents who maltreat their children: an educational deficit that pertains to child development. *J Clin Psychol* 1982;38:497-503.
13. Kairys SW, Johnson CF, Committee on Child Abuse and Neglect: The psychological maltreatment of children-technical report. *Pediatrics* 2002;109:e68.
14. American Academy of Child and Adolescent Psychiatry: Practice parameters for the assessment and treatment of children and adolescents with posttraumatic stress disorder. *J Am Acad Child Adolesc Psychiatry* 1998;37(suppl 10):4S-26S.
15. American Medical Association: American Medical Association diagnostic and treatment guidelines on child physical abuse and neglect. *Arch Fam Med* 1992;1:187-197.
16. Wright RJ, Wright RO, Isaac NE: Response to battered mothers in the pediatric emergency department: a call for an interdisciplinary approach to family violence. *Pediatrics* 1997;99:186-192.
17. Chang JJ, Theodore AD, Martin SL, et al: Psychological abuse between parents: associations with child maltreatment from a population-based sample. *Child Abuse Negl* 2008;32:819-829.
18. Knapp JF, Dowd MD: Family violence: implications for the pediatrician. *Pediatr Rev* 1998;19:316-321.
19. Milner JS, Murphy WD: Assessment of child physical and sexual abuse offenders. *Fam Relat* 1995;44:478-488.
20. Ibanez ES, Borrego J Jr, Pemberton JR, et al: Cultural factors in decision-making about child physical abuse: identifying reporter characteristics influencing reporting tendencies. *Child Abuse Negl* 2006;30:1365-1379.
21. Flaherty EG, Sege R: Barriers to physician identification and reporting of child abuse. *Pediatr Ann* 2005;34:349-356.
22. Jones R, Flaherty EG, Binns HJ, et al: Clinicians' description of factors influencing their reporting of suspected child abuse: report of the child abuse reporting experience study research group. *Pediatrics* 2008;122:259-266.
23. Flaherty EG, Jones R, Sege R: Telling their stories: primary care practitioners' experience evaluating and reporting injuries caused by child abuse. *Child Abuse Negl* 2004;28:939-945.
24. Jones PM, Appelbaum PS, Siegel DM: Law enforcement interviews of hospital patients: a conundrum for clinicians. *JAMA* 2006;295:822-825.
25. Leavitt WT, Armitage DT: The forensic role of the child psychiatrist in child abuse and neglect cases. *Child Adolesc Psychiatr Clin N Am* 2002;11:767-779.
26. Napier MR, Adams SH: Criminal confessions: overcoming the challenges. *FBI Law Enforc Bull* 2002;71:10-20. http://www.fbi.gov/publications/leb/2002/nov2002/nov02leb.htm#page_10. Accessed February 7, 2009.
27. Bross DC, Ballo N, Korfmacher J: Client evaluation of a consultation team on crimes against children. *Child Abuse Negl* 2000;24:71-84.
28. Lamberg L: Domestic violence: what to ask, what to do. *JAMA* 2000;284:554-556.
29. Zuravin SJ: Fertility patterns: their relationship to child physical abuse and child neglect. *J Marriage Fam* 1988;50:983-993.

30. Jenny C, Committee on Child Abuse and Neglect: Evaluating infants and young children with multiple fractures. *Pediatrics* 2006;118:1299-1303.
31. Chadwick DL, Chin S, Salerno C, et al: Deaths from falls in children: how far is fatal? *J Trauma* 1991;31:1353-1355.
32. Lyons TJ, Oates RK: Falling out of bed: a relatively benign occurrence. *Pediatrics* 1993;92:125-127.
33. Pierce MC, Bertocci GE, Vogeley E, et al: Evaluating long bone fractures in children: a biomechanical approach with illustrative cases. *Child Abuse Negl* 2004;28:505-524.
34. American Academy of Pediatrics Committee on Child Abuse and Neglect: When inflicted skin injuries constitute child abuse. *Pediatrics* 2002;110:644-645.
35. Leventhal JM, Thomas SA, Rosenfield SA, et al: Fractures in young children. Distinguishing child abuse from unintentional injuries. *Am J Dis Child* 1993;147:87-92.
36. Kellogg N, American Academy of Pediatrics Committee on Child Abuse and Neglect: The evaluation of sexual abuse in children. *Pediatrics* 2005;116:506-512.
37. Hymel KP, American Academy of Pediatrics Committee on Child Abuse and Neglect: When is lack of supervision neglect? *Pediatrics* 2006;118:1296-1298.
38. Dubowitz H, Giardino A, Gustavson E: Child neglect: guidance for pediatricians. *Pediatr Rev* 2000;21:111-116.
39. Stockhammer TF, Salzinger S, Feldman RS, et al: Assessment of the effect of physical child abuse within an ecological framework: measurement issues. *J Community Psychol* 2001;29:319-344.
40. Fraser JJ Jr, McAbee GN, American Academy of Pediatrics Committee on Medical Liability: Dealing with the parent whose judgment is impaired by alcohol or drugs: legal and ethical considerations. *Pediatrics* 2004;114:869-873.

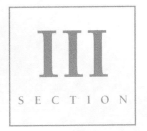

SEXUAL ABUSE OF CHILDREN

Nancy D. Kellogg, MD

9

THE PHYSICAL EXAMINATION OF THE CHILD WHEN SEXUAL ABUSE IS SUSPECTED

Reena Isaac, MD

INTRODUCTION

What was initially described as a "hidden pediatric problem" in 1977 has become an increasingly recognized phenomenon in subsequent decades.[1] Sexual abuse occurs when a child or adolescent is engaged in sexual activities that they cannot comprehend, for which they are developmentally unprepared and unable to give informed consent, and/or when there is violation of the legal or social taboos of society.[2] Sexual abuse includes a full spectrum of activities ranging from oral, genital, or anal contact, and fondling by or to the child, to noncontact abuses, such as exhibitionism, voyeurism, or various forms of child exploitation, such as pornography or prostitution. Child sexual abuse may involve one type of activity, or evolve over time into several other activities.

MEDICAL EVALUATION

When sexual abuse is suspected, the medical evaluation of the child serves a dual purpose: (1) to ensure the health of the child after an alleged abusive abuse; and (2) to document any injuries or other evidence that may support the allegation of child sexual abuse (CSA).[3] Children from abusive households are at greater risk for undiscovered and inadequately treated health problems. In a retrospective study, Girardet et al[4] found a medical or psychological condition requiring intervention in 123 (26%) of 473 children referred for sexual abuse evaluations. In 39 (8%) of those children, the diagnosis had the potential to result in significant patient morbidity if not immediately addressed.

Time should be taken in establishing a relationship and rapport with the child. Proper introductions and spending a few minutes in nonthreatening social conversation builds the patient's rapport and trust, and increases his or her comfort with the medical evaluation.

The interview of the child and caretaker begins the evaluation process (see chapters 7 and 8). The medical and psychological reviews of systems often reveal behavioral, emotional, and/or physical symptoms in the child. Information can be gathered from the child, the parent, or through standardized instruments such as the Trauma Symptom Checklist for Children.[5] In addition, information can also be gathered by a team of professionals, including the clinician, a mental health professional, a nurse, child life specialist, and/or a social worker. Medical and behavioral assessments often reveal symptoms important to the recovery and treatment of the child, but are usually not specific to the diagnosis of sexual abuse; most physical symptoms, for example, can be seen in other medical illnesses as well.[6,7] Table 9-1 lists common physical signs and symptoms commonly identified in sexually abused children.[6-9]

APPROACH TO THE PHYSICAL EXAMINATION

Timing of the Examination

The anogenital examination serves to identify and treat possible trauma and other sequelae of abuse and to gather physical evidence of sexual abuse. Additionally, the anogenital examination provides reassurance for the child. The physical examination in the majority of sexual abuse cases is normal.[10]

The date and time of the last incident should be obtained on initial presentation of a child for alleged sexual abuse. When and where the medical examination is conducted is crucial. Acute injuries and/or other physical findings must be appropriately documented, and evidence must be preserved. If the most recent assault of a child has occurred less than 72 hours before the child presents, and/or the history reveals the likelihood of transfer of biological evidence from the perpetrator (i.e., semen, saliva, or blood), forensic evidence collection should be done (see Chapter 13). The patient should immediately be assessed for potential life-threatening physical trauma in addition to evaluation of the sexual assault. When more than 72 hours has passed and no acute injuries are present, an emergency examination usually is not necessary. In these cases, if the parents and child agree, an evaluation should be scheduled at the earliest convenient time in a more appropriate setting such as an advocacy center or clinic. Clinicians should be familiar with regional protocols providing recommendations for forensic evidence collection timing and procedures.

An emergent medical evaluation should be done if the child complains of pain in the genital or anal area or if there is anal or genital bleeding or injury.[11] Genital and anal injuries in children heal quickly and may not persist if the examination is delayed. In some cases, the child will have emergent health issues (mental or physical) requiring immediate attention. In others, the child's disclosure might put them in imminent danger. The person triaging the child for examination must determine if the child should be examined

Table 9-1	Presenting Signs and Symptoms of Sexual Abuse

Early Warnings

Generalized statements about abuse
Sexualized play

Psychosomatic and Behavioral Changes

Sleep disturbances
Appetite disturbances
Neurotic or conduct disorders
Phobias, avoidance behavior
Withdrawal, depression
Guilt
Temper tantrums, aggressive behavior
Excessive masturbation
Suicidal behavior
Hysterical or conversion reactions

Physical Symptoms

Genital, anal, or urethra trauma
Genital discharge
Sexually transmitted infections
Recurrent UTI
Abdominal pain
Chronic genital or anal pain
Enuresis
Encopresis

Other Problems

Pregnancy
School problems
Promiscuity/ prostitution
Substance abuse
Sexual perpetration on other children

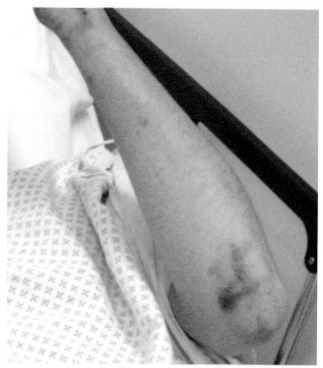

FIGURE 9-1 Defensive wounds on the volar surface of the forearm obtained when the victim attempted to thwart an attacker's blows by shielding his face with his arms.

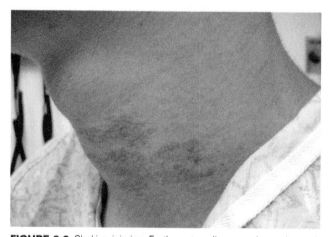

FIGURE 9-2 Choking injuries. Erythematous linear marks on the neck from attempted strangulation. The patient presented with a hoarse voice.

immediately or whether the child's examination can be deferred.

Preparing the Child for Examination

Taking time to explain the importance of the examination helps gain the child's confidence and trust. The child should have a feeling of control over what happens next to her body. Allowing her to have choices such as who should chaperone the examination helps give the child some control and demonstrates respect for her feelings. Propping up the head of the examining table so the child can see the physician during the examination will usually decrease the child's anxiety. The equipment used during the examination can appear intimidating and technical to the family and child. All procedures and equipment should be explained, including the colposcope. Distraction techniques, such as singing, counting, reciting nursery rhymes, or blowing bubbles will encourage the child to relax. Because abuse usually involves authority and control over the child, children should not be subjected to force during a medical examination. If an emergent evaluation is essential for the child's medical health and the child is unable to cooperate with the examination, use of anesthesia or conscious sedation is a reasonable alternative.[12,13]

THE MEDICAL EXAMINATION

The medical examination of the child should include a thorough "head-to-toe physical examination, leaving the anogenital examination until the end of the examination. In addition to evaluating for possible physical injuries or unmet health care needs of the child, the inclusion of the entire physical examination of the body relays to the child that all parts of his or her body are important. The examination should be unhurried and thorough, looking for physical abuse injuries such as defensive wounds (Figure 9-1), strangulation or choking injuries (Figure 9-2), ligature marks, or bruising. Photo-document, sketch, and measure any

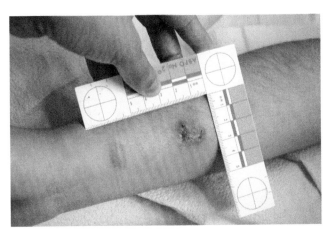

FIGURE 9-3 Self-inflicted injury. A sexually abused adolescent picked at her skin causing skin abrasions and erosions.

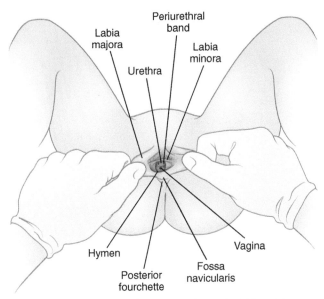

FIGURE 9-4 The anatomical structures of prepubertal female's anogenital area.

cutaneous injuries noted on the child's body. Bitemarks, if acute, should be swabbed for forensic evidence. Photographs of bitemarks should include a size standard and color bar (see Chapter 27). Self-inflicted injuries should be assessed and documented. Self-mutilation injuries such as "picking" (Figure 9-3) or "cutting" of the skin can be a sign of covert abuse or psychiatric disorders.

The physician should be competent and comfortable in identifying anatomical structures of the anogenital area correctly and conditions that may mimic sexual abuse.[14,15] Figure 9-4 illustrates the anatomical structures of the prepubertal female's anogenital area. The examination should include an estimate of sexual maturity, based on Tanner staging.[16] The sexual maturity rating tracks the normal appearance and pattern of pubic hair development in males and females, breast development in females, and testicle size, scrotum, and phallus development in males. These physical changes noted on inspection of children have been shown to correlate with the hormonal changes occurring during adolescent development.[16] A more recent and exhaustive study, the collection of data known as the National Health and Nutrition Examination Survey III (NHANES III),[17,18] has provided normative data on the sexual maturation of American boys and girls. The study, conducted over a 10-year period, included large samples of American girls and boys of different ethnic groups. Many factors can affect the timing of the onset and duration of puberty, including, genetics, nutrition, intercurrent illness, geographical conditions, and excessive exercise.[17-19]

When examining the anogenital area, the child should be placed in a position that is comfortable for both child and examiner, and that allows for the best visualization of anatomical structures. The liberal use of drapes safeguards the child's sense of modesty and preserves a sense of control for the child.

Examination Positions

A number of positions have been described for conducting the anogenital examination of the prepubertal child (Figure 9-5). Some positions work better than others for both the patient and the examiner. Often the use of more than one position is indicated. The supine frog-leg position offers the

child relative comfort and provides the examiner with a clear view of the anogenital region (Figure 9-5, *A*). This position can be assumed in the lap of a parent or a supporting adult, or on the examination table. Children are told their legs will represent a frog's legs or the wings of a butterfly, and the position can be demonstrated on a doll or stuffed animal. The use of a gynecological examination table with "stirrups" (the lithotomy position) can be used with older children and adolescents to ensure adequate abduction of the legs and optimal visualization of the genitalia.

When the patient is supine, the examiner can gently separate the labia by pulling the tissues downward and outward (labial separation, Figure 9-5, *B*). Another effective method of visualizing the internal genital structures is to use labial traction [Figure 9-5, *C*]. Here, the labia are lightly grasped by the examiners hand and pulled downward, outward, and anteriorly toward the examiner.

In the prone knee-chest position (Figure 9-5, *D*), the child is placed prone with her chest touching the examination table, her back in a lordotic posture, her thighs perpendicular to the examination table, and her knees apart. The anterior vaginal wall falls forward, allowing better viewing of the posterior hymen and upper vagina. This position should be used to confirm a suspected hymen injury. The knee-chest position is a particularly vulnerable position for the child, especially if the child had been victimized in this position. Anticipate and avoid adverse reactions by having a parent or other supportive person talk to the child when this position is used. The buttocks can then be gently pulled upward and outward to view the internal structures.

When there is redundancy or cohesion of the hymenal tissue, the use of saline to "float" the hymen is occasionally helpful. Sterile saline ampules (saline "bullets") can be used to squirt saline onto the hymenal opening. In more mature adolescents, the examiner can run a small-diameter, saline-moistened cotton swab along the internal edge of the hymen to more easily see the hymenal rim (Figure 9-6). The unestrogenized hymen is exquisitely sensitive to touch, so any

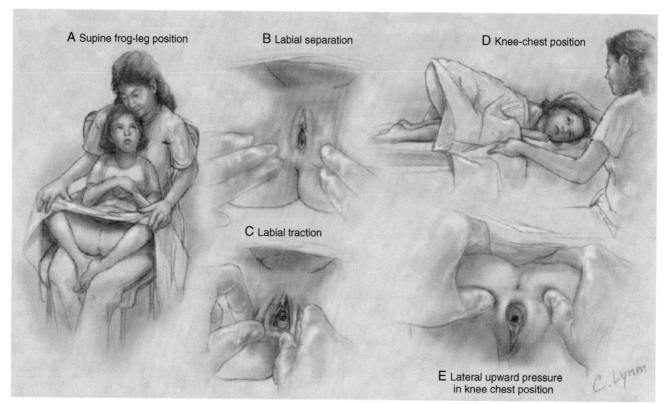

FIGURE 9-5 Examination positions and techniques used to evaluated the female genitalia of the prepubertal child. **A**, Supine frog-leg position. **B**, Labial separation. **C**, Labial traction. **D**, Knee-check position. **E**, Lateral upward pressure on the buttocks in knee-chest position. *(From Berkoff MC, Zolotor AJ, Makoroff KL, et al: Has this prepubertal girl been sexually abused? JAMA 2008;300:2779-2792. Copyright © 2008 American Medical Association. All rights reserved.)*

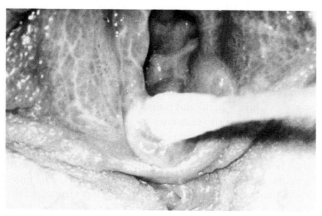

FIGURE 9-6 Use of a moistened swab to assess the hymenal rim.

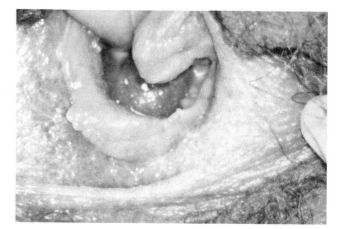

FIGURE 9-7 Using a Foley catheter to assess the adolescent hymenal rim.

direct manipulation with a swab should be avoided in a prepubertal child.

In adolescents, a Foley catheter can be used to confirm notches, clefts, and transections of the hymenal rim (Figure 9-7). An uninflated catheter is inserted into the vagina, inflated (with either air or 15 cc of water) and then the catheter bulb is slowly extracted. The posterior rim of the hymen is then stretched and fully revealed against the inflated balloon. This particular technique requires much skill and experience to manipulate the device and accurately assess examination findings.

The male penis and scrotum can be examined with the patient in the supine or upright position. Signs of trauma should be carefully documented by making detailed diagrams of the finding or by taking high quality photographs.

Examination Equipment

An optimal examination of the genitalia and anus requires proper lighting, privacy, adequate positioning, and patient cooperation. Colposcopy does not significantly increase the recognition of physical findings that are diagnostic of sexual abuse; however, it is an excellent tool for magnification of the anatomy and affords superb photodocumentation of the examination.[20] Photodocumentation allows for peer review of findings without subjecting the child to repeat examinations. If the child sustains an injury, the subsequent healing of the injury can be chronicled. The colposcope, when attached to a video monitor, can allow the child to observe what the examiner is doing throughout the examination. The child may achieve a sense of participation and control that enhances his or her cooperation.[21,22] Use video images rather than still photographs because the video allows for the viewing of the dynamic nature of the anogenital anatomy.

A speculum examination is not recommended for prepubertal children unless there is upper tract bleeding, raising concern for intravaginal injury. If vaginal injury is suspected, the child should be examined under anesthesia by a surgeon or gynecologist.

When there is a history of recent sexual contact, an alternate light source (ALS) may assist in detecting areas contaminated with semen. ALS can be used on skin surfaces and internal structures (vaginal, anal, pharyngeal). Investigators use ALS to examine clothing and bedding to locate forensically important materials. In the clinical setting, an appropriate ultraviolet light source would be the Bluemaxx 500™ (Sirche Finger Print Laboratores, Inc., Raleigh, N.C.), which emits light with a longer wave length where semen fluoresces (490 nm). The standard Wood's lamp often used during sexual assault examinations has been shown to be ineffective in identifying semen[23] because it emits light in the 320 to 400 nm spectrum.

Specific Anatomical Areas

The Vestibule. Injuries to the vestibule can include tissue edema, abrasions, lacerations, puncture wounds, hematomas, bruising, and/or bleeding. Acute injuries should be noted, described appropriately, and documented. Documentation should include the shape and contour of the hymenal orifice, the appearance of the external surface of the hymen (including any transections, distortions, redundancy, or signs of healed injury), and the appearance of the periurethral area, fossa navicularis, and the posterior fourchette. The location of physical findings can be described in terms of the face of a clock.

The Hymen. The shape, contour, and normal variations of the normal hymen have been well documented.[21,22] Normal and abnormal hymenal findings should be documented. Hymenal redundancy can make it difficult to delineate the rims of the hymen and various methods (swab, foley, valsalva, change in position) may aid in clarifying the findings.

The anus and perianal area. The anus and perianal area are examined with the child placed in any of the following positions: (1) supine with the legs flexed onto the abdomen; (2) lateral decubitus with buttocks separation (although this position provides a less optimal view); or (3) knee-chest position. When examining the external anal verge, the rugae usually have a symmetrical puckered appearance radiating from the anal orifice. Normal findings on the anus include diastasis ani (a flat, pale structure at 6 o'clock), anal tags in

the midline, sphincter relaxation when the ampulla contains stool or when the child is examined in the knee-chest position, and presence of the dentate line in the anal canal.[24] Documentation of normal and abnormal findings should be done carefully in the record.

DEBRIEFING THE CHILD AND CAREGIVERS AFTER THE EXAMINATION

The medical evaluation can be therapeutic for the child, and may confirm his or her sense of physical security and normalcy. One function of the medical examination is to alleviate the child's fears about being injured or "different" from other children. The physician should discuss with the child and parents the results of the examination in language appropriate for the child's age. A child with injuries can be reassured that his or her injuries will heal or have already healed. Older children are sometimes worried that their experience will affect their ability to have children or sexual relations. Most children can be reassured that there will be no long-term physical consequences from the abuse. The clinician should emphasize the need for mental health services for both child and parent as indicated.

The extent to which a child victim of suspected sexual abuse should be medically evaluated for the presence of sexually transmitted infections (STIs) should be determined on a case-by-case basis, based on the events of the assault, the child's age, the presence of symptoms, the prevalence of a STI in a community and any information available on the risk status of the perpetrator.[25] The yield of positive cultures is very low in asymptomatic prepubertal children, especially those whose history indicates fondling only.

DOCUMENTATION

All health care professionals who evaluate suspected victims of child sexual abuse should provide written and visual documentation of all aspects of their medical evaluation in a manner that meets acceptable medical records standards. Clear documentation of the child's statements and physical findings is an integral part of the sexual abuse evaluation. The medical record can best serve the interests of the child effectively if it accurately reflects the medical history and physical examination. Diagrams and photographs are essential tools for recording diagnostic findings. The preservation of such information is essential to child protection and legal proceedings.

INTERPRETATION OF MEDICAL FINDINGS

The appropriate interpretation of physical and laboratory findings in child victims of suspected sexual abuse requires the medical provider to be familiar with the results of research studies of abused and nonabused children. Published studies and recommendations that have been subjected to peer review and ongoing revision reflect current knowledge.[11] Ultimately, however, most physical examinations will be normal, even if the child gives a clear history of penetration or the perpetrator confesses to penetration.[10,26] A normal physical examination does not negate a history of sexual abuse. In contrast, a child sometimes has clear evidence of anogenital trauma without an adequate history. Although this is rare, a report to child protective services is necessary when abuse is suspected.

Clinicians should be cautious in opining that specific acute genital injuries are indicative of forceful, nonconsensual penetration, especially when dealing with adolescents. It is best to describe such injuries as "evidence of recent penetrating trauma." The physical findings in adolescent girls who have consenting sex with same-aged partners and in adolescent girls who are abused or assaulted are often similar.[27,28] The patient's history is important in determining if a crime has occurred. It is the obligation of the health care provider to formulate an opinion that is supported by science, with an understanding of the limitations of what can and cannot be said with certainty.[11]

In the courtroom, the physician's role is to explain and describe the clinical picture and provide medical testimony that is accurate and objective. A careful physical examination and excellent documentation will aid the physician when he or she is called upon to present evidence.

References

1. Kempe CH: Sexual abuse, another hidden pediatric problem: the 1977 C. Anderson Aldrich lecture. *Pediatrics* 1978;62:382-389.
2. Kellogg N, American Academy of Pediatrics Committee on Child Abuse and Neglect: The evaluation of sexual abuse in children. *Pediatrics* 2005;116:506-512.
3. Finkel MA, DeJong AR: Medical findings in sexual abuse. *In:* Reece RM, Ludwig S (eds): *Child Abuse: Medical Diagnosis and Management,* ed 2, Lippincott Williams & Wilkins, Philadelphia, 2002, pp 207-286.
4. Girardet RG, Giacobbe L, Bolton K, et al: Unmet health care needs among children evaluated for sexual assault. *Arch Pediatr Adolesc Med* 2006;160:70-73.
5. Briere J, Johnson K, Bissada A, et al: The trauma symptom checklist for young children (TSCYC): reliability and association with abuse exposure in a multi-site study. *Child Abuse Negl* 2001;25:1001-1014.
6. Krugman RD: Recognition of sexual abuse in children. *Pediatr Rev* 1986;8:25-30.
7. Mellon MW, Whiteside SP, Friedrich WN: The relevance of fecal soiling as an indicator of child sexual abuse: a preliminary analysis. *J Dev Behav Pediatr* 2006;27:25-32.
8. Friedrich WN, Dittner CA, Action R, et al: Child sexual behavior inventory: normative, psychiatric and sexual abuse comparisons. *Child Maltreat* 2001;6:37-49.
9. Hunter RS, Kilstrom N, Loda F: Sexually abused children: identifying masked presentations in a medical setting. *Child Abuse Negl* 1985; 9:17-25.
10. Adams J, Harper K, Knudson S, et al: Examination findings in legally confirmed cases of child sexual abuse: it's normal to be normal. *Pediatrics* 1994;94:310-317.
11. Adams JA, Kaplan RA, Starling SP, et al: Guidelines for medical care of children who may have been sexually abused. *J Pediatr Adolesc Gynecol* 2007;20:163-172.
12. Yaster M, Maxwell L: The pediatric sedation unit: a mechanism for safe pediatric sedation. *Pediatrics* 1999;103:198-201.
13. Parker RI, Mahan RA, Giugliano D, et al: Efficacy and safety of intravenous midazolam and ketamine as sedation for therapeutic and diagnostic procedures in children. *Pediatrics* 1997;99:427-431.
14. Finkel MA, Giardino AP: *Medical evaluation of child sexual abuse: a practical guide,* ed 2, Sage, Thousand Oaks, Calif, 2002.
15. Bays J, Jenny C: Genital and anal conditions confused with child sexual abuse trauma. *Am J Dis Child* 1990;144:1319-1322.
16. Tanner J: *Growth at adolescence,* ed 2, Blackwell Scientific, Oxford, UK, 1962.
17. Wu T, Mendola P, Buck GM: Ethnic differences in the presence of secondary sex characteristics and menarche among U.S. girls: the third national health and nutrition examination survey, 1988-1994. *Pediatrics* 2002;110:752-757.
18. Herman-Giddens ME, Wang L, Koch G: Secondary sexual characteristics in boys: estimates from the national health and nutrition examination survey III, 1988-1994. *Arch Pediatr Adolesc Med* 2001; 155:1022-1028.
19. Wang Y: Is obesity associated with early sexual maturation? A comparison of the association in American boys versus girls. *Pediatrics* 2002;110:903-910.
20. Adams JA, Girardino B, Faugno D: Adolescent sexual assault: documentation of acute injuries using photocolposcopy. *J Pediatr Adolesc Gynecol* 2001;14:175-180.
21. McCann J, Wells R, Simon M, et al: Genital findings in prepubertal girls selected for non-abuse: a descriptive study. *Pediatrics* 1990; 86:428-439.
22. Ricci LR: Medical forensic photography of the sexually abused child. *Child Abuse Negl* 1988;12:305-310.
23. Berenson AB, Heger AH, Hayes JM, et al: Appearance of the hymen in prepubertal girls. *Pediatrics* 1992;89:387-394.
24. McCann J, Voris J, Simon M, et al: Perianal findings in prepubertal children selected for nonabuse: a descriptive study. *Child Abuse Negl* 1989;13:179-193.
25. Ingram DM, Miller WC, Schoenbach VJ, et al: Risk assessment for gonococcal and chlamydial infections in young children undergoing evaluation for sexual abuse. *Pediatrics* 2001;107:e73.
26. Muram D: Child sexual abuse: relationship between sexual acts and genital findings. *Child Abuse Negl* 1989;13:211-216.
27. Hoffman RJ, Ganti SA: Vaginal laceration and perforation resulting from first coitus. *Pediatr Emerg Care* 2001;17:113-114.
28. Adams JA, Botash AS, Kellogg N: Differences in hymenal morphology between adolescent girls with and without a history of consensual sexual intercourse. *Arch Pediatr Adolesc Med* 2004;158:280-285.

NORMAL AND DEVELOPMENTAL VARIATIONS IN THE ANOGENITAL EXAMINATION OF CHILDREN

Nichole G. Wallace, MD, and Michelle Amaya, MD, MPH

Recognition and diagnosis of abnormal anogenital anatomy require the examiner to first master knowledge of normal male and female anatomy, including the variations that present during the process of child physical development. This has sometimes been a challenge in the field of child abuse pediatrics because use of high-grade magnification (colposcopy or digital imaging) typically reveals details that can mistakenly be attributed to trauma or disease. Studies of newborns and children selected for nonabuse provide important data that has defined normal anatomy. This chapter describes aspects of anogenital embryology and major anatomical structures assessed during child sexual abuse medical evaluations. This information provides a basis for accurate interpretation of injuries and diseases that can be associated with sexual abuse.

GENITAL EMBRYOLOGY

Early in development, the genital system is undifferentiated and has the capability of forming either male or female anatomy.[1] Three primary structures evolve to form the genital system: primordial germ cells, two sets of paired indifferent ducts, and the cloaca. Primordial germ cells from the embryonic endoderm migrate to a midregion, the urogenital ridge, becoming the "indifferent" gonads. By gestational week six, two symmetrical sets of paired ducts form near the urogenital ridge, the wolffian (mesonephric) ducts and the müllerian (paramesonephric) ducts. The ducts lengthen, descending into the future pelvis to join the cloaca (primitive bladder-rectum) at a cloacal protuberance called the müllerian tubercle. During this time, the ureteric buds form off the mesonephric (wolffian) ducts, eventually becoming the kidneys and ureters. If the fetus is male, the gonads become testes and produce AMH (anti-müllerian hormone), causing the müllerian ducts to regress and disappear. The testes produce testosterone, which maintains the growth of the wolffian ducts and promotes their further differentiation to form the spermatic ducts (vas deferens, epididymis).

Female gonads differentiate into ovaries. The ovary does not produce testosterone or AMH. In the absence of testosterone, the wolffian ducts regress. Wolffian duct remnants may remain as "rests" of tissue (epithelial inclusions). Paravaginal or paracervical wolffian remnants may form cysts called Gartner duct cysts.[1] Without AMH, the müllerian ducts flourish, fuse in the midline near the junction to the cloaca, and differentiate further to become the uterus, fallopian tubes, and upper (proximal) two thirds of the vagina.

The cloaca is the precursor for the external genitalia, the bladder, urethra, and the rectum. The urorectal septum forms by gestational week seven to separate the cloaca into two parts, the rectum and the urogenital sinus. In females, the müllerian tubercle (cephalic end of the urogenital sinus) joins to the fused müllerian ducts (now a primitive uterovaginal canal). The caudal side of the müllerian tubercle forms the vaginal plate and two sinovaginal bulbs, which elongate to reach the perineum. The perineal surface of the urogenital sinus is the urogenital membrane, flanked by swellings that form the urogenital folds, outer labioscrotal swellings, and the genital tubercle (different from the müllerian tubercle).

At this point, the external genitalia are "indifferent" genitals. With further growth and differentiation, the genital tubercle becomes either the glans penis (male) or the clitoris (female), the urogenital folds become the body of the penis (male) or the labia minora (female), and the labioscrotal swellings become the scrotum (male) or the labia majora (female). In males, the urogenital membrane first becomes a groove, then the penile urethra as the urogenital folds encircle it. In females, the urogenital membrane becomes the vestibule. The urogenital sinus separates into urethral and vaginal canals. The central cells of the solid vaginal canal break down caudally to form the vaginal lumen, extending to canalize the hymen.

The hymen contains fibrous connective tissue that is part elastic and part collagenous in nature. The inner surface of the hymen contains cells from the vagina (embryological vaginal plate) and the external surface of the hymen contains cells derived from the urogenital sinus.[2,3] Incomplete canalization of the hymen results in an imperforate, microperforate, or septated hymen.[1,4-6] Using animation, this embryological process is well illustrated on the Web site of The Hospital for Sick Children, Toronto, Canada, called "Sick Kids Child Physiology.[7]"

Recent studies challenge the accepted concept that the upper vagina is müllerian in origin and the lower vagina originates from the urogenital sinus (cloaca). Studies of wolffian structures in rat embryos demonstrate that the entire outer vagina is formed from wolffian duct cells and lined internally with müllerian tubercle (urogenital sinus) cells.[8,9] No studies have challenged the origin of hymenal tissues from the urogenital membrane (cloaca).

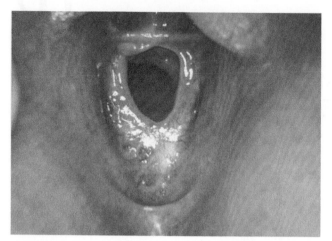

FIGURE 10-1 An annular hymen.

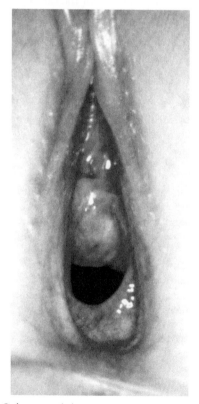

FIGURE 10-2 A crescentic hymen.

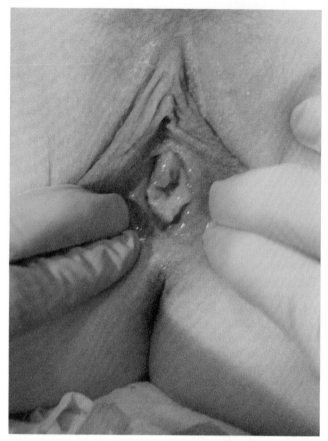

FIGURE 10-3 A fimbriated hymen. *(Courtesy of W. Darby, PhD, CRNP, and D. Colvard, MD, Cramer Children's Center, Florence, AL).*

VARIANTS IN FEMALE GENITAL ANATOMY

Hymenal Configurations

The hymen has several distinct anatomical configurations that are influenced by the child's age and physical maturation. The three most common configurations are annular, crescentic, and fimbriated.[10-17] An annular hymen has hymenal tissue present circumferentially and forms a doughnutlike appearance (Figure 10-1). A crescentic hymen has no definable hymenal tissue between approximately the 11 and 1 o'clock positions anteriorly (Figure 10-2). A fimbriated hymen has multiple folded areas of tissue along the hymenal edge (Figure 10-3). These redundant projections of tissue frequently overlap and obscure the hymenal orifice. A sleevelike hymen is a redundant or thickened hymen seen typically in infants with residual maternal estrogen (Figure 10-4). As estrogen resolves, annular hymens become more common. Crescentic hymens occur most commonly in girls aged 4 through 9 years.[13,14]

Other hymenal configurations such as septate and cribriform occur less frequently. A septate hymen has one or more nonrigid bands of hymenal membrane that cross the orifice and essentially create two (or more) separate openings (Figure 10-5). The septum often resolves as the child develops, or ruptures spontaneously. Septate hymens do not usually cause any problems, though if the septum persists at the time of menses, the use of tampons might be problematic.

Examination should differentiate a septate hymen from a vaginal septum. Vaginal septa divide the vaginal canal into two vaginal sections (Figure 10-6). The vaginal septum can be transverse or longitudinal. Differential diagnosis of a transverse septum includes imperforate hymen, vaginal atresia, or vaginal agenesis. Importantly, a longitudinal vaginal septum (which divides the vagina lengthwise) can occur in association with other genitourinary anomalies, especially uterine didelphys (duplication) or bicornuate uterus. A vaginal septum or complete vaginal duplication (with uterine didelphys) is thought to occur during fetal development when the müllerian ducts fail to fuse

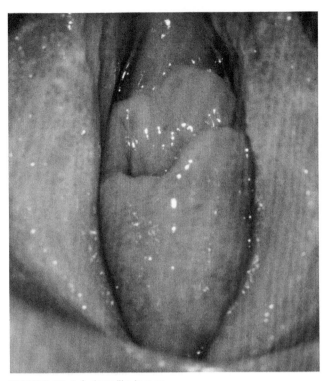

FIGURE 10-4 A sleevelike hymen.

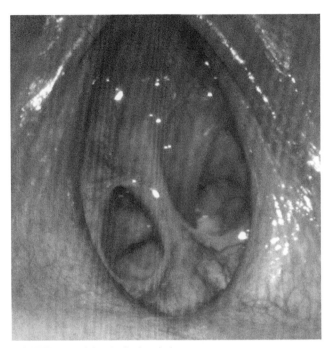

FIGURE 10-6 A longitudinal vaginal septum.

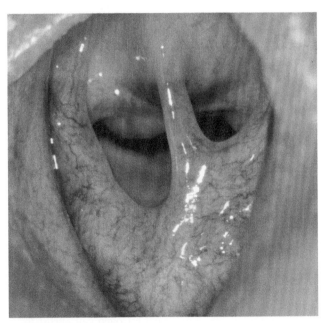

FIGURE 10-5 A septate hymen.

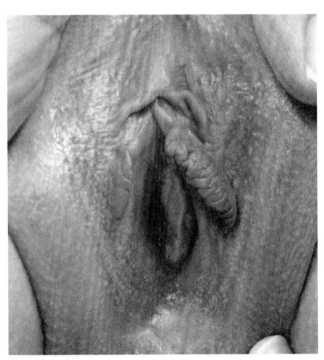

FIGURE 10-7 An imperforate hymen. *(Courtesy of L. C. Doggett, MD, Anniston Pediatrics, Anniston, AL).*

completely. Urological anomalies are found in 20% to 30% of females with uterine anomalies and in 50% with vaginal agenesis because ureteric bud formation (kidney and ureter development) occurs at the same stage of development. MRI is recommended as the optimal test to differentiate müllerian agenesis, cervical agenesis, transverse vaginal septum, imperforate hymen, and longitudinal septum.[18]

A cribriform (sievelike) hymen is defined by multiple small openings in the hymenal membrane. The hymen may have only a very small opening (microperforate) or no opening at all (imperforate) (Figure 10-7). Careful examination (with positioning to improve relaxation, application of saline drops, or use of a small swab) can differentiate a truly imperforate hymen from a normal one with adherent edges. An imperforate hymen should be followed yearly, but if it persists at the onset of puberty (sexual maturity level 2), the child should be referred to a gynecologist. Septate, cribriform, and imperforate hymenal variations result from failure of the urogenital membrane to completely canalize/perforate during embryogenesis.[18,19]

A number of variables affect the appearance of the hymen, particularly the child's developmental stage (sexual maturity rating) and presence of estrogen. Extrinsic factors such as examination position (supine versus prone knee-chest), the child's comfort and relaxation during the examination, and the examiner's experience and technique have been shown to affect the observed hymenal configuration and morphology. In one study of 93 prepubertal girls selected for nonabuse (ages 10 months to 10 years), hymens were more frequently characterized as crescentic when examined in the prone knee-chest position (54%) than the supine position with either labial separation (41%) or labial traction (44%).[10] This study also found that examination position and technique affected the relative redundancy, vascular patterns, and size of the hymenal orifice. Additional variables such as a child's comfort level and ability to cooperate with the anogenital examination often markedly affect the appearance of the hymen and surrounding structures.

The Newborn Hymen

The question of whether there is a congenital condition of "absent hymen" is sometimes raised when a child is examined for suspected sexual abuse. To address this question, Jenny et al[20] examined 1311 female newborns before discharge from their birth hospital; all had hymens. Jenny concluded "… in the absence of major genitourinary anomalies, one could expect hymenal tissue to be present in young female children." In addition, Mor and Merlob reported examinations of more than 25,000 female newborns. All had hymens,[21] effectively disproving the idea of congenital absence of the hymen in otherwise normal females. Several other studies have examined this question and all have confirmed that newborn females are born with hymens.[10,22]

Girls born with vaginal agenesis or atresia (for example Mayer-Rokitansky-Küster-Hauser syndrome) have normal external genitalia (Figure 10-8). Their condition develops from müllerian agenesis, resulting in absence or rudimentary formation of müllerian structures (uterus, fallopian tubes, and proximal vagina). This condition is the most common cause of primary amenorrhea (15%) and may be associated with renal and skeletal anomalies.[23-24] Abnormalities/absence of the hymen might be expected with significant cloacal anomalies, such as persistent cloaca (confluence of rectum, vagina, and urethra), imperforate anus with fistula, or cloacal extrophy. However, *absence of the* hymen associated with these or any other disorders has not been reported.

Developmental Changes to the Hymen

The hymenal configuration changes during different stages of growth and development, particularly with exposure to estrogen. Estrogen effect on the hymen is first apparent at birth due to maternal estrogen crossing the placenta during gestation. A newborn hymen appears thickened and pale, often associated with labial and clitoral prominence (Figure 10-9). Estrogen exposure produces a thick, white vaginal discharge, and in some cases, withdrawal vaginal bleeding occurs in the neonatal period as estrogen levels decrease. Once maternal (or exogenous) estrogen is eliminated, the

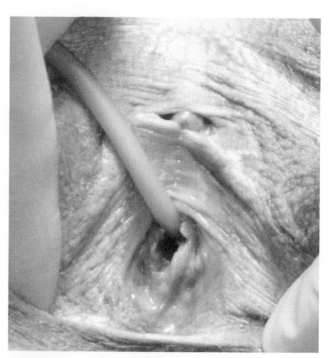

FIGURE 10-8 Mayer-Rokitansky-Küster-Hauser syndrome (vaginal agenesis). The catheter enters the urethra. The external genitalia appear normal except for the absence of the vagina. *(Courtesy of K. Morcel, MD, Rennes University Hospital Department of Obstetrics & Gynecology, Rennes, France).*

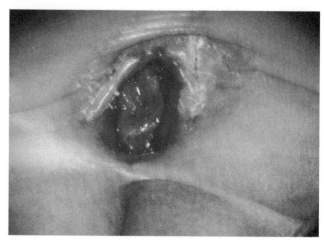

FIGURE 10-9 The typical appearance of the hymen of a newborn.

hymen gradually becomes thin and less redundant with sharp, well-defined edges. The labia also appear less prominent. This transition usually occurs within months after birth, but the effects of maternal estrogen can persist for 2 to 3 years in some cases.[12,13]

Hymenal changes in early childhood have been well documented by several longitudinal studies by Berenson et al.[12-14,22] They initially examined 468 female newborns and found that 80% had annular hymens, 19% had fimbriated hymens, and 1% had septate or cribriform hymens.[22] None of the newborns had crescentic hymens. In a follow-up study, Berenson reexamined 57 of these infants and noted that by 1 year of age, 42% of them had undergone a change in hymenal morphology since birth. At 1 year, 28% of subjects now had a crescentic hymenal configuration while 7% were fimbriated and only 54% remained annular.[12] Many

Table 10-1	**Overview of Longitudinal Studies of Hymenal Morphology by Berenson et al**[12-14,22]					
	Newborn **n = 468**	**1 Year** **n = 62**	**3 Years** **n = 42**	**5 Years** **n = 93**	**7 Years** **n = 80**	**9 Years** **n = 61**
Hymenal Configurations						
Annular	80%	54%	38%	23%	18%	10%
Crescentic	0%	28%	55%	77%	82%	90%
Fimbriated	19%	7%	2%	0%	0%	0%
Variations						
Clefts/notches	35%*	29%	12%	7%	9%	11%
Tags	13%	11%	10%	13%	10%	10%
External ridges	93%	14%	6%	3%	1%	0%
Longitudinal intravaginal ridges	56%	53%	81%	86%	90%	92%
Vestibular bands†	–	95%	100%	100%	100%	100%
Redundant/thickened‡	100%	42%	25%			

*Not recorded in newborns with fimbriated hymens.
†Not quantified for newborns due to difficulty with visualization; also includes periurethral bands.
‡Effects of maternal estrogen.

infants progressing from an annular to a crescentic hymen by age 1 had a hymenal notch at 12 o'clock (anterior) as a newborn. This finding lends support to the idea that crescentic hymens begin as annular or fimbriated configurations with a superior midline notch that widens to fill the 11:00 to 1:00 o'clock positions. Berenson also noted that by 1 year, 58% of subjects had a marked decrease in tissue redundancy, correlating with the expected decrease in serum estrogen levels after birth.

In a subsequent study, Berenson[13] examined a group of 134 female infants between birth and 2 months old and again at 3 years old. (Forty-two of these subjects were also examined near 1 year of age). At 3 years old, a majority of subjects (55%) now had crescentic hymens and 38% had annular configurations. Berenson observed that hymenal configuration changed in 65% of subjects between birth and 3 years of age, largely because of the increasing numbers of crescentic hymens. Maternal estrogen effects also resolved in 75% of 3-year-old subjects. As a result, hymenal edges transformed from thickened and redundant to sharp and well-defined.[13]

Subsequent examinations were conducted at 5, 7, and 9 years of age.[14] The percentage of hymens in the crescentic configuration continued to increase as prepubertal girls aged. By 9 years old, 90% of the 61 subjects had a crescentic hymen and only 10% remained annular (Table 10-1).

Like the effects of maternal estrogen at birth, increased serum estrogen during puberty causes a second period of change in hymenal morphology. In general, as girls develop secondary sexual characteristics, their hymens transition from a thin, translucent appearance to a redundant, elastic, and thickened hymen (Figure 10-10). The hymenal tissue also becomes less sensitive to touch, such that adolescents

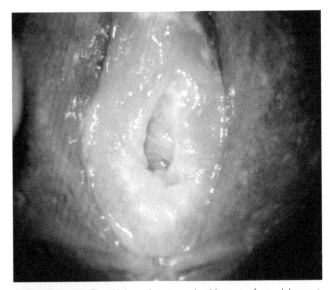

FIGURE 10-10 The thickened, estrogenized hymen of an adolescent.

are better able to tolerate examination aids, such as a swab or Foley catheter balloon.

Yordan and Yordan[25] conducted a cross-sectional study of 168 girls ages 7 to 17 years (sexual maturity ratings I-V) to determine if progressive genital changes could be correlated to sexual maturity ratings of the breasts. Subjects with sexual maturity rating (SMR) I breast development were noted to have very thin hymenal rims with small, thin, smooth labia minora. These girls also had a network of fine blood vessels in the fossa navicularis that extended to the hymenal rim. In SMR II subjects, there was a less

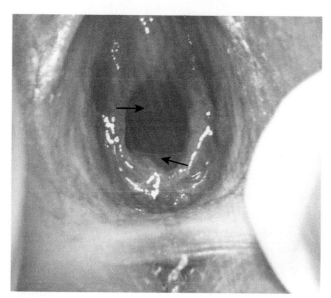

FIGURE 10-11 Longitudinal intravaginal ridges (at arrows).

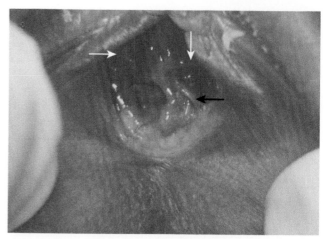

FIGURE 10-12 Vestibular bands, including a perihymenal band *(black arrow)* and periurethral bands *(white arrows)*.

pronounced vascular pattern and the hymenal rim remained thin. SMR III subjects demonstrated the beginnings of true estrogen effects on the genitals with hymenal thickening and still less prominence of superficial blood vessels. Clear vaginal secretions (physiological leukorrhea) appeared during this stage. SMR IV breast development was associated with hymens with thick, redundant projections and without visible blood vessels in the hymen or fossa navicularis. These subjects also had enlargement and darker pigmentation of the labia minora. SMR V subjects had further changes to the labia minora with elongation and development of rugae. While this cross-sectional study provides an important description of the hymen and surrounding tissues at different sexual maturity ratings of the breast, a longitudinal study further describing hymenal and genital tissue changes associated with progress through puberty would be an important contribution.

Longitudinal Intravaginal Ridges

Longitudinal intravaginal ridges are narrow, thickened ridges on the vaginal wall that often extend from the inner surface of the hymen into the vaginal vault (Figure 10-11). At the point where an intravaginal ridge attaches to the inner surface of the hymen, there is frequently a hymenal mound (bump). Intravaginal ridges have been noted to occur in 61% of newborns and appear to become more common with age.[13] Intravaginal ridges have been described in 89% to 94% of prepubertal females.[10,14,17] Children often appear to develop multiple intravaginal ridges as they age. Intravaginal columns are prominent intravaginal ridges that occur along the anterior and posterior vaginal walls.

External Ridges

External ridges are longitudinal ridges located on the *external* surface of the hymen. They are located superiorly from the hymenal edge to the urethra and inferiorly from the hymenal edge to the fossa navicularis. External ridges

are seen frequently in newborns (82%) but disappear with age.[12] Among infants initially examined at birth who were reexamined at 1 year old, only 14% had external ridges persistent since birth; by 3 years old 6% had persistent external ridges.[13] No children at age 3 years had external ridges not observed at birth. While this finding appears to be far more common in infants, external ridges can be present in some older children and should still be considered a normal variant.

Vestibular Bands

Vestibular bands are paired, thin bands of tissue generally located in the periurethral or perihymenal region that have the same color and texture as surrounding tissues (Figure 10-12).[12] Periurethral bands extend from the periurethral tissues to the wall of the vestibule such that a small, curved space is usually visible on both sides of the band. Perihymenal bands, also known as pubovaginal bands, connect the hymen to the lateral walls of the vestibule. Vestibular bands have been found in 92% to 98% of prepubertal girls selected for nonabuse.[11,12,17] In general, periurethral bands occur in 51% of prepubertal subjects.[10] A much higher frequency of periurethral bands was noted among Berenson's 3-year-old subjects; all had periurethral bands when the periurethral area could be visualized.[13]

Hymenal Tags and Mounds

Hymenal tags and mounds (bumps) are defined as elevations or projections of hymenal tissue that occur in any location along the inner hymenal rim (Figure 10-13). In the past, there have been efforts to distinguish a hymenal tag from a hymenal mound or bump, with a tag defined as an elongated projection of tissue arising from the hymenal rim and a mound or bump being at least as wide as it is long.[26] There appears to be no significant difference in terms of cause or clinical significance. McCann et al hypothesized that hymenal tags may be remnants of hymenal septa that cleave in utero or shortly after birth, a theory that might explain the presence of some tags.[10] However, many tags that have been noted in young children were not present at birth.[12,13]

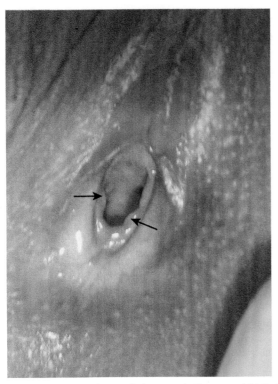

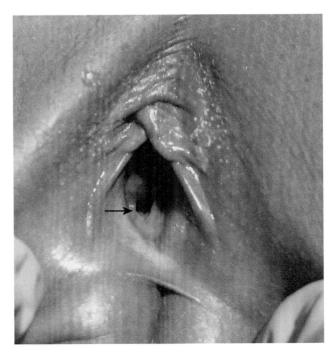

FIGURE 10-14 Hymenal notch (at arrow). *(Courtesy of W, Darby, PhD, CRNP, Cramer Children's Center, Florence, AL).*

FIGURE 10-13 Hymenal mounds (at arrows). *(Courtesy of W, Darby, PhD, CRNP, Cramer Children's Center, Florence, AL).*

Tags, like mounds and bumps, are sometimes associated with a longitudinal intravaginal ridge or an external hymenal ridge. Overall, hymenal tags, bumps, and mounds have been found in 10% to 24% of premenarchal females selected for nonabuse and should be considered a normal variant of the hymen.[10,11,15]

Notches/Clefts

A hymenal notch or cleft is an indentation or concavity in the edge of the hymenal margin (Figure 10-14). Notches and clefts differ from traumatic hymenal transections, which are interruptions of the hymenal margin that extends through the entire depth of the hymenal membrane to the vaginal wall. Hymenal transections, when located on the posterior hymen, are abnormal findings.

Of known variations in the hymenal rim, clefts and notches have perhaps received the most attention. In past years, posterior hymenal notches or clefts (from 3 to 9 o'clock posteriorly) that extended through more than 50% of the width of the hymenal rim were considered concerning for sexual abuse or trauma.[27,28] A number of other studies have contributed to our understanding of normal notches and clefts in nonabused females.[10-14,17]

In longitudinal studies of children selected for nonabuse, Berenson et al found that 38% of newborns had lateral or superior hymenal notches, which subsequently decreased to 29% of subjects at 1 year of age and then to 12% at 3 years of age.[12,13] Many of the superior notches had been noted from 11 o'clock to 1 o'clock in infants with annular hymens. These notches resolved as the hymenal configuration transitioned from annular to crescentic. Berenson et al also noted that some of these children who did not have notches

present at birth went on to have either lateral or superior notches at 1 and 3 years of age.[12,13]

In studies that examined prepubertal female subjects across a broad age group, superior and lateral hymenal notches were noted to be present in 2% to 8% of subjects.[10,11] In one study, the frequency of notches varied with examination position, with 6.6% of subjects noted to have a notch when in the supine position versus 2.2% of subjects in the prone knee-chest position.[10]

Posterior hymenal notches or clefts are still a topic of some debate regarding what constitutes normal and what suggests evidence of prior trauma. Berenson et al[12] noted in their longitudinal study of newborn and 1-year-olds that none of the infants had notches between 4 and 8 o'clock posteriorly and concluded that an inferior notch should "… continue to be considered an acquired, abnormal finding." Their prior cross-sectional study of 211 nonabused prepubertal girls also revealed no subjects with notches between 4 and 8 o'clock, lending further evidence to the idea that any posterior notch was abnormal and concerning.[11]

More recently, studies of girls selected for nonabuse have shown that certain types of posterior clefts appear to be a normal finding. Heger et al[17] examined 147 premenarchal girls who were referred for a gynecological examination to clarify findings noted on well-child examinations. In these cases there was no suspicion of abuse and 18% of subjects had a partial posterior hymenal cleft (an angular or v-shaped indentation) and 30% had a posterior hymenal concavity (curved or hollowed U-shaped depression). None of the subjects had a hymenal transection. In a case-control study of abuse with penetration, Berenson et al[28] examined 200 nonabused subjects and found that 7 of them (3.5%) had superficial posterior hymenal notches (involving less than or equal to half the hymenal rim), again suggesting that this finding can be seen outside the setting of abuse.

Transverse Hymenal Diameters

Measurement of transverse hymenal diameters in the evaluation of child sexual abuse has caused significant controversy in years past. In the 1980s, research focused on using this measurement as an objective, gold standard test for prior sexual abuse.[29,30] White et al[29] noted that 94% of children with an introital diameter greater than 4 mm had a history of sexual contact and concluded that this threshold was "highly associated with a history of sexual contact." More recent research has documented that measurements of transverse hymenal diameters vary with measuring technique and other factors such as age, developmental stage, hymenal configuration, subject's degree of relaxation, and examination technique.[10] In the nonabused population, diameters increase as children age and have been documented as large as 8 mm by the age of 3 years.[10,13,14] A more recent study of 147 premenarchal females selected for nonabuse showed that 30% had transverse hymenal diameters greater than 4 mm.[17] The measurement of the transverse diameter of the hymenal opening has become clinically irrelevant.[31]

Width of the Inferior Hymenal Rim

In recent years, the width of the inferior hymenal rim has been a focus in the examination of suspected sexual abuse victims. Several studies suggest that a narrow posterior rim is concerning for sexual abuse.[32-34] In order for this measurement to have clinical significance, normal values in nonabused females are necessary for comparison. Berenson's longitudinal studies of nonabused girls found that the inferior hymenal rim measured 2 mm or greater in all 1 and 3 year olds and did not vary with age.[13] By age 5 years, she noted a slight decrease in mean inferior rim depth in both supine (2.8 to 2.6 mm) and prone knee-chest (2.7 to 2.5 mm) examination positions.[14]

When comparing posterior hymenal width between adolescent subjects with and without a history of consensual sexual intercourse, Adams et al[35] found no significant difference between groups, with a mean of 2.5 versus 3 mm, respectively. They did note, however, that the admitted sexual intercourse group was more likely to have a posterior hymenal rim of less than or equal to 1 mm compared with the group with no consensual intercourse (22% versus 3%, respectively). "Narrow" hymenal rims (<1-2 mm) were also found in 22% of 147 premenarchal subjects selected for nonabuse. Heger[17] observed that 79% of this group was greater than the 75th percentile for weight for age. Heger also commented that measurements were often imprecise, raising concern about objectivity.

Measuring such a small area of tissue during an examination can be a challenge and many examiners simply use visual estimation to determine the posterior rim depth. Several studies have commented on the difficulty determining the width of the posterior hymen.[10,11] When considering variations of only a millimeter or less, this presents a challenge to the accuracy of the measurement and as such should raise appropriate concern about interpreting the significance of this measurement in clinical practice.

Vascularity and Erythema of the Hymen and Vestibule

The vascular pattern of the prepubertal hymen is generally described as lacy with multiple small vessels on the hymenal surface. In approximately 5% of prepubertal children, a single prominent vessel is superimposed on this finer vascular network.[11] Erythema of the hymen and surrounding tissues frequently causes parental concern for child sexual abuse. When examining a child, it is important to remember that erythema of the hymen and vestibule is a relatively subjective finding that is difficult to quantify. The determination of redness as abnormal could well differ from one examiner to the next. Studies that have examined the prevalence of erythema have noted this finding to be present in 3% to 56% of children.[10,17,28,32] Variables such as examination position have also been shown to affect the presence of erythema, seen more commonly in the supine than the prone knee-chest position.[10] To differentiate vascularity from erythema, two examinations performed days apart may be helpful; erythema would be expected to resolve or change whereas vascularity would likely remain consistent in appearance. In practice, however, this is rarely done because erythema is such a nonspecific finding.[28]

Linea Vestibularis

Linea vestibularis is another normal variant of female genital anatomy, characterized as white streaks that run from the inferior hymenal border to the posterior commissure (Figure 10-15).[36] Partial linea vestibularis is described as white spots rather than streaks in the same distribution. Linea vestibularis also has been described as "midline sparing" in a number of past studies.[10,11,15] In a study of 123 newborns, Kellogg et al[36] noted that 10% had white streaks, which they defined as linea vestibularis and another 14% had findings of partial linea vestibularis. Kellogg also noted that these findings are "... distinct from a median or perineal raphe, which is a flesh-colored, slightly raised, perineal structure whereas linea vestibularis is an avascular, flat, posterior vestibule structure." Among infants who were reexamined over time, some findings resolved and others became more prominent.[37] Linea vestibularis has also been found to occur in

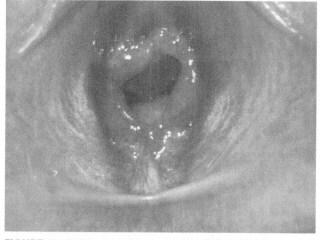

FIGURE 10-15 Linea vestibularis—a pale area in the fossa navicularis.

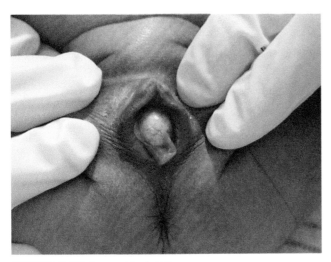

FIGURE 10-16 A paraurethral cyst.

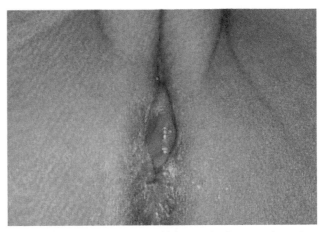

FIGURE 10-17 An infantile pyramidal protrusion between the vagina and the anus.

15% to 26% of premenarchal subjects across a wider age range.[10,15,17]

Lymphoid Follicles

Lymphoid follicles are a normal variant described as small 1 to 2 mm yellow or white papules on the hymen or surrounding tissues that represent follicular hyperplasia. They are found in approximately one third of girls.[3,10]

Paraurethral Cysts

Paraurethral cysts are uncommon findings that result from an obstruction or cystic degeneration of embryonic remnants of the urogenital sinus (Figure 10-16). Rarely, such cysts may obstruct the vagina or compress the urethra.[3] They usually resolve or rupture without requiring intervention.[38]

Imperforate Hymen

Imperforate hymen (Figure 10-7) is a congenital anomaly in which the hymenal membrane has no functional opening and occludes the entrance to the vagina. Most commonly this is an isolated finding with an incidence that ranges from 0.014% to 0.1% in term births.[38,39] Imperforate hymens are generally diagnosed as incidental findings in young females or later in adolescence when a girl remains amenorrheic despite age-appropriate breast and pubic hair development. Clinical symptoms in adolescents include primary amenorrhea and abdominal pain, which can accompany a midline lower abdominal mass on examination. Genital examination can reveal hydrometrocolpos, or a bulging, bluish vaginal mass that is caused by vaginal secretions and menstrual blood accumulating behind the imperforate hymen. In younger girls, hydrocolpos may be noted on examination, which is a tense and gray-white appearing vestibule caused by the accumulation of vaginal secretions behind the imperforate hymen.

A retrospective case series by Posner et al[40] of imperforate hymens found a bimodal distribution of age at diagnosis; 43% were diagnosed at less than 4 years of age and 57%

were not diagnosed until more than 10 years of age. Almost all of the younger patients were asymptomatic, unlike the older group where 100% were symptomatic at the time of diagnosis. These older girls presented with abdominal pain, urinary symptoms, or both. Almost half of the older patients were given an alternate diagnosis before imperforate hymen was discovered and 86% underwent unnecessary diagnostic evaluations such as blood work, urinalysis, and abdominal radiography. Posner concludes, "It can be surmised that if each older girl had undergone a complete examination of the genitalia as part of a routine well-child visit early in her life, then none would have had to endure the symptoms and diagnostic evaluations associated with late diagnosis.[40]" The treatment is surgical hymenectomy, which removes the obstruction.

PERINEAL VARIANTS

Infantile Pyramidal Protrusion

Infantile pyramidal protrusion is a perineal variant originally described in a series of case reports of fifteen Japanese children (Figure 10-17).[41] These children, 1 to 30 months of age, presented with a characteristic pyramidal area of smooth, pink or red tissue located in the midline and anterior to the anus. Of note, 14 of the 15 children were girls, which is similar to McCann's study of perianal anatomy where he found 18 similar cases, all females.[42] Mechanical irritation such as vigorous wiping has been suggested as a cause of swelling of the protrusions.[43]

Failure of Midline Fusion

Failure of midline fusion (Figure 10-18), also known as a perineal groove, is a congenital finding characterized by the presence of mucosal surface along the midline between the fossa navicularis and the anus (on the perineal body).[44] This impressive normal variant is often confused with traumatic injury, but can be distinguished by its persistent, unchanged appearance at follow-up examination. A traumatic injury is expected to change in a period of days to weeks. Failure of midline fusion has been noted to resolve at puberty.

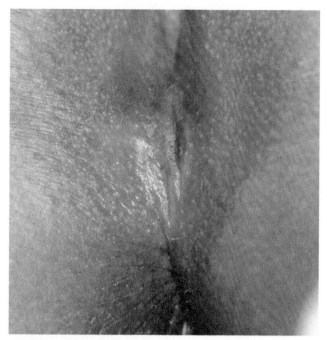

FIGURE 10-18 A failure of midline fusion on the perineum (perineal groove). *(From Fleet SL, Davis LS: Infantile perianal pyramidal protrusion: report of a case and review of the literature. Pediatr Dermatol 2005;22: 151-152.*

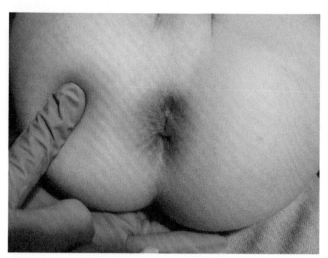

FIGURE 10-19 Diastasis ani at 12 and 6 o'clock.

Median Raphe

The median raphe is yet another midline structure in males and females that can sometimes be confused with trauma or scarring. This midline ridge from the female posterior commissure to the anus (or along the male penile shaft, scrotum, and perineum) denotes the junction of the two halves of the perineum.[26] In addition to being slightly raised, it can also have a subtle difference in coloration from surrounding perineal tissue.

PERIANAL VARIANTS

Diastasis Ani

Diastasis ani is a congenital variant characterized by an apparent absence of muscle fibers in the midline of the external anal sphincter (Figure 10-19). This results in a smooth, usually wedge-shaped area in the 12 or 6 o'clock positions that has been confused with anal scarring from prior trauma. In McCann's study of 266 healthy, prepubertal subjects selected for nonabuse, diastasis ani was found in 26% of subjects, was always located in the midline, and was associated with a midline depression in 47% of cases.[42] Berenson et al[45] studied 1 to 17 month olds and found that 26% of 89 subjects had similar smooth areas adjacent to the perianal folds in the midline only. The most common location for this finding was the 6 o'clock position (83%), with 26% in the 12 o'clock position. Some subjects had this finding in both positions. Diastasis ani occurred more frequently among white subjects (48%) than black (30%) or Hispanic (22%) subjects.

Prominent Skin Folds and the Pectinate Line

Anal skin folds appear due to contraction of the external anal sphincter. The skin folds can be very prominent and protrude from the surrounding skin, seen in approximately 4% to 7% of children.[46] The pectinate or dentate line is a demarcation between the distal portion of the anal valves and the smooth zone of stratified epithelium that extends to the anal verge. This line can be seen when the internal and external anal sphincters dilate, or upon traction of the perianal tissues during examination.

Anal Skin Tags

Anal skin tags are areas of redundant perianal skin (Figure 10-20). McCann et al[42] found skin tags in 11% of prepubertal children—present in equal distributions among preschool, school-aged, and preadolescent children with no difference among ethnic groups.[42] Berenson et al noted anal skin tags in 3% of their 89 subjects.[45] Another study of 305 children between 5 and 6.75 years of age found anal skin tags in 6.6%, all in the midline and mostly located in the 12 o'clock position.[46] They typically are located in the midline and their presence outside of this region should prompt consideration of other causes.

Anal Dilatation

The degree of anal dilatation during the anogenital examination has raised concern of anal abuse; however, multiple studies have confirmed that anal dilatation of the external sphincter is a normal occurrence. When both external and internal anal sphincters dilate without stool present, and in excess of 20 mm, concerns persist that this could be caused by anal penetration. Studies that consistently demonstrate an association with anal penetration in children are lacking, however. McCann et al[42] noted external anal sphincter dilatation in 49% of the nonabused children they examined. They found an anterior-posterior diameter of less than 20 mm in 91% of all children with anal dilatation. Among children with at least 20 millimeters dilatation, only 1.2%

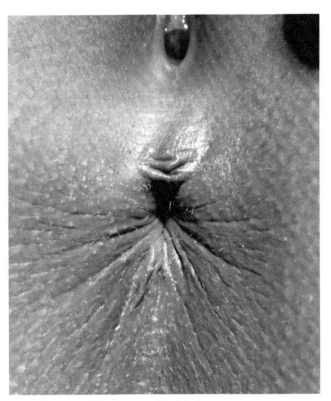

FIGURE 10-20 Anal skin tag at 12 o'clock.

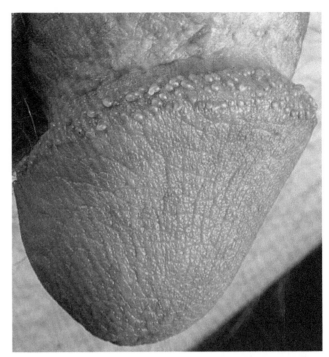

FIGURE 10-21 Pearly penile papules (at arrow). *(From Bylaite M, Ruzicka T: Images in clinical medicine: pearly penile papules. N Engl J Med 2007;357:691.Copyright © 2007 Massachusetts Medical Society. All rights reserved.)*

had no visible stool within the ampulla, suggesting that significant anal dilatation usually occurs in conjunction with the presence of stool. Among the children with anal dilatation, 38% remained dilated during the examination while 62% intermittently opened and closed. Myhre[46] noted external anal dilatation to occur in 11% of prepubertal non-abused children in the left lateral position and 19% in the prone knee-chest position. The difference in dilatation between positions was postulated to be due to differences in intraabdominal pressure and resulting external sphincter tone.

Anal dilatation can be affected by factors that alter muscle tone. Neuromuscular disorders such as myotonic dystrophy have been reported to cause external and internal anal sphincter laxity with reflex dilatation during examination, which thus might raise concern for sexual abuse.[47] Sedation and anesthesia are also noted to cause internal and external anal sphincter dilatation that resolves with the return of normal consciousness and muscle tone.

The most extreme example of muscle tone laxity occurs with death. McCann's study of postmortem subjects showed that anal dilatation was a common finding at autopsy with 77% of subjects having some degree of dilatation.[48] Ninety-four percent of these children died of natural causes or accidental mechanisms. McCann does note that children who died of a CNS injury or were severely brain damaged had an increased likelihood of a dilated anus.

Venous Congestion

Perianal venous congestion is a blue or purple discoloration around the anus that is thought to result from temporary obstruction of venous outflow. This nonspecific finding is positional in nature and has been noted to occur more frequently in the prone knee-chest examination position and with prolonged examinations. In McCann's study of prepubertal children selected for nonabuse, 7% of subjects had venous congestion at the beginning of the examination, 52% of subjects at the examination midpoint, and 73% by the end of the examination.[42] All of these examinations were performed in the knee-chest position. Mean examination time was almost 4 minutes, a duration that likely contributed to the substantial numbers of subjects with this finding. Myhre noted venous congestion in 17% of subjects in left lateral position and 20% of subjects in prone knee-chest position, with significantly more girls than boys with this finding.[46]

VARIANTS IN MALE GENITAL ANATOMY

Pearly Papules

Pearly penile papules are small (less than 1 mm), palpable lesions distributed circumferentially around the corona of the penis (Figure 10-21).[49] They may also be found on the penile shaft just proximal to the corona. These papules are small angiofibromas and are normal variants that require no treatment. They occur in 14% to 48% of young, postpubertal adults, but are relatively uncommon in preadolescent children. They have sometimes been observed more frequently in circumcised men. Pearly papules have also been confused with genital warts. Clinical distinction of this normal variant from HPV is important.

Hypospadias

Hypospadias is an abnormal ventral opening of the urethra that can occur anywhere along the penis, scrotum, or perineum and is caused by underdevelopment of the urogenital folds. It can be associated with ventral penile curvature (chordee). It occurs in 2 to 8 of 1000 live births.[50] Familial clustering has been noted with 6% to 8% of fathers and 14% of male siblings of affected children also having hypospadias.

Three types of hypospadias occur. In *first degree* hypospadias, the urethral meatus opens onto the glans penis. In *second degree* hypospadius, the urethra opens on the shaft of the penis, and in *third degree* hypospadius, the urethra opens on the perineum.[51] Hypospadias may be an isolated finding or part of a complex intersex condition. An isolated finding of hypospadias on an otherwise normal examination can also be associated with significant underlying urological abnormalities, so complete urological evaluation is required. Routine circumcision is contraindicated in children with hypospadias, as the foreskin is needed for repair. Surgical repair is recommended when there are impairments in urination, sexual intercourse, or effective insemination.[52]

Hydroceles

A hydrocele is a fluid collection that may occur anywhere along the path of testicular descent. The hydrocele may be communicating, with fluid of peritoneal origin, or noncommunicating, where fluid arises from the mesothelial lining of the tunica vaginalis. Hydroceles are common in newborns and usually resolve spontaneously by age 12 months. In older children and adolescents, hydroceles may be idiopathic but may also result from trauma, tumor, infection, or testicular torsion. Thorough testicular examination and often ultrasound are warranted to exclude these associated conditions.

A hydrocele usually presents as a painless, cystic scrotal mass. A communicating hydrocele may increase in size with standing or the Valsalva maneuver, whereas a noncommunicating hydrocele should have a fixed size. Diagnosis can be aided by transillumination of the scrotum, which reveals a fluid collection.

Hydrocele management in infants consists of watchful waiting. Surgical correction is recommended for hydroceles that persist beyond age 1 year. In older children, surgical repair is often indicated for communicating hydroceles because of risk of incarcerated inguinal hernia. It may be considered for some symptomatic hydroceles.[53]

Varicocele

A varicocele is the dilatation of the veins of the pampiniform plexus of the spermatic cord.[53] Rarely found before puberty, varicoceles are reported in approximately 15% of adolescent males and are seen in 15% to 20% of adult men. They are usually an asymptomatic scrotal mass or swelling that worsens with standing. On examination, a varicocele will often increase in size with the Valsalva maneuver and then decompress in the recumbent position. Palpation of a varicocele is often described as feeling like a "bag of worms." Assessment of testicular volume is a crucial component of the examination in order to identify varicoceles that are inhibiting testicular growth.

Most varicoceles occur on the left side as a result of the left spermatic vein draining into the left renal vein at a 90-degree angle, compared to the right spermatic vein, which drains more directly into the inferior vena cava. Bilateral or right-sided varicoceles should prompt consideration of an intraabdominal or retroperitoneal mass. Varicoceles are associated with infertility in some cases.

Varicoceles are usually managed conservatively with simple observation. Surgical ligation or testicular vein embolization are treatment options for symptomatic varicoceles, bilateral varicoceles, and varicoceles compromising testicular volume.

FUTURE RESEARCH

Understanding embryological development and the spectrum of normal anogenital variation is fundamental to accurately establishing a medical diagnosis of injuries caused by child sexual abuse. While recent studies provide compelling support that narrow hymenal rims (particularly in overweight premenarchal girls) and superficial posterior notches/clefts (less than or equal to half the hymenal width) may be seen in nonabused girls, studies are needed to further evaluate the significance of these findings. Studies elucidating standardized methods of measuring hymenal rim widths (perhaps from printed images) may be useful for achieving these goals. Other areas suggested for further research include exploring the usefulness of measuring antero-posterior diameters of anal dilatation to determine whether anal penetration has occurred. Again, methodological studies first standardizing these measurements to improve their accuracy and precision are suggested. Recent embryological studies in rats suggest an important role of the wolffian ducts in vaginal development. Confirmatory studies are needed along with specific descriptions of hymenal appearance in girls with cloacal developmental anomalies.

References

1. Crum CP: The female genital tract. *In*: Cotran RS, Kumar V, Collins T, et al *(eds)*: *Robbins Pathologic Basis of Disease*, ed 7, Elsevier Saunders, Philadelphia, 2005, pp 1059-1114.
2. Mahran M, Saleh AM: The microscopic anatomy of the hymen. *Anat Rec* 1964;149:313-318.
3. Reed WJ: Anogenital anatomy: developmental, normal, variant, and healing. *In*: Giardino AP (ed): *Sexual Assault: Victimization Across the Lifespan*. GW Medical, St Louis, 2003, pp 17-52.
4. Muram D: Anatomy. Embryology of the genital tract. *In*: Heger A, Emans SJ, Muram D (eds): *Evaluation of the Sexually Abused Child*, ed 2, Oxford University Press, New York, 2000, pp 95-104.
5. Laufer MR, Goldstein DP, Hendren WH: Structural abnormalities of the female reproductive tract. *In*: Emans SJ, Laufer MR, Goldstein DP (eds): *Pediatric and Adolescent Gynecology*, ed 5, Lippincott Williams & Wilkins, Philadelphia, 2005, pp 334-338.
6. Siegfried EC, Frasier LD: The spectrum of anogenital diseases in children. *Curr Probl Dermatol* 1997;9:33-80.
7. Wall S, Tait G: Sick kids child physiology, The Hospital for Sick Children (website): http://www.aboutkidshealth.ca/HowTheBodyWorks/Duct-Differentiation.aspx?articleID=7709&categoryID=XS-nh3-03 and http://www.aboutkidshealth.ca/HowTheBodyWorks/Genital-Development.aspx?articleID=7710&categoryID=XS-nh3-04. Accessed March 1, 2009.
8. Sánchez-Ferrer ML, Acién MI, Sánchez del Campo F, et al: Experimental contributions to the study of the embryology of the vagina. *Hum Reprod* 2006;21:1623-1628.

9. Drews U, Sulak O, Schenk PA: Androgens and the development of the vagina. *Biol Reprod* 2002;67:1353-1359.

10. McCann J, Wells R, Simon M, et al: Genital findings in prepubertal girls selected for nonabuse: a descriptive study. *Pediatrics* 1990; 86:428-439.

11. Berenson A, Heger A, Hayes J, et al: Appearance of the hymen in prepubertal girls. *Pediatrics* 1992;89:387-394.

12. Berenson A: Appearance of the hymen at birth and one year of age: a longitudinal study. *Pediatrics* 1993;91:820-825.

13. Berenson A: A longitudinal study of hymenal morphology in the first 3 years of life. *Pediatrics* 1995;95:490-496.

14. Berenson AB, Grady JJ: A longitudinal study of hymenal development from 3 to 9 years of age. *J Pediatr* 2002;140:600-607.

15. Gardner JJ: Descriptive study of genital variation in healthy, nonabused premenarchal girls. *J Pediatr* 1992;120:251-257.

16. Myhre AK: Genital anatomy in nonabused preschool girls. *Acta Paediatr* 2003;92:1453-1462.

17. Heger AH, Ticson L, Guerra L, et al: Appearance of the genitalia in girls selected for nonabuse: review of hymenal morphology and nonspecific findings. *J Pediatr Adolesc Gynecol* 2002;15:27-35.

18. Lin PC, Bhatnagar KP, Nettleton GS, et al: Female genital anomalies affecting reproduction. *Fertil Steril* 2002;78:899-915.

19. Edmonds DK: Congenital malformations of the genital tract and their management. *Best Pract Res Clin Obstet Gynaecol* 2003;17:19-40.

20. Jenny C, Kuhns ML, Arakawa F: Hymens in newborn female infants. *Pediatrics* 1987;80:399-400.

21. Mor N, Merlob P: Congenital absence of the hymen only a rumor? *Pediatrics* 1988;82:679.

22. Berenson A: Appearance of the hymen in newborns. *Pediatrics* 1991;87:458-465.

23. Pletcher JR, Slap GB: Menstrual disorders. Amenorrhea. *Pediatr Clin North Am* 1999;46:505-518.

24. Morcel K, Camborieux L, Programme de Recherches sur les Aplasies Mülleriennes, et al: Mayer-Rokitansky-Küster-Hauser (MRKH) syndrome. *Orphanet J Rare Dis* 2007;2:13.

25. Yordan EE, Yordan RA: The hymen and tanner staging of the breast. *Adolesc Pediatr Gynecol* 1992;5:76-79.

26. APSAC Task Force on Medical Evaluation of Suspected Child Abuse: *Practice guidelines: descriptive terminology in child sexual abuse medical evaluations.* American Professional Society on the Abuse of Children, Chicago, 1995.

27. Adams JA: Evolution of a classification scale: medical evaluation of suspected child sexual abuse. *Child Maltreat* 2001;6:31-36.

28. Berenson AB, Chacko MR, Wiemann CM, et al: A case-control study of anatomic changes resulting from sexual abuse. *Am J Obstet Gynecol* 2000;184:820-831.

29. White ST, Ingram DL, Lyna PR: Vaginal introital diameter in the evaluation of sexual abuse. *Child Abuse Negl* 1989;13:217-224.

30. Cantwell HB: Vaginal inspection as it relates to child sexual abuse in girls under thirteen. *Child Abuse Negl* 1983;7:171-176.

31. Berenson AB, Chacko MR, Wiemann CM, et al: Use of hymenal measurements in the diagnosis of previous penetration. *Pediatrics* 2002;109:228-235.

32. Emans S, Woods E, Flagg N, et al: Genital findings in sexually abused, symptomatic, and asymptomatic girls. *Pediatrics* 1987;79:778-785.

33. McCann J: Labial adhesions and posterior fourchette injuries in childhood sexual abuse. *Am J Dis Child* 1988;142:659-663.

34. Pokorny SF: Configuration and other anatomic detail of the prepubertal hymen. *Adolesc Pediatr Gynecol* 1988;1:97-103.

35. Adams JA, Botash AS, Kellogg N: Differences in hymenal morphology between adolescent girls with and without a history of consensual sexual intercourse. *Arch Pediatr Adolesc Med* 2004;158:280-285.

36. Kellogg ND, Parra JM: Linea vestibularis: a previously undescribed normal genital structure in female neonates. *Pediatrics* 1991;87: 926-929.

37. Kellogg ND, Parra JM: Linea vestibularis: follow-up of a normal genital structure. *Pediatrics* 1993;92:453-456.

38. Emans SJ: Vulvovaginal problems in the prepubertal child. *In:* Emans SJ, Laufer MR, Goldstein DP (eds): *Pediatric and Adolescent Gynecology*, ed 5, Lippincott, Williams & Wilkins, Philadelphia, 2005, pp 83-119.

39. El-Messidi A, Fleming NA: Congenital imperforate hymen and its life-threatening consequences in the neonatal period. *J Pediatr Adolesc Gynecol* 2006;19:99-103.

40. Posner JC, Spandorfer PR: Early detection of imperforate hymen prevents morbidity from delays in diagnosis. *Pediatrics* 2005;115: 1008-1012.

41. Kayashima K, Masato K, Tomomichi O: Infantile perianal pyramidal protrusion. *Arch Dermatol* 1996;132:1481-1484.

42. McCann J, Voris J, Simon M, et al: Perianal findings in prepubertal children selected for nonabuse: a descriptive study. *Child Abuse Negl* 1989;13:179-193.

43. Fleet SL, Davis LS: Infantile perianal pyramidal protrusion: report of a case and review of the literature. *Pediatr Dermatol* 2005;22:151-152.

44. Adams JA, Horton M: Is it sexual abuse? Confusion caused by a congenital anomaly of the genitalia. *Clin Pediatr (Phila)* 1989;28:146-148.

45. Berenson A, Somma-Garcia A, Barnett S: Perianal findings in infants 18 months of age or younger. *Pediatrics* 1993;91:838-840.

46. Myhre AK, Berntzen K, Bratlid D, et al: Perianal anatomy in nonabused preschool children. *Acta Paediatr* 2001;90:1321-1328.

47. Reardon W, Hughes HE, Green SH, et al: Anal abnormalities in childhood myotonic dystrophy—a possible source of confusion in child sexual abuse. *Arch Dis Child* 1992;67:527-528.

48. McCann J, Reay D, Siebert J, et al: Postmortem perianal findings in children. *Am J Forensic Med Pathol* 1996;17:289-298.

49. Bylaite M, Ruzicka T: Images in clinical medicine: pearly penile papules. *N Engl J Med* 2007;357:691.

50. MacLellan DL, Diamond DA: Recent advances in external genitalia. *Pediatr Clin North Am* 2006;53:449-464.

51. Duckett J Jr: Hypospadias. *Pediatr Rev* 1989;11:37-42.

52. Borer J, Retik AB: Hypospadias. *In:* Wein AJ, Kavoussi LR, Novick AC, et al (eds): *Campbell-Walsh Urology*, ed 9, Saunders, Philadelphia, 2007.

53. Schneck FX, Bellinger MF: Abnormalities of the testes and scrotum and their surgical management. *In:* Wein AJ, Kavoussi LR, Novick AC, et al (eds): *Campbell-Walsh Urology*, ed 9, Saunders, Philadelphia, 2007.

11

PHYSICAL FINDINGS IN CHILDREN AND ADOLESCENTS EXPERIENCING SEXUAL ABUSE OR ASSAULT

Deborah Stewart, MD, FAAP

INTRODUCTION

Since the early 1980s, medical care providers have played a major role in describing physical findings in children and adolescents where sexual abuse or assault is suspected. Initial studies suggested that tissue injury was commonly seen in these patients.[1-3] The early studies on abused children, however, were done before studies of nonabused children. It was soon discovered that many of these presumed post-traumatic findings were in fact normal or nonspecific findings commonly seen in nonabused children. Over the last 2 decades there have been several studies of genital and anal findings in children carefully screened for nonabuse using screening methods such as sexual behavior inventories, one on one interviews with the child, parental interviews, and medical records searches.[4-12] There has been a major effort to standardize medical terminology led by the American Professional Society on the Abuse of Children (APSAC), creating more rigorous definitions for anogenital findings in children and adolescents who are suspected victims of sexual abuse.[13]

IMPORTANCE OF STANDARDIZATION OF EXAMINATION TECHNIQUES

It has become increasingly clear that the use of various examination positions and the use of adjunct techniques affect the results of examinations of children and adolescents for suspected sexual abuse. A recent study by Boyle et al[14] emphasized the importance of using three examination positions: supine labial separation, supine labial traction, and prone knee chest when examining prepubertal and pubertal girls with genital injury. In this retrospective study of 46 prepubertal girls with genital injuries from various causes and 74 pubertal girls with injuries from sexual assault, the investigators found that the use of all three methods was necessary to the ensure successful and adequate visualization of the hymen and to detect all the injuries. No single technique consistently allowed the separation of the hymenal edges for adequate visualization of normal structures and hymenal lacerations and contusions. This was true in both the prepubertal and pubertal populations. The authors concluded that without the combined use of the three methods, a significant number of injuries, particularly hymenal lacerations, could be missed in the child and adolescent.

Studies of injuries have also been enhanced by the use of multiple adjunct techniques to assist in the delineation of injuries to the anogenital tissues, when necessary. This includes the use of cotton-tipped applicators to explore the edge of the hymen, the use of the water or saline to "float" the hymen, and the Foley catheter technique (see Chapter 9). Another technique that has been used is the staining of genital and perianal tissues with toluidine blue dye, a nuclear stain taken up by subepithelial layers of disrupted skin to accentuate subtle abrasions of the tissues.[15,16] While some practitioners find the use of toluidine blue very helpful in diagnosing acute trauma from assault, its use in children is not standard with all examiners.

Abnormal physical findings in sexually abused/assaulted children and adolescents remain rare. Normal examinations of the genitalia and anus are reported in up to 95% of children evaluated for abuse.[17]

ACUTE GENITAL FINDINGS FOLLOWING SEXUAL TRAUMA

If children are seen soon after an abusive episode, they are much more likely to have physical findings corroborating the abuse.[18] Children and adolescents can be exposed to multiple types of trauma during sexual abuse. Friction (rubbing or fondling) often leaves no findings or can result in tissue erythema, abrasions, scratches, bruising, or edema. Penetrating trauma can cause lacerations, fissures, transections, abrasions, or perforations of the vaginal or bowel wall. In some cases of known sexual penetration, no abnormal findings are noted on examination.[19] There also can be extragenital injuries such as bite marks, bruising, suction ecchymoses, and marks from ligatures or strangulation.

Studies of prepubertal victims of acute sexual assault have noted injuries including vaginal lacerations, complete hymenal transections, deep clefts, hymenal bruises, abrasions and tears, bruises or abrasions to the fossa navicularis and posterior fourchette (Figures 11-1, 11-2, and 11-3).[18,20-25] A study by Palusci et al of 190 children under the age of 13 seen urgently within 72 hours for evaluation for sexual abuse or assault found that 13.2% had positive examination findings that included a vaginal laceration (1), complete hymenal transections (4), acute hymenal transections through more than 50% of the hymenal width (9), hymenal abrasions (2), and perihymenal bruises (4).[26] Importantly, only vaginal

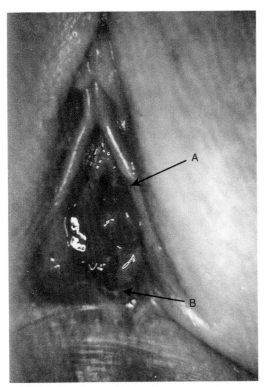

FIGURE 11-1 Genitalia of a one year old girl with acute genital and hymenal trauma. Arrow A indicates submucosal hemorrhage at 2 o'clock. Arrow B indicates acute laceration into posterior fourchette.

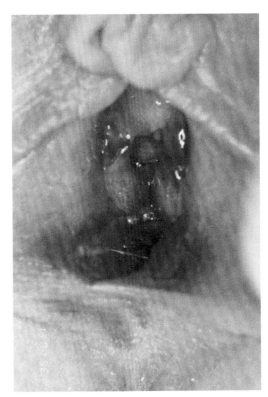

FIGURE 11-3 Exam of a 10 year old female with bruising of the posterior left labum, and laceration extending from the hymen throught the posterior fourchette onto the perineum.

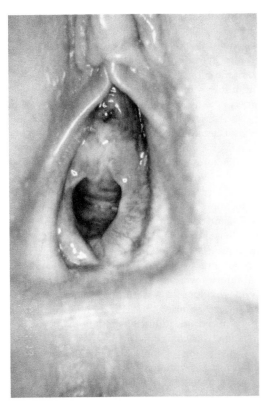

FIGURE 11-2 Same girl 3 years later with a healed transaction at 6 o'clock.

lacerations and hymenal transections greater than 50% of the width of the hymen were statistically associated with positive forensic evidence. In addition, children with positive examination findings were older (8.8 years versus 5.8 years), pubertal (Tanner stage III or greater), and disclosed a history of genital contact or perpetrator ejaculation. The proportion of positive findings was highest in the first 12 hours (29%).

In a study by Christian et al of 293 children younger than 10 years old,[18] most of whom (88%) were evaluated within 24 hours of suspected sexual assault, 23% had anogenital injuries. Injuries were seen in the anus (24%), hymen (16%), labia minora (16%), posterior fourchette (19%) and perineum (9%); 3% had intravaginal injuries. The types of injuries included lacerations or tears (55%), abrasions (38%), and bruises (7%). Erythema was noted in 38% of the acute examinations, as well. The presence of injury was predictive of identifying forensic evidence (odds ratio 3.23).

Another study by Heppenstall-Heger of 94 children with acute anogenital trauma, from both accidents and sexual abuse found 171 injuries[24]: 47 to the posterior fourchette, 37 to the hymen, 39 to the perihymenal tissue, 17 to the labia minora or majora, and 31 to the anus. The 24 children with a history of penile-vaginal penetration had the highest percentage of significant injuries. These included: 12 complete transections of the hymen, 14 injuries to the posterior fourchette, and 2 partial tears of the hymen. Comparing hymenal trauma from sexual assault and accidental injuries, hymenal trauma was associated with a history of sexual assault in 23 of 43 cases (53.4%) versus 8 of 25 accidental injuries (32%). Of the 17 complete hymenal transections, 12 were associated with a history of penile-vaginal penetration, 1 occurred in a preverbal child who gave no history, and 4 were associated with penetrating accidental injuries. All but one tear was located between 4 and 8 o'clock on the hymenal rim.

In the same study,[24] partial tears of the hymen were noted between 4 and 8 o'clock as well. Histories accompanying these injuries included 4 children with digital-vaginal contact, 2 children with penile-vaginal penetration, one child with a straddle injury, and one preverbal child with no history. Injury to the posterior fourchette was most common, found in 58.3% of prepubertal children having sexual abuse trauma, and 51.8% of those children having accidental trauma. Perihymenal injuries were commonly associated with straddle injuries or digital-vaginal penetration. Labia majora/minora trauma was associated with straddle injuries. Very significantly, of the 171 injuries, only 14.6% healed with findings diagnostic of previous trauma. The authors concluded, "There are usually no acute or chronic residua to sexual contact. Most examinations for possible sexual abuse are normal or nonspecific because of the nature of the abuse of children, the child's perception of the abuse, and a delay in disclosure that allows injuries to heal."[24] The study also demonstrates an overlap of injury patterns associated with sexual abuse and accidental injury. The history is important to distinguish between these two causes.

There have been multiple studies of acute examination findings in adolescents following genital trauma,[25,27-30] although some have included adult subjects.[31-34] Sugar et al[35] in their study of 819 women coming to an urban emergency department, found that 37% of 15- to 19-year-old female rape victims had bodily injuries other than anogenital trauma including bruises, abrasions, fractures, visceral injuries, attempted strangulation, and intracranial trauma. In the same group, 29% had trauma to the genitals or anus. Girls with no prior history of intercourse had a much higher frequency of genital injury (39.5%) than those who had had prior intercourse (19.3%). A recent study by Drockton et al[32] of colposcopic photos of 3356 acutely sexually assaulted females over 12 years old examined the risk variables that were predictive of acute genital injury. These variables include vaginal penetration or attempted penetration with a penis, finger, or object; alcohol use during the incident; virginal status; and lack of lubricant use. There also was an association between acute genital injury and the inability of the victim to recall a penetration history. Another study by White[30] of 224 adolescents ages 12 to 17 from the United Kingdom having a history of rape or sexual assault compared injury patterns in virginal and nonvirginal girls. Again, those reporting no prior intercourse had more genital injuries than those with prior sexual experience (53% versus 32%). Injuries included lacerations, bruises, and abrasions.

Most studies of adolescents (and adults) agree that the most common acutely injured site after sexual assault is the posterior fourchette and fossa navicularis.[32,35,36] Adams et al[36] studied 214 acutely assaulted 14-to 19-year old girls and found that 40% had tears of the posterior fourchette and/or fossa navicularis. This consistent pattern in acutely sexually assaulted adolescents (and adults) strongly suggests that when injury is seen in adolescent rape victims, it occurs as a result of an entry injury, resulting from insertion or attempts at insertion of the penis or other object into the vagina.

HEALING OF ACUTE ANOGENITAL INJURIES

Prepubertal children rarely present for medical examinations immediately following sexual assault. Although few studies[24,25] detail the timing and the morphological changes in the healing process following sexual assault, it is clear that healing of hymenal tissue occurs rapidly and often completely, and that hymenal scarring is rare.[24] In a study by Heger of 13 boys and 81 girls with a history of sexual assault or anogenital trauma,[24] there were 171 injuries noted, only 25 of which healed leaving any stigmata of previous trauma (including two hymenal tears requiring reparative surgery). Penile-vaginal penetration was associated with the most significant injuries. This study indicated the importance of prompt examination and the likelihood of complete healing, even in cases of injuries causing pain and bleeding.

John McCann[25] led a multicenter retrospective longitudinal study of 113 prepubertal and 126 pubertal girls with acute hymenal trauma. The healing process was examined in detail to determine factors that might determine the age of a hymenal injury. Prepubertal children had both accidental and assault injuries, while postpubertal children had only assault injuries. The healing patterns and timing of key acute hymenal injuries such as petechiae, blood blisters, contusions, and lacerations were followed using photographs.

Petechiae of the hymen were defined as "pinpoint, non-raised perfectly round, purplish red spots on the hymenal membrane," and were identified acutely in 60% of prepubertal and 50% of adolescent girls. The authors found that petechiae resolved quickly. None were detected beyond 48 hours in prepubertal girls, or beyond 72 hours in adolescent girls. Hematomas of the hymen were described in the study as a circumscribed area of blood. Hematomas quickly evolved into diffuse submucosal hemorrhages. The authors noted that the submucosal hemorrhages in both prepubertal girls and adolescents were primarily found in the posterior quadrants of the hymen. Hematomas were relatively uncommon (4% in prepubertal girls and 10% in adolescents). Submucosal hemorrhages were common, found in 51% of prepubertal girls and 53% of adolescents.

The McCann et al[25] study documented the healing process in 40 hymenal lacerations in prepubertal girls and 80 hymenal lacerations in adolescents. There was a difference in location of acute injuries between the prepubertal and adolescent population. Prepubertal girls had predominantly posterior injuries (88%), with 8% lateral and 5% anterior injuries. The majority of the posterior injuries in prepubertal girls were midline. Conversely, adolescents' hymenal injuries were posterior only 61% of the time, with 29% being midline; 23% were at the lateral hymenal wall and 15% were anterior. Visualization of all the anterior findings required an adjunct technique.[37] As healing took place, changes were noted in the depth of the laceration and in the configuration of the laceration. In the prepubertal children, most lacerations became more superficial with healing (e.g., transections with an extension evolved into transections without an extension, deep lacerations evolved into intermediate or superficial lesions). However, 15% of deep lacerations had accompanying swelling of the tissues, which obscured the initial depth of a transection. In adolescents, similar patterns of healing were noted, as some transections became more superficial with healing and other injuries were noted to be deeper after swelling subsided. With regard to timing, the healing of acute hymenal lacerations began quickly and was complete by approximately 3 weeks in the prepubertal girl and 4 weeks in the adolescent girl. In both prepubertal and adolescent girls, the healing process resulted in continuity of the hymenal rim with a smooth edge in all but those with the most severe initial lacerations. Importantly, no scar was noted on any hymens.

McCann's study[25] noted that the extent of the hymenal injury dictated the final outcome of the configuration of the hymen in both prepubertal girls and adolescents. That is, those who had sustained either a transection or transection with an extension were much more likely to heal into either a transection or into a deep appearing laceration. In 15% of the cases the reverse was seen. When the swelling subsided, deep lacerations were actually complete transections. In prepubertal girls with a superficial, intermediate, or deep laceration, 75% healed to result in smooth hymenal rims with no disruption in contour, and even those with a hymenal transection or transection with an extension, surprisingly resulted in a smooth rim (17%) and continuous hymenal membrane (22%) on healing. Adolescent girls who had a superficial, intermediate, or deep laceration healed 59% of the time to have normally appearing (scalloped) hymenal rims.

This paper[25] further helped clarify the significance of the hymenal rim width of 1 mm in the presence of the history of penetration. Among prepubertal children with acute transections to the base of the hymen or with extensions into the surrounding tissue, 72% eventually healed with a hymenal rim width of greater than 1 mm. In adolescents, only 13% of these transections healed leaving a hymenal rim of less than 1 mm.

The authors noted several findings from their study. First, the study corroborated previous findings that genital injuries heal "… remarkably well and tend to leave little, if any, evidence of the previous trauma." They also concluded that the presence of petechiae and blood blisters are helpful in determining the age of a genital injury. Finally, they concluded that the rapidity of the healing process reminds us that children and adolescents need to be examined as soon as possible following a suspected sexual assault.

Interestingly, the authors noted that there did not seem to be any difference in the healing process between prepubertal girls and adolescent girls with regards to their hymenal injuries. None of the subjects' injuries resulted in scar tissue on the hymen. The authors reminded examiners to "… exercise caution before calling a finding normal, without evidence of a previous injury."

NONACUTE EXAMINATIONS OF PREPUBERTAL CHILDREN

Most prepubertal children are examined long after the alleged assault. Recent studies have verified that few sexually abused children have abnormal physical findings on their anal and genital examinations.[20,21,23] The reasons for this include: (1) in many cases, no physical injury is sustained at the time of the assault; (2) in some cases the genital and anal tissues are sufficiently elastic to distend or stretch without discernible injury during episodes of penetration; and (3) injuries that do occur usually heal quickly and completely.

Occasionally, children will have physical evidence of sexual abuse/assault that occurred sometime in the past including complete hymenal tears, deep hymenal notches, marked narrowing of their hymens, or scars in the posterior fourchette or fossa navicularis (Figures 11-4, 11-5, 11-6, 11-7, and 11-8). Studies on genital and anal findings in normal, nonabused children have contributed greatly to the examiner's ability to interpret findings in the nonacute setting.[4-12,39-40] One case-control study by Berenson compared vulvar and hymenal features in 192 prepubertal girls

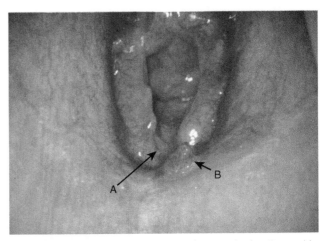

FIGURE 11-4 Arrow *A* indicates hymenal transection in a 2-year-old girl. Arrow *B* indicates condyloma in the child's fossa navicularis.

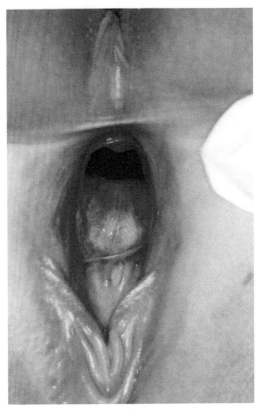

FIGURE 11-5 Marked narrowing of the hymenal tissue in a child who described ongoing sexual abuse, seen best in the knee chest position. Interpretation of this finding is controversial, and might be a normal or indeterminate finding.

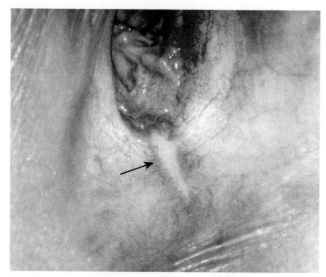

FIGURE 11-6 Scar on the posterior fourchette (at arrow) in a sexually abused child with a healed previous injury.

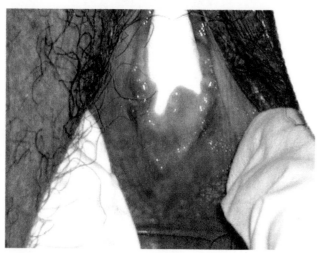

FIGURE 11-7 A deep hymenal cleft at 7 o'clock in a sexually abused girl.

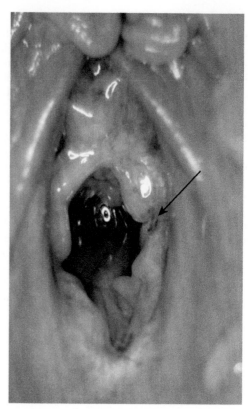

FIGURE 11-8 Seven-year-old girl described penile penetration over two years. Last incident was 48 hours before examination. Cleft at 6 o'clock indicates healed hymenal trauma. Arrow points to acute submucosal petechial hemorrhages.

ages 3 to 8 with a history of penetration and 200 children who denied prior abuse.[21] The median length of time between the last episode of the abuse and the examination was 42 days. The authors found physical findings strongly suggestive of sexual abuse in less than 5% of prepubertal girls. The findings from this study are detailed in Table 11-1. Of particular interest were the findings regarding hymenal notches. There was no difference between the abused and the nonabused group in the configuration of the notch ("U" vs. "V"). Likewise, there was no significant difference between these two groups in the prevalence of superficial hymenal notches. Children who reported three or more episodes of abuse were more likely to have a superficial notch (14%) than those who reported fewer episodes (0%) or no abuse (5%). However, deep notches and transections were observed only in abused children. The two deep notches were seen on the inferior rim of the hymen in children who were abused within 7 days of the examination. The authors concluded that a deep notch, a transection, or

a perforation on the inferior portion of the hymen could be considered as a definitive sign of sexual abuse or other trauma.

Based on this and other studies, child abuse pediatricians have developed an approach to the interpretation of findings, listed in Table 11-2.[42] It is important to realize that research in this field is ongoing, and guidelines might be modified as new information is obtained. Notable in the guidelines is the category of "Indeterminate Findings" based on insufficient or conflicting data from research studies. The authors note that these findings, "May require additional studies/evaluation to determine significance. These physical/laboratory findings may support a child's clear disclosure of sexual abuse if one is given, but should be interpreted with caution if the child gives no disclosure."[41] As an example of an indeterminate finding, the authors described the presence of deep clefts or notches in the posterior rim of the hymen, but have been rarely described in studies of nonabused girls. In the Berenson[21] study, no nonabused children had deep notches (greater than 50% of the width of the hymen), though notches less than 50% of the width of the hymen occurred equally in abused and nonabused children. Another finding listed as "indeterminate" is a hymenal rim of less than 1 mm in width. The rim is defined as the distance between the inner edge of the hymenal membrane and the attachment of the membrane to the muscular portion of the vaginal introitus, viewed in the coronal plane. It is accepted that an accurate measurement of the hymenal rim is quite difficult, and measurements may vary based on the child's

Table 11-1	Number and Percentage of Hymenal Findings in Abused *vs.* Nonabused Children		
Hymenal Feature	**Abused n = 192**	**Nonabused n = 200**	**Statistical Significance**
Prominent vessels	15 (8%)	13 (7%)	p = .70
Periurethral bands	180 (94%)	189 (95%)	p = .83
Vestibular bands	104 (55%)	120 (60%)	p = .31
Notches			
Superficial	13 (7%)	10 (5%)	p = .52
Deep	2 (1%)	0	p = .24
Transection	1 (1%)	0	p = .49
Perforation	1 (1%)	0	p = .49
Longitudinal intravaginal ridges	170 (89%)	174 (87%)	p = .65
External ridges	15 (8%)	16 (8%)	p = 1.0
Bumps	87 (46%)	92 (46%)	p = .92
Tags	5 (3%)	10 (5%)	p = .29

From Berenson AB, Chacko MR, Wiemann CM, et al: A case control study of anatomic changes resulting from sexual abuse, *Am J Obstet Gynecol* 2000;182:820-831.

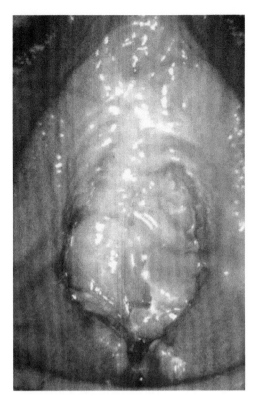

FIGURE 11-9 A 12-year-old female with a groove in the fossa navicularis, a normal finding in a well estrogenized female.

relaxation and the examiner's skill level. Thus the use of adjunct techniques such as "floating the hymen" with water and the use of multiple examination positions is often of critical importance in allowing complete visualization of the posterior rim of the hymen.

NONACUTE EXAMINATIONS OF ADOLESCENTS

Studies of healed injuries of adolescents presenting for forensic sexual abuse examinations include a retrospective case review by Kellogg et al of 36 pregnant adolescent girls presenting for forensic evaluations for suspected sexual abuse.[43] Only 2 of 36 (5.6%) were described as having clefts (transections) in the posterior rim of the hymen extending through to the base of the hymen. Overall, 22 (64%) had normal or nonspecific findings, 8 (22%) had inconclusive findings, 4(8%) had findings of abuse including deep notches and visible scars. All of the girls were examined at least one month following the most recent sexual contact. The authors reminded us that a "normal examination" does not mean that "nothing happened"[43] (see Figures 11-9 and 11-10).

A recent study (by Adams et al) of differences in hymenal morphology in adolescents ages 13 to 19 with (n = 27) and without (n = 58) a history of consensual intercourse found that 48% of the sexually active girls had deep notches or complete clefts in the lateral or posterior hymenal rim.[27] A

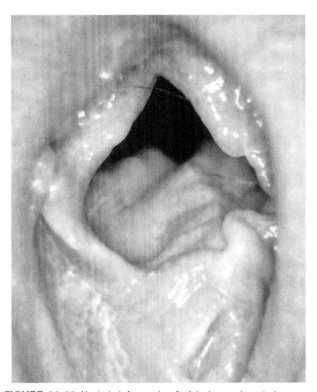

FIGURE 11-10 Healed cleft noted at 6 o'clock seen best in knee chest position.

Table 11-2	Approach to Interpreting Physical and Laboratory Findings in Suspected Child Sexual Abuse

Findings Documented in Newborns or Commonly Seen in Nonabused Children

(The presence of these findings generally neither confirms nor discounts a child's clear disclosure of sexual abuse.)

Normal Variants
1. Periurethral or vestibular bands
2. Intravaginal ridges or columns
3. Hymenal bumps or mounds
4. Hymenal tags or septal remnants
5. Linea vestibularis (midline avascular area)
6. Hymenal notch/cleft in the anterior (superior) half of the hymenal rim (prepubertal girls), on or above the 3 o'clock to 9 o'clock line, patient supine
7. Shallow/superficial notch or cleft in inferior rim of hymen (below 3 o'clock to 9 o'clock line)
8. External hymenal ridge
9. Congenital variants in appearance of hymen, including: cresentic, annular, redundant, septate, cribiform, microperforate, imperforate
10. Diastasis ani (smooth area)
11. Perianal skin tag
12. Hyperpigmentation of the skin of labia minora or perianal tissue of children of color
13. Dilatation of the urethral opening with application of labial traction
14. "Thickened" hymen (may be due to estrogen effect, folded edge of hymen, swelling from infection or swelling from trauma. The latter is difficult to assess unless follow-up examination is done.)

Findings Commonly Caused by Other Medical Conditions
15. Erythema (redness) of the vestibule, penis, scrotum, or perianal tissues (may be due to irritants, infection, or trauma)
16. Increased vascularity ("Dilatation of existing blood vessels") of vestibule and hymen may be due to local irritants or normal pattern in the nonestrogenized state.
17. Labial adhesions (may be due to irritation or rubbing)
18. Vaginal discharge (Many infectious and noninfectious causes, cultures must be taken to confirm if it is caused by sexually transmitted organism or other cause.)
19. Friability of the posterior fourchette or commissure (may be due to irritation, infection, or may be caused by examiners traction on the labia majora)
20. Excoriations/bleeding/vascular lesions. (These findings can be due to conditions such as lichen sclerosus eczema or seborrhea, vaginal/perianal group A streptococcus, urethral prolapse, hemangiomas.)
21. Perineal groove (failure of midline fusion), partial or complete
22. Anal fissures (usually due to constipation, perianal irritation)
23. Venous congestion or venous pooling in the perianal area (usually due to positioning, also seen with constipation)
24. Flattened anal folds (may be due to relaxation of the external sphincter or swelling of perianal tissues due to infection or trauma)
25. Partial or complete anal dilatation to less than 2 cm (A-P diameter), with or without stool visible (may be a normal reflex, or may have other causes, such as severe constipation or encopresis, sedation, anesthesia, neuromuscular conditions)

Indeterminate Findings: Insufficient or Conflicting Data from Research Studies
(May require additional studies/evaluation to determine significance. May support a child's clear disclosure of sexual abuse, if one is given, but should be interpreted with caution if the child gives no disclosure. In some cases, a report to child protective services may be indicated to further evaluate possible sexual abuse.)

Physical Examination Findings
26. Deep notches or clefts in the posterior/inferior rim of hymen in prepubertal girls, located between 4 and 8 o'clock, in contrast to transections (see 41)
27. Deep notches or complete clefts in the hymen at 3 or 9 o'clock in adolescent girls
28. Smooth, noninterrupted rim of hymen between 4 and 8 o'clock, which appears to be less than 1 mm wide, when examined in the prone knee-chest position, or using water to "float" the edge of the hymen when the child is in the supine position
29. Wartlike lesions in the genital or anal area (Biopsy and viral typing may be indicated in some cases if appearance is not typical of Condyloma accuminata.)
30. Vesicular lesions or ulcers in the genital or anal area (viral and/or bacterial cultures, or nucleic acid amplification tests may be needed for diagnosis)
31. Marked, immediate anal dilatation to an AP diameter of 2 cm or more in the absence of other predisposing factors

Lesions With Etiology Confirmed: Indeterminate Specificity for Sexual Transmission
32. Genital or anal condyloma in child, in the absence of any other indicators of abuse
33. Herpes Type 1 or 2 in the genital or anal area in a child with no other indicators of sexual abuse

Table 11-2	**Approach to Interpreting Physical and Laboratory Findings in Suspected Child Sexual Abuse—cont'd**

Findings Diagnostic of Trauma and/or Sexual Contact

(The following findings support a disclosure of sexual abuse, if one is given, and are highly suggestive of abuse even in the absence of a disclosure, unless the child and/or caregiver provide a clear, timely, plausible description of accidental injury. It is recommended that diagnostic quality photodocumentation of the examination findings be obtained and reviewed by an experienced medical provider before concluding that they represent acute or healed trauma. Follow-up examinations are also recommended.)

Acute Trauma to External Genital/Anal Tissues
34. Acute lacerations or extensive bruising of labia, penis, scrotum, perianal tissues, or perineum (may be from unwitnessed accidental trauma, or from physical or sexual abuse)
35. Fresh laceration of the posterior fourchette, not involving the hymen (must be differentiated from dehisced labial adhesion or failure of midline fusion; may also be caused by accidental injury or consensual sexual intercourse in adolescents)

Residual (Healing) Injuries
(These findings are difficult to assess unless an acute injury was previously documented at the same location.)
36. Perianal scar (rare, may be due to other medical conditions such as Crohn disease, accidental injuries, or previous medical procedures)
37. Scar of posterior fourchette or fossa (pale areas in midline may also be due to linea vestibularis or labial adhesions)

Injuries Indicative of Blunt Force Penetrating Trauma (or from Abdominal/Pelvic Compression Injury if such History is Given)
38. Laceration (tear, partial or complete) of the hymen, acute
39. Ecchymosis (bruising) on the hymen (in the absence of a known infectious process or coagulopathy)
40. Perianal lacerations extending deep to the external anal sphincter (not to be confused with partial failure of midline fusion)
41. Hymenal transection (healed): An area between 4 and 8 o'clock on the rim of the hymen where it appears to have been torn through, to or nearly to the base, so there appears to be virtually no hymenal tissue remaining at that location. This must be confirmed using additional examination techniques such as a swab, prone knee-chest position, or Foley catheter balloon, or water as appropriate. This finding has also been referred to as a "complete cleft" in sexually active adolescents and young adult women.
42. Missing segment of hymenal tissue: Area in the posterior (inferior) half of the hymen, wider than a transaction, with an absence of hymenal tissue extending to the base of the hymen, which is confirmed using additional positions/methods as described above

Presence of Infection Confirms Mucosal Contact With Infected and Infective Bodily Secretions, Contact most Likely to Have Been Sexual in Nature
43. Positive confirmed culture for gonorrhea, from genital area, anus, throat, in a child outside the neonatal period
44. Confirmed diagnosis of syphilis, if perinatal transmission is ruled out
45. Trichomonas vaginalis infection in a child older than 1 year of age, with organisms identified by culture or in vaginal secretions by wet mount examination by an experienced technician or clinician
46. Positive culture from genital or anal tissues for *Chlamydia*, if child is older than 3 years at time of diagnosis, and specimen was tested using cell culture or comparable method approved by the Centers for Disease Control and Prevention
47. Positive serology for HIV, if perinatal transmission, transmission from blood products, and needle contamination has been ruled out

Diagnostic of Sexual Contact
48. Pregnancy
49. Sperm identified in specimens taken directly from a child's body

From Adams JA, Kaplan FA, Starling SP, et al: Guidelines for medical care of children who may have been sexually abused. *J Pediatr Adolesc Gynecol* 2007;20:163-172 and Kellogg N, American Academy of Pediatrics Committee on Child Abuse and Neglect: Report to protective services recommended by AAP Guidelines, *Pediatrics* 2005;116:506-512.

deep notch was identified in 2 (3%) of subjects who denied prior intercourse. These subjects did describe prior painful insertion of a tampon but this phenomenon was seen in the nonsexually active group as well. In the girls who denied sexual intercourse, 52 of 58 used tampons, and 25 (48%) reported pain and difficulty with insertion of the tampon on the first attempt at using them. Emans et al addressed the issue of tampon use and hymenal anatomy in a prospective study of 300 girls and found that sexually active subjects were significantly more likely than nonsexually active tampon users and pad users to have complete clefts in the posterior hymen, and that the hymenal morphology of tampon users was not significantly different from pad users.[28]

The authors concluded that the presence of lateral or posterior deep notches or complete clefts of the hymen in adolescent girls should be strongly suggestive of previous penetration. They further concluded that 52% of the girls

who admitted past intercourse did not have deep notches or complete clefts in the lateral or posterior portion of the hymen and thus the absence of notches or clefts does not rule out previous penile-vaginal penetration in an adolescent.

Adolescents admitting to sexual intercourse were more likely to have a hymenal rim measurement less than or equal to 1 mm (22%) than adolescents who denied a history of previous intercourse (3%).[27] This study indicated that the absence of any injury to the hymen does not negate a history of penetration.

EVALUATION OF SERIOUS GENITAL INJURIES FROM SEXUAL ASSAULT

Acute injuries due to sexual assault in children and adolescents, though rare, sometimes require surgical consultation and management. The unestrogenized vaginal mucosa of prepubertal females is highly vascularized, leading to profuse bleeding with seemingly small vaginal injuries. Conversely, if there is a penetration through the vaginal wall, internal injury is possible in the presence or absence of bleeding and symptoms. Very forceful vaginal penetrating trauma can lead to severe lacerations along the lateral vaginal wall and posterior fornix. These patients can have vaginal bleeding that can lead to shock and are at risk of morbidity or death from exsanguination.

If the initial evaluation of the child or adolescent determines that the extent of the injury extends above the hymen, a further examination under anesthesia is usually necessary. Such an injury would preferably be handled by a team of specially trained clinicians, including surgeons and child abuse examiners experienced in collecting forensic evidence.

A recent study by Jones of genital and anorectal injuries requiring surgical repair in predominantly prepubertal females found that in comparison to accidental injuries, injuries from sexual abuse/assault were more likely to involve the internal vagina, anus, and rectum.[30] The severity of these injuries was second only to those found in motor vehicle accidents. Two older adolescent victims described their intercourse with older males as consenting, but had significant injuries (both had vaginal lacerations, one had an intraperitoneal extension of the tear, and the other presented in hemorrhagic shock). The authors suggest that the evaluation of children and adolescents with anal and genital injuries must be thorough and incorporate an assessment for sexual contact or abuse.

Genital and Anal Injuries in Sexual Abuse of Males

Far fewer sexual assaults are reported by boys compared to girls, particularly in adolescents. Finkelhor[44] found that boys were less likely to report than girls because of the fear of retribution, the social stigma against homosexual behavior, the desire to appear self-reliant, and the concern about loss of independence following disclosure. Types of abuse perpetrated on males includes forced anal penetration, oral-genital contact (either perpetrator on victim or victim on perpetrator), manual-genital contact by the perpetrator on the victim, or forced vaginal penetration of a female perpetrator.[45]

As is true for girls, when the boys are examined at a time distant from the traumatic event, the likelihood of physical findings decreases.[24] Occasionally male victims do have injuries such as genital bruises, burns, abrasions, lacerations, or "degloving" injuries (Figures 11-11, 11-12, and 11-13). In these types of injuries, it may be difficult to distinguish if the trauma was physical or sexual in nature.

There are few published studies on physical findings on pediatric male sexual assault. Reinhart[46] described 189 boys up to age 17 who were victims of sexual abuse. Five percent had genital abnormalities. All of the abnormalities were found in children under 12 years of age, and included bruising and bite marks, along with erythema, rashes, and urethral discharge, which may be more nonspecific in nature. A study of acute genital injuries in abused boys by Hobbs[47] suggested that injuries such as bruises and small petechial

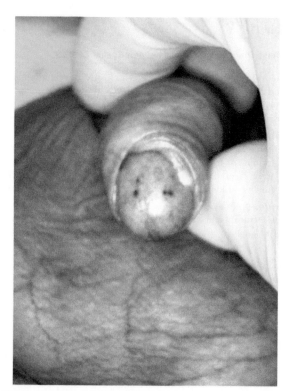

FIGURE 11-11 Twelve-year-old male with petichiae on glans of the penis. History of oral copulation.

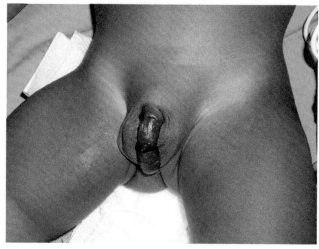

FIGURE 11-12 A "degloving injury" on the penis of a small boy.

hemorrhages, especially on the penile shaft, and tears of the delicate fold of skin at the ventral base of the foreskin, should raise concern for possible sexual abuse. He found that the most common site for injury was the prepuce or foreskin, suggesting forceful masturbation.

For a single episode of acute trauma in boys, anal findings are seen in 5% to 34%.[46,48,49] More recently, Heger[23] described abnormal findings in 1% of 177 boys who disclosed anal penetration. Most children were evaluated within 7 days of the last event. Another study of pediatric males with anogenital injuries seen in the emergency department found that accidental anogenital injuries were more

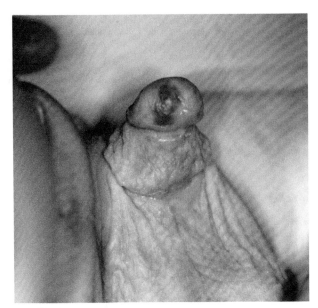

FIGURE 11-13 A bruise on a boy reporting being bitten on his penis.

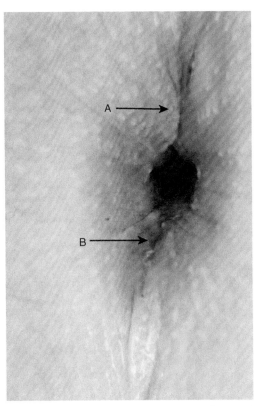

FIGURE 11-14 Anal lacerations extending out onto the normal squamous epithelium at 12 *(arrow A)* and 6 o'clock *(arrow B)*. Anal dilation can be a normal finding. History of sodomy 6 hours before examination. On follow up, the lacerations resolved.

likely to result in penile and scrotal injuries, and suspected victims of sexual abuse were much more likely to have rectal injury, which was usually midline.[48]

Anal Injuries

Children can experience both penetrating and nonpenetrating anal contact. Adolescents are more likely to report penetrating anal contact. Penetration can be by a penis, finger, or foreign object, and in rare cases, can lead to severe injuries.[50] Anal and rectal injuries are reported at about the same rate for males and females who report a history of anal penetration. Common anal injuries after penetration include lacerations, abrasions, and bruising (Figures 11-14).

In Heppenstall-Heger's longitudinal study of anal findings in assaulted and injured children,[24] anal trauma was documented in 30 of the 62 cases referred for sexual assault. There was one child with accidental trauma. There were 13 abrasions and 18 lacerations or tears; most of the acute trauma occurred at the midline at 12 and 6 o'clock. Four tears were transiently associated with changes in anal tone. Most acute trauma healed quickly and completely and only three cases (9.6%) healed with anatomic changes; one had an anal tag and two had scarring and hyperpigmentation after surgery for extensive tissue damage.

Anal findings indicative of trauma are rare in children who are *not* examined shortly after an assault. Adams et al[20] found anal lacerations ("clear evidence") in 2 of 213 (1%) of legally confirmed cases of childhood sexual abuse: Ninety-four percent had normal or nonspecific examinations.

DIRECTIONS FOR RESEARCH

Much research has been done in the area of delineating physical findings in both nonabused and nonsexually active prepubertal children and adolescents, along with children and adolescents who have been sexually abused and assaulted. However, further research is needed in multiple areas:

1. More large prospective multicenter studies are needed on the sequence and timing of the healing process of anogenital injuries in prepubertal children and adolescents. Such studies must use meticulously defined definitions of physical findings and be conducted in a blinded fashion. High quality photographs should be obtained, and examinations should be performed using standardized multimethod techniques for all examinations. Such data from larger studies will allow examiners to potentially interpret the presence and timing of healed anogenital injuries with a greater degree of accuracy and precision.

2. There are very few published studies of perianal injuries. Multicenter descriptive studies are badly needed that describe types of injuries seen and include follow-up examinations, as well as careful evaluations looking for any condition that could mimic an anogenital injury (e.g., constipation, Crohn's disease).

3. Critically, for this field, more studies of physical findings in populations of nonabused children and adolescents are needed. Such studies will help clarify indeterminate findings listed in consensus guidelines recently promulgated by a group of experts in child abuse pediatrics.[41] Further development of rigorous screening tools will be critical to further distinguish characteristics identifying a truly nonabused population. It has been the difficulty in obtaining a truly nonabused population that has made the interpretation of the normal studies challenging.

Although this field of research is relatively new, and surely challenged by the difficulties inherent in the subject and in the age of many of the children who present to our centers for examination, research in the field has progressed over the past 3 decades. The establishment of the many academic centers of excellence, and the multidisciplinary societies dedicated to the advancement of knowledge in child abuse and pediatric and adolescent gynecology have created fertile ground for future collaborative research in this area.

References

1. Cantwell HB: Vaginal inspection as it relates to child sexual abuse in girls under thirteen. *Child Abuse Negl* 1981;7:171-176.
2. Hobbs CJ, Wynne JM: Child sexual abuse; an increasing rate of diagnosis. *Lancet* 1987;1:837-841.
3. Hobbs CJ, Wynne JM: Sexual abuse of English boys and girls: the importance of anal examination. *Child Abuse Negl* 1989;13:195-210.
4. Jenny C, Kuhns ML, Arakawa F: Hymens in newborn females. *Pediatrics* 1987;80:399-400.
5. McCann J, Wells R, Simon M, et al: Genital findings in prepubertal girls selected for nonabuse: a descriptive study. *Pediatrics* 1990;86:428-439.
6. Berenson A, Heger A, Andrews S: Appearance of the hymen in newborns. *Pediatrics* 1991;87:458-465.
7. Gardner JJ: Descriptive study of genital variation in healthy, nonabused premenarchal girls. *J Pediatr* 1992;120:251-257.
8. Berenson AB, Heger AH, Hayes JM, et al: Appearance of the hymen in prepubertal girls. *Pediatrics* 1992;80:387-394.
9. Berenson AB: Appearance of the hymen at birth and one year of age: a longitudinal study. *Pediatrics* 1993;91:820-825.
10. Berenson AB: A longitudinal study of hymenal morphology in the first 3 years of life. *Pediatrics* 1995;95:490-496.
11. Myhre AK, Bemtzen K, Bratlid D: Genital anatomy in non-abused preschool girls. *Acta Paediatr* 2003;92:1453-1462.
12. Heger AH, Ticson L, Guerra L, et al: Appearance of the genitalia in girls selected for nonabuse: review of hymenal morphology and nonspecific findings. *J Pediatr Adolesc Gynecol* 2002;15:27-35.
13. American Professional Society on the Abuse of Children Task Force on Medical Evaluation of Suspected Child Abuse: *Descriptive terminology in child sexual abuse medical evaluations.* American Professional Society on the Abuse of Children, Chicago, 2003.
14. Boyle C, McCann J, Miyamoto S, et al: Comparison of examination methods used in the evaluation of prepubertal and pubertal female genitalia: a descriptive study. *Child Abuse Negl* 2008;32:229-243.
15. Lauber AA, Souma SM: Use of toluidine blue for documentation of traumatic intercourse. *Obstet Gynecol* 1982;60:644-648.
16. McCauley J, Guzinski G, Welch R, et al: Toluidine blue in the corroboration of rape in the adult victim. *Am J Emerg Med* 1987;5:105-108.
17. Heger A, Ticson L, Velasquez O, et al: Children referred for possible sexual abuse: medical findings in 2384 children. *Child Abuse Negl* 2002;26:645-659.
18. Christian CW, Lavelle JM, De Jong AR, et al: Forensic evidence findings in prepubertal victims of sexual assault. *Pediatrics* 2000;106:100-104.
19. Muram D: Child sexual abuse: relationship between sexual acts and genital findings. *Child Abuse Negl* 1989;13:211-216.
20. Adams JA, Harper K, Knudson S, et al: Examination findings in legally confirmed child sexual abuse: it's normal to be normal. *Pediatrics* 1994;94:310-317.
21. Berenson AB, Chacko MR, Wiemann CM, et al: A case control study of anatomic changes resulting from sexual abuse. *Am J Obstet Gynecol* 2000;182:820-831.
22. Finkel MA: Anogenital trauma in sexually abused children. *Pediatrics* 1989;84:317-322.
23. Heger A, Ticson L, Velasquez O, et al: Children referred for possible sexual abuse: medical findings in 2384 children. *Child Abuse Negl* 2002;26:645-659.
24. Heppenstall-Heger A, McConnell G, Ticson L, et al: Healing patterns in anogenital injuries: a longitudinal study of injuries associated with sexual abuse, accidental injuries, or genital surgery in the preadolescent child. *Pediatrics* 2003;112:829-837.
25. McCann J, Miyamoto S, Boyle C, et al: The healing of hymenal injuries in prepubertal and adolescent females: a descriptive study. *Pediatrics* 2007;110:e1094-e1106.
26. Palusci VJ, Cox EO, Shatz EM, et al: Urgent medical assessment after child sexual abuse. *Child Abuse Negl* 2006;30:367-380.
27. Adams JA, Botash AS, Kellogg N: Differences in hymenal morphology in adolescent girls with and without a history of consensual sexual intercourse. *Arch Pediatr Adolesc Med* 2004;158:280-285.
28. Emans SJ, Woods ER, Allred EN, et al: Hymenal findings in adolescent women; impact of tampon use and consensual sexual activity. *J Pediatr* 2004;125:153-160.
29. Jones J, Dunnuck C, Rossman L, et al: Adolescent Foley catheter technique for visualizing hymenal injuries in adolescent sexual assault. *Acad Emerg Med* 2003;10:1001-1004.
30. Jones JG, Worthington T: Genital and anal injuries requiring surgical repair in females less than 21 years of age. *J Pediatr Adolesc Gynecol* 2008;21:207-211.
31. White C, McLean I: Adolescent complainants of sexual assault; injury patterns in virgin and non-virgin groups. *J Clin Forensic Med* 2006;13:172-180.
32. Drockton P, Sachs C, Chu L, et al: Validation set correlates of anogenital injury after sexual assault. *Acad Emerg Med* 2008;15:231-238.
33. Slaughter L, Brown C, Crowley S, et al: Patterns of genital injury in female sexual assault victims. *Am J Obstet Gynecol* 1997;176:609-616.
34. Riggs N, Houry D, Long G, et al: Analysis of 1076 cases of sexual assault. *Ann Emerg Med* 2000;35:358-362.
35. Sugar NF, Fine DN, Eckert LO: Physical injury after sexual assault. *Am J Obstet Gynecol* 2004;190:71-76.
36. Adams JA, Giardin B, Faugno D: Adolescent sexual assault: documentation of acute injuries using photo-colposcopy. *J Pediatr Adolesc Gynecol* 2001;14:175-180.
37. Jones JS, Rossman L, Hartman M, et al: Anogenital injuries in adolescents after consensual sexual intercourse. *Acad Emerg Med* 2003;10:1378-1383.
38. Boyle C: Personal communication. August, 2008.
39. Berenson AB, Grady JJ: A longitudinal study of hymenal development from 3 to 9 years of age. *J Pediatr* 2002;140:600-607.
40. Berenson A, Heger A, Andrews S: Appearance of the hymen in newborns. *Pediatrics* 1991;87:458-465.
41. McCann J, Voris J, Simon M, et al: Perianal findings in prepubertal children selected for nonabuse: a descriptive study. *Child Abuse Negl* 1989;13:179-193.
42. Adams JA, Kaplan FA, Starling SP, et al: Guidelines for medical care of children who may have been sexually abused. *J Pediatr Adolesc Gynecol* 2007;20:163-172.
43. Kellogg ND, Menard SW, Santos A: Genital anatomy in pregnant adolescents: "normal" does not mean "nothing happened." *Pediatrics* 2004;113:67-69.
44. Finkelhor D, Hotaling G, Lewis IA, et al: Sexual abuse in a national survey of adult men and women: prevalence, characteristics, and risk factors. *Child Abuse Negl* 1990;14:19-28.
45. Holmes WC, Slap GB: Sexual abuse of boys. *JAMA* 1998;280:1855-1862.
46. Reinhart MA: Sexually abused boys. *Child Abuse Negl* 1987;11:229-235.
47. Hobbs CJ, Osman J: Genital injuries in boys and abuse. *Arch Dis Child* 2007;92:328-331.
48. Kadish JA, Schunk JE, Britton H: Pediatric male rectal and genital trauma: accidental and nonaccidental injuries. *Pediatr Emerg Care* 1998;14:95-98.
49. Muram D: Anal and perianal abnormalities in prepubertal victims of sexual abuse. *Am J Obstet Gynecol* 1989;161:278-281.
50. Orr CJ, Clark MA, Hawley CA, et al: Fatal anorectal injuries: a series of four cases. *J Forensic Sci* 1995;40:219-221.

12

MEDICAL CONDITIONS WITH GENITAL/ANAL FINDINGS THAT CAN BE CONFUSED WITH SEXUAL ABUSE

Mark J. Hudson, MD, Alice D. Swenson, MD, Rich Kaplan, MD, and Carolyn J. Levitt, MD

The medical evaluation of sexual abuse, while predominantly relying upon history, needs to include a thorough and specialized genital and anal examination. Examiners require a detailed understanding of physical findings that might be suggestive or even diagnostic of genital trauma or sexually transmitted infections. In addition, health professionals examining possible victims of sexual abuse must have a thorough knowledge of those medical conditions that can cause genital and/or anal findings that might be confused with abusive trauma or sexually transmitted infections. As the evidence base relating to the interpretation of genital and anal findings has grown, there has been a concurrent recognition of those medical conditions that can be confused with findings from abusive trauma. It is therefore critical that the examiner has up-to-date information on such clinical entities.

"Mimics" range from the relatively common finding of erythema to uncommon presentations such as genital ulcerations. In this chapter we review several of the more common conditions including those that are associated with inflammatory changes, other medical mimics, and non-sexual genital trauma.

IRRITANTS AND DERMATITIS

Vaginitis, vulvitis, and vulvovaginitis are nonspecific signs with a multitude of causes (Figure 12-1). Dermatitis is the most common vulvar condition in children and most often the result of atopy or irritants in nondiapered children.[1] The onset of symptoms related to vulvar atopic dermatitis can be after the child is toilet trained. Children often present with vulvar itching and the labia majora are dry, erythematous, and can be lichenified. The labia minora can be involved. Desquamation of the labia minora can lead to staining of the underwear, which is often interpreted as vaginal discharge. Treatment includes emollients and 1% hydrocortisone cream.[2]

A significant cause of genital discharge, pain, irritation, and redness in toilet trained children appears to be poor hygiene habits, which lead to an irritant contact dermatitis.[3] In fact, improved hygiene techniques are often curative in children without a history of trauma and with examination findings suggestive of poor hygiene habits.[4] Wiping the vulvo-perianal area from back to front has been implicated as a risk factor. Soaps, bubble baths, and shampoo can also lead to irritant contact dermatitis, as can prolonged wearing of wet swimming suits and shaving or plucking of pubic hair.[2,5] Allergic vulvar dermatitis is a rare finding in young children but has been reported as the result of the dyes, rubber chemicals, or glues in diapers.[6,7] Pinworms can be found in more than 30% of children presenting for medical care because of signs or symptoms of vulvovaginitis.[3] *Candida* can be seen in diapered children, but it is rarely a cause of vulvovaginitis in nondiapered children before puberty.[2,4]

Diaper dermatitis is the most common dermatological condition in diapered children. Though there are clear overlaps and a distinction is somewhat artificial, diaper dermatitis can be divided into primary and secondary types. Secondary diaper dermatitis is defined as an eruption that occurs in the diaper area with a defined cause. Causes of secondary diaper dermatitis include malaria rubra (the result of blockage of the eccrine ducts), seborrheic dermatitis, and allergic contact dermatitis and a variety of other infectious agents.[8]

Primary diaper dermatitis is ill defined and is primarily noninfectious and nonallergic. The cause is multifactorial and the most important factors are moisture, friction, urine, feces, and sometimes microorganisms. Persistent moisture and fecal enzymes disrupt skin integrity and cause the skin to be more susceptible to injury. The clinical presentation of primary diaper dermatitis can be varied, but often includes erythema and mild scaling of the gluteal cleft, buttocks, thighs, and lower abdomen (Figure 12-2). There may be maceration in the skin folds and areas rubbed by the diaper are often most severely affected. First line treatment of primary diaper dermatitis is elimination of the irritants. This includes daily baths, frequent diaper changes, and barrier creams such as zinc oxide. Second line treatment includes 1% hydrocortisone cream, antifungal cream, and mupirocin ointment.[8]

Children who have chronic incontinence of feces or urine can develop Jacquet erosive diaper dermatitis of the genital or perianal skin (Figure 12-3), "characterized by 2-5 mm well-demarcated papules and nodules with central umbilication or punched-out ulcers."[9,10] There have been other reports linking chronic incontinence of feces or urine to pseudoverrucous papules and nodules mimicking condyloma acuminatum (Figure 12-4).[10]

Though more likely mistaken for physical rather than sexual abuse, severe dermatitis resembling a scald burns have been reported in children who have ingested senna-containing laxatives. The exact pathogenic mechanism is

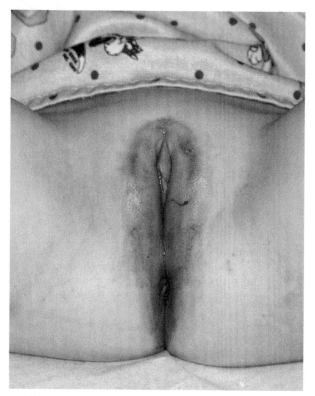

FIGURE 12-1 Five-year-old girl with vulvovaginitis secondary to a vaginal foreign body.

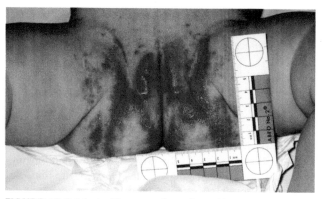

FIGURE 12-2 Infant with severe diaper dermatitis.

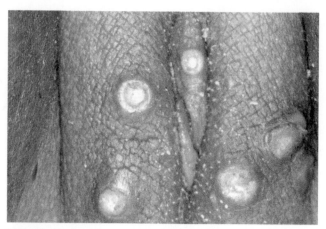

FIGURE 12-3 Close-up view of labia majora and minora of a 6-year-old girl with Jacquet erosive diaper dermatitis from chronic incontinence of urine. She had a congenital myelomeningocele and was awaiting ileal diversion.

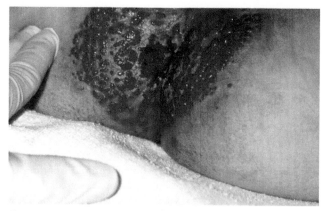

FIGURE 12-4 Prepubertal girl with ulcerated erythematous perianal pseudoverrucous papules and nodules mimicking HPV. She had continuous incontinence of watery feces.

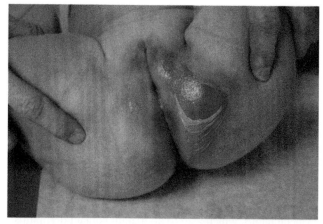

FIGURE 12-5 Diaper area burn caused by accidental ingestion of laxatives containing senna as the active ingredient. Initially the lesions were thought to be due to unexplained burns and the child was referred for a child abuse evaluation.

unclear but appears to be related to irritant effects of the senna (Figure 12-5).[11]

LABIAL ADHESIONS

Labial adhesions are often noted as an incidental finding (Figure 12-6). Less frequently they are discovered in the course of evaluation of genital complaints such as discomfort, dysuria, or recurrent vulvar or vaginal infections. They can also present with blood in the underwear if adhesions are lysed through the course of play or through minor genital trauma (Figure 12-7). The vestibule is sometimes obscured and patients present with a thin avascular line in the midline. The fusion can appear thin and filmy or dense and fibrous.

The true incidence of labial adhesions is unknown. Many girls with adhesions remain asymptomatic and never require

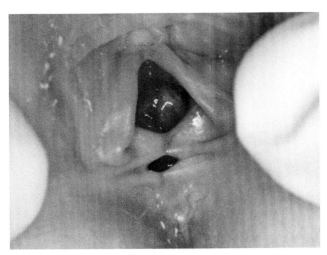

FIGURE 12-6 The labial adhesions found in this 6-year-old girl makes it difficult to assess the hymen.

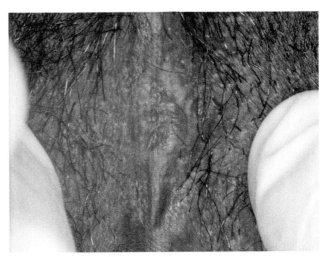

FIGURE 12-8 A 15-year-old girl with "ambiguous" genitalia because of female circumcision, resembling labial fusion. The labia were surgically sutured together in childhood.

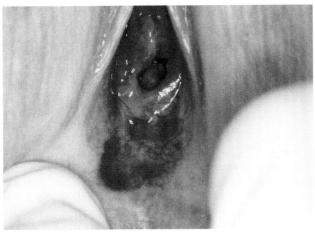

FIGURE 12-7 Labial adhesions were separated by recent minor accidental trauma that caused minimal bleeding and led to referral for a sexual abuse evaluation for unexplained genital bleeding. Note that the separation resulted in raw, denuded, red skin present on one side and not on the other.

medical intervention. The pediatric gynecologic literature reports an incidence of 0.6 to 3.0% in prepubertal girls; however, the sexual abuse literature focused on collecting normative values reports a much higher incidence.[12] McCann reported an incidence of 38.9% but many of these adhesions were 2 mm or less.[13] Berenson reported agglutination significant enough to obscure visualization of the hymen in 5% of girls less than 7 years old and partial agglutination in another 17%.[14]

The cause of labial adhesions remains unclear but is thought to be related to conditions that cause local irritation combined with the low estrogen level of childhood. Some suggest that the thin skin covering the labia is easily denuded as a result of local irritation which leads to the labia adhering in the midline. As re-epithelialization occurs on both sides the labial remain fused. The fact that labial adhesions are rarely seen during childbearing years supports a protective role for estrogen. The exact role of estrogen however is unclear and some authors argue that estrogen may not be a factor at all.[15] Female circumcision can mimic labial adhesions (Figure 12-8).

Treatment of labial adhesions is controversial and longitudinal studies are lacking. Many advocate for no treatment in children with asymptomatic adhesions. Most adhesions resolve without treatment and virtually all resolve with the onset of puberty. Adhesions that result in discomfort, dysuria, recurrent vulvar or vaginal infections, or urinary retention might require intervention. If adhesions obscure the hymen in a suspected sexual abuse victim, a history suggestive of hymenal injury should guide the decision to treat, given the low overall incidence of hymenal findings in sexually abused children. Estrogen cream is usually considered first line treatment but side effects such as local skin pigmentation and breast budding can occur. Estrogen cream should be used sparingly for a short period of time in prepubertal child. One study suggested a success rate with estrogen use of only about fifty percent.[16] Betamethasone 0.05% cream might also be an effective treatment, either as first line therapy or for patients that have failed previous therapy.[17] Mechanical separation can be effective. This can be done in the office very gently with or without local anesthetic using an examining finger, swab or probe. Dense adhesions causing symptoms might require surgical intervention Estrogen cream following mechanical separation helps prevent recurrence.

CROHN DISEASE

Crohn disease or regional enteritis is a chronic inflammatory bowel disease (IBD). Unlike ulcerative colitis, which presents as mucosal inflammation of only the colon, Crohn is characterized by transmural "skip lesions" that can occur anywhere in the gastrointestinal tract from the mouth to the anus. Such anal lesions have caused concern for abuse in clinical reports (Figure 12-9).[18,19] In addition to GI tract findings, several reports have described so-called "metastatic Crohn" with cutaneous and genital manifestations. Crohn vulvitis was first described by Parks in 1965.[20] A careful family history is important as approximately 20% of patients have an affected relative. Additionally, a complete history

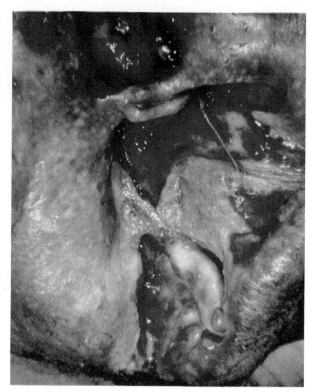

FIGURE 12-9 Ten-year-old girl recently diagnosed with Crohn disease. Perianal tissue is destroyed making it difficult to discern landmarks. Note the hymen at top of photo.

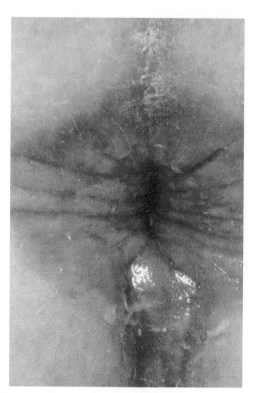

FIGURE 12-10 Six-year-old boy with perianal streptococcal cellulitis. He also had impetigo.

and physical evaluation will reveal characteristic findings, including poor growth, diarrhea, abdominal pain, and enteric blood loss.[21] The accurate diagnosis of Crohn disease can be critically important to a young patient.

GENITAL/ANAL INFECTIONS

There are a variety of bacteria that can cause significant genital or anal inflammation in children. In a study looking primarily at *Gardnerella vaginalis* in nonabused preschool children, Myhre and colleagues[22] cultured a wide variety of common pathogenic and nonpathogenic bacteria from the youngsters. Isolates included *Streptococcus pyogenes, Staphylococcus aureus, Streptococcus pneumonia, Escherichia coli,* and *Hemophilus influenzae.* Among those isolates, *Streptococcus pyogenes* and *Hemophilus influenzae* were commonly associated with inflammatory findings.[22] *Streptococcus pyogenes, Staphylococcus aureus,* and *Hemophilus influenzae* are well documented causes of vulvar and perianal infection. Though trained examiners rarely confuse such infections with abusive trauma, the child's caregivers and perhaps some less experienced examiners might attribute clinical findings of vulvovaginitis to trauma (Figure 12-10). In addition to the often-needed reassurance, identification and treatment are crucial as well. There is evidence, for example, that the reactive arthritis associated with group A streptococcal pharyngitis can also occur in association with genital infections.[23] There are reports of methicillin-resistant *Staphylococcus aureus* (MRSA) vulvar infections in women,[24] and scrotal ulceration in men.[25] A complete medical evaluation of these infections necessarily includes bacterial and viral cultures.

Finally, with respect to infectious mimics, warty growths such as *verruca vulgaris* and *molluscum contagiosum* can certainly be confused with human papillomavirus (HPV) infections and thus raise concern for the possibility of sexual contact (Figure 12-11). Because of the absence of clarity with respect to the transmission of HPV, these findings should be treated quite conservatively when there is no history for sexual contact. Verruca and molluscum are generally self-limiting infections.

FOREIGN BODIES

Vaginal foreign bodies have been reported in 4% to 10% of prepubertal girls who come in for evaluation of persistent vaginal discharge.[26,27] Vaginal bleeding and blood-stained, foul-smelling discharge are the primary symptoms mimicking sexually transmitted infections (STI) or trauma. The presence of blood is an important predictor and is found in at least 50% of children with a vaginal foreign body.[26-28] A recurrent or persistent discharge despite changes in hygiene habits and antibiotic treatment can be a clue to the diagnosis. Many times a detailed history will reveal that the child recalls the insertion of the item.[28] Retained toilet paper is common but any number of other objects are inserted. In some situations, foreign body insertion is associated with a history of sexual abuse. Symptoms usually resolve after the removal of the foreign body. Irrigation can be used but is unlikely to be effective unless the foreign body is in the distal vagina and can be visualized (Figure 12-12). Radiographic imaging can be helpful but a negative study does not rule out a foreign body. Vaginoscopy with anesthesia is indicated

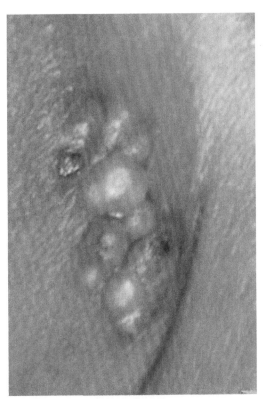

FIGURE 12-11 Lesions of molluscum contagiosum resembling genital warts found near the scrotum of an 18-month-old boy.

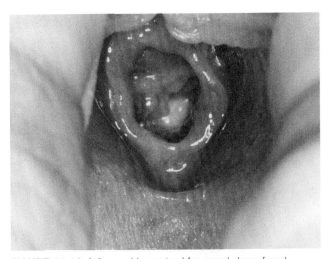

FIGURE 12-12 A 6-year-old examined for sexual abuse found incidentally to have a nonpurulent, watery vaginal discharge. A yellow foreign body (a thumbtack) was removed under anesthesia.

if suspicion of a foreign body is high or if the patient has persistent bloody vaginal discharge. Vaginoscopy allows the identification of foreign bodies and other pathology, such as malignancies and fistulas.[26,29]

VASCULAR PROBLEMS

Both vasculitides and vascular anomalies can raise concern for genital trauma. Apparent genital trauma, including acute scrotal hemorrhage and stenosing urethritis, have been described in association with Henoch-Schönlein purpura.[30,31] Levin and Selbst[32] described a case in which a vulvar hemangioma was thought to be a traumatic finding. Penile lymphangioma associated with cellulitis has also been described and can appear to be of traumatic origin.[33] While these conditions are most often confused with physical abuse, any time there is concern for inflicted genital trauma, the specter of sexual abuse is raised.

NEOPLASIA

Sarcomas, carcinomas, and germ cell tumors of the genitals have all been reported in childhood. Of these, the embryonal type of rhabdomyosarcoma, sarcoma botryoides, is far and away the most common.[34,35] It presents as a polypoid mass protruding from the vagina sometimes confused with urethral prolapse or human papillomavirus (HPV). Unexplained genital masses should, of course be referred for definitive diagnosis as soon as possible.

ANAL FINDINGS

Among parents and health professionals alike, the issue of fecal incontinence often raises concern for sexual abuse. There are some publications that describe an association of encopresis with sexual abuse.[36-38] These studies, however, have methodological shortcomings and do not confirm that fecal incontinence is a reliable indicator of sexual abuse. In one study that examined fecal soiling as a predictor of sexual abuse, children with a history of sexual abuse were compared with children referred for psychiatric evaluation and a normative sample.[39] While the sexually abused group did have significantly more incontinence than the normative sample, there was no significant difference compared with the group referred for psychiatric evaluation, indicating that soiling is not a reliable sign of sexual abuse.

Chronic constipation can be associated with marked anal dilatation on examination, and the dilatation should not be assumed to be a sign of sexual abuse.[40] Anal dilatation can also be seen as a normal variant when stool is not present in the rectal vault.[41] Anal fissures are a rare finding in the general pediatric population; however, they are seen in approximately 25% of children evaluated for constipation.[40-42]

Perianal erythema is common and is not a specific sign of sexual abuse. Perianal venous congestion can resemble a perianal bruise but is a common finding, particularly when children are in a knee-chest position for an extended time (Figure 12-13). Perianal skin tags are not an indicator of sexual abuse trauma and frequently are found in the midline.[42]

Rectal prolapse is rare in children, but when it does occur, the child is usually brought urgently to medical attention and this might raise concern for rectal trauma and sexual abuse. It is most common before age 4 and the incidence is highest in the first year of life. It can involve only the mucosa or all layers of the rectum. The latter condition is referred to as procidentia. Parents often note a dark, red mass and excess mucus emerging from the anal verge, but note that the child does not appear to be in pain. Often the prolapse resolves by the time the child comes for medical attention. Because up to 23% of cystic fibrosis patients can

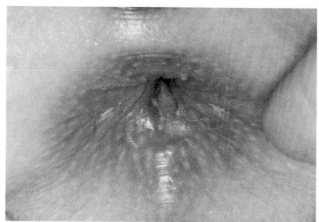

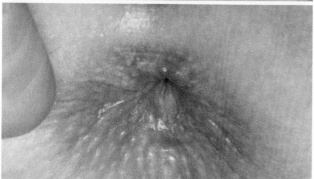

FIGURE 12-13 A 4-year-old girl whose examination demonstrates perianal venous engorgement mimicking a bruise (upper image). When the examiner's hands are removed from putting pressure on the ischium, the venous engorgement abates and the area becomes normal (lower image).

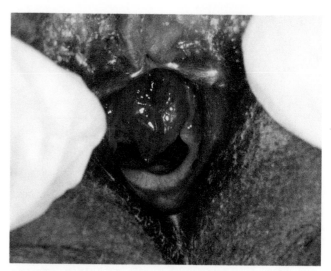

FIGURES 12-14 Urethral prolapse found incidentally in a 5-year-old girl on a colposcopic examination for suspected abuse.

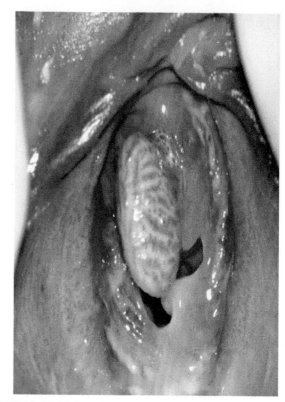

FIGURES 12-15 A urethral prolapse that mimics a condyloma acuminatum.

have rectal prolapse, sweat chloride testing is indicated in any child with rectal prolapse. Recurrent prolapse can require surgical intervention.[43]

Dilated hemorrhoid veins can be a source of rectal bleeding leading to the consideration of trauma. Hemorrhoids are rare in young children but more commonly effect teens and young adults. In children hemorrhoids are usually benign but the possibility of portal hypertension should be entertained. Treatment is often only symptomatic but any associated constipation or fecal impaction should be treated to avoid recurrence.[44]

URETHRAL PROLAPSE

Prolapse of the urethral mucosa in girls is an uncommon condition.[45,46] The prolapse appears as a friable rosette of bright red or cyanotic tissue in the urethral area (Figure 12-14). At times the prolapse is large enough to fill the vulvar introitus and obscure the hymen.[47] The disorder occurs most commonly in prepubertal girls between the ages of 1 to 10 years.[48] Usually there are no symptoms and the prolapse is visualized incidentally after bathing as a red-colored mass protruding from the labia. Bleeding from the genital area, which is generally minimal but commonly attributed to trauma, is often the first sign of urethral prolapse, and pain or tenderness are infrequent.[47,49,50] Rarely there can be urinary retention.[51,52]

Clinicians not experienced with urethral prolapse may mistake its presentation with that of sexual abuse, particularly when the presenting complaint is vaginal bleeding or the prolapse is hemorrhagic, thereby mimicking acute trauma to the hymen.[53] In addition urethral prolapse can resemble human papillomavirus (HPV) infection of the urethral area (Figure 12-15). Predisposing factors to this condition are thought to be perineal trauma, straining with constipation, diarrhea, or coughing.[47,49] Urethral prolapse is seen most commonly in African-American girls with some studies reporting as many as 89% to 100% of cases occurring in African-American girls.[45,47-49]

It is unclear whether urethral prolapse requires any treatment since most are asymptomatic before discovery. The literature is of little help, with most case series in pediatric urology, pediatric surgery, or gynecology journals describing simple resection as the favored mode of treatment. Those who treat all their patients surgically do it because they believe those treated medically might not gain complete resolution of the prolapse or are more prone to recurrent prolapse,[48] but this has not been clearly demonstrated.[50]

Medical management of urethral prolapse is suggested by several authors. Favored treatments include sitz baths, topical antibiotics, estrogen creams, bed-rest, topical steroids, or some combination of the above.[47,50,51] These approaches have varying degrees of success. Most or all patients have resolution of symptoms,[47,50] and in one study, either marked decrease in the size of the prolapse or complete absence of the protrusion was found on follow-up examination.[50] Within the child abuse pediatrics community, a "watchful waiting" approach has been advocated by many clinicians. Certainly if the presentation is benign with only mild spotting, it is reasonable to simply re-examine the patient several weeks after the initial presentation for evidence of resolution. Anecdotal evidence suggests that such an approach is viable and avoids some of the side effects of the medical management, such as systemic absorption of topical estrogen, and the morbidities associated with surgical management such as infection, stenosis, or complications of general anesthesia.

URETEROCELE

A ureterocele is a relatively rare urinary malformation in which a cystic dilatation of the terminal ureter extends into the bladder, urethra, or both.[54] The American Academy of Pediatrics classifies ureteroceles as either intravesical (within the bladder) or ectopic, in which the tissue can lie within the bladder neck or urethra. When the ureterocele extends into the distal urethra it can protrude through the urethral meatus and present as an erythematous, cystic introital mass (Figure 12-16).[55] Like urethral prolapse, the presenting symptoms, including protrusion or vaginal bleeding, can be confused with sexual abuse. A prolapsed ureterocele can be asymptomatic or can have symptoms of abdominal or pelvic pain, urinary tract infections, hematuria, obstruction, or in severe cases urosepsis.[54] Patients with prolapsed ureteroceles are often quite uncomfortable and describe a feeling of needing to strain or pass something from the perineal area. Ureteroceles are seen most commonly in Caucasians and are 4 to 6 times more common in girls than in boys.[54] Ureteroceles are frequently associated with other urinary tract abnormalities, such as ureteric duplication. Abdominal ultrasound is the initial diagnostic test of choice for ureterocele, and a voiding cystourethrogram can be complementary. Management of prolapsed ureterocele is surgical.

LICHEN SCLEROSUS ET ATROPHICUS

Lichen sclerosus et atrophicus (LS & A) is a dermatologic condition appearing in young girls and is diagnosed by a characteristic appearance of thinned, white, crinkly or wrinkled skin that often forms a figure of 8 appearance, including the perineum and the perianal tissues (Figure 12-17).[56,57] The skin appears bruised with small broken blood vessels. Fissuring is common in the perianal area and around the labia minora. Small hematomas are often present, but can involve the entire labia minora (Figure 12-18). Many of the children are asymptomatic and present when the apparent "injury" to the genital area is first noted by the child or parent. Most commonly in childhood LS & A symptoms are mild, including pruritus and dysuria along with constipation attributed to stool withholding because of painful defecation from the perianal fissuring.

LS & A is often mistaken for acute genital trauma because the involved skin is friable and prone to bleeding from minimal trauma. One young girl came in for evaluation with multiple small circular hematomas arranged symmetrically in a pattern on each side of the labia majora where the skin folds. She had reported that she had just begun to ride her bike that spring. Because findings resemble acute trauma and a history of trauma is denied, clinicians will sometimes suspect sexual abuse.

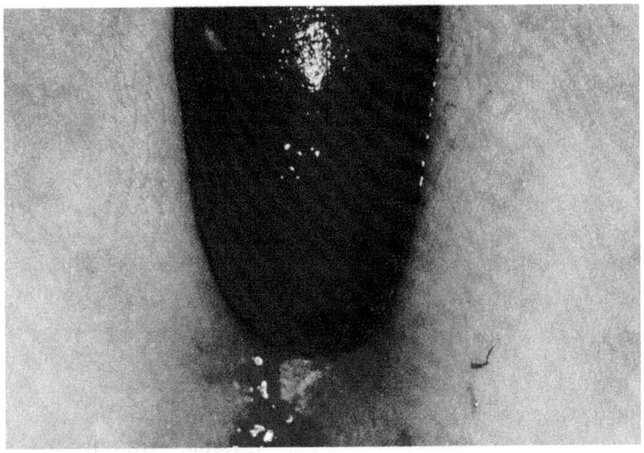

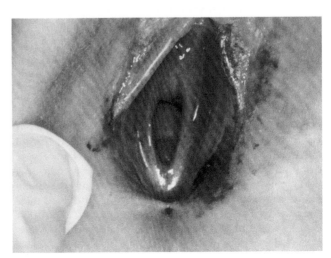

FIGURE 12-16 Prolapsed ureterocele noted in a toddler. A large cystic mass fills the introitus, obscuring the hymen and other landmarks.

FIGURE 12-17 Lichen sclerosus et atrophicus in a prepubertal girl. Note the thin, white, atrophic, friable skin on the genitals that bleeds with minimal trauma.

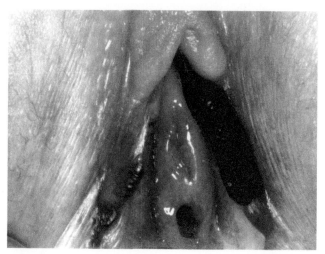

FIGURE 12-18 A prepubertal girl who came to the emergency department complaining of minimal genital pain. She had no history of trauma to explain the large hematomas on the labia minora. She was diagnosed with lichen sclerosus et atrophicus.

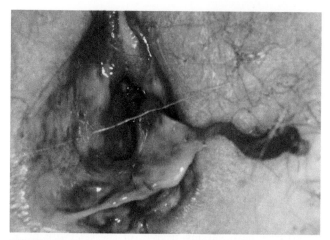

FIGURE 12-19 A 12-year-old girl with coalesced necrotic genital ulcers that were not due to herpes virus nor Behçet disease. When examined under anesthesia, she had no other findings. She was treated with antibiotics and the ulcers resolved over a 2-week period.

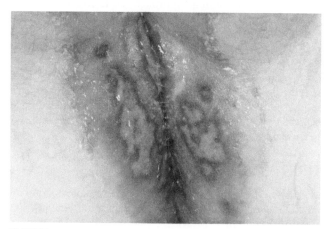

FIGURE 12-20 Genital herpes due to herpes virus type II.

The natural history of LS & A in the childhood population has not been well studied. Clearly, there have been concerns raised about the chronicity and morbidity of this condition in older women and men,[56,58-61] but the natural progression or remission and long-term outcome in children is unclear. There is no clear guidance from the literature regarding the effect of puberty on the course of this disease.[56] Some patients experience complete resolution of skin lesions,[62] while others have persistent vulvar changes but are symptom-free.[63] It is important to note that morphologic changes of the disease might be indistinguishable from disease activity.[56] It is also unknown whether aggressive therapy in children will have any therapeutic or preventative effects later in their life.

LS & A is associated with a 4% to 6% increased risk of vulvar squamous cell carcinoma in adult women.[56,58,59,64] As many as 18% of children reportedly develop other long-term sequelae including scarring, adhesions, and atrophy.[63,65-69] What is unclear from the review of the current literature is whether the chronicity of these more identifiable signs could have been prevented with treatment. In the literature, no study of the results of using "no treatment" has been done.

GENITAL ULCERS

Genital ulcers, whether painful or not, offer diagnostic challenges. Some types of genital ulcer disease, such as herpesvirus infections, can be associated with sexual activity or sexual abuse, and others are not. This increases the need for accuracy in the diagnosis. Genital ulcers can be single, multiple, coalescing, and necrotic (Figure 12-19). They can be painful or not painful, recurrent or occurring one time only.

The most common type of painful genital ulcers is due to herpes simplex virus (HSV) type-2. HSV type-1 is typically associated with oral infections and as many as 70% to 100% of the population are seropositive by adulthood.[70] Recently, HSV-1 has been reported to account for at least half of the first episodes of genital herpes.[70] HSV infections are commonly transmitted from those who are not aware that they are infected; the disease is lifelong, with intermittent reactivation, which can or cannot be apparent to the patient or on examination.[70] HSV-1 or HSV-2 lesions are generally clusters of erythematous papules and vesicles on the external genital and perianal regions, and upper thighs. They are associated with pain, itching, burning, dysuria, fever, headache, malaise, and myalgias. Over a 2 to 3 week period, new lesions form and existing lesions progress to vesicles or pustules, and can coalesce into ulcers (Figure 12-20). The majority of HSV-2 cases will reoccur within the first year of infection. Testing for type specific IgG glycoprotein G of HSV-1 and HSV-2 can distinguish between the two virus types.[70] It is recommended that antiviral therapy be initiated promptly without waiting for the results of the culture because antiviral therapy does decrease viral shedding, prevent development of new lesions and improve symptom resolution and healing of the current lesions.[70]

Very little is known about nonsexually transmitted vulvar ulcerations in the pediatric age group. There have been case reports of Epstein-Barr viral (EBV) infections, Crohn disease, Behçet syndrome, and leukemia causing genital ulcerations that mimic HSV infections.[71] In 2004, Deitch et al[72] described their experience with nine peripubertal girls with genital ulcers who denied sexual activity or abuse and had negative

HSV cultures. Six patients had no definitive final diagnosis, two were diagnosed with "possible Behçet," and one was diagnosed with Behçet. Huppert and colleagues[73] felt that none of their 20 adolescent girls met the criteria for other causes of vulvar ulcerations including Behçet and that these lesions may represent a systemic viral infection or an aphthous process developing in response to an acute illness.

Over the same period of time one of the authors (Levitt) cared for 12 almost identical patients, offering the same diagnostic and treatment challenges. Many of the patients had such severe pain, erosion, and necrosis along with tremendous swelling, that adequate examinations were nearly impossible. Treatment was focused on trying to maintain comfort, including placement of an indwelling Foley catheter as an outpatient and intravenous narcotic management for an inpatient. Currently this severe nonherpetic vulvar ulcerative condition seems to be occurring less frequently, supporting a viral cause.

Behçet syndrome is a chronic recurrent illness characterized by painful ulcerative lesions of mucosal surfaces, most commonly the mouth and the genital area, which affects multiple systems. The prevalence in Western countries is estimated at 0.12 to 0.64 per 100,000 people.[74] The diagnosis of Behçet is challenging because many neurological, ocular, and vascular manifestations occur long after the onset of the disease. The criteria for diagnosing Behçet were established in 1990 and includes having three episodes of oral aphthous ulcerations per year and any two of the following: skin lesions, eye lesions (uveitis or retinitis), genital ulcerations, and a positive pathergy test.[74-76] Systemic symptoms such as fever, malaise, headache, and myalgias, are common with Behçet, but are not required for the diagnosis nor are they specific to Behçet.[73]

The vulvar ulcers with Behçet typically involve the labia minora in females and the scrotum and penis in males.[74] On examination, the lesions are frequently multiple, shallow, with sharp erythematous borders. It is not uncommon for them to have overlying eschar or exudate described as yellowish to gray-brown.[74]

The treatment of Behçet disease is challenging and should be tailored to the severity and clinical manifestations of the disease in the individual patient. Those patients with primarily mucocutaneous lesions need not be treated as aggressively as those with ocular and/or other systemic manifestations.[77] Once a comprehensive assessment has been completed to determine other systems typically affected by Behçet, such as uveitis, patients should be followed at routine intervals for documentation of resolution or progression of symptoms and recurrences if any that might further clarify the diagnosis.

Aphthae can be diagnosed by disease type and can include simple aphthosis, which consists of recurrent episodes of herpetiform aphthae with distinct ulcer-free periods (also known as recurrent aphthous stomatitis), or complex aphthosis which consists of almost constant presence of greater than three oral aphthae or recurrent oral or genital aphthae, and exclusions of Behçet.[78] Pseudo-Behçet is a term used to describe patients referred for consultation with a diagnosis of possible Behçet, who do not have Behçet disease.[71]

All of the ulcerative conditions noted above can be mistaken for sexual abuse. The ulcerations seen in these patients can present as necrotic-appearing lesions, which may suggest a traumatic cause. In addition, any of the ulcerations can appear morphologically indistinguishable from sexually-transmitted herpetic lesions and, as such, can raise concern for sexual abuse. It is incumbent upon the clinician to obtain a full medical, social, and sexual history, and perform adequate diagnostic testing before diagnosing ulcerative lesions of the genitalia as secondary to child sexual abuse.

ACCIDENTAL ANOGENITAL INJURY

Accidental anogenital injury is a relatively uncommon phenomenon. It is important for the clinician to recognize the hallmarks of this occasionally dramatic injury and to differentiate it from sexual abuse.[79] Accidental hymenal injury, including a transection, is an even rarer event, but it does occur (Figure 12-21). As clinicians we must rely on detailed accounts from the children or reliable witnesses to validate these rare events. Additionally, whether the child or parent seeks help immediately does not help to differentiate accidental from abusive trauma.

The most common mechanism of accidental anogenital injury is the straddle injury, defined as a blow to the perineum from falling or striking a surface or object with the force of one's own body's weight. The most common history provided in these injuries is falling astride the crossbar of a bicycle (Figure 12-22).[80] Straddle injury can be further categorized as either due to blunt force trauma, which compresses the urogenital soft tissues against the bony margins of the pelvic outlet or due to penetrating trauma, in which a narrow sharp or round object directly and forcefully penetrates the perineum or vaginal or anorectal opening (Figure 12-23). The most common complaint for 106 girls representing three different studies at presentation to the emergency department with blunt urogenital trauma was blood noted in the underwear or on the perineum.[79-81] Bleeding can range from spotting associated with minor external injury, to frank, profuse bleeding from penetrating vaginal or anorectal trauma. Males with straddle injuries tend to have pain rather than bleeding.[80]

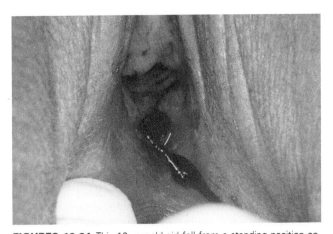

FIGURES 12-21 This 10-year-old girl fell from a standing position on a folding chair. She did not tell her mother about the accident until several hours later, during which time she experienced vaginal pain and bleeding. In the emergency department, she had a transection of her hymen at 6 o'clock that was somewhat obscured by the clotted blood overlying it.

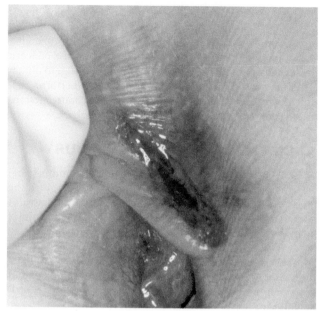

FIGURE 12-22 A 5-year-old girl had blood in her underwear after a straddle injury on a bicycle. On colposcopic examination, she had a dehiscence of adhesions between the labia minora and labia majora. There is also a shallow laceration in the base of the newly dehisced tissue.

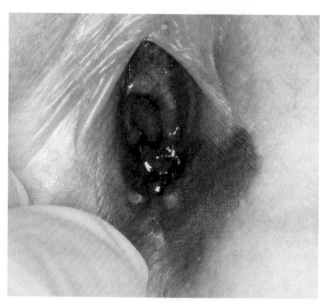

FIGURE 12-24 A 1-year-old girl fell from a slide. The hymen is bruised but not torn. The blunt force impact caused a small round hole where the hymen attaches to the fossa navicularis.

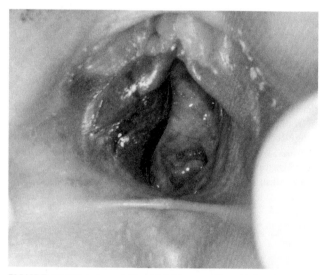

FIGURE 12-23 A 4-year-old girl fell from a recliner, hitting the handle on the side of the chair. Note bruising of labia minora and shallow laceration just medial to labia minora.

Blunt, nonpenetrating accidental anogenital injury generally involves the more superficial tissues of the perineum, and most commonly results in abrasions, bruising, or hematoma of the impacted surface. Areas most commonly impacted are the labia majora, mons pubis, external urethra, perineal body, and buttocks.[81] Lacerations are less common, occurring if the child falls onto an object or sharp edge. Case reports describe lacerations of the fossa navicularis extending into the base of the hymen secondary to blunt force trauma without involvement of a sharp object. In some cases, despite hymenal bruising or laceration of the fossa

navicularis and or vagina, the hymenal edge remained intact. In other girls it is speculated that the force of the trauma caused "splitting" or stretching of the relatively delicate tissues resulting in well-demarcated fenestration of the perihymenal tissue (Figure 12-24).[82] There are rare examples of activities such as in-line skating in which the child fell with sharply abducted legs (splits), resulting in deep perineal laceration with hymen bruising, but no laceration of the hymen.[83] Penetrating injuries of the anorectal, vaginal, and urethral orifices are somewhat less common. When they do occur, the presentation is often dramatic, with profuse bleeding and a clear history of impalement. Other presenting complaints include dysuria, pain on defecation, constipation, loss of bowel continence, or simply localized pain and tenderness. Structures commonly injured in such accidents include the hymen, posterior fourchette, anal sphincter, and, in more severe cases, internal structures such as the bowel or vagina. There are reports in the literature of boys incurring anorectal injury by accidental impalement on a pole, a broom handle, or toilet brush.[84] Kadish et al[85] compared boys injured accidentally with those injured nonaccidentally by abuse, and found that no patients suffering accidental impalement had isolated rectal injury; all had associated genital or perineal findings.[85]

Male straddle injuries involve the scrotum most commonly, and lacerations are the most common scrotal injury.[80] Penile trauma, including laceration or ecchymoses, is the next most common injury.[80] Common accidental injury mechanisms in boys include falling onto a sharp object, bicycle accidents, and, distinct from girls, zippers, toy box, or toilet seat accidents in which the penis or scrotum gets "caught" in the zipper or by the heavy cover. Strangulation injuries of the penis by hair tourniquet are usually considered accidental.

Perhaps the most important point for the clinician to appreciate is the relative rarity of hymen injury in accidental trauma. Reports of four large series of accidental genital trauma sustained by prepubertal girls published from 1989-1997, included 161 girls but only six hymen injuries. There were three accidental hymen transections in the 32 girls in one; 3 were from sliding down a tree trunk into a protruding stump, jumping on a plastic toy in a wading pool, or falling on a bicycle part.[86] Bond et al[87] reported that in their 56 girls with accidental perineal injuries, the only hymenal injury was a pinpoint abraded area. Dowd et al[80] reported injuries to the hymen in only 2 of 67 girls. One had minor bruising of the hymen from straddling the bicycle crossbar and the other had a 5 mm hymenal and vaginal tear with laceration of the posterior fourchette from falling on a plunger handle. These authors offered no description of external examination findings in these girls to assist in separating accidental from abusive hymenal trauma. Other examples demonstrate that hymen transections due to accidental trauma are not always witnessed by a parent or another adult. In these situations it is extremely important to take a detailed history from the injured child or another child witness. For example a 7-year-old girl who had vaginal bleeding was found on genital examination to have a hymenal transection. When questioned, she related a detailed, corroborated history of playing in the bathtub after a shower and falling onto her toy horse in the tub. She described experiencing immediate pain and bleeding.[88]

Not all nonabusive hymen transections are due to straddle injuries; some are iatrogenic. Pokorny[86] reported one hymenal transection caused by the doctor inadvertently putting his finger in the hymen as he was examining for rectal bleeding. One of the authors (Levitt) found an acute hymen tear after a nurse accidentally put a Tylenol suppository in the vagina instead of the anus. Another nurse caused a deep anal laceration while performing a routine procedure, blindly placing a Tylenol suppository into an anus following a surgical procedure. In addition there are four case reports of accidental anogenital injury occurring in conjunction with motor vehicle accidents where the child was run over at low speed; this compression mechanism likely lead to uterine pressure or shearing injury.[89]

It is important when evaluating acute accidental anogenital injury to fully appreciate the extent of the injury. The literature is rife with reports of perineal, vaginal, and anorectal impalement resulting in peritoneal signs and perforated viscus.[81,90,91] The initial medical examination may underestimate the extent of injury, and further examination under anesthesia is sometimes necessary.[81] The history is of utmost importance, not only to rule out sexual abuse, but also to get a good description of the traumatizing object. If possible, the object should be inspected in the emergency department to determine if any part of it is long enough to penetrate the pelvic floor.[90,91] A surgical consultation is not necessary if there is a reliable history of a straddle astride a nonpenetrating surface and the child has only minor bleeding or simply pain and tenderness of the perineal area. Blunt injury with significant bleeding might require examination under anesthesia, and vulvar hematomas can enlarge dramatically and require incision and evacuation (Figure 12-25).[90] Use of a colposcope is encouraged to help demonstrate and document the extent of injury. In addition, care should be taken to assess for urethral trauma and to assure that the child is able to void.[90]

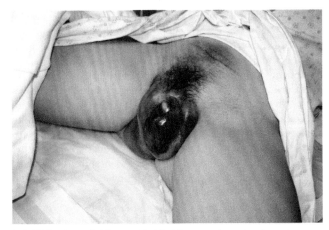

FIGURE 12-25 A 15-year-old girl with a massive vulvar hematoma due to her first episode of consensual penile-vaginal penetration.

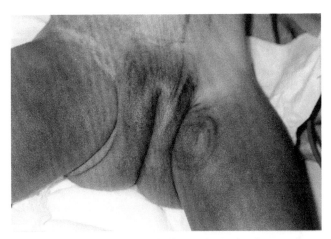

FIGURE 12-26 An 18-month-old girl with abusive head trauma has patterned bruising on the labia majora and inner thigh from being whipped using a belt.

Anal/Genital Injuries Due to Physical Abuse

At times children are the victims of abusive injury to the genital or anal area through burning, whipping, biting, or forceful penetration of fingers into the anus or vagina (Figure 12-26). In some cases it is difficult to determine whether these are injuries resulting from physical or sexual assault or whether the focus of the abuser's anger was the anogenital area because of the child's incontinence of urine or feces.

STRENGTH OF MEDICAL EVIDENCE AND DIRECTIONS FOR FUTURE RESEARCH

Some of the "mimics" of sexual abuse such as infection and diaper dermatitis are relatively common and are quite well studied. However, other conditions such as lichen sclerosus, genital ulcerations, urethral prolapse and accidental trauma are relatively rare and not well suited for prospective studies or large case series from any single center. Much of the knowledge at this time is anecdotal or based upon studies of adults. Anecdotal evidence has great value and is always the starting point in the development and advancement of medical knowledge. Child abuse pediatricians are in a unique situation to gather and evaluate reliable anecdotal evidence. Consideration of outliers or mimics of abuse and then looking for evidence to support or refute a hypothesis is central to the evaluation of child abuse. Perhaps more than any other group of physicians, we have access to community professionals such as law enforcement and social service workers who can investigate and can uncover corroborating evidence that confirms an unusual accidental history. Larger scale collaborative studies consolidating reliable anecdotal evidence is a reasonable next step.

Moving beyond anecdotal evidence, there is certainly a need for large prospective studies of rare conditions. For example at this time there are no studies addressing the long term outcome for children diagnosed with lichen sclerosus or urethral prolapse, and if treatment alters the outcome. Again collaboration of multiple centers will likely be a requirement to obtain the best data.

References

1. Fischer G, Rogers M: Vulvar disease in children: a clinical audit of 130 cases. *Pediatr Dermatol* 2000;17:1-6.
2. Fischer GO: Vulval disease in pre-pubertal girls. *Australas J Dermatol* 2001;42:225-236.
3. Pierce AM, Hart CA: Vulvovaginitis: causes and management. *Arch Dis Child* 1992;67:509-512.
4. Paradise JE, Campos JM, Friedman HM, et al: Vulvovaginitis in pre-menarcheal girls: clinical features and diagnostic evaluation. *Pediatrics* 1982;70:193-198.
5. Welsh BM, Berzins KN, Cook KA, et al: Management of common vulval conditions. *Med J Aust* 2003;178:391-395.
6. Alberta L, Sweeney SM, Wiss K: Diaper dye dermatitis. *Pediatrics* 2005;116:e450-e452.
7. Belhadjali H, Giordano-Labadie F, Rance F, et al: "Lucky Luke" contact dermatitis from diapers: a new allergen? *Contact Dermatitis* 2001;44:248.
8. Scheinfeld N: Diaper dermatitis: a review and brief survey of eruptions of the diaper area. *Am J Clin Dermatol* 2005;6:273-281.
9. Rodriguez-Poblador J, Gonzalez-Castro U, Herranz-Martinez S, et al: Jacquet erosive diaper dermatitis after surgery for Hirschsprung disease. *Pediatr Dermatol* 1998;15:46-47.
10. Silverberg NB, Laude TA: Jacquet diaper dermatitis: a diagnosis of etiology. *Pediatr Dermatol* 1998;15:489.
11. Leventhal JM, Griffin D, Duncan KO, et al: Laxative-induced dermatitis of the buttocks incorrectly suspected to be abusive burns. *Pediatrics* 2001;107:178-179.
12. Omar HA: Management of labial adhesions in prepubertal girls. *J Pediatr Adolesc Gynecol* 2000;13:183-185.
13. McCann J, Wells R, Simon M, et al: Genital findings in prepubertal girls selected for nonabuse: a descriptive study. *Pediatrics* 1990;86:428-439.
14. Berenson AB, Heger AH, Hayes JM, et al: Appearance of the hymen in prepubertal girls. *Pediatrics* 1992;89:387-394.
15. Caglar MK: Serum estradiol levels in infants with and without labial adhesions: the role of estrogen in the etiology and treatment. *J Pediatr Adolesc Gynecol* 2007;24:373-375.
16. Muram D: Treatment of prepubertal girls with labial adhesions. *J Pediatr Adolesc Gynecol* 1999;12:67-70.
17. Myers JB, Sorensen CM, Wisner BP, et al: Betamethasone cream for the treatment of pre-pubertal labial adhesions. *J Pediatr Adolesc Gynecol* 2006;19:407-411.
18. Stratakis CA, Graham W, DiPalma J, et al: Misdiagnosis of perianal manifestations of Crohn's disease. Two cases and a review of the literature. *Clin Pediatr (Phila)* 1994;33:631-633.
19. Sellman SP, Hupertz VF, Reece RM: Crohn's disease presenting as suspected abuse. *Pediatrics* 1996;97:272-274.
20. Parks AG, Morson BC, Pegum JS: Crohn's disease with cutaneous involvement. *Proc R Soc Med* 1965;58:241-242.
21. O'Gorman M, Lake AM: Chronic inflammatory bowel disease in childhood. *Pediatr Rev* 1993;14:475-480.
22. Myhre AK, Berntzen K, Bratlid D: Genital anatomy in non-abused preschool girls. *Acta Paediatr* 2003;92:1453-1462.
23. Roddy E, Jones AC: Reactive arthritis associated with genital tract group A streptococcal infection. *J Infect* 2002;45:208-209.
24. Andrews WW, Schelonka R, Waites K, et al: Genital tract methicillin-resistant *Staphylococcus aureus*: risk of vertical transmission in pregnant women. *Obstet Gynecol* 2008;111:113-118.
25. Al-Tawfiq JA, Aldaabil RA: Community-acquired MRSA bacteremic necrotizing pneumonia in a patient with scrotal ulceration. *J Infect* 2005;51:e241-e243.
26. Smith YR, Berman DR, Quint EH: Premenarchal vaginal discharge: findings of procedures to rule out foreign bodies. *J Pediatr Adolesc Gynecol* 2002;15:227-230.
27. Paradise JE, Willis ED: Probability of vaginal foreign body in girls with genital complaints. *Am J Dis Child* 1985;139:472-476.
28. Stricker T, Navratil F, Sennhauser FH: Vaginal foreign bodies. *J Paediatr Child Health* 2004;40:205-207.
29. Striegel AM, Myers JB, Sorensen MD, et al: Vaginal discharge and bleeding in girls younger than 6 years. *J Urol* 2006;176:2632-2635.
30. Soreide K: Surgical management of nonrenal genitourinary manifestations in children with Henoch-Schönlein purpura. *J Pediatr Surg* 2005;40:1243-1247.
31. Hara Y, Tajiri T, Matsuura K, et al: Acute scrotum caused by Henoch-Schönlein purpura. *Int J Urol* 2004;11:578-580.
32. Levin AV, Selbst SM: Vulvar hemangioma simulating child abuse. *Clin Pediatr (Phila)* 1988;27:213-215.
33. Swanson DL: Genital lymphangioma with recurrent cellulitis in men. *Int J Dermatol* 2006;45:800-804.
34. La Vecchia C, Draper GJ, Franceschi S: Childhood nonovarian female genital tract cancers in Britain, 1962-1978. Descriptive epidemiology and long-term survival. *Cancer* 1984;54:188-192.
35. Rescorla F, Billmire D, Vinocur C, et al: The effect of neoadjuvant chemotherapy and surgery in children with malignant germ cell tumors of the genital region: a pediatric intergroup trial. *J Pediatr Surg* 2003;38:910-912.
36. Dawson PM, Griffith K, Boeke KM: Combined medical and psychological treatment of hospitalized children with encopresis. *Child Psychiatry Hum Dev* 1990;20:181-190.
37. Boon F: Encopresis and sexual assault. *J Am Acad Child Adolesc Psychiatry* 1991;30:509-510.
38. Morrow J, Yeager CA, Lewis DO: Encopresis and sexual abuse in a sample of boys in residential treatment. *Child Abuse Negl* 1997;21:11-18.
39. Mellon MW, Whiteside SP, Friedrich WN: The relevance of fecal soiling as an indicator of child sexual abuse: a preliminary analysis. *J Dev Behav Pediatr* 2006;27:25-32.
40. Berenson AB: Normal anogenital anatomy. *Child Abuse Negl* 1998;22:589-596.
41. Agnarsson U, Warde C, McCarthy G, et al: Perianal appearances associated with constipation. *Arch Dis Child* 1990;65:1231-1234.
42. McCann J, Voris J, Simon M, et al: Perianal findings in prepubertal children selected for nonabuse: a descriptive study. *Child Abuse Negl* 1989;13:179-193.
43. Sialakas C, Vottler TP, Andersen JM: Rectal prolapse in pediatrics. *Clin Pediatr (Phila)* 1999;39:63-72.
44. Klein MD, Thomas RP: Surgical conditions of the anus, rectum and colon. *In:* Kliegman RH, Behrman RE, Jenson HB, et al (eds): *Nelson's Textbook of Pediatrics*, ed 18, Saunders Elsevier, Philadelphia, 2007, pp 1635-1641.
45. Jerkins GR, Verheeck K, Noe HN: Treatment of girls with urethral prolapse. *J Urol* 1984;132:732-733.
46. Venable DD, Markland C: Urethral prolapse in girls. *South Med J* 1982;75:951-953.
47. Richardson DA, Hajj SN, Herbst AL: Medical treatment of urethral prolapse in children. *Obstet Gynecol* 1982;59:69-74.
48. Valerie E, Gilchrist BF, Frischer J, et al: Diagnosis and treatment of urethral prolapse in children. *Urology* 1999;54:1082-1084.
49. Lowe FC, Hill GS, Jeffs RD, et al: Prolapse in children: insights into etiology and management. *J Urol* 1986;135:100-103.
50. Redman JF: Conservative management of urethral prolapse in female children. *Urology* 1982;19:505-506.
51. Rudin JE, Geldt VG, Alecseev EB: Prolapse of urethral mucosa in white female children: experience with 58 cases. *J Pediatr Surg* 1997;32:423-425.

52. Kisanga RE, Aboud MM: Urethral mucosa prolapse in young girls. *Cent Afr J Med* 1996;42:31-33.

53. Johnson CF: Prolapse of the urethra: confusion of clinical and anatomic characteristics with sexual abuse. *Pediatrics* 1991;87:722-725.

54. Shokeir AA, Nijman RJM: Ureterocele: an ongoing challenge in infancy and childhood. *BJU Int* 2002;90:777-783.

55. Pike SC, Cain MP, Rink RC: Ureterocele prolapse-rare presentation in an adolescent girl. *Urology* 2001;57:554.

56. Smith YR, Haefner HK: Vulvar lichen sclerosus: pathophysiology and treatment. *Am J Clin Dermatol* 2004;5:105-125.

57. Warrington SA, de San Lazaro C: Lichen sclerosus et atrophicus and sexual abuse. *Arch Dis Child* 1996;75:512-516.

58. Pugliese JM, Morey AF, Peterson AC: Lichen sclerosus: review of the literature and current recommendations for management. *J Urol* 2007;178:2268-2276.

59. Funaro D: Lichen sclerosus: a review and practical approach. *Dermatol Ther* 2004;17:28-37.

60. Cooper SM, Gao XH, Powell JJ, et al: Does treatment of vulvar lichen sclerosus influence its prognosis? *Arch Dermatol* 2004;140:702-706.

61. Powell J, Wojnarowska F: Childhood vulvar lichen sclerosus. The course after puberty. *J Reprod Med* 2002;47:706-709.

62. Clark JA, Muller SA: Lichen sclerosus et atrophicus in children. A report of 24 cases. *Arch Dermatol* 1967;95:476-482.

63. Ridley CM: Genital lichen sclerosus (lichen sclerosus et atrophicus) in childhood and adolescence. *J R Soc Med* 1993;86:69-75.

64. Poindexter G, Morrell DS: Anogenital pruritus: lichen sclerosus in children. *Pediatr Ann* 2007;36:785-791.

65. Cario G, House M, Paradinas F: Squamous cell carcinoma of the vulva in association with mixed vulvar dystrophy in an 18-year-old girl. Case report. *Br J Obstet Gynaecol* 1984;91:87-90.

66. Garzon MC, Paller AS: Ultrapotent topical corticosteroid treatment of childhood genital lichen sclerosus. *Arch Dermatol* 1999;135:525-528.

67. Wallace HJ: Lichen sclerosus et atrophicus. *Trans St Johns Hosp Dermatol Soc* 1971;57:9-30.

68. Meffert JJ, Davis BM, Grimwood RE: Lichen sclerosus. *J Am Acad Dermatol* 1995;32:393-416.

69. Helm KF, Gibson LE, Muller SA: Lichen sclerosus et atrophicus in children and young adults. *Pediatr Dermatol* 1991;8:97-101.

70. Gupta R, Warren T, Wald A: Genital herpes. *Lancet* 2008;370:2127-2137.

71. Rogers RS 3rd: Pseudo-Behçet's disease. *Dermatol Clin* 2003;21:49-61.

72. Deitch HR, Huppert J, Adams Hillard PJ: Unusual vulvar ulcerations in young adolescent females. *J Pediatr Adolesc Gynecol* 2004;17:13-16.

73. Huppert JS, Gerber MA, Deitch HR, et al: Vulvar ulcers in young females: a manifestation of aphthosis. *J Pediatr Adolesc Gynecol* 2006;19:195-204.

74. Sakane T, Takeno M, Suzuki N, et al: Behçet's disease. *N Engl J Med* 1999;341:1284-1291.

75. Haidopoulos D, Rodolakis A, Stefanidis K, et al: Behçet's disease: part of the differential diagnosis of the ulcerative vulva. *Clin Exp Obstet Gynecol* 2002;29:219-221.

76. Criteria for diagnosis of Behçet's disease. International study group for Behçet's disease. *Lancet* 1990;335:1078-1080.

77. McCarty MA, Garton RA, Jorizzo JL: Complex aphthosis and Behçet's disease. *Dermatol Clin* 2003;21:41-48.

78. Letsinger JA, McCarty MA, Jorizzo JL: Complex aphthosis: a large case series with evaluation algorithm and therapeutic ladder from topicals to thalidomide. *J Am Acad Dermatol* 2005;52:500-508.

79. Greaney H, Ryan J: Straddle injuries–is current practice safe? *Eur J Emerg Med* 1998;5:421-442.

80. Dowd MD, Fitzmaurice L, Knapp JF, et al: The interpretation of urogenital findings in children with straddle injuries. *J Pediatr Surg* 1994;29:7-10.

81. Lynch JM, Gardner MJ, Albanese CT: Blunt urogenital trauma in prepubescent female patients: more than meets the eye! *Pediatr Emerg Care* 1995;11:372-375.

82. Hostetler B, Muram D, Jones C: Sharp penetrating injuries to the hymen. *Adolesc Pediatr Gynecol* 1994;7:94-96.

83. Herrmann B, Crawford J: Genital injuries in prepubertal girls from inline skating accidents. *Pediatrics* 2002;110:e16.

84. Jona JZ: Accidental anorectal impalement in children. *Pediatr Emerg Care* 1997;13:40-43.

85. Kadish HA, Schunk JE, Britton H: Pediatric male rectal and genital trauma: accidental and nonaccidental injuries. *Pediatr Emerg Care* 1998;14:95-98.

86. Pokorny SF, Pokorny WJ, Kramer W: Acute genital injury in the prepubertal girl. *Am J Obstet Gynecol* 1992;166:1461-1466.

87. Bond GR, Dowd MD, Landsman I, et al: Unintentional perineal injury in prepubescent girls: a multicenter, prospective report of 56 girls. *Pediatrics* 1995;95:628-631.

88. Boos SC: Accidental hymenal injury mimicking sexual trauma. *Pediatrics* 1999;103:1287-1290.

89. Boos SC, Rosas AJ, Boyle C, et al: Anogenital injuries in child pedestrians run over by low-speed motor vehicles: four cases with findings that mimic child sexual abuse. *Pediatrics* 2003;112:e77-e84.

90. Pokorny S, Merrit D: Tips for clinicians: evaluating and managing acute genital trauma in premenarchal girls. *J Pediatr Adolesc Gynecol* 1999;12:237-238.

91. Pokorny SF: Genital trauma. *Clin Obstet Gynecol* 1997;40:219-225.

13

THE FORENSIC EVIDENCE KIT

James Anderst, MD, MSCI

INTRODUCTION

When examining a victim of sexual abuse, the medical professional has the dual duty of providing medical treatment to the victim and collecting forensic evidence to assist in legal handling of the case. The collection of forensic specimens from a victim of rape can provide definitive evidence of sexual contact. Policies and procedures vary by jurisdiction, and clinicians must comply with local state crime lab procedures regarding evidence collection, processing, storage, and chain of evidence.

Forensic evidence collected can include sperm, semen, blood, hair, DNA evidence, and saliva (see Chapter 14). The collection of this evidence, in addition to assessing physical findings, toxicology findings, and the history provided by the victim, optimizes the medical care of the child and legal handling of the case. Recovery rates of forensic materials differ between prepubertal and postpubertal victims. Protocols for collection procedures should reflect these age-specific variations; however, examiners often need to modify the examination and evidence collection based on the specific needs of the patient.

COLLECTING FORENSIC EVIDENCE

Consent

In sexual assault evaluations, two separate consent processes exist: consent for medical diagnosis and treatment and consent for forensic examination and evidence collection. It is recommended that health care professionals obtain both written and verbal consent before conducting a medical examination and forensic evidence collection in sexual assault victims. Patients must be provided with all relevant information regarding their examinations, and it must be provided in a way that is clearly understandable. Patients can decline all or any part of an examination. Examiners should inform the patient of the risks of refusing any part of the examination, including how their decisions might affect their medical treatment and the investigative process. Consent is required for forensic examination and evidence collection including the following: photographs, toxicology screening, and examination and evidence collection.[1]

Examiners must also refrain from any coercive practices when obtaining consent. If the child cannot tolerate the

examination, the importance of the examination and evidence collection should be reassessed. If deemed necessary for either medical or forensic reasons, sedation or anesthesia should be considered for the child. Policies regarding consent for medical evaluation and treatment are generally established by the treating facility. Aspects of the examination that require this type of consent include: general medical care, pregnancy testing, testing and prophylaxis for sexually transmitted infections (STI) and HIV, and release of medical information.

Typically, consent should be obtained from both the parent and the child. Different jurisdictions have different consent requirements. For example, in some jurisdictions, minors can give consent to receive care for STIs, but not a forensic examination. Other jurisdictions have laws that allow children to consent to both the examination and evidence collection. Some states permit physicians to evaluate minors for abuse without parental consent.

Collection and Handling of Evidence

Standardized protocols, typically established in conjunction with the local police department and forensic laboratory, eliminate the need for hospital personnel to testify at each trial about how the evidence was collected and how chain of custody was maintained. Protocols also can eliminate errors of omission in the process.

Before beginning the examination, all equipment, containers, and other necessary materials should be in the room, and if possible, covered before the child's entry. The following should be available[1]:

1. A copy of the jurisdiction's most current evidence collection protocol;
2. A private examination room with an obstetric/gynecological examination bed;
3. "Comfort supplies" such as a change of clothes for the victim or materials to distract a child during the examination;
4. Sexual assault evidence collection kit (see Figure 13-1) and related supplies;
5. A method or device to dry evidence;
6. A camera, ruler, and related supplies for forensic photography;
7. Testing and treatment supplies;
8. An alternate light source, if available;

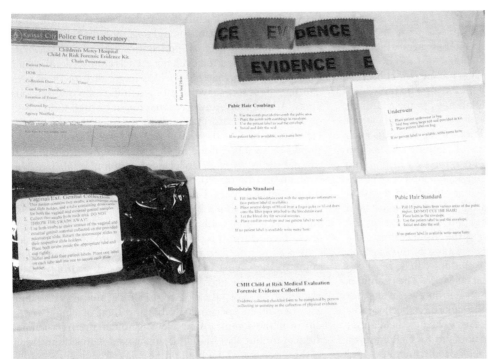

FIGURE 13-1 An example of a forensic medical evidence kit.

9. A colposcope with photographic ability or alternative method for detailed photodocumentation; and,

10. Written materials for patients on the sexual assault examination, counseling resources, STIs, and other medical and legal information.

The examiner should always wear gloves throughout the entire examination to avoid contamination of evidence. Evidence should be placed in paper bags rather than plastic to prevent mold, bacterial, and fungal overgrowth that can occur with moisture retention. Once collected, evidence in envelopes should be sealed with moistened gauze, as opposed to licking the envelopes, to prevent contamination. All swabs and other evidence collected should be completely air-dried in a clean environment, again, to prevent contamination. A drying box will facilitate the process.[1] Protocols should be established for handling specimens that will not dry immediately, such as tampons, condoms, wet clothing, or diapers. Collected specimens should be labeled with the child's name, date, and time of collection, site from which the specimen was taken, and name of the person collecting the evidence. Once evidence is appropriately processed, packaged, and labeled, it should be stored in designated locked cabinets, freezers, and refrigerators. Kits with wet evidence or drawn blood need to be refrigerated. Urine should be frozen or refrigerated. Previously, it was felt that any biological evidence possibly containing DNA should be stored at very low temperatures.[2] However, preliminary information from the National Institute of Standards and Technology suggests that DNA samples might not need refrigeration.[3]

Chain of Custody

Transfer of evidence to law enforcement must follow a "chain of custody." Examiners must ensure secure collection and storage of evidence during the examination, while drying, and until it is sealed. Then documentation of transfer of evidence should continue as it is moved from medical personnel to law enforcement and to the crime laboratory. Examiners should be mindful of keeping material collected for forensic purposes separate from that collected for medical purposes. Chain of custody is not necessary for medical specimens such as materials for STI testing.

Timing of Evidence Collection

Many jurisdictions previously considered it unnecessary to collect forensic evidence using a rape kit after 72 hours postassault. Reexamination of the literature that documents the recovery of useful evidence outside of this time frame has extended the recommended time period for forensic evidence collection in many jurisdictions.[4-6] Examiners should keep in mind that evidence might be recoverable in certain cases outside the recommended timeframe.

THE RAPE KIT

Minimal guidelines have been established for contents of a sexual assault evidence kit (Figure 13-1).[1] The minimum standards include:

1. A kit container with a label for identifying information and documenting chain of custody;
2. An instruction sheet or checklist that guides examiners in collecting evidence and maintaining the chain of custody;
3. Forms that facilitate evidence collection and analysis; and,
4. Materials for collecting and preserving evidence.

Evidence should be collected even if the examiner is unsure if it is necessary. It is better to have too much evidence than not enough.

Clothing

After consent is obtained and the materials needed for collection are organized, the victim should disrobe over two clean sheets of paper. The upper sheet allows for collection of any evidence that falls off the child as she/he undresses. The lower sheet prevents contamination from the examination room floor and should be discarded. If the child cannot undress on her own, or the condition of the victim is such that it is necessary to cut off items of clothing, do not cut through existing stains or tears. Tears or cuts in clothing might be evidence of a physical struggle. Each piece of clothing and the collection paper on which the victim disrobed should be placed in separate paper bags. These bags are then labeled, sealed and signed. If the child is not wearing the same clothing that she wore during the assault/abuse, the examiner should inquire about the location of this clothing and then notify investigators so the clothing can be retrieved before the degradation of biological evidence. The examiner should collect the clothing the child has on even if she has changed, as secretions on the child might have been deposited on the clothing in the interim. Any evidence that cannot be dried thoroughly at the collection site (wet clothing or tampons) should be packaged in leak-proof containers and separated from other evidence while being transported.[1]

Swabs

Some protocols call for collection of swabs from the mouth, body, vagina, perineum, and anus in all cases, regardless of the history provided by the victim. The rationale for this approach is that the victim's recollection of the event might not be complete or supportive of other evidence collected.[7] The totality of evidence must be carefully interpreted. For example, studies have documented the presence of sperm in the anal canal despite no history of anal penetration.[8] Large numbers of sperm were also reported in vaginal contents in these cases. The authors interpreted this as contamination of the anus with vaginal contents. Conversely, many victims, particularly children, find the examination uncomfortable and unsettling, and minimizing the trauma associated with evidence collection is appropriate. Additionally, internal vaginal swabs might not be necessary in prepubertal children who do not have apparent vaginal/hymenal injuries. Forensic evidence on these children is more likely to be in the vestibule or external surfaces, such as the perineum. In support of selective sampling of only high-yield sites, a recent national protocol recommends, "Specimens should be collected only from orifices and areas surrounding the orifices that the patients report to be involved in the assault.[1]"

When swabbing for forensic evidence, at least two swabs should be used at each site. One is reserved for the prosecution, the other for independent analysis.[2] Each swab should be lightly moistened with nonbacteriostatic saline. Cotton-tipped or Dacron swabs should be used.[9] The examiner should take special caution to prevent contamination of swabs with materials from other areas (such as vaginal secretions on a rectal swab), as the specific location of collected evidence is critical to the investigation.

Obtaining mouth swabs first allows the victim to rinse his or her mouth after specimen collection. Mouth swabs should include specimens from the buccal mucosa, the gum line, between the teeth, and underneath the tongue. Some protocols stipulate the use of dental floss for obtaining specimens from between the teeth. The victim's entire body and hair should be searched for evidence of secretions, blood, other stains, or foreign material such as grass, dirt, or fibers. An alternate light source will assist in identification of suspicious areas. Additionally, any areas that might be high yield based on the victim's history should be swabbed. General high-yield areas, such as the neck, external genitalia, and breasts, should be swabbed if the history is absent or incomplete. If vaginal swabs are to be collected in a prepubertal child, the swab should be placed through the hymenal opening and rotated several times. Care should be taken to avoid touching the hymen, which is uncomfortable for the prepubertal patient. A vaginal wash can sometimes yield assailant secretions. To perform this procedure, 2 to 3 ml of nonbacteriostatic saline is instilled into the vagina with a dropper. The saline in the vagina is then aspirated using a dropper and stored in a sterile glass tube. A wet mount can be done by placing a drop of saline on a glass slide, mixing the saline with one of the specimen swabs, and then placing a cover slip over the sample. After viewing under the microscope, the wet mount slide should be packaged, labeled, and sent to the forensics lab with all other collected evidence.

Swabs from both the vaginal vault and cervical os should be taken when a vaginal speculum examination is possible (only in postpubertal patients). Any contraceptive or sanitary devices identified should be collected and retained as evidence. To collect a rectal specimen, place the swab 1 inch into the rectum, rotate, and remove it. Using two slightly moistened swabs, swab the external genitalia area.

Blood, buccal swabs, or saliva "control" samples can be collected to distinguish the patient's DNA from that of the suspect. Use of a buccal swab or saliva is suggested as it is the least invasive method of DNA collection, although a buccal or saliva sample might be contaminated with the perpetrator's DNA as well. When oral-genital contact is suspected, a blood sample is preferred to confirm the victim's DNA typing. If blood is not being drawn for medical purposes, a dry blood sample should be considered. For this procedure, the victim's fingertip is cleaned with Betadine, and then pricked with a sterile lancet. Drops of blood are collected on a blood collection card, dried, and packaged.

For male patients, the presence of feces, vaginal secretions, or saliva on the penis can be used as evidence of assault or abuse. At least two swabs should be taken from the penile shaft and glans.

The examiner might identify secretions such as semen, saliva, or blood on other parts of the victim's body. If dry, this material should be collected by moistening a swab with sterile water and swabbing the identified area. Alternatively, dry secretions can be flaked off with a sterile instrument and collected. Moist secretions can be collected with a dry swab. Any head, facial, or pubic hair matted with dried secretions should be cut and placed into an evidence envelope.

Semen/sperm: Multiple factors must be considered when evaluating the presence of sperm or semen after an assault. Activities of the victim, such as running, walking, defecating, urinating, spitting, or brushing teeth, are thought to decrease the longevity of sperm. No sperm will be recovered if the assailant is azoospermic, impotent, or vasectomized. At the bedside, semen can be identified by microscopic examination of bodily fluids and the observation of motile sperm or nonmotile sperm. Motile sperm can be detected using a saline wet mount. Nonmotile sperm are detected by gram stain, Papanicolaou smear, or nuclear fast red-picroindigocarmine ("Christmas tree") stain.

Previous sources have documented time frames for the persistence of sperm and other markers in the vagina, oral cavity, and rectum.[10] However, motile and nonmotile sperm have been recovered from these sites well beyond the accepted timeframes. Typically, motile sperm rarely persist for longer than a few hours after intercourse.[5] Yet, motile sperm have been detected in the endocervix up to 7 days after intercourse,[11] and have been reported in vaginal samples up to 24 hours after intercourse.[1] Even in a controlled environment with volunteer couples, only 50% of women tested positive for motile sperm 3 hours after intercourse.[5] Nonmotile sperm can be found beyond 72 hours in vaginal samples from nearly 50% of postcoital women,[5] and have been detected up to 17 days after intercourse.[6] Vaginal douching was found to reduce the percentage of spermatozoa found in vaginal smears.[4]

Sperm persists for a shorter time in the rectum. It is uncommon to recover sperm from anal swabs beyond 6 hours.[12] Sperm is rarely found in the oral cavity beyond a few hours,[8] but has been documented up to 13 hours after an alleged offense.[13] Others report persistence of sperm up to 28 to 31 hours in the oral cavity[14]. Additionally, both saliva (obtained by having the patient expectorate saliva) and swab samples may be necessary to detect all sperm in the oral cavity.[14]

Bite Marks

Some victims of sexual assault have evidence of bite marks on their skin. Bite marks frequently contain useful forensic evidence (see Chapter 60 for a discussion on preserving and interpreting bite mark evidence).

Hair

Any hairs seen on the victim should be collected for forensic analysis. Hairs may be transferred via direct contact, clothing transfer, friction, or forcible removal during an assault. Hair, particularly head and pubic hair, can be compared to known samples from the victim and alleged perpetrator. The victim's hair should be combed over a piece of paper to collect any loose hairs or fibers. The comb and materials gathered from the combing are then folded into the paper, placed into an envelope, and labeled. This procedure should be repeated with the pubic hair. Many patients, if capable, prefer to do this procedure themselves to minimize embarrassment. Though combing is more comfortable for the patient, plucked hair is more likely to contain roots and is better for DNA analysis. Many jurisdictions do not collect victim hair samples routinely during the examination. However, samples of the victim's hair might be requested at a later time, depending on evidence found at a crime scene. The family and victim should be told to avoid having the victim's hair processed, colored, or cut before completion of the investigation. Protocols typically require hair to be collected from multiple areas of the scalp (sides, top, front, and back) with up to 100 hairs being collected.

Nails

If the patient states that he/she scratched the alleged perpetrator's body or clothing, or if material is noted under the patient's fingernails, the nails should be scraped individually with a solid implement or a cotton swab lightly moistened with sterile water. The nails from each hand should be scraped over a separate piece of paper, and the paper should be placed in an individual collection envelope along with the device used for scraping.

Toluidine Dye

Some previous rape kit protocols have suggested using toluidine dye on the perineum and posterior fourchette for detection of minor tissue injuries not readily visible with white light and/or magnification.[2,15] However, minor tissue injury to these regions is a nonspecific finding for trauma and can be caused by other irritative and infectious conditions. Toluidine dye is not a diagnostic tool, but rather accentuates minor epithelial damage that can then be photographed.

Alternative Light Sources

A Wood's lamp produces ultraviolet radiation emitting wavelengths of approximately 320 to 400 nm. Various substances fluoresce when viewed under a Wood's lamp. Semen placed on cotton fabric was not found to fluoresce using a Wood's lamp,[16] but was found to fluoresce at a wavelength outside of that emitted by a Wood's lamp. A different light source, the Bluemaxx 500 (Sirchie Finger Print Laboratories, Inc., Youngsville, N.C.) is a more appropriate tool for identifying semen on fabric by fluorescence. The Bluemaxx 500 used in conjunction with an added orange barrier filter has been reported to be 100% sensitive in detecting semen as a fluorescing agent on cotton fabric and this fluorescence persists for at least 16 months.[17] It should be noted, however, that other substances fluoresce under the Bluemaxx 500 in addition to semen (hand cream, castile soap, and bacitracin).

Detecting semen on skin by fluorescence is more difficult. Wawryk et al[18] found that the light source needed to be very close to the skin (less than 3 cm) to cause visible fluorescence of the semen. In fact, dried semen was noted to be more easily visible with the naked eye than with a number of alternative light sources and filters.[18] A Poliray light source (Rofin Forensic, Melbourne, Australia) with a filter and goggles documented semen fluorescing on various cloths and skin,[19] but still may not be as effective as the naked eye when looking for semen on skin.[18]

In summary, a Wood's lamp is not likely to be useful in detecting semen on skin or fabrics. Instead, other light sources (Bluemaxx 500 or Poliray), with appropriate filters, should be used with the understanding that relatively fresh, dried semen might be more easily seen with the naked eye than with an alternative light source.

Saliva

DNA evidence can be recovered from saliva deposition after biting, licking, kissing, and sucking. Saliva can be collected with the "double swab" technique as described for bite marks.[20]

FREQUENCY OF RECOVERABLE EVIDENCE

Several studies have evaluated forensic evidence collected in large numbers of adult and children sexual assault victims. The nature of the acts involved in the sexual abuse/assault of children is different than those involved in the assault of adults, so one cannot extrapolate all of the available data to children.

In a series of 1076 mostly adult victims of sexual assault, evidence of semen or sperm on vaginal, rectal, oral, and skin swabs was found in 48.3%.[21] Interestingly, 45% of cases with no semen or sperm identified in the emergency department (ED) by wet mount had positive identification by the crime lab using microscopy or acid phosphatase; however, in 7.5% of cases with semen or sperm identified by wet mount in the ED, no evidence was found in the crime lab.[21] A study of 418 adult and child victims of sexual assault showed evidence of sperm in approximately 30% of cases seen within 72 hours.[22] Other studies showed sperm and semen products were recovered from vaginal samples in 25% to 37% of rape victims.[23] Recovery from skin, oral, and anal samples is usually much lower, between 1% and 12%.[23] It should be noted that these studies contain large numbers of adult patients, and do not provide results specific to children.

Studies of volunteers after consensual sex have documented higher retrieval rates. Soules[5] reported 100% recovery of sperm heads up to 24 hours after intercourse. Another study reported recovery rates of 64% within 24 hours after voluntary intercourse.[4] The higher frequency of evidence recovery after voluntary intercourse versus rape cases is likely explained by the very different nature of the event and activities of the female after the event.

Although numerous studies have found the association of semen or sperm recovery with a history of penetration or ejaculation, victims of sexual assault/abuse often require forensic evidence collection even if this history is not provided. One study documented the presence of semen in several patients that denied ejaculation or penetration, or that stated a condom was used by the perpetrator.[7]

Frequency of Forensic Evidence in Children

Few studies have examined the frequency of recovery of forensic evidence from sexually abused children. Christian et al[24] reviewed 273 children younger than 10 years who were evaluated for sexual assault. Approximately 25% of those evaluated had forensic evidence identified, all of whom were examined within 44 hours of assault. Over 90% of those with forensic evidence present were seen within 24 hours of the assault, and 64% of the evidence was found on clothing and linens. However, only 35% had clothing collected for analysis. After 24 hours, all evidence, with the exception of 1 pubic hair, was recovered from clothing or linens. No swabs taken from the child's body were positive for blood after 13 hours or sperm or semen after 9 hours. Of the children evaluated, 23% had genital injuries. Genital injury and a history of ejaculation provided by the child were

associated with an increased likelihood of identifying forensic evidence, but the forensic evidence recovered in several children was unanticipated by the child's history. The authors concluded that swabbing a young child's body for evidence is probably unnecessary after 24 hours, but clothing and linens should be obtained for analysis whenever possible.

A 2006 study by Palusci et al[25] evaluated the presence of sperm or semen in children under the age of 13 evaluated within 72 hours of assault. Of 190 subjects, 9% had positive findings; 6.5% of body swabs and 12.5% of clothing analyzed had sperm or semen found. Semen or sperm was identified from body swabs only from female children older than 10 years who had not bathed since assault. All other semen or sperm was recovered from clothing or objects. No child under the age of 10 had a positive body swab, but some with negative body swabs had positive evidence on clothing. Factors that best predicted forensic evidence findings were: victim age greater than 10, older alleged perpetrator, pubertal status of victim, and victim with examination findings consistent with sexual assault. Factors that best predicted lack of forensic evidence were: alleged perpetrator less than 15 years old, victim less than 10 years old, prepubertal status, normal or nonspecific anogenital examination findings, and victim changing clothes before collection of evidence.

Young et al[26] reviewed 80 children evaluated within 72 hours of sexual abuse. Sixteen of the 80 cases had positive findings for semen. All 16 of those subjects presented for evaluation within 24 hours of the last assault or abuse. Of those older than 12 years, 13 of 31 had semen identified. Of those younger than 12 years, 3 of 49 were positive for semen, and in those 3 children, semen was recovered only from clothing or linens.

These studies indicate that younger children rarely have positive body swabs after sexual abuse, and clothing and linens should be collected and analyzed whenever possible. Additionally, although there are associations between the likelihood of forensic evidence recovery and several factors including ages of the involved parties, timing of the abuse relative to the examination, and other specific aspects of the abuse, each case requires individual considerations and careful assessment.

STRENGTH OF MEDICAL EVIDENCE AND DIRECTIONS FOR FUTURE RESEARCH

Medical evidence suggests that body swabs of prepubertal children after the immediate postassault period (12 to 24 hours) are rarely useful. Good evidence exists to support the collection of linens, clothing, and other articles from the scene of assault, particularly in cases involving young children. Evidence supporting the regular use of alternative light sources is only fair, as forensic material may frequently be seen with the naked eye, and alternative light sources are costly. Little research exists to substantiate claims that activities such as defecation, walking, running, or eating/drinking by the victim after an assault markedly decreases the presence of forensic material on the victim.

Future research evaluating the presence of DNA on victims is warranted, particularly as new technologies develop. Research evaluating the usefulness of swabbing specific body sites in children based on outcry, physical findings, and time since assault is needed, and could decrease the invasiveness of the examination for many victims. Additionally, research aimed at clarifying the specific effects of post-victim activity on the presence of forensic evidence is needed.

References

1. U.S. Department of Justice, Office of Violence Against Women: *A National protocol for sexual assault medical forensic examinations* (website): http://www.ncjrs.gov/pdffiles1/ovw/206554.pdf#search=%22OVW%20National%20Protocol%2. Accessed February 18, 2009.

2. Jenny C: Forensic examination: the role of the physician as "medical detective." *In*: Heger A, Emans SJ, Muram D (eds): *Evaluation of the Sexually Abused Child*, ed 2, Oxford University Press, New York, 2000, pp 79-94.

3. Kline MC, Redman JW: *DNA stability studies*, Chemical Science and Technology Laboratory (website): www.cstl.nist.gov/biotech/strbase/NIJ/DNAstability.htm. Accessed February 16, 2009.

4. Silverman EM, Silverman AG: Persistence of spermatozoa in the lower genital tracts of women. *JAMA* 1978;240:1875-1877.

5. Soules MR, Pollard AA, Brown KM, et al: The forensic laboratory evaluation of evidence in alleged rape. *Am J Obstet Gynecol* 1978;130:142-147.

6. Sharpe N: The significance of spermatozoa in sexual offenses. *Can Med Assoc J* 1963;89:513-514.

7. Hook S, Elliot D, Harbison S: Penetration and ejaculation; forensic aspects of rape. *N Z Med J* 1992;105:87-89.

8. Enos WF, Beyer JC: Spermatozoa in the anal canal and rectum and in the oral cavity of female rape victims. *J Forensic Sci* 1978;23:231-233.

9. Bernard D, Peters M, Makoroff K: The evaluation of suspected pediatric sexual abuse. *Clin Pediatr Emerg Med* 2006;7:161-169.

10. Lavelle J: Forensic evidence collection. *In*: Giardino AP, Alexander R (eds): *Child Maltreatment*, ed 3, GW Medical, St Louis, 2005, pp 853-860.

11. Perloff WH, Steinberger E: In vivo survival of spermatozoa in cervical mucus. *Am J Obstet Gynecol* 1964;88:439-432.

12. Willott GM, Allard JE: Spermatozoa-their persistence after sexual intercourse. *Forensic Sci Int* 1982;19:135-154.

13. Willott GM, Crosse MA: The detection of spermatozoa in the mouth. *J Forensic Sci Soc* 1986;26:125-128.

14. Rogers D: Evidence-based forensic sampling-more questions than answers. *J Clin Forensic Med* 2006;13:162-163.

15. McCauley J, Gorman RL, Guzinski G: Toluidine blue in the detection of perineal laceration in pediatric and adolescent sexual abuse victims. *Pediatrics* 1986;78:1039-1043.

16. Santucci KA, Nelson DG, McQuillen KK, et al: Wood's lamp utility in the identification of semen. *Pediatrics* 1999;104:1342-1344.

17. Nelson DG, Santucci KA: An alternate light source to detect semen. *Acad Emerg Med* 2002;9:1045-1048.

18. Wawryk J, Odell M: Fluorescent identification of biological and other stains on skin by the use of alternative light sources. *J Clin Forensic Med* 2005;12:296-301.

19. Lincoln CA, McBride PM, Turbett GR, et al: The use of alternative light source to detect semen in clinical forensic medical practice. *J Clin Forensic Med* 2006;13:215-218.

20. Sweet D, Lorente M, Lornte J, et al: An improved method to recover saliva from human skin: the double swab technique. *J Forensic Sci* 1997;42:320-322.

21. Riggs N, Houry D, Long G, et al: Analysis of 1076 cases of sexual assault. *Ann Emerg Med* 2000;35:358-362.

22. Grossin C, Bibille I, Lorin de la Grandmaison G, et al: Analysis of 418 cases of sexual assault. *Forensic Sci Int* 2003;28:125-130.

23. Ferris LE, Sandercock J: The sensitivity of forensic tests for rape. *Med Law* 1998;17:333-349.

24. Christian CW, Lavelle JM, DeJong AR, et al: Forensic evidence findings in prepubertal victims of sexual assault. *Pediatrics* 2000;106:100-104.

25. Palusci VJ, Cox EO, Shatz EM, et al: Urgent medical assessment after child sexual abuse. *Child Abuse Negl* 2006;30:367-380.

26. Young KL, Jones JG, Worthington T, et al: Forensic laboratory evidence in sexually abused children and adolescents. *Arch Pediatr Adolesc Med* 2006;160:585-588.

14

TESTS USED TO ANALYZE FORENSIC EVIDENCE IN CASES OF CHILD SEXUAL ABUSE AND ASSAULT

Allan R. De Jong, MD

INTRODUCTION

Forensic science is the application of a broad spectrum of scientific disciplines to assist in legal decision making. The modern use of forensic evidence in sexual assault cases has evolved over the past century. Forensic evidence collected in emergency departments and sexual assault centers focuses on the transfer of body fluids and other materials from perpetrator to victim during the sexual encounter. The primary focus of this evolving quest is to establish the identity of the perpetrator.

Serum proteins and antigens, particularly those that are highly polymorphic, (having multiple alleles) with varying distributions in the population, became essential to analyzing body fluids collected in sexual assault cases. By the mid 1970s, evidence samples were analyzed using multiple polymorphic blood group antigens plus a few serum proteins, and calculations were made of the probability of a random match between a suspect and the evidence sample based on the distribution of the genotypes in the general population.[1] These calculations often gave very small probabilities for a match between two unrelated individuals, but the sensitivity and specificity of the genetic markers were limited.[1] More powerful, stable, and reliable methods were desirable. Forensic identification technology changed abruptly in 1985 with the introduction of DNA methodology to criminal investigation, and use of DNA testing was widespread by the late 1990s.[1] Ultimately, the goal of any physical evidence examination is to perform presumptive testing through serological, chemical, or other methods to identify materials gathered from the victim, the suspected perpetrator, and the crime scene that have the greatest potential to yield valid DNA profiles.[2]

This chapter discusses the application of forensic evidence testing in cases of sexual assault (more specifically, in cases of *child* sexual abuse and assault), the role of trace evidence, and the scientific and legal interpretation of the results of laboratory testing of evidence. Two general types of forensic evidence are used in sexual assault cases, transfer evidence and identification evidence. Transfer or trace evidence includes foreign materials found on the surface of the victim's body or clothing that were transferred to the victim from the abuser or from the crime scene. Identification evidence includes biological materials primarily bodily fluids that can be used to identify the abuser.

ANALYSIS OF BODILY FLUIDS

Semen/Seminal Fluid

Semen, or seminal fluid, is a complex fluid derived from the prostate and other accessory sex glands. Semen is composed of two major components, the cellular fraction and the seminal plasma. The ejaculate is consists of up to 10% spermatozoa (220-300 million sperm cells) and 90% seminal plasma. The cellular fraction contains spermatozoa, plus other cellular elements including epithelial cells. The seminal plasma or fluid component of seminal fluid is derived primarily (65%-75%) from the seminal vesicles. It contains carbohydrates, proteins, citric acid, and zinc.[3] Screening tests for prostatic acid phosphatase (PAP), prostate specific antigen (PSA or p30), and semenogelin in seminal plasma have been used to detect the presence of seminal fluid. PSA has a higher sensitivity than semenogelin or PAP, but semenogelin has higher specificity.[4]

Alternate light sources (ALS) also are used in screening for the presence of semen, displaying a high sensitivity approaching that of the chemical tests, but a lower specificity due to common fluorescence of other materials.[5] ALS have the advantage of not consuming any of the sample. Maximal semen fluorescence is produced by visible blue light at wavelengths between 450 and 490 nm. Standard Wood's lamps or ultraviolet lamps with shorter wavelengths, including those with old bulbs, might not cause semen to fluoresce. Selecting alternative light sources that produce light with wavelengths between 450 and 490 nm will maximize sensitivity and specificity.[5,6]

The forensic application of DNA technology to biological evidence takes advantage of the greater stability of DNA compared with the enzymes and proteins used in serological testing. Compared with serological markers, DNA allows evidence to be extracted from much smaller amounts of material, and increases the specificity of the match between the evidence sample and the suspect's DNA.[7,8] DNA from every human except identical twins is unique because of polymorphisms, the occurrence of more than one allele of a genetic marker at the same locus on the DNA strand. On average, 3 million base pairs differ between any two individuals. Polymorphisms may be length-based or sequence-based. Length-based polymorphisms are repetitive DNA sequences found within 20% to 30% of noncoding DNA.

Many repetitive regions vary in the number of core repeats between different individuals, and are designated "variable number tandem repeats" or VNTR loci. The "short tandem repeats" or STR loci are particular repetitive regions that are used in nuclear DNA profiling. Sequence-based polymorphisms are differences in one or more base pairs in similar length DNA fragments at a particular location in the genome. These point mutations are also known as "single nucleotide polymorphisms" or SNP loci. SNP tests and mitochondrial DNA tests are examples of sequence-based tests.[9]

The VNTR loci had the advantage of having a large number of alleles to produce high discrimination power, but analysis was limited by requiring a relatively large amount of high quality DNA and by being very time consuming.[8] Polymerase chain reaction (PCR) amplification increased the sensitivity of DNA testing by allowing amplification of even very tiny amounts of degraded DNA into the quantities required for analysis. Smaller size variable areas, the STR loci, could be used increasing both sensitivity and specificity because STR loci are more numerous than VNTR loci. Automated technology has allowed for more efficient, rapid, and simultaneous analysis of multiple STR loci, known as "multiplexing," leading to the development of national DNA databases for use in criminal identification. The United States' Combined DNA Index System, or CODIS, uses 13 specific STI loci identified by the Federal Bureau of Investigation (FBI) to create a database for use in matching crime scene materials to previously typed individuals. "Single nucleotide polymorphisms" (SNP loci) represent single point mutations that are very numerous, but typically produce only two alleles. Therefore a relatively large number of SNP loci would have to be analyzed to provide significant discriminatory power for forensic purposes.[8]

Mitochondria contain their own small DNA genomes known as mitochondrial DNA (mtDNA). Normally mtDNA is inherited only from the mother. Cells contain only one nucleus with one copy of nuclear DNA, but the cytoplasm of each cell contains multiple mitochondria with up to thousands of copies of mtDNA. The forensic advantage is that specimens with absent or highly degraded nuclear DNA can be analyzed if mtDNA is present. The mtDNA units are smaller, containing only a fraction of the genome compared with nuclear DNA, so mtDNA lacks the discriminatory power or specificity of nuclear STR loci.[1] The resulting discriminatory power of mtDNA sequencing is on the order of one in a few hundred.[9]

The Y chromosome is transmitted as a single copy only from fathers to sons, and contains hundreds of recognized STR loci. Y chromosomal analysis is particularly useful in resolving mixtures of DNA from different males, when the male component of mixtures is completely masked by female DNA in sexual assault cases, and when some seminal fluid is present but no intact sperm remain.[8,10,11] The overall discriminating power of Y chromosomal DNA is compromised by the relatively limited portion of the genome on the Y chromosome and because the results are incompatible with the nuclear DNA databases.[8,9]

DNA analysis can result in three determinations regarding identity: exclusion, inconclusive, and match. "Exclusion" means the two DNA samples are different, "inconclusive" means the results cannot confirm similarity or difference, and a "match" means the DNA types are similar with no

significant differences. Somewhat less than half of DNA tests result in a match of the suspect to the crime.[9] The current technology for DNA typing has progressed to the point where the reliability and validity of properly collected, properly preserved,[12] and properly analyzed DNA data should not be in doubt. However, the analysis can only yield probabilities and absolute certainty is beyond the realm of science.[8,9]

Blood

Most screening tests for the presence of blood are based on the peroxidase-like reaction of the hemoglobin molecule with chemical agents including luminol, phenolphthalein, leucomalachite green, and several proprietary reagents. The specificity of the tests is limited by frequent cross-reactivity with iron and copper containing salts and certain vegetables and fruits containing peroxidase enzymes. When tested against five other agents, luminol had the highest sensitivity and specificity, and did not destroy the DNA contained in the samples.[13] Newer tests based on using anti-human hemoglobin antibodies to identify human blood have very high specificity, but they have a lower sensitivity than the chemical tests.[13] Alternate light sources (ALS) can also be used to detect blood, with blood having a strong narrow absorption band for fluorescence at about 415 nm. Luminol is significantly more sensitive than ALS in detecting blood.[14] Blood found on body surfaces, body orifices, or clothing of sexual assault victims often comes from the victim, but sometimes it can originate from the perpetrator. Although the density of DNA is lower in blood than in seminal fluid, the white blood cells are nucleated and provide a relatively good source of DNA evidence.

Identification using conventional serology is based on the fact that approximately 80% of the humans are "secretors"; all their bodily fluids including semen, saliva, vaginal secretions, and perspiration will contain the genetic markers found in their blood or serum. The frequencies of the various alleles of individual markers in the general population are known, and the probability of multiple markers occurring in a single person can be calculated for specific combinations of alleles. At one time the most commonly used genetic markers were the ABO blood group antigens, Lewis blood group antigens, phosphoglucomutase, glycooxalase I, and peptidase A, augmented with other blood group antigen systems and polymorphic enzymes to improve discrimination.[7]

DNA testing replaced serology because of the serology's significant limitations in both sensitivity and specificity. Approximately 20% of humans are "nonsecretors" with no genetic markers in body fluids other than blood. The effects of proteolytic enzymes present in semen, and bacterial and environmental degradation, can result in the rapid loss of markers in blood, semen, and saliva, leading to erroneous results. Furthermore, the genetic markers in semen are rapidly degraded in vaginal secretions after intercourse, usually after 6 hours, but can persist longer in dry stains.[1,7,9]

Saliva

Human saliva is 98% water, but also contains electrolytes, mucus, antibacterial compounds, α-amylase, lysozyme, lingular lipase, and cellular material. As many as 8 million human cells and 500 million bacterial cells are present per milliliter of saliva. Forensic testing of suspected saliva samples includes screening tests that typically identify the presence of α-amylase. The α-amylase in saliva hydrolyzes complex carbohydrates such as starch into oligosaccharides, and this reaction produces a characteristic color change, indicating a positive result.[15]

Obstacles in presumptive saliva screening include the innate variation of salivary amylase levels among humans, difficulties in interpreting color change-based tests, body fluid specificity issues, and relatively poor sensitivity compared to screening tests for blood and semen.[15] Salivary α-amylase is found in lower concentrations in other body fluids such as perspiration, tears, breast milk, urine, serum, feces, and semen. Pancreatic α-amylase can be found in vaginal secretions, urine, serum, fecal material, and semen. A ubiquitous enzyme, α-amylase also is found in many plants and in the saliva of pigs, rodents, elephants, and non-human primates.[15]

Screening for saliva in the clinical setting is often based on a history of oral contact or presence of bite marks; however, the use of multiwavelength or "tunable" alternate light sources are helpful in finding stains that might contain semen or saliva.[14,16] This technique can also be used in the laboratory for presumptive identification of saliva and semen stains on fabric. An advantage of this technique is the preservation of the original samples, allowing the entire specimen to be available for DNA processing.[5,6] Maximal saliva fluorescence is produced by visible blue light at wavelengths around 450 nm and saliva detection is poor at shorter wavelengths of 415 nm or less.[14] Selecting "ultraviolet lamps" or alternative light sources that produce light with wavelengths of 450 nm will maximize sensitivity.

Following a positive screening test for saliva, DNA testing can be performed on the cellular component of the saliva using STR analysis. The major limitations are the relative insensitivity of available tests for identifying potential saliva stains and the relatively low density of cellular material in saliva stains.[17]

TRACE EVIDENCE

Trace evidence includes hair, fibers, paint, polymers, glass, soil, plant materials, impressions, cosmetics, lubricants, other chemical residues, and even epithelial cells. Hair and fiber evidence are the predominant types of trace evidence analyzed in sexual assault cases. Locard's exchange principle states that whenever two objects come into contact, a transfer of material will occur.[9] Trace evidence that is transferred can be used to associate objects, individuals, or locations. The integrity and significance of trace material as associative evidence and as potential identity evidence relies on proper detection, collection, and preservation.

A variety of instruments and visualization tools are used to analyze trace evidence. Trace evidence analysis begins with microscopic techniques using visible, polarized, and ultraviolet light. Microspectrophotometry, infrared spectroscopy, thin-layer chromatography, liquid chromatography, and mass spectrometry supplement microscopy when appropriate.[9]

Scalp, pubic, or body hair from the perpetrator occasionally can be found on the victim's body. Scalp hairs have the most interpersonal variation, and facial, axillary and body hairs the least amount of interpersonal variation. Microscopic analysis of scalp and pubic hairs are often conducted, but comparisons of hair from other body regions are less significant and less frequently conducted.[18] Exline et al[19] studied the transfer of pubic hair during consenting sexual contact and found at least one hair transfer in 17.3% of pubic hair combings. Transfers to males (23.6%) were more common than transfers to females (10.9%).[19] Pubic hair transfer in actual sexual assault cases, however, show a much lower rate of transfer.[19,20] Mann reported only 4% of pubic hair combings submitted for forensic analysis revealed hair transfer from suspect to victim.[21] Examination of the undergarments of victims showed a transfer of head hair and pubic hair from the suspect in 4% and 3% of cases, respectively. Examination of the outer clothing of both victims and suspects indicated a transfer rate of head hair of approximately 14% and of pubic hair of 1% to 3%.[20]

Hair analysis requires the collection of suspicious "foreign" hair from the body of the victim, and collection of multiple specimens from the alleged perpetrator and the victim. Hair features such as color, shaft configuration, cross-sectional shape, pigment distribution, hair diameter, and cuticle can be used to classify a hair. Significant variation occurs in scalp hairs of a single individual. The use of dyes, rinses, permanents, and other chemical applications, and environmental exposure to excessive sunlight, wind, and dryness can cause even greater changes in microscopic appearance. Animal hairs can also be transferred as trace evidence, and can be determined to belong to a specific species using microscopy.

When the identity analysis of individual hairs with nuclear or mtDNA is compared with microscopy, a false positive rate of 11% to 20% is found with microscopy.[20] Associations between hairs using microscopy are helpful in determining which hairs to send for DNA analysis. In addition, 86% of hairs unsuitable for microscopic comparison or determined to be inconclusive had sufficient mtDNA available for analysis.[20] Microscopic analysis has limited specificity and the laboratory can only conclude in the majority of cases that the sample is a consistent, inconsistent, or inconclusive match when compared with the perpetrator's hair.[21]

Scalp hair transfer is a complicated process, including primary and secondary transfer, and can be influenced by many environmental and personal variables.[22] Individuals shed approximately 100 head hairs every day and can transfer them to other individuals. Secondary transfer from clothing or other surfaces, persistence of hair despite laundering, and known transfer during laundering, decreases the evidentiary value of hair when a suspect and victim live together or launder their clothing together, as is the case in many child sexual assaults.[23] Most shed hairs lack nucleated cells so they are not amenable to nuclear DNA analysis. These hairs might contain sufficient mitochondrial DNA for analysis of mitochondrial DNA.[20]

The transfer of fibers has been studied extensively, and fiber transfers or exchanges of fibers between garments occur with every contact between two pieces of clothing. Fiber transfers are dependent on a number of variables including the type of contact, the types of garments/fabrics making contact, and fiber length. Transferred fibers generally are lost rapidly, but some transferred fibers even persist on fabrics that have been washed or dry cleaned. Secondary transfer of fibers may occur from horizontal surfaces to clothing.[23] Microscopic comparison of fibers found on the victim's body with known fibers from the perpetrator's house can help confirm the location of the abuse unless they live in the same house. Proper handling of fiber evidence maximizes the value of fiber analysis.[24] Microscopic analysis has limited specificity and the laboratory can only conclude in the majority of cases that the sample is consistent, inconsistent, or inconclusive when compared with known fibers.

DNA containing materials including skin cells, blood, saliva, or semen from a perpetrator can be collected from fingernails, particularly if the victim has scratched the perpetrator during the assault. This material is often collected as part of the sexual assault forensic evidence kit by scraping under the nails, swabbing under the nails, or clipping the nails. Individual clinical casework commonly yields a mixture of perpetrator and victim DNA. However, experimental studies suggest clippings are minimally helpful and gentle scraping or swabbing beneath the nails is more likely to detect useful evidence. Gentle techniques appear to be superior to thorough scraping with a sharp instrument.[25-27]

Epithelial cells can also be transferred through physical contact, providing another potential source of DNA for analysis. The estimated detectible primary transfer between individuals or from an individual to a surface is approximately 20 to 1000 cells. A secondary transfer theoretically is possible but is considered unlikely.[28] The average human sheds approximately 400,000 skin cells every day, with each nucleated skin cell containing about 5 pg of nuclear DNA. Multiplex PCR DNA analysis can produce full DNA profiles to identify individuals at or below 100 pg of purified DNA, therefore as few as 20 cells may be sufficient to produce an individual's DNA profile.[28] Direct physical contact, however, is not the only way epithelial cells are transferred. Indoor dust is composed largely of epithelial cells, containing more than 10 μg (10 million pg) of total DNA per gram of dust, and the DNA is stable in the dry state. Environmental dust transfer can produce one or more DNA profiles from individuals not related to the crime being investigated.[29] Therefore, epithelial cell analysis is usually not done in sexual assault, other than from fingernail scrapings.[27]

CLINICAL CONSIDERATIONS

Protocols have long recommended forensic evidence collection to detect sperm, seminal fluid, and serological markers, when the examination occurs within 72 hours of acute sexual assault or sexual abuse.[25,30] The increasing sensitivity of DNA analysis and the increasing importance of DNA evidence in prosecution of acute sexual assault of adults and adolescents has prompted some centers to extend evidence collection timeframes from 72 to 96 up to 168 hours following a sexual assault.[25] There is little scientific evidence to support obtaining anal/rectal samples unless history or trauma support anal penetration, and when these samples can be collected within 24 hours of the sexual penetration[25] (see Chapter 13). Studies do not support an extended timeline for collection of evidence in young children,[31-33] and there is no other published data assessing the utility of any

DNA testing in prepubertal or young pubertal children. The reasons that young children have significantly lower rates of positive tests for forensic evidence than adults might include differences in the dynamics of the assault and physiological differences. Certainly, the collection of clothing and linens should be performed beyond 24 hours in children.

Common reasons for unprocessed materials or uninterpretable results from clinical specimens from sexual assault cases include insufficient sample quantity, sample degradation (through action of bacteria, enzymes, and environmental factors), and sample purity (including impurities present within the sample and contamination during or subsequent to obtaining the sample).[9] The primary reason for unprocessed materials, however, is the limited availability of proper equipment and technicians for processing of DNA evidence, leaving public laboratories with the resources to analyze only "the most serious cases." The ability to introduce findings in court is greatly impacted by the evidence collection process itself and documentation of evidence collection and evidence handling. Improper collection techniques, lack of proper documentation of collection and processing, and not maintaining a chain of custody of the samples from time of collection through completion of laboratory analysis can result in uninterpretable or unreliable results.

LEGAL ISSUES

Before 1985, legal issues related to identity evidence concerned the relative lack of specificity of serological testing methods.[1,8] During the initial years of DNA analysis, the admissibility of DNA as an accepted scientific methodology was a major question. As DNA evidence has become widely accepted in the legal setting, the challenges have shifted from admissibility to reliability of collection, preservation, and handling of the biological evidence on which DNA analysis is performed. DNA evidence is accepted as being reliable in theory, but legal challenges now focus on suggesting critical mistakes were made from the time of collection through completion of the analysis that invalidate the results.[9] Other authors[34] suggest the principal problems in forensic science in general involve issues of judgment, ethics, and attitude, not inadequate technology or poor quality control. The real challenge is finding ways to preserve the impartiality and independence of both private and public laboratories within an intentionally adversarial legal system. Meeting this challenge could require a cultural change.

A second legal issue is the potential for misinterpreting trace evidence from the environment. Theoretically, low copy-number or low-template DNA processing could replicate a limited size DNA sample from a single cell into samples that allow DNA analysis. Despite the high sensitivity of this process, the resulting DNA profiles have lower specificity than conventional DNA analysis. The high number of replication cycles increase the risk of creation of false alleles and allele drop out if one allele of a heterozygote locus in amplified while the other is not. Unfortunately, the increased sensitivity of this process also increases the potential for analyzing trace DNA from a person unrelated to the crime or the crime scene, or from contamination of evidence following the crime. Furthermore, it is impossible to determine of the type of cell from which the DNA originated, when that sample was deposited, or when or how the DNA became a part of the sample.[1,27,28] Since many children are sexually abused by individuals who are well known to them, those same individuals are likely to contribute trace DNA to the environment if they live in the same house or frequently visit, sleep in the same bed, sit on the same couches, and use the same or adjacent towels in the bathroom. The same concern can be raised about the presence of other trace evidence from household or other frequent contacts collected in cases involving child victims.

A third issue is the interpretation of the results in the courtroom. A full conventional DNA profile (13 STR loci) will have a match probability to a randomly selected member of the general population of approximately 1 in 1 billion to 1 in 1 trillion.[1] Partial profiles from degraded or limited cellular material will not allow comparison of as many STR loci, decreasing the match probability. Matching a sample from the crime scene with a smaller, selected population, such as those individuals contained in the CODIS data base also decreases the match probability because the size of the comparison population is much smaller. Using likelihood ratios rather than a profile probability in these cases more accurately represents the probability of the sample DNA coming from an individual in a data base.[1,8]

A final legal issue is the expectations of the judge or jury regarding the presence of forensic evidence, particularly in cases of sexual assault involving children. The limited clinical data on young children suggest they have significantly lower rates of sperm or seminal fluid identification from forensic examination than adults, and there is little data on DNA evidence in children. Popular media suggests forensic evidence is everywhere and forensic evidence is essential, raising inappropriate expectations in juries hearing cases involving children.

STRENGTH OF THE MEDICAL EVIDENCE

Eyewitness testimony was a factor in three quarters of cases involving 158 previously convicted individuals proven innocent using postconviction DNA testing. About two thirds of these convictions were also related to some misapplication of forensic science, with 40% of the convictions related in part to identification using conventional serology and about 20% related in part to hair comparisons.[35] The transfer of trace evidence including hair, fibers, or foreign materials can suggest possible or probable association but usually provide only weak evidence for the identity of the perpetrator. Identification evidence, primarily body fluids, can provide stronger evidence of sexual acts and the identity of the perpetrator. The presence of sperm, acid phosphatase, PSA, and screening tests for saliva and blood are helpful in supporting the history of sexual contact and in identifying possible substances to submit for DNA analysis. Conventional serology can play a limited role in identity, but it is more helpful in excluding possible suspects than confirming actual perpetrators. DNA analysis provides a more sensitive and more specific approach to the identity of the offender than conventional serology, seminal fluid markers, and trace evidence testing, but there is little published data about the performance of DNA analysis in child and adolescent sexual assault cases.

SUGGESTED DIRECTIONS FOR FUTURE RESEARCH

Two major areas of research are anticipated: one basic science and one clinical in nature. The first area will focus on improvements in DNA technology with increased use of Y chromosomal STR loci, mtDNA loci, SNP loci, and phenotypic DNA profiling.[8,9] This research will involve both improving the specificity of these techniques and improving speed and automation using biochemical tools including DNA microarrays, miniaturization, and "expert systems."[1,8] A major clinical area of research is the utility of forensic evidence collection in both adults and children on obtaining usable DNA materials. There have been no large studies of DNA evidence in sexual assault victims of any age. Studies are needed on the effect of evidence collection methods used in adults on DNA analysis results. In addition, prepubertal children should be studied to determine whether the time limits and techniques for evidence collection used for adults and adolescents are valid in children, or whether modifications are needed in the forensic evidence protocols for children.

References

1. Gill P: DNA as evidence - the technology of identification. *N Engl J Med* 2005;352:2669-2671.
2. Myers JR, Adkins WK: Comparison of modern techniques for saliva screening. *J Forensic Sci* 2008;53:862-867.
3. Duncan MW, Thompson HS: Proteomics of semen and its constituents. *Proteomics Clin Appl* 2007;1:861-875.
4. Sato I, Barni F, Yoshiike M, et al: Applicability of Nanotrap SG as a semen detection kit before male-specific profiling in sexual assaults. *Int J Legal Med* 2007;121:315-319.
5. Nelson DG, Santucci KA: An alternate light source to detect semen. *Acad Emerg Med* 2002;9:1045-1048.
6. Lincoln CA, McBride PM, Turbett GR, et al: The use of an alternative light source to detect semen in clinical forensic medicine practice. *J Clin Forensic Med* 2006;13:215-218.
7. Gill P, Jeffreys AJ, Werrett DJ: Forensic application of DNA "fingerprints." *Nature* 1985;318:577-579.
8. National Commission on the Future of DNA Evidence: *The future of forensic DNA testing.* U.S. Department of Justice, National Institute of Justice, Washington, DC, 2000, pp 1-83.
9. Polesky HF, Roby RK: Identity analysis: use of DNA polymorphisms in parentage and forensic testing. *In:* McPherson RA, Pincus MR (eds): *Henry's Clinical Diagnosis and Management by Laboratory Methods,* ed 21, Saunders Elsevier, Philadelphia, 2007, pp 1340-1349.
10. Johnson CL, Giles RC, Warren JH, et al: Analysis of non-suspect samples lacing visually identifiable sperm using a Y-STR 10-plex. *J Forensic Sci* 2005;50:1116-1118.
11. Sibille I, Duverneuil C, Lorin de la Grandmaison G, et al: Y-STR DNA amplification as biological evidence in sexually assaulted female victims with no cytological detection of spermatozoa. *Forensic Sci Int* 2002;125:212-216.
12. National Academy of Science: The evaluation of forensic DNA evidence: excerpt from the executive summary of the National Research Council report. *Proc Natl Acad Sci U S A* 1997;94:5498-5500.
13. Tobe SS, Watson N, Daeid NN: Evaluation of six presumptive tests for blood, their specificity, sensitivity, and effect on high molecular-weight DNA. *J Forensic Sci* 2007;52:102-109.
14. Johnston E, Ames CE, Dagnall KE, et al: Comparison of presumptive blood test kits including Hexagon OBTI. *J Forensic Sci* 2008;53:687-689.
15. Vandenberg N, van Oorschot RA: The use of Polilight(r) in the detection of seminal fluid, saliva, and bloodstains and comparison with conventional chemical-based screening tests. *J Forensic Sci* 2006;51:361-370.

16. Pang BC, Cheung BK: Applicability of two commercially available kits for forensic identification of saliva stains. *J Forensic Sci* 2008;53:1117-1122.

17. Wawryk J, Odell M: Fluorescent identification of biological and other stains on skin by the use of alternative light sources. *J Clin Forensic Med* 2005;12:296-301.

18. Sweet D, Loprente JA, Valenzuela A, et al: PCR-based DNA typing of saliva stains recovered from human skin. *J Forensic Sci* 1997;42:320-322.

19. Exline DL, Smith FP, Drexler SG: Frequency of pubic hair transfer during sexual intercourse. *J Forensic Sci* 1998;43:505-508.

20. Houck MM, Bodowle B: Correlation of microscopic and mitochondrial DNA hair comparisons. *J Forensic Sci* 2002;47:964-967.

21. Mann M: Hair transfers in sexual assault: a six year study. *J Forensic Sci* 1990;34:951-955.

22. Kolowski JC, Petraco N, Wallace MM, et al: A comparison study of hair examination methodologies. *J Forensic Sci* 2004;49:1253-1255.

23 Gaudette BD, Tessarolo AA: Secondary transfer of human scalp hair. *J Forensic Sci* 1987;32:1241-1253.

24. Grieve MC, Wiggins KG: Fibers under fire: suggestions for improving their use to provide forensic evidence. *J Forensic Sci* 2001;46:835-843.

25. U.S. Department of Justice: *A national protocol for sexual assault medical forensic examinations: adults/adolescents.* U.S. Department of Justice, Office on Violence Against Women, Washington DC, 2004, pp 1-130.

26. Wiegand P, Bajanowski T, Brinkmann B: DNA typing of debris from fingernails. *J Forensic Sci* 2008;106:81-83.

27. Oz C, Zamir A: An evaluation of the relevance of routine DNA typing of fingernail clippings in forensic casework. *J Forensic Sci* 2000;45:158-160.

28. Wickenhauser RA: Trace DNA: a review, discussion of theory and application of the transfer of trace quantities of DNA through skin contact. *J Forensic Sci* 2002;47:442-450.

29. Toothman MH, Kester KM, Champagne J, et al: Characterization of human DNA in environmental samples. *Forensic Sci Int* 2008;178:7-15.

30. American College of Emergency Physicians: *Evaluation and management of the sexually assaulted or sexually abused patient.* American College of Emergency Physicians, Dallas, 1999, pp 1-82.

31. Christian CW, Lavelle JM, De Jong AR, et al: Forensic evidence findings in prepubertal victims of sexual assault. *Pediatrics* 2000;106:100-104.

32. Young KL, Jones JG, Worthington T, et al: Forensic laboratory evidence in sexually abused children and adolescents. *Arch Pediatr Adolesc Med* 2006;160:585-588.

33. Palusci VJ, Cox EO, Shatz EM, et al: Urgent medical assessment after child sexual abuse. *Child Abuse Negl* 2006;30:367-380.

34. Bromwich MR: Justice Department investigation of FBI laboratory: executive summary. Department of Justice Office of the Inspector General. *Crim Law Reporter* 1997;61:2017-2039.

35. Neufeld PJ: The (near) irrelevance of Daubert to criminal justice and some suggestions for reform. *Am J Public Health* 2005;95:S107-S113.

15

DRUG-FACILITATED SEXUAL ASSAULT

Nancy S. Harper, MD

OCCURRENCE AND CHARACTERISTICS OF DRUG-FACILITATED SEXUAL ASSAULT

Media attention in the 1990s popularized the term "date-rape drugs." Drugs, however, have been used to facilitate other crimes such as robbery or physical assault for centuries. "Micky Finns" ("knock-out drops") were named after a Chicago bartender who mixed chloral hydrate into drinks he served his customers so he could rob them.[1,2] "Date-rape drugging" is more accurately referred to as drug-facilitated sexual assault (DFSA), defined as "… offenses in which victims are subjected to nonconsensual acts while they are incapacitated or unconscious due to the effects of alcohol and/or drugs, and are therefore prevented from resisting and/or are unable to consent.[3]"

A recent study found that 1.6% of teens ages 12 to 17 reported serious dating violence, with 0.9% reporting sexual assault. Just more than 10% of those sexual assaults were DFSA.[4] The prevalence of DFSA is lower among younger adolescents. In a 2010 survey, almost 1% of 12-14 year-olds reported DFSA versus 4% of 15-17 year-olds.[5] The Roofie Foundation was established in 1996 in the United Kingdom to serve as a helpline for victims of DFSA. As of October 2006, there had been 9887 reports to the helpline. Adolescents ages 14 to 18 years accounted for 7.3% of these cases.[6] In an almost 10-year retrospective study of individuals seen for sexual assault in Canada, 15.4% of 1594 sexual assaults met criteria for DFSA, not including alcohol overuse and forcible injection of drugs.[7] Adolescents had the highest baseline incidence rate, which rose from 15/100,000 in the first study period (1993 to 1998) to 59.3/100,000 in the second study period (1999 to 2000). Whether the increase in incidence is due to an increased in DFSA or improved recognition by law enforcement and clinicians is not known.[7]

The true incidence of DFSA is difficult to determine since not all victims present for timely medical care or receive drug screening. Due to the nature of the assault, delayed reporting is common. Victims of drug-facilitated sexual assault often have limited memory of events occurring after drug ingestion (anterograde amnesia).[8] Brief periods of awakening ("cameo appearances") often occur in response to loud noises or pain. The victim might remember being unable to move or speak or might recall witnessing part of the assault.[8] Once the victim sleeps off the drug, she is sometimes ambivalent about reporting the assault to law enforcement or accessing health care.[9] In one study of DFSA, 24% of the victims had no recollection of events and 59% had unclear or "patchy" memories.[10] Only 15% had "clear and concise" memories of the event. This worsens the crime, leaving victims unable to provide a history and powerless to fight back.[8] Victims of DFSA are less likely than other sexual assault victims to report the crime to the police, are more likely to delay medical care, and are less likely to have genital and nongenital trauma.[9] Cases with forensic evidence and victim injury are more likely to be prosecuted, so DFSA victims are less likely to see a just resolution of the crime.[11-14] The ideal drug for surreptitious administration and facilitation of a crime should be colorless, odorless, tasteless, easily obtained, and have a rapid onset of action. The drug's clinical effects should include sedation, disinhibition, relaxation of voluntary muscles, and anterograde amnesia.[15] Anterograde amnesia involves impairment of acquisition, consolidation, and storage of memory, and can occur with little change in the victim's outward behaviors.[16] A list of drugs commonly reported as being used in DFSA is found in Table 15-1.

Reports of "drink spiking" and "date rape" have focused largely on flunitrazepam (Rohypnol), gamma hydroxybutyrate (GHB), and ketamine (Ketanest, Ketaset, or Ketalar). Yet, flunitrazepam is rarely found in toxicological studies of DFSA, representing less than 1% of the drugs detected in these cases. Alcohol is much more common, and is found in 40% and 70% of cases, either alone or combined with other drugs.[19-22]

A program was established in the United States in the late 1990s to provide independent testing of urine samples in cases of suspected DFSA.[19] Patient samples were submitted from 49 states. Of the 3303 urine samples tested, 73% were collected within 24 hours of drug ingestion and 98.8% by 72 hours. Samples were screened by immunoassay and confirmed by gas chromatography-mass spectrometry (GC-MS). Additional testing for benzodiazepines and GHB was performed. More than 60% of the samples were positive for one or more drugs, with an average of 1.6 drugs per sample.[19] Alcohol was found in 67% of the positive samples. Alcohol and cannabis was the most frequent combination found, followed by alcohol and benzodiazepines. Benzodiazepines

Table 15-1	Drugs Often Cited as Being Used in Drug-Facilitated Sexual Assaults[2,3,17,18]		
Category	**Names of Drugs (Generic and Trade)**	**Category**	**Names of Drugs (Generic and Trade)**
Alcohol		Opiates and analgesics	Codeine
			Hydrocodone (Vicodin, Lortab)
Benzodiazepines	Alprazolam (Xanax)		Hydromorphone (Dilaudid)
	Chlordiazepoxide (Librium)		Meperidine (Demerol)
	Clonazepam (Klonopin)		Methadone
	Diazepam (Valium)		Morphine
	Flunitrazepam (Rohypnol)		Oxycodone (Percodan)
	Lorazepam (Ativan)		Propoxyphene (Darvocet)
	Nordiazepam (Calmday)	Over-the-counter	Brompheniramine
	Oxazepam (Serax)		Chlorpheniramine
	Temazepam (Restoril)		Diphenhydramine
	Triazolam (Halcion)		Doxylamine
Cannabis	Marijuana		Dextromethorphan
Stimulants and related substances	Amphetamine	Anti-cholinergics	Scopolamine
	Methamphetamine		Atropine
	Cocaine	Miscellaneous	Carisoprodol (Soma)
	Methylenedioxymethamphetamine (Ecstasy)		Clonidine (Catapres)
			Chloral Hydrate
Non-benzodiazepine hypnotics	Zolpidem (Ambien)		Cyclobenzaprine (Flexeril)
	Eszopiclone (Lunesta)		Doxepin
	Zaleplon (Sonata)		Ketamine
			Meprobamate (Miltown)
Barbiturates	Amobarbital		Valproic Acid (Depakene)
	Butalbital	Antidepressants	Amitryptiline
	Pentobarbital		Citalopram Hydrobromide (Celexa)
	Secobarbital		Fluoxetine (Prozac)
GHB and related substances	Gamma-hydroxybutyric acid (GHB)		Imipramine
	Gamma-butyrolactone (GBL)		Nortriptyline
	1,4-butanediol (1,4-BD)		Sertraline (Zoloft)

were found in 15.4% of the positive samples. GHB was not found in samples with detectable alcohol, but did occur in 4.9% of the positive samples. GHB might have been underestimated in this study due to its short half-life. Investigators found benzodiazepines alone in 98 samples (4.8%), but there was no medical or recreational drug history recorded in the study.[20]

In an attempt to better answer the question of voluntary versus involuntary drug use, Hurley et al[10] studied the drug screens of 76 cases of DFSA. Voluntary alcohol use was reported by 77% of subjects, with the consumption of at least four drinks in 71%. Prescription drug use was reported in 49%, and 26% reported recreational drug use. Unexpected drugs not knowingly consumed were found in 20% of the 76 subjects. While DFSA can occur through involuntary ingestion, voluntary ingestion, or a combination of both,[3] the majority of cases of DFSA occur after the voluntary ingestion of recreational drugs and alcohol.[18] It can be difficult to separate cases of surreptitious administration from voluntary ingestion. Regardless, incapacitation through drugs and alcohol eliminates the ability to consent. Careful history taking is essential to determine which drug might be contributing to the clinical symptoms. Table 15-2 lists the common historical and clinical features in DFSA.

Table 15-2	Common Physical Effects and Common Clinical Patterns Seen in Drug-Facilitated Sexual Assault[2,15,28,30]	
Common Clinical Effects		**Common Clinical Patterns**
Nausea, vomiting		Sudden intoxication
Headache		Intoxication out of proportion to alcohol consumed
Confusion		
Dizziness		
Drowsiness		Unattended beverage
Reduced inhibitions		Attending a party or rave
Impaired judgment		Waking in unexpected location
Impaired concentration		
Lack of muscle coordination		Waking with an unexpected person
Ataxia		
Loss of consciousness		Clothing removed
Hypotension, bradycardia		Clothing on inside out
Respiratory depression		Semen stains on clothing
		Genital/rectal soreness or trauma
		"Cameo appearances" or flashes of memory
		No memory of events

SUBSTANCES COMMONLY USED IN DFSA

Ethyl Alcohol

Ethyl alcohol is the most common drug detected in cases of alleged sexual assault, with a prevalence rate ranging from 40% to 70%.[19-23] Among college students surveyed for rape and sexual assault, 1 in 20 women reported rape and in 72% of those cases, the rape occurred while the victim was intoxicated.[24] Surveys of adolescents in grades 7 through 12 report that alcohol is involved in 12% to 20% of sexual assaults, with higher rates occurring in female adolescents 16 years of age or older. Alcohol-related assaults were more likely to occur at parties or at someone else's home.[25]

In a prospective study of patients presenting to emergency departments for suspected DFSA, 94% of the blood samples collected were positive for alcohol and 65% had blood alcohol concentrations greater than 160 mg/dL.[26] In the study by Hurley et al,[10] the average blood alcohol level in suspected DFSA victims was 0.11% (110 mg/dL). Based on the delay between the assault and the sampling, the authors estimated the average blood alcohol concentration at the time of the assault was from 0.22% to 0.33%. Performing back calculations of blood alcohol levels in victims of suspected DFSA can be helpful in understanding the degree of impairment at the time of the assault. Back calculations assume that no alcoholic beverages were consumed between the assault and the examination, and that the victim metabolizes alcohol with zero-order (linear) kinetics. Rates of alcohol metabolism can vary with gender, tolerance (social versus chronic drinkers), and phenotypic differences in alcohol dehydrogenase.[2,27] Alcohol has a half-life of approximately 4 hours and elimination rates can vary between 10 and 25 mg/dL/hr.[28]

In one study of alleged DFSA, investigators recorded blood and urine alcohol concentrations and performed back calculations assuming an elimination rate of 18 mg/dL.[28] Of the 391 samples obtained within 12 hours of assault, 81% were positive for alcohol. Sixty percent of those positive had back-calculated levels greater than 150 mg/dL (sufficient to cause drunkenness in a social drinker), 36% percent had levels greater than 200 mg/dL ("heavy drunkenness"), and 4% had levels greater than 300 mg/dL ("extreme drunkenness").[28]

The symptoms seen in alcohol intoxication can progress from nausea and vomiting to respiratory depression and loss of consciousness, depending on blood levels and on an individual's tolerance level (Table 15-3). Alcohol is hydrophilic and absorbed through the gastrointestinal system with simple diffusion. Absorption rates and peak blood alcohol concentrations (BAC) vary depending on the alcohol content of the beverage and whether food was ingested simultaneously.[3] Calculators are available online to estimate BAC based on gender, weight, number of standard drinks, and length of time over which the drinks were consumed (http://www.ou.edu/oupd/bac.htm).[29]

Benzodiazepines and Flunitrazepam

Benzodiazepines are central nervous system (CNS) depressants that cause dizziness, disorientation, lack of coor-

Table 15-3	The Progression of Clinical Impairment and Effects with Increasing Blood Alcohol Content[29-31]	
Blood Alcohol Content (%)	**Clinical Effects**	**Psychomotor Impairment**
0.02	Relaxation, lightheaded	No loss coordination
0.05	Lowered inhibitions, euphoria, feelings of well-being, warmth	Reduced coordination Minor impairments attention, memory and judgment
0.08	Blunted emotions Disinhibited	Legally impaired, illegal to drive Impairment of memory, speech, comprehension, perception
0.10	Loss of inhibition Loss of euphoria	Loss of coordination and judgment Ataxia
0.15	Emotional lability Nausea Dysphoria	Severe impairment of motor (staggering), speech (slurred), vision (blurring), judgment
0.20	Confusion, disoriented Needs help walking, standing Nausea, vomiting	Loss of balance Gag reflex impaired
0.25	Vomiting, choking Sudden blackouts	Risk of aspiration Risk of injury and falls
0.30	Stupor Pass out suddenly	Loss of consciousness Loss of bladder control
0.35	Difficult to arouse	Equivalent to surgical anesthesia Coma possible
0.40 or greater	Respiratory depression Respiratory arrest	Coma Death

dination, slurred speech, loss of consciousness, flaccid muscle tone, nystagmus, and anterograde amnesia due to their effects on specific neurotransmitter receptor sites for gamma-aminobutyric acid (GABA).[2] Twenty-six different classes of benzodiazepines have different affinities for the receptor. Flunitrazepam, a member of the 7-nitrobenzodiazepine class, has a high affinity for the receptor.[2,3]

Benzodiazepines are ideal agents for drug-facilitated sexual assault. In combination with alcohol, smaller doses are needed and the effects are synergistic. As a single drug, benzodiazepines are found less frequently in DFSA patients than alcohol, marijuana, or cocaine,[21] but in one large study,

58% of the victims with more than one substance detected were positive for benzodiapezines.[21] Used in combination with alcohol, benzodiazepines were second only to marijuana. Flunitrazepam was seen in very few samples (7 out of 2003). Oxazepam, diazepam, lorazepam, and clonazepam represented the majority of benzodiazepines detected.[21]

Sexually active females between the ages of 14 to 26 years were surveyed at family planning clinics about voluntary use of flunitrazepam;[32] 5.9% reported using the drug at some time. First use occurred on average at 17 years, with some using the drug at as young as 11 years of age. Seventy-four percent reported taking the drug with alcohol; 10% of users reported physical or sexual assaults after voluntary use.[32]

In the United States importation of flunitrazepam was banned 1996, but it is still available and popular in Europe and Latin America.[2] It is tasteless, odorless, and colorless, and dissolves easily in alcohol. The manufacturer has recently reformulated the drug to give a blue color when dissolved in clear drinks and to cause haziness in colored beverages.[33]

"Roached out" is slang for being under the influence of flunitrazepam. Other street names of the drug include roofies, rophies, roopies, rib, rope, pappas, peanuts, pastas, forget pills, row-shays, roaches, Mexican valium, circles, rubies, and roche 2.[2,34] The hypnotic effects of flunitrazepam predominate over the sedative and anxiolytic effects. It has been used as a sleep-inducing drug at the 2 mg dose with little psychomotor impairment (hangover effects) in the morning. It has a high-affinity for the GABA receptor, with 10 times the potency of diazepam and longer amnesia.[35] More than 80% of the drug is absorbed from the gastrointestinal tract. Clinical effects occur in 20 minutes and can persist up to 24 hours. Flunitrazepam metabolizes to 7-aminoflunitrazepam and norflunitrazepam. It is detectable up to 2 days in blood and 4 days in urine, but is not captured by traditional immunoassay urine drug screening. Other testing such as GC-ECD (electron capture detection) and GC-MS are quite sensitive in detecting its metabolites.[36]

The prevalence of flunitrazepam use has diminished as the use of clonazepam (Klonopin) has risen.[37] Clonazepam also is sold under the street name of "roofies" with clinical effects quite similar to flunitrazepam. It has been found twice as often as flunitrazepam in suspected DFSA victims.[21] Dowd et al[38] compared the behavioral and cognitive effects of flunitrazepam and clonazepam in two groups of volunteers. Cognitive testing was performed at baseline and repeated after drug exposure. Subjects appeared disinhibited to the investigators. The groups reported "patchy amnesia" for what occurred after drug ingestion. Six of 10 subjects exposed to clonazepam had no memory of a second set of evaluations. Clonazepam had a longer half-life than flunitrazepam and a longer period of impairment.[38] Effects are experienced 30 to 60 minutes after ingestion and last up to 12 hours. It is metabolized by the liver to 7-aminoclonazepam. Clonazepam has been detected up to 14 to 21 days in urine with targeted testing.[39]

Although they are rapid and inexpensive, immunoassay urine drug screening tests using competitive binding between an antibody and a drug antigen are limited in their ability to detect benzodiazepines. The antibody is most specific and sensitive to the drug used to generate the antibody. For benzodiazepines, oxazepam is commonly used as the antigen. Benzodiazepines that do not metabolize to oxazepam (e.g., clonazepam, lorazepam, alprazolam, and triazolam) will not be detected. In addition, a small amount of drug might not produce sufficient metabolites to yield a positive screen. False-negative urine screens for benzodiazepines often occur.[2,40] If a patient's clinical symptoms are concerning for DFSA, urine drug confirmation for benzodiazepines is necessary even if the screen is negative.

Cannabis

Marijuana is perhaps the most common illicit drug found in urine samples analyzed for suspected DFSA, and is found in 18% to 26% of samples analyzed. It is found as a solitary agent in 7% to 11% of cases.[19-22] Clinical effects include relaxation, an altered sense of time, euphoria, drowsiness, and impairment of short-term memory. Unique cannabinoid receptors are present in the brain, the peripheral nervous system, and the immune system. Onset of action can occur within 15 to 30 minutes when smoked and the effects can last 4 to 6 hours. It is extremely lipid soluble and has a half-life of several days, which may contribute to its high prevalence in samples.[41] In one study of 260 samples positive for cannabinoids, 63 subjects (24%) admitted to voluntary use.[22] Cannabinoids are detected by routine immunoassay urine drug screening, and is present in urine for several days after acute ingestion and for weeks in chronic users. Its persistence can make it difficult to determine its role in an acute assault.

Cocaine

Cocaine is a CNS stimulant producing generalized nervous system activation and reuptake inhibition of multiple neurotransmitters including dopamine, norepinephrine, and serotonin. In addition to tachycardia, hyperactivity, and restlessness, clinical effects include euphoria, increased energy, appetite suppression, and increased self-confidence and libido.[41] Cocaine can be inhaled, smoked, and injected. "Speed-balling" is the street term for the intravenous injection of heroine and cocaine. A "liquid lady" refers to the combination of alcohol and cocaine. It is frequently found in combination with alcohol and other drugs, perhaps to attenuate the abrupt onset and cessation of clinical effects. In toxicological studies of DFSA, the most common illicit drug found in combination with cocaine is cannabis.[20,22] The prevalence of cocaine in samples submitted for analysis for DFSA ranges from 8% to 11%.[19-22] As the sole drug, it is present in just less than 2% of cases.[20-22]

Cocaine and its primary metabolite, benzoylecgonine is routinely detected on immunoassay urine drug screens. Metabolism of cocaine to benzoylecgonine occurs through hepatic carboxylesterase enzymes, which are inhibited if alcohol ingestion precedes cocaine use.[41] Depending on dosing, metabolites of cocaine can be detected for 2 to 3 days in urine and up to a week at higher doses.[40] There is little cross-reactivity with other substances and few false positives. False negatives occur with very low drug levels. Despite the high positive predictive value of the urine drug screen for cocaine, drug confirmation is still recommended for legal purposes.

Amphetamines/Methamphetamines

Amphetamine and methamphetamine is found in 4% to 7% of samples from DFSA cases.[19,20] They are often found in combination with other drugs such as alcohol, cocaine, benzodiazepines, and marijuana. They are found as the solitary drug in DFSA in less than 2% of cases. This class of drugs is often used at "raves" (drug-fueled dance parties), and is called crystal meth, speed, crys, jip, and meth. Methamphetamines come in powder form and are easily taken orally, smoked, or inhaled. Clinical effects include tachycardia, hypertension, hyperthermia, and sweating.[42] Amphetamines and methamphetamines are detected by routine drug screening, but drug screens have cut-off thresholds for positive tests that are quite high. Another rave favorite, ecstasy (3,4-methylenedioxymethamphetamine or MDMA), has both stimulant and hallucinogenic effects with a toxicity similar to amphetamines and cocaine.[42] Ecstasy is often used in combination with alcohol, cocaine, GHB, cannabis, and amphetamines. Clinical symptoms of intoxication are largely related to sympathetic activation including palpitations, dizziness, weakness, and anxiety. When ecstasy is used in combination with other drugs, clinical symptom patterns can change dramatically. For example, when ecstasy is combined with GHB ingestion, coma and hypothermia can be seen. Severe medical complications of ecstasy, especially when combined with other drugs, include cardiac arrest, hyperthermia, rhabdomyolysis, disseminated intravascular coagulation, renal insufficiency, and liver failure.[43] The use of ecstasy in DFSA has been rarely studied, as most investigators group amphetamines and methamphetamines as a class. In one study screening for ecstasy in 1014 DFSA cases, it was detected in 5%.[22] Ecstasy in high doses can be detected on routine urine drug screening as amphetamines, but in low doses it is undetectable.[42] Ecstasy is notorious for being impure, which affects toxicological analyses.

GHB (Gamma-Hydroxybutyric Acid), GBL (Gamma-Butyrolactone), and 1,4 BD (1,4-Butanediol)

Grievous bodily harm, Georgia home boy, liquid ecstasy, liquid X, liquid E, GBH, soap, scoop, easy lay, salty water, g-riffick, cherry meth, organic quaalude, natural sleep-500, and somatomax are just a few of the street names for gamma-hydroxybutyric acid (GHB).[2,44] Over the years GHB has been marketed as a sleep aid, weight aid, performance enhancer, and sex enhancer, and it has been used for the treatment of depression, anxiety, and alcohol and opiate withdrawal.[6,8,45-47] In 2000, GHB was declared a Schedule I controlled substance by the U.S. Food and Drug Administration. GHB in the form of sodium oxybutyrate (Xyrem) is still available by prescription as a Schedule III orphan drug for use in the treatment of narcolepsy and cataplexy.[48]

GHB is a naturally occurring metabolite of gamma-aminobutyric acid (GABA). It is present in both the peripheral and central nervous systems at concentrations less than 1.0 μg/ml.[47] It is reversibly metabolized to GABA in the central nervous system. GABA is metabolized to succinic semialdehyde (SSA) and enters the Krebs cycle. A small portion of SSA is then metabolized back to GHB.[3] GBL and 1,4-BD enter the process as precursors for GHB. Recipes for the home-based manufacture of GHB from GBL and sodium hydroxide are easily located on the Internet. GBL is available as an industrial solvent. Both GBL (called renew trient, blue nitro, or revivarant) and 1,4-BD (with street names of weight belt cleaner, soma, inner G) can be ingested without laboratory conversion to GHB.[3,15] GBL has a greater bioavailability and is rapidly converted to GHB by enzymes in the blood and liver.[47,49] All three drugs come in a white powder or tablet form and dissolve easily in water. GHB is a sodium salt, hence the terminology "salty water."[3,45,49]

GHB crosses the blood-brain barrier, affects the endogenous opioid system, and increases dopamine levels. GHB has an affinity for both the GHB-specific receptor and the GABA type B receptor. Ingestion of GHB causes CNS depression, sedation, nausea, drowsiness, dizziness, decreased inhibitions, euphoria, and increased sensuality. Effects are easily confused with those of alcohol ingestion and are synergistic with alcohol. Dose dependent effects occur within 15 to 30 minutes,[34,50] and range from amnesia and hypotonia at 10 mg/kg, rapid eye movement (REM) and non-REM sleep at 20 to 30 mg/kg, anesthesia at 50 mg/kg, and severe respiratory depression and coma at doses exceeding 50 mg/kg.[44] A recreational dose of 1 g can produce amnesia and hypotonia, 2 g deep sleep, and 4 g coma.[43] Effects can last several hours. Patients with GHB intoxication and overdose have clinical effects lasting from 20 minutes to as long as 10 hours. Coma in nonintubated patients rarely lasts longer than 4 hours.[51] Victims often recover spontaneously in as little as 1 to 2 hours.[2,34] Coingestion of alcohol and other drugs can alter the symptom pattern and increase the depth and length of a coma.[52]

Routine immunoassay urine drug screening does not include GHB. GHB is an endogenous substance and is excreted in urine. A forensic threshold of 10 μg/mL has been suggested as the lower limit for a positive test.[3] Urine GHB levels ranged from 0.9 to 3.5 μg/mL in volunteers not taking the drug.[53]

The prevalence of GHB in suspected DFSA is approximately 3% to 4%.[19-21] Reported prevalence rates of GHB are quite likely underestimated as the metabolism and clearance is so rapid.

Table 15-4 summarizes other drugs that are uncommonly reported to be associated with DFSA.[2,3,17,18]

RECOMMENDATIONS

Victims of suspected DFSA sometimes come to emergency departments with altered mental status and no known history of sexual assault. Initial medical management consists of supportive care (airway, breathing, circulation) and monitoring. It is not uncommon for victims with GHB intoxication to have a Glasgow Coma Scale of 3. Coma in GHB intoxication can last 4 to 6 hours, or longer if intubation is required for respiratory failure.[51] Initial laboratory studies should include rapid glucose testing, a complete blood count, comprehensive metabolic panel, serum osmolality, urinalysis, pregnancy testing, toxicology screening, an electrocardiogram, and cultures as indicated. Sexual assault victims with altered mental status should be carefully examined for coexisting head and abdominal injuries. Depending on the drug detected, helpful medications can include glucose/thiamine

Table 15-4 Less Commonly Encountered Drugs Used in Drug-Facilitated Sexual Assault (DFSA)

Drug Class	Drug Name	Street Name	Prevalence in DFSA	Mechanism	Clinical Effects	Timing	Urine Drug Screening
Opiates	Codeine Heroin Hydrocodone (Vicodin, Lortab) Hydromorphone (Dilaudid) Meperidine (Demerol) Methadone Morphine Oxycodone (Percodan) Propoxyphene (Darvocet)	Smack, Horse, Hard Stuff, Junk, Hairy, Harry, M, Morf	2-10%[19,22] 1% heroin (targeted testing for 6-acetylmorphine)[22]		Analgesia Sedation	Onset: 5 min INH/IM to 30-60 min PO	Detected Limitations: Routine immunoassays detect naturally occurring opiates such as morphine and codeine False negatives occur with semi-synthetics (hydrocodone, hydromorphone, oxycodone, fentanyl); recommend urine drug confirmation with GC-MS to improve detection synthetic opiates and confirm positive results Targeted Testing: Methadone, Propoxyphene[2]
Non-benzodiazepine hypnotics	Zolpidem (Ambien) Zaleplon (Sonata) Eszopiclone (Lunesta) Zopiclone (Imovane)	A-Tic-Tacs	6/1014 samples, 1 attributed to DFSA[22]	GABA Receptor (selective for receptors in the brain)	Anterograde Amnesia Benzodiazepine effects	Onset: 10-30 min Half-Life: 1 (Ambien) to 6 (Lunesta) hrs	Not detected
Barbiturates	Amobarbital Butalbital Pentobarbital Phenobarbital Secobarbital Thiopental	Barbs, barbies, sleepers, blue bullets, nembies, pink ladies, red devils	1% or less[19,20]	GABA Receptor (distinct receptor sites)	CNS depression Sedation Anesthesia Hypnosis Anxiolysis	Ultrashort-acting (thiopental) to Long-acting (Phenobarbital)[3] Half-Life: 80-120 hrs (Phenobarbital)	1-4 days urine[2]
Non-barbiturate hypnotics	Chloral Hydrate	"Mickey Finn"			Effects similar to alcohol, benzodiazepines, barbiturates Amnesia at higher doses[3]	Onset: 30 min Half-Life: 4-12 hrs[22]	Not detected Metabolites: trichloroethanol TCE-glucuronide Trichloroacetic acid[22]

Continued

Table 15-4 **Less Commonly Encountered Drugs Used in Drug-Facilitated Sexual Assault (DFSA)—cont'd**

Drug Class	Drug Name	Street Name	Prevalence in DFSA	Mechanism	Clinical Effects	Timing	Urine Drug Screening
Other	Ketamine	K, Special K, Ket Super Acid, Super C, Vitamin K, Smack K, Kit-kat, Keller, HOSS, Kiddie, Special LA Coke, Wonk[2,33]	0.5%[22]		Delirium Amnesia Analgesia Hallucinations Hypersalivation Nystagmus Dissociative Anesthesia (at higher doses)[2,34]	Onset: 20 sec IM to 20 min PO Half-Life: 2-3 hrs[2]	Not detected Metabolites: Norketamine dehydronorketamine[2]
Anticholinergics	Atropine Scopolamine	Nightshade CIA Drug Jimsonweed Stinkweed			Sedation Amnesia Confusion Anticholinergic	Onset: 15-30 min Duration: up to 2-3 days[2]	Not detected
Antihistamine	Diphenhydramine Chlorpheniramine		1.4%[21]		CNS depression Anticholinergic	Onset: 15-60 min Duration: 4-6 hrs[2]	Not detected
Antitussives	Dextromethorphan	Dex, DXM, Tuss, Robo, Skittles, Triple-C, Syrup[2]		NMDA glutamate receptor: non-competitive antagonist[2]	Euphoria Analgesia Sedation Dissociation		Detected: cross reacts with opiates Targeted testing Metabolite: dextrorphan[2]
Miscellaneous	Tetrahydrozoline (Visine)		Case Report— Adult male utilized Visine drops to incapacitate and sexually abuse/ assault children and spouse[57]	Alpha-agonist (presynaptic alpha-2 receptors, spinal cord)[57]	Effects similar to clonidine Hypotonia Muscle flaccidity[57]		Not detected

(alcohol intoxication), naloxone (opiate ingestion), flumazenil (benzodiazepine ingestion), and activated charcoal.

If DFSA is suspected, collect blood and urine samples as soon as possible, using strict documentation of the chain of custody of the samples. If the victim presents within 24 hours of drug exposure, a blood sample at least 7 to 10 mL in grey-top tubes (sodium fluoride and potassium oxalate) should be collected.[2,3,18] Urine samples should be collected up to 96 hours after drug exposure.[19] Samples should contain at least 100 mL of urine.[54]

A detailed history of prescription and recreational drug use is essential for proper interpretation of test results, covering drugs ingested in the days to weeks before the alleged assault. Alcohol consumption should be documented including the type of alcohol, and the number and size of drinks, and the number of hours over which the alcohol was consumed. Record any drugs the suspected assailant might have accessed.[18] Containers for urine and blood samples are often included in forensic evidence kits. Kits containing blood or urine should be refrigerated.

When patients have clinical symptoms concerning for DFSA, obtain blood alcohol levels and a urine drug screen. Urine drug confirmation should be performed on positive drug classes. False-negative screening test can occur. The clinician should determine the need for additional confirmation of benzodiazepines or other drug classes based on clinical history and presentation. While commercial laboratories offer comprehensive DFSA panels, they are quite expensive.

Coasters and cards are sold that detect "date rape drugs," such as The Drink Safe Coaster (Drink Safe Technologies, Victoria, Australia), Drink Guard (Access Diagnostic Tests UK, Ltd., Halam, UK) and Drink Detective (Bloomsbury Inovations, Ltd., London). These have been tested and found to have limited usefulness. Few drugs were detected and false negatives and false positives frequently occured.[3,55,56]

Adolescents should be educated about DFSA and how to prevent it, including the association between sexual assault and the voluntary use of drugs and alcohol. Adolescents and young adults should be educated on the volume of alcohol in popular drinks and cocktails, and the effects of multiple drinks on decision making and the ability to self-protect. Potential victims of DFSA should be encouraged to report any incidents, and to quickly seek medical attention for evaluation and forensic evidence collection. Counseling should be encouraged for all victims, with the understanding that many victims will not know what happened to them.[33] Continued support is even more crucial for a crime that leaves its victim powerless to know and report its details.

References

1. Asbury H: *Gem of the prairie.* AA Knopf, New York, 1940.
2. Bechtel LK, Holstege CP: Criminal poisoning: drug-facilitated sexual assault. *Emerg Med Clin North Am* 2007;25:499-525.
3. LeBeau MA: *Drug-facilitated sexual assault: a forensic handbook.* Academic Press, San Diego, 2001.
4. Wolitzky-Taylor KB, Ruggiero KJ, Danielson CK, et al: Prevalence and correlates of dating violence in a national sample of adolescents. *J Am Acad Child Adolesc Psychiatry* 2008;47:755-762.
5. The Roofie Foundation: Roofie foundation statistics: updated Oct 2008 (website): http://www.roofie.com/index.php?option=com_content&task=view&id=21&Itemid=46. Accessed March 4, 2009.
6. McCauley JL, Conoscenti LM, Ruggiero KJ, et al: Prevalence and correlates of drug/alcohol-faciliated and incapacitated sexual assault in a nationally representative sample of adolescent girls. *J Clin Child Adolesc Psychol* 2009;38:295-300.
7. McGregor MJ, Ericksen J, Ronald LA, et al: Rising incidence of hospital-reported drug-facilitated sexual assault in a large urban community in Canada. Retrospective population-based study. *Can J Public Health* 2004;95:441-445.
8. Fitzgerald N, Riley KJ: Drug-facilitated rape: looking for the missing pieces. *Natl Inst Justice J* 2000;4:8-15. http://www.ncjrs.gov/pdffiles1/jr000243c.pdf. Accessed on March 4, 2009.
9. McGregor MJ, Lipowska M, Shah S, et al: An exploratory analysis of suspected drug-facilitated sexual assault seen in a hospital emergency department. *Women Health* 2003;37:71-80.
10. Hurley M, Parker H, Wells DL: The epidemiology of drug facilitated sexual assault. *J Clin Forensic Med* 2006;13:181-185.
11. McGregor MJ, Le G, Marion SA, et al: Examination for sexual assault: is the documentation of physical injury associated with the laying of charges? A retrospective cohort study. *CMAJ* 1999;160:1565-1569.
12. McGregor MJ, Du Mont J, Myhr TL: Sexual assault forensic medical examination: is evidence related to successful prosecution? *Ann Emerg Med* 2002;39:639-647.
13. Rambow B, Adkinson C, Frost TH, et al: Female sexual assault: medical and legal implications. *Ann Emerg Med* 1992;21:727-731.
14. McGregor MJ, Wiebe E, Marion SA, et al: Why don't more women report sexual assault to the police? *CMAJ* 2000;162:659-660.
15. Schwartz RH, Milteer R, LeBeau MA: Drug-facilitated sexual assault ("date rape"). *South Med J* 2000;93:558-561.
16. Goulle JP, Anger JP: Drug-facilitated robbery or sexual assault: problems associated with amnesia. *Ther Drug Monit* 2004;26:206-210.
17. LeBeau M, Andollo W, Hearn WL, et al: Recommendations for toxicological investigations of drug-facilitated sexual assaults. *J Forensic Sci* 1999;44:227-230.
18. LeBeau MA: Guidance for improved detection of drugs used to facilitate crimes. *Ther Drug Monit* 2008;30:229-233.
19. ElSohly MA, Salamone SJ: Prevalence of drugs used in cases of alleged sexual assault. *J Anal Toxicol* 1999;23:141-146.
20. Hindmarch I, ElSohly M, Gambles J, et al: Forensic urinalysis of drug use in cases of alleged sexual assault. *J Clin Forensic Med* 2001;8:197-205.
21. Slaughter L: Involvement of drugs in sexual assault. *J Reprod Med* 2000;45:425-430.
22. Scott-Ham M, Burton FC: Toxicological findings in cases of alleged drug-facilitated sexual assault in the United Kingdom over a 3-year period. *J Clin Forensic Med* 2005;12:175-186.
23. Ledray LE: The clinical care and documentation for victims of drug-facilitated sexual assault. *J Emerg Nurs* 2001;27:301-305.
24. Mohler-Kuo M, Dowdall GW, Koss MP, et al: Correlates of rape while intoxicated in a national sample of college women. *J Stud Alcohol* 2004;65:37-45.
25. Young A, Grey M, Abbey A, et al: Alcohol-related sexual assault victimization among adolescents: prevalence, characteristics, and correlates. *J Stud Alcohol Drugs* 2008;69:39-48.
26. Hughes H, Peters R, Davies G, et al: A study of patients presenting to an emergency department having had a "spiked drink." *Emerg Med J* 2007;24:89-91.
27. Smith GD, Shaw LJ, Maini PK, et al: Mathematical modelling of ethanol metabolism in normal subjects and chronic alcohol misusers. *Alcohol Alcohol* 1993;28:25-32.
28. Scott-Ham M, Burton FC: A study of blood and urine alcohol concentrations in cases of alleged drug-facilitated sexual assault in the United Kingdom over a 3-year period. *J Clin Forensic Med* 2006;13:107-111.
29. University of Oklahoma Police Department: Blood alcohol calculator (website): http://www.ou.edu/oupd/bac.htm. Accessed March 5, 2009.
30. National Highway Traffic Safety Administration: The ABCs of BAC: a guide to understanding blood alcohol concentration and alcohol impairment (website): http://www.nhtsa.dot.gov/people/injury/alcohol/stopimpaired/ABCsBACWeb/page2.htm. Accessed March 5, 2009.
31. Virginia Polytechnic Institute and State University: Students. Alcohol's effects (website): http://www.alcohol.vt.edu/students/alcoholEffects/index.htm. Accessed March 5, 2009.
32. Rickert VI, Wiemann CM, Berenson AB: Prevalence, patterns, and correlates of voluntary flunitrazepam use. *Pediatrics* 1999;103:E6.

33. Schwartz RH, Weaver AB: Rohypnol, the date rape drug. *Clin Pediatr (Phila)* 1998;37:321.

34. Smith KM: Drugs used in acquaintance rape. *J Am Pharm Assoc (Wash)* 1999;39:519-525.

35. Mattila MA, Larni HML: Flunitrazepam: a review of its pharmacological properties and therapeutic use. *Drugs* 1980;20:353-374.

36. LeBeau MA, Montgomery MA, Wagner JR, et al: Analysis of biofluids for flunitrazepam and metabolites by electrospray liquid chromatography/mass spectrometry. *J Forensic Sci* 2000;45:1133-1141.

37. Raymon LP, Steele BW, Walls HC: Benzodiazepines in Miami-Dade County, Florida driving under the influence (DUI) cases (1995-1998) with emphasis on Rohypnol: GC-MS confirmation, patterns of use, psychomotor impairment, and results of Florida legislation. *J Anal Toxicol* 1999;23:490-499.

38. Dowd SM, Strong MJ, Janicak PG, et al: The behavioral and cognitive effects of two benzodiazepines associated with drug-facilitated sexual assault. *J Forensic Sci* 2002;47:1101-1107.

39. Negrusz A, Bowen AM, Moore CM, et al: Elimination of 7-aminoclonazepam in urine after a single dose of clonazepam. *Anal Bioanal Chem* 2003;376:1198-1204.

40. Gourlay DL, Caplan YH, Heit HA: *Urine drug testing in clinical practice: dispelling the myths & designing strategies.* PharmaCom Group, Stamford, Conn, 2006.

41. O'Brien CP: Drug addiction and drug abuse. *In:* Brunton L, Lazo J, Parker KL (eds): *Goodman & Gilman's the pharmacological basis of therapeutics,* ed 11, McGraw-Hill, New York, 2005, pp 607-627.

42. Jamieson MA, Weir E, Rickert VI, et al: Rave culture and drug rape. *J Pediatr Adolesc Gynecol* 2002;15:251-257.

43. Liechti ME, Kunz I, Kupferschmidt H: Acute medical problems due to ecstasy use. Case-series of emergency department visits. *Swiss Med Wkly* 2005;135:652-657.

44. Centers for Disease control and Prevention (CDC): Gamma hydroxy butyrate use–New York and Texas, 1995-1996. *MMWR Morb Mortal Wkly Rep* 1997;46:281-283.

45. Centers for Disease Control and Prevention (CDC): Multistate outbreak of poisonings associated with illicit use of gamma hydroxy butyrate. *MMWR Morb Mortal Wkly Rep* 1990;39:861-863.

46. Sumnall HR, Woolfall K, Edwards S, et al: Use, function, and subjective experiences of gamma-hydroxybutyrate (GHB). *Drug Alcohol Depend* 2008;92:286-290.

47. Stillwell ME: Drug-facilitated sexual assault involving gamma-hydroxybutyric acid. *J Forensic Sci* 2002;47:1133-1134.

48. Orphan Medical Announces FDA Approval of Xyrem (website): http://www.projectghb.org/orphan_medical.htm. Accessed February 8, 2010.

49. Centers for Disease Control and Prevention (CDC): Adverse events associated with ingestion of gamma-butyrolactone–Minnesota, New Mexico, and Texas, 1998-1999. *MMWR Morb Mortal Wkly Rep* 1999;48:137-140.

50. Bismuth C, Dally S, Borron SW: Chemical submission: GHB, benzodiazepines, and other knock out drops. *J Toxicol Clin Toxicol* 1997;35:595-598.

51. Liechti ME, Kupferschmidt H: Gamma-hydroxybutyrate (GHB) and gamma-butyrolactone (GBL): analysis of overdose cases reported to the Swiss Toxicological Information Centre. *Swiss Med Wkly* 2004;134:534-537.

52. Liechti ME, Kunz I, Greminger P, et al: Clinical features of gamma-hydroxybutyrate and gamma-butyrolactone toxicity and concomitant drug and alcohol use. *Drug Alcohol Depend* 2006;81:323-326.

53. Yeatman DT, Reid K: A study of urinary endogenous gamma-hydroxybutyrate (GHB) levels. *J Anal Toxicol* 2003;27:40-42.

54. Ledray LE, Kraft J: Evidentiary examination without a police report: should it be done? Are delayed reporters and nonreporters unique? *J Emerg Nurs* 2001;27:396-400.

55. Meyers JE, Almirall JR: A study of the effectiveness of commercially available drink test coasters for the detection of "date rape" drugs in beverages. *J Anal Toxicol* 2004;28:685-688.

56. Beynon CM, Sumnall HR, McVeigh J, et al: The ability of two commercially available quick test kits to detect drug-facilitated sexual assault drugs in beverages. *Addiction* 2006;101:1394-1395.

57. Spiller HA, Rogers J, Sawyer TS: Drug facilitated sexual assault using an over-the-counter ocular solution containing tetrahydrozoline (Visine). *Leg Med (Tokyo)* 2007;9:192-195.

16

Adolescent Sexual Assault and Statutory Rape

Martin A. Finkel, DO, and Mark V. Sapp, MD

Adolescent sexual assault and abuse are some of the last frontiers within the field of child abuse still in great need of enhanced research and services. Although reports of sexual abuse of younger children have decreased steadily over the past several years, adolescent females continue to have the highest rates of sexual assault compared to all other age groups. An estimated 46% of women with a history of sexual assault say they were first assaulted before the age 18. One third of the women assaulted before age 18 say their assault occurred between ages 12 and 17 years.[1,2]

A national survey of adolescents found 8% overall prevalence among 4023 participants reporting being victims of at least one sexual assault.[3,4] Many young victims are particularly reluctant to report sexual assault because of embarrassment, fear of retribution, feelings of guilt or a lack of knowledge regarding victim's rights. The adolescent victim can also feel he or she contributed to the abuse or they might not identify what happened to them as rape because their experience did not fit the popular conception of sexual assault.[5] A better understanding of adolescents' vulnerability and response to sexual abuse and assault is needed for improved outcomes for victims.

ADOLESCENT PERCEPTIONS AND ATTITUDES

Adolescence is a time of rapid physical growth and social development. Many teens have not yet acquired the skills needed to recognize and avoid potentially dangerous social situations. Cassidy and Hurrell[6] found that when adolescents were presented with a vignette of unwanted sexual activity accompanied by a photograph of the victim dressed in provocative clothing, they were more likely to conclude that the victim was in part responsible for the assault, were more likely to view the assailant's behavior as justified, and were less likely to interpret the unwanted sexual experience as rape.[6] In another study, 32% of the adolescent girls surveyed believed forced sex was acceptable if the couple had been dating a long time, 31% believed the unwanted sexual activity was acceptable if the girl agreed to have sex with her partner but later changed her mind, and 27% of the girls believed forced sex was acceptable if the female "led him on."[7] In the same study, 54% of the adolescent boys questioned believed that forced sex was acceptable if his date initially said "yes" even though she later changed her mind.

Forty percent of the boys also believed that forced sex was acceptable if the male had spent a lot of money on the date.[7] These attitudes and perceptions should serve as a wake-up call for increased education and guidance surrounding adolescent physical, sexual, and social behavior and development.

Changes in behavior noted by parents, friends, and teachers can raise concerns for possible sexual abuse. Worrisome behaviors include sudden changes in clothes or make-up, falling grades, dropping out of school, avoiding or changing friends, sudden changes in mood, sudden changes in sleeping or eating habits, depression, anxiety, suicidal ideations and suicide attempts, and high-risk sexual behavior.[8,9] Concerning behaviors can be markedly different depending on the age and the developmental and cognitive levels of the child. While none of these behaviors are diagnostic of abuse, clinicians should be mindful of the need to explore abuse issues with adolescents as part of a work-up for behavior problems.[10]

POPULATIONS AT RISK

Adolescent "runaways" often leave dysfunctional and abusive families hoping to find jobs and new lives. Life on the street, however, is often characterized by hunger, prostitution, chronic illness, violence, and the threat of HIV/AIDS.[11] Research on street youth 12 to 19 years of age in three cities (Denver, New York, and San Francisco) found prevalence rates of sexual abuse of 35% in females and 24% in males.[12] The mean age of first sexual abuse was 9.0 years for females and 9.9 for males. Respondents were more likely to report sexual abuse while living at home than while living on the street. Of the abused youth, 52% were abused at home, 15% on the street, and 33% both at home and on the street. Significantly higher rates of suicide attempts were noted among homeless youth who were sexually or physically abused before leaving home.[12] Compelling research begs for enhanced medical and social interventions to decrease the long-term medical and mental health sequelae of homeless and runaway adolescents.[13]

Other groups with a high prevalence of sexual abuse include intravenous drug users, incarcerated youth, and teens exploited through the sex industry and prostitution. Studies evaluating both prevalence of sexual assault and factors associated with sexual violence found that IV drug-using men and women had a 36% reported lifetime history of sexual violence, with 21% reporting sexual assault during the adolescent years (33% for women and 13% for men).[14] Among incarcerated youth, victimization and perpetration rates of sexual abuse also were found to be higher than the general population.[15]

Teenage prostitution is one of the nation's least recognized public health epidemics.[16] At any given time an estimated 325,000 children nationwide are being sexually exploited through prostitution and/or pornography.[17-20] Criminal justice data estimates that 25% of all individuals involved in sex work are under the age of 18, with an estimated age of entry into sexual exploitation as young at 13.[17] Research suggests that nearly one third of this nation's runaway youth (yearly estimate of 1.5 million) have had some involvement or exposure to prostitution or pornography.[18] This sector of America's youth is a diverse group representing all racial, economic, and cultural backgrounds. They are seriously underserved medically, with limited resources available to them.[18,21-24]

The health problems associated with child prostitution include infectious diseases, pregnancy, mental illness, substance abuse, violence, and malnutrition.[21] Prostituted children contract an estimated 300,000 cases of human immunodeficiency virus (HIV), 500,000 cases of hepatitis B virus (HBV), and 4.5 million new cases of human papilloma virus (HPV) annually.[19,20,21,25] The morbidity and mortality associated with these infections are staggering and are likely increased because of inadequate and inaccessible medical services. The United States accounts for approximately 15% of the world's exploited children and youth, and thus we are facing a health care crisis in our own backyard. The crisis is not only limited to developing countries.

THE CLINICAL IMPLICATIONS OF SEXUAL ASSAULT AND ABUSE

It is important to understand and differentiate sexual abuse from sexual assault. Both forms of inappropriate adolescent sexual experiences have much in common but they differ in many ways. Sexual abuse is ongoing sexual activity with an adolescent, often by someone in the victim's family or social network. Sexual assault by definition involves the use of force and restraint to engage the victim in sexual acts (rape). Rape involves forceful vaginal, anal, or oral penetration by the offender. The penetrating object can be a penis, a finger, or a foreign object. In some cases, the victim's ability to give consent is compromised by intoxication or developmental disability.[26,27] A large percentage of rapes are never reported to the police and greater than 50% of rape victims tell no one about their experiences. Only 5% of rape victims visit rape crisis centers.[28,29] Fifty percent of all rape victims are under the age of 18 and 16% are under the age of 12.[30] More than 75% of adolescent rapes are committed by an acquaintance of the victim, with less than 25% committed by a stranger.[31,32]

Historically, the definition of rape has been gender specific, referring to the forced penetration of a female by a male assailant. Many states have now abandoned this concept in favor of the gender-neutral term of sexual assault. Thus the legal definition of criminal sexual assault is any genital, oral, or anal penetration by a part of the accused's body or by an object, using force or without the victim's consent.[33]

As a general rule, adolescents are more likely to be assaulted by someone they do not know compared to adults and younger children. Stranger assaults are also less likely to be repeated events. Stranger assaults are more likely to result in genital/anal and extragenital trauma, and have the potential for serious bodily harm. The extent to which injuries are incurred depends on the degree of force, the size differential between the victim and the assailant, the degree of resistance on the part of the victim, and whether drugs and alcohol played a part. Stranger assault has the potential for serious long-term physical and mental health sequelae. Victims of sexual assault are not only frightened by the event itself, they are frequently told if they tell anyone about the assault they will experience further harm or even be killed. Consequently many sexually assaulted adolescents never disclose their experiences, or if they do, they do so long after the event occurred when they feel safe. Adolescent victims frequently blame themselves for what happened and harbor feelings of shame, stigmatization, and embarrassment. In stranger assaults, victims will not feel safe nor likely be able to begin the process of recovery until the assailant is apprehended.

INTIMATE PARTNER VIOLENCE

Adolescents are not immune to intimate partner violence, and approximately 45.5% of female and 43.2% of male high school students report they have been victims of physical aggression by dating partners at least once.[34,35] Other studies conducted in U.S. high schools report that a substantial number of adolescents have experienced some form of sexual assault in a dating relationship. The Sexual Experience Survey, administered to 6159 women and men enrolled in 32 higher-education institutions across the United States, revealed that since the age of 14 years, 27.5% of college women had experienced an act that met the legal definition of rape and 7.7% of college men had committed such an act.[36] The vast majority of sexual assaults committed on college campuses are perpetrated by boyfriends, friends, or acquaintances of the victim, with more than 59% occurring on a date.[37] Acquaintance rape among younger adolescents is frequently incestuous. The United States Bureau of Justice Statistics reported that 20% of rape victims aged 12 to 17 years were attacked by family members.[30] By definition, acquaintance rape refers to sexual abuse committed by someone known to the victim, such as a date, teacher, employer, or family member. Assault by a perpetrator related to the victim is defined as incest. Although incest refers to sexual intercourse among family members (those legally barred from marriage), this definition has been broadened also to include step relatives and parental figures living in the home.[38] The highest incidence of acquaintance rape is among girls in the 12th grade and young women in the first year of college.

Date rape is considered a subset of acquaintance rape and generally refers to forced or unwanted sexual activity that occurs within a dating relationship.[38] Adolescent girls intentionally hurt by a date or intimate partner in the previous year were found to be more likely to experience sexual heath risks, including increased vulnerability to human immunodeficiency virus infections and other sexually transmitted infections.[39] Other studies found similar results regarding the associations of both severe dating violence and sexual abuse histories with pregnancy and sexual risks among adolescents.[40-42] Adolescent victims of dating violence were less likely to use condoms consistently or to negotiate condom use, suggesting a possible coercive role on the part of the male dating partner resulting in an increased incidence of unsafe sex practices.[43]

A significant percentage of sexually abused adolescents are abused by someone whom they know, love, and trust. The identity of the perpetrator is rarely an issue. Force and restraint are less likely to be involved. Instead, coercion, deceit, intimidation, bribery, threats, and misrepresentation of moral standards are more likely to be used by the perpetrator. Most perpetrators will avoid causing physical injury because they intend to engage the adolescent in the acts repeatedly over time. Threats are used to maintain secrecy, and the intrusiveness of the sexual acts often increase over time. Adolescents who are victims of sexual abuse are more vulnerable to sexual assault than adolescents who have not been previously sexually abused.

STATUTORY RAPE

Statutory rape is defined as sexual intercourse between a person 18 years or older and a person under the age of legal consent.[26] Statutory rape laws are based on the premise that until a person reaches a certain age, he or she is legally incapable of consenting to sexual intercourse. The age at which an adolescent may consent to sexual intercourse varies from state to state and ranges from 14 to 18 years. Data from the National Maternal and Infant Health Survey indicate that 24% of births to 17-year-old women, 27% of births to 16-year-old girls and 40% of births to 14 year olds were fathered by men at least 5 years older than the mother.[44,45]

Earlier concerns over a possible link between statutory rape and teen pregnancy led many states to enact legislation requiring mandatory reporting of statutory rape as child abuse. In 1996, Congress enacted amendments to the federal Child Abuse Prevention and Treatment Act (CAPTA), which changed the definition of rape to include some forms of statutory rape. Clinicians and health care providers have voiced concern about the impact that statutory rape reporting and enforcement might have on the adolescent's access to health care. Researchers have looked at the effects of increased criminalization of statutory rape and have not found any associated improvement in the child welfare system response or health care access for adolescents following reporting. Furthermore, researchers have not found any proven link or relationship between expanded statutory rape laws, increased mandatory reporting, and a reduction in the incidence of teenage pregnancy.[46] Concern remains that the new laws and mandatory reporting statutes could have a significant impact on the interaction between the health care providers and the adolescent patient. Some adolescents might refuse to seek medical care or disclose personal risk information because of the possible reporting of their sexual partner.[45,47]

Medical and Psychological Consequences of Sexual Abuse and Assault

Sexual victimization is often accompanied by wide-ranging physical and mental health adverse outcomes. A strong relationship exists between sexual abuse and the development of pain disorders, infectious diseases, and multiple psychiatric conditions such as depression, anxiety, sleep disturbances, low self-esteem, suicidality, cutting, and alcohol and substance abuse.[48] In the United States the incidence of psychiatric diagnoses occurring over a lifetime is 56% for women and 47% for men who report histories of childhood sexual abuse. The rates of psychiatric diagnoses when no history of child sexual abuse is reported are significantly lower at 32% for women and 34% for men.[49] The prevalence of women with lifetime alcohol dependence was 15.6% among those reporting child sexual abuse, compared with 7.6% among those not reporting abuse. The equivalent percentages among men were 38.7% and 19.2%.[50] Unwanted sexual experiences in adolescence have also led to gender-reversal patterns such as internalizing behaviors in males (e.g., bulimia) and externalizing behaviors such as fighting in females.[40] Other associations between adolescent rape and behavioral changes include younger age of first voluntary sexual intercourse, increased seeking and receipt of psychological services, and greater amounts of illegal drug use.[51,52]

SEXUAL ABUSE AND ASSAULT AND PREGNANCY

The risk of pregnancy following sexual assault is estimated to be as high as 5% and thus postassault pregnancy prophylaxis is recommended.[53] Pregnancy prevention and postcoital contraception should be addressed with every adolescent female sexual abuse and assault victim. Several forms of emergency contraception are available for women who are victims of sexual assault. Intrauterine devices are not recommended because of the risk of complications. Hormonal therapy is the safest option for emergency contraception. Multiple drug combination regimens are available, but more recently, high-dose progesterone has been used with a reported decrease in adverse side effects and an 89% efficacy rate in prevention of unwanted pregnancy. Plan B (Duramed Pharmacueticals, Inc., Cincinnati), for example, is an FDA-approved high-dose progesterone-only emergency contraceptive that can prevent a pregnancy after contraceptive failure, unprotected sex, and in cases of sexual assault, if taken within 72 hours of the sexual contact. Plan B is not the "abortion pill" (RU498 or misoprostal [Mifeprex, Danco Laboratories, New York]) and does not work if you are already pregnant. Plan B, like other hormone preparations, does not protect against HIV and other sexually transmitted diseases, but when used as instructed, it serves as an effective method for prevention of unwanted pregnancies resulting from sexual assault and abuse.[54] (Information is available at http://www.go2planb.com.)

Discussions with victims should include risks of failure of contraception, side effects of medication, and options for pregnancy management. Always obtain a baseline urine pregnancy test during the initial abuse evaluation because the adolescent could be pregnant from sexual activity that occurred before the assault.[55-57]

RAPE TRAUMA SYNDROME

Posttraumatic stress disorder occurs in up to 80% of rape victims.[58] Results from The National Survey of Adolescents indicated that sexual assault was a significant risk factor for a range of comorbid disorders, including posttraumatic stress disorder (PTSD), major depression, and substance abuse.[59] Many rape and sexual assault survivors will experience the condition known as rape trauma syndrome. This syndrome is characterized by an initial phase lasting days to weeks during which the victim experiences disbelief, anxiety, fear, emotional lability, and guilt. The reorganization phase can last months to years, where the victim progresses through a period of adjustment, integration, and recovery.[56] In general, adolescents often feel that their trust has been violated. They also experience increased self-blame, less positive self-esteem, anxiety, alcohol abuse, and adverse effects on sexual activity, including increased sexual risk behaviors.[60,61]

EXAMINATION OF THE SEXUALLY ASSAULTED ADOLESCENT PATIENT

Every adolescent who discloses inappropriate sexual contact should receive a comprehensive medical evaluation. The evaluation has many purposes: (1) to diagnose any injuries; (2) to screen for sexually transmitted infections (STIs); (3) to collect forensic evidence of the assault; (4) to screen for pregnancy; (5) to offer prophylaxis to prevent STI and pregnancy if indicated; and (6) to assess the adolescents mental status, to offer reassurance, to assure the ongoing safety of the patient, and to offer resources for counseling. Minimizing physical and psychological trauma throughout the medical examination is essential, using a patient/adolescent centered approach that is both age and developmentally appropriate. Patients should never be rushed during the medical examination and they should be provided sufficient time to ask questions and receive clear and concise explanations of the procedures used during the examination.

Issues of patient confidentiality should be addressed. The adolescent is to remain in control of his or her body and have control over the timing and speed at which the examination proceeds. A detailed description of the examination is found in Chapter 9.

Establishing Adolescent Rapport and Confidentiality

Confidentiality is critical to adolescents sharing information with health care professionals. One of the significant adverse consequences of abuse and assault on adolescents is the development of an inability to trust and of a sense of betrayal, especially if the abuser is a friend of family member. The inability to trust can become generalized, and can inhibit the development of future meaningful, healthy relationships. The clinician should have a dialogue with the adolescent that acknowledges the trust and betrayal issues while emphasizing that it was the individual(s) who committed those acts who are not trustworthy. Explain to the adolescent that their need for confidentiality will be respected and honored, but explain legally required limitations to confidentiality as well. When adolescents understand the "ground rules" of open communication, the potential to obtain a complete history is increased. Ford et al[62] surveyed students to find out about their preferences for communicating on the issue of confidentiality. Based on their research, they made the following recommendations: (1) Emphasize the protections of confidentiality; (2) explain the limits of confidentiality within the context of caring rather than the law; (3) be very specific about what can and cannot be managed confidentially; (4) avoid the word "except"; (5) consider using the phrase, "I promise"; (6) act trustworthy; and, (7) communicate how you will manage the "gray" areas.[62]

Professionals are required to report any disclosure of physical or sexual abuse of a child or adolescent, as well and disclosure by patients indicating potential risk of harm to themselves or others. When confidentiality must be breached for either ethical or legal reasons, adolescents should be informed and told what to expect, and they should be assured the clinician will help them through the process.[63]

Encouraging the Adolescent to Cooperate with the Examination

The potential to enhance the cooperativeness of the adolescent patient during a complete head-to-toe examination is in direct proportion to the rapport that has been developed with the patient. When adolescents view clinicians as nonjudgmental and empathetic, they are more comfortable sharing their anxiety and fears. Ask adolescents to voice their concerns no matter how embarrassing, disturbing, or worrisome they might be, so that their concerns can be addressed during the physical examination. When they understand the benefits of the examination they are more likely to cooperate. For many adolescents, the anogenital and pelvic examination following their disclosure will be their first. They might think the examination will be painful and that they will not be in control of their bodies.[64,65] Overcoming their anxieties and fears by open communication will demystify the examination. Whenever possible during the examination, give the patient choices. Respect their need for personal space and privacy. Where video colposcopy is available, some adolescents will find observation of the examination on a monitor to be reassuring. It will provide them with knowledge about their bodies.[66]

When adolescents refuse an examination it is never appropriate to force, coerce, or threaten them for not cooperating. Some adolescents are emotionally unable to cooperate and require counseling before they are examined. If adolescents refuse examination, tell them you respect their desire for privacy and that you will be available to help them when they are ready to be examined. Laboratory testing for STIs and pregnancy can be done before the physical examination if necessary. If the adolescent refuses the examination, clothes, linens, and other objects in the environment can be collected for evidence. In the rare event where the adolescent could have serious internal injuries, an examination under anesthesia will be required.

Adolescents' Understanding of "Sex"

"I did not have sex" can mean different things to different people.[67] As adolescents grapple with the emotionally charged issue of virginity, their definition of "not having sex" could be misinterpreted. For some adolescents, they can engage in various sexual acts such as oral or anal sex and still consider themselves to be abstinent. A survey of 1101 college students found that anal intercourse, oral sex, and stimulating a partner to orgasm where all behaviors that could be defined as abstinent behaviors.[68] Those individuals who engage in a spectrum of sexual acts short of vaginal intercourse consider themselves to be "technical virgins." When adolescents deny having sex, the clinician should ask them what that means. When an adolescent says they are "not sexually active," they might be saying they have not had penile-vaginal intercourse. Clinicians should take a sexual history that specifically addresses genital touching, oral sex, and anal sex in a nonjudgmental way.[69] The clinician can then provide anticipatory guidance and answer adolescents' questions and concerns. When adolescents see their physician as a resource rather than a source of information for their parents, they will be more likely to engage in a dialogue. Adolescents should also be asked about high-risk behaviors, such as multiple sexual partners, and alcohol and substance abuse, and about sexual victimization, intimate partner violence, eating disorders, depression, suicidal ideation, and self-mutilation or cutting. These can all be signs of psychological trauma.[70]

MANAGING THE SYSTEM'S RESPONSE TO ADOLESCENT SEXUAL ASSAULT AND ABUSE

When child protective services (CPS) and/or law enforcement agencies are notified about child maltreatment, their response is critical to assure the safety of the adolescent and to apprehend the perpetrator. When adolescents disclose they have little knowledge of the cascade of events that will follow. Often adolescents disclose assault because they are worried about their bodies or are fearful of pregnancy or STI. In cases of intrafamilial abuse the most common reason for disclosure is for the abuse to stop and for their family member to get help. The adolescent is often surprised by the very different objectives of the police and CPS. The system's response that follows can be intrusive and traumatic if not managed in a manner that puts the adolescent's best interests ahead of the system's needs. The unanticipated consequences of a disclosure might include not being believed, being rejected, being intimidated, or being abandoned by the family of origin. The adolescent might then recant the allegation to avoid further victimization.

The desire to collect evidence should never trump the best interests of the adolescent. Adolescents who experience assault/abuse were not given a choice about that experience and they should not feel pressured by medical, CPS, or law enforcement professionals to undergo an evidentiary examination. The key to seeking the cooperation of an adolescent lies in the clinician's ability to engage the adolescent in an empathetic dialogue that identifies and addresses her fears and anxiety. Rapport building occurs when the clinician has an opportunity to take a complete medical history from the adolescent about their experience independent of the caretaker. In this context adolescents are more likely to engage in open conversation and share their worries and concerns if approached correctly. Adolescent victims often feel isolated, responsible for the sexual assault, and afraid of the consequences of their disclosure. These factors combined with worries and concerns about their body can be immobilizing. Some adolescents are also afraid that an examination might detect prior consensual sexual acts they do not want their parent to know about.

WHEN A PARENT REQUESTS AN EXAMINATION TO DETERMINE IF THEIR CHILD IS A VIRGIN

After an adolescent discloses sexual abuse or assault, parents often want to know if their daughter is still a "virgin." Or, when an adolescent's behavior suggests that she is engaging in consensual sexual intercourse, the parent might want "proof" from the physician that she is being truthful. Occasionally parents will request an examination of their daughter to determine if she is a virgin. Often the girl is threatened that the physician will examine her (against her will).

Parents usually want their adolescents to delay sexual activity as long as possible. In reality, most adolescents do not ask their parents for permission to have sex. When a parent wants to find out what their adolescent will not tell them, the clinician should refocus the issue away from the "virginity check" to issues about communication between parents and adolescents. Adolescents are much better served when parents are equipped to face the reality of unapproved activities and provide education and medical care (including contraception) for their children rather than denying the reality of the adolescents' behavior. Parents should know that in most cases, clinicians will not be able to provide an opinion about "loss" of virginity unless there is an acute hymenal injury or a healed hymenal transection. Kellogg et al[71] examined 36 pregnant adolescents. Only two had morphological hymenal changes that could be attributed to vaginal penetration.[71] There is no absolute test for virginity, even though societal myths and Internet resources promulgate a myriad of misinformation about the subject.

The most accurate way to determine if adolescents are "virgins" is through confidential dialogues with them that recognize and address their emerging sexuality. These conversations allow opportunities to provide guidance about their right to personal space and privacy, to help them understand what consenting to sexual activities means, and what they can do when they find themselves in uncomfortable or dangerous situations.

CONCLUSIONS

Clinicians who assess adolescent victims of sexual abuse/assault should help them address the medical, emotional, and body image concerns that follow their experiences. When adolescents refuse to cooperate, let them know that you understand and respect their decisions, but reinforce the value of the examination and discuss your willingness to limit the examination to the components they feel emotionally ready to experience. Tell them that the most significant impact of their experience will be psychological and reinforce the importance of seeing a mental health clinician. Emphasize that although many adolescents might want to forget about the experience, the only effective way to move beyond the trauma is to talk about the experience with someone who understands and can help professionally. By talking to a mental health clinician, the adolescent sexual assault victim is paving the way to recovery. Posttraumatic stress disorder is the most common psychological sequelae to sexual victimization and screening for it should be routine. Trauma-focused cognitive behavioral therapy has shown to be effective in treating adolescent victims of sexual abuse and assault.[72,73] Ideally, adolescents will leave the evaluation appointment with a sense of hope that they are connected with professionals who care about them and who want to help them.

References

1. Livingston JA, Hequembourg A, Testa M, et al: Unique aspects of adolescent sexual victimization experiences. *Psychol Women Q* 2007; 31:331-343.
2. Snyder HN: *Sexual assault of young children as reported to law enforcement: victims, incident, and offender characteristics*, Bureau of Justice Statistics, U.S. Department of Justice (website): http://www.ojp.usdoj.gov/bjs/pub/pdf/saycrle.pdf. Accessed March 24, 2009.
3. Gorey KM, Leslie DR: The prevalence of child sexual abuse: integrative review adjustment for potential response and measurement biases. *Child Abuse Negl* 1997;21:391-398.
4. Kilpatrick DG, Acierno R, Saunders B, et al: Risk factors for adolescent substance abuse and dependence: data from a national sample. *J Consult Clin Psychol* 2000;68:19-30.
5. Commonwealth Fund: *In their own words: adolescent girls discuss health and health care issues.* Louis Harris & Associates, New York, 1997.
6. Cassidy L, Hurrell RM: The influence of victim's attire on adolescents' judgments of date rape. *Adolescence* 1995;30:319-323.
7. Parrot A: Acquaintance rape among adolescents: identifying risk groups and intervention strategies. *J Soc Work Hum Sex* 1989;8:47-61.
8. American Academy of Pediatrics Committee on Child Abuse and Neglect: Guidelines for the evaluation of sexual abuse of children: subject review. *Pediatrics* 1999;103:186-191.
9. Nicoletti A: Perspectives on pediatric and adolescent gynecology from the allied health care professional. Recognizing teen dating violence. *J Pediatr Adolesc Gynecol* 2000;13:79-80.
10. Hornor G: Sexual behavior in children: normal or not? *J Pediatr Health Care* 2004;18:57-64.
11. Shane PG: Changing patterns among homeless and runaway youth. *Am J Orthopsychiatry* 1989;59:208-214.
12. Kral AH, Molnar BE, Booth RE, et al: Prevalence of sexual risk behaviour and substance use among runaway and homeless adolescents in San Francisco, Denver and New York City. *Int J STD AIDS* 1997;8:109-117.
13. Molnar BE, Shade SB, Kral AH, et al: Suicidal behavior and sexual/physical abuse among street youth. *Child Abuse Negl* 1998;22:213-222.
14. Braitstein P, Li K, Tyndall M, et al: Sexual violence among a cohort of injection drug users. *Soc Sci Med* 2003;57:561-569.
15. Morris RE, Anderson MM, Knox GW: Incarcerated adolescents' experiences as perpetrators of sexual assault. *Arch Pediatr Adolesc Med* 2002;156:831-835.
16. Wurzbacher KV, Evans ED, Moore EJ: Effects of alternative street school on youth involved in prostitution. *J Adolesc Health* 1991; 12:549-554.
17. Nadon SM, Koverola C, Schludermann EH: Antecedents to prostitution: childhood victimization. *J Interpers Violence* 1998;13:206-221.
18. English B: Leaving "the life." *The Boston Globe*, June 21, 2006.
19. Yates GL, Mackenzie RG, Pennbridge J, et al: A risk profile comparison of homeless youth involved in prostitution and homeless youth not involved. *J Adolesc Health* 1991;12:545-548.
20. Yates GL, Pennbridge J, Swofford A, et al: The Los Angeles system of care for runaway/homeless youth. *J Adolesc Health* 1991;12:555-560.
21. Willis BM, Levy BS: Child prostitution: global health burden, research needs, and interventions. *Lancet* 2002;359:1417-1422.
22. Barrett D: Reaching out to child prostitutes. *Nurs Stand* 1999; 13:22-23.
23. Roy E, Haley N, Leclerc P, et al: Mortality in a cohort of street youth in Montreal. *JAMA* 2004;292:569-574.
24. Unger JB, Simon TR, Newman TL, et al: Early adolescent street youth: an overlooked population with unique problems and service needs. *J Early Adolesc* 1998;18:325-348.
25. Tyler KA, Whitbeck LB, Hoyt DR, et al: Risk factors for sexual victimization among male and female homeless and runaway youth. *J Interpers Violence* 2004;19:503-520.
26. American Academy of Pediatrics Committee on Adolescence: Sexual assault and the adolescent. *Pediatrics* 1994;94:761-765.
27. Greenfeld RA, Rand MR, Craven D, et al: *Violence by intimates. Analysis of data on crimes by current or former spouses, boyfriends, and girlfriends*, U.S. Department of Justice, Office of Justice Programs (website): http://www.ojp.usdoj.gov/bjs/pub/pdf/vi.pdf. Accessed March 6, 2009.
28. Perkins C, Klaus P: *Criminal victimization 1994.* Bureau of Justice Statistics, Washington, DC, 1996.
29. Koss MP, Harvey MR: *The rape victim: clinical and community interventions.* Sage, Newbury Park, Calif, 1991.
30. Langan PA, Harlow CW: *Child rape victims*, 1992, U.S. Dept of Justice, Bureau of Justice Statistics (website): http://www.ojp.usdoj.gov/bjs/pub/pdf/crv92.pdf. Accessed March 6, 2009.
31. Kilpatrick DG, Edmunds CN, Seymour AK: *Rape in America: a report to the nation*, National Victim Center & Medical University of South Carolina (website): http://colleges.musc.edu/ncvc/resources_prof/rape_in_america.pdf. Accessed March 7, 2009.
32. Heise LL: Reproductive freedom and violence against women: where are the intersections? *J Law Med Ethics* 1993;21:206-216.
33. American Medical Association: *Strategies for the treatment and prevention of sexual assault.* American Medical Association, Chicago, 1995.
34. O'Keeffe NK, Brockopp K, Chew E: Teen dating violence. *Soc Work* 1986;31:465-468.
35. O'Keefe M, Treister L: Victims of dating violence among high school students: are the predictors different for males and females? *Violence Against Women* 1998;4:195-223.
36. Koss MP, Gidycz CA, Wisniewski N: The scope of rape: incidence and prevalence of sexual aggression and victimization in a national sample of higher education students. *J Consult Clin Psychol* 1987;55:162-170.
37. Abbey A: Acquaintance rape and alcohol consumption on college campuses: how are they linked? *J Am Coll Health* 1991;39:165-169.
38. Hibbard RA, Orr DP: Incest and sexual abuse. *Semin Adolesc Med* 1985;1:153-164.
39. Silverman JG, Raj A, Mucci LA, et al: Dating violence against adolescent girls and associated substance use, unhealthy weight control, sexual risk behavior, pregnancy, and suicidality. *JAMA* 2001; 286:572-579.
40. Shrier LA, Pierce JD, Emans SJ, et al: Gender differences in risk behaviors associated with forced or pressured sex. *Arch Pediatr Adolesc Med* 1998;152:57-63.
41. Coker AL, McKeown RE, Sanderson M, et al: Severe dating violence and quality of life among South Carolina high school students. *Am J Prev Med* 2000;19:220-227.
42. Raj A, Silverman JG, Amaro H: The relationship between sexual abuse and sexual risk among high school students: findings from the 1997 Massachusetts youth risk behavior survey. *Matern Child Health J* 2000;4:125-134.
43. Wingood GM, DiClemente RJ, McCree DH, et al: Dating violence and the sexual health of black adolescent females. *Pediatrics* 2001; 2001:e72.
44. Small S, Kerns D: Unwanted sexual activity among peers during early and middle adolescence: incidence and risk factors. *J Marriage Fam* 1993;55:941-952.
45. Donovan P: Can statutory rape laws be effective in preventing adolescent pregnancy? *Fam Plann Perspect* 1997;29:30-34.
46. Teare C, English A: Nursing practice and statutory rape. Effects of reporting and enforcement on access to care for adolescents. *Nurs Clin North Am* 2002;37:393-404.

47. Ford CA, Millstein SG: Delivery of confidentiality assurances to adolescents by primary care physicians. *Arch Pediatr Adolesc Med* 1997;151:505-509.

48. Beautrais AL: Risk factors for suicide and attempted suicide among young people. *Aust N Z J Psychiatry* 2000;34:420-436.

49. Martin G, Bergen HA, Richardson AS, et al: Sexual abuse and suicidality: gender differences in a large community sample of adolescents. *Child Abuse Negl* 2004;28:491-503.

50. Kessler RC, McGonagle KA, Zhao S, et al: Lifetime and 12-month prevalence of DSM-III-R psychiatric disorders in the United States. Results from the national comorbidity survey. *Arch Gen Psychiatry* 1994;51:8-19.

51. Miller BC, Monson BH, Norton MC: The effects of forced sexual intercourse on white female adolescents. *Child Abuse Negl* 1995; 19:1289-1301.

52. Nagy S, DiClemente R, Adcock AG: Adverse factors associated with forced sex among southern adolescent girls. *Pediatrics* 1995;96: 944-946.

53. Schludermann EH, Holmes MM, Resnick HS, et al: Rape-related pregnancy: estimates and descriptive characteristics from a national sample of women. *Am J Obstet Gynecol* 1996;175:320-324.

54. Trussell J, Ellertson C, Rodriguez G: The Yuzpe regimen of emergency contraception: how long after the morning after? *Obstet Gynecol* 1996;88:150-154.

55. Linden JA: Sexual assault. *Emerg Med Clin North Am* 1999;17:685-697.

56. Petter LM, Whitehill DL: Management of female sexual assault. *Am Fam Physician* 1998;58:920-926.

57. Hampton HL: Care of the woman who has been raped. *N Engl J Med* 1995;332:234-237.

58. Pynoos R, Nader K: Post traumatic stress disorder. *In*: McAnarney E, Kreipe R, Orr D, et al *(eds): Textbook of Adolescent Medicine.* WB Saunders, Philadelphia, 1992, pp 1003-1009.

59. Kilpatrick DG, Ruggiero KJ, Acierno R, et al: Violence and risk of PTSD, major depression, substance abuse/dependence, and comorbidity: results from the national survey of adolescents. *J Consult Clin Psychol* 2003;71:692-700.

60. Laumann EO: *Early sexual experiences: how voluntary? How violent?* Henry J Kaiser Family Foundation, Menlo Park, Calif, 1996.

61. Moore KA, Nord CW, Peterson JL: Nonvoluntary sexual activity among adolescents. *Fam Plann Perspect* 1989;21:110-114.

62. Ford CA, Thomsen SL, Compton B: Adolescents' interpretations of conditional confidentiality assurances. *J Adolesc Health* 2001; 29:156-159.

63. Sigman G, Silber TJ, English A, et al: Confidential health care for adolescents: position paper of the Society for Adolescent Medicine. *J Adolesc Health* 1997;21:408-415.

64. Larsen SB, Kragstrup J: Experiences of the first pelvic examination in a random sample of Danish teenagers. *Acta Obstet Gynecol Scand* 1995;74:137-141.

65. Bodden-Heidrich R, Walter S, Teutenberger S, et al: What does a young girl experience in her first gynecological examination? Study on the relationship between anxiety and pain. *J Pediatr Adolesc Gynecol* 2000;13:139-142.

66. Mears CJ, Heflin AH, Finkel MA, et al: Adolescents' responses to sexual abuse evaluation including the use of video colposcopy. *J Adolesc Health* 2003;33:18-24.

67. Carpenter LM: The ambiguity of "having sex": the subjective experience of virginity loss in the United States. *J Sex Res* 2001;38:127-139.

68. Medley-Rath SR: "Am I still a virgin?": what counts as sex in 20 years of Seventeen. *Sex Cult* 2007;11:24-38.

69. Bersamin MM, Fisher DA, Walker S, et al: Virginity and abstinence: adolescents' interpretations of sexual behaviors. *J Adolesc Health* 2007;41:182-188.

70. Nock MK, Teper R, Hollander M: Psychological treatment of self-injury among adolescents. *J Clin Psychol* 2007;63:1081-1089.

71. Kellogg ND, Menard SW, Santos A: Genital anatomy in pregnant adolescents: "normal" does not mean "nothing happened." *Pediatrics* 2004;113:e67-e69.

72. Cohen JA, Mannarino AP, Deblinger E: *Treating trauma and traumatic grief in children and adolescents.* Guilford Press, New York, 2006.

73. Deblinger E, Behl L, Glickman AR: Treating children who have experienced sexual abuse. *In*: Kendall PC (ed): *Child and Adolescent Therapy: Cognitive-Behavioral Procedures,* ed 3, Guilford Press, New York, 2005, pp 383-416.

17

FEMALE GENITAL MUTILATION/CUTTING

Susan Bennett, MB, ChB, FRCP

TERMINOLOGY

The term "female genital mutilation/cutting" (FGM/C) refers to all procedures involving partial or total removal of the external female genitalia or other injury to the female genital organs for nonmedical reasons.[1] The terminology for these procedures has undergone various changes over the last few decades. The term "female circumcision" was widely used for many years to describe the practice; it has been largely abandoned, however, as it implies an analogy with the circumcision of newborn boys, a low-risk procedure with medical benefits.[2,3] The expression "female genital mutilation" gained growing support from women's rights and health advocates in the late 1970s to emphasize the serious harm associated with the practice and to define it as a violation of girls' and women's human rights. The World Health Organization (WHO) recommended that the United Nations (UN) adopt this term in 1991 and it has subsequently been widely used by WHO and in other UN documents.

In the mid-1990s many practicing communities and activists decided to use a more neutral term, "female genital cutting" (FGC), because they considered the term FGM to be stigmatizing to those who had undergone the procedure. In addition, it appeared that the word was estranging practicing communities and perhaps hindering the process of social change necessary for the elimination of FGM.

While the UN continues to use FGM in official documents, some of its agencies (United Nations Children's Fund [UNICEF] and United Nations Population Fund [UNFPA]) have started to use the combined term female genital mutilation/cutting (FGM/C) to capture the significance of the term "mutilation" at the policy level and at the same time to use less judgmental terminology for practicing communities.[4] It is important that health care providers use culturally sensitive terms with patients when discussing this practice and its consequences.

PREVALENCE AND GEOGRAPHIC DISTRIBUTION

The World Health Organization estimates that between 100 million and 140 million girls and women worldwide have undergone some type of FGM, and that currently, about 3 million girls, most of them under 15 years of age, undergo the procedure every year.[4] The great majority of affected women live in 28 countries in Africa, but the practice has also been reported in parts of the Middle East, Asia, and Latin America. Countries on the African continent with the highest likelihood of FGM being practiced are Djibouti, Egypt, Eritrea, Ethiopia, Gambia, Guinea, Mali, Sierra Leone, Somalia, and Sudan.

Growing migration has increased the number of girls and women living outside their country of origin; many who now live in Europe, the United States, Canada, New Zealand, and Australia have undergone FGM or may be at risk of being subjected to the practice.[5-7] Some families arrange for their daughters to undergo FGM while on vacation in their home countries.

Female genital mutilation is practiced by people from all education levels and social classes, including urban and rural residents, and different religious and ethnic groups. It is generally practiced on girls between the ages of 4 and 10 years, although in some communities it is performed shortly after birth, during adolescence, just before marriage, during first pregnancy, or after the first birth. In some practicing cultures, women are re-infibulated (re-stitched) following childbirth as a matter of routine. The age at which female genital mutilation is performed varies with local traditions and circumstances, and is reported to be decreasing in some countries.[4]

The procedure is usually performed by traditional birth attendants or older women in the community who do not have formal training. It is often carried out using primitive instruments, razor blades or pieces of glass, and without anesthetic or attention to hygiene.[8] The child can be subjected to the procedure unexpectedly and held down on the floor by several attendants. Often a number of girls undergo the procedure during a single ritual ceremony and in these cases the same instrument is commonly used on all the girls. Increasingly, in some communities, FGM is being "medicalized" and performed in modern clinical settings by a physician or other health professional in the belief that complications occur less frequently.[4]

TYPES OF FEMALE GENITAL MUTILATION

Recognition of the different types of FGM is important because the complications differ with the severity of the procedure.

Table 17-1	World Health Organization Classification of Female Genital Mutilation[4]

- Type I: Clitoridectomy: Partial or total removal of the clitoris and/or the prepuce (Figure 17-2)
  - Type Ia, removal of the clitoral hood or prepuce only
  - Type Ib, removal of the clitoris with the prepuce
- Type II: Excision*: Partial or total removal of the clitoris and the labia minora with or without excision of the labia majora (Figure 17-3).
  - Type IIa, removal of the labia minora only
  - Type IIb, partial or total removal of the clitoris and the labia minora
  - Type IIc, partial or total removal of the clitoris, the labia minora, and the labia majora
- Type III: Infibulation[†]: narrowing of the vaginal orifice with creation of a covering seal by cutting and appositioning the labia minora and/or the labia majora, with or without excision of the clitoris (Figures 17-4 and 17-5).
  - Type IIIa: removal and apposition of the labia minora
  - Type IIIb: removal and apposition of the labia majora
- Type IV: Unclassified: All other harmful procedures to the female genitalia for nonmedical purposes, for example, pricking, piercing, incising, scraping, and cauterization

*Note that in French the term "excision" is often used as a general term covering all types of female genital mutilation.
[†]Reinfibulation is covered under this definition. This is a procedure to recreate an infibulation usually after childbirth in which defibulation was necessary.

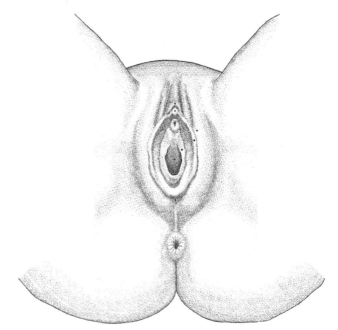

FIGURE 17-1 Normal, unmutilated female genitalia. *(From Cooper SW, Estes RJ, Girardino AP, et al: Child sexual exploitation, ed 1, GW Medical Publishing, Inc, St Louis, 2005.)*

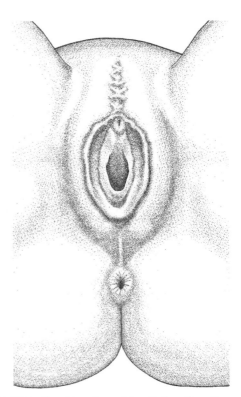

FIGURE 17-2 Type I female genital mutilation. *(From Cooper SW, Estes RJ, Girardino AP, et al: Child sexual exploitation, ed 1, GW Medical Publishing, Inc, St Louis, 2005.)*

The WHO/UNICEF/UNFPA 1997 Joint Statement classifies FGM into four types based on the severity of structural disfigurement.[1] This was slightly modified in 2008.[4] Within each type of FGM there will be variation with respect to the amount of tissue removed. Table 17-1 lists the classifications of FGM. Figure 17-1 represents normal, unmutilated female genitalia. Figures 17-2, 17-3, and 17-4 represent various types of FGM. Current estimates indicate that about 90% of female genital mutilation cases include Types I or II and IV and about 10% are Type III.

The type of FGM varies by region and ethnicity.[9] In reality, the extent of cutting and stitching varies considerably since the excisor is usually a layperson with limited knowledge of anatomy and surgical technique. With local or no anesthesia, the girls often move to the extent that cutting cannot be accurately controlled.

CULTURAL ISSUES

It is not known when or where the tradition of FGM originated. Evidence from Egyptian mummies suggests that infibulation (also known as the pharaonic procedure) was practiced there some 5000 years ago.[10] Cliteroidectomy was used in western medicine up to the late 1950s as a treatment for nymphomania, promiscuity, and masturbation.[11,12]

FGM continues within a complex web of social, cultural, and economic justification and is deeply embedded in local traditional belief systems. These beliefs involve continuing long-standing custom and tradition, maintaining virginity, enhancement of girls' ability to marry, promotion of fidelity in married women, enhancement of male sexual pleasure, increasing fertility and child survival, upholding family honor, perceived religious dictates, and contributing to social stability.[4]

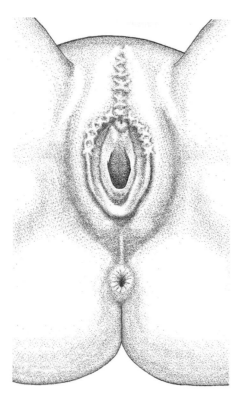

FIGURE 17-3 Type II female genital mutilation. *(From Cooper SW, Estes RJ, Girardino AP, et al:* Child sexual exploitation, *ed 1, GW Medical Publishing, Inc, St Louis, 2005.)*

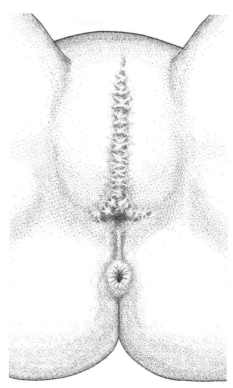

FIGURE 17-4 Type III female genital mutilation. *(From Cooper SW, Estes RJ, Girardino AP, et al:* Child sexual exploitation, *ed 1, GW Medical Publishing, Inc, St Louis, 2005.)*

Preservation of Cultural Identity

In communities where it is widely practiced, FGM is considered an honorable tradition that is an important part of the cultural identity of girls and women. In some societies, the practice is embedded in coming-of-age rituals and girls who undergo the procedure are given rewards such as celebrations, public recognition, and gifts.

Marriage

Some of the other justifications offered for FGM are also linked to girls' marriage prospects. Marriage is essential to the social and economic security for women in FGM practicing communities. FGM becomes a physical sign of virginity and is regarded in many societies as a prerequisite for an honorable marriage. In some communities, it is thought to restrain sexual desire, thereby ensuring marital fidelity. A belief sometimes expressed is that FGM enhances a man's sexual pleasure.

Religion

While religious duty is commonly cited as justification for the practice of FGM, it is important to note that FGM is a cultural and not a religious requirement. Even though the practice can be found among Christians, Jews, and Muslims, none of the holy texts of any of these religions prescribes FGM and the practice predates both Christianity and Islam.

Health

FGM is thought to improve fertility and prevent infant and maternal mortality.

Hygiene and Aesthetic Reasons

FGM is also considered to promote cleanliness. In some cultures it is believed that a girl who has not undergone FGM is unclean and not able to handle food or drink. Removal of genital parts is thought of as eliminating "masculine" parts such as the clitoris or in the case of infibulations, to achieve smoothness which is considered to be beautiful.

Contributing to Social Stability

The practice of FGM is often upheld by local structures of power and authority such as traditional leaders, religious leaders, circumcisers, elders, and even some medical personnel. It can be a lucrative source of income in some communities. It is often practiced even when known to inflict harm upon girls because the perceived social benefits of the practice are deemed higher than its disadvantages. Parents who support the practice of FGM say that they are acting in the child's best interests and risk their child's marriage prospects and being ostracized by their community should they resist the practice.

HEALTH COMPLICATIONS

A wide range of complications of FGM are documented, including short-term and long-term physical, sexual, and psychosocial problems.[13] The type and severity of the consequences vary according to the type of procedure performed; the extent of the cutting; the skill of the incisor; the hygienic conditions; the physical and mental health of the girl undergoing the procedure; the child's access to adequate health care; and particular characteristics of the child, including age, ethnicity, and family and societal support.

For many women the most difficult physical problems coincide with various life cycle events such as immediately after cutting, at menstruation, at time of marriage, and during childbirth. The physical complications are summarized in Table 17-2.

Findings from a recent large scale WHO multicountry study confirm that women who had undergone FGM had significantly increased risks for adverse events during childbirth.[15] Higher incidences of cesarean section and postpartum hemorrhage were found in women with type I, II, and III FGM compared to those who had not undergone FGM, and the risk increased with the severity of the procedure.

A striking new finding from the study is that the FGM of mothers has negative effects on their newborn babies. Most seriously, death rates among babies, during and immediately after birth, were higher for those born to mothers who had undergone FGM compared with those who had not: 15% higher for those whose mothers had type I, 32% higher for those with Type II, and 55% higher for those with type III FGM. The consequences of FGM for most women who deliver outside the hospital setting are expected to be even more severe. The high incidence of postpartum hemorrhage, a life-threatening condition, is of particular concern where health services are poor or inaccessible to women.

In contrast to numerous studies and case reports on the physical complications of FGM, little scientific research is available on the sexual and psychosocial consequences of the practice. This is partly due to difficulties in measuring psychological distress and partly due to women's reluctance to discuss these issues.

For many girls and women, FGM is an acutely traumatic experience that leaves a lasting psychological mark and may adversely affect full emotional development. Girls are generally conscious when the operation is performed and for many it is a shocking experience marked by acute pain, fear, and confusion. The experience of FGM has been related to a range of psychological and psychosomatic disturbances, including changes in eating and sleeping habits, loss of appetite, weight loss or excessive weight gain, panic attacks, difficulties in concentrating and learning, and symptoms of posttraumatic stress disorder.[4,16] In many cases, women and girls who have been traumatized by FGM remain silent about their experience. In some cultures they have no socially acceptable means of expressing their feelings or distress.

There may be additional psychological implications for immigrant women who live in western societies where FGM is not traditionally practiced. These women confront the conflicting attitudes of their traditional culture and of western culture towards FGM, sexuality, and women's rights. Some community groups and agencies have reported girls

Table 17-2	Possible Complications of Female Genital Mutilation

- Short-term complications*
  - Severe pain
  - Severe hemorrhage
  - Shock
  - Injury to adjacent tissues (e.g., urethra)
  - Injury due to restraint (e.g., fractures, dislocations)
  - Acute retention of urine
  - Infections after use of contaminated instruments and during the healing period (wound infections, septicemia, tetanus, pelvic inflammatory disease, urinary tract infections, HIV, hepatitis B and C)
  - Death from hemorrhagic shock, neurogenic shock as a result of extreme pain and trauma, or severe, overwhelming infection and septicemia
- Long-term complications
  - Girls and women undergoing FGM Type III are particularly likely to suffer serious and long-term complications; the stitching of the labia majora to create a flap of skin covering the vaginal opening causes a direct mechanical barrier to urination, menstruation, sexual intercourse, and to delivery of infants.
  - Local vulval problems: retention cysts, abscesses, keloids, excess scar tissue at site of cutting, and painful neuromas as a result of the entrapment of nerve endings in the scar
  - Chronic upper and lower urinary tract infection potentially resulting in renal failure, septicemia, and death
  - Calculus formation in the vagina
  - Chronic vaginal and pelvic infections leading to scarring and infertility
  - Increased risk of HIV
    - From the use of the same instruments used for other initiates
    - Secondary to increased need for blood transfusions due to hemorrhages either when the procedure is performed, at childbirth or as a result of vaginal tearing during defibulation and injurious sexual intercourse[14]
  - Dysmenorrhea and blocked menstrual flow with hematocolpos, which can lead to endometriosis
  - Hemorrhage due to recurrent trauma, possibly resulting in anemia
  - Complications in pregnancy and childbirth
    - Prolonged and obstructed labor due to unyielding scar tissue
    - Tearing of the perineum, hemorrhage, fistula formation (vesico-vaginal or recto-vaginal)
    - Uterine inertia, rupture, or prolapse
  - Postpartum wound infection and retention of lochia may lead to puerperal sepsis
  - Neonatal problems from obstructed or prolonged labor. If deinfibulation is not performed and delivery of the head is delayed, anoxia and fetal death can occur.

*Immediate consequences are usually only documented when hospital treatment is sought, therefore the true extent of immediate complications is unknown.

experiencing difficulties with their peer group (e.g., a young man rejecting a girlfriend when he discovers she was subjected to FGM as a child, or a girl discovering that other girls have not been subjected to FGM).[5]

Much of the qualitative research regarding the effects of FGM on the sexuality of women has suggested that all types of FGM inhibit sexual fulfillment and pleasure for women. The physical damage resulting from FGM combined with the psychological trauma and pain can compromise an adult woman's sexual life. Moreover, women who have been infibulated may be defibulated upon marriage, a process that is a source of both pain and further psychological trauma. Marital problems can arise and can eventually lead to divorce, which in turn jeopardizes women's social and economic status and that of their children.[16]

MANAGEMENT OF FGM

The influx of refugees and immigrants from different parts of Africa to North America, Europe, and Australasia in the past two decades requires that physicians and other health professionals familiarize themselves with the practice of FGM, its causes, cultural meanings, and health and legal ramifications. Health professionals play a key role in the prevention of FGM, including educating patients and communities about the harmful consequences and promoting the benefits in eliminating the practice, along with providing early identification and treatment of complications of the procedure. The training of health professionals has been identified as a priority strategy for the elimination of FGM.[4]

The World Health Assembly (the highest authority of the WHO),[17] the World Medical Association,[18] and the International Federation of Gynecology,[19] and medical associations in many countries have opposed FGM as a medically unnecessary practice with serious, potentially life-threatening complications. These organizations have issued statements condemning the practice as harmful and calling for coalitions to abolish it. Performing FGM in pain-free and sterile conditions does not alleviate the long-term detrimental effects and can wrongly legitimize the practice as medically sound or beneficial for girls' or women's health, thereby perpetuating rather than preventing or reducing the practice.

A number of professional bodies have published guidelines for medical professionals such as nurses, midwives, and obstetricians and gynecologists for the provision of antenatal, delivery, and postpartum care for women who have undergone FGM. Such guidelines include management of specific procedures such as deinfibulation and care of women with complications from the practice, including compromises in menstrual and sexual health.[20-29]

Multiagency child protection guidelines have also been developed for professionals from the health, social services, law enforcement, and education sectors in the developed world to respond to children at risk and to children and women who have undergone FGM.[30-33]

Child Protection Management

There are two circumstances relating to FGM that require identification and intervention. The first is to identify children at risk of being subjected to FGM and responding

Table 17-3	Indicators of Girls at Risk of FGM

Indicators that FGM Might Soon Occur

- The family comes from a community that is known to practice FGM.
- Any female child born to a woman who has been subjected to FGM or who has existing daughters who have undergone FGM.
- Parents state that they or a relative will take the girl out of country for a prolonged period.
- A girl who talks about a long holiday to her country of origin or another country where the practice is prevalent.
- A girl who confides that she is to have a special procedure or attend a special celebration for her.

Indicators that FGM May Have Already Occurred

- Prolonged absence from school with noticeable behavior change on her return
- Long periods away from classes or other activities, possibly with bladder or menstrual problems

appropriately to protect them. The second is to identify children who have been subjected to FGM and providing appropriate support for them. Table 17-3 lists indicators of girls at risk for FGM.

Clinicians and child protection professionals should discuss the issue of FGM with parents who wish to continue the practice and educate them about the health consequences and legal restrictions. Every attempt should be made to work with parents on a voluntary basis to prevent FGM and includes the use of community organizations and/or community leaders to facilitate the work with parents and families. Suspicion of intent to perform FGM should be addressed immediately as there is the risk that the child could suddenly disappear or be sent abroad. A report should be made to child protection services if a child is in need of protection.

On physical examination of a girl who has undergone FGM, there can be little or no evidence of genital scarring or only attenuation of clitoral tissue, as many FGM procedures do not involve removal of significant amounts of tissue. Minor changes are difficult to evaluate when no history is available. However, the physical findings in girls who have had procedures involving extensive removal of tissue and major changes in the size of the introitus are sufficiently dramatic not to be missed on careful examination.[34] Procedures are often performed under less-than-sterile conditions and carry a risk of viral and bacterial infection transmitted by instruments used in surgery. Serology for HIV, hepatitis B, and hepatitis C are indicated in children who have evidence of FGM.

Young immigrant women who come from cultures and communities where FGM is commonly performed are likely to face conflicting cultural messages about the meaning of FGM as they grow up. Their families may be concerned primarily about the social consequences of noncompliance with the tradition. Conflicting messages are a potential source of confusion and distress. The psychosocial needs of children and adolescents who have undergone FGM should be recognized specifically and appropriate counselors and networks identified.

Medical Management

Defibulation is a surgical procedure to reverse infibulations. Defibulation can be performed before marriage, before or during pregnancy, or at childbirth. Adolescents who have undergone some form of FGM in childhood might wish to have the procedure reversed at a time other than that which is culturally preferred or acceptable.[35] The procedure allows them to use vaginal tampons, have penetrative sex, reduces the likelihood of complications with a vaginal delivery at a later date, and may satisfy their body image concerns. Like all operative procedures, it is obviously most desirable that the procedure is sanctioned by the young woman's parents. In most cases the girl should be encouraged to involve her parents and there should be detailed consideration of the most extreme possible consequences of not involving them. Justification of reversal of FGM on medical grounds might potentially be less threatening to parents and community members.

Women with FGM Type III require special care during pregnancy and childbirth, especially if it is the first pregnancy or the woman has had a previous caesarian section or past reinfibulation. Elective defibulation during the antenatal period, ideally around 20 weeks, reduces lacerations and avoids the necessity of performing defibulation or anterior episiotomy during labor, thereby reducing the risk of caesarian section. The operation should be carried out under adequate anesthesia, which can be general or spinal. Inadequate pain relief could cause traumatic flashbacks.

Obstetricians and midwives might be asked to reinfibulate (re-stitch) a woman following a vaginal delivery. While legal in some countries, requests by women in western countries for reinfibulation following childbirth are outlawed on the grounds that this is damaging to their health and well-being. Any repair carried out after birth, whether following spontaneous laceration or deliberate defibulation to facilitate delivery, must not be to the degree that makes intercourse difficult or impossible.

Culturally competent and compassionate care for women and their partners is important to dissuade them from resorting to illegal community practitioners who may operate under inadequate and unhygienic conditions. Health care professionals should be aware of the mental health needs of women who have experienced FGM and refer them (where necessary) to culturally appropriate services.

INTERNATIONAL RESPONSE

Over the last several decades there has been a shift from the perspective of FGM as a cultural and health issue to recognizing it as a pressing human rights and public health issue among governments, the international community, and professional health organizations.[16] FGM is a practice that is discriminatory on the basis of sex and violates women's rights in many ways including: (1) The right to the highest attainable standard of physical and mental health; (2) the right to security; (3) the right to freedom from all forms of physical and mental violence; (4) the right to freedom from cruel, inhuman, or degrading treatment; (5) the right to protection from harmful traditional practices; and, (6) the right to life when the procedure results in death. These rights are protected in international law. A number of human rights conventions and declarations are directly or indirectly violated by the practice of FGM, including the Universal Declaration of Human Rights (1948),[36] the UN Convention on the Elimination of All Forms of Discrimination against Women (1979),[37] the UN Convention on the Rights of the Child (1990),[38] and the Beijing Declaration and Platform for Action of the Fourth World Conference on Women (1995).[39] Signatory states have an obligation under these standards to take legal action against FGM.

In 1997, a joint statement was issued by WHO, UNICEF, and UNFPA expressing commitment from all three organizations towards abolition of the practice.[1] A new 2008 Interagency Statement, based on new evidence over the last decade, has been signed by a wider group of United Nations agencies than the previous one.[4]

Nongovernmental organizations (NGOs) play a central role in generating national and international commitment to end the practice of FGM. At a regional level the Inter-African Committee on Traditional Practices Affecting the Health of Women and Children (IAC)[40] is the oldest NGO network dedicated to the abandonment of FGM in Africa. In other parts of the World, other NGOs have been involved with the work of abolishing FGM, including the Foundation for Women's Health Research and Development (FORWARD),[41] the Research, Action and Information Network for the Bodily Integrity of Women (Rainbo),[42] and the European Network for the prevention of FGM (euronet-FGM).[43]

Laws pertaining to FGM include both criminal and child protection laws. In some countries, the existing provision of criminal codes have been or can be applied to FGM. In Africa and in the Middle East, a large number of countries have introduced specific legislation to address FGM. Laws prohibiting FGM have also been introduced in a number of countries where the issue has arisen among immigrant communities including Australia, New Zealand, Canada, the United States, and several countries in Western Europe. Many countries have recognized the right to asylum for women and girls at risk of FGM.[6,44]

A number of countries have declared the applicability of their child protection laws to FGM while others have enacted and applied specific provisions for the elimination of harmful practices including FGM. Child protection laws provide for state intervention in cases in which the state has reason to believe that child abuse has occurred or might occur.

Despite the existence of laws forbidding the practice, enforcement of the laws can be lax or nonexistent. Furthermore, cultural norms in these countries or regions render women unwilling to seek protection or compensation under the law. Imposing sanctions alone runs the risk of driving the practice underground and having a very limited impact on the occurrence of FGM.

Clearly, the elimination of FGM is not simply a law enforcement issue. FGM is acknowledged as a unique, deeply rooted cultural practice and ending FGM requires a long-term commitment to establishing a foundation for sustained behavior change. Gender discrimination underlies the practice of FGM and the most effective strategies for dealing with FGM involve empowering and educating women and girls within their own communities and cultures. In addition, recognition that the support of men and community leaders, both religious and secular, is vital to ending the practice. The approach to FGM is part of a larger commitment to combat violence against women and children around the world.[45-47]

Actions taken at international, regional, and national levels over the past decade or more have begun to bear fruit and, in some areas, the prevalence of female genital mutilation has decreased. Key lessons learned are that actions and interventions must be multisectoral, sustained, and community led.[16,48]

The Millennium Development Goals[49] establish measurable targets and indicators of development that are relevant to ending FGM; namely, to promote gender equality and empower women, to reduce child mortality, and to improve maternal health. A World Fit for Children,[50] the outcome document of the 2002 UN General Assembly Special Session on Children, explicitly calls for an end to harmful traditional or customary practices such as female genital mutilation. The UN Study on Violence against Children[45] report provides another important opportunity to highlight the issue and generate action to realize the goal of the abandonment of FGM.

Processes of social change leading to abandonment of the practice, while ensuring the marriageability of daughters and the social status of families who do not cut their girls, are underway in a number of countries, creating a new social norm that does not harm girls or violate their rights. With global support, it is conceivable that FGM can be abandoned in practicing communities within a single generation.[16] The United Nations has designated February 6 as the International Day of Zero Tolerance of Female Genital Mutilation.

References

1. Female Genital Mutilation: A Joint WHO/UNICEF/UNFPA statement. World Health Organization, Geneva, 1997. http://www.childinfo.org/files/fgmc_WHOUNICEFJointdeclaration1997.pdf. Accessed March 7, 2009.
2. American Academy of Pediatrics: Report of the task force on circumcision. *Pediatrics* 1989;84:388-391.
3. Klausner JD, Wamai RG, Bowa K, et al: Is male circumcision as good as the HIV vaccine we've been waiting for? *Futur HIV Ther* 2008; 2:1-7.
4. Eliminating Female Genital Mutilation: An interagency statement. World Health Organization, Geneva, 2008. http://www.unfpa.org/webdav/site/global/shared/documents/publications/2008/eliminating_fgm.pdf. Accessed March 7, 2009.
5. Lockhat H: *Female genital mutilation: treating the tears.* Middlesex University Press, London, 2004.
6. Momoh C (ed): *Female genital mutilation.* Radcliffe Publishing, Oxford, UK, 2005.
7. Bosch X: Female genital mutilation in developed countries. *Lancet* 2001;358:1177-1179.
8. Toubia N: *Female genital mutilation: a call for global action.* Women's Ink, New York, 1995.
9. Nour NM: Female genital cutting: clinical and cultural guidelines. *Obstet Gynecol Surv* 2004;59:272-279.
10. Izett S, Toubia N: *A research and evaluation guidebook using female circumcision as a case study: learning about social changes.* RAINBO, New York, 1999.
11. Toubia N: Female circumcision as a public health issue. *N Engl J Med* 1994;331:712-716.
12. Kandela P: Sketches from the *Lancet*: clitoridectomy. *Lancet* 1999; 353:1453.
13. Lovel H, McGettigan C, Mohammed Z: *A systematic review of the health complications of female genital mutilation including sequelae in childbirth,* World Health Organization (website): http://www.who.int/reproductive-health/docs/systematic_review_health_complications_fgm.pdf. Accessed March 7, 2009.
14. Brady M: Female genital mutilation: complications and risk of HIV transmission. *AIDS Patient Care STDS* 1999;13:709-716.
15. WHO Study Group on Female Genital Mutilation and Obstetric Outcome: Female genital mutilation and obstetric outcome: WHO collaborative prospective study in six African countries. *Lancet* 2006;367:1835-1841.
16. Lewnes A (ed.): Changing a harmful social convention: female genital mutilation/cutting. *Innocenti Digest* 12, Florence, Italy, 2005; http://www.unicef-irc.org/publications/pdf/fgm_eng.pdf. Accessed March 6, 2010.
17. World Health Assembly resolution on female genital mutilation, May 2008. http://www.iac-ciaf.com/Documentation/UN%20and%20UN%20agencies/WHO%20FGM%20resolution%20May%202008.pdf. Accessed March 7, 2009.
18. World Medical Association: Statement on condemnation of female genital mutilation. Adopted by the 45th World Medical Assembly, Budapest, October 1993 (revised 2005).
19. World Health Organization, International Federation of Gynecology and Obstetrics (FIGO): Female circumcision. Female genital mutilation. *Eur J Obstet Gynecol Reprod Biol* 1992;45:153-154.
20. WHO: *Management of pregnancy, childbirth and the postpartum period in the presence of female genital mutilation: report of a WHO technical consultation* (website): http://www.who.int/reproductive-health/publications/mngt_pregnancy_childbirth_fgm/text.pdf. Accessed March 7, 2009.
21. WHO: Female genital mutilation. The prevention and the management of the health complications. Policy guidelines for nurses and midwives (website): http://www.who.int/reproductive-health/publications/rhr_01_18_fgm_policy_guidelines/fgm_policy_guidelines.pdf. Accessed March 7, 2009.
22. Buck P: RCOG statement No 3. Female genital mutilation, Royal Collage of Obstetricians and Gynecologists (website): http://www.rcog.org.uk/files/rcog-corp/uploaded-files/RCOGStatement3FemalegenitalMutilation2003.pdf. Accessed March 7, 2009.
23. American College of Obstetricians and Gynaecologists: *Female genital cutting: clinical management of circumcised women,* ed 2, ACOG, Washington, DC, 2007.
24. The College of Physicians and Surgeons of Ontario: Policy on female circumcision, excision and infibulation (website): http://www.cpso.on.ca/policies/policies/default.aspx?ID=1596. Accessed March 7, 2009.
25. The Royal Australian and New Zealand College of Obstetricians & Gynaecologists: Female genital mutilation: information for the Australian health professional (website): www.ranzcog.edu.au/publications/pdfs/FGM-booklet-sept2001.pdf. Accessed March 7, 2009.
26. Royal College of Nursing: Female genital mutilation royal college of nursing educational resource for nurses and midwives (website): http://www.rcn.org.uk/__data/assets/pdf_file/0012/78699/003037.pdf. Accessed March 7, 2009.
27. Adamson F: *Female genital mutilation information for counseling professionals.* FORWARD, London, 1997.
28. Mwangi-Powell F: *Holistic care for women. A practical guide for midwives.* FORWARD, London, 2001.
29. Toubia N: *Caring for women with circumcision: a technical manual for health care providers.* RAINBO, New York, 1999.
30. London Safeguarding Children Board: Safeguarding children at risk of abuse through female genital mutilation (website): http://www.london-scb.gov.uk/files/procedures/LondonFGMProcedureFinalDoc.doc. Accessed March 7, 2009.
31. British Medical Association: Female genital mutilation: caring for patients and child protection (website): http://www.bma.org.uk/images/FGMJuly06_tcm41-146715.pdf. Accessed March 7, 2009.
32. Dorkenoo E, Hedley R: *Child protection and female genital mutilation: advice for health, education and social work professionals.* FORWARD, London, 1996.
33. Committee on Bioethics: Female genital mutilation. *Pediatrics* 1998; 102:153-156.
34. Sugar NF, Graham EA: Common gynecologic problems in prepubertal girls. *Pediatr Rev* 2006;27:213-223.
35. Strickland JL: Female circumcision/female genital mutilation. *J Pediatr Adolesc Gynecol* 2001;14:109-112.

36. General Assembly of the United Nations: *Universal declaration of human rights*. United Nations General Assembly, New York, 1948. http://www.un.org/Overview/rights.html. Accessed March 7, 2009.

37. General Assembly of the United Nations: Convention on the elimination of all forms of discrimination against women. United Nations General Assembly, New York, 1979. http://un.org/womenwatch/daw/cedaw/text/econvention.htm. Accessed March 7, 2009.

38. The United Nations convention on the rights of the child. United Nations General Assembly, New York, 1989. http://www.unhchr.ch/html/menu3/b/k2crc.htm. Accessed March 7, 2009.

39. Fourth World Conference on Women: Beijing declaration and platform for action. Fourth World Conference on Women, Beijing, 1995. http://www.un.org/womenwatch/daw/beijing/platform/declar.htm. Accessed March 7, 2009.

40. Inter-African committee on traditional practices affecting the health of women and children (IAC). Available at www.iac-ciaf.net. Accessed March 6, 2010.

41. Foundation for Women's Health Research and Development (website): Available at http://www.forwarduk.org.uk. Accessed March 7, 2009.

42. RAINBO. The Research, Action and Information Network for the Bodily Integrity of Women (website): http://www.charitycommission.gov.uk/registeredcharities/ScannedAccounts/Ends91%5C0001095691_AC_20061231_E_C.PDF. Accessed March 6, 2010.

43. European Network for the Prevention of FGM (website): www.euronet-fgm.org. Accessed March 7, 2009.

44. Toubia N: *Female genital mutilation: a guide to laws and policies worldwide.* Zed Books, London, 2000.

45. UN Division for the Advancement of Women: UN study on violence against children (website): http://www.violencestudy.org/IMG/pdf/English-2-2.pdf. Accessed March 7, 2009.

46. UN WomenWatch: UN study on violence against women (website): www.un.org/womenwatch/daw/vaw/panel2.htm. Accessed March 7, 2009.

47. Watts C, Zimmerman C: Violence against women: global scope and magnitude. *Lancet* 2002;359:1232-1237.

48. World Health Organization: Female genital mutilation. Programmes to date: what works and what doesn't: a report (website): http://www.who.int/reproductive-health/publications/fgm/fgm_programmes_review.pdf. Accessed March 7, 2009.

49. United Nations: Millennium goals (website): www.un.org/millenniumgoals. Accessed March 7, 2009.

50. UN General Assembly: A world fit for children: resolution adopted by the General Assembly. United Nations, New York, 2002.

18

INTERNET CHILD SEXUAL EXPLOITATION

Daniel D. Broughton, MD

CHILDREN ON THE INTERNET

The Internet has become one of the most important and available resources to people everywhere. There are an estimated 1.4 billion Internet users worldwide with 248 million in North America in 2008, an increase from 360 million users worldwide and 108 million in North America in 2000.[1] The Internet is an amazing avenue for communication, an incredible repository of information. In the United States more than 90% of young people have been online by the time they are 9 years old.[2]

In addition to providing opportunities for learning, the Internet is an effective communication network and provides an infrastructure for group discussions among people from every corner of the planet. Likewise there are boundless sources of entertainment including interactive venues where games can be played with others, and sites that demonstrate ways to learn tools and skills. Children are expected to have Internet access to have a reasonable chance of reaching their full potential.

While the positive value of the Internet is undeniable, there also are concerns, especially as it relates to children. Advertisers are using the Internet to promote and to sell products to this age group. Some sites promote dangerous behavior such as anorexia by providing helpful hints to limit intake, purge, and exercise excessively. Sites also can include offensive language, ideas, or images, including pornography and obscenity. Online pornography is a multibillion dollar industry with an estimated 4.2 million pornographic websites in 2006.[3] In addition, cyber-bullying has become a significant problem and can be extremely harmful to those who are targeted in this way.[4]

There are many ways that young people communicate electronically. E-mail was the earliest form of Internet communication. This new technology suddenly allowed people to connect electronically with relatives and friends and even to meet people with efficiency and ease that never existed previously. While young people tend to consider many of these new contacts as "new friends," they often have no idea who is at the other end of an electronic message. A 30-year-old man can become a 13-year-old boy or girl. An extension of e-mail is instant messaging where several individuals are involved in a single electronic conversation similar to a conference call.

The simplest form of electronic communication is by text messaging using cell phones. Since many cell phones now are equipped with cameras, images can be sent as quickly and effortlessly as a text message. Text messaging can be safe by limiting contacts to telephone numbers of known individuals. However, messages and images from unknown sources can be easily forwarded to anyone, anywhere with a cell phone. Also, many cell phones now are connected to the Internet, thus increasing the reach and potential circulation of cell phone messages. In this way a private message, which may include photos not intended to be shared beyond a single recipient, can end up anywhere in the world accessible through cyberspace.

A chat room is a virtual place set up by individuals or web pages to facilitate discussion of a specific subject or to bring together people with similar interests. For example, a chat room can provide a forum for individuals or family members with a serious but uncommon illness to connect with others in a similar situation. Many chat rooms are monitored, meaning that there is a leader who controls and participates in the discussion, ensuring that inappropriate topics are not introduced or that the forum is not otherwise misused. However, other chat rooms are unmonitored and there is no way to know exactly who is participating in a given discussion.

Predators often use chat rooms as a mechanism to meet vulnerable youth. For example, an adult could join a discussion intended for young people by posing as a teenager in a chat room about cheer leading or teen fashion. This person can then initiate direct contact with other chat room members outside of the chat room. Once a relationship is initiated with other participants, the predator will search for opportunities to continue and develop it. As another example, a person could participate in a discussion about science or architecture that would not be expected to specifically attract young people. Once a young person identifies him/herself, the predator will use this opportunity to portray himself as having similar interests and pursue a direct correspondence.

The newest type of electronic communication comes from social networking sites such as Facebook and MySpace, each with more than 100 million users.[5] These sites allow customers or users to create web pages where personal information is shared. Some sites are general but others aim toward specific groups such as BlackPlanet (African Americans, with 20 million users), specific interests such as Flixster (movie buffs, 63 million users) and for specialized groups such as BTMS (actors and filmmakers, 15,000 users).[5]

Unfortunately, many teens use poor judgment in managing their sites and include personal information or provocative images. One study found that nearly two thirds of adolescents post photos or videos of themselves, almost 60% list the city in which they live, and half give the name of their school.[2] Nearly 60% do not feel that posting a photo or video on public networking sites is dangerous and half are unconcerned that posting private information might affect their future.[2] When armed with the personal information and anonymity, a potential predator has an opportunity to begin a relationship that can progress to face-to-face contact. In one study, 14% of teens have met someone face-to-face after meeting the person online while 30% have considered doing so.[2] Of those receiving messages from unknown people, 40% said they usually would respond and chat with that person. Older teens were more likely to allow a meeting. Only 18% said they would tell a parent. Younger users (8-12 years old) are much more likely to tell their parents. Ninety-six percent of this age group tells their mother and father about at least some of what they do online; 76% tell parents everything. Of those who tell someone when they receive online messages from unknown senders, the vast majority reach out to their mother (91%).[2]

Most reputable social networking sites have built in safeguards that protect clients from unwanted or unknown contacts. For example, MySpace has a list of safety tips that include warnings such as:

"MySpace profiles and forums are public."
"People online are not always who they say they are."
"It is not safe or appropriate to pretend to be older or younger."

Most sites have an age limit (usually 14 years old) for those registering and setting up sites. They also provide mechanisms allowing a site holder to limit access to those to whom specific permission has been granted. Sadly, despite the best efforts, there have been many examples of criminals, including sexual predators, registering under false names with false profiles.

In a survey of child Internet users, Wolak et al found that one in seven children had been solicited online for sex over a 1-year period.[6] They also found that one in 25 youth had been aggressively solicited by a predator trying to arrange a meeting, calling the youth on the phone, or sending correspondence that may have included money or gifts. Roughly 80% of the solicitations occurred while the children were using their home computers. Only about one fourth of the children who were victims of solicitations told their parents. This type of sexual predation is not limited to adult perpetrators. More than 40% of all solicitations, including aggressive solicitations, were by individuals younger than 18 years.[7] Nearly 10% of young people have been harassed through online contacts and more than a third found the episodes distressing.[7] Children face danger in the presumed safety of their own homes and usually without their parents' knowledge.

CASE EXAMPLES

A 12-year-old boy is chatting with a 12-year-old girl via e-mail. The conversation becomes increasingly provocative with sexual undertones. Eventually the boy asks the girl if she has a web camera. She says she can borrow one from a friend and asks why. He asks for a picture of her, initially fairly playfully but eventually requesting one of her with no clothes on. The boy is actually 27-years-old. If the girl provides such a photo, it can become part of the network of child pornography without her knowledge. This is carried out in the privacy of the child's own bedroom in complete secrecy from parents.

A series of messages are exchanged between a 13-year-old boy and a 12-year-old girl who met online. Over time the girl tells her new friend that she and her family will be staying at a resort for their vacation at the end of the month. The boy excitedly points out to her that in an amazing coincidence, his father will be at the same resort at the same time attending a business meeting. He then tells her that he is going to send a gift for her with his father. The gift is to be a secret and she is not to tell anyone, not even her parents. The boy is actually 42-years-old and poses as "his father" at the resort.

In response to the Internet enticement of children and child pornography cases, the Justice Appropriations Act passed in 1998 directed the Office of Juvenile Justice and Delinquency Prevention (OJJDP) to create the Internet Crimes Against Children Task Force (ICAC), a national network of state and local law enforcement units to investigate cases of child sexual exploitation (Pub. L. No. 105-119). As of 2007 each state now has an ICAC Task Force to investigate and coordinate cases involving computers and the sexual exploitation of children. Because of the utility of the Internet, several jurisdictions often are involved, possibly from different states or countries. The ICAC task forces facilitate communication between the various agencies that are involved in the investigation of specific cases. Among techniques used are "sting" efforts where law enforcement officers pose as children and try to arrange meetings with predators, leading to the predators' arrests. In 2006, ICAC investigations led to more than 2040 arrests and more than 9600 forensic examinations of children.

CHILD PORNOGRAPHY

The Internet provides a unique environment in which child pornography can proliferate. Early photographic child pornography had significant limitations for those producing the material. Film had to be developed and printed, which was time consuming, and required specialized equipment and space for a darkroom. Sending it out to be developed was extremely risky because of the possibility of discovery. The advent of Polaroid cameras and eventually camcorders made production much easier and quicker. However, distribution continued to be a problem. The material has to be transported, adding significant risk of being caught. Using the mail for distribution of child pornography adds the possibility of federal charges in addition to the violation of state laws. All of this changed with the introduction of digital photography and even more significantly with the explosion of the Internet. Suddenly it was possible to produce high quality photos and videos in secure places with minimal expense and then distribute them via the Internet with ease, anonymity, and relative safety from exposure.

Child pornography long has been an important and effective tool for those who sexually prey on children. It can aid in coercing children to perform sexual acts, it can be a powerful tool to ensure silence of the victims by threat of exposure. Perhaps most damaging, the images become a permanent record of the abuse. The Internet exacerbates this concern. Once these images hit the Internet, they never go away. Literally, they may show up again at any time and any place with the potential to cause great embarrassment or harm to the victim.

While the Internet has been a great boon to child sex abusers, others have used it as a stunningly successful avenue to distribute child pornography as a commercial venture with profits of billions dollars a year. The Internet Watch Foundation estimated that in 2006 there were more than 10,000 known child pornography domains with more than half housed within the United States alone.[7] The estimated number of U.S. sites might be artificially high because of the disproportionate numbers of Internet Service Providers (ISP) and Electronic Service Providers (ESP) located in the United States. Child pornography sites can be incredibly profitable. One such site called Landslide Productions, managed by a couple in Texas, was identified with a list of more than 300,000 customers in 37 states and 60 countries.[8] Customers were paying $20 to $30 a month to access the images. At one point this highly successful enterprise was taking in over $1.4 million per month.

There has been a concerted and coordinated effort to combat the growing problem of child pornography on the Internet. In 1998, the United States Congress authorized the establishment of the CyberTipline. Housed at the National Center for Missing and Exploited Children (NCMEC) in Alexandria, Va., analysts joined with federal law enforcement officers from the Federal Bureau of Investigation (FBI), Immigration and Customs Enforcement (ICE), and the U.S. Postal Service to collect tips about crimes involving child pornography and other sexual exploitation of children on the Internet. These agents work closely with other federal agents, state programs (such as ICAC), local law enforcement, and internationally with foreign agencies, such as Interpol and Scotland Yard. ISPs and ESPs now are required to immediately report child pornography found on their servers to the CyberTipline. More than 600,000 reports have been processed, which included more than 5 million images and video files. There has been a 250% increase in reports between 2004 and 2007 with more than 5 million images processed in 2007 alone. While many of these images are of individual children, many have more than one victim and in some cases the same victims have been identified serially at different ages over time.[9]

Another important tool in the fight against commercial child pornography has been developed through the Financial Coalition to Combat Child Pornography,[10] developed in cooperation with the International Centre for Missing and Exploited Children and law enforcement agencies throughout the world. Credit card companies and financial institutions in the United States and Europe have come together to work with law enforcement to effectively stop the flow of money, thus interrupting the normal conduct of business transactions that involve child pornography. Countless sites have been shut down as a result of this effort. While it is more difficult to deal with the primary producers of child pornography and those who molest children, this assault on the financial aspect of child pornography had significant impact on the commercial capability of this illegal industry.

In 2002 the Child Victim Identification Program (CVIP) was initiated at NCMEC to assist local and federal law enforcement to identify victims who appear in the photos. CVIP has reviewed more than 15 million images submitted by law enforcement agencies. Using sophisticated technology and sharpened analytic skills, clues collected from the pictures are used to track the location where they were taken. Often it is possible to approximate the time that the photos were taken. By narrowing the search to a specific city or region, it often is possible to locate the victims and ultimately the perpetrators. According to Michelle Collins and Jennifer Lee of the NCMEC (oral communication November 2008), more than 1500 victims have been identified. Of this number 72% were girls and 28% were boys. Age demographics indicate that 54% of the victims are classified as prepubescent, 40% as pubescent, and 6% as infant/toddler.

As in other forms of child abuse, those who produce most of the child pornography are close to the children they exploit. Twenty-eight percent of those producing pornographic images are parents, 4% the partner of the child's guardian, and 11% other relatives. Others are trusted family friends and neighbors (25%) and 5% baby sitters and coaches. Perpetrators who the children met online accounted for 13% of the images. Only 2% of victims of child pornography were identified as child prostitutes. Four percent of the images were produced by people that were unknown to the victim.

The most shocking statistic about those who produce child pornography is that 8% of the images were produced and distributed by the victims themselves. In April 2006, 16-year-old Justin Berry testified before the U.S. House of Representatives Subcommittee on Oversight and Investigation about his operation of a child pornography site beginning at age 13, featuring himself and other teenage boys.[11] In Victoria, Australia, investigators found that it was not uncommon for young people to possess child pornography, including youths as young as 10 to 14 years old. In one sting operation, Victoria Police found the most common age group possessing pornography was 15 to 19 years.[12]

The involvement of young people in child pornography raises other important issues. Children are not immune to prosecution for posting such material. In many jurisdictions the underage possessors and producers of child pornography run the risk of having to register as sex offenders, and can face devastating consequences. In 2006 a 16-year-old boy was convicted of child pornography for posting a sexually explicit photo of two younger teens.[13] He was sentenced to 2 years probation and 120 hours of community service. In another case in 2007, the Florida Appeals Court upheld the conviction of two girls (ages 16 and 17) for taking sexually explicit pictures of themselves and sending them via e-mail to each other.[14] A 17-year-old boy was charged with a felony in May 2008 for having posted graphic pictures of his former girlfriend on his MySpace account. His former girlfriend had taken the photos herself and sent them to him via her cell phone. He said he was venting because she broke up with him.[15] For these adolescents facing criminal charges, it is difficult to assess risk to others and to provide appropriate treatment, particularly if the youthful perpetrator also has been a victim previously. These are difficult questions that require careful study and considerable discussion in the future.

Virtual child pornography is another important facet of Internet child sexual exploitation. Using inexpensive software, it is possible to produce lifelike images of children from scratch or to manipulate actual photographs in a way to change the appearance of the victims. In this way the producers of the material can hide the identity of the victims or claim that the images are not real. This is particularly significant when the child victim has not yet been identified. Perpetrators and their attorneys can claim that if the subject has not been identified, the photo must be considered to be "virtual" and not within the scope of child pornography.

Congress enacted the Child Pornography Prevention Act of 1996 (CPPA) in an attempt to deal with this problem. There were significant first amendment arguments regarding infringement of free speech. Some were concerned that mainstream art forms, including movies, could be cited for using young adult actors in provocative roles. In *Ashcroft v. The Free Speech Coalition*, the U.S. Supreme Court held that the government may not criminalize such action because the production of "virtual child" pornography does not sexually abuse an actual child.[16]

Congress subsequently passed the PROTECT Act of 2003. This bill was a comprehensive, multipurpose law aimed at addressing and preventing child abuse. In an attempt to address the Supreme Court's concerns about the CPPA, one section dealt with virtual child pornography. In May 2008, the U.S. Supreme Court upheld that part of the legislation specifically dealing with virtual child pornography.[17]

CYBERSEX

Another example of online exploitation of youth is called "cybersex" or computer sex. This issue relates to "virtual" sexual encounters between two or more people on at least two different computers. People send each other sexually explicit messages via the Internet, often describing sexual acts or pretending to be having sexual relations with the person on the other end of the line. Masturbation can be involved. This activity commonly takes place in chat rooms or via instant messaging or e-mail. Probably the most notorious example of cybersex involving an adult and teenager was the case of Representative Mark Foley who carried on sexually explicit conversations over the Internet with underage Congressional pages.[18] Ultimately, Mr. Foley was forced to resign from Congress in disgrace. Cybersex can lead to sharing of sexually explicit photos or even to personal encounters between the predator and victim. In an interesting twist, law enforcement has found cybersex to be a useful tool in the fight against child molesters. Officers will masquerade as underage participants and engage in sexually explicit communications with adults, often resulting in arrests and convictions.

A new type of sexual exploitation of teenagers has arisen in the last few years called "sexting." When "sexting," teens send nude pictures or videos of themselves to their boyfriends or girlfriends. This is a form of self-exploitation. In some cases, the friends then send the images on to other people. Both of these actions can lead to criminal convictions of the teens providing or forwarding the material.[19] One online survey found that 20% of teens reported sending nude or semi-nude pictures of themselves via the internet.[20]

RECOMMENDATIONS

To protect our children from these concerns, we must equip them and their parents with the skills needed to navigate the Internet safely and comfortably. It is common for children, especially teens, to know much more about computer technology and use than their parents. It is important to stress to parents that they need to learn about computers and Internet use if they are to help their children be as safe as possible when they are online. They also need to be aware that the Internet has expanded well beyond home, school, and work computers. Cell phones and PDAs effectively have become miniature computers that easily can connect to the Internet at any time and at any place.

Parental supervision of computer use is the single most important step. Parents need to be involved in all aspects of their children's computer use from games to online activities. Home computers, including laptops, should be kept in a public part of the house where parents can access it at all times. It should not be in a child's room and never in a room where a door can be closed and locked. The amount of time spent on the computer should be limited. The American Academy of Pediatrics[21] recommends that children and teens average no more than 2 hours a day using screens, including computer games, Internet, television, videos, and video games. Some flexibility may be permitted for homework. Parents should be aware of the sites that are visited by their children. Most computers are equipped to allow at least a limited look back in time at sites visited, and software is available to enhance this monitoring.

Use of e-mail, chat rooms, and social networking sites also must be followed closely. It is valuable to enter into a "safe computering" contract in which children agree to abide by certain rules and to allow parent access to their personal sites. Children and teens should not be allowed to have accounts to which parents do not have access. Parents should know their children's user names and passwords. Additionally, filtering software can limit the sites that a specific computer can access. This tool can be particularly useful for younger children, although parents need to be aware that these filters can be indiscriminate and might be more restrictive than desired.

Specific recommendations that are particularly useful for social networking sites or blogs include:

- Never post personal information
- Never give out a password (except to parents)
- Only add people you know well in person to your lists
- Check safety settings frequently
- Photos can have identifying information on them that will make it easy for someone to find you. Do not post personal photos.
- Protect your friends and do not say things about them that you would not want to hear from you.

Professionals have a responsibility as well. We need to understand the issue and be sure we keep up-to-date on the nuances. We need to educate our patients and their families about the value of the Internet, the concerns and dangers, and equip them with resources to ensure safety. We need to talk to our colleagues and professional societies to be sure that they understand the importance of the issue and the need to stay current and involved. We also have to use our influence to help change society to be more protective of children and young people. In addition to trying to make individuals safer, we must encourage society to understand the complexity of child exploitation and change attitudes so that this exploitation is no longer acceptable in any form.

References

1. Internet Worlds Stats Usage and Population Statistics. Internet Coaching Library (website): http://www.internetworldstats.com/. Accessed March 8, 2009.
2. Cox Communications: *Tweens and internet safety* (website): http://www.cox.com/takeCharge/includes/docs/survey_results_2008.pdf. Accessed March 6, 2010.
3. Internet Pornography Statistics TopTenReviews (website): http://www.internet-filter-review.toptenreviews.com/internet-pornography-statistics.html. Accessed March 8, 2009.
4. Wolak J, Mitchell KJ, Finkelhor D: Does online harassment constitute bullying? An exploration of online harassment by known peers and online only contacts. *J Adolesc Health* 2007;41:S51-S58.
5. Wikipedia: *List of social networking websites* (website): http://en.wikipedia.org/wiki/List_of_social_networking_websites. Accessed March 8, 2009.
6. Wolak J, Mitchell K, Finkelhor D: *Online victimization of youth: five years later*, National Center for Missing & Exploited children (website): http://www.missingkids.com/en_US/publications/NC167.pdf. Accessed March 8, 2009.
7. Internet Watch Foundation: *Trend analysis*, Internet Watch Foundation annual report 2006 (website): http://www.iwf.org.uk/documents/20070412_iwf_annual_report_2006_(web).pdf. Accessed March 8, 2009.
8. CBS News, the Fifth Estate: *Landslide. Profile of a pornographer* (website): http://www.cbc.ca/fifth/landslide/profile.html. Accessed March 6, 2010.
9. National Center on Missing & Exploited Children: *CyberTipline fact sheet* (website): http://www.missingkids.com/en_US/documents/CyberTiplineFactSheet.pdf. Accessed March 8, 2009.
10. Testimony of Jodi Golinshy before the Committee on Banking, Housing, and Urban Affairs, United States Senate, September 19, 2006, Washington, DC. http://banking.senate.gov/public/_files/golinsky.pdf. Accessed March 8, 2009.
11. Testimony of Justin Berry before the United States House of Representatives, Committee on Energy and Commerce, April 4, 2006, Washington, DC. http://archives.energycommerce.house.gov/reparchives/108/Hearings/04042006hearing1820/Berry.pdf. Accessed March 8, 2009.
12. Crawford C, Wilkinson G: *Making child pornography is now kids' stuff.* Herald Sun, July 2, 2008. Available at http://www.heraldsun.com.au/news/victoria/making-porn-is-now-kids-stuff/story-e6frf7kx-1111116794353. Accessed March 6, 2010.
13. Evane Brown: *Sixteen-year-old girl criminally liable for child pornography*, Internet Cases (website): http://blog.internetcases.com/2007/01/23/sixteen-year-old-girl-criminally-liable-for-child-pornography/. Accessed March 8, 2009.
14. First District Court of Appeal: *A.H., a Child, Appellant v. State of Florida, Appellee* (website): http://opinions.1dca.org/written/opinions2007/1-19-07/06-0162.pdf. Accessed March 8, 2009.
15. James SD: *Child porn charge for MySpace revenge pics*, ABC News (website): http://abcnews.go.com/TheLaw/Story?id=4912041&page=1. Accessed March 8, 2009.
16. *Ashcroft v. Free Speech Coalition* (00-795) US 234 (2002) 198 F.3d.1083, affirmed. http://www.law.cornell.edu/supct/html/00-795.ZS.html. Accessed March 8, 2009.
17. *United States v. Williams* (06-694) 444 F. 3rd 1286, reversed. http://www.law.cornell.edu/supct/html/06-694.ZS.html. Accessed March 8, 2009.
18. Babington C, Weisman J: *Rep Foley quits in page scandal*, Washington Post (website): http://www.washingtonpost.com/wp-dyn/content/article/2006/09/29/AR2006092901574.html. Accessed March 8, 2009.
19. Walker JT, Moak S: Child's play or child pornography: The need for better laws regarding sexting. *ACJS Today* XXXV(1), February, 2010. Available at http://www.acjs.org/pubs/uploads/ACJSToday_February_2010.pdf. Accesed March 6, 2010.
20. The National Campaign to Prevent Teen and Unwanted Pregnancy and *CosmoGirl.com*: Sex and Tech: Results of a Survey of Teens and Young Adults. Washington, DC, 2008. Available at http://www.thenationalcampaign.org/sextech/PDF/SexTech_Summary.pdf. Accessed March 6, 2010.
21. American Academy of Pediatrics Committee on Public Education: Children, adolescents, and television. *Pediatrics* 2001;107:423-426.

19

Evaluating Images in Child Pornography

Shelly D. Martin, MD[1]

INTRODUCTION

The production, collection, distribution, and use of child pornography in this country are major issues affecting many children. The purpose of this chapter is to aid clinicians in assessing the images and videos that are distributed as child pornography, and to provide guidance about making a determination that a person depicted in an image is less than 18 years of age.

Controversy exists regarding morphed or virtual images of child pornography. Advances in technology make it easier to produce images of children that appear real, but may not depict actual children. Virtual child pornography would include modified photographs of real children, images of people older than 18 years of age who appear younger or are made to look younger, and fully computer-generated images.

Computer generated images take a file in one format and use software to manipulate the lighting, reflections, and other features to create a photorealistic image. Age progression and regression software is also used. Current laws attempt to protect children by imposing limits on technological advances that perpetuate child pornography.

The evaluation of an image should include an assessment and documentation of whether the image appears altered or morphed. It is usually difficult to make this determination strictly by viewing the image, though one may consider shadowing, coloring, and proportions which may not appear consistent throughout the image and look obviously mismatched. Computer experts are trained to make determinations regarding the alteration of computer images.[1]

The National Center for Missing and Exploited Children maintains a database of known child pornography victims. This database contains all identified series of a particular victim categorized, indexed, and described in detail.[2] The database is updated annually and can be accessed by law enforcement and other investigative entities to compare seized collections with known underage victims for identification purposes.

NORMATIVE STUDIES OF PHYSICAL AND SEXUAL MATURATION

The Third National Health and Nutrition Examination Survey (NHANES III), conducted from 1988 to 1994, was a study of the health of a nationwide representative sample of children in the United States.[3] Some of the papers generated from this study provide data on the timing of puberty in American children. A second large scale study was conducted in the office-based network of pediatricians participating in research known as the Pediatric Research in the Office Setting Network (PROS). This study specifically looked at sexual maturity ratings (Tanner stages) in girls 3 to 12 years old. All girls presenting to a participating pediatrician's office for a physical examination or for illnesses requiring a full physical examination were included. Participating providers received special training in assessing sexual maturity rating (SMR).

The aforementioned studies provided valuable datasets that have established a basis for relating SMR to age. For example, the PROS study, which includes more than 17,000 females, shows more than 95% of females have begun breast development by the age of 12 and more than 90% will have at least Tanner stage 2 pubic hair by age 12.[4] These studies established that a white American girl with Tanner 2 breast development is 99.9% likely to be younger than 17.5 years old (and 99.7% likely to be less than 14 years old). The PROS study provided 95% confidence intervals for SMR in girls by mean age. Standard deviations provide the age range for each stage of development African American females are listed separately since they tend to reach puberty earlier than non-Hispanic white American girls.

Papers derived from the NHANES study provide important information for pubertal thresholds in boys and girls. For example, the study reports that the average American boy enters puberty at 9 to 10 years of age and attains full sexual maturity by 14 to 16 years of age.[5] Information is provided for white, African-American, and Hispanic-American males, demonstrating differences in pubertal development. Tables are provided that list the percentage of boys by age that are in a particular stage of sexual development.

Although information from these studies is important in the analysis of pornographic images, SMR were not designed to age children, but to provide a descriptive means of quantifying the development of secondary sexual characteristics.

[1]The opinion and assertions herein are the private views of the author and are not to be construed as those of the Department of Defense, Air Force, Army, or Navy; the Armed Forces Center for Child Protection; the National Naval Medical Center; or Walter Reed Army Medical Center.

The development of secondary sexual characteristics is an important marker for the transition between childhood, through adolescence, into adulthood. Other factors, discussed below, are also important indicators and supporting factors, but the progression through puberty is an identifiable and quantifiable process. If the person in question has not begun to develop secondary sexual characteristics, then the above studies provide supportive data to assert the person is less than 18 years of age.

It is often argued, particularly in court, that SMR cannot be used to age children. If the provider who is attempting to determine whether a child is less than 18 years old is doing so correctly, that argument has no merit. SMR is not used to determine a child's *age*, but to describe the stage of sexual development of an individual depicted in an image. Other studies have correlated the stages of sexual development with age. Therefore, the provider is using SMR as a descriptive means of assessing sexual maturity, and comparing the SMR with population-based data on development by age. SRM is simply a tool, one of many, that aids the provider in making a developmental assessment, which in turn helps determine the likelihood that an individual is less than 18 years old.

REVIEWING IMAGES AND VIDEOS

When asked to evaluate a series of images or videos of suspected child pornography, the provider should first assess the quality of the material being provided. Size and overall image quality are important considerations. Often images will be salvaged from computers in a thumbnail format. These can vary in size, but are usually very small and difficult to assess. The people in the images are often so small that it is difficult to make any assessments regarding sexual development or other characteristics. Because most images are digital, an attempt can be made to enlarge the image, but quality and resolution is usually lost as the image becomes blurred and pixilated. Even when images are of sufficient size, quality might still be poor. An image should be clear and not blurred or pixilated to an extent that makes it difficult to assess.

Shadows, lighting, and positioning of the individuals in the image can affect the ability to make determinations of sexual and physical maturity. Often body parts that need to be evaluated are covered or not fully seen and determinations cannot be made.

Physical Characteristics and Age Ranges

A variety of physical characteristics can be used to assist in determining whether a child is less than 18 years old. When first assessing an image or video, the overall appearance of the individual in question should be considered. Overall health, nutrition, and the presence of characteristics associated with medical conditions and genetic disorders can affect the appearance of an individual and also affect the onset of puberty. For example, development can be delayed in children who are malnourished, who exercise excessively, or who have severe chronic illnesses. Chromosomal abnormalities can also affect the onset of puberty. Females with Turner syndrome are missing an X chromosome and most will not

begin sexual maturation unless hormone replacement is initiated. Girls with Turner syndrome have distinct physical characteristics including short stature, a broad chest with wide spaced nipples, and a webbed neck.[6] Males with Klinefelter syndrome have an extra female chromosome and tend to be tall with small testicles and gynecomastia.[7] The conditions tend to have with characteristic physical features that are easily discernable in an image or video and would not confuse an experienced clinician.

Other physical characteristics that change significantly from childhood to adulthood can be used to support a conclusion that an individual is less than 18 years old. For example, teeth go through a characteristic progression as the smaller baby teeth are lost and replaced by the larger permanent teeth. Size, proportion, and spacing are all obviously different as teeth mature. Age ranges for when particular teeth are lost and permanent teeth erupt are also established. Baby teeth are lost beginning at about 6 years of age until about 12 years of age. Permanent teeth erupt immediately after loss of baby teeth or lag by 4 to 5 months.[8]

Body size and shape change dramatically as children develop. At birth, the head is large compared to the body. As a child grows, the body lengthens and the head becomes less prominent. Leg length also varies considerably with growth. From the age of 1 year, the legs grow faster than the trunk of the body up until puberty. At puberty the trunk then grows more rapidly. Tables have been derived to compare the normal leg length to body length ratios at various ages.[9] For example, in boys at 1 year of age, leg length is 38% of body length, and at 13 years it is 49% of body length.

Body shape also undergoes considerable change. Before the onset of puberty, boys and girls have similar body shapes and proportions with cylindrical trunks and minimal waist indentation. Viewing body habitus from the back, it would be difficult to tell a boy from a girl before puberty. As females go through puberty, the pelvis widens and becomes broader than the shoulders, hips become rounder, and the indentation at the waist becomes obvious. In males the shoulders widen more than the hips and there is not pronounced indentation of the waist.[10]

Muscle development is also a marker of puberty with muscle mass increasing dramatically with puberty. This is much more pronounced in males. Body fat distribution also changes. Female body fat content increases from about 16% to 27% as females go through puberty. Male body fat content increases from about 4% to 11%.[11]

Body hair growth and distribution patterns also vary with age. Younger children have soft downy hair on their bodies that is not particularly visible. With androgens and puberty, hair becomes coarser and darker. In males hair growth is most prominent on the chest, underarms, and face. Hair growth is not as dramatic in females, but changes in axillary and leg hair are obvious. In one study, pubertal changes related to hair growth were noted for American boys and girls. The onset of axillary hair was reported to occur in females between 12 and 14 years of age and in males between 13 and 15 years of age.[12] Facial hair growth in males was reported to first occur between 13.8 and 16 years of age.[12]

Facial characteristics also change with puberty. The jaw becomes longer and thicker. The chin progresses from being small and recessed in childhood to more prominent and adultlike with a larger mouth.[13] The rounded baby-faced appearance disappears to form a more adultlike profile. The nose projects more in adults and sits lower on the face compared with children. In younger children, the nose is smaller in proportion to the rest of the face and turns upright.[14] Facial growth can continue until 21 years of age.[15]

Progression of body changes, such as those listed, can be difficult to assess based on one image. Providers rarely have additional photographs showing changes in an individual with the progression of time. These physical features can be used as an important adjunct with other factors in assessing images, but should not be used as the sole determining factor.

Secondary Sexual Characteristics

Sexual maturity rating (SMR) is a useful tool in evaluating the development of secondary sexual characteristics.[14] SMR in males describes the development of pubic hair and changes in genitalia. In females, pubic hair and breast development are assessed (Figure 19-1).

Pubic hair in both males and females progresses through stages from puberty to adulthood.[16] In the prepubertal stage, or SMR 1, there is no pubic hair. In stage 2, the pubic hair is scant, long, and may be straight or slightly curly. In males

the hair is primarily seen at the base of the penis. In females, hair growth begins around the edges of the labia majora. Stage 3 pubic hair becomes darker, coarser, and starts to curl. In males, hair growth extends over the junction of the pubic bones above the penis and in females there is further extension over the labia. Maturity continues in stage 4 with the hair now appearing adultlike in color, curl, and coarseness in both sexes. Pubic hair is distributed incompletely over the pubic area. Stage 5 pubic hair has full adult quantity and distribution with extension to the inner surface of the thighs. In males, there is a classic pattern of an inverted triangle, and in females there is full coverage over the labia.

SMR in males also classifies the development of the male testes, scrotum, and penis. SMR 1 genitalia have the same size and proportion seen in early childhood. With progression to stage 2, the scrotum and testes enlarge and the scrotal sac reddens and becomes thinner, coarser, and larger. There is little to no change in penis size. The testes and scrotum continue to grow in stage 3, as the penis initially grows in length rather than width. In stage 4, growth continues with darkening of the scrotal skin. Penile growth continues both in breadth and length, and there is development of the glans. In Tanner stage 5, the penis reaches full maturity in size and shape and no further growth occurs. Studies have shown

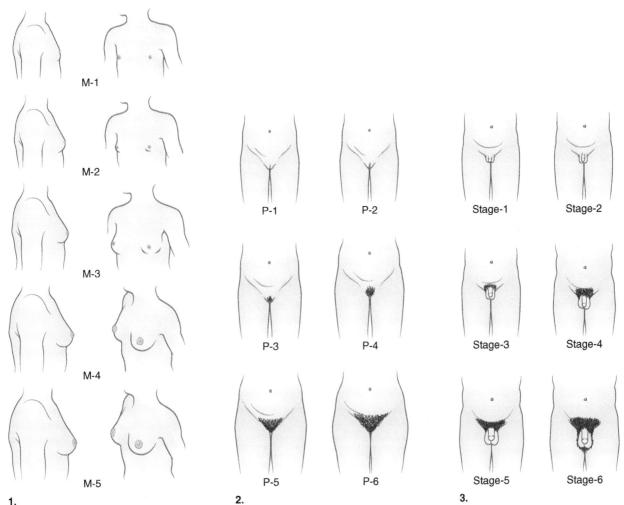

1. 2. 3.

FIGURE 19-1 Sexual maturity rating (SMR) stages, based on the work of Tanner et al. *(From Tanner JM: Growth and maturation during adolescence. Nutr Rev 1981;39:43-55.)*

good concordance between pubic hair and genital development in boys so that with normal hormonal production the stage of pubic hair correlates closely to the stage of genital growth.[17]

In females, SMR classifies the different stages of breast and areolar development. In Tanner stage 1, there is no breast development. The infantile stage of breast development persists until the onset of puberty. No breast tissue is seen or palpated and the areola is flat. Estrogen from the mother affects female breast tissue and a breast bud may be palpable until about 4 months of age, but beyond that there is no palpable breast tissue until puberty in most girls.[18] The first sign of breast development is seen in stage 2 with the development of the breast bud. This is a small mound of breast tissue under the areola, which is not larger than the areola. In stage 3, the breast and areola continue to grow and enlarge. The areola has the same contour as the breast tissue with no separation. In stage 4, the areola and nipple increase in size forming a secondary mound that protrudes from the breast tissue. At full maturity, SMR stage 5, there is a prominent nipple and the areola is again in the same contour with the breast and is not a separate mound.

Supplemental Secondary Sexual Characteristics

Other secondary sexual characteristics in females can also be used to assess development. There are changes in the labia, nipple, and hymen. The nipple development is mentioned in some descriptions of SMR, but is not consistently incorporated into the analysis. The nipple of the immature breast is small and does not protrude. It grows larger and wider with breast growth. The diameter of the nipple does not change much between stages 1 and 3. Increases are seen after breast stage 3 with a final diameter of approximately 9 mm.[19] The mons pubis increases in size due to fat deposition and the labia majora become larger.[20] Wrinkles (or rugae) develop on both labia that become more prominent following menarche. The labia minora also thickens and will usually protrude beyond the labia majora.

The hymen also undergoes significant changes with the onset of puberty and increased estrogen. The hymen is not visible in most images of child pornography, but there are occasionally images and videos with close-ups that allow for the hymen to be evaluated. In these cases, the prepubertal, nonestrogenized hymen can be easily distinguished from the estrogenized form that is seen with puberty. The immature hymen is often flat and thin (Figures 10-1 and 10-2). With the onset of estrogen stimulation in early puberty, the hymen thickens. In fully developed adolescents, the hymen is thick, redundant, and paler (Figure 10-10).

By combining assessments of secondary sexual characteristics and other physical characteristics, it is possible to form a medical opinion as to whether or not the person depicted in an image is less than 18 years of age. Most images will not show every characteristic that can be assessed. When evaluating images as many secondary sexual and physical factors as possible should be used in each image or video. Documentation should include the features evaluated in each image. For example, an image containing what appears to be a young female could be documented as: Breasts—SMR 1 to 2, pubic hair—SRM 1 to 2, minimal to no breast/

nipple development, immature genitalia, immature dentition, and body size and habitus of a child.

When physical and sexual characteristics are inconsistent with the apparent age range, image or individual alteration should be suspected. For example, a female with a mature body habitus with prominent hips and an indented waist, might appear to have SMR 1 or 2 breasts. Since it does not make sense for mature hips to be associated with stage 1 breasts, the image has likely been altered. The maturity of the labia might confirm that the person depicted is mature. Evaluating images can be difficult. Often it is evident that pubic hair has been shaved, but in some photos or videos, the image quality or positioning of the subjects makes it difficult to be certain. Sometimes, the legs are held close together so that female genitalia appear more immature than they actually are. Care should be taken to ensure all aspects of the image fit together when making a determination. If something does not fit, then the image should be rated as "cannot determine SMR."

Ratings Based on Body Size and Habitus in Smaller Children

Sometimes an image will depict a child participating in a sex act while clothed. For younger children, it is possible to rate that child as less than 18 years old based on body size and habitus. An infant, toddler, or preschool age child has a characteristic body size and habitus that is usually obvious enough to determine that the person depicted is less than 18. The size of a young child can be determined relative to other people or objects in the image. Some images will contain body parts that can be used for comparison. For example, the image showing an apparent adult sized hand along with the hand of a small child clearly demonstrates differences in size and maturity. This may be applied to early school age children as well, but age estimates of older children should not be attempted without the corroborating secondary sexual characteristics and other physical characteristics. It is important to clearly visualize most or all of the body to ensure a reasonable estimation with appropriate consideration of factors related to photographic technique and quality, and scale.

Challenges in Assessing Age and Maturity of Photographic Subjects

Several factors may impact the clinician's ability to provide age estimation data. For example, penis size varies considerably with erection, and variations among individuals further compromise the assessment of size. There is no data to associate penile size with age. There is also a wide variation in the size and shape of the adult female breast. Areolar size and coloring varies as does the amount of breast tissue. It can be difficult to rate a breast in a two dimensional image, especially if body position is not optimal to examine the breasts. Sometimes only part of the breast is visualized or it is seen from angles that preclude adequate assessment. Lying supine flattens breast tissue and can distort the contours of the breast.

There is also a wide variation in final adult body size and shape. Muscle mass progresses with age, particularly in males, but many adult males do not have a lot of muscle mass. Final adult height is also widely variable. In addition, many people shave pubic and body hair. As mentioned, this may be evident if photo quality is good. Females are more likely to shave pubic hair, but it does occur in males. Some males may also shave their chest or other body hair for various reasons. Since the development of body hair corresponds to pubertal growth, the lack of pubic or body hair can make the individual appear younger.

Thin individuals can also be difficult to assess as they can appear younger due to decreased muscle mass and perhaps smaller breast size. Again other factors of breast maturity such as nipple and areolar development can differentiate between a small breast and an immature one. Also, genital development and other signs of physical maturity can be used to distinguish the thin individual from the immature male or female. Malnutrition is also a consideration when looking at thin individual as poor nutrition can delay puberty. Nonetheless, genitals and breasts will have the immature appearance of early puberty.

The rate of pubertal development varies. Some males and females have fully developed secondary sexual characteristics at a younger age. These individuals appear older than actual age. Conversely, someone who develops more slowly appears younger. This makes a conservative approach in rating children very important. Often an image will depict someone who is most likely in their mid teens but with mature sexual development. Because the secondary sexual development is mature, such individuals cannot reliably be rated as less than 18 years old using the objective medical criteria outlined. On average males begin puberty at 11.6 years of age with a range from 9.5 to 13.5 years. The average length of time for puberty is 3 years, but ranges from 2 to 5 years, and most are fully developed by 14. 5 years (range 11.5 to 18 years).[21] Females begin puberty on average at 11.2 years of age with a range from 9.0 to 13.4 years. The average time to completion of puberty is 4 years with a range of 1.5 to 8 years; most are fully developed by 15 years of age.[21] The variability of progression through puberty and variations in body size and shape, make it difficult to rate a mid to late teenager with a reasonable degree of medical certainty. When there is any doubt that the subject is less than 18 based on image quality, the body parts visualized, or the positioning of the individuals, caution should be exercised and the person rated as "cannot determine SMR." It should be noted that both males and females can achieve full adult sexual and physical maturity before age 18.

Providers may be asked to assert whether or not people depicted in an image are clearly adult. The above criteria and knowledge of development can be used to assert that an individual is older than 18 years of age and does not have the characteristics of a child.

Many images reviewed will be placed in an "indeterminate" or "cannot determine" category. The factors and issues addressed above attest to the wide variations in development and associated problems in image quality that make it difficult to determine an individual to be less than 18 years old by viewing an image. Only individuals at the earliest stages of puberty can be determined to be less than 18 years old with medical certainty. Older children, though less than 18, are more difficult to assess.

The guidelines addressed in this chapter support a conservative approach when assessing whether or not underage children are depicted in pornographic images. There is good medical evidence to support limiting specific opinions unless the children are in very early stages of puberty. As children mature, it is more difficult due to the wide variations found. Child abuse specialists and other experienced health care providers can use the combination of physical and sexual development, with knowledge of the supporting literature, to assess pornographic images and determine the presence of minors to a reasonable degree of medical certainty.

References

1. Farid H: Digital image forensics. *Sci Am* 2008;298:66-71.
2. National Center for Missing & Exploited Children: *Child victim identification program* (website): http://www.missingkids.com/en_US/publications/NC166.pdf. Accessed March 8, 2009.
3. Plan and operation of the third national health and nutrition examination survey, 1988-1994. Series 1: programs and collection procedures. *Vital Health Stat* 1994;1:1-407.
4. Herman-Giddens ME, Slora EJ, Wasserman RC, et al: Secondary sexual characteristics and menses in young girls seen in office practice: a study from the Pediatric Research in Office Settings network. *Pediatrics* 1997;99:505-512.
5. Herman-Giddens ME, Wang L, Koch G: Secondary sexual characteristics in boys: estimates from the national health and nutrition examination survey III, 1988-1994. *Arch Pediatr Adolesc Med* 2001;155:1022-1028.
6. Jones KL: Chromosomal abnormality syndromes, 45X syndrome. *In*: Jones KL (ed): *Smith's Recognizable Patterns of Human Malformation*, ed 6, Saunders, Philadelphia, 2006, pp 76-81.
7. Jones KL: Chromosomal abnormality syndromes, XXY syndrome, Klinefelter syndrome. *In*: Jones KL (ed): *Smith's Recognizable Patterns of Human Malformation*, ed 6, Saunders, Philadelphia, 2006, pp 68-69.
8. Behrman RE, Kleigman RM, Jenson HB: Assessment of growth. *In*: Behrman RE, Kleigman RM, Jenson HB (eds): *Nelson Textbook of Pediatrics*, ed 17, Saunders, Philadelphia, 2004, p 61.
9. Bayer LM, Bayley N: *Growth diagnosis*, ed 2, University of Chicago Press, Chicago, 1976.
10. Wheeler MD: Physical changes of puberty. *Endocrinol Metab Clin North Am* 1991;20:1-14.
11. Slap GB: Normal physiological and psychosocial growth in the adolescent. *J Adolesc Heath Care* 1986;7(suppl 6):13S-23S.
12. Lee PA: Normal age of pubertal events in American males and females. *J Adolesc Heath Care* 1980;1:26-29.
13. Melson B: Palatal growth studied on human autopsy material. A histologic microradiographic study. *Am J Orthod* 1975;68:42-54.
14. Tanner JM: Growth and maturation during adolescence. *Nutr Rev* 1981;39:43-55.
15. Krogman WM: Maturation age of the growing child in relation to the timing of statural and facial growth at puberty. *Trans Stud Coll Physicians Phila* 1979;1:33-42.
16. Behrman RE, Kleigman RM, Jenson HB: Adolescence. *In*: Behrman RE, Kleigman RM, Jenson HB (eds): *Nelson Textbook of Pediatrics*, ed 17, Saunders, Philadelphia, 2004, pp 53-55.
17. Wheeler MD: Physical changes of puberty. *Endocrinol Metab Clin North Am* 1991;20:1-14.
18. Sucato GS: Breast disorders. *In*: McMillan J, Reigin RD, DeAngelis CA (eds): *Oski's Pediatrics: Principles and Practice*, ed 4, Lippincott Williams & Wilkins, Philadelphia, 2006, p 558.
19. Grumback MM, Styne DM: Puberty: ontogeny, neuroendocrinology, physiology, and disorders. *In*: Kronenberg HM, Melmed S, Polonsky KS, et al *(eds)*: *Williams Textbook of Endocrinology*, ed 10, Saunders, Philadelphia, 2003, p 1118.
20. Wheeler MD: Physical changes of puberty. *Endocrinol Metab Clin North Am* 1991;20:1-14.
21. Neinstein LS, Kaufman FR: Normal physical growth and development. *In*: Neinstein LS (ed): *Adolescent Health Care, A Practical Guide*, ed 2, Williams & Wilkins, Baltimore, 1996, p 22.

20

CHILD MOLESTERS

Nathan W. Galbreath, PhD, MFS

INTRODUCTION

A twenty-four year-old man volunteers as a karate coach and part-time sitter for families on the team. Children on the team complain of having to go skinny-dipping and getting their photographs taken while undressed. Investigators eventually discover hundreds of images of children in the man's possession; some documenting his sexual exploits with blonde-haired, blue-eyed boys on the team.

Police apprehend a 12-year-old boy for shoplifting. He tells police that his biological mother has been having sexual intercourse with him since he was the age of nine. The mother confesses to the sexual acts and explains that she perpetrated them out of anger at her husband for his frequent absences on military deployments. She tells police, "I used my son as I would a man."

A 30-year-old man with three daughters, aged 5, 9, and 12, is accused by his eldest daughter of sexual abuse while she sleeps at night. Interviews of the younger children disclose the father has also sexually touched the 9 year old. The 5 year old denies any inappropriate contact by her father. The mother accuses the 12-year-old of lying and kicks her out of the family home.

A twice prior convicted child molester and former youth minister arranges to meet an undercover postal inspector via the Internet for videos of child pornography and sex with two 14- year-old boys. During his arrest, postal inspectors discover dozens of videos of preteen child pornography.

This book has thus far focused on the recognition and recovery of evidence in cases of child sexual abuse and exploitation. This chapter will address the molesters and the manner by which they perpetrate such crimes. Any discussion of child molesters must begin with the fact that they are a heterogeneous group.[1] While each of the case vignettes above has a common thread of child sexual exploitation, the characteristics of the child molesters described are very different. Some molesters have common methods of accessing and exploiting children. Yet, they often lack commonality in victim preference, victim accessibility, offenses perpetrated, means of perpetration, etiology, risk of reoffense, and many other aspects that make broad discussions of them challenging. In addition, the tendency to aggregate all offenders into one homogenous group by the media, the public, and lawmakers can also lead to false assumptions about dangerousness, recidivism, and treatment potential.

From an investigative viewpoint, there is great utility in understanding common or prevalent behaviors of child molesters. Understanding their individual differences, however, often yields more evidence for additional victim identification and prosecution. This chapter will focus on the investigation of people who are suspected of directly or indirectly victimizing children, while using the scientific literature as a foundation for investigative and clinical decision making.

At the outset of any investigation, little might be known about a child molester. Sometimes the victim might not be familiar with the molester or even know that he or she was victimized, which is often the case in Internet crimes. But in the majority of sex offenses involving children, the victim likely knows the perpetrator. Of the children in the United States who were reported to be sexually abused in 2006, 26.2% were abused by a parent, 29.1% were abused by a relative other than a parent, 6.1% were abused by an unmarried partner of a parent, and 4.4% were abused by a friend or neighbor.[2]

While these statistics can certainly guide investigative activity, they also indicate that in roughly one third of cases the relationship between the victim and the perpetrator might be unknown or not readily apparent. Nevertheless, children are more likely to be sexually exploited by someone they know than by a stranger.[3]

Men are much more likely than women to perpetrate sex crimes against children.[4] The actual number of men and women who find children to be sexually attractive, however, remains unknown. No epidemiological study has been conducted to establish the extent of sexual interest in children. Seto[5] found that a number of studies suggest that less than 3% of men report children as a focus of sexual interest. This number is likely to be an upper limit estimate, given the limitations of the research that he reviewed. Other methods used to estimate the number of individuals who are sexually interested in children are likely to be equally imprecise for a variety of reasons. For example, 8.8% of child abuse victims reported to authorities in 2006 were sexually abused, which accounted for more than 78,000 children.[2] However, research indicates that most sexual contact with children is not reported, especially when the victim is male.[6] Retrospective studies of adults who were abused as children also indicate that sexual abuse is underreported.[7] Studies of molesters have found that a relatively small number of men might be involved with several thousand victims and tens of thousands of incidents over the lifetime. In her summary of Abel and associates' research in the 1980s, Salter[8] notes that 232 men reported responsibility for 38,000 incidents of abuse, involving more than 17,000 child victims. Men who molested out-of-home girls reported an average of 20 victims. Though perpetrators were fewer in number, men who molested out-of-home boys averaged 150 victims each.

DEFINITIONS

Child Molesters

For the purposes of this chapter, a child molester is anyone who perpetrates a sexual crime against a child. This includes contact offenses where the molester has a personal encounter with the victim, and also child molesters who do not directly touch their victims, but commit exhibitionistic or voyeuristic crimes with children, inappropriately photograph children, or obtain or disseminate child pornography.

From an investigative perspective, child molesters can be viewed on a continuum of behaviors. On one end of the continuum are the individuals who find children of sexual interest, but have yet to act upon their feelings in any overt way. At the other end of the continuum lie people who are involved in full sexual contact with children. In this view, a willingness to assume risk moves the individual across the continuum, from no contact to full contact. Initial forays into using children as sex objects often rely on low risk means, such as using legally available and mental imagery of children. In males, these types of imagery are a likely focus for masturbatory activity. When the individual's interest promotes greater sexual risk taking, he or she may resort to obtaining more sexualized images of children, participating in activities that provide frequent access to children, and expanding the kinds of social and physical contact made with children. (The process of facilitating sexual contact with children is called "grooming.") Some molesters never become sufficiently comfortable with their desires or gain the kind of access to children that leads to a contact offense. Yet, there is limited research that indicates that some child molesters eventually move from fantasy or noncontact offenses (such as downloading child pornography or covert photography of children in various stages of undress) to contact offenses. In some child molesters, there might even be a "feedback loop" involving deviant arousal fantasies of children leading to a first contact offense, which subsequently leads to greater deviant arousal fantasies, and so on.[9]

Despite the heterogeneity of child molesters, such men tend to fall into two broad categories based on their offense behavior. These two groups have been described in several ways in the scientific literature. Groth[10] described the two groups as "regressed" and "fixated" molesters. Others have described them as "situational" and "preferential" child molesters.[11] Both attempt to capture the concept that some molesters victimize children sexually, but only under certain circumstances, while other molesters prefer children as their primary source of sexual gratification. There is some support for these broad categories in the literature, but the two groups are hardly mutually exclusive. Nevertheless, there is benefit in describing child molesters with these terms, both clinically and investigatively. No typology, however, has been thoroughly validated. Consequently, all typologies of child molesters should only be used as a heuristic to consider broad clusters of offender behaviors.

Situational child molesters perpetrate the majority of the offenses referred to child protective services in the United States. They are often family members of the victim, or simply living in the home. Consequently, most familial offenses typically fall into this category. Lanning[12] suggests that situational molesters do not have a true sexual preference for children. Rather, they select children for sexual activity using wide-ranging rationales, including ease of access, a belief they will not be caught, insecurity about their sexuality, curiosity, and lack of a willing adult partner. Situational molesters' behavior typically emerges in adulthood and tends to be influenced greatly by external stressors and opportunities for victim access. Increased stress brought on by significant life change (such as unemployment, relationship problems, and loss of social support) or by negative mood state (such as loneliness, depression, and anxiety) often precedes a sexual act with a child.[1] In comparison to preferential molesters, situational molesters typically have fewer victims because opportunity plays heavily in offense decision making. Many situational child molesters rely on institutional (schools, churches) or public (parks or other facilities) means to access children. Their offenses do not always involve the same victim repeatedly. However, other situational child molesters have long-term relationships with or access to their victims, causing sexual abuse to occur over many years.

Preferential child molesters are almost exclusively sexually involved with children. Their sexual interest in children begins in adolescence,[13] but never matures to a sexual interest in age mates or other adults. Preferential molesters might have had a few sexual relationships with peers, and tend to spend a majority of their social time with children and/or individuals much younger than they are. These molesters often have a great many victims across their lifetime. Most of their sexual energy is directed toward making contact with children, assessing children as potential sexual partners, and facilitating sexual activity with them. In recent years, preferential molesters have made great use of the Internet for trading information about where to meet children, downloading child pornography or erotica, and as a means for potential victim identification and selection.

Pedophilia, Paraphilia, and Hebephilia

Many preferential child molesters and relatively fewer situational child molesters are likely to meet the diagnostic criteria for pedophilia as described in the Diagnostic and Statistical Manual (DSM-IV) of the American Psychiatric Association.[14] According to the DSM-IV, pedophilia is defined as a mental disorder that involves persistent sexual interest in prepubescent children, manifested in thoughts, fantasies, urges, sexual arousal, or sexual behavior (Table 20-1).[14] The term pedophilia comes from a term coined by Krafft-Ebing, *pedophilia erotica*, which means the erotic love of children.[4] The pubertal status of the child or children who are of sexual interest is important in diagnosis.[5] Individuals qualify for the diagnosis when they show a marked sexual interest in prepubertal children who are usually under the age of 13. Child molesters that are attracted to children aged 13 and over qualify for a diagnosis of "Paraphilia, Not Otherwise Specified." Hebephilia is also a term that has sometimes been used to describe sexual attraction to children that are developing secondary sexual characteristics, usually between the ages of 11 to 14. It should be noted that all groups of children are minors under the law, and cannot consent to sexual activity with an adult. However, pedophilia is not a criminal offense; it is a mental disorder. Sexual

Table 20-1 DSM-IV Criteria for Pedophilia

- Over a period of at least 6 months, recurrent, intense sexually arousing fantasies, sexual urges or behaviors involving sexual activity with a pre-pubescent child or children (generally age 13 or younger)
- The fantasies, sexual urges, or behaviors cause clinically significant distress or impairment in social, occupation, or other important areas of functioning
- The person is at least age 16 years and at least 5 years older than the child or children in Criterion A. Note: Do not include an individual in late adolescence involved in an ongoing sexual relationship with a 12- or 13-year-old

contact with a child and possession of child pornography are criminal offenses in which pedophiles often engage.

Not all pedophiles are child molesters. There are a few examples in the scientific literature,[15] and in clinical practice,[16] of individuals who have sexual interests in children, but yet do not act on them. Given the associated stigma, these individuals rarely present clinically, and when they do, are likely to be regarded with suspicion and concern. These patients present considerable legal and ethical challenges for clinicians, especially when the presenting patient has legitimate, regular access to or involvement with children.

Likewise, not all child molesters are pedophiles. In fact, only those individuals who have demonstrated a marked sexual interest to children and meet the requisite criteria should be diagnosed with the disorder. As indicated above, situational molesters might not exhibit the recurrent thoughts, urges, or behaviors required for a diagnosis of pedophilia. A man who has had a single sexual contact with a child and lacks observable, persistent sexual interests in children would not meet DSM-IV diagnostic criteria. Nevertheless, the sexual contact with the child would no doubt be of both clinical and legal interest.

INTERNET CHILD MOLESTERS

The growth of the Internet has influenced what we know about men who use technology to identify and access child victims for sexual exploitation and abuse. In the early 1990s, law enforcement in the United States was making relatively few arrests for child pornography. Evidence seized from suspects often consisted of decades-old naturist magazine photographs, or series of photographs that were well known to investigators. However, the Internet's accessibility, affordability, and perceived anonymity are likely factors, if not the causes, of the upsurge of arrests and prosecution for child pornography and sex transportation cases in the past decade.[17] The primary sexual exploitation offense referred to U.S. attorneys has shifted from sexual abuse to child pornography. Child pornography matters accounted for 82% of the growth in sexual exploitation matters referred from 1994 to 2006. During 2006, 3661 suspects were referred and 2039 suspects were prosecuted for federal sex offenses, with the latter representing about 2.5% of the approximate 80,000 suspects prosecuted in federal courts.[18]

Research indicates that men involved in the Internet sexual exploitation of children have several common characteristics. In a representative sample of approximately 1700 child pornography offenders, Wolak and associates[19] found that nearly all were male (more than 99%) and white (95%). While their ages ranged between 15 and 90, the vast majority were older than 25 (86%). Most were unmarried at the time of the crime because they had never married (41%) or were separated, divorced, or widowed (21%). However, 38% of the offenders were living with partners. About one third of offenders had minor children living at home, while nearly half had direct access to minors because they lived with them or had contact with them in a job or organized youth activity. At the time of the crime, few offenders in the study had been *previously* diagnosed with a mental or sexual disorder, few exhibited past evidence of other deviant sexual behaviors, and less than one fifth of them had known alcohol or drug problems. Only 11% had a known incident of violence in their past, and only 22% had a prior arrest for a nonsexual offense. Eleven percent had a prior arrest for a sexual offense against a minor.[19] Clinical samples of offenders are likely to be similar, but might have a higher incidence of diagnosed mental and sexual disorders.[16]

ETIOLOGY OF CHILD MOLESTERS

Sexual orientation and interests are generally thought to be discovered rather than decided. That is, a person does not wake up one morning and decide what will arouse him or her sexually. Rather, finding out about one's own sexual interests is a process of discovery that starts in early life.[20] As an individual matures, new sexual stimuli are incorporated into his or her repertoire of sexual interests. However, in most cases sexual interests appear to be known to oneself —though perhaps not acted upon—early in life. There is some evidence to indicate that pedophiles discover their sexual attraction to children during adolescence. Self-report studies over the past 20 years have found that a significant portion of pedophiles recall having their first deviant fantasies before the age of 18. Pedophiles and nonpedophiles alike might share a sexual curiosity about other children when they were children themselves. However, a pedophile's sexual attraction never grows beyond children. Why this occurs during adolescence has yet to be established empirically. However, puberty appears to be a critical time in the emergence of all sexual interests and preferences.[5]

There have been a number of theories offered to explain pedophilia and the development of sexual interest in children generally. Unfortunately, scientific support for them is limited, and significant gaps remain in our understanding of how pedophilia and related problematic behavior develops. Pathogenic risk factors that contribute to pedophilia early in the individual's life are different from the risk factors that maintain the disorder. From a biological perspective, elevated neurotransmitter levels, developmental delay, brain structure abnormalities, and hormonal anomalies have all been suggested as possible risk factors.[4] Seto,[5] however, contends that there is consistent evidence that pedophilia, at least for some men, is a neurodevelopmental disorder. He bases this conclusion on reviews of studies of neuropsychological testing, educational histories, head injury history, and structural neuroimaging. For example, samples of child molesters score significantly lower on measures of intelligence than samples of sex offenders who don't abuse children. In addition, men who offended against younger children tended to have lower average IQ scores than men who offended against older children.[21] Head injury before the age of 13, abnormalities in the frontal and temporal regions of the brain, and differences in the volume of white matter connecting structures in the frontal and occipital regions of the brain have also been found in samples of pedophiles. Why these neurodevelopmental disorders express themselves in some men as pedophilia and not as other paraphilias or disorders has yet to be explained.

Environmental risk factors have also been implicated in the development of pedophilia and sexual interest in children. A history of childhood sexual abuse has long been associated with adult sexual offending against children. Yet, Hanson and Slater[22] found that only about one quarter of 1700 adult sexual offenders in 25 different studies admitted they had been sexually victimized as children. Unfortunately, numerous methodological problems in this area make it difficult to be certain about the impact of childhood sexual victimization on child molesters. While other lines of research have found similar rates of victimization in adult sex offenders,[23] the number of molesters and the kind of child molestation in which they engaged was not always specified in the studies. Burton and associates[24] found that male sex offenders in general with a history of childhood victimization were more likely to have had a closer relationship with their perpetrator, had a male perpetrator, had a longer duration of sexual abuse, experienced more forceful sexual abuse, and had been penetrated as part of the abuse. A more sophisticated statistical analysis of their sample actually showed that having perpetrators of both sexes and a experiencing a high level of force were the best predictors of later sexual offending against children.

Maladaptive childhood experience in a dysfunctional family has also been cited as a risk factor for perpetration of child molestation.[25] The families of offenders have been reported as violent, unstable, and disorganized. While this may be common in many individuals who perpetrate crime, child molesters' homes seem to be most often characterized by instability, poor emotional bonds between parent and child, early exposure to sexual material and behavior, high risk for sexual abuse or exploitation by another adult, and minimal resources to cope with the effects of sexual abuse once it has been disclosed by the victim.

Situational or dynamic risk factors are likely to be of particular importance in the maintenance of a molester's sexual abuse of children, and are likely to precipitate an incident of abuse. Interpersonal conflict, emotional identification with children, unresponsiveness to treatment, lack of personal support, noncompliance with previous treatment, symptoms of major mental illness, impulsivity, negative attitude towards treatment, lack of insight, unrealistic planning, stress in the environment, and exposure to destabilizing influences (e.g., drugs and alcohol) all have been identified as dynamic factors related to offending and reoffending.[26] When one or more of these dynamic factors is present to a sufficient level when the molester has live or Internet-mediated access to children, an offense is likely to follow.

OBTAINING EVIDENCE

Physical evidence of crime and victim statements are valuable sources of evidence to be considered in any case involving the sexual abuse of a child. The molester's behavior and the thought processes supporting the decisions made in committing the crime can also be of great value, especially when the victim cannot be an effective witness. Statements, behaviors, and the possible rationalizations behind them are useful in supporting probable cause statements, identifying additional victims, discovering additional physical evidence, and linking together cases by the same molester.

Cognitive Evidence

Finkelhor's precondition model[13] for the sexual abuse of children lays an excellent foundation for understanding molester behavior. Finkelhor's purpose was to construct a model that would address both the perpetrator's internal thought process and the situational aspects of child sexual abuse that are present in both familial and nonfamilial incidents. He proposed that four preconditions must be met before sexual abuse can occur: motivation to sexually abuse; overcoming internal inhibitors; overcoming external inhibitors; and overcoming the resistance of the child.[27] Each of the four concepts is briefly described below.

Motivation to sexually abuse. A particular child must meet an emotional need for a molester. The needs for each perpetrator are different, but include such things as attention, admiration, control or even "love." The molester also must be sexually aroused by the child. Many misinterpret a child's need for affection or attention as a sign of sexual seduction. Child pornography or deviant fantasies can further sexualize children in the eyes of a molester. Motivation will also be driven by self-esteem problems, and a belief that sexual relationships with those his own age are impossible or undesirable.

Overcoming internal inhibitors. The molester must learn how to discount any reservations he might have about acting out sexually with a child. Many times, alcohol provides a quick way to lower inhibitions. Other molesters have psychosis, a psychological disorder, or impulse control problems. A molester's inability to appropriately empathize with the experience of the victim also impacts his ability to self-regulate his behavior.

Overcoming external inhibitors. The presence of a child's parents, both physically and emotionally, has been found to be a protective factor in preventing the abuse of children. Absent, ill, or emotionally unavailable parents tend to be less of a deterrent. Molesters often manipulate children into situations where they are unsupervised, many times with the approval or consent of the unsuspecting parent.

Overcoming the resistance of the child. Molesters often use persuasion, lies, gifts, and coercion to convince children that sex between adults and minors is not only acceptable but something they should or must do. Children are usually powerless to resist, and typically submit, especially when they have a close relationship with the molester. Victims can be so taken with the molester that they become regularly compliant with sexual activity, sometimes in exchange for special gifts and privileges. Violent molesters sometimes sexually and physically assault victims who resist.

Motivation and overcoming the internal and external barriers described by Finkelhor[13] are largely dependent on the molester's cognitive distortions, or thinking errors. Such distortions are used by perpetrators to deny, justify, rationalize, or minimize their offending behavior.[28] Often times these errors can provide insight that will allow an investigator to successfully interview and obtain a statement from a molester. Cognitive distortions are also helpful clinically, as they suggest a starting point for a variety of psychological interventions. Evidence of the cognitive distortions used by a particular molester can be obtained from the interviews of the molester himself, his victims, and from people who know the molester, even if they do not have first hand knowledge of the crime. A molester will often try to ensure or coerce secrecy from the victim by telling the child his reasons for their sexual activity. What follows are a few of the more commonly held cognitive distortions, supported by research,[29] and investigative experience. The interviewing "themes" associated with each cognitive distortion mesh with techniques and training similar to that offered by Reid and Associates.[30]

Children are sexual beings. Preferential molesters, and some situational molesters, believe that children are sexual creatures that have a need to express themselves sexually, especially with adults. Because this kind of behavior is "natural," they believe little harm can come from adult-child sexual interaction. This cognitive distortion allows the molester to view common child behaviors in an overtly sexual way. Innocent requests for affection and attention from a child are often interpreted as solicitation for and consent to sex. Molesters sometimes appoint themselves as teachers or mentors that selflessly help children discover their "true" sexual self. Molesters who have incorporated this distortion into their thinking might respond to investigative interviewing themes that center on the behavior of the child as an invitation to sex, the "service" being provided by the molester as a trusted mentor, and the "natural" and "loving" nature of sex between children and adults. The following was drawn from the website of the North American Man-Boy Love Association (NAMBLA), a group that advocates for the repeal of age of consent laws and physical relationships between men and minor boys:[31]

"…The manifold nature of our humanity appears in the emotional, spiritual, and physical attractions between people. Attractions between men and boys can be found in every society, crossing lines of race, age, temperament and occupation. They form a sure basis for mentoring and friendship traditions the world over. Man/boy love is exceptional only for the degree to which it is still misunderstood in cultures derived from Northwestern Europe. Most man/boy relationships are based on mutual respect and affection, and strongly desired by both partners. Such relationships do not harm anyone, and often entail many benefits for both man and boy. Boy-lovers and boys alike respond to the needs of those they love—needs for affection, understanding, and freedom."[31]

Sex with children isn't harmful. Some molesters believe that their behavior with children is only harmful when the sexual contact is physically aggressive. Others believe that sex with adults is not detrimental to a child, as sex is a "natural" act. Molesters who subscribe to this distortion believe that children have the full knowledge and ability to consent to sex, and society "just doesn't understand" how beneficial an adult sexual relationship can be for a child. These molesters might respond to interviewing themes that focus on how "enlightened" the molester must be given his knowledge about the nature of children, how "fortunate" the child was to have the molester in his or her life, how children can be "willing" sex partners, and how no real harm was done because the child was not wounded. In the absence of physical injury to the victim, these molesters are unlikely to acquiesce to suggestions that they ever caused harm to a child. Rather, their likely counter is that they would never *hurt* a child, because they *love* children.

The world is a dangerous place. Molesters might subscribe to one of two distortions about the potential for rejection in a world they perceive as hostile. Some molesters believe that society and the children that come from it are all potential sources of derision and ridicule. Consequently, a molester can put such children "in their place" by controlling and abusing them. This distortion might be part of an overall antisocial or sadistic personality. Such molesters can be emotionally or physically brutal in their interactions with children. A molester with this distortion might find it arousing to recall and describe his abusive behavior. While investigators find great utility in this kind of disclosure, clinicians consider it counterproductive for treatment. Interventions that focus on building victim empathy with this molester are likely to be ineffective. Conversely, a molester might view relationships with children as the sole source of safety and acceptance in a world that scorns him. This latter viewpoint is likely to be much more common. Interview themes should focus on the unjust nature of the molester's history of social rejection and how accepting and loving children can be to adults.

Adults are entitled. Some molesters prioritize their needs over the needs of anyone less worthy, including children. In this way of thinking, molesters believe they are entitled to meet their sexual needs whenever they choose, with whomever they choose. Some perpetrators might use this distortion to justify covert photography of nude children in a locker room, or even overt photography of children at the beach or a pool. Interviewing themes might be productive if centered on the benefits of being assertive, that children are there to learn from or serve the needs of adults, and how the molester *deserves* sex/love/relationships just like anyone else.

Some things are uncontrollable. Molesters can believe that they cannot control powerful urges when they are faced with their "triggers"—specific situations or conditions that increase the likelihood that the molester will offend or reoffend. Alcohol, drugs, sex drive, and stress are often things that child molesters cite as reasons for perpetrating sexual abuse. The molester might even view himself as a victim of his family, society, or his biology. Interviews might be productive if an investigator shows some kind of sympathy for the problems encountered by the molester throughout his life.

Behavioral Evidence

How a child molester accesses, selects, and trains his target to become a victim is directly influenced by his cognitions. Investigators and clinicians alike will find great overlap in how the molester thinks and how he has offended in his past.

If the individual in question has indeed molested a child or perpetrated some form of Internet-mediated offense related to children, then evidence of his behavior leading up to the incident will exist. Some molesters are savvier than others and take great pains to perpetrate secretly. Those who facilitate their crimes with the use of technology might even have elaborate systems set up to obfuscate or destroy evidence. One such molester had a series of powerful magnets set up covertly around a doorway, arranged so that any attempt to remove his computers from the room would degauss the hard drives inside the machines. Other molesters have been known to keep their collections of pornography and victims' personal articles in hidden locations far from their homes. One molester's travel to such a location was by a circuitous route and involved the employment of advanced counter-surveillance techniques. While not all molesters are this cautious, some are quite prepared for the possibility that they could be discovered by law enforcement. A few of the more hardcore molesters are well armed and are likely to resist returning to prison, especially if they have two prior convictions in states with "three-strikes" laws.

Victim Access

Preferential molesters often show considerable planning and effort in identifying and employing multiple methods to access potential victims. Situational molesters are less likely to show evidence of planning. Before widespread use of the Internet, most molesters accessed potential victims in person or had to obtain child pornography through the mail, from other molesters, or from bookstores that secretly carried such materials. Historically, preferential molesters have been known to enter employment where they have daily contact with children, have volunteered as sponsors or coaches for children's activities, and have frequented parks, beaches, and recreation centers where children are abundant. Most all forms of contact with children are sexually arousing to a preferential molester. Brushing up against children in public places, photographing children overtly or covertly, hearing children speak or sing, and olfactory cues have all been reported by molesters as potential sources for arousal.

Once a molester decides to make physical contact with a child, the victims he chooses are likely to relate to his individual interests and sexual desires. Interests can take the form of hobbies, sports, and other avocations in which he participates. A molester's interests often provide the means by which he accesses children. The molester's sexual desires largely reflect the kinds of children he finds to be sexually arousing. These desires can be widely inclusive (all children under a certain age) or very exclusive (school-aged, red-haired, green-eyed girls without any secondary sexual characteristics). The intersection of the molester's interests and sexual desires produces his target group. For example, one search of a molester's home revealed a variety of karate, skateboarding, and rollerblading equipment. Interviews of the man's victims disclosed that he often made contact with boys at karate practice or at recreational facilities where boarding and blading were featured. While the man had spoken and shown interest in a number of children at these facilities, only blonde-haired, blue-eyed boys between the ages of 9 and 12 reported any kind of inappropriate behavior with the man (skinny-dipping, photography during bathing).

Ironically, none of the children reported any kind of sexual touching. Only film negatives in the man's photograph collection showed that the boys had been touched on their genitals while they slept.

Preferential molesters that have well-defined target groups require investigations that involve hundreds of interviews of potential victims. Given the time-intensive nature of child interviews and the associated alarm likely to be raised by parents or the media, use of a victim matrix can help an investigator rapidly sort through which children are likely to be victims. While this technique can initially narrow the initial scope of interviews, all children might eventually need to be interviewed. This is especially true when further investigation shows that the preferential molester's target group is not as well defined as initially believed. A victim matrix is constructed by combining information about the means of access and common physical or personality features from a group of known victims. Often times, a white board, a wall covered in butcher paper, or a computerized spreadsheet is used to set up the matrix. Names of potential victims are listed down the rows of a single column. To the right across the top of the matrix are additional columns that contain the various methods of access and physical characteristics known to relevant to the molester. Check marks are placed in the rows next to the names of those children who are known to have the kind of access or characteristic favored by the molester. Those children who meet most of the known requirements of the molester's target group are interviewed first. Information from additional investigative activity and subsequent victim interviews might expand or limit the number of potential victims in the matrix.

For example, the victim matrix from the case described above was developed based on the common characteristics of three known victims. It was then used to identify all boys between the ages of 9 and 12 enrolled at the karate school and recreational facility. Once those boys were identified, investigators worked quietly with instructors and attendants to identify the boys' physical characteristics. Once all the blonde-haired, blue-eyed boys were identified, only those seen talking with the suspect were interviewed with a structured set of screening questions, so as not to cause alarm. Subsequent interviews disclosed that the suspect even had favorites in this group of boys. Those interviews disclosed that the suspect had befriended those boys' mothers and had often volunteered to baby sit for each family. The mothers, who were mostly single or separated from their husbands, had been eager to let the suspect stay with their children, especially since they knew the suspect was a military police officer. While none of the children in these families disclosed sexual contact by the man, the boys did disclose the fact that he had often taken their photographs while bathing or swimming nude at a nearby lake. This information was used to execute a search warrant on the man's home. The man had collected hundreds of photographs of children; however, none of them contained any evidence of inappropriate contact. Upon close review of the film negatives also in the box, 10 photographs were discovered that showed the man had taken pictures of the "favorite" boys bathing at home and at the lake. A few of the photos showed that the man had pulled down the boys' underwear while they were asleep and fondled them. Finally, one photograph was found on the negative roll that showed the suspect naked at the lake with the boys. This photograph corroborated one of the victim's accounts that the suspect made them all go skinny-dipping at the lake, or else he would make them walk the 125 miles home.

Unfortunately, many victims experience much more violent means of access. Some molesters engage in high-risk attempts to coerce children into cars or away from safety by telling elaborate stories to gain trust. A minority of molesters kidnap, sexually mutilate, and kill victims. Some molesters pay to join Web sites on the Internet to access child pornography or watch live through a webcam while a child masturbates or is sexually abused by another adult. Others travel to countries where sex tourism includes having child prostitutes brought to a hotel room. However, most molesters simply walk to a room in their home and sexually abuse a child they know.

Grooming. Child molesters are not only skilled at accessing children, but also at convincing and coercing their victims to engage in sexual activity. Grooming is a process whereby a child molester overcomes a child's resistance to sex and elicits cooperation. The molester's techniques for grooming are likely to have a significant relationship with his individual interests and sexual desires, similar to his methods for victim access. Preferential and situational molesters alike can show evidence of grooming. Grooming typically occurs gradually. Initial steps might involve simply seeing how open a child is to conversation. The child's response to a smile or a subtle touch can signal to the molester how open the child might be to further contact. As the relationship between the molester and the child grows, so does the possibility for additional touching and interaction between the two. Eventually, sexual talk or an "accidental" touch of the breasts or genitals of a victim during play might act as a gateway to more sexual activity. Alternatively, the molester might purposefully leave sexually explicit material where the child might find it. This constructed situation can elicit an opportunity to ignite the child's curiosity about sex. Other techniques involve frequent nudity by the molester around the child and genital exposure or the "accidental" discovery of the molester with an erection. Well-versed molesters have an explanation ready for just about any situation, justifying their inappropriate behavior as "natural" or "acceptable" between people who are close. Once the child appears ready, the molester moves to more involved sexual activity with the child. Again, "effective" grooming is the molester's assurance the victim will not only comply, but keep the activity secret as well.

Grooming can also be used as a method of victim selection from a group of potential victims. One such case involved a molester from a small southwestern town who volunteered at his church as the boys' junior high school youth group leader. The small religious sect fully trusted the molester with the group of six or seven boys for unsupervised meetings at his home in a rural area. The boys would often have youth group sleepovers at the molester's home on Saturday nights and then attend church together on Sunday morning. While at his home, the molester would convince the boys to play sexually themed games. One such game was "strip basketball," which involved removing an article of clothing every time a shot was missed. The molester also engaged the children in wrestling matches. However, the man encouraged the boys to wrestle in their briefs while he

wore very small, tight-fitting nylon jogging shorts. During the matches the boys often noticed the molester's erection under or protruding from the shorts. The molester would also offer some of the boys back rubs. The boys that accepted were usually the boys whom the molester would later target for additional sexual abuse. Once the molester determined that a boy might be receptive, he would then take the boy aside for what he called an "attitude check" in his home's bathroom. He often used false empathy to gain the boy's trust by acknowledging the difficulties of being an adolescent. The man would then tell the boy his "secret" to further cement the relationship with sympathy: the molester disclosed that he was born "without a scrotum," which caused many to make fun of him in school locker rooms when the molester was a teenager. The molester would then expose himself and show the child in great detail how physicians had taken a skin graft from his upper leg and fashioned a scrotum for him later on as an adult. The molester would excuse his erection during this process by saying that it was a "natural" byproduct of being a healthy man in his sexual prime. During interviews, none of the boys believed the man had been sexually inappropriate with them. Even the boys who had received back rubs and felt the molester's erection on their backs only thought the man was being "weird" and "gross." The boys had all been convinced the games were normal, despite their use to identify which of them was most receptive to further sexual contact from the molester.

Groth classifies grooming methods according to the technique employed.[32] "Pressured sex" involves enticement or entrapment. This molester, or "groomer," entices the child into sex through persuasion or cajoling. Entrapment makes the child feel obligated or indebted by asking for sex in exchange for some favor or gift. Molesters using this method, however, do not resort to more forceful means to obtain sex because a "willing" or "consenting" partner is the desired goal.

"Forced sex" means using threats or physical aggression in the commission of the offense. This molester, or "grabber," may exploit the child's relative weakness or naïveté and intimidate the child into having sex. Should that not work, the molester might simply overpower the child and engage in the kind of sexual activity desired. For some molesters, the use of force is instrumental in obtaining sex; for others, however, the use of force itself is sexually gratifying.

Once the victim has been engaged in sex, the molester uses grooming to ensure secrecy and continued access to the child. Lies, gifts, and guilt are frequently used to maintain the sexual relationship. Some molesters purchase expensive gifts for the child, and make the victim have sex a number of times to charge off the "debt." Other molesters provide alcohol or drugs to their victims, telling them that should their sexual behavior be discovered they would both go to prison for using substances illegally. Some even anesthetize victims through the use of alcohol and drugs to ensure that there is no or minimal memory of the abuse. Molesters also employ threats of harm to family, friends, pets, and possessions to coerce secrecy from the victim.

The molester's home and decor are sometimes themselves evidence of grooming. While instrumentalities used in sexual activity with the child are always relevant (e.g., sex toys, pornography, photographic equipment, etc.), attention should be given to items in the home and how they are arranged. For example, a large number of children's movies, games, and toys in the home of a 40-year-old single male who has no children of his own might be of interest to a court, especially when such items are made relevant through expert testimony. Posters, furniture, food, and reading materials that appeal to children can also be important. Photography of the interior and exterior of the suspect's home before search and seizure is always recommended. Before widespread knowledge of the techniques of child molesters, many such men would set up their homes with the latest video games, electronics, movies, and toys so that children in the neighborhood would naturally flock to the home to play. While this has become less common, some unsuspecting and trusting individuals still allow their children to unknowingly associate with molesters in this way.

Digital evidence is becoming increasingly important in the identification, investigation, and prosecution of child molesters. Most home computers now contain everything about the individual, from financial status, to hobbies, to a photographic record of the individual's life, to what he or she does when they believe no one else is looking. Camera phones can now take both still and motion photography surreptitiously. Higher quality digital video cameras can be secreted in bags, clothing, air vents, and behind screens. Small, wireless webcams can now be placed anywhere within reach of a Wi-Fi network. Technology has made it increasingly easy for molesters to access child victims without their knowledge. Images are often rapidly distributed via the Internet to trusted customers and other molesters. Digital evidence requires special skill and training for proper recovery and presentation in court. Well-meaning investigators can unwittingly destroy or alter such evidence very easily and make it inadmissible. There are a growing number of resources available to aid the investigator in this rapidly growing and changing area.[33] Use of the Internet for child exploitation is addressed in greater detail in another chapter of this book (see Chapter 18).

CHILD MOLESTERS: OTHER POPULATIONS

There is growing knowledge about the behaviors of molesters other than adult males. These groups are described briefly below.

Juvenile Child Molesters

Adolescent males perpetrate approximately 20% of rapes and between 30% and 50% of child molestations.[34] Juvenile molesters occupy the middle ground between childhood and adulthood. Most children below the age of 12 are not considered to be "offenders" because in Western courts they cannot be held accountable for a crime. Individuals older than age 18 are typically considered to be adults. Therefore, most of the data about this group comes from juvenile sex offenders ages 12 to 17. From 1985 to 2003, just less than 92% of the accused standing trial in juvenile court for sexual offenses against persons were between these ages.[35]

As with adult offenders, juvenile sex offenders are a heterogeneous group. There are numerous challenges in making firm conclusions about the nature of juvenile child molesters, largely due to definitions of offender, offense, victim, and the methodology of studies in this area. In most of the literature reviewed, a "child" is someone who is at least 5 years younger than the juvenile molester. One of the commonly held assumptions about juvenile child molesters that *is not supported* by the research is that they are similar to adult child molesters in etiology, cognition, behavior, and offense history. Rather, our concept of juvenile child molesters' behavior is mediated by a variety of factors, chief of which appears to be the effects of growth and development. Nevertheless, there are a few trends emerging in the data available on juvenile child molesters that might be helpful to clinicians and investigators alike.

When compared with juvenile rapists, juvenile child molesters appear to exhibit more socially inadequate behavior, to be more socially isolated, and to have more often been victims of sexual abuse themselves.[36] Juvenile rapists show more evidence of *externalizing* problem behavior (e.g., behaviors where the child acts negatively on the external environment, usually defined as aggression, delinquency, and hyperactivity). Juvenile child molesters tend to show more evidence of internalizing problem behavior (e.g., behaviors where the child reacts negatively on the self, and can include such problems as being withdrawn, anxious, inhibited, and depressed).[37] Juvenile child molesters often have a history of problems with social confidence, childhood depression, and anxiety. Another study found preliminary evidence that juvenile child molesters have greater psychosocial deficits, more aggression in their sexual offending, and are more likely to victimize a relative than those offenders who sexually abuse peers.[38] In a meta-analysis of studies describing conduct problems and juvenile sexual offending, Seto and Lalumière[39] found that study samples containing more juvenile sex offenders who abused children had fewer conduct problems relative to non–sex-offending juveniles. In fact, the authors believed this finding supported the possibility that juvenile child molesters might be a subgroup of juvenile sex offenders who show few conduct problems and restrict their antisocial conduct to just sexual behavior. They surmised that these juvenile child molesters might have a pedophilic interest that motivates their offense behavior. However, Seto and Lalumiére[39] found one exception to these results. Juvenile child molesters were more likely to engage in fire setting than those juvenile sex offenders who targeted peers or adults. They speculated that fire setting might be an expression of an atypical sexual interest, but also acknowledged that it might be a sign of lower intelligence, neurodevelopmental problems, or assertiveness deficits.

A study of 116 Dutch juvenile sex offenders supports several of the trends in the literature described previously. Hendriks and Bijleveld[40] compared a sample of 58 juvenile child molesters to a sample of 54 juvenile peer abusers. Juvenile child molesters started sexually offending at a younger age and had relatively more victims. The child molesters also had more psychological problems than the offenders who victimized peers or older people. Both groups experienced parenting problems, early abuse, victimization by bullies, and poor relationships with peers. Juvenile child molesters, however, tended to prefer male victims and used little or no violence to subdue their victims. The authors cautioned that their study was limited in that it only involved young males charged with a criminal offense.

Female Child Molesters

The amount and quality of information about female molesters has increased over the past decade. Nevertheless, most information in the literature is based on very small samples of women, drawn from a very limited number of settings (e.g., prisons, treatment cohorts). Consequently, what is known about women who molest children is very preliminary. Given the limited data, we do not yet have a full representation of kinds of behaviors employed when women molest children. Women traditionally have not been viewed as molesters by society, which might stem from the fact that they account for very few *reported* sex crimes in relation to men. Until the case of Mary Kay Letourneau and Vili Fualaau (which, ironically, occurred at the author's elementary school in Burien, Washington), relatively little public attention was paid to women who molest boys. Since that time, female teacher-male student molestations have become a topic of greater discussion in the media. Despite the fact that most sexual assaults perpetrated by women involve children,[41] they are rarely diagnosed with pedophilia.

Based on a variety of estimates, women likely account for 4% to 5% of all sexual abuse annually.[41,42] While initial data indicated that women primarily molested boys, there is a growing body of evidence to indicate that girls, or both girls and boys constitute a significant portion of a female molesters' victims.[42] Women also tend to abuse children with whom they have a caretaking relationship of some sort, and rarely perpetrate against a child unknown to them.[43] Whom a female molester abuses appears to be related to the manner in which the abuse is perpetrated. Female molesters that abuse with a comolester tend to have more than one victim, are more likely to molest both boys and girls, are more likely to be related to the victim and have a nonsexual criminal offense in their history in addition to the instant sex offense.[43] Early research also suggested that women only tended to abuse very young children, but newer studies are indicating fairly consistently that women molest children of all ages.[41] However, study sampling appears to directly influence victim demographics. One recent study compared the victims from a sample of female molesters referred to Child Protective Services (CPS) to the victims of a sample of female molesters taken from the criminal justice system (CJS).[44] In the CPS sample, most victims were female, under age 12, and from intrafamilial cases. In the CJS sample, the victims were mostly male, between the ages of 13 and 18, and involved extrafamilial cases.

Most female child molesters appear to share a history of child abuse. A significant number of female molesters have been sexually abused, with many studies reporting the proportion to be more than 70%.[42] A recent study that compared female sex offenders to female non-sex offenders found that the sex offender group reported significantly more frequent incidents of childhood sexual abuse for a greater duration of time than the non-sex offender group.[45] This finding is consistent with what Grayston and De Luca[42] found in their review of the literature on female perpetrators of sexual abuse. In fact, there is a great deal of data to indicate that female perpetrators might have experienced particularly invasive and severe forms of sexual abuse, and physical and emotional abuse.[42]

Again, the research on female child molesters is still too limited to be able to construct a valid typology to reliably inform clinical and investigative decision-making. Grayston and DeLuca's summary of the research through 1999 provides an informational context and motivational themes for female child molesters. Much of the research since that time has been supportive of their summary:[42]

"Although female perpetrators of sexual abuse are a rather heterogeneous mix, it is possible to draw some very general and preliminary conclusions regarding the "typical" female offender based on the previous literature review. Given, however, that the bulk of existing data regarding abusive women is derived from uncontrolled studies and very small samples of perpetrators who have come to professional attention, considerable caution must be used in interpreting these summary statements. While studies of identified offenders may yield a range of in-depth information regarding women who sexually abuse, they are not likely to represent the full spectrum of female-perpetrated victimization because very few offenders of either gender find their way to prison or treatment. Indeed, it may be true that cases involving identified female offenders (i.e., those women convicted of sexual abuse or receiving offender treatment) represent the most serious and unusual of all incidents of child sexual abuse.

With these caveats in mind, it would appear that several tentative conclusions can be made regarding female sex offenders. First, the "typical" or "modal" perpetrator of child sexual abuse may be a young woman falling somewhere in her 20s or 30s. She is likely to have come from a dysfunctional family of origin, and, in many cases, may have experienced physical, emotional, and/or sexual abuse as a child, adolescent, or adult. Very often, her experiences of abuse will have been extensive and severe, involving invasive sexual and physical activities, and multiple offenders. Although it is likely that most of the sexual abuse will have been perpetrated against the woman by familiar and trusted males, in some cases, the woman may have been molested by one or more female offenders.

As an adult, the literature suggests that the "typical" female perpetrator is likely to be experiencing problems in many areas of her life. Although she may have an average level of education, for example, she is likely to be centralized in the lower socioeconomic strata, and, if employed, may occupy poorly paid and stereotypically feminine occupational roles.

Very often, marital and peer relationships will be absent in the woman's life, and those which do exist may be dysfunctional, abusive, or otherwise distressed. In many cases, the offender may be isolated from social supports and may suffer from a range of mental health problems. While it is unlikely that she will be psychotic or otherwise grossly disturbed, the literature suggests that she may experience a range of other problems, including difficulties with depression, suicidal ideation, chemical dependency, and/or low self-esteem. Existing data also indicate that, in some cases, the offender may have one or more psychiatric disorders (e.g., posttraumatic stress disorder, borderline personality disorder), and that she may be very likely to have poorly developed or inadequate coping skills.

With respect to motives for committing sexual abuse, the literature would suggest no consistent or typical pattern.

While some female offenders may have deviant arousal and interest patterns and may derive some sexual gratification from their abusive behavior, current data also indicate that abusive women may act out for a number of other reasons. Some women, for example, appear to have distorted perceptions regarding the inappropriateness of their acts, viewing abuse as a "normal" expression of affection for a child or a spouse, and denying or minimizing the seriousness of their sexually aggressive acts.

Some offenders appear to molest children, at least in part, in response to environmental stressors (e.g., domestic violence, male coercion), while still others appear to use abuse as a means (albeit inappropriate) of addressing various feelings and unmet needs (e.g., feelings of anger and loneliness, needs for attention and affection). Many offenders appear to experience considerable guilt and shame for engaging in acts of abuse.

In terms of actual sexual offenses, the "typical" or "modal" female offender is most likely to abuse a female child, although male children, and youngsters of both genders may also be commonly abused. While the offender may molest only a single child, in many cases, the abuse may be widespread, involving multiple victims. Typically, the woman will abuse children with whom she has an enduring or familiar relationship, and youngsters who fall within the preschool and school-age range.

The "modal" offender is very likely to act in concert with another adult (usually male), although she may initiate independent acts of sexual abuse instead of, or in addition to, acts of coperpetration. Typically, offenses will involve abuse of moderate intensity, without the use of force or threats. Nevertheless, in many instances, the sexual abuse may coexist with other forms of maltreatment (e.g., neglect or physical abuse).[42]"

Organized Groups

Affinity groups that support and advocate the sexual abuse of children have become rather irrelevant since Internet use became widespread in the late 1990s. In the 1970s and 1980s, these groups gained a great deal of public attention for where they met and who comprised their membership. Of the North American Man-Boy Love Association (NAMBLA), The Pedophile Information Exchange, the Rene Guyon Society, the Child Sensuality Circle, and other such groups, only NAMBLA has remained somewhat of an on going concern on the Internet. Investigators, however, continue to encounter publications from all these groups in the possession of current molesters. Although the leadership of the groups claimed to have membership numbering in the thousands, their reason for existing—and public and police scrutiny—kept whatever members they had from seeking publicity. Nevertheless, the groups claimed to lobby for the repeal of age of consent laws because they believed such laws were "harmful" to the full expression of a child's sexual behavior. The Federal Bureau of Investigation, Scotland Yard, and other national and international law enforcement agencies targeted the more vocal members of the groups for investigation. In fact, a Fairfax County, Va., law enforcement officer went undercover in the 1990s and joined NAMBLA's governing board, discovering the group had approximately 1100 members.[46] Another group, the Diaper Pail Friends (DPF), has never officially advocated repeal of age of consent laws. The group advocates that it is solely a meeting point for individuals with an interest in infantilism or a diaper fetish. The author has investigated cases, however, where the offenders were self-proclaimed members of the DPF and possessed child pornography or ordered it through the mail.

Given the significant law enforcement interest in such groups, the perceived anonymity of the Internet offered a more covert method for sharing interests, experiences, writings, and child pornography. Consequently, organized child molester groups have largely dissipated—with only NAMBLA and the DPF actively maintaining Web sites at the time of this writing. While affinity groups sometimes facilitated the sharing of information and materials that aided the exploitation of children, their prominence has given way to groups organized by criminal intent. Aided by the distribution capabilities of the Internet, organized crime groups with an international reach have found that technology offers a cheap means for production and dissemination of child pornography and other sexually exploitative products. Eastern Europe is now one of the largest suppliers and distributors of child pornography in the world. For example, in 2004, the officers of a Minsk, Belarus company pleaded guilty to providing billing services worth $3 million to more than 50 Web sites containing child pornography.[47] Current production of child pornography is supported by a kidnapping and human trafficking operation that spans a number of countries in Central and Eastern Europe. Additional child pornography production, and sex tourism involving child prostitution, continues in the Philippines, Thailand, and Central America.

Perhaps the least organized—but potentially the most destructive—groups involved in child sexual exploitation are the parents of children who photograph and videotape their children and then sell or trade the images online to others. This "home-grown" porn covers a wide range of material, from scantily clad children in provocative poses to full-on child/child or adult/child sex. The former, also called "gray market child pornography," is viewed as legal in some jurisdictions because the children are not photographed nude. Other groups of child molesters, connected only by technology, have been known to "take an order" from the membership, kidnap a child meeting that description, and then sexually abuse or otherwise exploit the child live on a webcam for the group's members. Consequently, child molester organizations that failed to launch a movement for public acceptance of adult/child sex have fallen by the wayside as other profit-driven criminal organizations successfully expanded the worldwide supply of child pornography via the Internet.

ASSOCIATED PROBLEMS OF CHILD MOLESTERS

Child molesters can experience a variety of psychological problems that influence their offending behavior. Other Axis I and Axis II disorders should be expected in this population because comorbidity rates are high. Raymond et al[48] found that in a mostly outpatient group of 45 men who were diagnosed with pedophilia more than half of the men met criteria for at least five or more other comorbid diagnoses in addition to pedophilia. Sixty-seven percent of the men had a history of a mood disorder, 64% had a history of an anxiety disorder, 60% had a history of substance abuse, 53% had a history of at least one additional paraphilia, and 30% had some form of impulse control disorder. Sixty percent of this sample also met criteria for some other Axis II disorder as well. In an incarcerated group of 45 child molesters, Eher and associates[49] found that 81% met the criteria for pedophilia, 42% had a history of substance abuse and/or dependence, 33% had a history of a mood disorder, 17% had an additional paraphilia, and 12% had a history of an anxiety disorder. Child molesters who are also psychopaths are at high risk for sexual and physical violence.[50]

Mental health problems play a complex part in the molestation of children. First, mood, anxiety, and other neurological or psychological disorders throughout the lifetime can be influential factors for some in the development of a sexual interest in children. Second, current psychological symptoms are a common precursor to an incident of child sexual exploitation. For example, a child molester with a mood disorder might be more prone to sexually gratify himself with a child during periods of symptom exacerbation. Likewise, an individual with pedophilia and an antisocial personality disorder likely feels entitled to have sex with children and has very little guilt or concern over how his behavior impacts his victims. Third, psychological disorders can substantially impact or complicate treatment for child molesters. Any assessment and treatment plan for a molester must include a functional analysis of how the individual's offense cycle is influenced by his or her mental illness. For example, an alcohol abuse diagnosis can complicate care substantially, particularly when the individual drinks to overcome inhibitions about the perpetration of a sex crime on a child.

A substantial portion of child molesters experiences a variety of family and societal problems associated with their behavior. Molesters living with others can experience stress and domestic violence when their offensive behavior is discovered. A molester might be expelled from the home and forced to live in a less than stable environment while the issue is being resolved within the family. Employers might also move the individual to temporary duties if the matter is before some kind of family or criminal court. Other companies are hesitant to change the status or terminate the employment of a molester until a case has been fully adjudicated. Still other companies and organizations dismiss the individual summarily. Financial stress, alienation of friends and family, loss of employment, and contact with the criminal justice system should all be considered as part of any treatment plan, and any safety plan for victims.

TREATMENT

The desired goal of any treatment is to prevent recidivism by the child molester. Treatment can consist of psychological therapies, medical interventions, or a combination of the two. The psychological therapies that have been most studied for child molesters have been cognitive behavioral therapy (CBT) and relapse prevention (RP). CBT addresses the thoughts and behaviors that support or perpetuate the molester's offending. Cognitive treatment components typically target those cognitive distortions, maladaptive beliefs, and schemas that give rise to offending. Behavioral compo-

nents typically focus on employing these new thoughts and beliefs to redirect sexual behavior away from children. RP focuses on maintaining treatment gains. This therapy helps the individual identify those situations, thoughts, and emotions that precede offending, and teaches alternative methods for coping with the stressors. Both CBT and RP can be delivered either individually or in a group setting.

Medical treatments are used to reduce sexual arousal in general by changing the availability of sex hormones in the system or by altering brain chemistry. While reducing sexual arousal does not change a molester's sexual interest in children, it is believed that a reduction in sex drive might lead to reduced offending as well. Historically, surgical castration was an option used to decrease testosterone. However, given the invasive and irreversible nature of the surgery and the presence of new alternatives, surgical castration is rarely performed as a treatment. California, Florida, Iowa, Louisiana, and Texas still permit voluntary surgical castration for individuals who have been convicted of a sex offense and are being considered for parole or probation.[51] Medical treatments more commonly rely on sex hormone altering medications such as medroxyprogesterone acetate (Depo-Provera), leuprolide acetate (Lupron Depot), and outside the United States, cyproterone acetate (Cyprostat). Sex offender treatment with these medications is not approved by the U.S. Food and Drug Administration. Consequently their use as a treatment for child molestation is "off label," and not often covered by insurance. While these drugs are effective at reducing serum testosterone, they do not eliminate sex drive or make men incapable of erections. The medications do, however, make sexual thoughts and behaviors less frequent and more difficult to produce. Other investigators have used fluoxetine, paroxetine, and other selective serotonin reuptake inhibitors (SSRIs) to reduce sex drive.[52] While abnormal levels of serotonin have not been causally linked to child molestation or paraphilias, the general reduction in libido associated with the SSRIs is thought reduce the likelihood of recidivism. Many clinics pair libido–reducing medications with CBT and/or RP as way to provide the individual with an opportunity to more effectively employ newly learned cognitive and behavioral interventions. One of the prime challenges with medical interventions, however, is that once the medication is terminated, sexual drive and the potential to re-offend return. In addition, there is a significant drop out rate with medication and a number of potentially harmful side effects, including hyperglycemia, hypertension, and osteoporosis.

There is great debate about the efficacy of treatment for child molesters. Public perception is that few molesters benefit from care. Clinicians have been more optimistic about treatment.[4,53] A number of studies and meta-analyses of studies have shown a modest effect for the treatment of sex offenders in general. In one of the most well regarded meta-analyses, Hanson and associates[54] found that psychological treatment was associated with reduced recidivism rates of sexual crimes for treatment groups (12.3%) when compared with "no treatment" comparison groups (16.8%). Recidivism for any crime was also lower for those who received psychological treatment (treatment 27.9%, comparison 39.2%). For child molesters, the findings are not quite as clear. Camilleri and Quinsey[55] found that the treatment effects specifically for child molesters in Hanson's meta-analysis are not quite as robust, and that any further analysis of the effects of treatment for molesters has been prevented by the quality of the studies reviewed.[55] In fact, in their comprehensive and rather stark review of pedophilia treatment and recidivism, Camilleri and Quinsey[55] contend that treatment has not shown to produce a change in molesters' sexual preference for children, has minor to no impact on recidivism, and has not demonstrated an improvement in results over the past several decades. This is not the final word, however, about the treatment of pedophilia. Camilleri and Quinsey[55] suggest that both current psychological and medical treatments have been ineffective for pedophiles because the treatments do not address the primary criminogenic need factor in pedophilia—a sexual preference for children. They suggest that *preventive* interventions might be more beneficial for pedophilia, rather than "cures" for the condition once it is established.

While there is yet little evidence to demonstrate treatment efficacy for pedophiles, other child molesters might indeed benefit from treatment. As stated at the outset of this chapter, not all individuals who molest children qualify for a diagnosis of pedophilia. Different groups of molesters are likely to show differential rates of treatment benefit and recidivism.[56] In fact, juvenile child molesters are a group that has shown considerably more promise than adults. Adolescents who complete comprehensive programs that combine a strong family-relationship component with offense specific interventions are less likely to commit further sex and non-sex crimes than those who have not completed treatment.[57] Despite the many limitations of studies in this area, a number of studies have shown sufficient evidence for the efficacy of treatment intervention for juvenile sex offenders.[58]

FUTURE DIRECTIONS

Good quality child molester research is comparatively new. A large portion of research currently underway focuses on means to assess child molesters. There have been no psychological instruments developed that can reliably and validly identify a child molester from a non-"child molester," including well-researched psychological tests such as the Minnesota Multiphasic Personality Inventory (MMPI-2), the California Personality Inventory (CPI), or the Milon Multiaxial Personality Inventory (MCMI-III). Sexual assessment instruments that are face-valid, and therefore easy for the subject to manipulate, are not useful, especially when the subject is being assessed in a forensic context. In addition, clinical judgment alone is also extremely unreliable with this population. The author has reviewed a large number of assessments from "expert" clinicians who have rendered opinions about the innocence of a suspect because he did not "look like someone who had just molested his daughter"; because he did not have the "spiritual wherewithal to have committed such a sin"; or because he "assured me that he would never have done such a thing." Experience working directly with this population is highly recommended, but still not a guarantor of full accuracy in assessment.

Nevertheless, there are some promising instruments that might be of use to a clinician in assessment and treatment of child molesters. Certainly, the psychological tests named above can be used to assess the individual's test taking attitude, tendency to malinger, and psychological state. Likewise, the Abel Assessment for Sexual Interest[59] has demonstrated some reliability in differentiating child molesters from nonchild molesters. This test uses a combination of two components, a screening tool using visual stimuli and a questionnaire with a number of scales to indicate the individual's sexual interest and test-taking approach. For psychological assessment purposes, the Abel Assessment has great utility. However, for forensic purposes—like any other test or assessment instrument—it cannot determine whether or not an individual perpetrated a crime, regardless of the individual's demonstrated sexual interest. Consequently, some courts have found it to be an impermissible comment on the defendant's credibility. In addition, some courts have found it to be inadmissible under Daubert, while a few others have allowed it.[60] When used correctly and ethically, penile plethysmographs, polygraphs, and other such instruments can also be of clinical use in the assessment and treatment of child molesters. However, like the Abel Assessment, they cannot be used forensically to determine guilt or innocence in any offense.

Other instruments are being developed to assess the risk for recidivism of child molesters. Actuarial risk scales, such as the Sex Offender Risk Appraisal Guide (SORAG),[61] the Minnesota Sex Offender Screening Tool-Revised (MnSOST-R),[62] the Rapid Risk Assessment for Sex Offense Recidivism (RRASOR),[63] and the Static-99[64] have all been developed to classify the predictive risk of reoffense of an individual based on the presence of certain static (or unchanging) risk factors in the person's history. For example, the strongest static predictors of sex offense recidivism are factors related to sexual deviancy, such as deviant sexual preferences, a history of sex offenses, and a history of childhood or juvenile sexual offenses.[65] Such instruments often are used in child molester evaluations for civil commitment, probation and parole hearings, and for other forensic applications. There is relatively much less research, however, on the dynamic (or changing) factors that impact sex offense recidivism. As described earlier in the chapter, the offender's mood at the time, access to victims, and previous treatment can play a part in reoffense. Consequently, Hanson[65] suggests that there is much more evidence to justify committing offenders than there is for releasing them.

Another problem is that actuarial risk instruments cannot predict accurately when or if an offender will actually recidivate. Instruments can only estimate a probability of reoffense. No actuarial instrument can reliably predict the behavior or occurrence of disease in a single individual.[66] Consequently, such instruments should only be part of a full battery of tests to inform expert opinion. Finally, actuarial instruments underestimate the risk of recidivism for some populations of offenders. For example, military sexual offenders were not included in the groups of offenders assessed in the development of such instruments. Many of the behaviors used to assess an individual for reoffense would be prejudicial to good order and discipline in the armed forces, and as such, are grounds for nonacceptance into uniformed service, discharge from the service, or court martial. Consequently, the factors commonly assessed by the actuarial instruments to develop a prediction would be absent from a military offender's history. Likewise, other forms of disciplinary action used solely by the military (nonjudicial punishment under Article 15 of the Uniformed Code of Military Justice, administrative actions, and service discharges) were not assessed as indicators of recidivism in any of the actuarial instruments currently in use. Consequently, use of an actuarial to predict the reoffense risk of a military member during the sentencing portion of a court martial would underestimate risk or otherwise be inaccurate and inappropriate. Similarly, use of such actuarials may underestimate the risk of any offender with a military history.

Acknowledgments

Special thanks goes to:

- U.S. Postal Inspector Michael J. Corricelli, who provided a scenario and other investigative background material for this chapter.
- Investigative psychologist, Dr. Nancy Slicner, who developed the victim matrix.
- Forensic psychiatrist, Dr. Fred S. Berlin, who provided the author experience working with pharmacological and psychological treatments for sexual offenders at the National Institute for the Study, Prevention, and Treatment of Sexual Trauma, in Baltimore.

References

1. Robertiello G, Terry KJ: Can we profile sex offenders? A review of sex offender typologies. *Aggress Violent Behav* 2007;12:508-518.
2. Gaudiosi JA: *Child maltreatment 2006*, U.S. Department of Health and Human Services, Administration for Children and Families (website): http://www.acf.hhs.gov/programs/cb/pubs/cm06/cm06.pdf. Accessed December 27, 2008.
3. Finkelhor D, Ormrod RK: Factors in the underreporting of crimes against juveniles. *Child Maltreat* 2001;6:219-229.
4. Fagan PJ, Wise TN, Schmidt CW, et al: Pedophilia. *JAMA* 2002;288:2458-2465.
5. Seto MC: Pedophilia: psychopathology and theory. *In*: Laws DR, O'Donohue WT (eds): *Sexual Deviance: Theory Assessment, and Treatment*, ed 2, Guilford, New York, 2008.
6. Holmes WC, Slap GB: Sexual abuse of boys: definition, prevalence, correlates, sequelae, and management. *JAMA* 1998;280:1855-1862.
7. Kendall-Tackett K, Becker-Blease K: The importance of retrospective findings in child maltreatment research. *Child Abuse Negl* 2004;28:723-727.
8. Salter AC: *Predators: pedophiles, rapists, and other sex offenders*. Basic Books, New York, 2003.
9. Dandescu A, Wolfe R: Considerations on fantasy use by child molesters and exhibitionists. *Sex Abuse* 2003;15:297-305.
10. Groth N, Birnbaum J: Adult sexual orientation and attraction to under-age persons. *Arch Sex Behav* 1978;7:175-181.
11. Lanyon RI: Theory and treatment in child molestation. *J Consult Clin Psychol* 1986;54:176-182.
12. Lanning KV: *Child molesters: a behavioral analysis*, ed 4, National Center for Missing & Exploited Children, Alexandria, Va, 2001.
13. Finkelhor D: *Child sexual abuse. New theory and research*. Free Press, New York, 1984.
14. American Psychiatric Association: *Diagnostic and statistical manual of mental disorders*, ed 4, American Psychiatric Association, Washington, DC, 2000.
15. Seto MC, Cantor JM, Blanchard R: Child pornography offenses are a valid diagnostic indicator of pedophilia. *J Abnorm Psychol* 2006;115:610-615.
16. Galbreath NW, Berlin FS, Sawyer D: Paraphilias and the Internet. *In*: Cooper A (ed): *Sex and the Internet: A Guidebook for Clinicians*. Brunner-Routledge, New York, 2002.
17. Cooper A: Sexuality and the Internet: surfing into the new millennium. *Cyberpsychol Behav* 1998;1:187-193.
18. Motivans M, Kyckelhahn T: *Federal prosecution of child sex exploitation offenders, 2006*, Bureau of Justice Statistics, U.S. Department of Justice (website): http://www.ojp.gov/bjs/pub/pdf/fpcseo06.pdf. Accessed March 23, 2009.
19. Wolak J, Finkelhor D, Mitchell K: *Child pornography possessors arrested in Internet-related crimes: findings from the national juvenile online victimization study*, National Center for Missing & Exploited Children (website): http://www.missingkids.com/en_US/publications/NC144.pdf. Accessed March 24, 2009.
20. Berlin FS: Issues in the exploration of biological factors contributing to the etiology of the "sex offender," plus some ethical considerations. *Ann N Y Acad Sci* 1988;528:183-192.
21. Cantor JM, Blanchard R, Robichaud LK, et al: Quantitative reanalysis of aggregate data on IQ in sexual offenders. *Psychol Bull* 2005;131:555-568.
22. Hanson R, Slater S: Sexual victimization in the history of child sexual abusers: a review. *Ann Sex Res* 1988;1:485-499.
23. United States General Accounting Office: *Cycle of sexual abuse. Research inconclusive about whether child victims become adult abusers*, United States General Accounting Office (website): http://www.gao.gov/archive/1996/gg96178.pdf. Accessed March 24, 2009.
24. Burton DL, Miller DL, Shill TC: A social learning theory comparison of the sexual victimization of adolescent sexual offenders and nonsexual offending male delinquents. *Child Abuse Negl* 2002;26:893-907.
25. Barbaree HE, Langton CM: The effects of child sexual abuse and family environment. *In*: Barbaree HE, Marshall WL (eds): *The Juvenile Sex Offender*, ed 2, Guilford Press, New York, 2006.
26. Studer LH, Aylwin AS: Male victims and post treatment risk assessment among adult male sex offenders. *Int J Law Psychiatry* 2008;31:60-65.
27. Howells K: Child sexual abuse: Finkelhor's precondition model revisited. *Psychol Crime Law* 1995;1:210-214.
28. Murphy WD: Assessment and modification of cognitive distortions in sex offenders. *In*: Marshall WT, Laws DR, Barbaree HE (eds): *Handbook of Sexual Assault: Issues, Theory and Treatment of Offenders*. Plenum Press, New York, 1990.
29. Gannon TA, Ward T, Collie R: Cognitive distortions in child molesters: theoretical and research developments over the past two decades. *Aggress Violent Behav* 2007;12:402-416.
30. Reid JE Associates: *The Reid technique of interviewing and interrogation*. John E Reid & Associates, Chicago, 2000.
31. The North American Man-Boy Love Association: *What is man/boy love?* (website): http://www.nambla.org/whatis.htm. Accessed March 6, 2010.
32. Burgess A, Groth AN, Holstrom L, et al: *Sexual assault of children and adolescents*. Lexington Books, Lexington, Mass, 1978.
33. Ferraro MM, Casey E: *Investigating child exploitation and pornography: the Internet, the law, and forensic science*. Elsevier Academic Press, New York, 2005.
34. Barbaree HE, Marshall WL: An introduction to the juvenile sex offender: terms, concepts, and definitions. *In*: Barbaree HE, Marshall WL (eds): *The Juvenile Sex Offender*, ed 2, Guilford Press, New York, 2006.
35. Stahl A, Finnegan T, Kang W: *Easy access to juvenile court statistics: 1985-2005*, U.S. Department of Justice Office of Juvenile Justice and Delinquency Prevention (website): http://ojjdp.ncjrs.org/ojstatbb/ezajcs/asp/aboutJCS.asp. Accessed March 25, 2009.
36. VanWijk A, Vermeiren R, Loeber R, et al: Juvenile sex offenders compared to non-sex offenders: a review of the literature 1995-2005. *Trauma Violence Abuse* 2006;7:227-243.
37. Becker JV, Hunter JA: Understanding and treating child and adolescent sexual offenders. *Adv Clin Child Psychol* 1997;19:177-197.
38. Hunter JA, Figueredo AJ, Malamuth NM, et al: Juvenile sex offenders: toward the development of a typology. *Sex Abuse* 2003;15:27-48.
39. Seto MC, Lalumiére ML: Conduct problems and juvenile sexual offending. *In*: Barbaree HE, Marshall WL (eds): *The Juvenile Sex Offender*, ed 2, Guilford Press, New York, 2006.
40. Hendriks J, Bijleveld CC: Juvenile sexual delinquents: contrasting child abusers with peer abusers. *Crim Behav Ment Health* 2004;14:238-250.
41. Logan C: Sexual deviance in females: psychopathology and theory. *In*: Laws DR, O'Donohue WT (eds): *Sexual Deviance: Theory Assessment, and Treatment*, ed 2, Guilford, New York, 2008, pp 486-507.
42. Grayston AD, DeLuca RV: Female perpetrators of child sexual abuse: a review of the clinical and empirical literature. *Aggress Violent Behav* 1999;4:93-106.
43. Vandiver DM: Female sex offenders: a comparison of solo offenders and co-offenders. *Violence Vict* 2006;21:339-354.
44. Bader SM, Scalora MJ, Casady TK, et al: Female sexual abuse and criminal justice intervention: a comparison of child protective service and criminal justice samples. *Child Abuse Negl* 2008;32:111-119.

45. Christopher K, Lutz-Zois CJ, Reinhardt AR: Female sexual-offenders: personality pathology as a mediator of the relationship between childhood sexual abuse history and sexual abuse perpetration against others. *Child Abuse Negl* 2007;31:871-883.

46. Soto OR: *FBI targets pedophilia advocates*, San Diego Union-Tribune (website): http://www.signonsandiego.com/uniontrib/20050218/news_1n18manboy.html. Accessed March 25, 2009.

47. U.S. Department of Justice: *Florida company pleads guilty to laundering funds for child pornography* (website): http://www.usdoj.gov/usao/nj/press/files/conn0503_r.htm. Accessed March 25, 2009.

48. Raymond NC, Coleman E, Ohlerking F, et al: Psychiatric comorbidity in pedophilic sex offenders. *Am J Psychiatry* 1999;156:786-788.

49. Eher R, Grunhut C, Fruhwald S, et al: Psychiatric comorbidity, typology and amount of violence in extrafamilial sexual child molesters. *Recht & Psychiatrie* 2001;19:97-101.

50. Seto MC, Barbaree HE: Psychopathy, treatment, behavior, and sex offender recidivism. *J Interpers Violence* 1999;14:1235-1248.

51. Scott CL, Holmberg T: Castration of sex offenders: prisoners' rights versus public safety. *J Am Acad Psychiatry Law* 2003;31:502-509.

52. Guay DR: Drug treatment of paraphilic and nonparaphilic sexual disorders. *Clin Ther* 2009;31:1-31.

53. Greenberg DM, DaSilva JA, Lob N: *Evaluation of the western Australian sex offender treatment unit (1987-1999).* Forensic Research Unit, Department of Psychiatry and Behavioural Sciences, University of Western Australia, Perth, Australia, 2002.

54. Hanson RK, Gordon A, Harris AJ, et al: First report of the collaborative outcome data project on the effectiveness of psychological treatment for sex offenders. *Sex Abuse* 2002;14:169-194.

55. Camilleri JA, Quinsey VL: Pedophilia: assessment and treatment. *In*: Laws DR, O'Donohue WT (eds): *Sexual Deviance: Theory Assessment, and Treatment*, ed 2, Guilford, New York, 2008, pp 183-212.

56. Harris AJR, Hanson RK: *Sex offender recidivism: a simple question, Public Safety and Emergency Preparedness*, Canada (website): http://ww2.ps-sp.gc.ca/publications/corrections/pdf/200403-2_e.pdf. Accessed March 25, 2009.

57. Worling JR, Langstrom N: Risk of sexual recidivism in adolescents who offend sexually: correlates and assessment. *In*: Barbaree HE, Marshall, WL (eds): *The Juvenile Sex Offender*, ed 2, Guilford Press, New York, 2006.

58. Waite D, Keller A, McGarvey EL, et al: Juvenile sex offender re-arrest rates for sexual, violent nonsexual and property crimes: a 10-year follow-up. *Sex Abuse* 2005;17:313-331.

59. Abel GG, Jordan A, Hand CG, et al: Classification models of child molesters utilizing the Abel assessment for sexual interest. *Child Abuse Negl* 2001;25:703-718.

60. Peters JM: *Using the Abel assessment for sexual interest to infer lack of culpability in a criminal case*, American Prosecutors Research Institute (website): http://www.ndaa.org/publications/newsletters/update_volume_14_number_12_2001.html. Accessed March 25, 2009.

61. Hanson RK, Harris AJ: A structured approach to evaluating change among sexual offenders. *Sex Abuse* 2001;13:105-122.

62. Epperson DL, Kaul JD, Huot S, et al: *Minnesota sex offender screening tool-revised (MnSOST-R) technical paper: development, validation, and recommended risk level cut scores.* http://www.psychology.iastate.edu/~dle/TechUpdatePaper12-03.pdf. Accessed March 25, 2009.

63. Hanson RK: *The development of a brief actuarial risk scale for sexual offense recidivism.* Department of the Solicitor General of Canada, Ottawa, 1997.

64. Hanson RK, Thornton D: *Static-99: improving actuarial risk assessments for sex offenders.* Department of the Solicitor General of Canada, Ottawa, 1999.

65. Hanson RK: Who is dangerous and when are they safe? Risk assessment with sexual offenders. *In*: Winick BJ, LaFond JQ (eds): *Protecting Society From Sexually Dangerous Offenders: Law, Justice, and Therapy.* American Psychological Association, Washington, DC, 2003.

66. Berlin FS, Galbreath NW, Geary B, et al: The use of actuarials at civil commitment hearings to predict the likelihood of future sexual violence. *Sex Abuse* 2003;14:377-382.

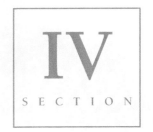

SEXUALLY TRANSMITTED INFECTIONS IN CHILDREN—EPIDEMIOLOGY, DIAGNOSIS, AND TREATMENT

Lori D. Frasier, MD, FAAP

21

Nonsexually Transmitted Infections of the Genitalia and Anus of Prepubertal Children

Andrew P. Sirotnak, MD, FAAP

In the evaluation of child sexual abuse, nonsexually transmitted infections of the genitalia and anus can be mistaken for sexually transmitted infection and thus for abuse. These infections can be encountered during routine pediatric primary care, or as a co-morbid finding in the child who has confirmed sexual abuse. The differential diagnosis of nonsexually transmitted infections is grounded in the knowledge of children's genital anatomy, vaginal flora changes, vulvovaginitis, and perianal infections.

NORMAL VAGINAL FLORA AND NONSPECIFIC VULVOVAGINITIS

Vulvovaginitis is the most common childhood and adolescent gynecological problem evaluated by pediatricians. It has those symptoms that can also be seen as a chief complaint in sexual abuse cases: discharge, erythema, pain, urinary frequency, dysuria, itchiness, odors, and less commonly, bleeding. Vulvitis has dysuria, pruritus, and vulvar erythema. Vaginitis predominantly has a discharge. Vulvovaginitis involves both manifestations. Not every genital discharge indicates infection. For example, physiologic leukorrhea related to increasing estrogen levels in older girls is a normal occurrence.

The lower genital tract is colonized by nonpathogenic bacteria from birth, and with growth and development, this environment changes over time. In prepubertal girls, gram-negative bacteria and enterococci predominate as the main flora before toilet training is completed. In adolescence, anaerobes gain greater prevalence. Aerobic colonization increases with age and onset of intercourse, with *Lactobacilli* the predominant flora in adolescents and adults.

The low estrogen state of prepuberty, the thin, atrophic vaginal mucosa with a neutral pH, and the natural warmth and moist nature of the vulvovaginal area all provide an excellent environment for bacterial growth. With puberty, estrogen increases, the pH of the vagina becomes acidic (in part from the increased production of acetic and lactic acid), accompanied by an increase in superficial cell proliferation, glycogen production, and normal bacterial flora enhancement.[1] Infectious vulvovaginitis usually begins in the vulva during childhood and in the vaginal canal during adolescence, particularly after onset of intercourse.

The epidemiology and etiology of vulvovaginitis is multifactorial. In children, vulvovaginal irritation results from the lack of labial fat pads and pubic hair, which protect the external genitalia after puberty. The prepubertal genitalia are more readily exposed to chemical irritants and bacteria. The close proximity of the anus to this tissue can allow transfer of bacteria. Poor hygiene, even after completion of toilet training, can exacerbate the irritant or infectious contacts, particularly in the child who wipes too quickly, inadequately, or who does not wash hands after toileting. More commonly, nonspecific vulvovaginitis is caused by direct irritation by tight fitting clothing (synthetic fiber and nonabsorbent underwear, bathing suits), chemicals (bubble-baths, deodorant sprays, detergents, soaps, medications or other contact allergens), physical agents (dirt, sand), or even prolonged urine and stool contact (unchanged diapers or underpants). The anal tissue is less frequently affected by poor hygiene or irritant contacts.

Constipation has been reported as a possible underlying related condition of recurrent vulvovaginitis.[2] Up to 75% of vulvovaginitis is nonspecific from the above causes, and treatment involves improved hygiene, avoidance of contact irritants, sitz baths, or bland emollients.[3]

Bacterial infectious causes of nonspecific vulvovaginitis are usually coliform bacteria from fecal contamination, or hemolytic streptococcus or coagulase positive staphylococcus transmitted from the nasopharynx.[1] Treatment with oral or topical antibiotics can be helpful for recurrent infections in addition to the above treatments.

Miscellaneous Causes

Overaggressive wiping by caregivers can cause additional irritation. Intravaginal foreign bodies (the most common is toilet paper remnants) have discharge and odor, and can be related to hygiene techniques or developmentally age appropriate body exploration with insertion of small toy objects or a coin. Recurrence of foreign bodies, progression of exploratory behaviors that are age inappropriate or that are associated with sexualized behaviors should lead to more direct evaluation for sexual abuse. Obesity can contribute to vulvovaginitis in the child with poor hygiene, urinary pooling, or tight fitting clothing. Finally, masturbation can cause erythema or irritation to the vulva and clitoral area.

SPECIFIC VULVOVAGINITIS

There are many specific bacterial and nonbacterial, nonsexually transmitted infectious causes of vulvovaginitis.

Many review studies have summarized epidemiology, presentations, and treatment options.[4-10] The American Academy of Pediatrics Red Book, Report of the Committee on Infectious Disease[11] has detailed and up-to-date information on these organisms.

Group A β-hemolytic Streptococcus (*S. pyogenes*)

Group A β-hemolytic *Streptococcus* (GAS) is a gram-positive coccoid that grows in chains. The M serotypes are the most common cause of pharyngitis and skin infections, including perianal disease and vulvovaginitis. The spectrum of skin disease itself ranges from classic scarlet fever, erysipelas, and impetigo and bullous impetigo to more invasive disease. Severe systemic disease with or without the signs of toxic shock, necrotizing fasciitis, or multisystem organ involvement is not usually seen with local infections of the vulva or anus.

Perianal streptococcal disease is characterized by well demarcated perianal erythema, with pruritus, pain with defecation, and blood streaked stools. Examination often shows a flat, beefy-red perianal erythema with sharp margins (Figure 12-10). Tenderness and fissures and bleeding are not uncommon. In vulvovaginitis, there can be nonspecific serous discharge and dramatic scarlet dermatitis of the vulva. The patient sometimes complains of discomfort with walking and difficulty with urination. These presentations can be mistaken for sexual abuse trauma by an inexperienced examiner. There is often a history of or examination consistent with concurrent or recent pharyngitis, and some practitioners will culture the pharynx and vulva or perianal area.[12] A recent case report has shown that rapid antigen testing can quicken the diagnosis and aid antimicrobial choice.[13] Severe invasive disease is rare, but the nonsuppurative complication of acute glomerulonephritis has been reported with GAS vulvovaginitis.[14] The differential diagnosis for infectious causes includes *Staphylococcus aureus* because this can cause similar signs and symptoms. Localized *S. aureus* infections can present as impetigo, cellulitis, and furuncles in adolescent patients. With the increasing incidence of methicillin resistant *S. aureus* (MRSA), cultures of pustular lesions are indicated and antibiotic therapy should be directed by results. Most GAS is sensitive to penicillins, cephalosporins, or clindamycin, as is most *S. aureus*. With MRSA, vancomycin, trimethoprim-sulfamethoxazole or clindamycin might be needed.

Shigella

Shigella sp. are the most common enteric pathogens that cause vulvovaginitis, and most often, *Shigella flexneri*.[15-18] In one series, *S. flexneri* followed by *S. sonnei* and *S. boydii* were most commonly identified as pathogenic species.[17] Infection is the result of contamination of the area by infected stool and presents as mucopurulent bloody discharge. It often can be chronic with intermittent bloody, foul smelling discharge and dysuria if antibiotic resistance is present.[16] Concurrent gastrointestinal infection may be present but in most cases it is absent, and evaluation of household members for similar symptoms might lead to consideration of this pathogen. This infection should also be considered in the context of recurrent evaluations for vaginal foreign bodies. Cultures of the discharge for enteric pathogens including antibiotic sensitivities would be prudent if this organism is suspected.

Topical treatment with triple sulfa cream has been reported as clearing some infections,[17] but the optimal treatment is a course of oral antibiotic. With present day *Shigella* frequently resistant to both ampicillin and trimethoprim/sulfamethoxazole, cefixime, ciprofloxacin, and azithromycin are alternatives to consider depending upon age of the child.[19] Good hygiene is important to prevent recurrence. There are no reports of severe complications of *S. flexneri* vulvovaginitis.

Other Less Common Bacteria

Haemophilus influenzae and *Moraxella catarrhalis* can be part of the normal vaginal flora but can also cause infections.[3,10] *Haemophilus influenzae* is another causative organism that is often associated with a preceding upper respiratory infection, and can be autoinoculated to the genital area. In one United Kingdom series, *H influenzae* was the second most common isolate after *S. pyogenes*,[20] and in a subsequent series in the same prepubertal population, *H. influenzae* biotype II was the most commonly associated biotype.[21] *Streptococcus pneumoniae* has also been reported to cause vulvar abscesses.[22]

Escherichia coli has been associated with vulvovaginitis and salpingitis in a prepubertal child with an ascending urinary infection.[23] *Yersinia enterocolitica* has also been associated with vulvovaginitis[24] and with labial abscess in a household with a co-infected dog.[25] The history of recent or concomitant gastrointestinal complaints and vaginitis symptoms should prompt a culture for enteric pathogens.

Nongonorrheal *Neisseria* species can occasionally be causes of vulvovaginitis as well. *N. sicca* and *N. meningitidis* have both been reported to cause vulvovaginitis.[26-28] Both are sensitive to penicillin but culture and sensitivities testing, and careful confirmation of the species, are warranted.

Anaerobic and Mixed Anaerobic Infections

Infections due to anaerobes and facultative anaerobes occur adjacent to mucosal surfaces, often as mixed infections with aerobes, but overall are uncommon nonsexually transmitted infections in prepubertal children. Vaginitis can be caused by an overgrowth of anaerobes and in adolescents and adults, and pelvic inflammatory disease and tubo-ovarian abscess can be caused by these mixed floras. Organisms specific to the female genital tract that can cause infections include *Bacteroides fragilis*, which is commonly found in appendicitis and tubo-ovarian abscesses; *Fusobacterium* sp., which also inhabit the gut and respiratory tracts; and very rarely, *Veillonella* organisms, which are normal flora of the mouth, upper respiratory, gut, and vagina.[29]

Peptococcus and *Peptostreptococcus*, *Eubacterium*, and *Propionibacterium* are all uncommon bacteria that have been cultured in prepubertal and adolescent vulvovaginitis,[1] and some of these have stronger associations with internal female genital tract diseases such as endometritis and salpingitis. Finally, *Clostridium perfringens* can cause perirectal cellulitis with myonecrosis in association with abdominal wounds. All of these rare infections are commonly associated with conditions that are unrelated to sexual abuse, such as crush injuries and trauma that devascularize skin and compromise tissue viability, or in the context of impaired host immunity.[29] Identification and treatment is best accomplished in collaboration with infectious disease experts.

Miscellaneous Bacteria

Other organisms have been reported to infect the female genitalia, usually associated with other primary diseases. The vulva and vagina can be the primary site of infection for *Corynebacterium diphtheriae*, but most often vaginitis is reported as secondary to a respiratory infection.[30,31] *Mycobacterium tuberculosis* causing either the scrofulous type or primary vulvar infection type of infection with localized painless, slowly developing nodular or ulcerative lesions is quite rare today.[31,32]

Fungal Causes of Vulvovaginitis

Candida albicans is a common cause of vulvovaginitis and in some series, more common than bacterial causes.[4,5] In prepubertal children, it is associated with wet diapers or poor hygiene, and can be seen secondary to predisposing factors such as recent antibiotic medication, diabetes mellitus, or immunodeficiency.[3] One adult series reported changes in the epidemiologic patterns of mycotic vulvovaginitis in adolescents and adults secondary to changing antimycotic regimens, with organisms such as *C. tropicalis*, *Prototheca wickerhamii*, and *Cryptococcus albidus*, among others, as cultured causes.[33]

Complaints of nonodorous white discharge, pruritus, and dysuria are common with typical findings of erythematous and edematous vulvar tissue and vaginal mucosa. The infant and young children sometimes have the classic erythematous perineal rash with satellite lesions. Severe or neglected infections can have fissures and excoriations. Although the examination is often diagnostic, a wet mount of discharge with 10% potassium hydroxide shows classic pseudohyphae. Topical antifungal creams for children and intravaginal preparations for adolescents are curative in most cases, but oral antifungals might be needed in severe cases. Finally, recurrence of infection or difficulty in treatment could be signs of immunodeficiency.

Malassezia furfur (previously known as *Pityrosporum orbiculare*) is a rare cause of skin conditions seen with scaly macules on the trunk. Lesions have been reported in the genital area. Diagnosis requires identification of hyphae and spores on wet prep with potassium hydroxide, and treatment is with topical clotrimazole.

Viral Causes of Vulvovaginitis

There are two common, direct viral causes of vulvovaginitis and several viruses that cause genital area signs and symptoms as part of systemic diseases. Molluscum contagiosum virus (MCV) is one of the most common viral infections of the skin that can be seen with vulvar lesions.[34,35] Infections of the mucous membranes and skin of infants, children, and adolescents are easily spread via direct nonsexual or sexual contacts by infected fomites, or by autoinoculation from another part of the body. MCV is a large DNA virus of the Poxviridae family, which also includes monkeypox and smallpox (which, long ago, was also a cause of vulvar lesions). MCV type 1 causes most skin infections, whereas MCV type 2 is the more likely to be sexually transmitted type. Incubation period is 2 to 7 weeks. Spread can be promoted by contact sports, shared bathtubs, pools, and towels. Children with atopic dermatitis or various immunosuppressed states including HIV, are predisposed to MVC, causing protracted infection and difficulty eradicating the virus.

Lesions appear as pearly papules 2 to 5 mm in size with a central dimple or umbilication (Figure 12-11), and occur commonly in the axillas and on the inner arms, chest, and trunk, with the antecubital fossa involved especially in the presence of eczema. Linear clustering of lesions (Koebner phenomenon) occurs when the child scratches and autoinoculates. Genital area lesions are common in the diaper distribution. Erythematous changes develop over time as a result of immune response and superinfection. Local superinfections can form abscesses. Lichenoid papules can develop as a result of allergic (id) reaction to the virus or because of their destruction during treatment.

Diagnosis is confirmed by the microscopic visualization of viral inclusion bodies in the central core. Skin biopsy is usually not needed except in the context of disseminated lesions. If there is concern about immune status, further immune work up is indicated.

Molluscum can resolve spontaneously, but can last from 6 months to 4 years, and can rarely heal with pitted scarring. Up to a third of infected children experience prolonged, significant discomfort and bacterial complications. Expectant treatment, with no intervention or curettage of lesions, has been the classic approach to molluscum. Reducing secondary skin symptoms and treating underlying atopic dermatitis are important. In recent years, a more aggressive approach has been advocated. Corticosteroids for dermatitis and topical and oral antibiotics for superinfections are common practice. Destructive therapies destroy lesions directly (e.g., curettage, topical nitrite application, cryotherapy, or hydroxy acids). Immune modulators such as imiquimod, and antiviral therapies such as cidofovir can be used in immunocompromised patients.[34,35] The optimum treatment is one that the parent and clinician agree upon that causes the least discomfort, has fewer side effects, and addresses any underlying disease.

Herpes simplex virus (HSV) is discussed in another chapter (see Chapter 23). Both HSV types 1 and 2 can involve the vulva, although neither is exclusively site specific. Autoinoculation of the vulva of HSV type 1 from the facial-oral area can occur. The appearance of painful vesicles, often in groups on an erythematous base is the typical presentation. The differential diagnosis also includes varicella zoster, and in adolescents, herpes zoster. Treatment with topical acyclovir reduces viral shedding and improves the rate of healing. Topical emollients and sitz baths can provide symptomatic relief. Oral acyclovir is used more commonly in sexually active adolescents.

Other viruses that cause genital signs and symptoms are enteroviruses and Epstein-Barr virus. Enteroviruses are small RNA viruses in the Picornaviridae family which includes poliovirus, Coxsackie, and echovirus subgroups. Spread person to person by the fecal-oral and respiratory route and vertically from mother to newborn, they cause a broad spectrum of disease. The nonspecific, more benign, febrile illness with typical viral symptoms of the respiratory and gastrointestinal tract lasts 4 to 7 days. These types of infections can cause macular, maculopapular, and petechial eruptions or vesicular or pustular lesions of the buttocks and groin, such as hand-foot-and-mouth disease caused by Coxsackie A viruses 5,7,9,10, and 16, Coxsackie B viruses 2 and 5, and or enterovirus 71.[36] Rashes of the genital area and buttock caused by enterovirus are, therefore, associated with other signs and symptoms and are self-limited, requiring no treatment. Finally, Epstein-Barr virus (EBV), as part of a systemic infection such as mononucleosis can cause genital secretions and rashes.

Helminths, Parasites, Protozoa, Lice, and Mites

Pinworms *(Enterobius vermicularis)* are helminths that commonly cause vulvar and perirectal pruritus. Female pinworms lay eggs at night around the anus and vulva. The mature worms, which are ½ inch long, white, and threadlike, can carry colonic bacteria to the perineum, causing recurrent vulvovaginitis. Nocturnal itchiness and variable gastrointestinal symptoms are reported by the child. Touching transparent adhesive tape to the perianal area to look for microscopic eggs is a well known diagnostic technique. Treatment consists of pyrantel pamoate or metronidazole, repeated in 2 to 3 weeks to ensure eradication, while simultaneously washing bedding and night clothing.

Giardia lamblia is a flagellate protozoan that can present as an asymptomatic fecal contaminant, or with a cramping diarrhea malabsorption syndrome (giardiasis). It also can cause vaginal discharge. Diagnosis is made by stool confirmation of the cyst or trophozoite phase of the organism. Metronidazole or quinacrine are drugs used for therapy.

Sarcoptes scabiei, subspecies *hominis,* are mites that have an incubation period of 4 to 6 weeks and cause nocturnal pruritus and vesicles or pustules in linear distributions, often in interdigital folds, flexor, and extensor surfaces of extremities, buttocks, and genital areas. Classic scabies burrows appear as gray or white threadlike lines, but most become excoriated with scratching. Mites might be seen on microscopic examination of scraped burrows, but more commonly black ova and dots of mites' feces (scybala) are seen. Treatment is topical with 5% permethrin cream, 10% crotamiton, or ivermectin in infants or children. Lindane 1% is used only with precautions in patients who fail treatment.

There is also a recent single case report of a possible association of the dust mite *Dermatophagoides* spp. and non-specific vulvovaginitis in a young child with perennial allergic rhinitis. This child, who had elevated IgE levels, had a skin test positive for this mite. Both symptoms were responsive to oral antihistamines and environmental control measures.[37]

Phthirus pubis (pediculosis pubis) are lice that cause intense pruritus and excoriations of the local skin. Pubic lice attach to hair shafts of groin, inner thigh, perineum, and perianal areas. Slate blue macules (maculae ceruleae) on chest, thighs, or abdomen are often a diagnostic clue. Incubation period from egg to hatching is 6 to 10 days with mature lice appearing in 2 to 3 weeks. Nymphs and adults feed on human blood. Although most commonly sexually transmitted, direct nonsexual and fomite contact, such as through towels and bedding, can transmit the organism. Nits on hair shafts or actual lice can be seen in hair or on clothing if magnified. There are a number of pediculicides that are effective including permethrin 1%, malathion 0.5%, and lindane 1%, and if over-the-counter preparations are ineffective, prescriptive treatment should be monitored by a clinician. Treatment should be repeated in 1 to 2 weeks to kill any lice that have hatched. As with scalp hair lice, removal of nits with a fine mesh comb and washing bedding and clothing is required.

Finally, there are other more uncommon protozoa and parasite diseases that have associated vulvovaginitis or perianal signs and symptoms. *Entamoeba histolytica, Ascaris lumbricoides, Trichuris trichiura,* schistosomiasis, and vaginal hirudiniasis (a condition resulting from leeches attaching themselves to the skin or being taken into the mouth or nose while drinking) have been reported in the literature.[31]

SUMMARY

It is important that medical care providers diagnosing or treating children with suspected sexual abuse be familiar with *nonsexually* transmitted infections of the genitals and anus. This will avoid misdiagnosis of infections attributed to sexual contact.

References

1. Sanfillipo JS: Vulvovaginitis. In: Kliegman RM, Behrman RE, Jenson HB, et al *(eds): Nelson Textbook of Pediatrics,* ed 18, Saunders, Philadelphia, 2004, pp 2274-2278.
2. vanNeer PA, Korver CR: Constipation presenting as recurrent vulvovaginitis in prepubertal children. *J Am Acad Dermatol* 2000;43: 718-719.
3. Kokotos F: Vulvovaginitis. *Pediatr Rev* 2006;27:116-118.
4. Deligeoroglou E, Salakos N, Makrakis E, et al: Infections of the lower female genital tract during childhood and adolescence. *Clin Exp Obstet Gynecol* 2004;31:175-178.
5. Koumantakis EE, Hassan EA, Deligeoroglou EK, et al: Vulvovaginitis during childhood and adolescence. *J Pediatr Adolesc Gynecol* 1997;10: 39-43.
6. Jones R: Childhood vulvovaginitis and vaginal discharge in general practice. *Fam Pract* 1996;13:369-372.
7. Nyirjesy P: Vaginitis in the adolescent patient. *Pediatr Clin North Am* 1999;46:733-745.
8. Farrington PF: Pediatric vulvo-vaginitis. *Clin Obstet Gynecol* 1997;40: 135-140.
9. Joishy M, Ashtekar CS, Jain A, et al: Do we need to treat vulvovaginitis in prepubertal girls? *BMJ* 2005;330:186-188.
10. Cuadros J, Mazon A, Martinez R, et al: The aetiology of paediatric inflammatory vulvovaginitis. *Eur J Pediatr* 2004;163:105-107.
11. Pickering LK, Baker CJ, Long SS, et al *(eds): Red book. 2006 Report of the committee on infectious diseases,* ed 27, American Academy of Pediatrics, Elk Grove Village, Ill, 2006.
12. Hansen MT, Sanchez VT, Eyster KM, et al: *Streptococcus pyogenes* pharyngeal colonization resulting in recurrent, prepubertal vulvovaginitis. *J Pediatr Adolesc Gynecol* 2007;20:315-317.
13. Muller WJ, Schmitt BD: Group A beta-hemolytic streptococcal vulvovaginitis: diagnosis by rapid antigen testing. *Clin Pediatr (Phila)* 2004;43:179-183.
14. Nair S, Schoeneman SJ: Acute glomerulonephritis with group A streptococcal vulvovaginitis. *Clin Pediatr* 2000;39(12):721-722.
15. Jasper JM, Ward MA: Shigella vulvovaginitis in a prepubertal child. *Pediatr Emerg Care* 2006;22:585-586.
16. Baiulescu M, Hannon PR, Marcinak JF, et al: Chronic vulvovaginitis caused by antibiotic-resistant *Shigella flexneri* in prepubertal child. *Pediatr Infect Dis J* 2002;21:170-172.

17. Murphy TV, Nelson JD: Shigella vaginitis: report in 38 patients and review of literature. *Pediatrics* 1979;63:511-516.

18. Bogaerts J, Lepage P, De Clercq A, et al: Shigella and gonococcal vulvovaginitis in prepubertal central African girls. *Pediatr Infect Dis J* 1992;1:890-892.

19. Basualdo W, Arbo A: Randomized comparison of azithromycin versus cefixime for treatment of shigellosis in children. *Pediatr Infect Dis J* 2003;22:374-377.

20. Cox RA, Slack MP: Clinical and microbiological features of *Haemophilus influenzae* vulvovaginitis in young children. *J Clin Pathol* 2002;55:961-964.

21. Cox RA: *Haemophilus influenzae:* an underrated cause of vulvovaginitis in young girls. *J Clin Pathol* 1997;50:765-768.

22. Zeiguer NJ, Galvano A, Comparato MR, et al: Vulvar abscesses caused by *Streptococcus pneumoniae*. *Pediatr Infect Dis J* 1992;11:335-336.

23. Touloukian RJ: Acute coliform salpingitis in a premenstrual child with severe vulvovaginitis. *J Pediatr* 1974;85:281.

24. Watkins S, Quan L: Vulvovaginitis caused by *Yersinia enterocolitica*. *Pediatr Infect Dis J* 1984;3:444-445.

25. Wilson HD, McCormick JB, Feeley JC: *Yersinia enterocolitica* infection in a 4-month-old infant associated with infection in household dogs. *J Pediatr* 1976;89:767-769.

26. Fallon P, Robinson ET: Meningococcal vulvovaginitis. *Scand J Infect Dis* 1974;6:295-296.

27. Gregory JE, Abramson E: Meningococci in vaginitis. *Am J Dis Child* 1971;121:423.

28. Weaver J: Non-gonorrheal vulvovaginitis due to gram-negative intracellular diplococci. *Am J Obstet Gynecol* 1950;60:257-260.

29. Fischer MC: Other anaerobic infections. *In*: Kliegman RM, Behrman RE, Jenson HB, et al *(eds): Nelson Textbook of Pediatrics*, ed 18, Saunders, Philadelphia, 2004, pp 1232-1240.

30. Eigen L: Vaginal diphtheria. *J Med Soc N J* 1932;29:778-780.

31. Chacko MR, Staat MA, Woods CR: Genital infections in childhood and adolescence. *In*: Feigen RD, Cherry JD, Demmler GJ, et al *(eds): Textbook of Pediatric Infectious Disease*, ed 5, Saunders, Philadelphia, 2004, pp 562-604.

32. Schaefer G: Tuberculosis of the female genital tract. *Clin Obstet Gynecol* 1970;13:965-998.

33. Jackson ST, Mullings AM, Rainford L, et al: The epidemiology of mycotic vulvovaginitis and the use of antifungal agents in suspected mycotic vulvovaginitis and its implications for clinical practice. *West Indian Med J* 2005;54:192-195.

34. Silverberg NB: A practical approach to molluscum contagiosum, part 1. *Contemp Pediatr* 2007;24:73-81.

35. Silverberg NB: A practical approach to molluscum contagiosum, part 2. *Contemp Pediatr* 2007;24:63-72.

36. Abzug M: Nonpolio enteroviruses. *In*: Kliegman RM, Behrman RE, Jenson HB, et al *(eds): Nelson Textbook of Pediatrics*, ed 18, Saunders, Philadelphia, 2004, pp 1350-1356.

37. Garcia-Aviles C, Caravalho N, Fernandez-Benitez M: Allergic vulvovaginitis in infancy: a study of a case. *Allergol Immunopathol (Madr)* 2001;29:137-140.

22

BACTERIAL SEXUALLY TRANSMITTED INFECTIONS IN CHILDREN

Rebecca Girardet, MD

EPIDEMIOLOGY

In the past three decades, reported rates of sexually transmitted infections in sexually abused children have been low. In their study of 1538 prepubertal children presenting for a complaint of sexual assault, Ingram et al[1] detected *Neisseria gonorrhoeae* in 2.8%, *Chlamydia trachomatis* in 1.2%, and *Treponema pallidum* (syphilis) in 0.1%. Siegel et al[2] reported an overall STI prevalence of 3.2% among prepubertal girls versus 14.6% among adolescents presenting for sexual assault. Both teams of investigators used cultures (not nucleic acid amplification tests) for diagnosis of *N. gonorrhoeae* and *C. trachomatis*. Similarly low prevalence rates for bacterial STIs among sexually abused prepubertal children were reported by other investigators from the United States and elsewhere using only non-DNA tests.[3-5] An investigation of 536 children (485 girls) presenting for a complaint of sexual abuse in four U.S. cities detected *C. trachomatis* by culture for 7 girls, *N. gonorrhoeae* by culture for 12 girls, syphilis in one girl, and *T. vaginalis* in 5 girls.[6] The use of nucleic acid amplification tests (NAATs) for *C. trachomatis* and *N. gonorrhoeae* in this study increased detection rates, but the overall prevalence of these organisms remained less than 4%.

The reasons for low prevalence rates of STIs in sexually abused children are unclear. It has been suggested that young girls are at increased risk of infection with HIV and *N. gonorrhoeae* due to the thinness and lack of estrogen in prepubertal vaginal epithelium.[7,8] The challenges inherent in eliciting an accurate abuse history and obtaining adequate anogenital specimens in young children might also contribute to low STI detection rates.

The low prevalence of STIs in sexually abused children also likely reflects declines in the numbers of reported cases of these diseases in the U.S. adult population that began in the mid-1970s. The decline was particularly steep for gonorrhea, which in 2004 reached its lowest rate since reporting began in 1941. Numbers of primary and secondary syphilis cases reached an all-time low in 2000, though they began to rise again subsequently, particularly among men having sex with men. Chlamydia prevalence rates increased modestly from 1999 to 2004, but the contributions of improved reporting and increased use of more sensitive diagnostic tests to these rates is unclear. Actual rates of both gonorrhea and chlamydia are estimated to be significantly higher than reported rates, due to both underdiagnosis and underreporting.[9]

CLINICAL MANIFESTATIONS

Infection with *N. gonorrhea* occurs via direct contact with secretions from infected mucosal tissues.[10] Infections of the male urethra and prepubertal vagina almost always cause a green purulent discharge, but genital tract infections in adolescent women are often asymptomatic. Even when asymptomatic, genital infection in adolescent women can progress to pelvic inflammatory disease (PID) with tubal scarring and resultant risk of infertility and ectopic pregnancy. Infection of the anus or pharynx in both sexes is often asymptomatic. Bacterial dissemination occurs more commonly in adolescent females who are infected within 1 week of menstruation. Dissemination can be manifested as a maculopapular rash with necrosis, tenosynovitis, and migratory arthritis (arthritis-dermatitis syndrome), or rarely, meningitis or endocarditis. Concurrent infection with *C. trachomatis* is common. The incubation period for gonorrhea is usually 2 to 7 days.[10,11]

Genital and anal infections with *C. trachomatis* can be asymptomatic in boys and girls of any age. Prepubertal girls can complain of vaginitis, adolescent females can develop inflammation anywhere along the genital tract, and males can develop epididymitis. Reiter syndrome, characterized by arthritis, urethritis, and bilateral conjunctivitis, can also occur. Infected adolescent girls are at risk for pelvic inflammatory disease (PID) even when asymptomatic, with scarring leading to infertility or ectopic pregnancy. Hemorrhagic proctocolitis can be severe and resemble inflammatory bowel disease. Chlamydial infection can also cause an ulcerative genital lesion and tender, suppurative, inguinal and/or femoral lymphadenopathy (lymphogranuloma venereum). Repeat infection with chlamydia in girls previously infected confers an elevated risk for PID and other complications compared with the initial infection. Infection can persist unnoticed for months to years, hence the caveat that a *Chlamydia* infection in a child less than 3 years of age can denote congenital infection rather than sexual contact.[12] The incubation period for chlamydia is typically at least 1 week.[10]

Because of its low prevalence in the United States, pediatricians rarely witness the clinical manifestations of syphilis, and then usually only in its congenital form. Infection with *Treponema pallidum* beyond the neonatal period causes distinct states of disease. The primary phase is characterized by painless chancres that occur at the site of inoculation, most commonly the genitals. Secondary syphilis begins 1 to 2 months following the appearance of chancres, and causes a maculopapular rash that involves the palms and soles. Hypertrophic lesions (condylomata lata) can appear on the genitalia and anus. The secondary phase is characterized by fever, malaise, generalized lymphadenopathy, splenomegaly, pharyngitis, headache, and/or arthralgias. The symptoms of secondary syphilis usually ebb and reappear for a period of years, followed by a latent period, where the patient remains seroreactive but has no clinical signs of disease. Tertiary syphilis refers to gumma formation and cardiovascular disease, and can begin years to decades following primary infection. Neurosyphilis occurs during any stage of infection, and is more likely to occur among persons infected with HIV. The incubation period is usually 3 weeks, but can range from 10 to 90 days.[10,11]

Diagnosis

Guidelines concerning sexual abuse by the American Academy of Pediatrics (AAP)[13] and the Centers for Disease Control and Prevention (CDC)[11] recommend testing children for STIs when the child discloses contact that might have involved transfer of genital secretions; when the child's symptoms or physical examination findings suggest the presence of an STI, penetrative trauma or ejaculation; when the abuser is thought to be at risk for STI infection; when community prevalence of an STI is high; when a family member is infected; and/or when the child or family requests testing. Studies of more restrictive testing criteria reported the highest predictive values for genital discharge, abnormal anogenital findings, suspected perpetrator STI infection, and child disclosure of genital-genital or genital-rectal contact.[14] The diagnosis of gonorrhea, in particular, appears to be highly associated with vaginal discharge in prepubertal girls with and without disclosure of sexual abuse,[14-16] although vaginal gonorrhea in girls without discharge has been reported.[14] Restrictive criteria for STI testing are not applicable to adolescent sexual abuse victims, nor do they apply to STI infection at nongenital sites.[14]

Chapter 25 discusses laboratory methods used in diagnosing STIs in sexually abused children and adolescents.

Forensic Applications

The use of molecular typing has been reported to be potentially helpful in forensic cases involving a positive test for gonorrhea. Martin et al[17] compared the genotypes from a culture isolate collected from a prepubertal child to an amplified DNA specimen extracted from purulent stains from the accused adult male's underwear. The isolates matched, and the perpetrator later confessed to the abuse. DeMattia et al[18] compared the genotypes of an isolate obtained from the vaginal discharge of a 3-year-old girl to that obtained from her 17-year-old half-brother, who became a suspect only after the diagnosis in his sister. The genotypes in this case did not match, and the 17 year old was exonerated.[18] The authors of these studies caution that gonorrhea genotyping is more typically used for epidemiological purposes and has not been validated for forensic purposes.

Treatment

Treatment of STIs in children and adolescents can be divided into two categories: cure of diagnosed disease, and prophylaxis following recent sexual contact. The Centers for Disease Control and Prevention regularly publish updated guidelines for management of STIs that address both issues, and these can be accessed online.[11] A summary of the most recent guidelines as they relate to uncomplicated infections in children and adolescents is provided in Table 22-1. It is important to note that since publication of the CDC STD 2006 Treatment Guidelines, quinolone antibiotics are no longer recommended for treatment of infection with *N. gonorrhoeae* in the United States due to widespread antibiotic resistance.[19]

Treatment of STIs in children and adolescents requires a few considerations that are not generally relevant to adults. First is the imperative of ensuring the accuracy of the diagnosis for any child or adolescent with a suspected STI before initiating treatment. This is important not only for the legal implications, but more immediately for the psychological welfare of the children and their families, and for the safety of the children and any siblings. Another treatment consideration is the age and weight of the child. For example, tetracyclines are contraindicated in children younger than 9 years of age due to their potential adverse effects on connective tissue. Most pediatric drug doses are titrated by the weight of the child.

Prophylactic antibiotics are recommended following sexual assault in adults and adolescents to prevent *N. gonorrhoeae*, *C. trachomatis*, and *Trichomonas vaginalis*. Prophylactic medications are also routinely provided to females to prevent pregnancy, and consideration should be given to the appropriateness of antiretroviral prophylaxis to protect against HIV. These topics are covered in other chapters in this book. Adolescent patients given prophylactic medications require follow-up testing only if they report symptoms or if there is uncertainty as to compliance with the medications. (An exception is prophylaxis for HIV, discussed in Chapter 24.) Prophylactic medications are generally not recommended for prepubertal children in the acute setting, primarily because of the low likelihood of STI, and the importance of making the diagnosis of an STI in this group, should one occur. If the child is thought to have been abused over a period of time by the same perpetrator, specimens for STI tests can be obtained at the time of the initial medical acute physical evaluation. Children who are thought to have been abused within a few days preceding examination should be tested acutely and again at 2 weeks post assault.

Follow-Up Considerations

Sexually abused children require close physical and psychological support following their initial medical evaluation. A second physical examination 1 to 2 weeks after the original evaluation is warranted if injuries were previously noted, or if STI testing needs to be repeated. Repeat serologies for syphilis and HIV (and hepatitis B in unimmunized children) should be obtained at 6 weeks, 3 months, and 6 months following the most recent sexual exposure. Each follow-up visit is an opportunity for the clinician to assess the patient's

Table 22-1	Treatment Guidelines for Uncomplicated Sexually Transmitted Infections[19]
	Adolescent	**Prepubertal Child**
C. trachomatis	Azithromycin 1 g PO one time or doxycycline 100 mg PO bid for 7 days*	Weight <45 kg: erythromycin base or ethylsuccinate 50 mg/kg/day PO divided qid for 14 days
		Weight >45 kg but age <8 years: Azithromycin 1 g PO one time
		Age >8 years: Azithromycin 1 g PO one time or doxycycline 100 mg PO bid for 7 days
N. gonorrhoeae	Ceftriaxone 125 mg IM one time or cefixime 400 mg PO one time*†‡	Weight <45 kg, anogenital or pharyngeal infection: ceftriaxone 125 mg IM one time
Syphilis	Parenteral penicillin G. Preparation, dose, and length of treatment depend on the stage of disease, clinical manifestations, and age/weight of the child; consider consultation with an infectious disease specialist	Parenteral penicillin G. Preparation, dose, and length of treatment depend on the stage of disease, clinical manifestations, and age/weight of the child; consider consultation with an infectious disease specialist
Trichomoniasis	Metronidazole 2 g PO one time*	N/A
Bacterial vaginosis	Metronidazole 500 mg PO bid for 7 days or metronidazole gel 0.75% intravaginally qd for 5 days, or clindamycin cream 2% intravaginally q.h.s. for 7 days	N/A

*For a list of alternative regimens, refer to CDC guidelines.
†Ceftriaxone is the only antimicrobial recommended for uncomplicated pharyngeal infection.
‡Quinolone antibiotics are no longer recommended for treatment of *N. gonorrhoeae* in the United States due to widespread resistance.

psychological and social well-being, and to consider additional interventions if current treatment resources are insufficient.

Tests of cure are not routinely required for nonpregnant patients diagnosed with chlamydia or gonorrhea, but should be performed if compliance with therapy is in question, if symptoms persist, or if reinfection is suspected. For persistent symptoms following a nonculture diagnosis of gonorrhea, the repeat test should be a true culture so that drug sensitivities can be determined. Partners of sexually active adolescents should be treated. Infections should be reported to state health departments when indicated. Because of the high rates of reinfection for chlamydia and gonorrhea, consideration should be given to repeat testing approximately 3 months following the initial infection. For patients with primary or secondary syphilis, repeat serologic tests and examination are performed 2 and 6 months following treatment. More intensive follow-up is required for patients with other stages of disease, and for pregnant adolescents and those coinfected with HIV. Consultation with an infectious disease specialist is recommended for children and adolescents infected with syphilis or HIV.

Another important purpose of ongoing medical care following sexual assault is to assess the child for unmet health care needs that might not be related to the episode(s) of abuse. Girardet et al documented that among 473 children presenting for a complaint of sexual assault, 26% had one or more unmet health care needs, as compared with 9% who had physical findings supporting the diagnosis of sexual abuse.[20] Ensuring ongoing, comprehensive health care to sexual abuse victims meets children's needs and obviates allegations that the clinician is purely concerned with documentation and collection of evidence.

STRENGTH OF THE EVIDENCE

While the diagnosis of a bacterial STI in an adult is generally interpreted as evidence of sexual acquisition, other explanations are often sought when these diseases are diagnosed in children. Although a history of sexual contact is not elicited from all infected children, the problem of incomplete disclosure is a recognized phenomenon in this age group.[21] An initial diagnosis of an STI must be confirmed by a qualified laboratory, as even standard tests are subject to misinterpretation, particularly in populations with a low prevalence of disease.[22] The possibility of previously unrecognized congenital infection must be entertained in infants and in toddlers up to 3 years of age, particularly for *C. trachomatis*.

Apart from congenitally acquired infections, sexual contact is considered the only mode of transmission for syphilis, gonorrhea, and chlamydia, except in rare circumstances, and it is considered to be the most likely mode of transmission for trichomonas.[13] Statements by the AAP and the CDC regarding sexual transmission of these organisms are supported by studies demonstrating a history of sexual contact among children diagnosed with these diseases and the lack of proof of transmission of these organisms to children from inanimate objects.[16,23-25] Proponents of arguments for nonsexual transmission of STIs point to a number of poorly investigated case reports in the medical literature, the majority of which are quite old, and to the possibility that unestrogenized vaginal epithelium might be more favorable to infection with *N. gonorrhoeae* than estrogenized tissue. Reports in the medical literature of recovery of *N. gonorrhoeae* and *T. vaginalis* from inanimate objects following inoculation (30 minutes to 3 days, depending on the organism and object) are also cited, but this ignores the fact that infection appears to require introduction of organisms into an orifice.[23,26-28]

An argument for nonsexual transmission of an STI can be made for individual cases on statistical grounds considering that the positive predictive value (PPV) for a diagnostic test (defined as the likelihood that a positive test result represents the presence of true disease in the person tested) is dependent on the prevalence of the condition in the population being tested. Because the prevalence of STIs in sexually abused children is quite low, even laboratory tests with sensitivities and specificities above 95% yield only moderate PPV values.

Low PPV values for diagnosis of STIs in children merely illustrate what is intuitively known by most clinicians, which is that in the case of a rare condition, all possible indicators of that condition must be carefully considered, documented, and investigated. For children presenting for suspected sexual abuse, this means that positive diagnostic tests must be confirmed, and that disclosures, physical findings, and scene investigation findings all must be approached with utmost care to arrive at an accurate diagnosis and render appropriate treatment.

SUGGESTED DIRECTIONS FOR FUTURE RESEARCH

Study of the diagnosis and management of bacterial STIs in sexually abused children is challenging because of the low prevalence rates of infection in this population. Early investigations of nucleic acid amplification tests for detection of *N. gonorrhoeae* and *C. trachomatis* in sexually abused children did not achieve statistical significance,[30-32] but served as catalysts for a multicenter investigation.[6,29] As more diagnostic tests for STIs become approved for use in children, further epidemiological studies will be required to ascertain the burden of disease in sexually abused children.

Systematic investigations of the management of children infected with bacterial STIs are not available. Further research regarding approaches for addressing the problem of poor follow-up for sexually abused children infected with bacterial STIs is warranted.

References

1. Ingram DL, Everett VD, Lyna PR, et al: Epidemiology of adult sexually transmitted disease agents in children being evaluated for sexual abuse. *Pediatr Infect Dis J* 1992;11:945-950.
2. Siegel R, Schubert CJ, Myers P, et al: The prevalence of sexually transmitted diseases in children and adolescents evaluated for sexual abuse in Cincinnati: rationale for limited STD testing in prepubertal girls. *Pediatrics* 1995;96:1090-1094.
3. Robinson AJ, Watkeys JEM, Ridgway GL: Sexually transmitted organisms in sexually abused children. *Arch Dis Child* 1998;79:356-358.
4. De Villiers FPR, Prentice MA, Bergh AM, et al: Sexually transmitted disease surveillance in a child abuse clinic. *S Afr Med J* 1992;81:84-86.
5. Kelly P, Koh J: Sexually transmitted infections in alleged sexual abuse of children and adolescents. *J Paediatr Child Health* 2006;42:434-440.
6. Girardet RG, Lahoti S, Howard LA, et al: The epidemiology of sexually transmitted infections in suspected child victims of sexual assault. *Pediatrics* 2009;124:79-86.
7. Dominguez KL: Management of HIV-infected children in the home and institutional settings. Care of children and infections control in schools, day care, hospital settings, home foster care, and adoption. *Pediatr Clin North Am* 2000;47:203-239.
8. Altchek A: Pediatric vulvovaginitis. *Pediatr Clin North Am* 1972;19:559-580.
9. Centers for Disease Control and Prevention: *Trends in reportable sexually transmitted diseases in the United States, 2006.* National surveillance data for chlamydia, gonorrhea, and syphilis. Centers for Disease Control and Prevention, Atlanta, Ga, 2007. http://www.obgyn.net/news/2006_STD_Surveillance_Report_Fact_Sheet.pdf. Accessed April 4, 2009.
10. Pickering LK, Baker CJ, Long SS, et al (eds): *Red book: 2006 report of the committee on infectious diseases,* ed 27, American Academy of Pediatrics, Elk Grove Village, Ill, 2006, pp 301-309, 252-257, 631-644.
11. Centers for Disease Control and Prevention, Workowski KA, Berman SM: Sexually transmitted diseases treatment guidelines, 2006. *MMWR Recomm Rep* 2006;55:1-94.
12. Bell TA, Stamm WE, Wang SP, et al: Chronic *Chlamydia trachomatis* infections in infants. *JAMA* 1992;15:400-402.
13. Kellogg N, Committee on Child Abuse and Neglect: The evaluation of sexual abuse in children. *Pediatrics* 2005;116:506-512.
14. Ingram DM, Miller WC, Schoenbach VJ, et al: Risk assessment for gonococcal and chlamydial infections in young children undergoing evaluation for sexual abuse. *Pediatrics* 2001;107:e73.
15. Shapiro RA, Schubert CJ, Siegel RM: *Neisseria gonorrhoeae* infections in girls younger than 12 years of age evaluated for vaginitis. *Pediatrics* 1999;104:e72.
16. Argent AC, Lachman PI: Sexually transmitted diseases in children and evidence of sexual abuse. *Child Abuse Negl* 1995;19:1303-1310.
17. Martin IM, Foreman E, Hall V, et al: Non-cultural detection and molecular genotyping of *Neisseria gonorrhoeae* from a piece of clothing. *J Med Microbiol* 2007;56:487-490.
18. DeMattia A, Kornblum JS, Hoffman-Rosenfeld J, et al: The use of combination subtyping in the forensic evaluation of a three-year-old girl with gonorrhea. *Pediatr Infect Dis J* 2006;25:461-463.
19. Centers for Disease Control and Prevention: *Updated recommended treatment regimens for gonococcal infections and associated conditions—United States, April 2007* (website): http://www.cdc.gov/std/treatment/2006/updated-regimens.htm. Accessed July 1, 2008.
20. Girardet R, Giacobbe L, Bolton K, et al: Unmet health care needs among children evaluated for sexual assault. *Arch Pediatr Adolesc Med* 2006;160:70-73.
21. Sjöberg RL, Lindblad F: Limited disclosure of sexual abuse in children whose experiences were documented by videotape. *Am J Psychiatry* 2002;159:312-314.
22. Whittington WL, Rice RJ, Biddle JW, et al: Incorrect identification of *Neisseria gonorrhoeae* from infants and children. *Pediatr Infect Dis J* 1988;7:3-10.
23. Ingram DL, White ST, Durfee MF, et al: Sexual contact in children with gonorrhea. *Am J Dis Child* 1982;136:994-996.
24. Neinstein LS, Goldenring J, Carpenter S: Nonsexual transmission of sexually transmitted diseases: an infrequent occurrence. *Pediatrics* 1984;74:67-76.
25. Bump RC, Sachs LA, Buesching WJ: Sexually transmissible infectious agents in sexually active and virginal asymptomatic adolescent girls. *Pediatrics* 1986;77:488-493.
26. Goodyear-Smith F: What is the evidence for non-sexual transmission of gonorrhoea in children after the neonatal period? A systematic review. *J Forensic Leg Med* 2007;14:489-502.
27. Kellogg N, Anderst J: Evidence-based or evidence-biased? *J Forensic Leg Med* 2008;15:471-472.
28. Perez JL, Gómez E, Sauca G: Survival of gonococci from urethral discharge on fomites. *Eur J Clin Microbiol Infect Dis* 1990;1:54-55.
29. Black CM, Driebe EM, Howard LA, et al: Multicenter study of nucleic acid amplification tests for detection of *Chlamydia trachomatis* and *Neisseria gonorrhoeae* in children being evaluated for sexual abuse. *Pediatr Infect Dis J* 2009;28:608-13.

30. Mathews-Greer J, Sloop G, Springer A, et al: Comparison of detection methods for Chlamydia trachomatis in specimens obtained from pediatric victims of suspected sexual abuse. *Pediatr Infect Dis J* 1999;18:165-167.

31. Girardet RG, McClain N, Lahoti S, et al: Comparison of the urine-based ligase chain reaction test to culture for detection of *Chlamydia trachomatis* and *Neisseria gonorrhoeae* in pediatric sexual abuse victims. *Pediatr Infect Dis J* 2001;20:144-147.

32. Kellogg ND, Baillargeon J, Lukefahr JL, et al: Comparison of nucleic acid amplification tests and culture techniques in the detection of *Neisseria gonorrhoeae* and *Chlamydia trachomatis* in victims of suspected child sexual abuse. *J Pediatr Adolesc Gynecol* 2004;17:331-339.

23

VIRAL AND PARASITIC SEXUALLY TRANSMITTED INFECTIONS IN CHILDREN

Arne H. Graff, MD, and Laurie D. Frasier, MD, FAAP

Viral diseases are among the most common sexually transmitted infections in humans. These infections have varied presentations and varying degrees of specificity for sexual abuse in children. Conditions to be addressed in this chapter include human papillomavirus, herpes viruses, viruses causing hepatitis, and molluscum contagiosum. HIV and AIDS are addressed in Chapter 24. Parasitic diseases such as trichomoniasis, scabies, and pediculosis also will be discussed.

HUMAN PAPILLOMAVIRUS (HPV)

The human papillomavirus is a DNA virus that consists of more than 100 subtypes, of which more than 40 are capable of infecting the genitals and anuses of humans.[1] Common sites of infection include the penis, rectum, vagina, cervix, urethra, perianal area, vulva, oral cavity and respiratory system, and skin. Fifteen subtypes are associated with dysplastic skin changes and an increased risk of oral, anal, or genital cancer. Types 16 and 18 are most commonly associated with oncogenic changes. Types 6 and 11 are most often associated with clinically apparent warts. It is estimated that 76% of the sexually active population will become infected during their life time. Currently approximately 20 million people are infected in the United States.[2] It is considered to be the most common sexually transmitted disease in the country.

HPV causes the development of epithelial tumors (condylomatous warts). It can remain latent in the epithelium, resulting in subclinical infections of normal epithelium. This could explain the high rate of relapse after treatment of warts. Transmission occurs from person to person during close contact, including sexual activity. Mechanical damage to the skin causes disturbance of the epithelial barrier and exposure of basal cells to infectious virus. The virus replicates in the nucleus of the cells causing typical changes of koilocytosis, or nuclear clearing, seen on microscopy.

Transmission can be vertical (during pregnancy and delivery) or horizontal (digital inoculation/autoinoculation, fomite contact, or sexual). Little is known about the acquisition of and the normal course of HPV genital and anal infections in children. Controversy exists over the length of time for incubation in infants/children. The time from vertical transmission to clinical infection, once considered possibly up to 2 years after delivery, is now questioned, with evidence that this time frame is unknown and could be extended. Other types of HPV infections acquired at birth

can present later than 2 years, however. For example, juvenile respiratory papillomatosis is usually seen within 5 years after the exposure to the virus during the birth process.[3,4] The general consensus, however, is that HPV acquired after 2 years of age are not likely to be from birth.[5]

HPV infections of genitals, oral cavity, or digital warts, in the parent or other children can play a significant role in the transmission of HPV to infants/children. Studies have demonstrated both genital and nongenital subtypes of HPV present in warts in the mouth and on hands and feet.[6,7] Nongenital subtypes 1,2, have been described in lesions on the genital area, suggesting transmission of a nonsexual nature, especially in flat warts occurring on the skin rather than condylomatous warts on the mucous membranes. Unfortunately these studies did not address the possibility that sexual transmission was due to digital genital contact.[2,8] Fomite transmission has been suggested to occur during the use of surgical instruments and gloves. Additional evidence of fomite transmission comes from a study linking the development of plantar warts to the use of public showers,[6] although a search for HPV DNA on floors, seats, and surfaces of humid dwellings (including indoor swimming pools, bathing resorts, and private homes) failed to identify any evidence of the virus.[9] Some studies appear to support nonsexual transmission of HPV between household members, further suggesting that some infections in children might not be the result of sexual abuse.[7]

When a child has anogenital warts, a concern of sexual abuse should be raised. The problem confronting the clinician is to balance the possibility of innocent versus sexual transmission. A study by Sinclair et al[10] compared the assessment of children with anogenital lesions referred to a sexual abuse clinic to the assessment of children with juvenile laryngeal papillomatosis evaluated in an otolaryngology clinic. The study highlights the difficulty in determining the source of HPV infections, particularly in young children. Thirty-one percent of the children with anogenital warts who were seen in a specialty clinic for children who were suspected as being victims of sexual abuse were actually found to have experienced abuse. None of the children seen in the otolaryngology clinic were assessed for possible abuse because the cause of the laryngeal lesions was assumed to be perinatal acquisition of the virus.

The risk factors for acquiring the infection in teens and adults include: increased number of sexual partners, young age of first sexual activity, and having a partner who has had multiple sexual partners.[11] Other potential factors include smoking, oral contraceptive use, and the presence of immunosuppressive conditions and medications.

Active infections can cause typical flat-topped, hyperpigmented, or cauliflower-shaped lesions that can cause pruritus, bleeding, or burning. The lesions range in size from a few millimeters to several centimeters. HPV can also cause respiratory symptoms when infecting the vocal cords and/or tracheal-bronchial tree. HPV lesions can develop into precancerous or cancerous lesions in squamous epithelial tissues.[12,13] Most HPV infections are asymptomatic and resolve within 2 years.[14]

Diagnosis is made by clinical examination. In adults, detection of lesions can be enhanced by soaking the skin or mucous membranes with mild (3%-5%) acetic acid solution for 3 to 5 minutes before colposcopic examination. Biopsy is indicated of any wart with an atypical appearance. Polymerase chain reaction (PCR) testing can be used to demonstrate HPV DNA within lesions. Androscopy in male partners is not routinely suggested unless high-risk HPV is found.

Localized destructive treatment such as cautery, cryotherapy, laser ablation, or use of caustic topical agents can be used on external warts by the treating health care provider. Patient-applied treatments include the use of podofilox 0.5% solution or gel (Condolox), or imiquimod cream (Aldera). For asymptomatic warts, no treatment (observation) is acceptable care. This is especially true in children where the disease often remits spontaneously and where all treatments cause some pain and irritation.[1] There are few studies in the literature comparing the effectiveness of the various treatment modalities for anogenital warts in children.

HPV quadrivalent vaccine (Gardasil and Cervarix) is available and recommended for people ages 9 to 26. It offers protection against subtypes 6, 11, 16, and 18.[15]

In sexual abuse evaluations, determination of the source of HPV in an infant/child can be elusive. The diagnosis of anogenital HPV infection, however, should prompt a medical evaluation that includes a thorough social history, history of previous HPV infection (common or genital), age-appropriate interview of the child, careful physical examination of the genitals and anus, and testing for other sexually transmitted infections. The decision whether to refer the case to a child protection agency should be made on a case-by-case basis.

VIRAL HEPATITIS

Viral hepatitis is an infection of the liver. There are six defined subtypes, hepatitis A through E, and G. Hepatitis A, B, and C are the most common subtypes seen in the United States. The actual incidence of these subtypes is thought to be underestimated due to the number of unreported and asymptomatic cases that occur. Overall the number of cases have decreased for hepatitis A (HAV) and hepatitis B (HBV) due to public health campaigns, vaccination policies, and public awareness, while a slight increase in hepatitis C (HCV) was noted in 2006.[16,17] The hepatitis viruses all share tropism for liver tissue, although the viruses all have different physical structures, pathobiology, and epidemiology.[18]

The clinical signs and symptoms of acute infection with hepatitis A, B, C, D, and E are similar, and include fever, light-colored stools, dark urine, jaundice, nausea, vomiting, and fatigue. Symptoms can persist for up to 2 months. Serum liver enzymes are initially elevated. The persistence of enzyme elevation varies depending on the type of hepatitis contracted. Asymptomatic infections do occur, particularly in children under the age of 6 years.[19]

Hepatitis A

Hepatitis A virus (HAV) is primarily transmitted by the fecal-oral route, occurring with ingestion of contaminated food or by contact with household members or sexual partners who are infected. Risk factors include: Men who have sex with men, users of illegal drugs, travel to endemic areas, working with primates that can be infected, and persons with clotting disorders. Diagnosis is made by demonstration of the IgM antibody to HAV, which can persist up to 6 months after the initial infection.[20] Incubation is from 15 to 50 days and lifelong immunity occurs following infection. Chronic infection does not occur with HAV.

Treatment is symptomatic. Preventative care includes good hygiene measures. Acutely exposed people can avert infection by receiving immune globulin within 2 weeks of exposure. Immune globulin is recommended after household or sexual exposure, and is 80% to 90% effective in protecting against infection.[21] Hepatitis A vaccine is available and provides immunity within 2 to 4 weeks of administration.

In cases of child sexual abuse, the risk of potential infection should be decided on a case-by-case basis (depending on the risk factors). Since hepatitis A is so commonly transmitted by nonsexual modes, sexual transmission, especially in children, cannot be assumed.

Hepatitis B

Viral Hepatitis B (HBV) is transmitted by sexual contact and by percutaneous contact with infected fluids.[18] While blood and all body fluids are considered potential sources of infection, only semen, blood, and saliva have been demonstrated to cause infections. Also, the presence of these fluids on surfaces of inanimate objects can be a source of infectious material. Risk factors for infection with HBV include skin injury with a contaminated instrument such as a needle, infants born to infected mothers, sexual contact with infected partners (posing a 40% risk of transmission with heterosexual sexual activity),[22] contact with wounds, or sharing of hygiene products of infected patients. The incubation period is from 60 to 150 days and the symptoms can last up to 6 months (typically lasting several weeks). The symptoms range from none at all (asymptomatic infection) to fulminate hepatitis. Chronic infection occurs more frequently in infants born to infected mothers (90%) and in children ages 1 to 5 (30% to 60%) than in adults.[17] Chronic infection is associated with hepatocellular carcinoma and cirrhosis, resulting in premature death.[23]

Testing includes liver function testing and HBV serologic markers.[24] A positive hepatitis B surface antigen (HBsAg) demonstrates active infection, either acute or chronic, and is positive by 3 to 5 weeks after infection. Positive hepatitis B surface antibody (HBsAb) indicates immunity, either from vaccine or infection. It should be noted that it can be negative in patients with declining immunologic-memory or in a nonresponding vaccine recipient. There is a window of time that both HBsAg and HBsAb both might be negative in an acute infection. For this reason, repeat testing in 3 months is recommended if disease is suspected. Anti-HBc IgM cannot be used to determine acute versus chronic infection because it can be positive in both. In prenatally acquired HBV, this test is negative.

Highly effective HBV vaccines are available for children and adults. A three-injection series is now recommended for all children, beginning shortly after birth.[25]

Hepatitis C

Viral Hepatitis C (HCV) is the most common cause of chronic liver disease in children of industrialized countries.[26] It is transmitted by exposure to infected blood products and body fluids (instruments, needles, and sexual contact), and by delivery of infants of infected mothers. Newborns are at increased risk if membranes rupture over 6 hours before delivery, if they are exposed to excessive amounts of maternal blood, and if their mothers' peripheral mononuclear blood cells are infected with HCV. Transmission is frequent among intravenous drug abusers, and also has been reported to be transmitted during tattooing and body piercing when infected needles are used.[27] Incarcerated juveniles have higher rates of infection compared with other children.[28] Other people at risk for infection with HCV include those who received organ donation or blood products before 1987.

Symptoms can develop from 2 weeks to 6 months after exposure, but many cases are asymptomatic. Many who become infected with HCV develop chronic hepatitis.[29] Testing is done for anti-HCV, but is often negative early in the infection and repeat testing should be considered. Treatment is symptomatic but if testing is positive, consultation with an infectious disease specialist or hepatologist is recommended for long-term follow-up.

Other Types of Viral Hepatitis

Viral hepatitis D (HDV) only exists as a coinfection with HBV. Transmission is by percutaneous or sexual contact with infected sources. With acute or chronic infections, the clinical course and the disease process (including development of cirrhosis and carcinoma) is often more severe than that of patients infected with HBV alone.[30] Antibody testing is used for confirmation, and management is similar to HBV.

Viral hepatitis E (HEV) is rare in the United States and also is transmitted by the fecal-oral route. Infection is confirmed by antibody testing. No chronic infection occurs and no vaccine is currently available in the United States.[31]

Viral hepatitis G (HGV) is transmitted by transfusions, by sexual activity, and during delivery. A mother's viral load and the mode of delivery influence the newborn's risk of infection. Chronic carriage of the virus can develop, but the virus has not been linked to a specific disease state.[32]

Hepatitis Viruses and Sexual Assault and Abuse

Hepatitis evaluation, in sexually abused/assaulted patients, is primarily for the identification, treatment, and potential long-term management of the disease. Identification of the source using genotypic methods at this time is not possible. The U.S. Centers for Disease Control and Prevention recommends screening unvaccinated victims for hepatitis B at the time of evaluation, and then administering the hepatitis B vaccine, followed by readministration of the vaccine at 1 to 2 months and 6 months after the first dose to complete the vaccine series. In the setting of acute sexual assault, when the risk of transmission of HBV is likely (offender has risk factors, mucosal injury, etc.) and the immunization status of the victim is unknown, HBV vaccine should be carefully considered. If the offender is known to be HBV-positive (infectious) and the victim is not previously immunized, hepatitis B immune globulin (HBIG) also should be considered. If given, it should be administered within 14 days of the contact.[17] Consultation with an infectious disease specialist or hepatologist is recommended in hepatitis B virus positive cases.

HERPES SIMPLEX VIRUS (HSV 1 AND HSV 2)

The herpes family consists of HSV1, HSV2, cytomegalovirus, Epstein-Barr virus, herpes zoster, and three other human herpes viruses. These viruses have a unique characteristic for harboring a latent infection (remaining in the sensory ganglion) after the clinical infections resolves, remaining there for the life of the patient. Reactivation can occur resulting in recurring clinical disease. Infections can also be asymptomatic. While both HSV1 and HSV2 can be identified in both genital and nongenital infections, HSV1 is more commonly found in nongenital infections. Epidemiological studies have shown that an increasing number of genital infections are due to HSV1 (up to 40% of new cases),[33] which might reflect a change in sexual practices. By age 5 years, approximately 40% to 60% of children will test positive for HSV 1, and by adolescence the number increases to 90%.

Transmission is by direct contact with lesions or contact with droplets from infected sites. Since the virus is quickly inactivated at room temperature or by drying, fomite spread is unusual.[34] Transmission of the virus can occur in the absence of active lesions, since the virus can be shed by the anogenital tract between outbreaks. During delivery, the chance that an infant will become infected is 30% to 50% if the mother has a new HSV infection, and less than 1% if the mother has an established infection.[35] Risk factors for acquiring the infection include damage to the skin that is exposed to an infectious source (for example, by eczema), sporting activities involving skin-to-skin or skin-to-inanimate object contact, and sexual contact. Increased risk related to sexual activity occurs with an increased numbers of sexual partners, early age of beginning sexual activity, and a history of other sexual transmitted diseases.[36] The risk of a child acquiring HSV through sexual abuse in unknown. Most infections in adults are transmitted from asymptomatic individuals. It is possible that a child could be infected by a person who does not know he or she has the disease.

The infection produces a microscopic picture of intranuclear inclusions within cells. Recurrences are generally site specific, with HSV-1 recurring more frequently in the oral cavity and HSV-2 recurring more frequently in the anogenital region. Incubation ranges from 1 to 14 days, and recurrent episodes tend to be shorter in duration, have fewer lesions, and less viral shedding with HSV-1. Symptoms can include lesions that progress from vesicular to granulated ulcers with a red base, and can be accompanied by lymphadenopathy, pain at the site of lesions (or region), dysuria, and headache. Lesions can be preceded by nonspecific complaints of tingling, fever, and malaise. Both HSV1 and HSV2 may have symptoms or be asymptomatic (for both primary and recurrent episodes).[37] Diseases associated include vulvovaginitis, gingivostomatitis, skin lesions, viral meningitis, and anal-genital infections.

Diagnosis should not be made based only on clinical presence of ulcers or vesicles. While HSV is the most common cause of genital ulcers, the differential must include other causes such as: drug eruptions, bullous erosive diseases, erythema multiforme, HIV, and Crohn disease.[38] Identification by use of Tzank smears is insensitive and is not recommended. The use of tests using nucleic acid amplification technologies (NAAT) to diagnose herpes infections is currently available.[39] NAAT might also have a role in the identification of the patient with asymptomatic shedding. Early studies indicate that NAAT for identifying HSV have nearly 100% sensitivity and specificity, and detect 25% more HSV-positive lesions than culture alone.[40]

Viral culture is considered the "gold standard" for the diagnosis of HSV[41]; however, sensitivity is low and likelihood of positive testing depends on the lesion used for collecting sample (>90% from vesicular and 24% with granulated lesion).[42] Therefore, obtaining material for culture from the freshest lesion is essential. The vesicle must be unroofed, and the base swabbed vigorously, with inoculation into appropriate viral transport media.

Type-specific serologic testing is available.[42] Type-specific tests have used glycoproteins (gG1 or gG2) to differentiate HSV1 from HSV2 and have 80% to 90% sensitivity and >96% specificity. Early in the infection a false-negative test can occur due to low viral loads. Also, in populations with a low prevalence for HSV, there is a higher likelihood of a false-positive test result. Type specific testing does not identify when the infection occurred; only that it has occurred in the past. Type specific serology is helpful in identifying HSV infection in high-risk individuals, but should not be used as a screening test in a low prevalence population such as children.[43] The forensic value of this test has also not been adequately determined. Also it is important to remember that antibody development can take up to 6 months to become positive (seroconvert) and that spontaneous reversion (to a negative test) can occur.[42]

Nucleoside analogs offer effective treatment for acute or recurrent HSV infections.[44] Available drugs include acyclovir, valacyclovir, and famciclovir, although data on the use of valacyclovir and famciclovir in children is limited. Patient education should include: risk of transmission (including during asymptomatic periods), suppressive therapy options, natural history (risk of recurrence), and risks for future pregnancy.

Genital HSV infections have been reported in sexually abused children.[45] Autoinoculation from oral lesions by children is also a possibility. A child with genital ulcers positive for HSV should receive a complete sexual abuse evaluation and testing for other sexually transmitted infections. The decision to refer a case to the appropriate child protection authorities should be done if abuse is suspected.

MOLLUSCUM CONTAGIOSUM

Molluscum contagiosum is caused by a virus in the poxvirus family. In adults it is often transmitted by skin-to-skin contact.[46] The condition is commonly contracted by children, however, and is not considered to be a sexually transmitted infection. It is more commonly found in tropical areas and where living conditions are overcrowded and hygiene is poor.[47] The overall incidence is unknown due to the lack of reporting, but it does appear to be increasing. It is a difficult infection to treat in immune compromised individuals. It is highly contagious and transmitted by both direct and indirect contact (shared clothing, contact sports, swimming pools, and by autoinoculation).[48] The typical molluscum lesion is flesh-colored or pearly white, dome shaped, approximately 1 to 5 mm in diameter with a central umbilication. Clinically, it often has multiple lesions and can appear on any part of the body. Incubation is unclear but can take up to 6 months to appear and the lesions often last up to 9 months, although some infections last for years. Mild pruritus and eczematous irritation can be associated, although the course of the illness is usually benign. As lesions crust over, small pitted scars may occur. The differential diagnosis should include all soft tissue tumors of the skin and other infectious causes. While diagnosis is usually made on clinical grounds, a crushed specimen (of the central plug) often shows intracytoplasmic inclusions (molluscum bodies) on microscopic examination. Upon biopsy, lesions have a typical appearance, with epidermal hyperplasia surrounding a cystic lobule.[46]

Treatment includes observation alone or mechanical destruction of lesions using methods such as curettage or cryotherapy, or topical application of cytotoxic agents such as cantharidin, retinoic acid, or podophyllin.[49]

TRICHOMONAS VAGINALIS (TV)

Trichomonas vaginalis is a flagellated protozoa that can be identified microscopically by its undulating membrane. It is a common sexually transmitted disease. The U.S. Centers for Disease Control estimates that 7.4 million new cases occur in the United States each year.[50] Unlike gonorrhea and chlamydia, TV's incidence appears to increase in middle-aged women.[51] Factors that may increase the chance of acquiring the disease include: increased number of sexual partners, adolescents whose partner is older by 4 or more years, and the presence of other sexually transmitted diseases.[52]

Trichomoniasis is a self-limited disease in less than 40% of men and less than 20% of women, where recovery occurs without treatment. The presence of a TV infection increases the risk of contracting HIV in women[53] and increases the shedding of HIV in semen of men.[54]

Transmission is primarily by sexual contact.[55] TV has been demonstrated to be viable on inanimate objects (e.g,. for 45 minutes on toilet seats[56] and up to 25 hours on damp towels[57]). The relationship between its presence and the risk of acquiring an infection from that source, however, is not well studied. Transmission can also occur during delivery, with disease being found in infants of infected mothers between 2% and 17% of the time.[50] Incubation ranges from 5 to 28 days. There is some indication that the prepubertal patient might be less likely to become infected after contact with the organism because of the high vaginal pH and lack of secretions in the vagina of the child.[58]

Diseases associated with TV include genital infections in newborns, vaginitis, vulvar cellulitis, nongonococcal urethritis, infertility in women, gestational trichomonas (low birth weight, premature rupture of membranes, preterm labor), and urethral strictures.[59] *Trichomonas vaginalis* has not been shown to affect the oral cavity or rectum, but women with vaginal infections can have urethral infections as well.[60] Trichomoniasis of the nose and respiratory tract sometimes occurs in newborn infants of infected mothers, potentially causing nasal congestion, pneumonia, and respiratory distress.[61]

Many infected females patients are asymptomatic.[62] Symptoms of trichomoniasis in females include discharge, odor, pruritus, bleeding, dyspareunia, dysuria, vulvar irritation, and abdominal discomfort. The presence of the "typical" yellow-green discharge with bubbles is found in less than half of the cases.

Males infected with TV are more commonly asymptomatic.[63] When symptomatic, men usually have dysuria and urethritis, although prostatitis and epididymitis have been described.

Most commonly, testing for trichomoniasis is done by direct microscopic examination of "wet preps" done on vaginal secretions. The test has been shown to detect 50% to 70% of infections in women, but is less sensitive in men.[59] The test must be performed promptly after the specimen is collected to detect viable organisms. Delays in performing wet preps leads to decreased diagnostic accuracy. Culture is currently the gold standard but requires up to 7 days for confirmation of the diagnosis. Point of care, rapid, nucleic acid probe tests are available for testing in women, with greater than 83% sensitivity and greater than 96% specificity noted.[64] Nucleic acid amplification tests are available, but are not as sensitive or specific as comparable tests are for other sexually transmitted infections such as gonorrhea and chlamydia.

TV is most commonly treated with metronidazole. If patients are sexually active, their partner should also be treated. Treatment failures are reported, but are often due to poor compliance or reinfection. When continued infections occur, culture should be done to confirm the presence of TV. Counseling regarding the potential increased risk of acquiring other STI should be provided.

The CDC recommends TV wet preps and cultures be done for routine screening of adult and adolescent victims of sexual assault.[65] For sexually abused children, the decision to test for STI should be made on a case-by-case basis, depending on the child's risk factors and clinical presentation. In children, the diagnosis is often coincidental, with the trichomonads being observed in the urine of a child. This raises the concern that the infection is sexually transmitted, and full assessment for sexual abuse should be undertaken. When TV is found in the urine, it must be differentiated from *Trichomonas hominis,* a common nonpathogenic contaminant from the gastrointestinal tract.

SCABIES

Scabies, an obligate parasite, is caused by a mite, *Sarcoptes scabiei*. It is a common disease in children and is found worldwide.[66] Transmission is skin-to-skin contact (not casual contact), including sexual partners, requiring close contact. Scabies are often transmitted between household contacts, however, possibly by fomites.[67] The mite can survive off the human body from 24 to 36 hours.[68] Clinical presentation includes typical subcutaneous burrows, pruritus (often worse at nighttime), and excoriated areas (due to the scratching). Occasional secondary skin infections may occur. Burrows can be difficult to identify due to the scratching or infections. Symptoms usually begin in 4 to 6 weeks, but may occur sooner in patients who have experienced a previous scabies infection. Symptoms are caused by an IgE-related hypersensitivity to the organism and its feces.[69]

Diagnosis is made with microscopic examination of a scraping of the burrow, looking to identify the mite, its eggs, or its feces. Treatment for infants older than 2 months and children includes the use of topical agents (5% permethrin) and careful laundering of clothing and bedding. Treatment of the pruritus might need to be continued for several weeks. Treatment of the entire household should be considered.

A diagnosis of scabies in a child or adolescent does not suggest sexual abuse.

PEDICULOSIS

Sucking lice that infect humans include *Phthirus pubis* (the crab louse or pubic louse), *Pediculus humanus humanus* (the body louse), and *Pediculus humanus capitis* (the head louse). These infections are worldwide, but the actual incidence is unknown. Conditions where poor hygiene and overcrowding occur are factors for an increased risk of transmission. Associated diseases include: epidemic typhus,[70] trench fever, relapsing fever,[71] secondary infections, and dermatitis.[72] Pruritis is the primary symptom associated with infections. The actual lice can be seen with the naked eye and examination often shows the nits attached to hairs. While scalp nits can, under Wood's lamp illumination, show yellow-green fluorescence, other body areas usually do not. One might also see louse feces (red-brown) on the skin during identification.

Treatment includes medications for pruritis, education for the family, cleaning of clothes and bedding, and topical medications. Topical permethrin cream 5% is most commonly used.[73] The identification of body louse does not require treatment, except for decontamination of clothing and house.

The presence of lice is not indicative of sexual abuse.

SUMMARY

The viral and parasitic infections noted here are some of the most prevalent. Herpes simplex virus and HPV have traditionally been considered indicative of sexual contact in children, however, other modes of transmission should be considered and neither disease is diagnostic of abuse. Sexual abuse is a possibility and should be considered carefully in the context of each situation. *Trichomonas vaginalis* has a higher likelihood of sexual transmission. Other parasitic infections such as scabies and lice might indicate an unhygienic environment, and might require intervention by a child protection agency if the infections persist following treatment and when evaluation of the social environment is indicated.

STRENGTH OF THE EVIDENCE

While the epidemiology of viral and parasitic sexually transmitted infections has been carefully researched in adults, children have received much less attention. Much of the information comes from clinical studies where the children's actual exposure to perpetrators is unknown.

AREAS FOR FUTURE RESEARCH

Future research is needed to more specifically define the normal flora of the prepubescent child's genitalia. Prospective studies of children born to HPV positive mothers will help determine if and when children exposed at birth will develop genital warts. Studies should also be done to determine if nucleic acid analysis would be helpful in matching organisms transmitted from offenders to victims.

References

1. Winer RL, Koutsky LA: Genital human papillomavirus infection. *In*: Holmes KK, Sparling PF, Stamm WE, et al: *Sexually Transmitted Diseases*, ed 4, McGraw-Hill, New York, 2008, pp 489-508.
2. Moscicki A: Impact of HPV infection in adolescent populations. *J Adolesc Health* 2005;37:S3-S9.
3. Mammas IN, Sourvinos G, Spandidos DA: Human papilloma virus (HPV) infection in children and adolescents. *Eur J Pediatr* 2009;168:267-273.
4. Derkay CS, Wistrak B: Recurrent respiratory papillomatosis: a review. *Laryngoscope* 2008;118:1236-1247.
5. Gutman LT, Herman-Giddens ME, Phelps WC: Transmission of human genital papillomavirus disease: comparison of data from adults and children. *Pediatrics* 1993;91:31-38.
6. Rintala M, Grénman SE, Puranen MH, et al: Transmission of high risk human papillomavirus between parents and infant: a prospective study of HPV in families in Finland. *J Clin Microbiol* 2005;43:376-381.
7. Sonnex C, Strauss S, Gray JJ: Detection of human papillomavirus DNA on the fingers of patients with genital warts. *Sex Transm Infect* 1999;75:317-319.
8. Ingram DL, Everette D, Lyna PR, et al: Epidemiology of adult sexually transmitted disease agents in children being evaluated for sexual abuse. *Pediatr Infect Dis J* 1992;11:945-950.
9. Puranen M, Syrjänen K, Syrjänen S: Transmission of genital human papillomavirus infections is unlikely through the floor and seats of humid dwellings in the countries of high-level hygiene. *Scand J Infect Dis* 1996;28:243-246.
10. Sinclair KA, Woods CR, Kirse DJ, et al: Anogenital and respiratory tract human papillomavirus infections among children: age, gender, and potential transmission through sexual abuse. *Pediatrics* 2005;116:815-825.
11. Ahmed AM, Madkan V, Tyring SK: Human papillomaviruses and genital disease. *Dermatol Clin* 2006;24:157-165.
12. Walboomers LM, Jacobs MV, Manos MM, et al: Human papillomavirus is a necessary cause of invasive cervical cancer worldwide. *J Pathol* 1999;189:12-19.
13. Daling JR, Sherman KJ: Relationship between human papillomavirus infection and tumours of anogenital sites other than the cervix. *IARC Sci Publ* 1992;119:223-241.
14. Ho GYF, Bierman R, Beardsley L, et al: Natural history of cervicovaginal papillomavirus infection in young women. *N Engl J Med* 1998;338:423-428.
15. Palmer KE, Jenson AB, Kouokam JC, et al: Recombinant vaccines for the prevention of human papillomavirus infection and cervical cancer. *Exp Mol Pathol* 2009;86:224-233.
16. Daniels D, Grytdal S, Wasley A, et al: Surveillance for acute viral hepatitis—United States, 2007. *MMWR Surveill Summ* 2009;58:1-27.
17. Centers for Disease Control and Prevention: *Guidelines for viral hepatitis surveillance and case management* (website): http://www.cdc.gov/Hepatitis/PDFs/2005Guidelines-Surv-CaseMngmt.pdf. Accessed July 21, 2009.
18. Lemon SM, Lok A, Alter MJ: Viral hepatitis. *In*: Holmes KK, Sparling PF, Stamm WE, et al: *Sexually Transmitted Diseases*, ed 4, McGraw-Hill, New York, 2008, pp 509-543.
19. Lednar WM, Lemon SM, Kirkpatrick JW, et al: Frequency of illness associated with epidemic hepatitis A virus in adults. *Am J Epidemiol* 1985;122:226-233.
20. Lemon SM, Brown CD, Brooks DS, et al: Specific immunoglobulin M response to hepatitis A virus determined by solid phase radioimmunoassay. *Infect Immun* 1980;28:927-936.
21. Winokur PL, Stapleton JT: Immunoglobulin prophylaxis for hepatitis A. *Clin Infect Dis* 1992;14:580-586.
22. Brook M: Sexually acquired hepatitis. *Sex Transm Infect* 2002;78:235-240.
23. Beasley RP, Hwang LY, Lin CC, et al: Hepatocellular carcinoma and hepatitis B virus: a prospective study of 22,707 men in Taiwan. *Lancet* 1981;2:1129-1133.
24. Chevaliez S, Pawlotsky JM: Diagnosis and management of chronic viral hepatitis: antigens, antibodies, and viral genomes. *Best Pract Res Clin Gastroenterol* 2008;22:1031-1048.
25. Lemon SM, Thomas DL: Vaccines to prevent viral hepatitis. *N Engl J Med* 1997;336:196-204.
26. Indolfi G, Resti M: Perinatal transmission of hepatitis C virus infection. *J Med Virol* 2009;81:836-843.
27. Baldo V, Baldovin T, Trivello R, et al: Epidemiology of HCV infection. *Curr Pharm Des* 2008;14:1646-1654.
28. Murray KF, Richardson LP, Morishima C, et al: Prevalence of hepatitis C virus infection and risk factors in an incarcerated juvenile population: a pilot study. *Pediatrics* 2003;111:153-157.
29. Ozaras R, Tahan V: Acute hepatitis C: prevention and treatment. *Expert Rev Anti Infect Ther* 2009;7:351-361.
30. Fattovich G, Giustina G, Christensen E, et al: Influence of hepatitis delta virus infection on morbidity and mortality in compensated cirrhosis type B. The European concerted action on viral hepatitis (EUROHEP). *Gut* 2000;46:420-426.
31. Mushahwar IK: Hepatitis E virus: molecular virology, clinical features, diagnosis, transmission, epidemiology, and prevention. *J Med Virol* 2008;80:646-658.
32. Sehgal R, Sharma A: Hepatitis G virus (HGV): current perspectives. *Indian J Pathol Microbiol* 2002;45:123-128.
33. Ross JD, Smith IW, Elton RA: The epidemiology of herpes simplex types 1 and 2 infection of the genital tract in Edinburgh 1978-1991. *Genitourin Med* 1993;69:381-383.
34. Cesario T, Poland J, Wulff H, et al: Six years experience with herpes simplex virus in a children's home. *Am J Epidemiol* 1969;90:416-422.
35. Brown ZA, Wald A, Morrow RA, et al: Effect of serologic status and cesarean delivery on transmission rates of herpes simplex virus from mother to infant. *JAMA* 2003;289:203-209.
36. Tideman RL, Taylor J, Marks C, et al: Sexual and demographic risk factors for herpes simplex type 1 and 2 in women attending an antenatal clinic. *Sex Transm Infect* 2001;77:413-415.
37. Gupta R, Warren T, Wald A: Genital herpes. *Lancet* 2007;370:2127-2137.
38. Bays J, Jenny C: Genital and anal conditions confused with child sexual abuse trauma. *Am J Dis Child* 1990;144:1319-1322.
39. Stellrecht KA: Nucleic acid amplification technology for the diagnosis of genital herpes infection. *Expert Rev Mol Diagn* 2004;4:485-493.
40. Filén F, Strand A, Allard A, et al: Duplex real-time polymerase chain reaction assay for detection and quantification of herpes simplex virus type 1 and herpes simplex virus type 2 in genital and cutaneous lesions. *Sex Transm Dis* 2004;31:331-336.
41. Scoular A: Using the evidence base on genital herpes: optimizing the use of diagnostic tests and information provision. *Sex Transm Infect* 2002;78:160-165.
42. Ashley RI: Performance and use of HSV type-specific serology test kits. *Herpes* 2002;9:38-45.
43. McCormack O, Carboy J, Nguyen L, et al: Clinical inquiries. What is the role of herpes virus serology in sexually transmitted disease screening? *J Fam Pract* 2006;55:451-452.

44. Cernik C, Gallina K, Brodell RT: The treatment of herpes simplex infections. An evidence-based review. *Arch Intern Med* 2008;168: 1137-1144.

45. Gardner M, Jones JG: Genital herpes acquired by sexual abuse of children. *J Pediatr* 1984;101:243-244.

46. Douglas JM Jr: Molluscum contagiosum. *In*: Holmes KK, Sparling PF, Stamm WE, et al: *Sexually Transmitted Diseases*, ed 4, McGraw-Hill, New York, 2008, pp 545-552.

47. Brown J, Janniger CK, Schwartz RA, et al: Childhood molluscum contagiosum. *Int J Dermatol* 2006;45:93-99.

48. Sladden MJ, Johnston GA: Common skin infections in children. *Br Med J* 2004;329:95-99.

49. Smolinski KN, Yan AC: How and when to treat molluscum contagiosum and warts in children. *Pediatr Ann* 2005;34:211-221.

50. Centers for Disease Control and Prevention: *Trichomonas CDC fact sheet* (website): http://www.cdc.gov/STD/Trichomonas/STDFact-Trichomoniasis.htm. Accessed July 21, 2009.

51. Miller WC, Swygard H, Hobbs MM, et al: The prevalence of trichomonas in young adults in the United States. *Sex Transm Dis* 2005;32: 593-598.

52. Johnston VJ, Mabey DC: Global epidemiology and control of *Trichomonas vaginalis*. *Curr Opin Infect Dis* 2008;21:56-64.

53. McClelland RS, Sangare L, Hassan WM, et al: Infection with Trichomonas vaginalis increases the risk of HIV-1 acquisition. *J Infect Dis* 2007;195:698-702.

54. Fleming DT, Wasserheit JN: From epidemiological synergy to public health policy and practice: the contribution of other sexually transmitted diseases to sexual transmission of HIV infection. *Sex Transm Infect* 1999;75:3-17.

55. Fouts AC, Kraus SJ: *Trichomonas vaginalis*: Reevaluation of its clinical presentation and laboratory diagnosis. *J Infect Dis* 1980;141:137-143.

56. Kessel JF, Thompson CF: Survival of Trichomonas vaginalis in vaginal discharge. *Proc Soc Exp Biol Med* 1950;74:755-758.

57. Burch TA, Rees CW, Reardon LV: Epidemiological studies on human trichomoniasis. *Am J Trop Med Hyg* 1959;8:312-318.

58. Jenny C: Sexually transmitted diseases and child abuse. *Pediatr Ann* 1992;21:497-503.

59. Hobbs MM, Seña AC, Swygard H, et al: *Trichomonas vaginalis* and trichomoniasis. *In*: Holmes KK, Sparling PF, Stamm WE, et al: *Sexually Transmitted Diseases*, ed 4, McGraw-Hill, New York, 2008, pp 771-793.

60. Wallin JE, Thompson SE, Zaidi A, et al: Urethritis in women attending an STD clinic. *Br J Vener Dis* 1981;57:50-54.

61. Temesvári P, Kerekes A: Newborn with suppurative nasal discharge and respiratory distress. *Pediatr Infect Dis J* 2004;23:282-283.

62. Romoren M, Velauthapillai M, Rahman M: Trichomoniasis and bacterial vaginosis in pregnancy: inadequately managed with the syndromic approach. *Bull World Health Organ* 2007;85:297-304.

63. Krieger JN, Jenny C, Verdon M, et al: Clinical manifestations of trichomoniasis in men. *Ann Intern Med* 1993;118:844-849.

64. Huppert J, Mortensen J, et al: Rapid antigen testing compares favorably with transcription-mediated amplification assay for the detection of trichomonas vaginalis in young women. *Clin Infect Dis* 2007;45: 194-198.

65. Centers for Disease Control and Prevention: Sexually transmitted diseases treatment guidelines, 2006. *MMWR* 2006;55(RR 11):1-94. http://www.cdc.std/treatment/2006/rr511.pdf. Accessed July 21, 2009.

66. Karthikeyan K: Scabies in children. *Arch Dis Child Educ Pract Ed* 2007;92:e65-e69.

67. Walton SF, Currie BJ: Problems in diagnosing scabies, a global disease in human and animal populations. *Clin Microbiol Rev* 2007;20: 268-279.

68. Arlian LG, Runyan RA, Achar S, et al: Survival and infectivity of *Sarcoptes scabiei* var. *canis* and var. *hominis*. *J Am Acad Dermatol* 1984;11:210-215.

69. Falk ES, Bolle R: In vitro demonstration of specific immunological hypersensitivity to scabies mite. *Br J Dermatol* 1980;103:367-373.

70. Bechah Y, Capo C, Megfe JL, et al: Epidemic typhus. *Lancet Infect Dis* 2008;8:417-426.

71. Fournier PE, Ndihokubwayo JB, Guidran J, et al: Human pathogens in body and head lice. *Emerg Infect Dis* 2002;8:1515-1518.

72. Leone PA: Scabies and pediculosis pubis: an update of treatment regimens and general review. *Clin Infect Dis* 2007;44:S153-S159.

73. Chosidow O: Scabies and pediculosis. *Lancet* 2000;355:819-826.

24

HIV AND AIDS IN CHILD AND ADOLESCENT VICTIMS OF SEXUAL ABUSE AND ASSAULT

Amy P. Goldberg, MD

INTRODUCTION

The incidence of human immunodeficiency virus (HIV) infection in children and adolescents resulting from sexual abuse and assault is unknown. Still, clinician's caring for pediatric victims of sexual abuse/assault must have a coherent approach to HIV risk assessment, screening, and management to meet the needs of patients and families.

HIV virus is a lentivirus, a member of the Retroviridae family, that can cause acquired immunodeficiency syndrome (AIDS).[1] HIV can be found as a free virus within infected immune system cells. It can be transmitted sexually via blood, semen, preejaculate, or vaginal secretions. HIV infects helper T cells, macrophages, and dendritic cells (found in the mucosa). Infection leads to low levels of CD4 T helper cells through three mechanisms: direct killing of infected cells, increased rates of apoptosis in infected cells, and killing of infected CD4 cells by CD8 cytotoxic lymphocytes. Cell-mediated immunity is depleted when CD4 helper T cells decline below critical levels, making the host vulnerable to opportunistic infection.[1]

INTERSECTION OF AIDS AND HIV WITH CHILD SEXUAL ABUSE AND ASSAULT

Children and adolescents are at risk for HIV/AIDS. Of the 35,963 newly diagnosed patients with AIDS-defining illness in the United States in the year 2007, 563 (15.7%) were children and adolescents less than 20 years of age.[2] Perinatal transmission accounted for greater than 90% of the 9209 AIDS cases in children less than 13 years of age documented through 2007.[2] Unlike younger children, adolescents primarily contract HIV via sexual transmission. Half of all new HIV infections in the United States occur in young people 13 to 24 years old.[3,4] The prevalence of HIV infection in high-risk adolescents evaluated in a sexually transmitted disease clinic was greater than 1%.[5]

The Centers for Disease Control and Prevention (CDC) estimates that 1% of children with AIDS lack an ascribable risk.[6] The CDC categorizes the transmission of these children's infection as "other/risk factor not reported or identified."[7] In other words a category to describe transmission from sexual abuse or assault is not used by the CDC; hence determination of an accurate rate of exposure from child

sexual abuse is not possible. Current statistics possibly underestimate prevalence of abuse-related HIV infections in children.

In 1998, Lindegren et al[8] published a case series using surveillance data that described 26 children under 13 years of age who were sexually abused and became HIV infected. The data expanded upon previous case reports of children who contracted HIV/AIDS from sexual abuse.[9-15] This study appropriately recommends the consideration of sexual exposure (and therefore sexual abuse) for all HIV-infected children less than 13 years of age, particularly for those whose mothers are HIV antibody negative after birth. Sexual abuse, however, as a potential cause of HIV infection should not be excluded if the mother is HIV seropositive. The risk factors for both HIV transmission and sexual abuse can co-occur within family settings.[12] The Lindegren et al data is limited in that only 29 states were included in the review and children older than 13 years of age were excluded, which likely underestimates the number of children who contracted HIV from sexual abuse or assault. The publication of these studies and case reports brought the issue of sexual abuse as a risk factor for HIV/AIDS to the forefront, encouraging clinicians to consider HIV screening during abuse evaluations.

After sexual abuse/assault occurs, it is critical to address both the victims' *current* and *subsequent* risks of contracting HIV. The risk of contracting HIV is known to be increased in individuals with a history of sexual abuse.[16] Brown et al[17] found that adolescents in an inpatient psychiatric facility with a history of sexual abuse had less knowledge of HIV, less frequent use of condoms, and poorer impulse control compared with their peers. They concluded that sexual abuse was associated with HIV risk-related behaviors in this population. In another study,[18] adult survivors with an early and chronic sexual abuse history had a sevenfold increase in HIV risk behaviors. Lambert et al[19] sought to determine the HIV seroprevalence of high-risk groups in Bolivia, a country with an overall low prevalence of HIV infection. They studied long-distance truck and bus drivers, commercial sex workers, and street youth, and found that street youth had the highest HIV seroprevalence. The youth frequently engaged in "survival sex" to obtain money or food. In addition, almost all the street youth reported being sexually abused as children.

These and other studies have established the association between child sexual abuse and increased HIV risk-taking behaviors, and have implications for early intervention aimed at vulnerable populations.[20,21] Given these findings, clinician's evaluating runaway adolescents must routinely assess HIV risk and understand the importance of screening for sexual abuse to mitigate future HIV risk-taking behaviors.

While the incidence of HIV infection acquired by children from sexual abuse and assault is unknown, an emergent literature describes the atrocity of child sex workers and their high rates of HIV infection. Each year 80% of the 600,000 to 800,000 individuals trafficked over global borders are girls and women.[22] It is estimated that 45,000 people are trafficked for sex across U.S. borders.[23] Some of these rescued women and girls describe the means by which they were lured into sex work. They describe false promises of employment, marriage, or dubious invitations to social or religious events, while others were kidnapped or drugged. Approximately half of victims were trafficked by strangers, while the remainder were trafficked by intimate partners, friends, or family members.[22,24]

Along with mental health and societal consequences of child trafficking, children are at elevated risk of contracting HIV compared with their adult counterparts.[25] One recent study assessed the prevalence of HIV infection in 287 repatriated Nepalese sex trafficked girls and women.[26] Thirty-three (14.7%) were less than 14 years old and 76 (33.8%) were 15 to 17 years old. The study found that very young age was associated with an increased risk of HIV infection, where 60.6% of the youngest aged victims were HIV seropositive. Other factors associated with increased rates of HIV were duration of forced prostitution and being forced to work in more than one brothel. Physically, the immature genitalia of children and the increased cervical ectopy of young adolescents are thought to put them at increased risk of becoming infected with HIV.[27]

Younger victims are treated differently than older trafficked sex workers, reflecting their increased value in the trade. Younger victims carry an increased monetary worth because some "clients" prefer young girls/virgins. Also, in many countries, a myth persists that having sex with a virgin can cure HIV and other maladies (the "virgin cure").[28] In South Africa it is estimated that "dozens" of babies have been raped due to this horrifying mendacity.[29] Due in part to the higher monetary value of these younger victims, they are moved among brothels to avoid detection by law enforcement, thereby increasing the time of exploitation and HIV risk.[26]

Theses studies establish the high rate of HIV infection in sex trafficked individuals and in particular identify that younger victims are at even greater risk for HIV infection. This larger population of sexually abused children in addition to the multiple reported cases of HIV contracted after sexual abuse and assault provide the clinician with a critical reference when confronted with HIV risk assessment of sexually abused/assaulted children or adolescents.

RISK ASSESSMENT

To estimate HIV risk in the sexually abused/assaulted pediatric patient, the clinician must consider patient and perpetrator factors along with the reported features of the abuse/assault. Biological factors and the histology of the vagina and cervix influence the likelihood of a child or adolescent contracting HIV and other sexually transmitted infections (STI). After birth, as maternally derived estrogen levels decrease, squamous cells in the vaginal lining are replaced with columnar epithelium. The resulting lining is thin and fragile and more easily traumatized. During puberty, rising circulating estrogen causes gradual squamous epithelialization of the vagina. Columnar epithelium, however, persists around the cervical os (cervical *ectopy*). In pubertal females, cervical ectopy increases the risk of STI such as *Chlamydia trachomatis*.[27,30,31] Other STIs are known to induce an immune response that can facilitate the transmission of HIV-1.[32] Factors that compromise the integrity of the anal or genital mucosa such as physical trauma,[33] alone or in combination with underlying infections, increase the risk of children acquiring HIV during sexual abuse/assault.

The assailant's seropositivity (including viral load and clinical state) greatly influences the risk of HIV transmission to the victim.[34] Studies estimate that 80% of children know the perpetrators of their abuse.[35] While as many as half of rape victims know their assailant, very few know the assailant's HIV status.[36] Given these facts, the clinician should ask the victim and his/her nonoffending caregiver what (if anything) is known about the perpetrator's health and habits. From this information, a risk profile can be developed (e.g., history of intravenous drug use, male assailant having sex with men, history of current or previous incarceration, history of infected partners, or assailant known to be infected with HIV). Determining the number of assailants is also important during risk assessment.

When detailed information about the perpetrator is unavailable, the seroprevalence of the relevant community where the abuse/assault occurred should be considered. Different states have different rates of HIV prevalence. For example, a clinician in the District of Columbia would take into account the fact that the rate of HIV infection there is 264.9/100,000 as compared with the clinician in North Dakota, who would consider the state rate of 1.9/100,000.[37] In addition, for assaults that either occur in prison or if the perpetrator is known to have been incarcerated, HIV infection is 14 times more prevalent in prisoners compared with the general U.S. population.[38]

In addition to quantifying the risk of HIV transmission based on the assailant's seropositivity or risk profile, the clinician can evaluate the level of risk based on the type of exposure. Studies estimate the relative risk of becoming infected from a single act of unprotected receptive anal intercourse with a man of unknown HIV status is 1/10,000.[34] For receptive vaginal intercourse, the relative risk per event is much lower, 2/100,000.[34] These numbers are generated from studies of consenting adults, and do not account for the unique risks to children and adolescents discussed above. Additionally, when multiple acts of abuse/assault occur, the risk increases. Finally, in assault (as compared with consenting sexual contact), risk of genital and anal trauma are increased,[39] most likely leading to increased risk of infection as well.

Commonly, child sexual abuse/assault victims will not be able to clearly describe the sexual contact that occurred. Factors that affect their ability to relate a history of the assault include level of maturity and language development, lack of knowledge about sexual acts, threats from the perpetrator, fear of their parents' reactions to the disclosure, and embarrassment or guilt. Even with adolescents, the history is often limited. In a 2006 study of 145 sexually abused adolescents,[40] 21% reported a "black-out" during the assault, 54% were unsure whether ejaculation occurred, and 27% were unsure whether a condom had been used. History should be supplemented with information from others (caretakers, investigators, etc.) to obtain as complete a risk profile as possible.

Other important information to consider is the time that elapsed since the abuse/assault occurred. Postexposure prophylaxis is not recommended if the event occurred over 72 hours ago. Another important factor is whether the victim has obvious physical trauma noted on examination, increasing the exposure to risk.

With information about the history of the event, characteristics of the perpetrator, results of the physical examination, and consideration of the vulnerabilities of the particular victim, risk assessment should be conducted and patients should be tested for and counseled about HIV. If the patient is found to be HIV seropositive, immediate referral to a pediatric infectious disease specialist is indicated.

The 2005 guidelines from the CDC recommend that postexposure prophylaxis (PEP) be considered on a case-by-case basis after sexual assault if the assailant's HIV status is unknown.[41] In some cases, it can take time for investigators to collect the information needed to assess risk. Initially starting HIV PEP could be considered, and later discontinued if the assailant is identified and found to be HIV negative. A sensitive discussion with victims and their families regarding HIV exposure can help alleviate emotional stress. Discussion of avoidance of high-risk sexual behaviors with adolescents should be deferred to a more appropriate time.

Table 24-1 provides suggested risk categories for the purposes of summarizing case information related to HIV risk in the context of acute sexual assault. The risk assessment tool has not been tested clinically, but contains important factors to consider when deciding whether to prescribe PEP. Table 24-2 contains another schema, used by Garcia et al[42] to assign victims' risk for HIV after sexual assault.

POSTEXPOSURE PROPHYLAXIS

Currently, highly active antiretroviral therapy is used to treat HIV infection and AIDS. Medications are classified by the phase of the retrovirus' lifecycle they inhibit. For example, nucleoside and nucleotide reverse transcriptase inhibitors inhibit reverse transcription by incorporating into the viral DNA and preventing elongation, while protease inhibitors target viral assembly by inhibiting the activity of protease, an enzyme used by HIV to cleave nascent protein for final assembly of new virons.[43]

The presumed mechanism of the prophylactic use of antiretrovirals is based on the fact that a period of time exists after the body is exposed to HIV when the viral load is low enough to be controlled by the host's immune system. Antiretrovirals given during this time period may diminish or end viral replication, enabling the body's defenses to manage the reduced viral inoculum. Animal and human tissue studies indicate that the window of opportunity after mucosal exposure might be up to 72 hours.[44] Studies evaluating the use of antiretrovirals prophylactically were first conducted in pregnant women infected with HIV. These studies revealed a substantial reduction in the risk of both vertical and perinatal transmission.[45]

Table 24-1	**Risk Categories for HIV PEP Consideration for Pediatric Patients Who Present Within 72 Hours* After Sexual Assault**
High risk Recommend PEP	Patient discloses penile-anal or penile-vaginal penetration by a known HIV positive perpetrator
High-moderate risk Offer PEP	Patient is unable to clearly disclose type of sexual contact by a perpetrator with unknown HIV status *but* anogenital trauma is present
Moderate risk Consider PEP	Patient discloses penile-anal or penile-vaginal penetration by a perpetrator with unknown HIV status *and* anogenital trauma is absent *but* factors exist that may modify the risk from the exposure such as: Multiple assailants were involved Perpetrator is known to be from a high risk population or engage in high risk behaviors[†] The patient and/or perpetrator has coexisting anogenital infection
Low risk No PEP	Patient discloses sexual assault that does not involve anal, vaginal, or oral penetration Patient is unable to clearly disclose type of sexual contact by a perpetrator with unknown HIV status *and* anogenital trauma is absent, *and* there are no factors that exist or are known that modify the risk from the exposure Patient discloses oral penetration without ejaculation The perpetrator is known to be HIV negative

*PEP is generally recommended within the 72 hours; however, within the pediatric setting time frame can be difficult to ascertain from a child historian. If the sexual assault was particularly severe (anogenital trauma, multiple modifying risk factors) then HIV PEP may be offered outside of the 72-hour recommended timeframe.
[†]High-risk populations include males who engage in sexual activity with other men, injection drug users, a perpetrator who has a history of previous incarceration, a perpetrator who has sex with a member of a high-risk population, a juvenile perpetrator who is known to have been sexually abused by an adult from a high risk population.

Table 24-2	Severity Grade of Sexual Assault When Evaluating for Antiretroviral Prophylaxis

Severity Grade	Type of Exposure
Low	Vaginal/oral intercourse without ejaculation and without visible trauma Ejaculation on intact skin Assailant uses of condom throughout the incident Assailant is known to be HIV negative at the time of the initial evaluation of the victim
Medium	Vaginal/oral intercourse with ejaculation but without trauma
High	Anal penetration Vaginal exposure with genital trauma Exposure to more than one assailant Presence of factors that increase risk (inflammation, ulcers, bleeding, trauma, presence of lacerations or menstruation) Assailant known to be HIV positive

From Garcia MT, Figueiredo RM, Moretti ML, et al: Postexposure prophylaxis after sexual assaults: a prospective cohort study. *Sex Transm Dis* 2005;34:214-219.

Animal studies that exposed primates to simian immunodeficiency virus with subsequent administration of various antiretroviral medicines also have supported the use of HIV PEP. These data have been instrumental in underscoring the importance of rapid administration of HIV PEP and in establishing the appropriate duration of treatment.[46]

The development of guidelines for when to provide nonoccupational HIV PEP are partially based on the provision of HIV PEP in the occupational setting where the risk of HIV transmission after percutaneous needlestick is 3.2/1000, similar to that for some sexual exposures from a source known to be HIV positive.[47] In 1997, Cardo et al[48] retrospectively studied 712 health care workers exposed to HIV through needlesticks. The group found that the probability of HIV seroconversion was reduced by 81% in those who took an antiretroviral zidovudine. Even despite the small sample taking zidovudine, the retrospective study design, and other limitations, this study along with perinatal and animal studies established much of the basis for providing nonoccupational HIV PEP.[49]

In 1998, an expert panel concluded that data were lacking to recommend for or against the use of PEP for nonoccupational exposures.[49] That same year, Katz and Gerberding[50] outlined reasons for considering nonoccupational HIV PEP after sexual and injection drug exposures, recommending its use in certain cases. Several individual states have developed guidelines recommending HIV PEP after sexual exposure.[51-54] The American Academy of Pediatrics 2003 Clinical Report on PEP in children and adolescents with nonoccupational exposures provided comprehensive guidance regarding risk assessment and treatment, but ultimately the AAP did not definitively recommend HIV PEP after sexual exposures.[55] In January 2005, the CDC released guidelines

recommending the use of HIV PEP in uninfected patients who have high-risk sexual exposures to people with *known* HIV infection and who present for treatment within 72 hours of the exposure.[41] These guidelines assume knowledge of the source's HIV status, rarely the situation in either adult or child acute sexual assault. To date there are no nationally accepted guidelines for providing HIV PEP after an acute sexual assault when the assailant's HIV serostatus is unknown. Despite this, published adult studies have shown increasing standardization of HIV PEP provision and successful follow-up.[56-59]

An example is a recent prospective study of 347 sexual assault victims (97.4% female, median age of 20 years with 4.6% of victims less than 13 years of age).[57] Victims were assigned to one of three groups, depending on their level of risk for exposure to HIV. PEP was offered to 278 of the medium- and high-risk victims, all of whom accepted the medication. Subjects received either a two- drug or three-drug regimen. Sixty-seven percent of subjects completed 28 days of medication. None of the study subjects seroconverted when tested at 6 month follow-up. The authors emphasized the importance of follow-up for sexual assault victims and noted factors that influenced patients' compliance with the drug regimen, including their level of education, a 2- versus 3-day regimen, their knowledge that the assailant was HIV positive, and being in the groups that actually received medication.[57]

While the adult literature is helpful, children and adolescent victims of sexual assault have unique issues complicating risk assessment, subsequent provision of drug regimens, and adherence to PEP. A study by Babl[59] et al reflects the lack of standardization as compared with the adult experience. The researchers surveyed pediatric infectious disease specialists and pediatric emergency medicine physicians regarding nonoccupational PEP for pediatric patients. They found that inconsistent risk assessment factors were considered and a variety of drug regimens prescribed. Merchant et al[60] recently confirmed the variability in the tests and prophylactic regimens offered to adolescent victims of sexual assault. PEP was offered less commonly than other types of antimicrobial prophylaxis and was found to be the least often accepted by patients. The study authors discuss that factors that might interfere with patients accepting HIV PEP, including the high cost (especially for uninsured patients), the recommended duration of treatment, the adverse side effects, and "discouragement from clinicians.[60]" In another study, children prescribed HIV PEP after sexual assaults have been shown to have poor rates of medical follow-up.[61]

An important justification for the provisions of HIV PEP even if the HIV status of the perpetrator is unknown is that the acquisition of a life-threatening and life-changing infection after a forced sexual encounter compounds the trauma inherent in sexual assault and leads to an ongoing violation of the victim's personal integrity and safety.

TREATMENT GUIDELINES

Before the provision of HIV PEP, a discussion with the patient and his/her family must include the lack of conclusive data on HIV PEP efficacy. It also must be stressed, however, that if the patient is prescribed and accepts HIV

PEP, compliance and follow-up are essential. Emergency departments should have protocols in place for the provision of HIV PEP, and hospitals should have follow-up protocols to ensure that medication can be obtained and that consultation with pediatric specialists is available to monitor toxicity and to provide medication compliance and the patient's level of psychological stress.[55] Ideally all patients on PEP should be seen within 72 hours of the first visit to answer questions and to address any reported side effects from medications. Careful telephone follow-up frequently throughout the course of treatment can increase patient adherence and successful completion of the course of therapy.[62]

HIV PEP should be started as soon as possible after exposure and continued for 28 days. It is only indicated for seronegative patients, so a rapid HIV test should be obtained during the initial evaluation. Initial provision of PEP should not be delayed pending the results of the rapid test. Postmenarchal female patients must have a pregnancy test before starting therapy as some regimens are contraindicated in pregnancy. At a minimum, in addition to HIV and pregnancy testing, laboratory assessment for potential drug toxicity should initially include a complete blood cell count (CBC), liver function studies (LFTs), and blood urea nitrogen and creatinine (BUN/Cr). Follow-up at 2 weeks and 4 weeks should include repeat CBC, LFTs, and BUN/Cr. At 4 weeks, 3 months and 6 months serologic testing for HIV should be repeated.[55]

There are few contraindications to prescribing nonoccupational HIV PEP, as it is generally well tolerated. Patients, however, should be informed about associated adverse reactions. Depending on the regimen, the most common side effects are nausea, fatigue, diarrhea, vomiting, and anorexia.[63] There have been case reports of more severe adverse events including death.[64] Patients should be informed that medication side effects generally diminish with time and that medications are best tolerated with food.

Data on the optimal choice and number of antiretrovirals to prescribe after sexual assault is largely empirical. The current CDC guidelines endorse a three-drug regimen for nonoccupational exposures to a *known* HIV infected source.[41] The efficacy of a three-drug regimen brings a higher level of toxicity and might reduce adherence to a full 28 days of PEP. Because this situation (sexual assault by a person known to be infected with HIV) is infrequent, a two-drug therapy for lower risk situations should be considered[51,56,65] (see Table 24-1). These two-drug regimens often include zidovudine and lamivudine because of their reduction in HIV transmission in occupational settings and because they are generally well tolerated. They are also available as syrups for younger children and as a coformulated tablet, increasing compliance for adolescents.

Before any regimen is adopted, consultation should be sought from experts in HIV treatment or should be administered in compliance with updated hospital protocols developed with HIV specialists. For the latest information on doses and side effects of antiretroviral drugs refer to the United States Department of Health and Human Services website, AIDSInfo at: http://www.aidsinfo.nih.gov/DrugsNew/Default.aspx?MenuItem=Drugs or refer to the most updated CDC guidelines for nonoccupational HIV PEP with specific regard for the section related to children and adolescents.

STRENGTH OF THE MEDICAL EVIDENCE

Estimation of the prevalence of HIV after child sexual abuse and assault is limited. Information on reports of both child sexual abuse and about people with HIV infection and AIDS are extremely sensitive and confidential. Even though the exact rate of transmission of HIV during sexual assault/abuse is unknown, the clinician still has a responsibility to conduct a risk assessment of HIV transmission during the child's evaluation and make informed choices about prescribing PEP.

The justification for providing HIV PEP after pediatric sexual assault is extrapolated from the adult experience. Unlike the adult setting, which has succeeded in conducting prospective studies to evaluate the use of HIV PEP, the pediatric community lacks prospective data on the use of HIV PEP after sexual assault of children. The adult literature is also limited in that it is based on primate studies, from information about PEP in the occupational setting, and from studies of vertical transmission.

SUGGESTED DIRECTIONS FOR FUTURE RESEARCH

A prospective study evaluating protocols for postexposure prophylaxis for pediatric patients is needed. Such data could help clinicians create effective protocols for risk assessment, taking into consideration difficult yet common variables such as dealing with preverbal patient or with patients who are unwilling to provide a detailed history because of fear of repercussions. Additionally prospective data comparing efficacy and acceptability of drug regimens in the pediatric context would be helpful. Perhaps of greatest importance would be a comprehensive prospective study of factors affecting access to and use of follow-up care by pediatric patients after sexual assault/abuse. Using the medical context after sexual abuse and assault to understand the complex factors that lead to the abuse is a venue with potential for primary and secondary prevention that should be further explored for patients prescribed HIV PEP or not.

An additional area that deserves future attention is the critical problem of trafficked child sex workers. There has been significant worldwide prevention efforts aimed at supporting commercial sex workers by empowering them to negotiate condom use with clients, eliminating legal actions against commercial sex workers, and improving their access to health care.[66] While these projects are important there should be care in understanding that children are never "workers" within this context. These children are being exploited and abused. Different language should be used, describing them as *victims* and their assailants as *perpetrators* (rather than *"clients"* as is done in several scientific papers). Efforts to prevent the occurrence of this atrocity from both a supply and a demand standpoint must be strengthened.

References

1. Harrington PR, Swanstrom R: The biology of HIV, SIV and other lentiviruses. *In:* Holmes KK, Sparling PF, Stamm WE, et al: *Sexually Transmitted Diseases,* ed 4, McGraw-Hill, New York, 2008, pp 323-339.

2. U.S. Centers for Disease Control and Prevention: *HIV/AIDS surveillance report*, 2007, (website): http://www.cdc.gov/hiv/topics/surveillance/resources/reports/. Accessed April 13, 2009.

3. Wright KL: HIV and adolescents. *Clin Fam Pract* 2000;2:945-966.

4. Futterman D, Chabon B, Hoffman ND: HIV and AIDS in adolescents. *Pediatr Clin North Am* 2000;47:171-188.

5. Rother-Borus MJ, Futterman D: Promoting early detection of human immunodeficiency virus infection among adolescents. *Arch Pediatr Adolesc Med* 2000;154:435-439.

6. Hammett TA, Bush TJ, Ciesielski CA: *Pediatric AIDS cases reported with no identified risks*. Paper presented at annual meeting of the American Public Health Association, San Francisco, October, 1993.

7. Centers for Disease Control and Prevention: *AIDS public information data set* (website): http://wonder.cdc.gov/wonder/help/AIDS/APIDS2002.pdf. Accessed April 13, 2009.

8. Lindegren ML, Hanson IC, Hammett TA, et al: Sexual abuse of children: intersection with the HIV epidemic. *Pediatrics* 1998;102:E46.

9. Claydon E, Murphy S, Osborne EM, et al: Rape and HIV. *Int J STD AIDS* 1991;2:200-201.

10. Albert J, Wahlberg J, Leitner T, et al: Analysis of a rape case by direct sequencing of the human immunodeficiency virus type 1 pol and gag genes. *J Virol* 1994;68:5918-5924.

11. Murphy S, Kitchen V, Harris JR, et al: Rape and subsequent seroconversion to HIV. *Br Med J* 1989;299:718.

12. Gellert GA, Durfee MJ, Berkowitz CD, et al: Situational and sociodemographic characteristics of children infected with human immunodeficiency virus from pediatric sexual abuse. *Pediatrics* 1993;91:39-44.

13. Gutman L, St Claire KK, Weedy C, et al: Human immunodeficiency virus transmission by child sexual abuse. *Am J Dis Child* 1991;145:137-141.

14. Persaud D, Chandwani S, Rigaud M, et al: Delayed recognition of human immunodeficiency virus infection in preadolescent children. *Pediatrics* 1992;90:688-691.

15. Leiderman IZ, Grimm KT: A child with HIV infection. *JAMA* 1986;256:1094.

16. Zierler S, Feingold L, Laufer D, et al: Adult survivors of childhood sexual abuse and subsequent risk of HIV infection. *Am J Public Health* 1991;81:572-575.

17. Brown L, Lourie KJ, Zlotnick C, et al: Impact of sexual abuse on the HIV-risk-related behavior of adolescents in intensive psychiatric treatment. *Am J Psychiatry* 2000;157:1413-1415.

18. Bensley LS, Van Eenwyk J, Simmons KW: Self-reported childhood sexual and physical abuse and adult HIV-risk behaviors and heavy drinking. *Am J Prev Med* 2000;18:151-158.

19. Lambert ML, Torrico F, Billot C, et al: Street youth are the only high-risk group for HIV in a low-prevalence South American country. *Sex Transm Dis* 2005;32:240-242.

20. Stoltz JA, Shannon K, Zhang R, et al: Association between childhood maltreatment and sex work in a cohort of youth. *Soc Sci Med* 2007;65:1214-1221.

21. Dickson-Gomez J, Bodnar G, Gueverra A, et al: Childhood sexual abuse and HIV risk among crack-using commercial sex workers in San Salvador, El Salvador: a qualitative analysis. *Med Anthropol Q* 2006;20;545-574.

22. Barrows J, Finger R: Human trafficking and the healthcare professional. *South Med J* 2008;101:521-524.

23. US Department of State: *Trafficking in persons report, June 2008* (website): http://www.state.gov/documents/organization/105501.pdf. Accessed April 13, 2009.

24. Beyrer C, Stachowiak J: Health consequences of trafficking of women and girls in Southeast Asia. *Brown J World Aff* 2003;10:105-117.

25. Sarkar K, Bal B, Mukherjee R, et al: Young age is a risk factor for HIV among sex workers- an experience from India. *J Infect* 2006;53:255-259.

26. Silverman JG, Decker MR, Gupta J, et al: HIV prevalence and predictors of infection in sex-trafficked Nepalese girls and women. *JAMA* 2007;298:536-542.

27. Moscicki A, Ma Y, Holland C, et al: Cervical ectopy in adolescent girls with and without human immunodeficiency virus infection. *J Infect Dis* 2001;183:865-870.

28. Meel BL: The myth of child rape as a cure for HIV/AIDS in Transkei: a case report. *Med Sci Law* 2003;43:85-88.

29. Sidley J: Doctor reprimanded for giving antiretroviral drug to baby who was raped. *Br Med J* 2002;324:191.

30. Berman SM, Ellen JM: Adolescents and STDs including HIV infection. In: Holmes Kk, Sparling PF, Stamm WE, et al: *Sexually Transmitted Diseases*, ed 4, McGraw-Hill, New York, 2008, pp 165-186.

31. Royce RA, Sena A, Cates W, et al: Sexual transmission of HIV. *N Eng J Med* 1997;336:1072-1078.

32. Fleming D, Wasserheit J: From epidemiological synergy to public health policy and practice: the contribution of other sexually transmitted diseases to sexual transmission of HIV infection. *Sex Transm Infect* 1999;75:3-17.

33. Lauber AA, Souma ML: Use of toluidine blue for documentation of traumatic intercourse. *Obstet Gynecol* 1982;60:644-648.

34. Varghese B, Maher JE, Peterman TA, et al: Reducing the risk of sexual HIV transmission: quantifying the per act risk for HIV on the basis of choice of partner, sex act, and condom use. *Sex Transm Dis* 2002;29:38-43.

35. Finkelhor D, Hammer H, Sedlak AJ: *Sexually assaulted children: national estimates and characteristics. National incidence studies of missing, abducted, runaway, and thrown away children*, Office of Juvenile Justice & Delinquency Prevention, U.S. Department of Justice (website): http://www.ncjrs.gov/pdffiles1/ojjdp/214383.pdf. Accessed April 14, 2009.

36. Du Mont J, Myhr TL, Husson H, et al: HIV postexposure prophylaxis use among Ontario female adolescent sexual assault victims: a prospective analysis. *Sex Transm Dis* 2008;35:973-978.

37. Henry Kaiser State Health Facts (website): http://www.statehealthfacts.org/comparecat.jsp?cat=11. Accessed March 10, 2010.

38. Gostin LO, Lazzarini Z, Alexander D, et al: HIV testing, counseling and prophylaxis after sexual assault. *JAMA* 1994;271:1436-1444.

39. Slaughter L, Brown CR, Crowley S, et al: Patterns of genital injury in female sexual assault victims. *Am J Obstet Gynecol* 1997;176:609-616.

40. Olshen E, Hsu K, Woods E, et al: Use of human immunodeficiency virus postexposure prophylaxis in adolescent sexual assault victims. *Arch Pediatr Adolesc Med* 2006;160:674-680.

41. Smith DK, Grohskopf LA, Black RJ, et al: Antiretroviral postexposure prophylaxis after sexual, injection drug-use, or other nonoccupational exposures to HIV in the United States: recommendations from the U.S. Department of Health and Human Services. *MMWR Recomm Rep* 2005;54:1-20.

42. Garcia MT, Figueiredo RM, Moretti ML, et al: Postexposure prophylaxis after sexual assaults: a prospective cohort study. *Sex Transm Dis* 2005;32:214-219.

43. Eron JJ, Hirsch MS: Antiviral therapy of human immunodeficiency virus infection. In: Holmes KK, Sparling PF, Stamm WE, et al: *Sexually Transmitted Diseases*, ed 4, McGraw-Hill, New York, 2008, pp 1393-1421.

44. Otten RA, Smith DK, Adams DR, et al: Efficacy of postexposure prophylaxis after intravaginal exposure to pig-tailed macaques to a human-derived retrovirus (human immunodeficiency virus type 2). *J Virol* 2000;74:9771-9775.

45. The Petra Study Team: Efficacy of three short-course regimens of zidovudine and lamivudine in preventing early and late transmission of HIV-1 from mother to child in Tanzania, South Africa, and Uganda (Petra study): a randomized, double blind, placebo-controlled trial. *Lancet* 2002;359:1178-1186.

46. Tsai CC, Emau P, Follis KE, et al: Effectiveness of postinoculation of (R)-9-(2 phosphonylmethoxypropyl) adenine treatment for prevention of persistent simian immunodeficiency virus SIV (mne) infection depends critically on timing of initiation and duration of treatment. *J Virol* 1998;72:4265-4273.

47. Gerberding JL: Prophylaxis for occupational exposure to HIV. *Ann Intern Med* 1996;125:497-501.

48. Cardo DM, Culver DH, Ciesielski CA, et al: A case-control study of HIV seroconversion in health care workers after percutaneous exposure. *N Engl J Med* 1997;331:1485-1490.

49. Centers for Disease Control and Prevention: Management of possible sexual, injecting drug-use, or other non-occupational exposure to HIV, including consideration related to antiretroviral therapy. Public health services statement. *MMWR Recomm Rep* 1998;47(RR-17):1-14.

50. Katz MH, Gerberding JL: The care of persons with recent sexual exposure to HIV. *Ann Intern Med* 1998;128:306-312.

51. NY State Department of Health AIDS Institute: *HIV prophylaxis following nonoccupational exposure including sexual assault*. New York State Coalition Against Sexual Assault, New York, 2008. Available at http://www.hivguidelines.org/GuideLine.aspx?guideLineID=2. Accessed April 14, 2009.

52. Merchant RC, Mayer KH, Browning CA: Nonoccupational HIV post-exposure prophylaxis: guidelines for Rhode Island from the Brown University AIDS program and the RI Department of Health. *Med Health R I* 2002;85:244-248.

53. Myles JE, Bamberger J, Housing and Urban Health of the San Francisco, Department of Public Health, California HIV PEP After Sexual Assault Task Force, California State Office of AIDS: *Offering HIV prophylaxis following sexual assault, 2001*, California Department of Health (website): http://www.dhs.ca.gov/ps/ooa/Reports/PDF/HIVProphylaxisFollowingSexualAssault. Accessed April 14, 2009.

54. Koh HK, De Maria A, McGuire JF: *HIV prophylaxis for nonoccupational exposures*, Office of Health and Human Services, Commonwealth of Massachusetts (website): http://www.mass.gov/dph/aids. Accessed April 14, 2009.

55. Havens P, Committee on Pediatric AIDS: Postexposure prophylaxis in children and adolescents for nonoccupational exposure to human immunodeficiency virus. *Pediatrics* 2003;111:1475-1489.

56. Gerard JB, Sonder MD, Van Den Hoek A, et al: Trends in HIV postexposure prophylaxis prescription and compliance after sexual exposure in Amsterdam, 2000-2004. *Sex Transm Dis* 2007;34:288-293.

57. Garcia MT, Figueiredo RM, Moretti ML, et al: Postexposure prophy-laxis after sexual assaults: a prospective cohort study. *Sex Transm Dis* 2005;32:214-219.

58. Schechter M, do Lago RF, Mendelsohn AB, et al: Behavioral impact, acceptability, and HIV incidence among homosexual men with access to postexposure chemoprophylaxis or HIV. *J Acquir Immune Defic Syndr* 2004;35:519-525.

59. Babl FE, Cooper ER, Kastner B, et al: Prophylaxis against human immunodeficiency virus exposure after nonoccupational needlestick injuries or sexual assaults in children and adolescents. *Arch Pediatr Adolesc Med* 2001;155:680-682.

60. Merchant RC, Kelly ET, Mayer K, et al: Compliance in Rhode Island emergency departments with American Academy of Pediatrics recom-mendations for adolescent sexual assaults. *Pediatrics* 2008;121:e1660-e1667.

61. Babl FE, Cooper ER, Damon B, et al: HIV postexposure prophylaxis for children and adolescents. *Am J Med* 2000;18:282-287.

62. Goldberg AP, Duffy SJ: Medical care for the sexual assault victim. *Med Health R I* 2003;86:390-394.

63. Luque A, Hulse S, Wang D, et al: Assessment of adverse events associ-ated with antiretroviral regimens for postexposure prophylaxis for occupational and nonoccupational exposures to prevent transmission of human immunodeficiency virus. *Infect Control Hosp Epidemiol* 2007;28:695-701.

64. Centers for Disease Control and Prevention: Serious adverse events attributed to nevirapine regimens for postexposure prophylaxis after HIV exposures -worldwide, 1997-2000. *MMWR Morb Mortal Wkly* 2001;49:1153-1156.

65. Merchant RC, Keshavarz R: HIV postexposure prophylaxis practices by U.S. ED practitioners. *Am J Emerg Med* 2003;21:309-312.

66. *Sex work and HIV/AIDS. UNAIDS technical update June, 2002*, UNAIDS (website): Available at http://data.unaids.org/Publications/IRC-pub02/jc705-sexwork-tu_en.pdf. Accessed April 15, 2009.

LABORATORY METHODS FOR DIAGNOSING SEXUALLY TRANSMITTED INFECTIONS IN CHILDREN AND ADOLESCENTS

Kimberle C. Chapin, MD

This chapter will address laboratory methods for diagnosing sexually transmitted infections (STIs). Both point-of-care tests (POCT) and laboratory performed tests can be used to identify the microbiological causes of sexually transmitted infections. Diagnostic methods can be separated by the specific pathogen, such as *Chlamydia trachomatis* and/or by the clinical presentation, such as cutaneous genital lesions or urethritis. Critical in potential sexual abuse or assault, the combination of attaining a detailed history of sexual victimization, recognizing significant symptoms and signs of STIs, and obtaining the appropriate specimens for testing are all required to optimize accurate STI diagnoses.

Table 25-1 lists the common STIs that are of note when identified in children and adolescents along with the test methods currently available for identification. Commentary on a test method is noted in the table or the text where appropriate. The methods listed should not be taken as a validation of the method compared with current recommended STI diagnostic testing guidelines specifically as they relate to children and sexual abuse/assault, but rather as a full menu from which to assess all methods. It should be recognized that diagnostic test methods are not specifically developed for detection of pathogens in children and that FDA-cleared tests for detection of STIs do not give a lower age limit in which patients they should be used. Most clinical trials for STIs, however, are performed in people older than 18 years of age. Which test methodology to use in evaluating children's specimens ultimately should be decided among the healthcare providers caring for these children in conjunction with the laboratory so that each is aware of issues relating to children and adolescents when sexual assault or abuse is considered.

The Centers for Disease Control and Prevention (CDC) have recently reported sequential yearly increases for cases of the three major reportable STIs, *Chlamydia trachomatis* (CT), *Neisseria gonorrhoeae* (GC), and syphilis, by 6%, 6%, and 14%, respectively, and an increase in cases of human immunodeficiency virus (HIV).[1,2] Nonreportable infections, including herpes simplex virus (HSV), *Trichomonas vaginalis,* and human papilloma virus (HPV), are likely to have increased as well. Thus the presence of STIs in the general population is high with more than 19 million occurring annually in the United States.[2,3]

Routine screening for STIs in sexually victimized children younger than 15 years old is under debate.[1,4-7] The most recently published general references in pediatrics on sexual abuse in children state approximately 5% of sexually abused children acquire an STI, but numbers of reported cases vary depending on age, gender, and test methodology.[6-10] This percentage is higher than what would be seen in a low-risk population for STIs.[1,2] Data on the incidence of STIs in children to date is based almost exclusively on culture methodologies for the most common STI pathogens, including bacterial, viral, and parasitic. In addition, not all children who have an STI show signs of infection (e.g., vaginal discharge) or claim they have been victimized.[4,5,10] Thus these patients might not even be among those being considered for testing. As has been noted in sexually active adolescents and adults where more sensitive test methods, specifically nucleic acid amplification tests (NAATs) are the recommended methodology (chlamydia*)*, the majority of patients are asymptomatic.[1] Thus it might stand to reason that more infections in children might be identified with the use of NAATs as well. A significant body of data remains to be provided.

SPECIMEN COLLECTION

In those children where specimens will be collected for culture, all specimens should be obtained at the initial visit if prophylactic therapy will be provided. Specimen sites for collection are recommended to be done selectively based on the patient's history; evidence of genital, oral, or anal penetration; or actual signs of STIs, such as ulcers or lesions. If one STI is detected, others should be assessed for as well.[1] Timing for serological tests depends on the probable duration of abuse. Most infectious diseases will take up to 2 weeks to have sufficient concentration for culture techniques (CT and GC) and up to 12 weeks for antibody response (HIV, HBV, syphilis).[11-15] Thus follow-up visits and testing are usually required. If abuse is suspected to have been long term, fewer visits might be required because of initial STI test positivity. Typically, an initial visit and a 2-week follow-up visit with visual inspection and collection of cultures are warranted from all vesicular or ulcerative lesions and any discharge. Treatment and testing guidelines currently available from the Centers for Disease Control[1] and Prevention (CDC) and the American Academy of Pediatrics (AAP)[7] differ slightly in their emphasis on preferred testing

Text continued on p. 198

Table 25-1 Diagnostic Tests for Sexually Transmitted Infections

Organism	Diagnostic Procedures	Test Names	Optimal Specimens	Transport Temperature/Time to Laboratory	Special Considerations for Test Method
Chlamydia trachomatis	NAAT*	Roche Amplicor CT and GC (Roche Molecular Diagnostics, Indianapolis); APTIMA Combo2 (Gen-Probe, Inc., San Diego), and BD ProbeTec (Becton Dickinson, Sparks, Md.)	Urine, endocervical, vaginal, and/or urethral swab	RT†/days	NAATs for CT do not distinguish between CT serovars. Sensitivity better than culture; may be considered in children when culture is not available. NAAT is not an FDA-cleared test for rectal or pharyngeal sources; availability is laboratory specific. NAAT recommended for patients >15.
	Hybridization probe	Digene Hybrid Capture II test CT/GC test (Digene, Silver Spring, Md.) and PACE 2C (CT/GC) (Gen-Probe, Inc., San Diego)	Endocervical or urethral swab	RT/days	Less sensitive than NAATs. Not cleared by FDA for urine specimens. Digene test not cleared for males.
	Cultures		Endocervical, urethral, or conjunctival swab	Refrigerate/<2 hours	Less sensitive that NAATs. Pharynx and rectal swab cultures have very poor sensitivity.
	DFA‡		Endocervical, urethral, or conjunctival swabs	RT/2 hours	Sensitivity equal to culture. Allows for assessment of adequacy of specimen.
Neisseria gonorrhoeae	Gram stain		Urethral discharge	RT/2 hours	For males with discharge. In sexual abuse cases, culture discharge.
	NAAT	Roche Amplicor CT and GC (Roche Molecular Diagnostics, Indianapolis); APTIMA Combo2 (Gen-Probe, Inc., San Diego), and BD ProbeTec (Becton Dickinson, Sparks Md.)	Urine, endocervical, and/or urethral swabs	RT/days	NAATs for CT do not distinguish between CT serovars. Sensitivity better than culture; may be considered in children when culture is not available. NAAT is not an FDA-cleared test for rectal or pharyngeal sources; availability is laboratory specific. Provider should check with laboratory for optimal specimen source. NAAT recommended for patients >15. More sensitive than culture in pharyngeal and rectal specimens.

Organism	Method	Specimen	Transport/storage	Comments
	Hybridization probe	Endocervical or urethral swab	RT/days	Not sensitive enough for primary screen test in sexual assault. Neither test FDA cleared for urine specimens; Digene test not cleared for males.
	Digene Hybrid Capture II test CT/GC test (Qiagen, Inc, Valencia, Calif.) and PACE 2C (CT/GC) (Gen-Probe, Inc., San Diego, Calif.)			
	Culture, direct inoculation onto media, optimal with CO_2 tablet	Endocervical, urethral, conjunctival, pharyngeal, or rectal swab	RT/≤6 hours; do not refrigerate specimen	Vancomycin in media inhibits some GC strains. Culture allows for antimicrobial susceptibility testing.
Herpes simplex virus types 1 and 2	DFA	Scraping of lesion base; swab rolled directly onto slide	RT/2 hours	Need epithelial cells for adequate examination.
	Culture	Scraping of lesion base and placed in VTM§; in infants, swab throat, nasopharynx, eyes, and rectum	VTM at RT/ refrigerated or on ice	Some samples can be maintained and shipped at RT, and other labs use a universal transport media adequate for CT and viruses. Check with laboratory for details.
	NAAT	Swab of lesion in VTM	RT/2 hours	Not cleared by FDA; availability is laboratory specific. Check with laboratory for optimal specimen source.
	Serology	Blood	None	Serology should be limited to patients with clinical presentation consistent with HSV but with negative cultures. For determination of asymptomatic carriers request type-specific glycoprotein based assays that differentiate between HSV-1 and HSV-2. See text for specific indications.
Treponema pallidum (syphilis)	Dark field microscopy	Cleanse lesion with gauze and saline. Swab lesion base directly to slide.	RT/immediately to laboratory	Not widely available. Must see motile spirochetes.

Continued

Table 25-1 Diagnostic Tests for Sexually Transmitted Infections—cont'd

Organism	Diagnostic Procedures	Test Names	Optimal Specimens	Transport Temperature/ Time to Laboratory	Special Considerations for Test Method
	DFA—Treponema pallidum (DFA-TP) slide test		Cleanse lesion with gauze and saline; swab lesion base	RT/days	Viable organisms not required. Limited availability; is offered in some public health laboratories.
	Serology—Nontreponemal	Rapid reagin (RPR) and Venereal Disease Research Laboratory (VDRL)	Serum	RT/2 hours	Less sensitive in early and late disease. Becomes negative after treatment.
	Serology—Treponemal	Enzyme immunoassay (EIA) formats, T. pallidum particle agglutination (TP-PA), and fluorescent treponemal antibody absorbed (FTA-ABS)	Serum	RT/2 hours	Follow titers using same test and/or lab. Positive for life after infection.
	NAAT		Lesion swab	RT/2 hours	Not an FDA-cleared specimen source or test; availability is laboratory specific. Check with laboratory for optimal specimen source. Currently only for research use.
Yeast	Wet mount and 10% potassium hydroxide (KOH)/pH strip		Swab of vaginal discharge submitted in 5 mL saline or culturette	RT/1-2 hours	Sensitivity of wet mount is 40% to 90%. Can visualize yeast mycelial elements. pH <4.5.
	Culture		Swab of vaginal discharge submitted in culturette	RT/12 hours	Consider when smear is negative or with history of antibiotics.
	Hybridization probe	Affirm VP III Assay (Becton Dickinson, Sparks, Md.)	Swab of vaginal discharge	RT/days	Special transport tube required. Does not rely on viable organisms for optimal test performance. Not recommended in children.
Bacterial vaginosis	Wet mount with 10% KOH/pH strip		Swab of vaginal discharge submitted in 0.5 mL saline or culturette	RT/2 hours	Visualize clue cells in wet mount. Amine odor detected when 10% KOH is added. pH >4.5. Culture not recommended.

	Method	Product	Specimen	Transport/Time	Comments
	Quantitative gram stain using Nugent criteria		Swab of vaginal discharge into culturette	RT/12 hours	Most specific stain procedure for BV. Culture not recommended.
	Hybridization probe	Affirm VP III Assay (Becton Dickinson, Sparks, Md.)	Swab of vaginal discharge	RT/days	Does not rely on viable organisms for optimal test performance. Special transport tube required. Specificity is limited. Not recommended in children.
Trichomonas vaginalis	Wet mount and 10% KOH/pH strip		Swab of vaginal discharge submitted in saline	RT/30 minutes to 1 hour	Smear sensitivity 50% to 70%. Trichomonads exhibit jerky motion. Amine odor detected when 10% KOH is added. pH >4.5.
	Rapid antigen test	OSOM Trichomonas Rapid Test (Genzyme, Diagnostics, Cambridge, Mass.)	Swab of vaginal discharge in culturette or saline	RT/24 hours	Does not require live organisms for optimal test performance. Sensitivity 70% to 80% compared with culture. Performance tested only in symptomatic women.
	Hybridization probe	Affirm VP III Assay (Becton Dickinson, Sparks, Md.)	Swab of vaginal discharge	RT/days	Special transport tube required. Does not rely on viable organisms for optimal test performance. Not recommended in children.
	Culture	InPouch TV culture system (Biomed Diagnostics) or Empyrean Diagnostics	Swab of vaginal discharge into culture pouch system	RT/48 hours	Allows both immediate smear and subsequent culture. Not widely available. Sensitivity approximately 70%.
	NAAT				Not FDA cleared. Availability is laboratory specific. Check with laboratory for optimal specimen source. Sensitivity greater than culture.
Lice	Macroscopic and microscopic visualization		Collect parasite into clean container	RT/24 hours	Body lice and pubic lice are distinguishable microscopically.

*NAAT, Nucleic acid amplification test.
†RT, Room temperature.
‡DFA, Direct fluorescent antibody.
§VTM, Viral transport media.

methodologies. The AAP guideline lists the common STIs that should be considered and the sexual abuse interpretation and suggested action if the patient is found to have the pathogen from specimens tested. The CDC STD guidelines outline specific test methodologies and follow-up testing schedules. Because some pathogens can be acquired perinatally or by vertical transmission, this possibility should be excluded before making an assessment of sexual abuse based on the identification of the pathogen.[1,7]

Chlamydia trachomatis (CT) and Neisseria gonorrhoeae (GC)

CT and GC are the most commonly identified bacterial STIs as causes of urethritis and cervicitis in the United States in patients that are sexually active. In prepubertal children and adolescents that have been sexually assaulted, these are the most common bacterial STIs identified as well.[1,7]

Typical sites infected include the urethra in males, the endocervix with concomitant urethral infection occurring in 70% to 90% in postpubescent females, and the vaginal orifice and urethra in prepubertal girls. Asymptomatic infection is common at all sites. Recent increased infections identified for CT and GC from oropharyngeal and rectal specimens have also identified that males, females, and children are more commonly asymptomatic at these sites as well.[11,12] Conjunctival or pharyngeal infection can occur in newborns of infected women, but beyond the perinatal period both CT and GC infections are considered to be infections of probable sexual abuse. In consideration of specimen collection sites for children specifically, GC and CT preferentially infect the columnar epithelium, thus in prepubertal children the urethra, vagina, pharynx, and rectum are at risk and in postpubertal children, the endocervix rather than the vagina is more appropriate to consider for testing.[11,12]

Many methods exist for laboratory detection of GC and CT. Testing for both organisms are typically requested simultaneously and for those test systems where both are assessed from a single specimen both pathogens will be discussed. Overall, NAATs are the preferred assays for detection of CT and GC in most patient settings because of increased sensitivity while retaining specificity even in low prevalence populations and the ability to screen with noninvasive specimens.[1,16] While culture is still the recommended test for detection of GC and CT in sexually assaulted and/or abused children when available,[1,7] recent literature suggests that noninvasive urine testing by NAATs in female victims is both adequate and preferred.[17] All diagnostic methods for these two STIs are presented since guidelines in testing postpubertal females and males recommend a variety of methods for screening, diagnosis, and treatment. Specifically, in cases where a previous sexual history is identified, and because the risk of STIs is highest among 15 to 19 year olds, the more sensitive CT/GC NAAT methods are likely to be more appropriate for treatment purposes in adolescents.[1]

For GC culture, swab specimens should be either Dacron or rayon, as calcium alginate and cotton can be toxic to the organism. Lubricants other than water or saline in obtaining speculum samples should not be used as they can be toxic to organisms as well. Specimens in prepubertal females should be collected at the vaginal orifice or vaginal walls and left for

10 to 15 seconds to absorb any secretions. For optimal detection of GC by culture, swabs should be directly inoculated onto growth medium (such as JEMBEC plates [Remel, Inc., Lenexa, Kan.], Gono-Pak [BD Biosciences, San Jose, Calif.], or the InTray GC System [BioMed Diagnostics, Inc., San Jose, Calif.]) Each of these systems uses a bicarbonate citric acid pellet that optimizes organism growth for GC when CO_2 is generated. Swabs inoculated in nonnutritive transport systems, such as Stuart's or Aime's buffered media, can also be used. Viable organisms decrease after 6 hours and significantly at 24 hours and if the specimens are refrigerated.[12] Culture in the laboratory is done using selective media that inhibit normal flora but allow the pathogenic Neisseria spp. to grow. Media plates are held for 72 hours before discarding. Initial suspicious colonies, presumptively identified as GC-based on gram stain, positive oxidase, and growth on selective media, are subsequently identified by at least two other specific identification methods in patient isolates where sexual abuse or assault is a consideration. These methods include acid production from carbohydrates, chromogenic substrate tests, monoclonal antibody tests, and the direct hybridization GC probe (Accuprobe N. gonorrhoeae Culture Confirmation Test [Gen-Probe, Inc.] Tests that detect acid production from glucose and the probe confirmation test provide the least equivocal results. A unique advantage of culture is the ability to perform susceptibility testing on the recovered isolate when necessary.[12] While GC culture is quite sensitive and specific with invasive urogenital specimens, issues with organism viability due to delay in transport, the presence of vancomycin in the media that may be inhibitory to the organism, the inability to use urine specimens, and the poor sensitivity in rectal and pharyngeal specimens, have made nonculture amplified molecular methods preferred by most health care providers and laboratories.[12]

Not all NAATs are equal in sensitivity or specificity from all specimen sites for GC. The first generation NAAT PCR test, Amplicor, (Roche Diagnostics) was not FDA-cleared for detection of GC from urine in women due to low sensitivity. In addition, this same assay has been shown to have false positive results due to other nonpathogenic Neisseria spp. as well as the BD ProbeTec.[18,19] The APTIMA Combo 2 has not been shown to yield false positive results in women with a low prevalence of GC to date.[12,20]

POCTs used in sexually active males that have urethritis, such as the gram stain and leukocyte esterase dipstick, are not recommended in children.

Chlamydia are obligate intracellular pathogens and specimens for culture must be transported and inoculated into a susceptible cell line as soon as possible. Optimally, specimens should be refrigerated for transport and processed within 24 hours.[11] As with GC, swabs tips should be Dacron and not be calcium alginate or wooden-shafted, which are inhibitory to chlamydia. Specimens are typically collected into a media with antibiotics that inhibit other bacterial flora, such as 2-sucrose-phosphate (2-SP). Some laboratories use a universal transport media that allows detection of both viruses and chlamydia. Optimally, if invasive specimens will be collected from the urethra, endocervix, or even the vagina, purulent discharge should be removed first because these may be inhibitory to CT culture. Performance parameters of CT culture yield excellent specificity but poor sensitivity (40%-70%) when compared with NAATs. Presently, both the availability of cell culture and ability to provide well-performed culture technique is limited.[11]

The CDC recommends that specimens for CT culture be collected from the vagina in prepubescent children and the urethra of boys, with meatal discharge in males being adequate if present.[1] Culture confirmation by a specific CT monoclonal antibody test is required. Amplified test methods, with the use of a second confirmatory NAAT, may be an alternative where culture is not available.[1] CDC does not recommend obtaining rectal or pharyngeal specimens for CT culture because the yield is so poor. Recent evaluations of molecular methods from these specimen sites has also identified the asymptomatic nature of many pharyngeal and rectal infections.[21,22]

The direct fluorescent antibody test (DFA) can be used to detect the presence of intracytoplasmic inclusions in epithelial cells in smears from specimens collected for CT and uses a monoclonal antibody directed at a *C. trachomatis*-specific epitope of the major outer membrane protein (MOMP). The specimen can be assessed for adequacy of the sample by looking for columnar epithelial cells on the slide. The DFA test is used as an alternative to culture for rectal, pharyngeal, and/or conjunctival specimen sites where culture has very poor sensitivity. Overall sensitivity is 75% to 85% compared with culture for invasive specimens.[11]

Current enzyme immunoassay (EIA) formats use monoclonal or polyclonal antibodies to detect CT lipopolysaccharide (LPS). Both laboratory and point-of-care formats exist. Sensitivity ranges from 62% to 72% compared with culture. Many false-positive results occur with the EIA formats because of the cross-reactivity with the LPS of other microorganisms. These tests should not be used in children where sexual assault or abuse is a concern.[23]

Two molecular hybridization formats exist for detection of GC and CT, the Digene Hybrid Capture II CT/GC test (Qiagen, Inc., Valencia, Calif.) and the PACE 2C (CT/GC), (Gen-Probe, Inc, San Diego). These tests offer the advantage of detection of both pathogens from one sample, but require an invasive specimen (urethral/endocervical swabs only). The Digene test is not approved for testing in men but is approved for testing of GC/CT and HPV from a liquid cytology specimen, which may offer convenience in limited settings. The PACE test is FDA-cleared for conjunctival specimens in newborns for both CT and GC. Importantly,

while hybridization tests are equal to culture sensitivity for detection of GC they are not as sensitive as NAAT for CT. The tests are neither sensitive enough nor have the ability to be confirmed by a secondary probe methodology and should not be used in sexual abuse or assault cases.[3,24]

Currently, three FDA-cleared NAATs exist for GC and CT in the United States, each using a different molecular strategy; Roche Amplicor CT and GC (Roche Molecular Diagnostics, Indianapolis), APTIMA Combo2 (Gen-Probe, San Diego), and BD ProbeTec (Becton Dickinson [BD], Sparks, Md.). See Table 25-2. Performance is fairly equivalent in comparison studies between the three methods for CT (Table 25-3). False-positive results for GC have been reported with both the Roche PCR and BD ProbeTec assays. A second FDA-cleared NAAT exists for both CT and GC from Gen-Probe (APTIMA-CT, and APTIMA-GC) that detect alternate targets from the APTIMA Combo2 test. These APTIMA alternate probe tests have been found to be useful in confirming the presence of CT and GC in low prevalence populations, sexual assault cases, and from alternate site specimens (conjunctiva, pharynx, rectal).[3,17,21,24-27]

Except for reference laboratories, most labs typically offer one NAAT for both pathogens. Routine practice for laboratories typically includes an equivocal range where positive specimens automatically get repeated.[28] Confirmation of an original NAAT positive result is different. Providers should be aware of what the laboratory policy entails. A number of options are currently acceptable and can be performed from the original specimen or a recollected specimen: (1) Repeat testing using the NAAT performed originally; (2) use of a second NAAT methodology; and (3) use of the same NAAT technology but a different target site. Recent data shows that reliability of NAAT confirmation can be dependent on the technology, where the APTIMA test appears to offer the most consistent results.[29,30] Use of NAATs from non-FDA-cleared sites, such as rectum, pharynx, and conjunctiva are dependent on validation and verification performed according to guidelines and laboratory availability, but NAATs have shown improved sensitivity over culture for both CT and GC from these sites.[3,21]

The use of amplified methods and false-positive results have been reported in relation to potential environmental contamination for CT.[31] While a positive result may occur because of gross contamination of positive specimen on

Table 25-2	FDA-Cleared Amplification Assays for *Chlamydia Trachomatis* (CT) and *Neisseria Gonorrhoeae* (GC)					
Assay	**Manufacturer**	**Organisms**	**Amplification Method**	**Target Nucleic Acid**	**Specimen Types (FDA Cleared)**	**Confirmatory Probe Available**
Amplicor CT/NG test	Roche	CT GC	Polymerase chain reaction	DNA	Endocervical, first void urine—males only	No
ProbeTec CT and GC	Becton-Dickenson	CT GC	Strand displacement amplification	DNA	Endocervical, first void urine, vaginal swab	No
APTIMA Combo 2	Gen-Probe, Inc.	CT GC	Transcription-mediated amplification	rRNA	Endocervical, first void urine, vaginal swab	Separate CT and GC alternate probe tests FDA cleared

Table 25-3 Reported Sensitivity Ranges for Molecular Methods for CT with Various Specimen Types			
	Endocervical	**First-void Urine**	**Vaginal**
Amplicor	≥70%	60%-90%	Not applicable
ProbeTec	≥80%	70-90%	Not applicable
APTIMA	≥95%	≥90%	≥95%
PACE 2C*	50%-80%	Not applicable	Not applicable
Hybrid Capture II*	50%-80%	Not applicable	Not applicable

*Hybridization formats, specifically PACE 2C by Gen-Probe, Inc. and Hybrid Capture II by Qiagen, Inc., are not sensitive enough to consider as primary methods for STIs in sexual abuse cases compared with amplification methods.

environmental surfaces at the site of collection, false-positive results are most likely to occur because of crossover contamination after amplification in the laboratory. However, routine laboratory protocol monitors drift and incidence of positive results that would identify this as a possibility. In addition, sexual assault samples are typically evaluated as a group, such that even two positive patients in a single assay analysis might be considered suspect. Specifically related to amplification methods, careful patient and health care provider instruction about collection and transferring of specimens to collection vials should be addressed.

In general, retesting patients with a follow-up NAAT for CT or GC (test of cure) is not recommended unless special circumstances exist (pregnancy). NAATs will remain positive for approximately 2 to 3 weeks with effective treatment. Patients that are at higher risk for STIs (15 to 19 year olds), should be screened in the next 3 to 12 months for possible reinfection because those patients with repeat infections are at higher risk for PID.[1]

Herpes Simplex Virus

Herpes simplex virus, types 1 and 2 (HSV-1 and HSV-2) are DNA viruses that result in life-long infections that occur worldwide with no seasonal distribution. They are extremely common, with at least 50 million people in the United States being infected. HSV is the most common cause of mucocutaneous genital lesions. The virus is transmitted by direct contact with virus in secretions with an incubation period to presentation of lesions, 1 to 26 days. Asymptomatic carriage is common and thought to range from 25% to 90%, as people with antibody to both HSV-1 and HSV-2 do not recall oral-labial or genital lesions. Thus subclinical transmission accounts for the majority of transmissions. Both genital and oral-labial lesions can be caused by either HSV-1 or HSV-2 and are clinically indistinguishable. In children less than 12 years of age, the occurrence of HSV-2 as a primary lesion is less common than that seen in sexually active adolescents (ages 12-18), but has increased over the past 10 years. In addition, there has been an increase in HSV-1 as a primary genital lesion.[14]

Detection of HSV is very dependent on appropriate specimen collection, timing of specimen collection relative to presentation of vesicles, and subsequent transport and processing in the laboratory. Specimens should not be collected with wooden-shafted or calcium alginate swabs because these will interfere with virus isolation. Dacron or rayon swabs should be submitted in viral transport media (VTM), which is specifically devised for viruses and contains antibiotics to control for bacterial overgrowth. Some studies have shown enhanced recovery when specimens are submitted on ice but some transport media can be stored and transported at room temperature. Providers should check with their individual laboratory for recommended optimal collection parameters.[14]

Viral culture and/or immunofluorescent antibody (FA) testing from lesion material are still the mainstays for diagnosis. Exudative material or necrotic debris should be removed with a cotton swab before sampling the lesion. An FA test may be performed directly from the slide obtained at the bedside or submitted in VTM. Specimen collection should entail removing the surface of the vesicle lesion and collection of not only the fluid but the skin cells at the base of the lesion. Care should be taken not to cause bleeding because this may interfere with performance of some assays. Neutralizing antibody in the blood can interfere with some assays as well. The FA slide test offers the benefits of assessing the quality of the specimen submitted (epithelial cells need to be present) and performance of the test the same day as specimen acquisition. The test is 10% to 87% sensitive compared with the culture.[14]

HSV causes cytopathic effect (CPE) in susceptible cell culture lines rapidly, typically within 24 to 48 hours and 90% of cultures are positive by day 5. Culture has excellent sensitivity when lesions are present and is more likely to be positive in patients that have vesicular versus ulcerative lesions and in patients where specimens are obtained from a first episodic lesion versus a recurrent lesion. Isolates should be typed to determine if they are HSV-1 or 2 since 12-month recurrence rates are more common with HSV-2 (90%) than HSV-1 (55%). While the presence of HSV-2 might result more commonly in a child from sexual assault, results for both HSV-1 and HSV-2 should be reviewed cautiously.[9,14] Enzyme immunoassay methods (EIA) are not sensitive enough in asymptomatic patients to be used with reliability and should not be performed in children where abuse is suspected. A Tzanck smear preparation that assesses cytologic changes associated with HSV infection is neither specific nor sensitive enough to use as a test for diagnosis of HSV.

NAATs, such as PCR, have been shown to be more sensitive than culture, especially from crusted lesions and in patients with asymptomatic infection.[14] However, no NAAT is currently FDA-cleared for detection of HSV from any source. Some laboratories have validated skin/lesion specimens for NAAT and providers should check with their individual reference laboratory for availability.

Antibody testing has limited uses but might be helpful in the diagnosis in someone with primary disease if a fourfold rise in titer is seen, especially in a patient where the perpetrator is known to have a history of HSV or other STIs and genital lesions are not noted at the time of examination or at follow-up. Importantly, type-specific glycoprotein G-based assays should be requested because they are the only reliable assays that differentiate between HSV-1 and HSV-2. Currently available point-of-care tests (POCT) for HSV-2 can yield false positive results in patient populations with a low likelihood of HSV infection, in early stages of infection, and yield false-negative results for patients with HSV-2 infection where they have had prior HSV-1 infections. Seroconversion typically is 2 to 3 weeks before these tests can be accurately interpreted.[1,14]

Human Papilloma Virus

Human papilloma virus (HPV) is a DNA virus with more than 115 types, of which at least 30 have been identified to infect the genital area. HPV is one of the most common STIs in sexually active individuals with more than 5.5 million new cases occurring per year in the United States.[24] Thus when anogenital infection is noted beyond infancy and in a prepubertal child, sexual abuse should be considered. Infections are often transient and subclinical. High-risk HPV types are associated with cervical dysplasia (including 16, 18, 31, and 33) but routine testing for high-risk HPV by DNA testing is only recommended in women over the age of 30, typically in conjunction with an abnormal Pap smear or as a primary screening test for cervical dysplasia. Guidelines, however, are continuously changing with the availability of the HPV vaccine for girls as early as age 11 and HPV genotyping tests. Anogenital warts, also called condylomata acuminata, are typically caused by HPV types other than those known to cause cervical and anogenital cancers, or "low-risk" HPV types (including 6, 11, 42, and 43). The diagnosis of genital warts is most commonly made by visual inspection, where skin-colored cauliflower like growths are noted on the mucous membranes of the genital, perianal, and/or anal areas either alone or in groups. HPV DNA or mRNA tests are not warranted in the routine diagnosis or management of genital warts since not every HPV type can be assessed with accuracy.[1] Confirmation of genital HPV infection can be performed by biopsy of the lesion and pathology interpretation.

Trichomonas Vaginalis and Other Causes of Vaginitis/Vaginosis

Vaginosis and vaginitis are infections characterized by vaginal discharge and/or pruritus. The diagnoses of bacterial vaginosis (BV), and vaginitis caused by fungal organisms (vulvovaginal candidiasis, VVC) or *T. vaginalis* are difficult because of overlapping signs and symptoms along with the possibility of dual infections. All entities are typically considered clinically and diagnostically at the same time.

BV is not an infection per se, but a disorder attributed to overgrowth of mixed vaginal flora including multiple anaerobes, *Gardnerella vaginalis*, and *Mycoplasma* spp. in addition to the loss of the normal lactobacilli. The change in flora results in an increase in volatile amines and increased vaginal pH (alkaline >4.5) that produces the typical "fishy" odor when 10% potassium hydroxide (KOH) is added to a smear of the vaginal discharge. The condition is most commonly seen in sexually active individuals; in those patients where BV is identified, the recommendation is to screen for other STIs. Thus the presence of BV in a child is not indicative of sexual abuse.[7]

Vulvovaginal candidiasis (VVC) is the second most common cause of vaginal symptoms in females presenting to health care providers; 20% to 30% of females have *Candida* spp. as part of their vaginal flora and seed urogenital areas from the gastrointestinal tract and perianal area. While vaginitis caused by yeast is not considered a STI, yeast vaginitis is identified in children that complain of vaginal discharge due to other bacterial causes. When children are out of diapers, typically this condition is seen in children who have received antibiotics.[10]

T. vaginalis is a flagellate parasite that infects the urogenital tract, commonly causing vaginitis, cervicitis, and urethritis. While there often is a discharge noted, an estimated 50% of infections in females are asymptomatic and in men nearly all infections are asymptomatic.[13] Trichomonas is one of the most common STIs worldwide, with 7.4 million cases identified in the U.S. each year. Neonates can acquire the organisms during passage through the infected birth canal by direct vulvovaginal contamination.[13] The overall estimated infection rate is likely to be grossly underestimated because of nonsensitive and nonspecific test methods routinely used for diagnosis, the nonreportable status to public health laboratories, and the high prevalence of asymptomatic infections. Presence of this organism in a child beyond 2 years old typically suggests sexual abuse.[7]

A number of POCTs can be performed from a vaginal discharge specimen while the patient is in the healthcare setting. These include a pH strip test and a wet mount smear examination. The wet mount microscopic examination uses a drop of physiological saline and material from a swab of the vaginal discharge. The specimen should be examined microscopically within 1 hour and performed under low power magnification with reduced illumination to view motile trichomonads. A drop of 10% KOH can be added to a slide of the vaginal discharge and evaluated for the detection of the pungent "fishy" odor that is given off from the volatile amines of anaerobic organisms associated with BV or for detection of mycelial fungal elements. In prepubescent children, the pH test is not reliable and this is not recommended to help define the diagnosis of BV or trichomonas.[4] Proficiency in microscopic examination is essential given infections may be mixed and/or patients may have atypical manifestations.

The following are general presentations with use of the wet mount for each of these conditions. In a postpubescent female, normal vaginal pH is 4.5 and vaginal discharge is typically scant, clear, or white. A wet mount will show minimal white blood cells (WBCs), normal epithelial cells, and a predominance of lactobacilli.

For yeast vaginitis, the pH is usually normal as well (4.5), but the discharge is moderate and is most commonly white and clumping without an offensive odor. Observation of a wet mount will show yeast forms and mycelial elements that will be enhanced by the addition of 10% KOH to eliminate other cellular material. An amine odor is not noted upon addition of the KOH.

For BV, the discharge is moderate and coats the vaginal walls. Typically the discharge is white to gray, may show bubbles, and is malodorous. The pH is >4.5 (alkaline). The wet mount may show clue cells, which are squamous epithelial cells coated with bacteria such that the borders are not clearly recognized. Compared with other disorders, there is a lack of WBCs. Addition of 10% KOH will give an amine or fishy odor ("whiff" test).

Trichomoniasis may produce a profuse purulent discharge. The discharge is typically yellow-green, bubbly, and will yield a pH >4.5. A wet mount will show trichomonads with a jerky motility and many WBCs. Sensitivity of the wet mount to diagnose trichomoniasis is typically reported to be only 50% to 70%.[13]

When examining wet mounts, it is important to remember that the columnar epithelial cells of the normal prepubertal vaginal wall appear quite different microscopically than the flat, irregular squamous epithelial cells of the adult vagina.

Two rapid antigen POCTs are available for the detection of *Trichomonas*, the OSOM Trichomonas Rapid Test (Genzyme Diagnostics, Cambridge, Mass.), which is an immunochromatographic dipstick antigen test and the Xenostrip Tv *T. vaginalis* test (Xenotope Diagnostics, Inc., San Antonio, Tex.). They can be performed in about 15 minutes using a swab from the vaginal discharge. In symptomatic patients, these tests yield about the same sensitivity compared with a wet mount (60% to 80%), with specificities >98%.[13] The advantage of these tests is the elimination for the requirement for viable organisms and/or the ability to perform a rapid wet mount microscopic examination. Studies have not been conducted on the tests in asymptomatic patients, males, and children. A positive rapid antigen test might offer the ability to identify when subsequent culture tests and/or NAATs should be performed in children where abuse is suspected.

For specimens that will be sent to the microbiology laboratory, swabs from the vaginal discharge should be placed in a tube of 0.9% physiological saline or in a swab collection system where the laboratory will subsequently perform a wet mount and/or KOH tests, quantitative gram stains, and culture if requested.

A graded gram stain of vaginal discharge, using the Nugent criteria, can be a highly sensitive and specific test for the detection of BV when the microscopist is experienced with the interpretation.[32] This graded gram stain relies on the quantitation of lactobacilli, *Gardnerella/Bacteroides* spp. and curved gram-variable rods (*Mobiluncus* spp.) per high power oil immersion field. The scoring is from 0 to 10 with zero to 3 being consistent with normal vaginal flora, 4 to 6 intermediate and 7 to 10 consistent with BV. Many laboratories perform this graded gram stain with difficulty. For BV, cultures are not recommended since there is not one specific pathogen that can be identified as the cause of BV. The presence of *G. vaginalis* alone does not indicate an STI because this can be normal vaginal flora.

For trichomoniasis, culture is somewhat limited in availability but is considered the standard to measure other tests and is recommended in circumstances of sexual assault or abuse, for the present time. Recent data comparing cuture to NAATs, however, shows culture is only 70% sensitive.[33] Specific culture systems, the InPouch TV culture system (Biomed Diagnostics, San Jose, Calif.), or the system of Empyrean Diagnostics, Inc. (Mountain View, Calif.) offer an alternative approach to testing for *Trichomonas* for off-site facilities that will have inherent delays in transport of the specimen or are unable to perform wet mounts. The patient specimen is directly inoculated into the culture system. These culture systems allow immediate direct examination using a special viewing clip, and the pouch of media subsequently serves as the transport container and growth chamber during incubation. *Trichomonas* is rarely identified in infected male patients unless a smear is prepared before any urination has occurred during the day. Urethral cultures directly inoculated into these culture media are preferred for increased sensitivity. Urine sediments are not recommended for visual evaluation of *T. vaginalis* because other nonsexually transmitted nonvaginalis species, such as *T. hominis*—a normal gastrointestinal flagellate—might be identified due to fecal contamination.[13]

The Affirm VP III Assay (Becton Dickinson, Sparks, Md.), is a DNA hybridization probe test that is unique in that it identifies organisms associated with each of the three entities of vaginosis/vaginitis; *G. vaginalis*, *Trichomonas*, and *C. albicans*, respectively. Organism quantity = 10^4 is the determined cut-off for a positive, which allows for greater specificity but may reduce sensitivity compared with culture methods. Specimens are submitted in a manufacturer specific collection device and transport is not an issue since the test does not rely on organism viability. Recent studies have shown that in symptomatic women, the Affirm test is more sensitive than wet mount and 10% KOH. Specificity is high when compared with the culture for *Trichomonas*, but the test is read subjectively.[13] This DNA hybridization probe test cannot be recommended for use in children and sexual assault victims, but is mentioned here to clarify that although it is molecular in nature, the poor specificity and sensitivity compared with NAATs, does not allow it to be used with certainty in this population.

An FDA-cleared NAAT is currently unavailable for *T. vaginalis*, but some laboratories have validated various molecular technologies with both vaginal swabs and urine specimens.[32] NAATs have been shown to be more sensitive than culture when discrepant results are resolved using infected patient status as delineated by two positive amplification results using two different methods and/or probes.[13,33,34]

Lice

Phthirus pubis, the pubic louse, is a sucking arthropod transferred from hosts by close physical contact. Bites can result in intense irritation for several days with each bite causing a red papule. The parasites are easily identified by nits and/or upon visual inspection of the organism in the laboratory. Submission of the parasite in a clean container and observation by light microscopy will yield the specific diagnosis. The predilection of pubic lice and body lice for their particular niches has to do with the length of the parasite legs with attached claws and ability to grasp the specific hair at that body site. Pubic lice, because of their shorter leg/claw length compared with body lice, are only able to attach to hair in the genital area or eyelashes. Lice identified in either of these areas denote a probable sexually transmitted infection that should be investigated. Lice in children are common and transmission occurs among household members and school-mates. Thus corroborating evidence for significance of this pathogen as an STI is necessary.[7]

SEROLOGICAL TESTING

Serological baseline tests (frozen from initial visit) include those for HIV, HBV, and syphilis. If these tests are negative at baseline, evaluations should be performed at 6 weeks, 3 months, and 6 months when indicated.[1,4,7]

Syphilis is a systemic disease that is caused by the spirochete, *Treponema pallidum*, and has recently seen an increase in incidence in some areas. A darkfield microscopic examination from a primary or secondary lesion swab specimen performed on site in the laboratory or a direct fluorescent antibody—*T. pallidum* (DFA-TP) slide test are definitive methods for diagnosis. Unfortunately, these tests are not readily available and in the case of the dark-field slide examination, requires immediate visualization to observe motile spirochetes. Most patients with syphilis are diagnosed by serological tests. The different serological tests are based upon the detection of antibodies that are produced following treponeme infection and are classified based on the type of antigen used in the test system. Nontreponemal tests (rapid reagin [RPR] and Venereal Disease Research Laboratory [VDRL]) use a mixture of cardiolipin with lipids to detect reagin, which is present in patients with syphilis. Treponemal tests, the enzyme immunoassay (EIA) formats, *T. pallidum* particle agglutination (TP-PA), and the fluorescent treponemal antibody absorbed (FTA-ABS) test, use *T. pallidum* or recombinant proteins as the antigen source to detect *T. pallidum* antibodies. Some of the EIA tests can be used as either a screening test or a confirmatory test and are being used more commonly because of increased specificity, sensitivity, and objective interpretation by instrumentation.[35]

Both types of serological tests need to be performed if a nontreponemal test is being used as the screening test, as a high percentage of false-positive results occur in many medical conditions unrelated to syphilis (Lyme disease, rheumatoid arthritis) and can be negative in early and late disease.[35,36] For subsequent testing, the same nontreponemal test should be performed for a legitimate comparison of titers and monitoring treatment.[35] Treponemal tests are usually positive for life and titers are not typically helpful in treatment decisions. Rare false-positive tests have been reported with the treponemal assays as well.[36]

Diagnosis of HIV is typically accomplished using an antibody screening test with positive results confirmed by a second assay such as a Western blot before considered a true positive. Serum is the routine specimen, but plasma can also be used. Specimens should be collected and cellular elements separated within 2 hours of collection and subsequently refrigerated. A NAAT can be used to diagnose acute HIV before the typical 6-week conversion period, but this test should be performed only on consultation with the laboratory. POCTs, such as the Oraquick test (Abbott), that use

serum, have been shown to be equal to EIA methods used in laboratories but POCTs using oral fluid (Orasure, Abbott) have resulted in more indeterminate Western blots.[15,37]

Serological markers for the detection of hepatitis B are very stable. Plasma or serum should be separated from blood within 24 hours and stored at 2° C to 8° C if testing will take place within 5 days. Both surface antigen and surface antibody to HBV are the most common tests employed for detection of viral exposure. Hepatitis B surface antigen (HBsAg) is used for the determination of acute disease but providers should recognize that HBsAg can be positive after vaccination and might not indicate infection. The other test commonly employed is for determination of vaccine success, antibody to hepatitis B surface antigen (anti-HBs). The protective level as determined by CDC and World Health Organization (WHO) is considered 10 IU/mL. Many FDA-cleared assays are available for both tests with volume needed for testing as little 10 μL to 35 μL in some assays. The HBV immunization series is required for most children in the United States by 7th grade. However, if exposure to blood has occurred, as may have occurred in a sexual assault, postvaccination testing for anti-HBs is recommended.[1] HBsAg can occur due to exposures other than sexual transmission. In fact, most transmissions occur in the setting of a household with a chronic HBV carrier.[38]

Reporting of STIs

All GC, CT, syphilis, HBV, and HIV are required to be reported from the laboratory testing site to the state public health laboratory in all the U.S. states and territories. Trichomoniasis, BV, herpes, and genital warts are not on this reportable list. The reporting by the laboratory to the state should not be confused with the reporting of the infection and/or the suspected child abuse that may also be required by the health care provider to the appropriate agencies.[1]

STRENGTH OF MEDICAL EVIDENCE

In determination of a true STI result from a child or adolescent, culture is the most specific test methodology for most of the pathogens discussed. If a STI organism grows and is not perinatally or vertically transmitted to the child, the organism presence raises concern for sexual abuse and requires reporting. Current data, however, in all other patient groups and other specimen sites, has repeatedly shown the lack of sensitivity for culture methods.[11-13,25] Lack of viability of the organism in the specimen by the time it is received in the laboratory, too low an organism load to result in detection, and inhibition by other normal flora contaminating the specimen all contribute. So what is the best test method? The strength of medical evidence for the use of NAATS is just starting to accrue and become available in children and adolescents being evaluated for sexual abuse or assault.[25] The use of molecular methods in adolescents and adults for STIs in other medical situations has become standard of care for screening, diagnosis, and treatment for the most prevalent STIs, CT, and GC.[1] Data on *Trichomonas* in these patient populations also shows that amplification assays might soon become the standard of care for optimal detection of this pathogen as well.[13,34] The benefits are clear for the use of molecular technology for diagnosing the most common STIs in children and adolescents being assessed for sexual abuse or assault: increased sensitivity compared with culture, the ability to use noninvasive specimens, specimen stability, collection of a single specimen per site for both CT/ GC, ability to reliably detect these pathogens at alternate sites compared with culture and rapid turnaround time. The real issue in converting from culture to NAAT is reliability of a positive result or concern about false positive tests. Reliability of any method is dependent on the correct use of the recommended specimen collection/transport containers and the recommended procedure. In addition, as with any test, even with a specificity of 99%, the positive predictive value of a single test performance in a low prevalence population will not be optimal.[18] Thus it is imperative for laboratories to have some confirmatory procedure in place to address positive results in this population and providers must understand the merits and disadvantages of each NAAT in their current formats.[3,24,29,30]

The use of NAATs, with the appropriate precautions as stated previously, will likely allow a better assessment of true STI transmission to abused victims earlier, allow a better understanding of pathogenesis in young children, identify more victims where appropriate treatment can be addressed, and improve prosecution of cases. More data needs to be collected and research presented for these methods in children less than 12 or prepubertal victims and male victims specifically from alternate sites (pharyngeal and rectal), as most data on all test methods are predominantly in females and vaginal or endocervical specimens. In addition, the medical community needs to specifically address the evidence to support or refute the benefits of NAATs in a written guideline so that use of this technology can be correctly interpreted and used appropriately.

References

1. Centers for Disease Control and Prevention: Sexually transmitted diseases treatment guidelines, 2006. *MMWR Morb Mortal Wkly Rep* 2006;55:1-136.
2. Centers for Disease Control and Prevention: Screening tests to detect *Chlamydia trachomatis* and *Neisseria gonorrhoeae* infections-2002. *MMWR Morb Mortal Wkly Rep* 2002;51(RR-15):1-38.
3. Chapin KC: Molecular tests for detection of the sexually-transmitted pathogens *Neisseria Gonorrhoeae* and *Chlamydia trachomatis*. *Med Health R I* 2006;89:202-204.
4. Groth SJ, Goldman PL, Burns-Smith G, et al: *Evaluation and management of the sexually assaulted or sexually abused patient*, American College of Emergency Physicians (website): http://www.acep.org/workarea/downloadasset.aspx?id=8984. Accessed April 4, 2009.
5. Holmes WC, Slap GB: Sexual abuse of boys. *JAMA* 1998;280:1855-1862.
6. Ingram DM, Miller WC, Schoenbach VJ, et al: Risk assessment for gonococcal and chlamydial infections in young children undergoing evaluation for sexual abuse. *Pediatrics* 2001;107:e73.
7. Kellogg N: The evaluation of sexual abuse in children. *Pediatrics* 2005;116:506-512.
8. Siegel RM, Schubert CJ, Myers MSW, et al: The prevalence of sexually transmitted diseases in children and adolescents evaluated for sexual abuse in Cincinnati: rationale for limited STD testing in prepubertal girls. *Pediatrics* 1995;96:1090-1094.
9. Reading R, Rannan-Eliya Y: Evidence for sexual transmission of genital herpes in children. *Arch Dis Child* 2007;92:608-613.
10. Shapiro RA, Schubert CJ, Siegel RM: *Neisseria gonorrhea* infections in girls younger than 12 years of age evaluated for vaginitis. *Pediatrics* 1999;104:e72.
11. Essig A: Chlamydia and chlamydophila. *In*: Murray PR (ed): *Manual of Clinical Microbiology*, ed 9, ASM Press, Washington, DC, 2007, pp 1024-1029.
12. Janda WM, Gaydos CA: Neisseria. *In*: Murray PR (ed): *Manual of Clinical Microbiology*, ed 9, ASM Press, Washington, DC 2007, pp 601-620.
13. Leber AL, Novak-Weekley S: Intestinal and urogenital amebae, flagellates, and ciliates. *In*: Murray PR (ed): *Manual of Clinical Microbiology*, ed 9, ASM Press, Washington, DC, 2007, pp 2092-2112.
14. Jerome KR, Morrow RA: Herpes simplex viruses and herpes B virus. *In*: Murray PR (ed): *Manual of Clinical Microbiology*, ed 9, ASM Press, Washington DC, 2007, pp 1523-1536.
15. Griffith BP, Campbell S, Mayo DR: Human immunodeficiency viruses. *In*: Murray PR (ed): *Manual of Clinical Microbiology*, ed 9, ASM Press, Washington, DC, 2007, pp 1308-1329.
16. Cook RL, Hutchinson SL, Østergaard L, et al: Systematic review: noninvasive testing for *Chlamydia trachomatis* and *Neisseria gonorrhoeae*. *Ann Intern Med* 2005;142:914-925.
17. Black CM, Driebe EM, Howard LA, et al: Multicenter study of nucleic acid amplification tests for detection of Chlamydia trachomatis and Neisseria gonorrhoeae in children being evaluated for sexual abuse. *Pediatr Infect Dis J* 2009;28:608-613.
18. Katz AR, Effler PV, Ohye RG, et al: False-positive gonorrhea test results with a nucleic acid amplification test: the impact of low prevalence on positive predictive value. *Clin Infect Dis* 2004;38:814-819.
19. Palmer HM, Mallinson H, Wood RL, et al: Evaluation of the specificities of five DNA amplification methods for the detection of *Neisseria gonorrhoeae*. *J Clin Microbiol* 2003;41:835-837.
20. Golden MR, Hughes JP, Cles K, et al: Positive predictive value of Gen-Probe APTIMA Combo 2 testing for *Neisseria gonorrhoeae* in a population of women with low prevalence of *N. gonorrhoeae* infection. *Clin Infect Dis* 2004;39:1387-1390.
21. Renault CA, Hall C, Kent CK, et al: Use of NAATs for STD diagnosis of GC and CT in non-FDA-cleared anatomic specimens. *MLO Med Lab Obs* 2006;38:10-22.
22. Lister NA, Tabrizi SN, Fairley CK, et al: Validation of Roche COBAS Amplicor Assay for detection of *Chlamydia trachomatis* in rectal and pharyngeal specimens by a PCR assay. *J Clin Microbiol* 2004;42:239-241.
23. Centers for Disease Control and Prevention (CDC): False-positive results with the use of chlamydia tests in the evaluation of suspected sexual abuse-Ohio, 1990. *MMWR Morb Mortal Wkly Rep* 1991;39:932-935.
24. Hill CS: Appendix V: molecular diagnostic tests for sexually transmitted infections in women. *In*: Monif GRG, Baker DA (eds): *Infectious Diseases in Obstetrics and Gynecology*, ed 6, Informa Healthcare, New York, 2008, pp 517-528.
25. Leder MR, Scribano PV, Marcon MJ: Comparison of NAAT on genital swabs and urine in the detection of *Neisseria gonorrhoeae* and *Chlamydia trachomatis* in child sexual abuse survivors (abstract). Pediatric Academic Societies' Annual Meeting, Toronto, 2007.
26. Chapin KC, Andrea SC, Jenny C, et al: Four year history of APTIMA GC/CT nucleic acid amplification testing (NAAT) in children seen for sexual abuse (abstract). National STD Prevention Conference, Atlanta, 2010.
27. Girardet RG, Lahoti SM, Howard LA, et al: Epidemiology of sexually transmitted infections in suspected child victims of sexual assault. *Pediatrics* 2009;123:79-86.
28. Van Der Pol BDH, Martin J, Schachter TC, et al: Enhancing the specificity of the COBAS AMPLICOR CT/NG test for *Neisseria gonorrheae* by retesting specimens with equivocal results. *J Clin Microbiol* 2001;39:3092-3098.
29. Chernesky M, Jang D, Luinstra K, et al: High analytical sensitivity and low rates of inhibition may contribute to detection of *Chlamydia trachomatis* in significantly more women by the APTIMA Combo 2 Assay. *J Clin Microbiol* 2006;44:400-405.
30. Schachter J, Hook EW, Martin DH, et al: Confirming positive results of nucleic acid amplification tests (NAATs) for *Chlamydia trachomatis:* all NAATs are not created equal. *J Clin Microbiol* 2005;43:1372-1373.
31. Meader E, Waters J, Sillis M: *Chlamydia trachomatis* RNA in the environment: is there potential for false-positive nucleic acid amplification test results? *Sex Transm Infect* 2008;84:107-110.
32. Nugent RP, Krohn MA, Hillier SA: Reliability of diagnosing bacterial vaginosis is improved by a standardized method of Gram stain interpretation. *J Clin Microbiol* 1991;29:297-301.
33. Nye MD, Schwebke JR, Body BA: Comparison of APTIMA Trichomonas vaginalis transcription-mediated amplification to wet mount microscopy, culture, and polymerase chain reaction for diagnosis of trichomoniasis in men and women. *Am J Obstet Gynecol* 2009;200:188. e1-188.e7.

34. Caliendo AM, Jordan JA, Green AM, et al: Real-time PCR improves detection of *Trichomonas vaginalis* infection compared with culture using self-collected vaginal swabs. *Infect Dis Obstet Gynecol* 2005;13:145-150.

35. Pope V, Norris SJ, Johnson RE: Treponema and other human host-associated spirochetes. *In*: Murray PR (ed): *Manual of Clinical Microbiology*, ed 9, ASM Press, Washington, DC, 2007, pp 987-994.

36. de Larrañaga G, Trinbetta L, Perés S, et al: False positive reactions in confirmatory tests for syphilis in presence of antiphospholipid antibodies: misdiagnosis with prognostic and social consequences. *Dermatol Online J* 2006;12(4):22-27.

37. Bulterys M, Jamieson DJ, O'Sullivan MJ, et al: 2004 Mother-Infant rapid intervention at delivery (MIRIAD) study group. Rapid HIV-1 testing during labor: a multicenter study. *JAMA* 2004;292:219-223.

38. Horvat RT, Tegtmeier GE: Hepatitis B and D viruses. *In*: Murray PR (ed): *Manual of Clinical Microbiology*, ed 9, ASM Press, Washington, DC, 2007, pp 1641-1659.

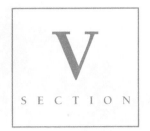

PHYSICAL ABUSE OF CHILDREN

Mary Clyde Pierce, MD

26

DOCUMENTING THE MEDICAL HISTORY IN CASES OF POSSIBLE PHYSICAL CHILD ABUSE

Allison M. Jackson, MD, MPH, and Brian M. Jackson, MD

The clinician's responsibility to document cases where child abuse is in the differential diagnosis is a critical aspect of providing effective patient care. The medical record can serve as an important tool for ensuring the immediate safety of the child and ongoing effective medical care. The medical record should be complete and thorough to provide the maximum benefit to those treating and safeguarding the child.

For years it has been known that the answer to the patient's medical condition is usually revealed by a comprehensive medical history.[1,2] Child physical abuse is no exception. The history is usually provided by the parent or caregiver, particularly when a child is preverbal or too ill to speak.[3] While a third party history is the norm in pediatric care, when possible a history should also be obtained from the child. Unlike other medical conditions, nonmedical professionals are often involved in obtaining historical information in cases of suspected abuse. The medical history, however, serves as a separate record from that obtained by nonmedical investigators. It is important that the medical record be unbiased. When documenting physical abuse of children, the clinician should maintain the attitude of a scientist and educator. The clinician is not a "child advocate" in terms of the individual case.[4] The patient will be best served when the medical record is unbiased, fact-oriented, and formatted to provide the best medical care for the child.

Recent studies have confirmed that current documentation practices in cases of suspected child abuse are often inadequate, lacking details about how the injury occurred, when and where the injury occurred, if witnesses were present at the time of the injury, the child's developmental abilities at the time of injury, and descriptions of past injuries.[5,6] Two studies from U.S. emergency departments showed medical records to be incomplete in at least one third of cases where abuse was suspected. While most clinicians effectively document the victim's age, injury type, and child protective services (CPS) involvement, few appropriately documented a developmental history, included an illustration of the injury location, or noted the presence of witnesses to the injury.[6-9] A comparison to documentation in 1980 showed minimal improvement in charting despite increased efforts to train clinicians.[6] A comparable Australian study of fractures in the emergency department found similar deficiencies.[10] There is a clear need for improved documentation of these cases.

The medical record is not only a means of communication among medical providers, but is also a legal document. Proper documentation is therefore important for several reasons. It records victims' statements for legal proceedings. The judicial system uses the medical history as recorded in the medical record as a factor in weighing the credibility of a child witness.[11] In most jurisdictions, a child's statement to an adult is hearsay and therefore inadmissible in legal proceedings. An exception often exists for statements made to medical professionals, exercised at the discretion of the presiding judge. One factor judges consider is whether the physician's testimony about the child's statement is consistent with the medical record.[12] Sometimes a complete medical record will allow a clinician to testify in place of a child, sparing the child significant emotional and psychological trauma.[10]

While physician testimony can be critical in child abuse cases, an adequate record often prevents the need for the physician to appear in court at all. Subpoenas for physicians are issued in about 15% of abuse cases, and physicians testify in fewer than 5% of cases.[13] Clear and complete documentation can be used by the legal system in place of in-person testimony, particularly in pretrial and/or presettlement negotiations.[14] Because physicians will not often testify in person in these cases, their documentation becomes extremely important.

Complete documentation helps prevent future episodes of abuse. Without clear documentation, it is difficult to distinguish abuse from nonabuse should the patient subsequently have a new complaint.[15] A full record of information also enables accurate data collection for child maltreatment research.

THE MEDICAL RECORD

The Interview Circumstances

Before delving into the substance of the history, the clinician should document the circumstances under which the interview took place. Documentation begins with a notation of the date, time, and location of the interview. This allows for an impartial observer to determine the elapsed time between the injury and the interview, and also allows for a chronology of the caregiver and/or child's statement. The reports in the medical record can be used in conjunction with police and social work reports. The time of documentation determines if the notes are contemporaneous. In general contemporaneous notes are considered more reliable than notes written after a significant amount of time has elapsed.[16]

The sources of the history should include the child, if developmentally and medically capable, and the parents/caregivers. Additional sources for the history might include other medical personnel, such as emergency medical services providers, nurses, and primary and specialty care providers. These professionals' documentation can be informative and should be included, when available, in the medical record. Thus clinicians should document the source(s) of the history and whether the participants were interviewed together or separately. If law enforcement, child protective services (CPS), or other personnel are present, this should be noted as well. Because the clinician's interview is primarily for medical purposes, statements made to medical staff alone are often given more weight in court than statements made to law enforcement or CPS. It may be useful to document the history from each historian separately, just as they should be interviewed separately.

Demographic information should also be included in the introductory section. The child's age and gender should be listed in the medical record. There is a dispute about the inclusion of race in the medical record because its inclusion may be used to infer bias on the part of the interviewer. Several authorities, including the World Health Organization, recommend including race in child abuse documentation.[17] If race is included, it should always be documented as the patient or guardian states.

Elicited and spontaneous statements should be noted as such in the record. If the statements are elicited, the record should indicate what questions were asked to evoke the responses.[9] Using open-ended questions, such as "Can you tell me what happened to bring you to the hospital?" can yield a narrative history from the caregiver and/or child. More direct questions might be necessary to clarify portions of the historian's narrative. Recent reports suggest that interviewers have a tendency to systematically misattribute elicited details of abuse to open-ended rather than closed-ended questions.[18] Using preplanned or standardized questions might help to ensure that questions and answers are recorded accurately. This should not, however, be so automated as to compromise the establishment of rapport with the patient and family or to limit further questioning based on the parent's or patient's responses. It should be clear whether information obtained from witnesses comes from their own first-hand observation or whether it comes from information relayed from another source (the latter is considered less reliable). All information should be documented verbatim or as close to verbatim as possible, using quotation marks around direct quotes from the source.

The History of Present Illness

The information gathered in the history of present illness (HPI) is critical to determining injury plausibility. The answer to the simple question, "Tell me what happened?" lies in this section. As in most medical conditions, the HPI will likely be the largest section of the medical record. In cases of suspected physical abuse, the HPI is often particularly lengthy as the history is provided from each parent, the child when possible, other health care providers, and the

Table 26-1	Questions to Ask in History of Present Illness

- What happened?
- Who was there when it happened?
- Where did it happen?
- When did it happen?
- What happened afterwards?
- When was the child noticed to be ill or injured? How did the child respond? When did symptoms start? How did you respond?
- What made you bring your child to the doctor/hospital?

medical record. Before delving into the history itself, the chief complaint should be noted in the parent's or patient's own words. This allows for documentation of the reason the child presented for care. There are two general portions of the HPI in most abuse cases (Table 26-1). The first portion includes the history of the injury event: what happened, when it happened, where it happened, and who was present. The second is how the child responded or behaved after the injury, including the development of medical signs, symptoms, and conditions relevant to the child's condition and care.[19,20] This information, particularly when documented chronologically, can be quite useful in establishing a timeline of events, in identifying inconsistencies with explanations, and in determining the mechanism and plausibility of the injury.

The history should include all details provided by the victim or other witnesses. Details that initially might seem irrelevant sometimes become relevant later. For example, a report of prior symptoms such as irritability or vomiting might correlate with newly discovered injuries that are not acute. The explanation of what happened, to include what was seen and heard, should be as extensive as possible. Eliciting and documenting a detailed description of the injury event, including how a child was discovered to be ill or injured, provide essential data for understanding the mechanism of injury.[21-23] The level of detail provided or omitted can be useful in assessing the believability of the explanation. Unknown details might be pertinent negatives in the history that should be documented. For example, it should be documented if the caregiver reports no traumatic incidents, accidental or otherwise, have occurred for the child. The date and time of the injury event and evolution of symptoms should be included with as much detail as possible. In some cases it is necessary or preferable to include a range of times of onset of symptoms if the child's status is not clearly described. If several discrete episodes of symptoms occurred, the record should indicate times for each with as much precision as possible. The location where the events took place should also be noted.

If abuse is suspected, a report should be made to the authorities in the appropriate jurisdiction. If the caregiver or patient says that abuse has occurred, the identity of the suspected abuser should be documented. If the child is unable to identify a person by name or title, a description of the person can be used. Additionally, any other people who were present during the injury event should be identified.

In addition to documenting the injury event, a thorough history of the condition(s) causing the child to present to a clinician and any attempts made by the caregiver to treat the injury or condition must be documented, as well as timing of onset of symptoms. Each sign or symptom reported should, when possible, have an onset time recorded and the documentation should also indicate the evolution of that symptom. Any sign or symptom reported to the medical professional must be documented even if it does not seem relevant to the current injury. These signs and symptoms can be indicators that suggest a diagnosis. Signs and symptoms should be recorded in as much detail as possible. If accounts of signs or symptoms differ among historians, this fact should be noted and the history provided by each person should be documented separately.

As the medical findings of the patient are revealed through the evaluation, the parent's and/or patient's explanation for the injuries should be sought and documented. The HPI should document all findings using the historian's own terms. While a physical examination might alter the clinician's impression of an injury, the documented history should be consistent with what the clinician is actually told by the caregiver or patient. Attempts to "clean-up" the story or to clarify terms (for example changing the report of a "cut" to a "laceration" or correcting the grammar of direct quotes) might undermine the credibility of the medical record.

Past Medical History and Review of Systems

There are several sources that should be referenced when documenting the past medical history (PMH) and review of systems (ROS). The first is clearly the victim and parent or guardian. The PMH and ROS should include explicit questions about previous injuries (accidental and abusive) and illnesses. Medication taken by the patient should also be documented because some medications can provide explanations for the child's condition. Specific mention should be made in the record of questions and answers that rule out medical diagnoses causing the presenting signs and symptoms. Noting pertinent negatives makes it clear to the reader that the clinician considered all diagnoses before reaching conclusions. Additionally, it is important that the clinician note any chronic conditions that afflict the child. Children with chronic disease, preterm infants, and twins are at significantly increased risk for abuse, and are also at risk for a host of unfortunate medical conditions and complications.[24] Some chronic diseases can mimic abuse. Having a detailed medical history can often provide elucidation.

In addition to direct history-taking, the documentation of the child's past medical history should include a review of notes from previous visits to other health care providers (Table 26-2). Obtaining birth and other medical records might reveal injuries or illnesses not reported or recalled by the patient and caregiver. It should be clearly noted in documentation when historical items are obtained from records and not from the patient or guardian. In addition, record reviews provide important information about growth patterns, nutritional parameters, immunizations, and adequacy of medical care. Similarly, if the patient is accompanied by a social worker, police officer, or CPS agent who provides

Table 26-2	Past Medical History and Review of Systems

- Birth history: planned or unplanned pregnancy, mode of delivery, use of instruments to aid delivery, perinatal complications
- Prior emergency visits and hospitalizations
- Tendency to bleed or bruise (nosebleeds, gums bleeding, easy bruising, prolonged nosebleeds, bleeding after invasive procedures such as circumcision, immunization, blood draws, phlebotomy, dental procedures)
- Prior injuries: falls, fractures, burns, lacerations, etc.
- Dietary history: vitamin supplementation, appetite changes, intolerance to foods
- Seizures
- Irritability
- General temperament
- Medications
- Immunizations
- Primary care practitioner (name and phone number)

additional information regarding the history, that information can be included in the medical record, but its source should be clearly identified.

The Developmental History

Perhaps the most overlooked aspect of medical documentation is the developmental history. The patient's developmental abilities are pertinent to understanding the mechanism of injury and the plausibility of the injury explanation, and it is therefore essential data when evaluating a child for suspected physical abuse (Table 26-3). A 1995 emergency department study did not a find a single medical record that had an adequate developmental history when physical abuse was suspected.[6] The history should document objective measures used to evaluate whether a child is at an appropriate developmental level. Whenever possible, the developmental milestones should be documented by direct observation. If developmental milestones are deemed met by patient or parent report, this source of information should be noted in the record. The clinician should state whether the child appears to have comparable chronological and developmental ages or if these measures are discrepant, but the focus should be on objectively documenting the child's developmental milestones. If the developmental history is missing, it is difficult or impossible to assess whether an injury is consistent with the history reported by the patient and his/her family. Furthermore, an accurate developmental history might reveal conditions that mimic abuse or that put the child at increased risk for abuse.

In some settings such as the emergency department, efficiency is paramount. In this setting it is still important to gather as much information as possible. While the developmental history might seem less important than the HPI, it is critical to determining whether the injury explanation is developmentally congruent. At a minimum, the provider should cross check the child's developmental accomplishments with the explanation provided.

Table 26-3 Developmental History
Developmental History
• Prior developmental concerns
• Loss of developmental milestones
• Motor landmarks—rolling, sitting, standing, walking, running, climbing stairs, ability to turn things off and on, grasp, visual tracking
• Social landmarks—feeds self, puts on clothes, washes and dries hands, toilet training
• Language skills—coos, laughs, babbles, imitates, says words (how many, examples), clarity of speech

The Social History

Child maltreatment occurs within all ethnicities, cultures, and classes. Knowing the social history of a child is important to identifying family factors putting the child at risk and family strengths that provide opportunities for the child to thrive. The clinician can also identify opportunities for health and safety prevention services that can reinforce family integrity (Table 26-3).[18,25] To that end, the living situation of the child should be documented. All persons, both children and adults living in the child's home should be noted in the record. The child's primary address and any temporary or shared addresses should be included in the history. Any other location where the child spends a significant amount of time (e.g., day care, relatives' homes) should also be noted, as should any alternative caregivers (e.g., babysitters). The use or lack of use of substances, including alcohol and drugs, should be noted. Parental substance abuse is a major stressor on family stability and can put children at risk.[26] A parental, patient, or sibling history of social service involvement and placement in foster care or other temporary living arrangements should be included in the social history as should any history of prior police involvement or incarceration. A statement of the family's socioeconomic status, including highest educational level completed by the parents and employment status, should be obtained. Other sources of support for the family such as food stamps, subsidized housing, and health insurance coverage should be noted as strengths that promote family stability.[22] Any history of domestic violence should also be noted because this puts children at risk for injury and emotional damage.[22] Ask about social supports such as extended family and friends to assess the family's degree of social isolation and connection. The source of all information included in the social history should be documented.

Some clinicians find an ecological model of reporting the social history to be beneficial.[16] In this model, the family dynamics are recorded on four levels. The first level reports the status of the individual within the family, including age, sex, and unique personal characteristics that strengthen or weaken family safety and cohesion. For the child, personal characteristics include temperament, birth order, status as a twin, or developmental challenges. The second level is of close social relationships with family members or friends. These factors include strength of parent-child bond, physical or developmental problems of family members, mental illness or substance abuse in family members, and a history of intimate partner violence. These relationships may be

Table 26-4 Social Risk Factors
Individual (Patient)
Temperament
Medical limitations
Cognitive limitations
Psychiatric diagnoses
Family
Poverty
Medical limitations
Cognitive limitations
Psychiatric diagnoses
Substance abuse
Interpersonal violence
History of abuse/victimization
Isolation
Community
Violence
Poverty
High unemployment
Isolation
Society
Poor economy
Glorification of violence
Normalization of sexual harm
Attitudes toward child discipline

protective or unprotective. The third level is the community, including factors like the availability of alcohol and drugs of abuse, high levels of unemployment, and lack of adequate housing, or positive factors such as adequate schools, safe neighborhoods, and available playgrounds, community centers, or outdoor spaces. Finally, societal factors such as social norms that promote or discourage violence toward others, social policies that lead to inequality or equality, and social norms that diminish or enhance the status of children contribute to this part of the history. Clearly, there is overlap between these realms, but by approaching the social history in this way lapses in documentation may be minimized (Table 26-4).

The Family History

The history of illness within the family should be specifically documented in the medical record (Table 26-5). Genetic illnesses that can mimic abuse should be asked about and documented. Any history of unexplained illness, injury, or death in siblings or other children residing in the same residence as the patient should be included or reported as a pertinent negative. A history of psychiatric illness in the patient's family members or caregivers should be sought.[27] A positive family history of abuse should also be noted.[16]

THE USE OF STANDARDIZED FORMS TO RECORD THE MEDICAL HISTORY

With the current emphasis on establishing computerized medical records, many practices use structured clinical

Table 26-5	Family History

- Sudden infant death syndrome/sudden unexplained infant deaths
- Seizures
- Developmental delays
- Hearing impairment
- Frequent fractures or fragile bones
- Dental problems (dentinogenesis imperfects)
- Bleeding/bruising tendency (ease of bruising, bleeding gums, nose bleeds, very heavy menses, excessive bleeding with childbirth or surgeries, need for transfusions
- Mental illness including substance abuse
- Child abuse/family violence

encounter forms designed for use by medical professionals and included in the patient's chart. Structured clinical encounter forms that are used in cases where child abuse is in the differential diagnosis have advantages and disadvantages. These forms are a part of the medical record and are often designed by child protection teams. They generally include space for all aspects of the history as outlined above, and they can help remind clinicians of important facts to document, providing clinicians with questions for better documentation of the history. Recent research, however, has shown mixed results with the introduction of these forms. A 1995 study showed no improvement in abuse documentation despite the introduction of a structured clinical form.[6] Other studies do show an improvement in documentation with well-designed clinical encounter forms.[28,29] If these forms are to be used, it is important that adequate space is given to elaborate on pertinent positives and negatives. Forms that are overly structured (e.g., many checkboxes) can result in the recording of less information. Including flow charts in the patient chart is another tool to augment documentation.[30] Further study is needed before widespread use of these forms can be recommended.

FINAL REPORTS

The documentation of the information discussed above is essential for the immediate treatment of injured children. Information should be recorded quickly so that it can be used as medical care is transitioned between health care professionals. In many cases, clinicians also are asked to provide final reports to child protection or law enforcement agencies for legal action affecting the child if abuse is suspected. It is important that medical records be clear and understandable, using accessible language and defining obscure medical terms.[31] Nonmedical and medical people often have different interpretations of the same term.[32] Medical providers are objective practitioners, and this objectivity should be reflected in the documentation. Final reports should express the tone of a scientist or educator rather than that of an advocate. Adopting these conventions makes it more likely that the report will be viewed as credible by the criminal and civil justice systems.

TOWARD THE FUTURE

The current shortcomings in documenting the history in cases of where physical abuse is in the differential diagnosis demonstrate a need for systemic improvement. First, additional studies of interventions aimed to improve documentation should be undertaken. While studies have found mixed results for structured clinical records and for individualized feedback based on chart reviews,[27] other interventions should also be tested. The advent of electronic medical records provides opportunities for newly structured forms and offers methods to improve documentation. These systems can facilitate rapid, legal, and appropriate release of information to authorities and can help reduce duplicative and sometimes illegible documentation. Many hospitals, especially pediatric hospitals, have developed specialized child protection teams that are better situated to handle documentation in these cases, and access to these teams is becoming the standard of care in all hospitals with a pediatric service.[33] These teams include members of the medical staff, social workers, and other professionals who work to coordinate their services to improve outcomes for the child. Above all, a conscious decision on the part of clinicians and researchers to address the challenges of accurate documentation should help to ensure that children and families are protected, and that the appropriate systems designated to take that responsibility make just and fair decisions.

References

1. Short D: History taking. *Br J Hosp Med* 1993;50:337-339.
2. Hampton JR, Harrison MJG, Mitchell JRA, et al: Relative contributions of history taking, physical examination, and laboratory investigation to diagnosis and management of medical outpatients. *Br Med J* 1975;270:486-489.
3. Gillis J: Taking a medical history in childhood illness: representations of parents in pediatric texts since 1850. *Bull Hist Med* 2005;79:393-429.
4. Chiocca EM: Documenting suspected child abuse, part II. *Nursing* 1998;28:25.
5. Christopher NC, Anderson D, Gaertner L, et al: Childhood injuries and the importance of documentation in the emergency department. *Pediatr Emerg Care* 1995;11:52-57.
6. Limbos MA, Berkowitz CD: Documentation of child physical abuse: how far have we come? *Pediatrics* 1998;102:53-58.
7. Anderst JD: Assessment of factors resulting in abuse evaluations in young children with minor head trauma. *Child Abuse Negl* 2008;32:405-413.
8. Boyce MD, Melhorn KJ, Vargo G: Pediatric trauma documentation: adequacy for assessment of child abuse. *Arch Pediatr Adolesc Med* 1996;150:730-732.
9. Johnson CF, Apolo J, Joseph JA, et al: Child abuse diagnosis and the emergency department chart. *Pediatr Emerg Care* 1986;2:6-9.
10. Ziegler DS, Sammut J, Piper AC: Assessment and follow-up of suspected child abuse in preschool children with fractures seen in a general hospital emergency department. *J Paediatr Child Health* 2005;41:251-255.
11. Jenny C: *Medical evaluation of physically and sexually abused children.* Sage, Thousand Oaks, Calif, 1996, pp 86-87.
12. Reece RM, Ludwig S (eds): *Child abuse: medical diagnosis and management,* ed 2, Lippincott, Williams, & Wilkins, Baltimore, 1996, p 545.
13. Palusci VJ, Hicks RA, Vandervort FE: "You are hereby commanded to appear": pediatrician subpoena and court appearance in child maltreatment. *Pediatrics* 2001;107:1427-1430.
14. Kellogg ND, Committee on Child Abuse and Neglect: Evaluation of suspected child physical abuse. *Pediatrics* 2007;119:1232-1241.
15. Zuckerman NS, Powell EC, Sheehan KM, et al: Community childhood injury surveillance: an emergency department based model. *Pediatr Emerg Care* 2004;20:361-366.

16. Hobbs CJ, Hanks HGI, Wynne JM: *Child abuse and neglect: a clinician's handbook*, ed 2, Churchill Livingstone, London, 1999.

17. Butchart A, Harvey AP, Mian M, et al: *Preventing child maltreatment: a guide to taking action and generating evidence*, World Health Organization (website): http://www.who.int/violence_injury_prevention/publications/violence/child_maltreatment/en/index.html. Accessed April 19, 2009.

18. Lamb ME, Orbach Y, Sternberg KJ, et al: Accuracy of investigators' verbatim notes of their forensic interviews with alleged child abuse victims. *Law Hum Behav* 2000;24:699-708.

19. Dubowitz H, Bross DC: The pediatrician's documentation of child maltreatment. *Am Dis Child* 1992;146:596-599.

20. Jackson AM, Rucker AR, Hinds T, et al: Let the record speak: medicolegal documentation in cases of child maltreatment. *Clin Pediatr Emerg Med* 2006;7:181-185.

21. Solomons G: Trauma and child abuse: the importance of the medical record. *Am J Dis Child* 1980;134:503-505.

22. Pierce MC, Bertocci GE, Janosky J, et al: Femur fractures resulting from stair falls in children: an injury plausibility model. *Pediatrics* 2005;115:1712-1722.

23. Hettler J, Greenes DS: Can the initial history predict whether a child with a head injury has been abused? *Pediatrics* 2003;111:602-607.

24. Krug EG, Dahlberg LL, Mercy JA, et al: *World report on violence and health*, World Health Organization (website): http://whqlibdoc.who.int/publications/2002/9241545615_eng.pdf. Accessed April 19, 2009.

25. Green J, Sullivan AL, Jureidini J: Shortcomings in psychosocial history taking in a paediatric emergency department. *J Paediatr Child Health* 1998;34:188-191.

26. Widom CS, Hiller-Sturmhofel S: Alcohol abuse as a risk factor for and consequence of child abuse. *Alcohol Res Health* 2001;25:52-57.

27. Shay NL, Knutson JF: Maternal depression and trait anger as risk factors for escalated physical discipline. *Child Maltreat* 2008;13:39-49.

28. Bar-On ME, Zanga JR: Child abuse: a model for the use of structured clinical forms. *Pediatrics* 1996;98:429-433.

29. Socolar RR, Raines B, Chen-Mok M, et al: Intervention to improve physician documentation and knowledge of child abuse: a randomized, controlled trial. *Pediatrics* 1998;101:817-824.

30. Benger JR, Pearce AV: Quality improvement report: simple intervention to improve detection of child abuse in emergency departments. *Br Med J* 2002;324:780-782.

31. David TJ: Avoidable pitfalls when writing medical reports for court proceedings in cases of suspected child abuse. *Arch Dis Child* 2004;89:799-804.

32. Mertz E: Translating science into family law: an overview. *De Paul Law Rev* 2007;56:799ff.

33. Committee on Pediatric Emergency Medicine: Guidelines for pediatric emergency care facilities. *Pediatrics* 1995;96:526-537.

27

PHOTODOCUMENTATION IN CHILD ABUSE CASES

Lawrence R. Ricci, MD, FAAP

INTRODUCTION

Over the past 20 years the need for expert medical evaluation of abused children and the benefits of high-quality photographs of significant physical findings have been recognized. This has placed demands on clinicians to familiarize themselves with medical forensic photographic techniques. Indeed, all medical providers who offer evaluations of abused children should have ready access to adequate photographic equipment and basic knowledge of camera operation, photographic composition, and the medical legal implications of photodocumentation.[1,2] Since there is already an extensive literature on the technical aspects of photodocumentation in child abuse and other forensic fields,[3-10] this chapter will highlight only the most important clinical elements.

Although a written description of physical findings remains an important aspect of child abuse injury documentation, if at all possible it is incumbent on the medical provider to obtain adequate photographic documentation of visible lesions. Some states require that reasonable efforts be made by providers "... to take or cause to be taken" color photographs of any areas of visible trauma on a child.[9,11]

The reasons for documenting evidence through the use of high-quality photography include:

1. Photographs can be reviewed after the examination to confirm findings and determine if previously unnoticed findings are present.
2. Photographs serve to enhance testimony by refreshing the examiner's memory of specific findings.
3. Photographic findings can be discussed among colleagues and consultants or can be compared with recent published data.[12]
4. Photographs allow improved communication for peer review with other child abuse physicians as a mechanism of education and accountability.[13]
5. Photographs of lesions can be compared, even overlaid with implements, if the magnification is precisely known (Figure 27-1).[14]
6. Imaging during a first visit will allow comparison with findings during a subsequent follow-up visit, or to compare findings with future visits should new allegations arise.
7. Photographs can be obtained of the child in a normal, uninjured state to establish a baseline reference if there is reason to believe that the child might be at future risk of injury.

8. Photographs allow quality control. It is recommended that new examiners photograph all examinations for adequate training and peer review.
9. Carefully acquired photographs and/or videos may save the child from the trauma of a repeat examination should a second opinion be requested of a particular child's findings.
10. Images provide an excellent tool for research and to teach normal and abnormal anatomy.[15]
11. Still photographs and videos are useful in court to illustrate significant findings to the judge and jury.
12. Digitized images can be transmitted electronically to colleagues for discussion. The use of telemedicine communication has emerged as a powerful tool in child abuse consultation and education.[16]

EQUIPMENT

Systems recommended in the past for photographing abuse victims have ranged from expensive colposcopes[17-21] to sophisticated but less expensive 35 mm close-up systems,[10] to even less expensive instant or self-developing camera systems.[1] With the emergence of the colposcope as a tool for obtaining close up photographs in child sexual abuse cases, the quality of documentation improved considerably.[13,15,17,19-24] Colposcopy enhanced the ability to examine genitalia with excellent magnification and lighting in a non-invasive manner. Perhaps most important, it allowed for close-up photographic documentation of findings. This high-quality documentation has supported the development of a common anatomic language, peer consultation, consensus building, and research. Alternatives to colposcopes have been introduced.[25] In general, these alternatives incorporate a close-up video camera attached to a stand with the image projected onto a monitor and saved on videotape (Figure 27-2). These systems are less expensive than colposcopes, provide the same quality of video documentation, and allow viewing of the findings on a monitor rather than through the eyepiece of the colposcope. Other forms of macrophotography have also emerged, first using macro lenses and ring flashes, and most recently using high definition digital video cameras.

Newer modalities of digital video and digital still imaging have virtually replaced 35 mm slide and print photography for image documentation. The newer digital still cameras are simple and easy to use. They are relatively inexpensive and fully automatic. They incorporate telephoto and limited

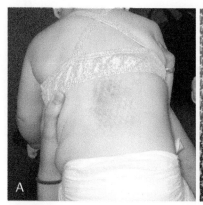
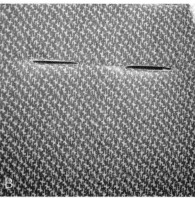
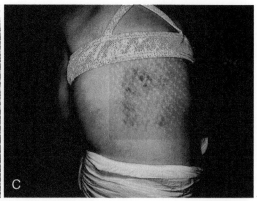

FIGURE 27-1 A, The infant has an unusual burn on the back. **B,** Her mother says they were riding in the car on a hot day. The car seat has a patterned surface noted in this photograph. **C,** Using Adobe Photoshop layer feature and making the photo of the car seat less opaque (more transparent) it was possible to superimpose the car seat on the burn demonstrating that the car seat pattern was, in fact, consistent with the burn pattern. For the purposes of this analysis the image of the infant was enhanced using Photoshop by increasing contrast and decreasing brightness.

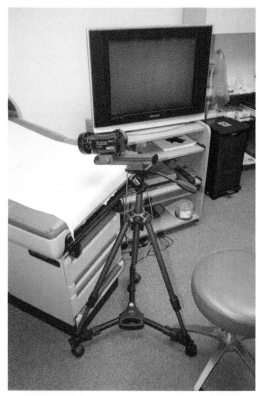

FIGURE 27-2 As an alternative to a colposcope, a high definition digital video camera with 6 megapixel digital still capability, set on a wheeled tripod with macro extender that allows the camera to reach over the table end. Camera has an attached video ring light and connects to a high definition video monitor via a HDMI cable.

macro or close-up (up to 0.25x) capability, built-in integrated flash, and auto focus. Digital single lens reflex (SLR) cameras combined with a 1x macro lens and ring flash compare favorably to and are significantly less expensive than colposcopic cameras for photographing the sexually abused child.[3] More recent digital cameras have incorporated image stabilization technology either in the camera body or in the lens. This allows for improved depth of field and/or faster shutter speeds by decreasing blurring (Figure 27-3).

Obtaining a photograph that adequately represents genital and rectal findings can be challenging, given both the inherent dynamic variability of these structures and the motion of the child.[17] This problem has led to the use of video photographic techniques for both documentation and teaching.[17]

Video provides a number of advantages over still photography when documenting anal and genital findings:

1. The dynamic variability of anogenital anatomy can be documented with greater ease.

2. Viewing the findings on a monitor, rather than through an eyepiece on the colposcope, allows the examiner to maintain visual contact with the child and quickly respond to the child.

3. An unanticipated advantage of the monitor is a reduction in anxiety for many children who are able to view the examination along with the examiner.

4. The examination can be recorded in its entirety for future reference.

5. Video recordings can be made available for opposing expert review, thus saving the child a repeat examination.

VHS and 8-mm video record approximately 200 lines of resolution, S-video and high 8 record 400 lines, and digital video records 500 lines.[16] The newer high definition (HD) digital video cameras further boost the resolution of the video image and allow even higher resolution still capture from video. For example, current HD cameras allow 720 lines or, depending on the format, up to 1080 lines of horizontal resolution. Although lines of resolution is a video construct not directly translatable to pixels, one can see that increasing the number of lines of horizontal resolution by as much as 100% over standard digital video should not only increase the resolution of the video but should significantly increase the resolution of a still later grabbed from the video.

A drawback of older video documentation systems has been the lack of high-quality images for publication, courtroom use, or teaching. This problem can be solved, albeit awkwardly, by recording the examination with both a

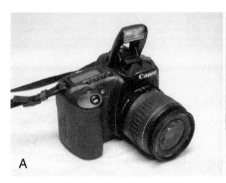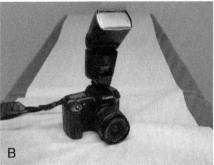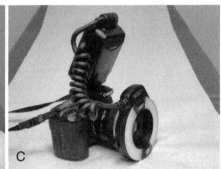

A   B   C

FIGURE 27-3 Examples of digital SLR camera setups. **A,** Digital single lens reflex camera with included flash. **B,** Same camera with hotshoe-mounted flash allowing bounce and/or diffusion screen to decrease glares. **C,** Same camera with a ring flash and 60 mm 1x macro lens for close-up photography.

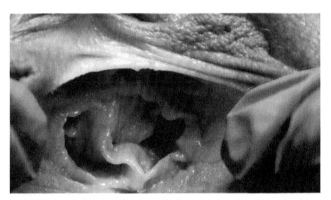

FIGURE 27-4 An example of a still photograph grabbed from a video using Pinnacle Studio software.

video camera and a still camera. With digital processing techniques, however, a video image can be converted to a digital image and then into a photograph of reasonable quality using commercial video editing software, such as Adobe Premiere or Pinnacle Studio. Newer high definition video cameras with upwards of 6 megapixel built in still cameras have virtually solved the problem (Figure 27-4). It should be mentioned, however, that a 6 megapixel still from a video camera is not currently of the same quality as a 6 megapixel still from a dedicated still camera primarily due to differing lens properties. In addition, compressed video shot through a still camera is markedly inferior to video shot by a dedicated video camera. Relatively inexpensive systems using digital video cameras mounted on a wheeled tripod produce equal if not better photodocumentation compared with significantly more expensive colposcopic systems (see Figure 27-3). When using photodocumentation, care should be taken to ensure that the child and parent are comfortable with the process. This can be a more difficult issue with children who have been involved in the creation of pornography.

Additional useful equipment includes spare batteries, USB cables to connect the camera to a computer to transfer images, and video cables to watch video on a monitor rather than the included LCD screen. Also recommended is an ABFO (American Board of Forensic Odontology) ruler. The size of lesions can be documented on the photograph by positioning such a measuring device adjacent to the lesion.[9,10,18]

It is difficult to recommend specific camera systems since any current recommendation will be out of date in a year. For many, a decision on whether to use a particular brand of colposcope or another form of imaging equipment should be based on cost, ease of use, compatibility with existing systems, and availability of technical assistance.[26-29]

COMPOSITION

Much can be learned from nonmedical texts on crime scene photography.[6,7] The goal of good crime scene photography is to capture all the relevant information as realistically as possible while excluding as much irrelevant information as possible. The photographer should think in terms of using the images to tell a story in such a way that someone looking at the photographs can mentally reproduce the scene. Composition, the arrangement of the visual elements in an image, must accurately show the primary subject. Viewpoint or perspective should exclude as many irrelevant items as possible. Viewpoint, whether horizontal or vertical, is contingent on the subject. For the most part, horizontal viewpoint is preferred with the subject composed in normal anatomic alignment if at all possible, recognizing the special limitations of photographing a moving child. Before snapping a picture the photographer must ensure, whether looking through a viewfinder or at an LCD display, that the subject is properly composed and the image is in focus. The single greatest difference between a skilled photographer and an unskilled one is that the skilled photographer pays close attention to foreground and background clutter.

According to Robinson,[6] the cardinal rules for crime scene photography are:

1. Fill the frame with the subject of interest. This is easily done either by physically moving closer or farther away or by zooming in or out. It is important to note that digital zoom is different than the lens zoom and the quality of the image is compromised. Avoid using digital zoom, which is calculated by the camera rather than the lens and although seeming to make things closer significantly degrades the image. A particular danger of moving the camera too close, however, is that the camera might not properly focus, producing a frame-filling, unfocused subject.
2. Maximize depth of field. This usually means using adequate ancillary lighting either constant (video lighting) or

intermittent (flash). With good lighting and standard film speed or digital film speed equivalent, most automatic cameras will use the smallest aperture and hence maximize the depth of focus. With digital cameras, sensor "speed" can be varied by using a higher ISO number leading to a smaller aperture. Some loss of detail, however, can occur at the highest ISO settings.

3. Keep the film plane parallel. This means that the back of the camera is parallel to the plane of the subject being photographed, avoiding if at all possible distorting viewpoints. (Sometimes angled viewpoints are useful, however, in creating contour-revealing shadows or eliminating flash glare, particularly on dark skin.)
4. Shoot distant, midrange, and close up pictures.
5. Be constantly aware of lighting and focus.

When photographing children, explain to them what is going to happen in language they will understand.[5,30] A significant benefit of videocolposcopy over simple still photography is that the child can actually watch the examination on the video monitor. The ability to observe what the examiner is doing might demystify the experience for the child, reduce his or her anxiety, and increase his or her cooperation. Although having the child in optimal photographic position would be ideal, it is better to have a cooperative, still child in a less optimal photographic position than an uncooperative, moving child. Infants and toddlers are usually photographed more easily if they are held in the lap of someone they know and trust.[31] Some children refuse photographic documentation despite the examiner's best effort. If possible, this refusal should be respected.[30,32,33]

The compositional principles for video are the same as for still photography with the addition that panning from side to side and up and down should be agonizingly slow with long pauses at significant pathology. Each finding should be videotaped using a distant, midrange, and close up view, again, both without and with a measuring ruler.

For an overview of technique, see Table 27-1.

STORAGE

Self-processing Polaroid film is expensive, difficult to reproduce, and difficult to store. Polaroid images and prints can be mechanically damaged and/or deteriorate, especially if exposed to light. Videotape, both analogue and digital, can be affected by magnets while the iron oxide matrix that makes up the tape has been known to deteriorate over time. CDs and DVDs store data using optical laser technology. CDs and DVDs will not deteriorate but they can be mechanically damaged. Hard drives can crash.

Because of these problems the best storage uses a redundant system, for example, filing the digital stills and/or video on optical media in the chart or in a secure location and storing them on a secure server with appropriate backup and/or redundancy such as an offsite server. Commercially available hard drives in the 1-plus terabyte storage range set up in a redundant array can now safely and easily store even the most massive digital video files.

Images can be viewed and sorted using standard commercial photo album software such as Adobe Photoshop Album. If proprietary medical image management software is used, it is important to be sure that images are not altered

| Table 27-1 | Shooting Tips |

- Familiarize yourself with the camera and its operation before attempting to use it clinically
- Generally shoot in automatic mode. Program mode is available for more experienced photographers. For example, aperture priority settings can be used to enhance depth of field while black and white settings can be used to photograph x-ray film and bite marks.
- Be sure the camera is set to its highest resolution and lowest compression. RAW format is available in many cameras but is of use primarily by professional photographers.
- Use the highest capacity storage media in the camera possible to assure sufficient space for multiple pictures.
- Always use a flash or ancillary full spectrum light source such as a video ringlight, and eliminate distracting shadow-producing light such as operative lights or sunlight, both of which can adversely affect exposure balance.
- Shoot at least three views of each finding: overview or distant, midrange, and close-up.
- Arrange the subject and/or the camera so that the surface of interest is parallel to the film plane. Do not be afraid to shoot from differing perspectives, which can enhance revealing shadows or eliminate flash glare.
- Compose the picture the way you would normally look at the area.
- Try to avoid a cluttered background and foreground.
- Take a photo of the child's name.
- Take several shots of each finding from several angles and distances.
- Take a set of photos without and then with an appropriate ruler such as an ABFO forensic ruler in the same plane as the injury. With modern auto white-balanced digital cameras color reference scales have become unnecessary for most child abuse photography. Even with a scale, color should be interpreted with great caution as so many factors such as lighting, printer quality, monitor quality and settings can affect the apparent color of an image.
- It is useful to photograph burns, dirty abrasions, or even unkempt children both before and after cleaning. Before and after photographs of children with failure to thrive can be particularly compelling. As conditions change over time, lesions should be re-photographed.
- Bite mark photography is a specialized branch of forensic photography and is best left to the forensic expert. (See Chapter 61.)
- When shooting video start with a patient identifier. Eliminate audio recording either in the camera software or by putting a dummy jack into the audio input. If at all possible, particularly with sexual abuse cases, use a tripod. Pan very slowly and pause for several seconds at each finding of significance. Video each finding using a distant, midrange and close-up view both without and with a measuring ruler.

or compressed by the software when stored, and are available in an unaltered original state for copying and viewing.

Whatever storage medium is used, images should be stored and released according to specific institutional policies. Guidelines should be consulted such as those developed by the American Professional Society on the Abuse of Children and the U.S. Department of Justice.[34]

COMMON ERRORS

Errors occur when the photographs do not show the pathology adequately because the composition is either too far away, too close, or because the photographer did not take enough pictures from different perspectives and distances. With modern digital technology it is always best to take many more pictures than needed rather than fewer.

The single most common error in photodocumentation is blurring of the image. This is much less of a problem with newer autofocused cameras. However, out of focus images can still occur when the camera is too close to the subject, or when the photographer does not wait for the camera to autofocus, or takes the picture even when the camera indicates it cannot autofocus. If the subject being photographed has few distinguishing contours or edges such as when photographing a close-up image of skin, the camera might not be able to find the autofocus point. One solution is to switch to manual focus; another is to focus on another object at equal distance by partially pressing the shutter then moving the camera over to the subject of interest and completing the shot.

Blur introduced by child movement is hard to control for except by using good lighting and fast shutter speeds. In some cases blur in the image is due to camera movement. This can be minimized by using a tripod or at the very least, using good camera technique with two hands holding the camera, the left bracing the elbow against the chest while the right snaps the picture.

Yet another problem occurs when the image has distorted color, often yellow or green. This most commonly occurs because a flash has not been used or has not recycled before the next picture was taken. Always use a flash indoors even if the room is very bright, allowing the flash sufficient time to recycle. If flash reflection is a problem, try shooting without a flash, or use of an adjustable bounce flash to both maintain color temperature balance and avoid flash reflection. Fresh, fully charged batteries shorten flash recycle time. Finally, lenses should be cleaned regularly.

ALTERNATE LIGHT SOURCE PHOTOGRAPHY

Alternate light source photography (ultraviolet or infrared) is widely used in forensic crime scene photography to reveal trace evidence such as blood and fingerprints.[7,36-42] It has not gained wide acceptance in child abuse photography, principally because of the cost and complexity of the equipment and the technical expertise required.

Reflected UV (ultraviolet) photography can reveal long-healed bite marks, belt imprints, and wound remnants. Vogeley et al[41] report the use of Wood's lamp illumination in digital photography in the documentation of bruises. They used direct UV illumination as an alternative to reflected UV. They reported on three patients whose bruises were only visible using the wood light. They used a Sony digital Mavica camera in low ambient light with illumination from the Wood's lamp held 10 cm from the skin. Images were contrast enhanced 10% to 40% using Adobe Photoshop software.

LEGAL ISSUES

The principal requirements for courtroom admission of a photograph into evidence are relevance and authentication.[42,43] Unless the photograph is admitted by stipulation, the party attempting to admit the photograph into evidence must be prepared to offer testimony that the photograph is an accurate representation of the scene. This usually means that someone must testify that the photograph is an accurate portrayal of the scene.[9] To help verify that the photographs are actually of a particular child, an identifying sign can be placed in front of the patient for each picture or at the very least at the beginning of the image sequence. The inclusion of such signs or labels in each photograph, however, is time-consuming and distracting.[44,45] In the end, it is the examiner who must verify that a photograph or video is of a particular child.

Photographs are generally considered admissible if they shed light on the issue, enable the witness to better describe the objects portrayed, permit the jury to better understand the testimony, or corroborate testimony. Courts generally permit medical providers to explain and illustrate their testimony with a photograph. A simple explanation by the photographer that the images are needed to adequately describe the complexity and extent of the injuries is all that is usually necessary.

When copying still images for legal purposes, it is important to create as exact a copy as possible. This means that the image should not be modified or cropped. If it is converted to a print, that print should be on high-quality photographic paper using a high-quality color printer. Black and white or even color copies on plain laser paper are virtually worthless. When copying video, the copy (and the original) should be made using the highest quality media at the best recording and copying settings. At the very least this means using standard play rather than extended play for recording and copying to tape or disk.

A particular legal concern about digital photographs is the potential for images to be digitally manipulated and, hence, not accepted in court. To date, there has been no legal precedent excluding the use of digitally obtained images. The Federal Rules of Evidence define writings and recordings to include magnetic, mechanical, or electronic recordings. If data is stored in a computer or similar device, any printout or other output shown to reflect the data accurately is an original. The rules go on to state that a duplicate, an accurate reproduction of the original, is admissible to the same extent as an original. This means that a photograph or video stored digitally in a computer is considered an original and an exact copy of the digital photograph is admissible as evidence. Original images for courtroom use should, of course, never be altered. If a copy is changed to improve viewing, such as by brightening or darkening, these changes should be noted clearly. The original digital image must be preserved in the original file format, ideally a lossless format such as TIFF or uncompressed JPG.[46]

Chain of evidence, critical when analyzing trace evidence, is less important in photodocumentation. Photos taken by medical providers, law enforcement, or child protective services can be verified as accurately representing the scene if these professionals attest to the accuracy of the photographs. Photos taken by nonprofessionals, for example, family members or day care providers, are less reliable unless the findings can be corroborated by a professional involved in the case. Digital images contain within the file so called "metadata." which notes date and time of photo (assuming the time on the camera was set accurately), camera and lens, shutter speed, f-stop, flash, and whether the image has been altered or modified.

Although many child abuse laws state that permission is not needed for photographs if photographs are obtained as part of a child abuse evaluation, going through the process of obtaining consent can establish an alliance with the family. A variety of consent forms are available, including a model form drafted by the American Medical Association.[11,44,47] Each institution should have a policy for the handling and release of photographs.

Child abuse medical specialists are often called on to review photographs of injuries and/or crime scenes they have not seen themselves. David[48] has noted that a professional reviewing photographs should insist on good quality glossy prints of original photographs (perhaps even better, copies of original digital files). Photographs of the scene, if available, also should be reviewed. Photographs, however, of suspected injuries can be misleading. Photographs might fail to show lesions that were present or might suggest the presence of lesions or injuries that do not exist. David reports on a case where five experts incorrectly diagnosed abuse because the two-dimensional color photographs failed to accurately reflect a three-dimensional normal variant.

CONCLUSION

The evidence base for techniques for and the value of photodocumentation is well established. Less well established is the effect of image quality on expert interpretation. Child abuse photodocumentation would benefit from research on the ability of observers to interpret findings using media of different types and quality, varying resolution still images, high definition vs. standard definition video, differing printer and print paper quality, and differing monitor resolution and color balance. Future research should also focus on even easier systems of photodocumentation for the unskilled photographer.

References

1. Baum E, Grodin MA, Alpert JJ, et al: Child sexual abuse, criminal justice, and the pediatrician. *Pediatrics* 1987;79:437-439.
2. American Medical Association: AMA diagnostic and treatment guidelines concerning child abuse and neglect. *JAMA* 1985;254:796-800.
3. Ricci LR: Medical forensic photography of the sexually abused child. *Child Abuse Negl* 1988;12:305-310.
4. Ricci LR: Photographing the physically abused child: principles and practice. *Am J Dis Child* 1991;145:275-281.
5. Ricci LR: Photodocumentation of the abused child. *In*: Reece RM (ed): *Child Abuse: Medical Diagnosis and Management*. Lea & Febiger, Philadelphia, 1994, pp 248-264.
6. Robinson EM, Witzke D: *Crime scene photography*. Academic Press, Burlington, Mass, 2007.
7. Weiss SL: *Forensic photography. The importance of accuracy*. Pearson Education Prentice Hall, Upper Saddle River NJ, 2008.
8. Dove SL: Non-accidental injury: photography and procedures. *J Audiov Media Med* 1992;15:138-142.
9. Smistek S: Photography of the abused and neglected child. *In*: Ludwig S, Kornberg AE (eds): *Child Abuse: A Medical Reference*. Churchill Livingstone, New York, 1992, pp 467-477.
10. Cordell W, Zollman W, Karlson H: A photographic system for the emergency department. *Ann Emerg Med* 1980;9:210-214.
11. Spring GE: Evidence photography: an overview. *J Biol Photogr* 1987;55:129-132.
12. Roberts I, Moran K: Inter-rater reliability in the medical diagnosis of child sexual abuse. *J Paediatr Child Health* 1995;31:290-291.
13. Adams JA, Phillips P, Ahmad M: The usefulness of colposcopic photographs in the evaluation of suspected child sexual abuse. *Adolesc Pediatr Gynecol* 1990;3:75-82.
14. Patno KC, Jenny C: Who slapped that child? *Child Maltreat* 2008;13:298-300.
15. Berenson AB, Grady JJ: A longitudinal study of hymenal development from 3 to 9 years of age. *J Pediatr* 2002;140:600-607.
16. Alexander R, Farst K: Telemedicine and child abuse examinations. *Pediatr Ann* 2009;38:574-578.
17. McCann J: Use of the colposcope in childhood sexual abuse examinations. *Pediatr Clin North Am* 1990;37:863-880.
18. Soderstrom RM: Colposcopic documentation. An objective approach to assessing sexual abuse of girls. *J Reprod Med* 1994;39:6-8.
19. Teixeira WRG: Hymenal colposcopic examination in sexual offenses. *Am J Forensic Med Pathol* 1981;2:209-215.
20. Woodling BA, Kossoris P: Sexual misuse: rape, molestation and incest. *Pediatr Clin North Am* 1981;28:481-499.
21. Woodling BA, Heger A: The use of the colposcope in the diagnosis of sexual abuse in the pediatric age group. *Child Abuse Negl* 1986;10:111-114.
22. Finkel MA: Anogenital trauma in sexually abused children. *Pediatrics* 1989;84:317-322.
23. Hobbs CJ, Wynne JM, Thomas AJ: Colposcopic genital findings in prepubertal girls assessed for sexual abuse. *Arch Dis Child* 1995;73:465-469.
24. Muram D, Arheart KL, Jennings SG: Diagnostic accuracy of colposcopic photographs in child sexual abuse evaluations. *J Pediatr Adolesc Gynecol* 1999;12:58-61.
25. Siegel RM, Hill TD, Henderson VA, et al: Comparison of an intraoral camera with colposcopy in sexually abused children. *Clin Pediatr* 1999;38:375-376.
26. Atabaki S, Paradise JE: The medical evaluation of the sexually abused child: lessons from a decade of research. *Pediatrics* 1999;104:178-186.
27. Brayden RM, Altemeier WA, Yeager T, et al: Interpretations of colposcopic photographs: evidence for competence in assessing sexual abuse. *Child Abuse Negl* 1991;15:69-76.
28. Norvell MK, Benrubi GI, Thompson RJ: Investigation of microtrauma after sexual intercourse. *J Reprod Med* 1984;29:269-271.
29. Sinal SH, Lawless MR, Rainey DY, et al: Clinician agreement on physical findings in child sexual abuse cases. *Arch Pediatr Adolesc Med* 1997;151:497-501.
30. Steward MS, Schmitz M, Steward DS, et al: Children's anticipation of and response to colposcopic examination. *Child Abuse Negl* 1995;19:997-1005.
31. Reeves C: Pediatric photography. *J Audiov Media Med* 1986;9:131-134.
32. Muram D, Aiken MM, Strong C: Children's refusal of gynecologic examinations for suspected sexual abuse. *J Clin Ethics* 1997;8:158-164.
33. Mears CJ, Heflin AH, Finkel MA, et al: Adolescents' responses to sexual abuse evaluation including the use of video colposcopy. *J Adolesc Health* 2003;33:18-24.
34. *Photodocumentation in the investigation of child abuse*. U.S. Department of Justice, Office of Juvenile Justice Programs, Washington, DC, 1996.
35. Photodocumentation Subcommittee of the APSAC Task Force on Medical Evaluation of Suspected Child Abuse: *Practice Guidelines: Photographic Documentation of Child Abuse*. American Professional Society on the Abuse of Children, Chicago, 1995. Available at http://www.reidwriting.com/images/PDF8.pdf. Accessed March 7. 2010.
36. Krauss TC, Warlen SC: The forensic science use of reflective ultraviolet photography. *J Forensic Sci* 1985;30:262-268.
37. Barsley RE, West MH, Fair JA: Forensic photography: ultraviolet imaging of wounds on skin. *Am J Forensic Med Pathol* 1990;11:300-308.
38. David TJ, Sobel MN: Recapturing a five-month-old bite mark by means of reflective ultraviolet photography. *J Forensic Sci* 1994;39:1560-1567.

39. West MH, Barsley RE, Hall JE, et al: The detection and documentation of trace wound patterns by use of an alternative light source. *J Forensic Sci* 1992;37:1480-1488.

40. West M, Barsley RE, Frair J, et al: Ultraviolet radiation and its role in wound pattern documentation. *J Forensic Sci* 1992;37:1466-1479.

41. Vogeley E, Pierce MC, Bertocci G: Experience with wood lamp illumination and digital photography in the documentation of bruises on human skin. *Arch Pediatr Adolesc Med* 2002;156:265-268.

42. Flower MS: Photographs in the courtroom. "Getting it straight between you and your professional photographer." *North Ky State Law Forum* 1974;2:184-211.

43. Myers JEB: *Legal issues in child abuse and neglect.* Sage, Newbury Park, Calif, 1992.

44. Sebben JE: Office photography. *Adv Dermatol* 1990;5:53-73.

45. Sebben JE: Office photography from the surgical viewpoint. *J Dermatol Surg Oncol* 1983;9:763-768.

46. Scientific Working Group on Imaging Technologies (SWIGIT): *Draft recommendations and guidelines for the use of digital image processing in the criminal justice system,* International Association for Identification (website): www.fdiai.org/images/SWGIT%20guidelines.pdf. Accessed April 19, 2009.

47. Weiss CH: Dermatologic photography of nail pathologies. *Dermatol Clin* 1985;3:543-556.

48. David TJ: Avoidable pitfalls when writing medical reports for court proceedings in cases of suspected child abuse. *Arch Dis Child* 2004;89:799-804.

28

ABUSIVE BURNS

Barbara L. Knox, MD, FAAP, and Suzanne P. Starling, MD

EPIDEMIOLOGY AND DEMOGRAPHICS OF CHILD ABUSE BY BURNING

The incidence of burns secondary to abuse in hospitalized burned children has been reported from low estimates of less than 11%[1-8] to high estimates of 16%[9,10] to 25%.[11] For burned children coming to emergency departments, the frequency of abuse or neglect has ranged from 0%[12] to 19.5%.[13] The variability in incidence estimation is due to differences in study methodology and inclusion criteria.[14] For instance, definitions for abusive burning in some studies include burns secondary to neglect,[1] while others include suspicious but unproven abuse cases.[15] Other variables include duration of time evaluated and sample size,[6] urban versus rural geographic location,[16] socioeconomic status of the community,[12,14,17] ability of medical personnel to recognize abuse, variations in reporting practices,[6] and availability of trained investigators.[6]

Abusive burns typically occur in children younger than age 6,[18,19] with most studies documenting a mean age of injury between 2 to 4 years.* Of the children admitted to the hospital for treatment secondary to abusive burns, infants and toddlers represent the greatest percentage of cases.† Children with abusive burns require longer hospital admissions than those with accidental burns,[6,7,15] have increased morbidity,[6,23] consume more resources during treatment and follow-up,[25] and are more likely to die from their injuries.[2,6,8,15] Scalding is the most frequent type of inflicted burn in childhood,[6,20,26,27] with hot water immersion being the most common mechanism reported.[11,19,28] Childhood abusive burn victims are more likely to have previous or concomitant signs of abuse/neglect and previous reports to child protective services.[3,9,16,23,29-31] Many studies report that boys are more frequently victims of abusive burns,‡ however, some have noted equal gender distribution.[11,13,21] The ethnic composition of burned children generally mirrors that of the community.[16] When siblings are present in a home, the youngest child is at greatest risk of victimization by abusive burning.[11,21,29,30]

Hammond et al[32] documented both receptive (comprehension and memory) and expressive (naming and descriptive) language deficits in 81% of children who were victims of abuse by burning compared with 42% of accidentally burned children. The authors hypothesized that caretaker frustration with verbally delayed children leads to increased incidence of abuse in this population.

Barillo et al[33] found an increased incidence of suspected/known intentional burn injury in boys who were small for their age. The authors found that 28% of boys at or below the 5th percentile for weight and 15.1% of males at or below the 5th percentile for height were victims of burn injury.

CHARACTERISTICS OF ABUSIVE BURN PERPETRATORS

Abusive pediatric burns occur more commonly in families with a single, young, socially isolated parent from a lower socioeconomic class.* The Hummel[17] study found that most parents of burn-abused children were unemployed with incomes of less than $20,000 per year. Children abused by scald or thermal contact burning were most likely to come from impoverished, welfare-dependent homes.[36] Hummel et al[17] reported that the abusive perpetrator was most frequently the child's parent or the mother's boyfriend.[17] Stepparents, siblings, and other relatives accounted for a lesser number of cases while only three abusive perpetrators in the study were nonrelative babysitters of the child victim.[17] Showers[30] found that women are the most frequent perpetrators in abusive childhood burn cases, contrasting Ojo et al[21] who documented all male perpetrators, identified as the biological mother's boyfriends.[21] Compliance with follow-up burn care and rehabilitation is also worse for children abused by burning compared to those with accidental burns.[17]

Classification of Burns

Skin consists of the epidermis, dermis, and the subcutaneous tissue. Figure 28-1 shows a cross section of skin anatomy. Each skin layer performs a specific function. The outermost skin layer, the epidermis, is made up of three sublayers, and its primary function is to serve as a protective barrier for the body. Melanocytes, cells which produce skin pigment, are located at the base of the epidermis. Underlying the

---

*References 2, 4, 5, 8, 9, 16, 20.
†References 2, 6, 8, 9, 16, 21-24.
‡References 2, 4-6, 8, 9, 14, 22, 23, 29, 30.

---

*References 2, 9, 13, 15, 17, 21, 22, 29, 30, 34, 35.

THICK (HAIRLESS) SKIN | THIN (HAIRY) SKIN

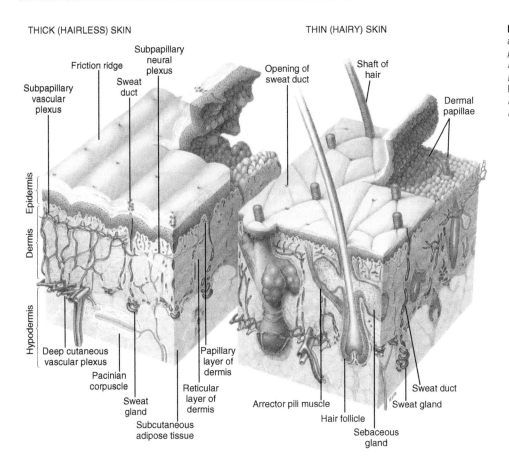

FIGURE 28-1 Cross sectional anatomy of the skin. *(Reprinted with permission from Standring S: Skin and its appendages. In Standring S [ed]: Gray's Anatomy: the Anatomical Basis of Clinical Practice, ed 39, Elsevier Churchill Livingstone, Edinburgh, 2005, p 158.)*

epidermis is the dermis, containing blood vessels, hair follicles, sweat glands, and lymph vessels. Beneath the dermis is the subcutaneous tissue, which contains collagen and fat cells.

Burns are primarily classified based upon the degree/depth of tissue injury. Historically, burn injury has been reported as first-, second-, third-, or fourth-degree injury. Most medical providers now use a classification system based upon partial or full-thickness tissue injury. Partial-thickness burns can be subdivided into superficial and deep partial-thickness injury. Superficial partial-thickness burn injury results in damage to the epidermal skin layer only, and correlates with the older first-degree burn classification system. The skin is characterized by localized erythema and these burns heal without treatment. Tissue damage that progresses into the dermal skin layer is reported as superficial partial thickness to deep partial-thickness burn injury, depending upon depth of tissue damage. These burns result in blister formation and correlate with the older second-degree burn classification. If the dermal tissue is only superficially injured, the damaged tissue will be replaced by the underlying healthy tissue. If the injury produces a deeper partial-thickness burn, these burns still heal without scarring, as long as other complicating factors, such as infection, are absent. When tissue damage penetrates to deeper layers of the dermis, deep partial-thickness burns result and scarring occurs. Full-thickness burns cause injury through the dermis into the subcutaneous tissue layer and correspond to the older third-degree burn. If injury penetrates through the subcutaneous tissue layer into the underlying muscle, fat,

and bone, this full-thickness burn injury correlates with the older fourth-degree burn classification. Full-thickness burns will not heal by tissue regeneration. If very small, the lesion can heal with scar formation by secondary intention. The majority of full-thickness burn injuries, however, require skin grafting.

Burns can result in production of hyperpigmented or hypopigmented scarring.[37] The pathophysiological role of melanocytes, their response to burn injury, and effect on scarring is not understood at this time. Therefore medical providers are currently unable to predict which pediatric patients will develop pigment abnormalities within the burn scar.[37]

TYPES OF BURNS AND MEDICAL EVIDENCE SUGGESTING MALTREATMENT

Burns also are classified by the source of damage to the skin and are divided into thermal, chemical, electrical, radiation, and friction/pressure tissue injury categories.

Thermal Burns

Thermal burns are the most common form of accidental and nonaccidental burns in children and consist of tissue damage from scalds, contact, flame, or radiation injury. Scald burns are further subdivided into immersion, flowing liquid, splash, and splatter injury. The majority of all scald burns are

FIGURE 28-2 The common distribution of inflicted and accidental immersion burns on young children. *(Reprinted with permission from Daria S, Sugar NF, Feldman KW, et al: Into hot water head first: distribution of intentional and unintentional immersion burns. Pediatr Emerg Care 2004;20:302-310.)*

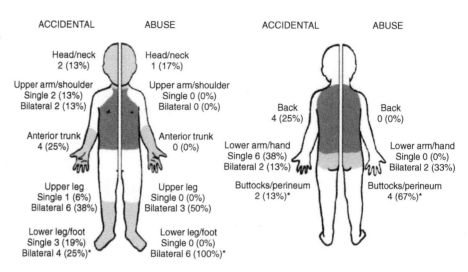

accidental and due to splash/spill injury by fluids other than tapwater,[28] such as soups,[38] hot beverages, and other cooking liquids,[39] and occur in the home environment.[40] For abusive burn injuries, scalding by immersion in hot tap water is most frequently reported.[11,19,28] Both accidental and abusive scald injuries account for the majority of pediatric burn hospital admissions,[20,40,41] and up to 14% of all scald burns are secondary to abuse.[36,42-44] Scald injury from hot tap water requires hospitalization in 39% of cases, and of these, 12% to 45% are considered to be abusive in nature.[19,20,34,45,46] Purdue et al[8] found that 82% of children admitted with abusive burns had scald injuries present and of these, 83% were secondary to tap water and 59% had an immersion patterns present. In contrast, only 15.7% of nonabused children had hot tap water scald burns. The mortality rate for abusive hot water immersion burns in Purdue's study was 10%.[8]

For suspected immersion scald injury, the pattern of injury present greatly assists both the medical provider and investigators in analyzing the case for accidental versus inflicted mechanisms. Burn patterns demonstrating uniformity of burn depth suggest the child was restrained or not moving during the time of injury occurrence,[23] and bilateral burn symmetry in the absence of splash marks suggests forced immersion.[23,28] Daria et al[28] reported that bilateral, symmetric lower extremity burn distribution pattern occurred more frequently in abused children. Figure 28-2 shows the distribution of inflicted and accidental immersion burns on young children.

Immersion burns typically have patterned injury demonstrating uniform burn depth, flexion sparing, linear contour between the burned and unburned skin areas, absence of splash marks, and can have skin sparing in areas where the skin was in contact with cooler surfaces, such as sink or tub bottoms. Absence of burning where the child came in contact with cooler surfaces represents doughnut burns often seen in inflicted immersion injuries. The presence of uniform burn line demarcation also suggests that a child was restrained while being immersed in the hot liquid,[47] and therefore unable to generate splash patterns in an attempt to get away from the painful stimulus.[19,47] Patterned injury demonstrating skin sparing in areas of flexion where skin-skin apposition occurs also suggests that the child was

withdrawing from painful stimuli at the time of the injury. This latter pattern can be seen in both accidental and inflicted scald burns. Figure 28-3 demonstrates some immersion injury patterns.

Titus et al[41] presented a case series of accidental scald burns in sinks occurring in ambulatory children 18 to 19 months of age. The injury patterns in the children demonstrated asymmetry with one extremity being significantly more injured than the other. The authors also noted splash marks to be *absent* in some cases of accidental immersion burns occurring in sinks.

There is a paucity of information in the medical literature regarding how rapidly burn injury occurs to children's skin. Table 28-1 documents minimum times and temperatures causing scald burns in children and adults. Children comfortably bathe at a temperature of 101° F (38° C), whereas hot tubs typically have temperatures fluctuating between 102° F to 104° F (39-40° C).[47] Adults sense water as painfully hot between temperatures of 112° F to 114° F (43-45° C).[47,48]

Moritz' and Henriques' research[49-53] represents the majority of published data regarding time-temperature burn associations. The authors evaluated the thresholds for development of first-degree and deep second-degree burning of adult skin. Production of a deep second-degree burn to both adult and child skin requires a water temperature of at least 113° F (45° C).[50,54,55] Both adult and premature infant skin would take a minimum of 6 hours continuous contact with this degree water temperature to induce a deep partial-thickness burn.[47,50,54,55] Water temperature of 120° F (49° C) produces deep second-degree burning of the skin after 10 minutes of contact.[19,50,56] Water temperatures must reach 130° F (54° C) before a difference is noted between adult and child skin burn times.[54] Children's skin is thinner, and there is an inverse relationship seen between thickness of the skin and temperature and time necessary to induce burning at this threshold. Feldman[54] reported that when temperatures exceed 130° F (54° C), children sustain burn injury in only a quarter of the time it takes adult skin to burn.

There have been many cases in which the caretaker has described the child climbing into a tub or sink after which the child becomes immobilized by pain, thereby creating a situation in which the child is unable to escape

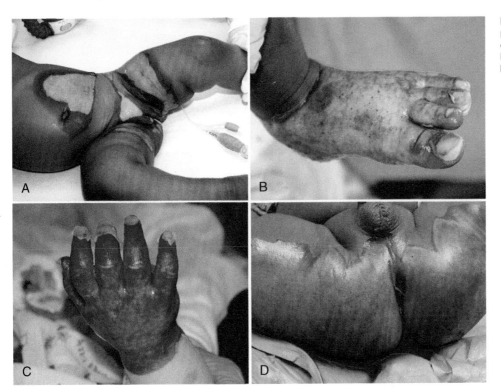

FIGURE 28-3 Immersion injury patterns. **A,** Sparing of the flexor creases. **B,** Immersion "stocking" burn. **C,** Immersion "glove" burn. **D,** Immersion buttocks burn.

Table 28-1	Minimum Times and Temperatures Cusing Scald Burns in Children and Adults						
Full Thickness Burn(s)*				**Subthreshold(s)†**			
‡Adult Calculated[1]	Adult Experimental[2]	§Child Calculated[3]	**Temperature**	‡Adult Calculated[1]	Adult Experimental[2]	§Child Calculated[3]
0.5	1	—	70°C (158°F)	0.4	—	—
1.0	2	0.5	65°C (149°F)	1.0	0.7	0.3
3.0	5	1.0	60°C (140°F)	2.3	2.6	0.5
—	—	4.0	57°C (135°F)	—	—	2.0
13.0	16	—	56°C (133°F)	8.1	8.3	—
31.0	35	10.0	54°C (130°F)	19.0	18	6.0

Reprinted with permission from Feldman KW: Help needed on hot water burns. *Pediatrics* 1983;71:145-146.
*As used in original paper, corresponds to minimum time and temperature causing deep second degree burns
†Corresponds to minimum time and temperature causing first degree burns
‡Based on adult thigh skin thickness of 2.5 mm[3]
§Based on 0-5 year old female child medial thigh skin thickness of 0.56 mm[3]
[1]Mortiz AR, Henriques FC: Studies of thermal injury, II. *Am J Pathol* 1947;23:695
[2]Henriques FC: Studies of thermal injury, V. *Arch Pathol* 1947;43:489
[3]International Commission of Radiological Protection (Snyder WS [Chairman]): *Report on the Task Group on Reference Man.* Oxford, Pergamon Press, 1975, pp 48.

from the hot water. This explanation is offered to account for the symmetrical uniform contour burn injury on the child's bilateral lower extremities. If this history presents itself, the multidisciplinary team must investigate if the developmental level of the child is inconsistent with the child's ability to extricate himself from the painful hot

water stimulus. Allasio et al[57] studied 176 children between the ages of 10 to 18 months presenting to a general pediatric office to determine at what age infant and toddler children could climb into a 14-inch tall bathtub. The authors reported 35% of the children studied were able to perform this climbing skill with older age improving success. One

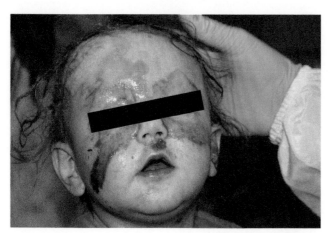

FIGURE 28-4 A 13-month-old female with facial burns caused by hot grease spilled from a frying pan.

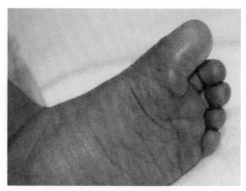

FIGURE 28-5 Blistering distal dactylitis. *(Photo courtesy Ron Paul, MD, Louisville, Ky).*

10-month-old infant was able to crawl in the tub despite not yet walking. By 18 months, nearly 80% of children were able to climb in the tub.

Hot water splash burn injuries require a minimum temperature of 140° F (60° C) to produce tissue injury; lower water temperatures will cool to a point where thermal cutaneous injury will not occur.[47] Scald patterns due to splash or flowing liquid can be altered based upon the presence or absence of clothing. In addition, the type of liquid present may significantly affect the burn. Scald injuries resulting from liquids other than water, such as hot beverages, foods, grease, oils, or wax, can reach temperatures much greater than the boiling point of water (212° F) and have a greater viscosity, which results in a deeper, more significant burn due to the higher heat source and prolonged contact with the skin.[58] Figure 28-4 shows a 13-month-old female with facial burns caused by hot grease spilling from a frying pan. Pull-down splash burns typically have a "triangular" appearance with the area of greatest burn injury occurring at the area of immediate skin contact. The scalding liquid then typically has a trickle-down drip pattern present. The majority of hot oil/hot grease burns in the pediatric population is secondary to accidental mechanisms.[59] Hankins et al[60] documented that children in the toddler and preschool age ranges are at greatest risk of sustaining scald burns from hot oil. Ninety-two percent of the children studied sustained hot oil scald burns after pulling the hot oil down onto themselves. The literature only documents a few cases of inflicted hot oil/hot grease burns in children. Murphy et al[59] reported only one case over a 20-year time span of regional burn center admissions in which abusive injury was secondary to a source of hot grease. Mukadam et al[61] reported on inflicted hot oil burns to a 7-year-old child, which produced contact and scald burns caused by a metal spatula heated in hot cooking oil.

Colombo et al[62] reported on cases of vaporizer-related thermal burn injuries in the pediatric population. These steam vaporizers resulted in severe facial burns and some cases of inhalation of hot steam producing severe pulmonary tissue injury. Scald burns also were reported after children spilled steamed vaporizer contents onto themselves. Vaporizers used today typically produce only cool mist. Wallis et al,[63] however, reported 27 children treated for scald injury secondary to breathing warm humidified air for treatment of upper respiratory infections between 2001 to 2006.[63]

Abusive Thermal Burn Mimics

Toxic epidermal necrolysis produces peeling of the skin in sheet layers and sloughing of the mucosal surfaces. It is typically associated with an infectious etiology or hypersensitivity to medications. The onset of its effect typically occurs within 21 days of medication use.[64] Both toxic epidermal necrolysis and Stevens-Johnson syndrome can present as mimics of abusive burn injury.

Murphy[65] reported on a case of a 15-month-old girl with three, well-circumscribed areas of skin loss on the posterior aspect of both lower limbs and right thigh with underlying, erythematous wet patches. These lesions, given the lack of historical explanation and concerning features were evaluated for abusive injury. They were later found to be the result of staphylococcal scalded skin syndrome. This produces blistering of the skin with subsequent exfoliation secondary to exfoliative toxins produced by *Staphylococcus aureus* bacteria. It is most commonly seen in infants and young children. Historical information allowing the medical provider to differentiate staphylococcal scalded skin syndrome from burns includes the fact that staphylococcal scalded skin syndrome is typically preceded by febrile illness and skin erythema. The toxin induces skin splitting of the epidermal tissue resulting in a wet erythematous epidermal base being left behind after sloughing occurs.[65]

Blistering distal dactylitis,[66] caused by group A beta-hemolytic streptococcal infection, presents as a superficial blistering lesion over the distal portion of a digit and may mimic thermal or flame injury.[67] Figure 28-5 demonstrates a child with blistering distal dactylitis.

Contact Burns

Contact burns result in thermal injury to the skin secondary to prolonged contact with the hot solid or smoldering source.[68] Abusive contact burns typically produce a branding injury characterized by distinct margins, grouped burn lesions, clearly inscribed patterns, and injuries on parts of the body normally covered by clothing.[69] Contact burns initially present as erythematous injury with subsequent hyperpigmented or hypopigmented cutaneous changes as

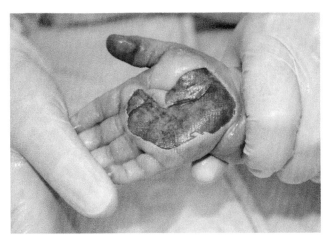

FIGURE 28-6 A burn to the hand from contact with a hot metal grill lid.

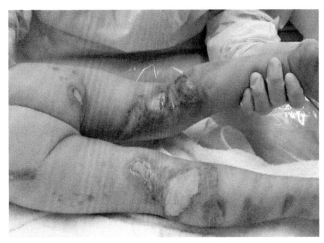

FIGURE 28-8 Fire pit grill grate marks on the posterior legs of a child.

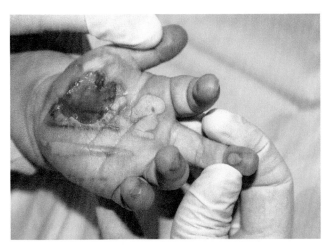

FIGURE 28-7 A contact burn from a radiator.

tissue healing occurs.[70] Figure 28-6 demonstrates a burn to the hand from contact with a hot metal grill lid, while Figure 28-7 shows a contact burn from a radiator. Figure 28-8 depicts fire pit grill grate marks on the posterior legs of a child.

Dry contact burns may include injuries resulting from objects such as a curling iron, steam iron, flat iron, radiator/grill grate, cigarette lighter, or various kitchen utensils. Figure 28-9 shows examples of pattern burn injury. The pattern left on the skin by curling iron burns can help in differentiating accidental from abusive injury mechanisms. If the burn pattern demonstrates a smeared edge appearance suggesting that the child was attempting to flee from the painful source, an accidental mechanism is most likely.[47]

Accidental foot burns in children during summer months resulting from contact with heated pavements by high ambient temperatures are very common. Burns due to contact with naturally heated surfaces are more likely to be bilateral, second-degree burns primarily of the plantar surface of the foot.[71] Harrington et al[72] found that asphalt pavement temperatures in the Arizona region reach temperatures hot enough to cause childhood pedal burns between 9 AM and 7 PM during the summer. The authors also documented that asphalt produces a second-degree

burn within 35 seconds of contact from between 10 AM and 5 PM.[72] Partial-thickness burns from car seats also have been reported to mimic inflicted abusive injury.[73]

Simons et al[74] documented that the median age of children sustaining hot iron accidental burns was 17 months. The authors found that 44% of these accidental hot iron burns were caused by touching the iron, and an additional 38% were caused by pulling the iron cord; 74% of these children were supervised by an adult or older teen at the time that the burn occurred and in 34% of cases, the iron was turned off at the time of injury. Gaffney[75] found that iron contact burns caused 23.5% of all reported contact burns in children 5 years of age or younger. Of the 60 children in the study evaluated for contact iron burns, inflicted injury was suspected in 17% of cases and confirmed in 15%. The mean age of children affected was 24 months, with 55% being between 1 and 2 years of age and the primary site of the injury in 63% of the children was the hands.

The Prescott[76] and Sudikoff[97] studies found that hair dryers generate temperatures of at least 110° F and retain sufficient heat within the grills to induce full-thickness burns several minutes after disconnecting power. Darok and Reischle[78] reported a 2½-year-old girl with inflicted hair dryer buttock burn injuries. During a scene reenactment, the investigators were able to determine that after 60 seconds, the hair dryer air temperature was 110° C and with that a maximum air steam temperature of 115° C documented at 150 seconds.

Cigarette burn injury in children can be produced by accidental brush-by contact with the glowing tip of a cigarette when a child is in close contact with a smoking caregiver, or can result from deliberately inflicted injury. Brush-by contact with heated cigarette ashes results in a poorly defined oval or wedge-shaped lesions.[79] Accidentally induced cigarette burns typically occur on children in areas not covered by clothing. These accidental burns do not result in full-thickness skin injury because the child quickly withdraws from the painful stimulus.

Cigarette burns caused by abuse usually present as multiple grouped lesions and typically present on the hands and feet.[80] An inflicted cigarette burn produces a deep partial to full-thickness burn lesion that ranges from 5 to 10 mm in

FIGURE 28-9 Pattern burn injury. **A,** A hair straightening iron burn on the buttocks. **B,** A burn caused by a steam iron. **C,** A burn caused by fork tines. **D,** A burn caused by a cigarette lighter. **E,** A cigarette burn.

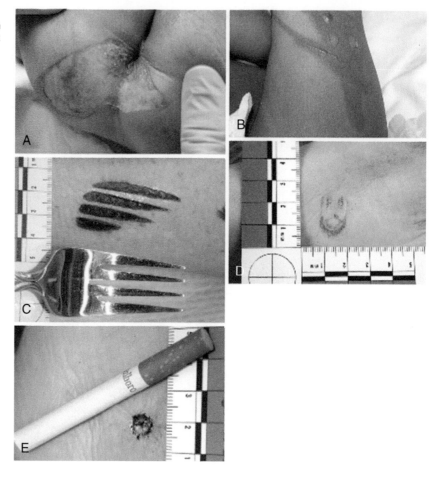

circumference and has a sharply defined punched out appearance.[79] If the cigarette had contact with the skin lasting greater than 1 second, it produces 5 to 10 mm circumferential to ovoid lesion, which can develop blistering. If untreated, the lesion heals gradually, resulting in a wrinkled appearing scar. Cigarette burns frequently can be confused with infectious skin conditions such as epidermolysis bullosa,[81,82] impetigo,[83,84] bullous impetigo,[85] focal pyoderma,[79] and ammoniacal diaper ulcerations seen in children who have prolonged skin contact with urine.[46,76] Chicken pox scars secondary to bacterial superinfection can also resemble cigarette burn lesions. Skin lesions caused by moxibustion (see section on Folk Practices below) can also be confused with cigarette burn scars.[47]

Heider et al[86] reported a case of punctate lesions of pediatric eczema mimicking inflicted thermal burn injury. Skin conditions such as eczema, bullous impetigo, epidermolysis bullosa, and others should be able to be differentiated from thermal injury by careful history. Chronic skin problems in pediatric patients are typically known to the caretakers. Insect bites present on eczematous skin typically have irregular margins and lack the typical crater appearance seen with cigarette burns.[86]

Chemical Burns

Chemical burns resulting from caustic ingestions can be the result of neglectful child supervision and intentional acts. Chemical injuries can result in deep burns as the agent continues to cause tissue damage until properly removed from the skin. Alkali burns are associated with deeper penetration and more extensive burns than acids.[87]

Adult drug use is a risk factor for pediatric caustic ingestions. Farst et al[88] reported two children who sustained oropharyngeal burns, esophageal injury resulting in stricture, and cutaneous partial-thickness burns after ingesting chemicals used in the production of methamphetamine. Massa and Ludemann[89] reported two toddlers who ingested a caustic liquid, which their parents had been using in the preparation of free-basing crack cocaine. Both had partial-thickness burns of the oral cavity, pharynx, and esophagus secondary to the ingestion. One child ingested ammonia from an unmarked container, and the other ingested potassium hydroxide.

Concentrated bleach does not immediately produce pain and therefore causes skin lesions that develop slowly and worsen with prolonged contact. Splash marks might be absent.[90] Howieson et al[91] found that exposure to microbial enzymes in biological laundry detergent resulted in partial-thickness burn injury in a 10-month-old child with a prolonged skin exposure time. The authors were able to reproduce this superficial partial-thickness burn injury after 12 hours' contact. Winek et al[92] reported a 2-year-old child who sustained a full-thickness chemical burn to his right thigh after prolonged contact with the chemical contents of damaged alkaline batteries, which had leaked from a CD player located on the toddler's car seat. The alkaline solution leaking from the batteries was absorbed into the child's pants

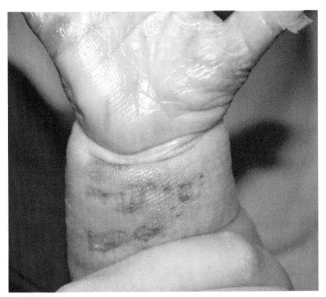

FIGURE 28-10 A chemical burn to the forearm and hand of an 8-month-old female who was placed in a snowsuit that had muriatic acid spilled onto the sleeve the preceding day.

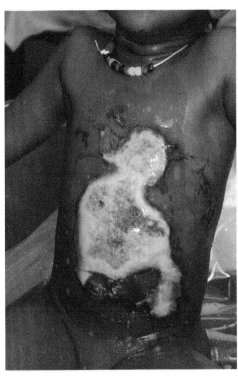

FIGURE 28-11 A 2-year-old child who sustained full-thickness burns to the chest and abdomen after her shirt caught fire when her sister was using it as traction while flicking a cigarette lighter.

and onto his skin, resulting in the full-thickness chemical burn. Figure 28-10 demonstrates a chemical burn to the forearm and hand of an 8-month-old female who was placed in a snowsuit that had muriatic acid spilled onto the sleeve the preceding day.

Laxative-induced buttock dermatitis frequently is confused with abusive immersion burns of the buttocks. Leventhal et al[93] reported on four children originally suspected of having immersion burns. The history in all cases was that the children had ingested Ex-Lax. The active ingredient, senna, produces diarrhea in cases of childhood overdose, leading to erythema and blister formation on the buttocks after prolonged exposure.

Flame Burns

Flame burn injury in the pediatric population is most often secondary to house fires. The leading cause of death from pediatric burns is from house fires. Abusive flame burn injury secondary to holding a child's skin in contact with a flame or to ignition of clothing as a consequence of abuse or neglect also occurs. Both Thombs[6] and Purdue[8] report approximately 10% of abusive pediatric burn admissions were caused by fire or flame.

Johnson et al[94] reported a 7-year-old developmentally delayed child with partial-thickness burns of the bilateral inner thighs, reported to be secondary to diaper ignition. A 12-year-old brother cooking near the patient caught a towel on fire on the stove, which reportedly landed on the patient's diaper and ignited it. The National Consumer Product Safety Commission reported nine known cases of childhood diaper ignition between 1980 and 1996 with three fatalities.

Figure 28-11 shows a 2-year-old child who sustained full-thickness burns to the chest and abdomen after her shirt caught fire when her sister was using it as traction while flicking a cigarette lighter.

Electrical Burn Injury

Electrical burns in children represent approximately 2% to 3% of all burns that require treatment in the emergency room.[95] The majority of all pediatric electrical burn injuries occur within the home setting,[95-97] and involve children less than 5 years old.[98] Low-voltage electrical injuries from sources less than 1000 volts are more common in younger children while high-voltage injuries are seen more frequently in the older pediatric population.[96] Children typically sustain localized burns when injured by electrical current,[97-99] most commonly from biting an electrical cord or placing an object into an electrical outlet.[95,96] Though most reported electrical injuries are not due to deliberate acts of child abuse, many typically occur in unattended or poorly supervised children. Therefore, electrical injuries in children might raise concern for neglect as a contributing factor to the injury.[96,97] Zubair et al[96] reported 127 children over a 25-year time span who were hospitalized with electrical burn injuries. Most burns in the study were associated with oral injury from biting an electrical cord (48/127), placing an object into an electrical socket (33/127), contact with a low-voltage wire or appliance within the home (25/127), contact with high-voltage outdoor wire (18/127), and being struck by lightening (3/127). Children suffering from oral burn injuries secondary to chewing on an electrical cord had a mean age of 2.7 years and a male to female ratio of 2:1. One patient included in the study was a victim of child abuse by use of an electrical current from a household wire/appliance. Garcia et al[98] reported 78 patients over a 6-year time period seen in the emergency department with electrical injuries. The authors found that the mean age of injury occurrence was 5.3 years, and that the majority occurred secondary to the child placing an object in an outlet, touching a cord while plugging it in, or placing a cord in the mouth.

High voltage electrical injuries most commonly occur in children outside of the home, with one study reporting the highest incidence in children who were climbing trees and had contact with main electrical power lines.[96] The mean age of high-voltage injuries was reported to be 11.3 years with a male to female ratio of 17:1.

Though most electrical burn injuries occur secondary to lack of supervision, frank child abuse has also been reported. Frechette and Rimsza[100] reported an 8-year-old boy with multiple 0.5 cm hypopigmented paired lesions present on his back, chest, abdomen, and thighs diagnosed as healing burn wounds. They were later determined to be inflicted by a stun gun as punishment. If recently inflicted, stun gun burns appear erythematous and slightly raised. Turner et al[101] reported the fatality of a 7-month-old infant, resulting from repeated shocking of the infant with a stun gun by his foster mother in an attempt to get the infant to stop crying. At autopsy, the paired lesions were reported to be macular, well-circumscribed, erythematous and with an appearance consistent with recent infliction.

Other lesions producing circular burn injuries in the pediatric population include cigarette burns, which typically do not present as paired lesions, and burns from enuresis alarms, which produce 0.4 to 0.6 cm linearly arranged circular burn patterns.[102]

Microwave Oven Burns

Alexander et al[103] reported two children who sustained full-thickness burns resulting from abuse after being placed in microwave ovens. The main effect of microwave radiation on living tissue is thermal in nature. A standard microwave oven causes 2 to 5 cm depth of thermal penetration.[104] Microwave radiation penetrates tissues with higher water content to a greater extent than other tissues and produces burns that are most severe on the skin, followed by the muscle due to its higher water content, and produces lesser damage to the subcutaneous fat. Physical findings suggesting microwave injury includes the presence of spared tissue levels noted on burn biopsy sites and well-demarcated cutaneous burns occurring on body areas closest to the microwave emission source.[103-105] For example, epidermal, dermal, and muscle tissue might demonstrate significant burned tissue while there is relative sparing of the subcutaneous fat layer. Microwave burns appear different than electrical burns in that charring of the skin is not present.[103,105]

Microwave ovens heat food and liquids unevenly and have also been associated with accidental pediatric scald injury resulting from food preparation. Sando et al[106] reported partial and full-thickness scald burns to the oropharynx of an infant after drinking formula heated in a microwave oven. Puczynski et al[107] described the case of a 1-week-old infant who sustained second-degree burns after the plastic baby bottle liner containing hot formula exploded several seconds after removal from the microwave oven. Palatal burns in an infant who had the baby bottle warmed in a microwave oven also has been reported.[108]

Lowell and Quinlan[39] found childhood access to a microwave oven increased the risk of accidental scald burns and

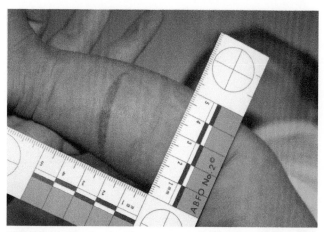

FIGURE 28-12 A pressure mark on an infant's posterior calf, *not* an inflicted injury.

most commonly resulted from children pulling overheated food or liquid onto themselves.

Friction/Pressure "Burns"

Innocent pressure injuries can be confused with dry contact burns as tissue ischemia resulting from constricting pressure (as seen with encircling elastic clothing) can produce similar findings. Johnson[109] first reported constricting bands from tight clothing as the cause of cutaneous pressure injuries resembling ligature mark, most often found on areas of the body where the tops of socks or clothing cuffs would be present. Feldman[70] documented four cases in which children ranging in age from 2 weeks to 3 years were evaluated for concerns of dry contact burns after erythematous, curvilinear 2 to 3 mm wide symmetric lesions were found on the bilateral calves, or brownish, hyperpigmented linear lesions more pronounced on the posterior calves were noted. Detailed history and medical evaluation in each case revealed the origin of these lesions was secondary to encircling elastic pressure. A noncircumferential injury can be produced if pressure from the constricting garment is augmented in a certain anatomic locations, which in Feldman's series was reported to be on posterior calf region.[70] Figure 28-12 demonstrates an infant with an innocent pressure injury to the posterior calf.

BURNS ASSOCIATED WITH CULTURAL MEDICINE PRACTICES

Cupping is a folk medicine therapy used to improve circulation and treat various ailments. The practice involves application of alcohol to the rim of a cup or glass, which is then heated and applied to the skin creating a suction effect resulting in production of an erythematous to ecchymotic lesion. The lesion can appear suspicious for circular patterned abusive burn injury,[110] or may result in superficial to deep partial-thickness burns of the skin if not properly used.[111,112] *Maquas* are small deep burns inflicted to the skin near diseased organs as part of a therapeutic process most often seen in the Arabic culture.[113] An 11-year-old Bedouin child was evaluated for child abuse after having bilateral dorsal hand burns with an unusual spiral configuration,[114] which were later determined to be a complication of treatment with a substance containing copper sulfate used by a traditional healer. Feldman reported on a series of children with multiple 0.5 to 1.0 cm circular or target-shaped burn scars present on the truncal or back region consistent with moxibustion.[115] Moxibustion treatment consists of heated object application to the skin at or near therapeutic points.[116] Kaplan[85] reported triangular-patterned burns to an 18-month-old Vietnamese child, which were determined to be consistent cao gio, the Vietnamese folk medicine treatment consisting of hot coin application to the skin.[116]

Garty[117] reported on a case of garlic burns on the wrists of a 6-month-old boy after garlic was used as a naturopathic remedy for aseptic meningitis. The family crushed garlic cloves and applied them to both of the infant's wrists, with adhesive bands over his pulse area for approximately 6 hours. The child developed lesions on both wrists with one wrist having a 1-cm circular area of ulceration surrounded by mildly elevated, erythematous borders and the other wrist having a superficial lesion. These lesions healed within 3 weeks' time. Parish et al[118] reported second-degree burns in a 17-month-old toddler following the application of garlic petroleum jelly plaster for an 8-hour time period.

Though not cited in the medical literature, the authors also have clinical experience a child having superficial partial-thickness burn injury to the neck resulting from application of a tomatillo as part of a Hispanic traditional healing practice to decrease swollen neck lymph nodes and treat a cough.

Although not considered abusive, in the United States when children sustain burns secondary to cultural practices, the family should be strongly discouraged from continuing use of folk medicine therapies for the child.

BURNS AND NEGLECT

Maltreatment by burning can be caused by either infliction of injury or by neglect due to a lack of adequate supervision. Andronicus et al[2] reported both neglect and inflicted injury as contributing to nonaccidental burn causation in children. Chester et al[14] performed a retrospective study on 440 hospitalized pediatric burn patients over a 2-year time period and found that 9.3% of the burn cases were diagnosed as occurring secondary to neglect. The authors reported delayed presentation, failure to care for the wound before seeking medical care, parental drug use, and single parent families were all more prevalent in children with burns secondary to neglect. Burns resulting from neglect are more likely to have deeper tissue injury requiring surgical intervention.[14] Of the neglected children, 82.9% had already been documented in the child protection system and nearly half of the neglected children were transferred into foster care at the time of the hospital discharge.[14]

PRESENTATION OF THE BURNED CHILD FOR MEDICAL CARE

A child presenting for medical care with burn injuries should be medically stabilized, followed by a physical examination noting the type of burn injury, severity of injury, and

Table 28-2	History to Obtain from Child/Caregiver Regarding Burn Injury[119]

- Anatomic location of the burn
- Source producing the injury
  - Hot tap water:
    - Water heater temperature
    - Water coming from the faucet
    - Free flowing or pooled water
  - Chemical:
    - Source contact time
- Explanation of the burn injury (Are there varying accounts?)
- Date/time the burn injury reportedly occurred
- Location of the child at the time of the burn
- Presence or absence of clothing
- Presence or absence of witnesses to the burn
- Time from burn occurrence to presentation for medical care
- Child and parent's reaction to the burn
- Developmental level of the child
- Prior injury or accidents
- Family composition and home environment

presence of other physical examination findings suggestive of abuse. The medical team should obtain separate histories from the child (if verbal) and caregiver regarding causation and time of the injury. The interviews should be conducted as soon as possible after presentation with a burn injury to document initial statements made by caregivers.[24] Concise documentation of the initial version of events is of utmost importance, as in many cases of child abuse, the perpetrator's accounting of events changes over time. Additional information regarding interviewing children and families about child maltreatment can be found in chapters 7, 8, and 26.

The key historical elements that should be obtained from the child and caregiver for pediatric burn cases are outlined in Table 28-2.[119] If the burn source was secondary to hot water, the medical provider should inquire about home water heater temperature and temperature of the water coming from the tap. It is also important to inquire about how long the child was in contact with the source of the burn and how the child gained access to the source.[119] Adult witnesses to the injury, or lack thereof, should also be determined, as many cases of pediatric burn injuries are the result of poor caretaker supervision. Information regarding the presence of existing medical conditions such as neurological, cognitive, or genetic disorders, which can impair the child's ability to perceive pain or alter the child's level of consciousness should also be collected.[120] Feldman reported handicapped children were at higher risk of tap water burns secondary to impaired sensory and motor capabilities in paralytic extremities.[121]

Clark et al[122] evaluated the use of a screening profile to enhance recognition of suspicious pediatric burn cases. Before initiation of the checklist, only 3% of childhood burn cases presenting to the emergency department were referred to social services for abuse investigation. After checklist implementation, 12.1% of cases were referred. The authors reported that burns with a history that is developmentally incompatible for the child, history of prior accidents involving the child, differing history, history incompatible with the physical findings, burns attributed to siblings, inappropriate parent affect, presence of other injuries, and mirror image burns were all correlated with inflicted injury to the child.[122]

After completing a detailed history, the medical provider should perform a more detailed physical examination of the child focusing on evaluating the patient for other signs of trauma, cutaneous findings or evidence of neglect such as malnutrition, failure to thrive, or poor hygiene. The provider should specifically document the location of the burn(s), depth of tissue injury, burn contours, and percent total body surface area affected by the burn.[119] Burn diagrams should be used in conjunction with photodocumentation of the injury. The medical provider should document the child's height and weight on admission, and plot this information on an age-appropriate growth curve. When possible, these data points should be compared with previously obtained height/weight data from previous medical examinations to evaluate for poor weight gain or abrupt weight loss, which might indicate a malnourished state. A cursory developmental examination should also be performed to determine if the child's developmental state is consistent with the reported causation of injury.

Based upon information obtained from the history of the burn injury and medical examination findings, case analysis is performed by the medical provider to determine if there are indications of abusive injury. Inconsistent history, social situation deemed as placing the child at risk, concerning pattern of injury, or extreme magnitude of injury when compared with the stated history are all concerning for child abuse. Table 28-3 outlines history and physical examination findings to consider in pediatric burn cases.[9,119,122,123] If abusive injury by burning is suspected, the medical provider can, when available, request consultation from the institutional child protection team. If the burn is determined to be suspicious for inflicted injury, the case must be reported to local child protective services and/or law enforcement for investigation and safety planning.

The role of the medical professional is to objectively evaluate, analyze, diagnose, and treat cases of suspected abuse by burning. To maintain objectivity in these cases, the medical provider should be nonjudgmental. Interactions with the family should focus on providing honest accurate information about the child's medical treatment. Determination of guilt and punishment in cases of child abuse by burning is the responsibility of law enforcement and prosecutors.

Yasti et al[119] evaluated 239 consecutively hospitalized pediatric burn patients to compare independent case diagnosis by the burn physician with that of a clinical forensic scientist (who in this study was also a general surgeon with burn experience) for accuracy in evaluating for nonaccidental mechanisms of injury including neglect. Overall, a difference in incident interpretation and diagnosis between the two doctors was seen in 16.3% (39/239) of patients. The burn physician diagnosed 41.4% of the incidents as accidental, while the forensic scientist documented only 27.6% of the same cases as an accident, leading the authors to conclude that the presence of a trained forensic scientist is needed for evaluation of pediatric burn cases to prevent false-negative and false-positive diagnoses from occurring.[124]

Table 28-3	Indicators of Concern for Abuse from History and Physical Examination Findings

History

- History reported not consistent with mechanism of the injury
- Unexplained delay in seeking medical care
- History of previous injury or repetitive accidents
- Presentation of coexisting injuries
- Presence of supervisory and/or environmental neglect
- Presentation for care with a nonrelated adult or nonparental relative
- Multiple/changing explanations for the injury
- Unwitnessed injury
- Injury attributed to siblings and/or pets
- Apathetic parents regarding the child's injury
- Unexplained burns in a delayed child
- Developmental level of the child inconsistent with reported mechanism of injury
- Submissive child with flat affect or lack of appropriate emotional response to pain

Areas Highly Concerning for Inflicted Injury
- Hands
- Feet
- Genital region
- Buttocks

Patterns of Injury Concerning for Abuse
- Large surface area of burn
- Uniform degree of burn injury
- Full-thickness burn
- Presence of sharply delineated burn margin
- Symmetrical burns
- Absence of burn in areas of skin flexion
- Sparing of skin with surrounding burn secondary to contact with cooler surfaces (doughnut burns)
- Scald injury without splash/drip marks

Other Findings Concerning for Abuse or Neglect
- Infected burns
- Chronic burns
- Burns in various stages of healing
- Burn appearance is older than stated history
- Concomitant cutaneous injuries

Adapted with permission from Farley RH, Reece RM: *Recognizing when a child's injury or illness is caused by abuse.* U.S. Department of Justice Office of Juvenile Justice and Delinquency Prevention, Washington, DC, 1996, pp 8-9.[9,121,124]

Discordant diagnoses were most likely to be associated with low socio-economic status, children between the ages of 3 and 6 years, and large family size.[124]

MEDICAL DOCUMENTATION

Due to the forensic issues surrounding cases of pediatric abusive burn injury, detailed medical documentation is important. The medical provider should inquire about and document a detailed account of the history including specifics regarding statements by the child or caregiver of burn location, description of the environment in which the burn

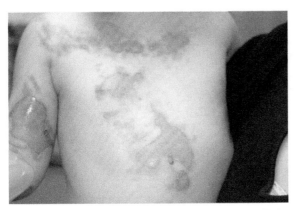

FIGURE 28-13 Splash burns that occurred when hot tea spilled over a child's clothing resulting in nonuniform burn injuries.

occurred, and temperature (if available) of the burn source. It is also important for the medical provider to document any clothing that the child may have been wearing during the time of the injury. Figure 28-13 demonstrates hot tea splash burns that occurred over clothing resulting in the nonuniform burn injury. Not only should the location of burn injury be clearly described, with inclusion of body diagram drawings, but it is also important to document areas that are free of injury.

The examining medical provider will, in situations when a child abuse specialist is not available, document a conclusion regarding the injury causation. When documenting a diagnosis, gradations of concern for suspicious burn cases can be used. If abusive injury by burning is suspected, but unable to be definitively proven at the time, the medical provider could include wording such as, "Concerning for abusive injury by burning based upon the following information:" then include supporting information such as, "The pattern of injury present does not appear to be consistent with the mechanism stated," or "The child's developmental level is not consistent with the injury mechanism stated." Cases in which the child gives a disclosure of abusive injury and physical examination findings are consistent with the disclosure, a diagnosis of definite physical abusive injury by burning can be made.

Photographs of burns are important to document visual evidence of the injury (see Chapter 27).

DATING OF BURN INJURIES IN THE MEDICAL RECORD

There are no studies documenting physician accuracy for dating burn injuries. However, physicians experienced in burns and wound healing should be able to make statements about injury timing. In cases where burn injury exists of varying ages, medical providers should be able to confidently say that one injury is older than another based upon differences noted in would healing between the lesions. Documenting that one burn injury is older than another would eliminate a caregiver's claim that the injury was secondary to accidental mechanisms occurring during a single event.

ADDITIONAL MEDICAL TESTING

Medical providers frequently question the necessity for obtaining a skeletal survey in children having a burn injury in the absence of other traumatic findings. In 1983, Merten et al[125] documented that children 2 years of age and younger with physical injury (including burn injury) were at greatest risk of occult fracture. Because 77% of the occult fractures were documented in this age group, the authors recommended the routine use of skeletal radiological imaging for this population. In 2001, Belfer et al[126] evaluated the incidence of clinically unsuspected fractures detected by skeletal survey in children with suspected physical abuse. The authors imaged 15 out of 75 (20%) children admitted with burn injury, with only a 10-month-old infant found to have an occult fracture. With such a small percentage of patients surveyed, these results might underestimate the true percentage of fractured patients with burns.

In 2007, Hicks and Stofli[127] evaluated the frequency of occult fractures in children with suspicious burns compared with children with other forms of physical abusive injury. The study documented 14% (5 of 36) of pediatric burn cases with positive skeletal surveys with occult fracture. The frequency of occult fracture in the nonburned abusive injury group was 34% (45 of 133 nonburn injuries). This study concluded that though children with abusive burns have a lower frequency of occult fractures than children with other physical abuse injuries, the 14% incidence of occult fractures supports a policy of routine imaging in this age group.

Degraw[128] in a study of children referred for subspecialty evaluation for physical abuse, found 16.3% (24/147) of children having burns also had fractures present. For children under 24 months of age with burns, 18.6% (18/97) had fractures identified on skeletal survey. This work further supports the need for skeletal survey imaging in children less than 2 years old with suspicious burns.

Skeletal surveys in pediatric burn patients should be obtained after the child has been adequately medicated for pain. If the critical nature of large burns or risk of infection takes precedent, the skeletal survey can be performed at the bedside or deferred until a later time.

SCENE INVESTIGATION

All suspicious burn injuries should be investigated by individuals experienced with scene assessment and evidence collection. Most burn scene investigations are conducted by trained law enforcement personnel with assistance from child protective services. In cases of hot water scald burn injury, a detailed scene investigation is necessary to assist with the critical analysis of the injury by a multidisciplinary team. Figure 28-14 provides investigators with an evidence collection worksheet for documentation of hot water burn scene information. Investigators should take a thermometer, tape measure, timer/stop watch, and camera equipment to the injury scene. A scientific thermometer designed to measure liquids and calibrated for accuracy should be used during these investigations. These thermometers typically can be purchased through a scientific catalogue or via the Internet. Most store bought thermometers are not significantly accurate for forensic purposes. Thermometers that do not specifically measure liquids, such as meat thermometers,

---

EVIDENCE WORKSHEET FOR HOT WATER BURNS

!

Items needed for scene investigation

☐ **Thermometer** (Use of a scientific thermometer designed to measure liquid temperatures and which as been calibrated for accuracy is recommended.)

Brand: _____

☐ Tape Measure
☐ Timer/Stopwatch
☐ Camera (film/digital)

A

Case No.

Present Date:

Suspect Name:

Victim's Name:

Incident Location (within dwelling):

Address:

City/State/Zip:

A1 Type of Burn: ☐ Immersion ☐ Splash ☐ Running water ☐ Other (spill, splatter, etc.)

B

Water Heater Temperature Measurement: (Electric – Disconnect power before removing plates!)

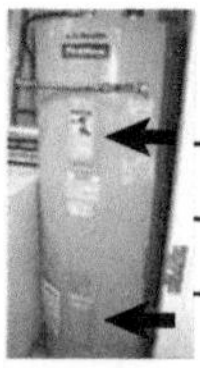

Electric Water Heater

Brand:

Capacity:

Upper plate temp:

Lower plate temp:

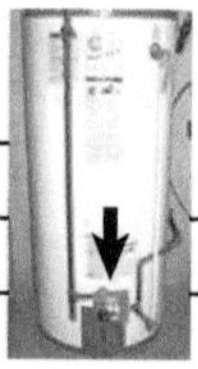

Gas Water Heater

Brand:

Capacity:

Temperature Setting:

C

Incident Location Measurements (in inches): ☐ Bathtub ☐ Basin/Sink ☐ Other

Width: _____ Inside Depth: _____ | *sketches*

Length: _____ Height from Floor: _____

Distance to faucet handles: _____ | Construction: (porcelain, fiberglass. etc.)

D

Running Water Temperatures (Hot) (in Fahrenheit or Celsius)				Standing Hot Water in Incident Location (temp. measured in middle of location, mid-depth)			
Seconds	Degrees	Seconds	Degrees	Inches	Min/Second	Minutes	Degrees
0	____	45	____			0	____
5	____	60	____	1	____	1	____
10	____	120	____	2	____	2	____
20	____	180	____	3	____	3	____
30	____	____	____	4	____	4	____
				5	____	5	____
				____	____	10	____
				____	____	30	____
						____	____

Maximum Temp

(Full hot running water) | **(Full H/C running water)***

Peak temp. | Seconds | Peak temp. | Seconds

_____ _____ | _____ _____

**(For a single handle faucet-use middle position)

E

_____ ran water in _____ identified as source of burn injury.

Results: _____ inches of water. One minute after water turned off the mid-depth temperature is _____ degrees F/C.

Investigator #1: _____ ID#: _____ Department: _____
Investigator #2: _____ ID#: _____ Department: _____

FIGURE 28-14 An evidence collection worksheet for documentation of hot water burn scene information. *(Adapted with permission from Phylip J. Peltier, District Attorney Investigator [retired], Paradise, Calif., and from Peltier PJ, Purdue G, Shepherd JR: Burn injuries in child abuse. U.S. Department of Justice Office of Juvenile Justice and Delinquency Prevention 1997; 19.)*

are inaccurate and should be avoided in burn scene investigations. Even scientific thermometers can lose accuracy over time and need to be recalibrated.

Before arrival at the scene, investigators should discuss the case with medical providers to determine the suspected mechanism of injury. In cases of suspected hot liquid burns, the investigators should record the water heater temperature. In the United States, most homes are heated with either an electric or gas water heater. If the scene has an electric water heater present, investigators need to examine and document the water temperature recordings from both the upper and lower water heater thermostats. The upper thermostat functions to heat only the top-most layer of water for replacement of water that has been drawn off. The lower thermostat functions to maintain a constant water temperature within the heating reservoir. To avoid electrocution, investigators must disconnect the power source to the electric water heater before investigation.[120] If the scene has a gas water heater, the thermostat is typically located on the outside near the base of the water heater unit.

Investigators should obtain a history from the caregiver regarding reported water usage in the time period preceding the injury. This information can be analyzed to determine if the burn injury occurred at a time when the water heater was at a constant temperature, or if the injury occurred during a time when the water heater was reheating following repeated withdrawal of hot water from the unit. For hot water burn injury occurring in an apartment complex or another area containing a central water heater source, it is important to determine if the water was mixing with another water heater, thereby potentially altering water temperature in relation to water heater temperature recordings. Information regarding scene location in relation to the water line should also be documented. Gas heaters have the potential to undergo water heater stacking, a phenomenon where the water may superheat after multiple small amounts of water have been removed in short succession.

The entire room in which the burn injury reportedly occurred should be photodocumented. Sinks and tubs should be measured, including width, height, length, inside depth, and construction material (i.e., porcelain, fiberglass, metal, etc.) and the distance from the basin to the faucet.

Investigators should clearly document the hot running water temperature at multiple time intervals including initial temperature, peak water temperature reached, and seconds required to reach this peak measurement. Note if the water is free flowing, or if the drain is plugged to some degree, thereby causing water to pool. Water should be collected in the tub or sink to the depth that is reported by history or documented on the physical examination. Temperature measurements from the collected water and the water fill rates should be documented.

Immersion burn injury patterns can be reconstructed on dolls or willing volunteers during investigations through use of fabric dyes.[120] Simulating the burn mechanism will leave dye on the skin in a pattern which could reflect the child's injury.

All information should be analyzed to correlate the child's burn injury with the caregiver's stated mechanism of injury (if available), developmental level of the child, size, and child's ability to turn on (or adjust) the water faucets. For nonwater burn injuries, scene investigation can provide the potential object causing the injury. Scene investigation also can identify unsafe and potentially neglectful situations that might have contributed to the injury or predispose the child to further injury.

PSYCHOLOGICAL ISSUES OF THE BURNED CHILD AND THE FAMILY

Antecedent psychopathology in the family unit of burned children is common. Long and Cope[129] found preexisting gross emotional disturbance within the family in 8 of 19 hospitalized burned children. Vigliano et al[130] suggested that chronic relationship problems can become overt at the time of the child's traumatic burn injury. Holter and Friedman[131] reported that 10 of 13 families studied with severely burned children had major psychological and social problems in the family unit which preceded the child's burn injury. Three of these cases were clearly abusive in nature and the mother was noted to suffer from disturbed personality in all cases. Two of the abuse cases reported "intact marriages," but both parents in each case were reported to have serious psychological problems. They also reported that for the three abusively scalded children in their study, parental responses to the child's injuries and treatment were void of concern or grief, and instead demonstrated annoyance, disgust, and lack of communication. The mother was suspected as the perpetrator of the abusive burns in two cases and the father in one.[131]

The literature is scant regarding the psychological sequelae of the burned child. Drake et al[132] reported that most young children between 12 to 48 months with acute burns exhibit multiple symptoms of posttraumatic stress disorder and that trauma severity correlates with increasing symptoms. Woodward et al[133] documented the presence of emotional disturbances consisting of fears, anxieties, management difficulties, lethargy, aggressiveness, and psychosomatic disorders including sleeping/feeding difficulties, enuresis, and stammering in approximately 80% of children who had recovered physically from severe burns. Stoddard et al[134] documented major depression in 26.6% of children between the ages of 7 to 19 years who had recovered from severe burns.

Treatment of the burn injury can be perceived as more distressing to the child than the burn injury itself. Kavanagh[135] reported that burned children (aged 2-12) who had control over the predictability of burn dressing change and took an active part in this process demonstrated significantly less depression and anxiety compared with children who participated in nurse-controlled dressing changes.

What the literature has failed to critically analyze at this point is psychological sequelae of the child who has been burned secondary to abuse versus the child who has been burned secondary to accidental means. A comprehensive answer regarding psychological sequelae in childhood victims of abuse by burning still remains unanswered.

BURN INJURY PREVENTION

Hot tap water scald burns remain a serious hazard to young children. Prevention efforts should focus on increasing educational ventures and public awareness about the hazards of hot tap water. Enhancing parent education by primary care providers and public health nurses about setting home water heater levels at 120° F should decrease the risk of hot water scald injuries by prolonging the time necessary to produce burn injury. Furthermore, encouraging retailers of this equipment to install the equipment set at safe levels will also assist with burn prevention. Legislative efforts requiring reduction in water heater settings showed a drop in the rate of hospitalizations from tap water scald injury.[136] Increased legislative efforts nationally to reduce water heater temperatures could result in even lower rates of scald burn injury. Prevention of scald burns from hot foods and beverages in the pediatric population can be achieved by preventing children in the kitchen while cooking, by using back burners on stoves, turning cooking handles inward, and by keeping young children away from foods and liquids recently heated in microwave ovens. Increased caregiver education about avoiding placing hot liquids on edges of countertops and tables (which frequently attract curious children) will also help to decrease scald injury. Thermal protective boxes to store irons and manufacturing irons with lower heat capacities and automatic shutoff switches would reduce accidental hot iron burn injury in children.[74] Since most accidental hot iron burns occur during the early morning hours, ironing at night when children are sleeping or ironing in a room without children present are strategies to prevent contact iron burns.[74] Parents and adult caregivers also should be counseled about the hazards of children placing electrical cords in their mouths as a means of preventing electrical burn injuries to young children. Simple home safety measures, such as safety-proofing electrical outlets will help prevent electrical injury in inquisitive toddlers. Increasing education regarding use of smoke detectors can help prevent serious morbidity and death in pediatric patients resulting from house fires.[137]

STRENGTH OF THE MEDICAL EVIDENCE

The literature has identified many factors that can help a multidisciplinary team determine if a burn injury is accidental or inflicted. Literature supports that a history of prior accidents, history incompatible with the physical examination findings, burns inconsistent with the developmental level of the child, differing or inconsistent historical accounts of the injury, inappropriate parental affect, and a delay in seeking care are concerning for abusive burn injury. In addition, certain patterns of injury, burns localized to the genitalia, perineum, buttocks, and bilateral lower extremities, presence of additional injuries, and older injuries are all reported frequently in inflicted injury. When presented with a suspicious burn, review of the injury using a multidisciplinary team is best practice to ensure thorough investigation, critical analysis, and accurate diagnosis of the case.

FUTURE DIRECTIONS FOR ABUSIVE BURN INJURY RESEARCH

As technology is enhanced, new types of water heaters are being produced. Little is currently known about the new energy efficient water heaters, which have the capability of heating water within a few seconds. As hot water burns cause a significant percentage of immersion burn injuries, more research is needed to determine how quickly burn injury occurs with this new model of water heater. In addition, research efforts are needed in the area of burn injury dating in order to present more scientifically based categories of wound healing times. Research also is needed to determine the psychological sequelae abusively burned children face to enhance successful trauma treatment programs.

References

1. Hobson MI, Evans J, Stewart IP: An audit of non-accidental injury in burned children. *Burns* 1994;20:442-445.
2. Andronicus M, Oates RK, Peat J, et al: Non-accidental burns in children. *Burns* 1998;24:552-558.
3. Keen JH, Lendrum J, Wolman B: Inflicted burns and scalds in children. *Br Med J* 1975;4:268-269.
4. Stone NH, Rinaldo L, Humphrey CR, et al: Child abuse by burning. *Surg Clin North Am* 1970;50:1419-1424.
5. Heaton PA: The pattern of burn injuries in childhood. *N Z Med J* 1989;102:584-586.
6. Thombs BD: Patient and injury characteristics, mortality risk, and length of stay related to child abuse by burning: evidence from a national sample of 15,802 pediatric admissions. *Ann Surg* 2008;247:519-523.
7. Hultman CS, Priolo D, Cairns BA, et al: Return to jeopardy: the fate of pediatric burn patients who are victims of abuse and neglect. *J Burn Care Rehabil* 1998;19:367-376.
8. Purdue GF, Hunt JL, Prescott PR: Child abuse by burning—an index of suspicion. *J Trauma* 1988;28:221-224.
9. Hight DW, Bakalar HR, Lloyd JR: Inflicted burns in children. Recognition and treatment. *JAMA* 1979;242:517-520.
10. Schanberger J: Inflicted burns in children. *Top Emerg Med* 1981;3:85-92.
11. Dietch E, Statts, M: Child abuse through burning. *J Burn Care Rehabil* 1982;3:89-94.
12. Rivara FP, Kamitsuka MD, Quan L: Injuries to children younger than 1 year of age. *Pediatrics* 1988;81:93-97.
13. Rosenberg NM, Marino D: Frequency of suspected abuse/neglect in burn patients. *Pediatr Emerg Care* 1989;5:219-221.
14. Chester DL, Jose RM, Aldlyami E, et al: Non-accidental burns in children—are we neglecting neglect? *Burns* 2006;32:222-228.
15. Kumar P: Child abuse by thermal injury—a retrospective survey. *Burns Incl Therm Inj* 1984;10:344-348.
16. Greenbaum AR, Donne J, Wilson D, et al: Intentional burn injury: an evidence-based, clinical and forensic review. *Burns* 2004;30:628-642.
17. Hummel RP 3rd, Greenhalgh DG, Barthel PP, et al: Outcome and socioeconomic aspects of suspected child abuse scald burns. *J Burn Care Rehabil* 1993;14:121-126.
18. Borland BL: Prevention of childhood burns: conclusions drawn from an epidemiologic study. *Clin Pediatr (Phila)* 1967;6:693-695.
19. Feldman KW, Schaller RT, Feldman JA, et al: Tap water scald burns in children. *Pediatrics* 1978;62:1-7.
20. Renz BM, Sherman R: Abusive scald burns in infants and children: a prospective study. *Am Surg* 1993;59:329-334.
21. Ojo P, Palmer J, Garvey R, et al: Pattern of burns in child abuse. *Am Surg* 2007;73:253-255.
22. Evasovich M, Klein R, Muakkassa F, et al: The economic effect of child abuse in the burn unit. *Burns* 1998;24:642-645.
23. Greenbaum AR, Horton JB, Williams CJ, et al: Burn injuries inflicted on children or the elderly: a framework for clinical and forensic assessment. *Plast Reconstr Surg* 2006;118:46e-58e.
24. Peck MD, Priolo-Kapel D: Child abuse by burning: a review of the literature and an algorithm for medical investigations. *J Trauma* 2002;53:1013-1022.
25. Allshouse MJ, Rouse T, Eichelberger MR: Childhood injury: a current perspective. *Pediatr Emerg Care* 1993;9:159-164.
26. Yeoh C, Nixon JW, Dickson W, et al: Patterns of scald injuries. *Arch Dis Child* 1994;71:156-158.
27. Lauer B, ten Broeck E, Grossman M: Battered child syndrome: review of 130 patients with controls. *Pediatrics* 1974;54:67-70.
28. Daria S, Sugar NF, Feldman KW, et al: Into hot water head first: distribution of intentional and unintentional immersion burns. *Pediatr Emerg Care* 2004;20:302-310.
29. Ayoub C, Pfeifer D: Burns as a manifestation of child abuse and neglect. *Am J Dis Child* 1979;133:910-914.
30. Showers J, Garrison KM: Burn abuse: a four-year study. *J Trauma* 1988;28:1581-1583.
31. Gillespie RW: The battered child syndrome: thermal and caustic manifestations. *J Trauma* 1965;5:523-534.
32. Hammond J, Nebel-Gould A, Brooks J: The value of speech-language assessment in the diagnosis of child abuse. *J Trauma* 1989;29:1258-1260.

33. Barillo DJ, Burge TS, Harrington DT, et al: Body habitus as a predictor of burn risk in children: do fat boys still get burned? *Burns* 1998;24:725-727.

34. Hobbs CJ: When are burns not accidental? *Arch Dis Child* 1986;61:357-361.

35. Bakalar HR, Moore JD, Hight DW: Psychosocial dynamics of pediatric burn abuse. *Health Soc Work* 1981;6:27-32.

36. Bennett B, Gamelli R: Profile of an abused burned child. *J Burn Care Rehabil* 1998;19:88-94; discussion 87.

37. Engrav LH, Garner WL, Tredget EE: Hypertrophic scar, wound contraction and hyper-hypopigmentation. *J Burn Care Res* 2007;28: 593-597.

38. Palmieri TL, Alderson TS, Ison D, et al: Pediatric soup scald burn injury: etiology and prevention. *J Burn Care Res* 2008;29:114-118.

39. Lowell G, Quinlan K: Unintentional scald burns in children under 5 years old: common mechanisms of injury. *J Trauma* 2007;63(suppl 3):S3.

40. Sie SD, van Rossum AM, Oudesluys-Murphy AM: Scald burns in the bathroom: accidental or inflicted? *Pediatrics* 2004;113:173-174.

41. Titus MO, Baxter AL, Starling SP: Accidental scald burns in sinks. *Pediatrics* 2003;111:E191-E194.

42. Raine PA, Azmy A: A review of thermal injuries in young children. *J Pediatr Surg* 1983;18:21-26.

43. Yiacoumettis A, Roberts M: An analysis of burns in children. *Burns* 1976;3:195-201.

44. Slater S, Slater H, Goldfarb, JW: Burned children: a socioeconomic profile for focused prevention programs. *J Burn Care Rehabil* 1987;8: 566-567.

45. Adams LE, Purdue GF, Hunt JL: Tap-water scald burns. Awareness is not the problem. *J Burn Care Rehabil* 1991;12:91-95.

46. Katcher ML: Scald burns from hot tap water. *JAMA* 1981;246:1219-1222.

47. Feldman KW: Burn injuries in child fatality review. *In*: Alexander RC (ed): *Child Fatality Review: an Interdisciplinary Guide and Photographic Reference*. GW Medical, St Louis, 2007, pp 281-296.

48. Stoll AM, Greene LC: Relationship between pain and tissue damage due to thermal radiation. *J Appl Physiol* 1959;14:373-382.

49. Henriques F, Moritz AR: Studies of thermal injuries. I. The conduction of heat to and through skin and temperatures attained therein. A theoretical and experimental investigation. *Am J Pathol* 1947;23:530-549.

50. Moritz A, Henriques FC: Studies of thermal injuries. II. The relative importance of time and surface temperature in the causation of cutaneous burns. *Am J Pathol* 1947;23:695-720.

51. Moritz A, Henriques FC: Studies of thermal injuries. III. The pathology and pathogenesis of cutaneous burns. An experimental study. *Am J Pathol* 1947;23:915-941.

52. Moritz A, Henriques FC, Dutra FR, et al: Studies of thermal injuries. IV. An exploration of the casualty-producing attributes of conflagration; local and systemic effects of general cutaneous exposure to excessive circumambient (air) and circumradiant heat of varying duration and intensity. *Arch Pathol* 1947;43:466-488.

53. Henriques F: Studies of thermal injuries. V. The predictability and the significance of thermally induced rate processes leading to irreversible epidermal injury. *Arch Pathol* 1947;43:489-502.

54. Feldman KW: Help needed on hot water burns. *Pediatrics* 1983;71:145-146.

55. Pollitzer MJ, Whitehead MD, Reynolds EO, et al: Effect of electrode temperature and in vivo calibration on accuracy of transcutaneous estimation of arterial oxygen tension in infants. *Pediatrics* 1980;65:515-522.

56. Feldman KW, Schaller RT, Feldman JA, et al: Tap water scald burns in children: 1997. *Inj Prev* 1998;4:238-242.

57. Allasio D, Fischer H: Immersion scald burns and the ability of young children to climb into a bathtub. *Pediatrics* 2005;115:1419-1421.

58. Chiu TW, Ng DC, Burd A: Properties of matter in assessment of scald injuries. *Burns* 2007;33:185-188.

59. Murphy JT, Purdue GF, Hunt JL: Pediatric grease burn injury. *Arch Surg* 1995;130:478-482.

60. Hankins CL, Tang XQ, Phipps A: Hot oil burns—a study of predisposing factors, clinical course and prevention strategies. *Burns* 2006;32:92-96.

61. Mukadam S, Gilles EE: Unusual inflicted hot oil burns in a 7-year-old. *Burns* 2003;29:83-86.

62. Colombo JL, Hopkins RL, Waring WW: Steam vaporizer injuries. *Pediatrics* 1981;67:661-663.

63. Wallis BA, Turner J, Pearn J, et al: Scalds as a result of vapour inhalation therapy in children. *Burns* 2008;34:560-564.

64. Schwartz RA: Toxic epidermal necrolysis. *Cutis* 1997;59:123-128.

65. Murphy S: Non accidental injury vs staphylococcal scalded skin syndrome. A case study. *Emerg Nurse* 2001;9:26-30.

66. Hays GC, Mullard JE: Blistering distal dactylitis: a clinically recognizable streptococcal infection. *Pediatrics* 1975;56:129-131.

67. Rhody C: Bacterial infections of the skin. *Prim Care* 2000;27: 459-473.

68. Johnson CF, French G: Bruises and burns in child maltreatment. *In*: Giardino A, Alexander RC (eds): *Child Maltreatment: a Clinical Guide and Reference*, ed 3, GW Medical, St Louis, 2005, pp 63-82.

69. Feldman KW: Child abuse by burning. *In*: Helfer RE, Kemp RS (eds): *The Battered Child*. University of Chicago Press, Chicago, 1987, pp 197-213.

70. Feldman KW: Confusion of innocent pressure injuries with inflicted dry contact burns. *Clin Pediatr (Phila)* 1995;34:114-115.

71. Sinha M, Salness R, Foster KN, et al: Accidental foot burns in children from contact with naturally heated surfaces during summer months: experience from a regional burn center. *J Trauma* 2006;61: 975-978.

72. Harrington WZ, Strohschein BL, Reedy D, et al: Pavement temperature and burns: streets of fire. *Ann Emerg Med* 1995;26:563-568.

73. Schmitt BD, Gray JD, Britton HL: Car seat burns in infants: avoiding confusion with inflicted burns. *Pediatrics* 1978;62:607-609.

74. Simons M, Brady D, McGrady M, et al: Hot iron burns in children. *Burns* 2002;28:587-590.

75. Gaffney P: The domestic iron. A danger to young children. *J Accid Emerg Med* 2000;17:199-200.

76. Prescott PR: Hair dryer burns in children. *Pediatrics* 1990;86: 692-697.

77. Sudikoff S, Young RS: Burn from hairdryer: accident or abuse? *Pediatrics* 1994;93:540.

78. Darok M, Reischle S: Burn injuries caused by a hair-dryer—an unusual case of child abuse. *Forensic Sci Int* 2001;115:143-146.

79. Faller-Marquardt M, Pollak S, Schmidt U: Cigarette burns in forensic medicine. *Forensic Sci Int* 2008;176:200-208.

80. Johnson CF: Inflicted injury versus accidental injury. *Pediatr Clin North Am* 1990;37:791-814.

81. Colver GB, Harris DW, Tidman MJ: Skin diseases that may mimic child abuse. *Br J Dermatol* 1990;123:129.

82. Winship IM, Winship WS: Epidermolysis bullosa misdiagnosed as child abuse. A report of 3 cases. *S Afr Med J* 1988;73:369-370.

83. Oates RK: Overturning the diagnosis of child abuse. *Arch Dis Child* 1984;59:665-666.

84. Wheeler DM, Hobbs CJ: Mistakes in diagnosing non-accidental injury: 10 years' experience. *Br Med J (Clin Res Ed)* 1988;296: 1233-1236.

85. Kaplan JM: Pseudoabuse—the misdiagnosis of child abuse. *J Forensic Sci* 1986;31:1420-1428.

86. Heider TR, Priolo D, Hultman CS, et al: Eczema mimicking child abuse: a case of mistaken identity. *J Burn Care Rehabil* 2002;23: 357-359.

87. Hettiaratchy S, Dziewulski P: ABC of burns: pathophysiology and types of burns. *Br Med J* 2004;328:1427-1429.

88. Farst K, Duncan JM, Moss M, et al: Methamphetamine exposure presenting as caustic ingestions in children. *Ann Emerg Med* 2007;49:341-343.

89. Massa N, Ludemann JP: Pediatric caustic ingestion and parental cocaine abuse. *Int J Pediatr Otorhinolaryngol* 2004;68:1513-1517.

90. Telmon N, Allery JP, Dorandeu A, et al: Concentrated bleach burns in a child. *J Forensic Sci* 2002;47:1060-1061.

91. Howieson AJ, Harley OJ, Tiernan EP: Laundry detergent and possible nonaccidental injury. *Eur J Emerg Med* 2007;14:163-164.

92. Winek CL, Wahba WW, Huston RM: Chemical burn from alkaline batteries—a case report. *Forensic Sci Int* 1999;100:101-104.

93. Leventhal JM, Griffin D, Duncan KO, et al: Laxative-induced dermatitis of the buttocks incorrectly suspected to be abusive burns. *Pediatrics* 2001;107:178-179.

94. Johnson CF, Oral R, Gullberg L: Diaper burn: accident, abuse, or neglect? *Pediatr Emerg Care* 2000;16:173-175.

95. Koumbourlis AC: Electrical injuries. *Crit Care Med* 2002;30: S424-S430.

96. Zubair M, Besner GE: Pediatric electrical burns: management strategies. *Burns* 1997;23:413-420.

97. Baker MD, Chiaviello C: Household electrical injuries in children. Epidemiology and identification of avoidable hazards. *Am J Dis Child* 1989;143:59-62.

98. Garcia CT, Smith GA, Cohen DM, et al: Electrical injuries in a pediatric emergency department. *Ann Emerg Med* 1995;26:604-608.

99. Young TL, Reisinger KS: Wall socket electrical burns: relevance to health education? *Pediatrics* 1980;65:825-827.

100. Frechette A, Rimsza ME: Stun gun injury: a new presentation of the battered child syndrome. *Pediatrics* 1992;89:898-901.

101. Turner MS, Jumbelic ML: Stun gun injuries in the abuse and death of a seven-month-old infant. *J Forensic Sci* 2003;48:180-182.

102. Diez F Jr, Berger TG: Scarring due to an enuresis blanket. *Pediatr Dermatol* 1988;5:58-60.

103. Alexander RC, Surrell JA, Cohle SD: Microwave oven burns to children: an unusual manifestation of child abuse. *Pediatrics* 1987;79:255-260.

104. Free J: The facts about microwave ovens. *Popul Sci* 1973;202:79-81,161-162.

105. Surrell JA, Alexander RC, Cohle SD, et al: Effects of microwave radiation on living tissues. *J Trauma* 1987;27:935-939.

106. Sando WC, Gallaher KJ, Rodgers BM: Risk factors for microwave scald injuries in infants. *J Pediatr* 1984;105:864-867.

107. Puczynski M, Rademaker D, Gatson RL: Burn injury related to the improper use of a microwave oven. *Pediatrics* 1983;72:714-715.

108. Hibbard RA, Blevins R: Palatal burn due to bottle warming in a microwave oven. *Pediatrics* 1988;82:382-384.

109. Johnson CF: Constricting bands. Manifestations of possible child abuse. Case reports and a review. *Clin Pediatr (Phila)* 1988;27:439-444.

110. Sandler AP, Haynes V: Nonaccidental trauma and medical folk belief: a case of cupping. *Pediatrics* 1978;61:921-922.

111. Sagi A, Ben-Meir P, Bibi C: Burn hazard from cupping—an ancient universal medication still in practice. *Burns Incl Therm Inj* 1988;14:323-325.

112. Kose AA, Karabagli Y, Cetin C: An unusual cause of burns due to cupping: complication of a folk medicine remedy. *Burns* 2006;32:126-127.

113. Rosenberg L, Sagi A, Stahl N, et al: Maqua (therapeutic burn) as an indicator of underlying disease. *Plast Reconstr Surg* 1988;82:277-280.

114. Lapid O: Copper sulfate burns to the hands, a complication of traditional medicine. *J Burn Care Rehabil* 2008;29:544-547.

115. Feldman KW: Pseudoabusive burns in Asian refugees. *Child Abuse Negl* 1995;19:657-658.

116. Bays J: Conditions mistaken for child abuse. *In*: Reece RM (ed): *Child Abuse: Medical Diagnosis and Management*. Lea & Febiger, Philadelphia, 1994, pp 358-385.

117. Garty BZ: Garlic burns. *Pediatrics* 1993;91:658-659.

118. Parish RA, McIntire S, Heimbach DM: Garlic burns: a naturopathic remedy gone awry. *Pediatr Emerg Care* 1987;3:258-260.

119. Richardson A: Cutaneous manifestations of abuse. *In*: Reece RM (ed): *Child Abuse: Medical Diagnosis and Management*. Lea & Febiger, Philadelphia, 1994, pp 167-184.

120. Feldman KW: Burn injuries: case studies. *In*: Alexander RC (ed): *Child Fatality Review: an Interdisciplinary Guide and Photographic Reference*. GW Medical, St Louis, 2007, pp 297-310.

121. Feldman KW, Clarren SK, McLaughlin JF: Tap water burns in handicapped children. *Pediatrics* 1981;67:560-562.

122. Clark KD, Tepper D, Jenny C: Effect of a screening profile on the diagnosis of nonaccidental burns in children. *Pediatr Emerg Care* 1997;13:259-261.

123. Farley RH, Reece RM: *Recognizing when a child's injury or illness is caused by abuse*. Portable Guides to Investigating Child Abuse, U.S. Department of Justice, Office of Juvenile Justice and Delinquency Prevention, Washington, DC, 2002.

124. Yasti AC, Tumer AR, Atli M, et al: A clinical forensic scientist in the burns unit: necessity or not? A prospective clinical study. *Burns* 2006;32:77-82.

125. Merten DF, Radkowski MA, Leonidas JC: The abused child: a radiological reappraisal. *Radiology* 1983;146:377-381.

126. Belfer RA, Klein BL, Orr L: Use of the skeletal survey in the evaluation of child maltreatment. *Am J Emerg Med* 2001;19:122-124.

127. Hicks RA, Stolfi A: Skeletal surveys in children with burns caused by child abuse. *Pediatr Emerg Care* 2007;23:308-313.

128. Degraw M: Relationship of burn injuries and the concomitant presence of fractures in children referred for concern of physical abuse, and implications for the usefulness of skeletal surveys in children who present with burns and concerns of physical abuse. Presented at the Ray E. Helfer Society Annual Meeting, Tucson, 2008.

129. Long RT, Cope O: Emotional problems of burned children. *N Engl J Med* 1961;264:1121-1127.

130. Vigliano A, Hart LW, Singer F: Psychiatric sequelae of old burns in children and their parents. *Am J Orthopsychiatry* 1964;34:753-761.

131. Holter JC, Friedman SB: Etiology and management of severely burned children. Psychosocial considerations. *Am J Dis Child* 1969;118:680-686.

132. Drake JE, Stoddard FJ Jr, Murphy JM, et al: Trauma severity influences acute stress in young burned children. *J Burn Care Res* 2006;27:174-182.

133. Woodward J, Jackson D: Emotional reactions in burned children and their mothers. *Br J Plast Surg* 1961;13:316-324.

134. Stoddard FJ, Stroud L, Murphy JM: Depression in children after recovery from severe burns. *J Burn Care Rehabil* 1992;13:340-347.

135. Kavanagh C: A new approach to dressing change in the severely burned child and its effect on burn-related psychopathology. *Heart Lung* 1983;12:612-619.

136. Erdmann TC, Feldman KW, Rivara FP, et al: Tap water burn prevention: the effect of legislation. *Pediatrics* 1991;88:572-577.

137. Squires T, Busuttil A: Child fatalities in Scottish house fires 1980-1990: a case of child neglect? *Child Abuse Negl* 1995;19:865-873.

29

BRUISES AND SKIN LESIONS

Tara L. Harris, MD, and Emalee G. Flaherty, MD

INTRODUCTION

The skin is one of the largest organs and perhaps one of the most complicated.[1] The skin has a multitude of functions and as many ways in which it can be injured. While skin injuries in childhood are common, they are also the most commonly seen manifestation of child abuse.[2-8] When McMahon et al[4] reviewed records of hospitalized children suspected to have been abused, they found that 92% had soft tissue injuries. Cutaneous manifestations of child abuse can include bruises, lacerations, abrasions, bites, and burns. We will discuss each of these modes of injury in detail, with the exception of bites and burns, which are covered in separate chapters. Understanding the skin's response to insult requires a basic review of skin structure and physiology.

Anatomy of the Skin

The outermost skin layer, the epidermis, is a compact, firm layer, composed primarily of keratinocytes (Figure 29-1). The keratinocytes migrate outward from the stratum basalis, through the stratum spinosum and stratum granulosum, to the outermost stratum corneum, composed of dead skin cells. From there, the dead cells are sloughed. This progression is completed in approximately 2 to 3 weeks.

Melanocytes, which provide pigmentation to the skin, are also found within the epidermis. Historically, it has been taught that an injury must affect the deeper levels of the epidermis, where the melanocytes reside, to cause scarring; the pale appearance of scars was thought to represent a decreased number or activity of melanocytes. Though there has been limited study of this issue, the research that has been done does not support these traditionally held beliefs. When the number of melanocytes and the production of melanin in scarred and adjacent healthy tissue were compared, they did not differ significantly.[9] Velangi and Rees postulated that instead the pale appearance of scars might be due to changes in the vascularity, organization of collagen fibers, lack of normal epithelial undulation, and/or epithelial thinning within the scar tissue.

The dermis is an easily deformed layer and underlies the epidermis. It is responsible for nourishing the epidermis and providing the structural integrity of the skin. The dermis is a matrix of collagen and elastin fibers embedded in amorphous ground substance. Blood vessels, nerves, and lymphatics course through this matrix. Collagen accounts for approximately 80% of the dry weight of skin and is responsible for maintaining the stiffness or structure of the skin. Elastin, in contrast, composes only 1% to 4% of the dry weight of the skin. It has long been thought that elastin is responsible for flexibility and the ability of the skin to return to its natural state after being deformed.[10] Some biomechanical research, however, suggests that the elastic properties of the skin are also attributable to the collagen content.[11] Proteoglycans, which bind water and therefore maintain skin turgor and contribute to the viscoelasticity of the skin, are found within the ground substance.[12] Sweat glands, sebaceous glands, and hair follicles are embedded within the dermal layer and project outward through the epidermis. The outer root sheath of hair follicles extends from the bottom of the hair bulb to the outer portion of the hair follicle, where it changes into epithelium;[13] hair follicles, therefore, can provide some regenerative potential to the epidermis if they remain intact after there is injury to the skin.

Underlying the dermis is the subcutaneous fat layer, which like the dermis, is readily deformed. This layer consists primarily of lobules of adipocytes. It also has an abundant supply of small blood vessels, which travel through the thin septae separating the lobules.[13] With trauma these capillaries can be damaged, causing blood to leak into the perivascular tissue. When bruises are visible externally, the bleeding has occurred most commonly in this layer.

Biomechanical Properties of the Skin

Skin demonstrates complicated viscoelastic behavior. The intrinsic properties of the skin partially govern its response to insult. Collagen provides stiffness and tensile strength to the skin. Human skin is under a constant level of resting tension; this tension causes the gaping seen between the edges of wounds. The skin's response to additional external tension is inversely related to the cross-sectional area across which a load is applied.[11] Hence, the skin will experience less tension (and less risk of injury) if a given load is applied over a large area of skin surface than it would if applied over a small area. Peak tensile strength is reached on average at age 8 years, where the mean is 21 N/mm.[2] Overall the tensile strength range of human skin is 5 to 30 N/mm^2. The elasticity of the skin, determined by elastin and collagen, provides

Cross Section of Skin

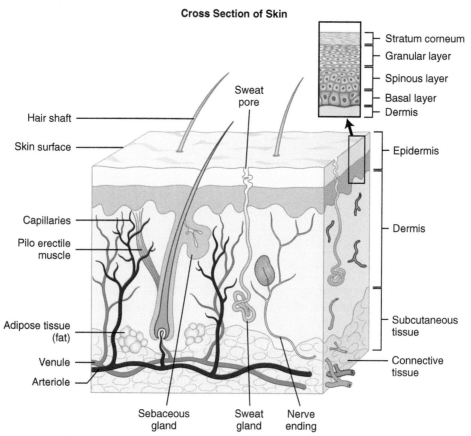

FIGURE 29-1 Anatomy of the skin.

resilience to the skin. In normal skin, maximal elasticity is reached at age 11 years at 70 N/mm², while the overall range is 15 to 150 N/mm².

Since both the tensile strength and elasticity decline with age and solar damage, the skin's response to trauma also changes. These losses do not factor into the assessment of possible child abuse, since there is no appreciable decline during the childhood years. Other factors that do affect the skin's intrinsic properties include underlying health status and certain medications. Examples of systemic health problems which can affect the skin include uremia, diabetes, shock, severe anemia, and malnutrition. Corticosteroids, which are commonly used in the general pediatric population, are an example of a medication that affects the skin by reducing the production of collagen. Anticoagulants, antiinflammatories, and antineoplastic agents are other medications that affect the skin's intrinsic properties, acting through a wide variety of mechanisms.[14]

When the skin is acted on by an outward force, the response is dependent on the specific region of skin involved. The volume of skin affected and thickness of underlying fat and muscle can have significant effect on the extent of injury sustained by the skin. Since the epidermal appendages, blood vessels, and nerves all serve to support and anchor the skin, the extent of injury also depends on the density of these structures in the injured area.

There may be differences in certain skin characteristics between racial groups. Wesley and Maibach[15] found in their meta-analysis that there is variation in blood vessel reactivity in the skin of different racial groups, and transepidermal water loss is increased in black skin compared with white skin. These differences in skin characteristics suggest the possibility that racial differences can cause minor variations in skin response to trauma. Further research is needed to investigate this possibility, since such differences may contribute to the finding, in some studies, that there are higher rates of bruising in white children compared with African American children.[16]

Ambient characteristics of the environment, such as temperature and humidity, will also affect the skin's response to trauma. For example, in a warm environment, the skin blood vessels will be dilated. For a 70 kg man, skin blood flow at normal indoor temperature is estimated to be 20 to 500 mL/min.[12] In contrast, when exercising in a warm environment, skin blood flow can increase to 2.1 to 3.5 L/min. The increase in blood vessel size, blood volume present, and rate of blood flow would all affect the appearance and extent of response to a trauma. Conversely, cold temperatures and shock may dramatically decrease the blood flow to the skin. In such situations, bruise formation could be delayed or diminished by the restricted blood flow to injured areas.

The characteristics of the external force acting on the skin are major determinants of the skin's response to trauma. The skin's resistance to stress is rate-dependent; a load applied quickly will cause skin failure (or breakage) at much lower stress levels than a load applied gradually.[11] The length of time during which a force is applied will also have impact on the resultant injury, as will the amount of force used.

Finally, the shape and composition of the impacting object will affect extent and type of injury.[14]

Repetitive handling or injury also affects the skin's responses. Edwards and Marks[11] noted that "the skin exhibits a 'memory,' so that the effects of strain are still obvious many hours after removal of the stretching force." Both in vivo and in vitro studies have shown that repeated strain alters the skin's responses. With repetitive strain, it takes progressively less force to extend the skin at low levels of extension, though this effect seems to be lost after approximately 40% extension.[10] Additionally, it has been shown in animal models that repetitive skin injury, in the form of bruising, leads to accelerated rates of bruise resolution with each successive injury.[17] Furthermore, this accelerated rate of healing could be passively transferred to another animal through whole blood transfusion, leading to the supposition that a humoral factor may be responsible for the quickened response. Though this has only been demonstrated in an animal model, it is possible that children who sustain a large number of bruises over time may develop factors which cause resolution of their bruises at an accelerated rate compared with other, less frequently injured, children.

While understanding of the biomechanical properties of skin and its associated responses is continually improving, this remains a difficult area to research. When studies are performed in vitro, the baseline resting tension of the skin in vivo is lost, and the surrounding support structures (including the subcutaneous fat) are often not included in the studied sample. However, data obtained from in vitro studies are usually more precise than that collected from in vivo studies.[11] There are also obvious challenges to studies in vivo. Only the top layers of the skin can be accessed easily, and there is not a way to measure stress/strain on the dermis without breaching the epidermis. Despite the challenges, extensive research in the area of skin biomechanics continues.

BRUISING

Definitions

A *bruise* can be defined as bleeding beneath intact skin due to trauma. A bruise occurs when the integrity of the vessel wall is compromised, allowing blood from the intravascular space to leak into the extravascular space. This can be caused by direct forces (e.g., blunt force trauma) or indirect forces (e.g., strangulation causing facial bruising). A variety of terms are used to describe bruises; these terms have different implications regarding morphology, and in some cases cause. *Petechiae*, the smallest bruises, are pinpoint-sized hemorrhages into the skin resulting from various processes. They can be differentiated from tiny vessels lying close to the surface of the skin because petechiae will not blanche with application of pressure. *Contusions* occur when a larger quantity of blood extravasates into the skin or subcutaneous tissue, again without breach of the overlying skin. The term contusion implies blunt trauma as the cause. In contrast, *ecchymoses* are not associated with blunt trauma. Ecchymoses occur when blood has dissected through tissue planes to become visible externally.[18] Both contusions and ecchymoses can be described as hematomas; *hematoma* is a more generalized term for a collection of extravasated blood under intact

Table 29-1	Factors Affecting the Development and Appearance of a Bruise

Properties of the impacting object or surface

Force of impact

Duration of impact

Properties of the body region impacted:
• Vascularization of the tissue bed at the impact site
• Tightness of the skin and connective tissue support
• Presence or absence of tissue planes
• Presence of underlying bone, such as tibia, spine, iliac crest

Quantity of blood extravasated

Distance of hemorrhage below the surface of the skin

Age and health status of the injured individual, including:
• Medications
• State of the coagulation system
• State of the immunological system (required to breakdown extravasated blood)

Color of the skin

Prior injury

skin. The term hematoma is often used when the extravasated blood presents as a localized area of bruising with palpable swelling.[19]

Bruise Evolution and the Myth of the Aging of Bruises

Many factors affect the development and appearance of a bruise, as shown in Table 29-1. Once an injury has been sustained which has disrupted blood vessels in or under the skin, a bruise may take minutes to days to appear. This is due to continued extravasation at the site of the injury and tracking of the blood through tissue planes. Mechanical irritation caused by the extravasated blood leads to release of histamine and neuropeptides, which then cause local vasodilatation.[20] Macrophages and neutrophils are recruited to the site of injury and begin to breakdown the erythrocytes. Hemoglobin within the erythrocytes is broken down into bilirubin, biliverdin, and hemosiderin. Biliverdin is rapidly metabolized to bilirubin by biliverdin reductase.[21] The progression of bruise appearance through various colors during resolution has long been attributed to this breakdown process, with red and blue being thought to represent hemoglobin and therefore "fresh" bruising, yellow/green to represent bilirubin and/or biliverdin and therefore older bruising, and brown to represent hemosiderin, which was expected for an old, resolving bruise. More recent studies evaluating the validity of this theory, however, have shown that determining the age of a bruise by its color is unreliable. Table 29-2 describes various bruising "myths" and actual facts about bruise identification and timing.

Table 29-2 Common Bruising Myths

Myth	Fact
Infants bruise easily	• Bruises in infants are rare • There is no evidence to support the idea that when impacted, an infant's skin bruises more readily than older children or adults
Different colored bruises are different ages	• Two bruises caused by a single event may be different colors and may change color at different rates
Presence of abrasions and/or swelling at the site of a bruise indicate that it is acute	• Though only assessed in one study, presence of abrasion or swelling was not a reliable indicator of injury age
The age of bruises can be determined based on their color	• Extensive research documents that color is not a reliable way to determine the age of bruises • Only consistent color indicator is that yellow has not been reported in bruises <18 hours old

Though many authors and texts have suggested that the age of a bruise could be determined based on appearance, Wilson in 1977 had already noted that such an estimation was "difficult and imprecise at best.[22]" In their landmark paper in 1991, Langlois and Gresham reviewed the literature available at that time regarding the aging of bruises.[23] They then examined 369 photographs of bruises from 89 subjects aged 10 to 100 years and found that the color progression previously described could not be supported scientifically. Red, previously thought to represent a fresh bruise, was common in bruises of all ages. The only relationship of color to time they observed was that yellow was not noted in any bruise less than 18 hours old. However, not all bruises developed yellow coloration after 18 hours. They also noted, importantly, that even two bruises on the same anatomic part, in the same patient, and from the same traumatic insult were not the same color and did not resolve at the same rate. Finally, they noted that some colors within a bruise would disappear and then reappear later. A subsequent study by Carpenter on normal bruising in infants also found no relation between the age of a bruise and color, except that yellow was only found in bruises greater than 48 hours old.[24]

Similar results were found by Stephenson and Bialas in 1996.[19] In this study, 50 photographs of 36 bruises on 23 children (ages 8 months to 13 years) were reviewed by one of the authors. Although the author believed he could determine whether the bruise was fresh (<48 hr), intermediate (48 hr-7 days), or old (>7 days) in 44 of the 50 photographed bruises, he was only correct in 24 of the 44 cases. Red was only seen in bruises up to 1 week old, but it was only seen in 15 of the 37 bruises in this group. Yellow was not noted in any of the bruises that were less than 1 day old, but it was only seen in 10 of the 42 bruises that were more than a day

old. Like Langlois and Gresham, they also noted that in one child with two different bruises from the same incident, the bruises were different colors.

The presence of other features accompanying bruising, such as swelling or abrasions, has not been shown to be useful in determination of the age of injuries. Bariciak et al[25] in 2003 reported on assessments of single bruises on 50 children, ages 1 week to 18 years. In this study, physicians and trainees were asked to estimate the age of a bruise based on physical examination, including notation of any swelling, abrasion, or tenderness. When asked to estimate the age of the injury within 24 hours, accuracy was less than 50% for all groups. However, when asked to categorize injuries to three timeframes (<48 hr, 48 hr to 7 days, or >7 days), accuracy improved significantly. There was, however, poor inter-rater reliability. Observers did not agree on color or the presence of accompanying features. Observers reported using color alone most often in their determinations, followed by color and tenderness, then color and swelling. None of these factors, however, were significantly correlated with accuracy.

Munang et al[26] also found poor interobserver reliability. Additionally, they found poor intraobserver reliability when bruises were photographed and the same observer was asked to assess the same injury again at a later date. In this study, 58 bruises on 44 children were assessed by three observers on two separate dates. The first assessment was done when the observer physically examined the child; the second assessment was of a photograph taken at the time of the first assessment. Two observers were in complete agreement on bruise color in only 27% of descriptions when the child was personally examined by the observers (in vivo) and 24% for photographed injuries. All three observers were in complete agreement in only 10% in vivo and 7% of photographs. At least one observer noted yellow in 30 of 174 interobserver comparisons in vivo; however, there was only agreement in 47% (14 of the 30). Similarly, yellow was noted in 52 of 174 interobserver comparisons photographically; agreement was observed for 31% (16 of 52). In addition, single observers frequently did not agree with their own previous assessments. When the observations of two different dates were compared, the observers only showed complete agreement for 31% (54 of 174) of their assessments. Yellow was noted in 42 of 174 assessments on at least one date; however, the same observer described yellow coloration in vivo and in the photograph for only 31% of those assessments (13 of 42).

Interestingly, Hughes et al[27] identified that observers have different, measurable thresholds for perceiving yellow. By digitally modifying photographs of bruises using Adobe Photoshop, they determined that the threshold for perceiving yellow, among their 50 subjects, ranged from 4% to 16%. Also of note, the threshold increased by 0.07% per year of subject's age, indicating that the ability to perceive yellow declines with age.

Schwartz and Ricci[28] identified several other problems in using color to determine the age of a bruise. They highlight that other features besides the color of the contusion itself, such as the patient's skin color and the ambient lighting, affect the way we perceive the color of the contusion. They also point out that most of the studies on bruise dating do not indicate whether the assessments are based on simple presence of a color within a bruise (even if in trace amounts) or whether that color is the predominant color within the bruise.

In recent years, there has been significant study in the assessment of skin injury using reflectance spectrophotometry in place of visual assessment. This is based on the concept that hemoglobin and its breakdown products can be identified by their specific absorption peaks. The absorption peak for hemoglobin is at 415 nm, bilirubin at 460 nm, and biliverdin at 660 to 620 nm.[21,29] This, however, is currently of little clinical utility due to the equipment required and the lack of reproducibility. Even within a single bruise, there is variation in color that produces different spectrophotometric readings.[21]

DEFINING OTHER SKIN INJURIES

While bruises are the most common skin injury seen in children,[30,31] there are a variety of other ways in which the skin can be injured. Abrasions occur when friction removes the superficial outer layers of the skin or mucous membranes. Scratches have the same mechanism but instead result in "light tearing of the skin,[30]" and usually refer to more linear areas of injury (e.g., those caused by finger nails). The term *scrape* has been used in the research literature referring to both abrasions and scratches, so its use will be avoided in this chapter. A *laceration* is the result of a shearing force and causes deeper skin tearing, through the epidermis and sometimes through the dermis and/or subcutaneous tissues. Avulsion injuries occur if skin is impacted at an acute angle (<90 degrees), often by a blunt or semiblunt object; the combination of the skin's resting tension and the impact interact to create this unique injury where the skin is torn away from the subcutaneous tissues but left with an attachment to an uninjured base of skin.[14] Avulsion injuries result in more extensive tissue damage than shear injuries, and they have a higher risk of infection and other complications with healing due to the disruption in vascular supply to the avulsed tissue.

EVALUATION OF CUTANEOUS INJURIES FOR POSSIBLE CHILD ABUSE

History

As with all evaluations for possible child abuse, obtaining a thorough history is critical. Table 29-3 lists important historical information to obtain in cases of skin injuries. No skin injury, by itself, is pathognomonic for either abuse or accidental injury. Factors that would indicate the need for more extensive investigation include absent, vague, implausible, or changing history, report of mechanism beyond a child's developmental ability, delay in seeking care, or other concerning injuries to the patient or siblings. For mobile children with small injuries, however, it is reasonable that the parent might not know the cause. In Carpenter's study of normal infants aged 6 to 12 months, the caretakers had no explanations for 9 of the 32 bruises (28%) observed; none of these bruises exceeded 10 mm in any direction.[24] The author states that she did not suspect abuse in any of these cases, though she does not state how this possibility was excluded. Another confounder to consider is that bleeding disorders

Table 29-3	Historical Information to Gather in Cases of Skin Injury

- Specific details of how the injury was sustained Characteristics of impacting surfaces/objects
  - Clothing child had on or other protective factors
  - Timing
  - Symptoms
- Presence of other injuries to the skin or other organ systems
- Developmental ability
- History of prior injuries to patient or siblings
- Extensive past medical history including recent medications and any abnormal bleeding
- Cultural background (especially if folk-medicine therapy is in the differential)

may also have bruising/bleeding that is out of proportion to the stated history.

Examination

Like a complete history, a thorough examination of the entire skin surface is also critical to ensure that all skin injuries have been noted and to elucidate any possible patterns. All infants and young children presenting for medical care should have a complete skin examination, regardless of any preexisting concern for abuse.[18] Areas that are unlikely to be bruised accidentally (e.g., behind the ears, the neck, trunk, and buttocks) should receive special attention. Sometimes it is necessary to perform serial examinations, since deeper bruising does not usually manifest immediately, and in some cases, observation of color change may be needed to confirm the diagnosis (e.g., differentiating bruise from Mongolian spot).

Sometimes, however, deep injury never becomes apparent externally. When children having fractures were examined for bruising in one study, only 8 of 93 had bruising in the overlying skin when they were first evaluated.[32] A total of 25 (28%) developed bruising during the first week after their injuries. Of note, all eight fractures that were associated with bruising at the time of initial evaluation were displaced and/or superficially located. None of the nondisplaced fractures or fractures well-covered by soft tissues had associated bruising. More recent studies have also supported the finding that abusive fractures are usually *not* accompanied by bruising, especially when skull fractures are excluded.[33,34]

Certain techniques can enhance our visual inspection of soft tissue injuries. For example, it may be helpful to examine the skin with an alternate light source, which employs a specific wavelength of light to illuminate the skin. One of the wavelengths used is infrared (IR), which has a longer wavelength than visible light (>700 nm). Infrared has the deepest penetration into tissues so has the potential to demonstrate deep soft tissue injury, though clinical use has not yet been scientifically established. Ultraviolet (UV) light is employed more commonly, for example with a Wood's lamp. UV wavelengths are shorter than those of visible light (<400 nm), and they penetrate only minimally into the epidermis. The use of UV light has been demonstrated to enhance the visualization of soft tissue injuries.[35] It is important, however, to note that fluorescence under UV light is nonspecific and is seen in the presence of semen, blood, gun powder, and certain other trace metals, in addition to bruises and healing skin.[36] Anecdotally, fluorescence under UV light has also been observed with some skin creams and organic fluids (such as fruit juices). Therefore, while alternate light sources might be a useful adjunct to the physical examination and can be used to support or refute proposed mechanisms of injury, they should not be interpreted as definitive evidence of injury by themselves.[35] With further research in this field, however, such evaluations might be improved. A technique called forensic diaphanoscopy, which used a small halogen lamp and a transparent ruler to transilluminate the skin, was found in one study to have high sensitivity (95%) and high specificity (97%) for identifying subcutaneous bruises, which were not visible externally.[37]

Documentation

Bruises should be documented as descriptively as possible, including the color, shape, size, site, whether they are palpable or flat, and any other notable characteristics. Whenever possible, photodocumentation is recommended (see Chapter 27).

Unfortunately, it does not appear that clinical practice meets current recommendations. In a study of all children aged 9 months and younger that were admitted to the general pediatrics service or pediatric intensive care unit at Carolinas Medical Center over 1 year, only 70% had a documented skin examination.[38] For children admitted with "nonaccidental trauma relevant diagnoses such as convulsions," presence or absence of bruising was noted in only 27%. Only 20% of admission notes included assessment of developmental ability (by parental report or direct observation). Clearly, if this is standard practice, many skin injuries in infants are being missed, and those that are being detected are likely not being adequately evaluated or their significance appreciated. Research by Pierce at al[39] also would support this. They found that among 18 victims of fatal or near-fatal child abuse, 7 (39%) had prior unexplained bruising that was specifically noted by medical providers but no further action had been taken.

Interpretation of Findings

Table 29-4 summarizes studies of bruise frequency, location, and cause. When interpreting the significance of skin injuries, there are many factors to consider. First, the patient's *age and developmental ability* should be taken into account. Counter to unsupported statements published in some earlier papers,[23,40,41] skin injuries in premobile infants are very uncommon, and therefore all should be thoroughly evaluated. Sugar et al, in their evaluation of normal children at well care visits, found that only 0.6% (2 of 366) of normal infants less than 6 months old had bruises.[16] The percentage increased significantly for 6- to 8-month-olds; 5.6% (6 of 107) had bruises. Only 2.2% (11 of 511) of children who could not yet cruise or walk had bruises. In contrast, this rate rose dramatically to 17.8% among cruisers and 51.9% among walkers. In Labbe's study[30] of 246 normal children, aged 0 to 8 months, 1.2% had bruises, 1.2% had

abrasions, and 11% had scratches. No other skin injuries were seen in this group. In Carpenter's study[24] of 6- to 12-month-old infants, 12.4% (22 of 177) had bruises. Separated out by developmental ability, bruises were seen in 4% (4 of 101) of infants who could only sit, 17% (9 of 52) of infants who could crawl, and 38% (9 of 24) of infants who could walk.

In contrast, after about 9 months of age, skin injuries are very common in normal children. Labbe,[30] who performed 2040 examinations on 1467 children, found that most children older than 9 months of age had 1 or more recent skin injuries. Injuries were more common in the summer and most frequently seen on the knees and shins. Bruises were the most common skin injury observed.

In conjunction with the age and development of the child, certain *types of injury* might also be helpful in determining the cause. Among premobile children, it is clear that bruises are not commonly seen. Scratches, however, might be common in this group. Labbe found that 11% of infants 0 to 8 months had scratches, which were thought to be self-inflicted via their own fingernails.[30] Among older children, lacerations may suggest an accidental cause. Pascoe et al[42] assessed soft tissue injuries in children 1 to 12 years old. They compared three groups: 154 suspected victims of child abuse or neglect, 91 children who had presented to the emergency department (ED) for accidental injuries, and 105 children seen in an outpatient clinic. Among the group presenting to the ED for accidental injury, 40% had lacerations, while only 6% of the abuse/neglect group and 10% of the ambulatory group had lacerations. In a study of 87 children under age 6 seen in an emergency department, Holter, too, found that while lacerations were common in accidentally injured children, they were not seen at all in the 10 children the investigators suspected were abused.[43] A final type of injury to consider is petechiae. Nayak et al found that among children with bruises, children with injuries caused by abuse more frequently had petechiae than children with injuries determined to be accidental (24% vs. 1.2%).[44] They found that the use of the presence of petechiae to diagnose nonaccidental injury has a sensitivity of only 22% but a specificity of 98%. Thus none of these types of injury are pathognomonic for either abuse or accident. Understanding their relative frequencies, however, is helpful in assessing the overall presentation and likelihood of abuse.

The *location* is also an important aspect of skin injury to consider (Tables 29-4 and 29-5). Maguire et al[45] reviewed 23 studies assessing the significance of bruising patterns. They found that in accidental injuries, bruises were usually located on the front of the body and were over bony prominences in almost all cases (93%-100%).[16,24] The most common sites of bruising in children able to walk were the knees and shins. When there was bruising on the head, it was usually on the forehead. Areas uncommonly bruised included the face, abdomen, hips, back, buttocks, upper arms, forearms, and posterior legs. There were *no* accidental bruises seen on the hands, feet, or ears.

Abusive bruises could be found anywhere on the body, but certain characteristics and locations were suggestive of an abusive cause.[45] Bruises in children who had been abused were more likely to be located in areas not overlying bony prominences and were more likely to be large, multiple (means ranged from 5.7 to 10 per child, with range 0 to 44,

Table 29-4 Injury Frequency by Location and Cause

Study Author, Year*	Population Studied	Neck/Face (Excluding Forehead)		Ears		Genitalia		Buttocks		Hands	
		Accidental	NAI	Accidental	NAI	Accidental	NAI	Accidental	NAI	Accidental	NAI
Herr,[46] 2003	14 days-17 years, children admitted for abusive trauma	—	—	—	21/95	—	—	—	—	—	—
Dunstan,[47] 2002	1-14 years, 133 physically abused and 189 controls	3% of 189† (face only)	65% of 133 (face only)	0 of 189	16% of 133	None reported	None reported	3% of 189	20% of 133	None reported	None reported
Labbe,[30] 2001	0-17 years, seen in clinic or emergency dept. for reasons other than trauma	3.9% of 2040	—	0.3% of 2040	—	—	—	1.6% of 2040	—	3.5 % of 2040	—
Carpenter,[24] 1999	6-12 months, hearing and developmental clinics	5/177	—	0/177	—	0/177	0/177	0/177	—	0 / 177	—
Sugar,[16] 1999	<36 months, at well care visits	7/973	—	None reported	—	None reported	—	0/973	—	0 / 973	—
Wedgwood,[48] 1990	<4 years, admitted for reasons other than NAI	—	—	—	—	<1% of 56 (combined with buttocks)	—	<1% of 56 (combined with genitals)	—	0 / 56	—
Mortimer,[49] 1983	<1 year, routine clinic visits	2/620	—	0/620	—	0/620	—	0/620	—	0 / 620	—

Continued

Table 29-4 Injury Frequency by Location and Cause—cont'd

Study Author, Year*	Population Studied	Neck / Face (Excluding Forehead) Accidental	Neck / Face (Excluding Forehead) NAI	Ears Accidental	Ears NAI	Genitalia Accidental	Genitalia NAI	Buttocks Accidental	Buttocks NAI	Hands Accidental	Hands NAI
Tush,[50] 1982	36-48 months, urban daycare centers	0 / 30	—	—	—	0 / 30	—	2 / 30	—	0 / 30	—
Roberton,[31] 1982	2 weeks to 11 years, control group seen for routine care, NAI group admitted or seen in emergency department	6.5% of 400 (includes entire head)	59.8% of 84	—	—	—	—	9.25% of 400 (combined with thighs)	41.7% of 84 (combined with thighs)	†Text says hands and feet were most common site of injury, but not included in data presented	—
Pascoe,[42] 1979	1-12 years, 3 groups: — suspected abuse/ neglect — accidents seen in emergency dept. — accidents seen in ambulatory clinic	2 / 196	66 / 154	1 / 196	10 / 154	0 / 196	11 / 154	3 / 196	41 / 154	—	—

*Some studies include all injuries, not just bruises.
†Totals are total number children examined, not number injured or number of bruises.
†"None reported" = able to deduce 0 from other numbers reported (e.g., If they stated there were seven bruises - two on the forehead and five on the shin – one can deduce that there were 0 on the buttocks.)

Table 29-5	Bruising Suggestive of Child Abuse

Bruising in a child <9 months or noncruising child

Bruises away from bony prominences

Bruises to the ears, face, abdomen, arms, back, buttocks, and hands

Multiple bruises in clusters

Multiple bruises of uniform shape

Bruises that have the shape of an object or a ligature

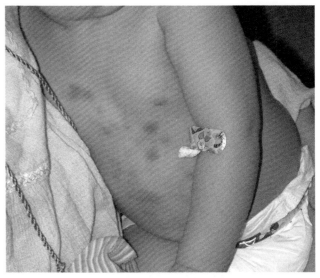

FIGURE 29-3 Bruising on the chest and abdomen.

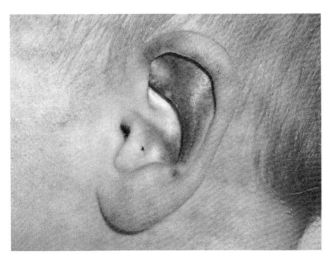

FIGURE 29-2 Bruising on the pinna.

in their study populations), and present in clusters. When clusters of bruises were seen on the upper arm, outside of the thigh, or on the trunk and adjacent extremity, they were often defensive bruises.[45]

Head and neck cutaneous injuries, particularly involving the face, require careful evaluation since they are more common in children who have been abused and are rare in nonabused children.* When Cairns reviewed available case records of 230 children who had been abused, 59% had signs of abuse on the head, face, or neck.[53] Of these, 95% had bruises and 33% had abrasions. In contrast, among Sugar's 930 nonabused children less than 36 months of age, bruises to the face (excluding the forehead) were only noted in one precruiser, one cruiser, and five walkers (0.8% of total study group); six were on the cheek and one was on the nose.[16]

Bruises around and on the ear (Figure 29-2) are also very concerning for abusive injury because they are seldom found in accidental injuries.† Dunstan[47] found ear bruises in 16% of the 133 children who had been abused and none of the 189 children who served as controls. Pascoe[42] found only 1 of 196 children, ages 1 to 12 years, with an accidental injury

to the ear, while 6% of the 154 children who had been abused had ear injuries. Herr et al[46] suggested that auricular bruising was a marker of severe abusive injury and that affected children had a high likelihood of significant morbidity and mortality.

Hand injuries are also concerning for abusive injury and are rarely caused by accidental injury.[16,24,30,47-50] The hands may be injured either as a primary target or as a secondary target as the child tries to shield other body parts.[54] Johnson,[54] who specifically studied abusive injuries to the hand, found that 94 (10%) of 944 physically abused children had injuries to the hand. Only 2% (19) had injury to the hand only; the remainder had additional injuries to other body parts. Notably, however, of the 94 children with abusive hand injuries (with or without other injuries), 18 (20%) required hospital admission. Of the 19 who had injury to the hand only, 5 (26%) required hospital admission. This would suggest that, like auricular bruising, injury to the hands may be a marker of severe physical abuse.

Bruising on the chest, abdomen, genitalia, buttocks, back, and posterior thighs should also raise suspicion for child abuse (Figures 29-3 and 29-4). Dunstan[47] found that 25% of abused children had bruises to the anterior chest and abdomen, while only 4% of his controls had bruises in those locations. In Pascoe's study,[42] abdominal bruising was seen only in children determined to have been abused. In addition, none of the 196 children he evaluated with accidental injuries had injuries to the genitalia, while 11 of 154 (7%) abused children had genital injuries. Bruising on the back, buttocks, and posterior thighs was also seen significantly more frequently in children who had been abused. Sugar et al[16] reported no bruising on the buttocks in the 973 children she studied.

The *total number of skin injuries* can also be helpful, though there is a wide range of normal in mobile children. In Labbe's study of normal children,[30] for example, the average number of skin injuries per child ranged from 1.3 for the 0- to 8-month-olds to 4.5 for 5- to 9-year-olds. The total range observed, however, went up to 21 for the 5- to 9-year-olds and up to 39 for the 9-month to 4-year-old group. Only

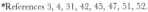

*References 3, 4, 31, 42, 45, 47, 51, 52.
†References 6, 24, 30, 42, 47, 49, 51.

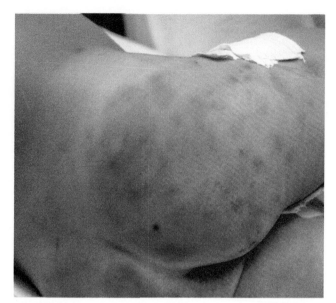

FIGURE 29-4 Bruising on the buttocks.

the range for 0- to 8-month-olds was uniformly low with a maximum of three injuries per child. Data from Sugar's study[16] is similar. For the 11 of 511 precruisers who did have bruises, the mean number of bruises per child was 1.3, with a range of 1 to 2. In contrast, for the 165 of 318 walkers who had bruises (ages 9-36 months), the average number of bruises per injured child increased to 2.4 with a range of 1 to 11. In Carpenter's study of 177 infants aged 6 to 12 months, the 22 infants with bruises had a mean of 1.5 bruises per child with a range of 1 to 4.[24] In contrast, Keen's early study of bruises in six normal 3- to 4-year-olds reported all the children had at least three bruises at each of the 60 examinations.[55]

A tool that may be more useful than total number of bruises for older children is a bruise score.[47,51] In a study of 133 abused children and 189 controls, age 1 to 13 years, the children were examined with measurement of the maximum dimension of all bruises. Total bruise lengths were then calculated for each of five different body regions. The authors used logistical regression to devise the following formula, weighted based on the probability that bruises in a given region are abusive (all lengths in cm):

$$\text{Score} = (2 \times \text{length on arms}) + (3 \times \text{length on legs}) + (4 \times \text{length on chest/abdomen/back}) + (5 \times \text{length on buttocks}) + (9 \times \text{length on head/neck})$$

The mean score for the abused children was 87.6 (SD 59.7), while the mean for controls was 5.9 (SD 9.0). The authors emphasize, however, that the usefulness of this score in determining the likelihood of abuse for any given child is highly dependent upon the pretest probability of abuse. Thus such a system must be used cautiously. The authors found that adding an element to weight bruises with identifiable shapes increased the specificity of the bruise score (for a given sensitivity). Table 29-5 summarizes characteristics of bruises that suggest an abusive cause.

There are several *other characteristics* of skin injuries which, when present, raise concern for abuse. For example, symmetric bilateral bruises rarely occur accidentally. In their study involving 20,896 examinations of 481 children under age 5 years, Laing and Buchan[56,57] observed 3709 injuries. Only one, however, was bilateral and was deemed by the authors to be clearly nonaccidental. Similarly, other injuries involving multiple planes of the body are not commonly accidental and should be assessed carefully.[18] If an appropriate history of trauma with multiple impacts is not forthcoming, the concern for abuse must be elevated. Additionally, observation of an old injury that should have received medical care but did not should raise concern.[58]

Observing a *pattern* to a bruise, abrasion, or scar is a final characteristic that is extremely concerning for physical abuse (Table 29-6). The pattern can reflect the shape of the impacting object, or it can result from something lying between the skin and object at the time of impact (e.g., a fabric pattern).[18] Patterns can also be influenced by underlying structures, and they may only appear in the skin overlying bony areas.[2] When there is rotational force on the impacting object (i.e., a whipping motion), the end of the object is moving at the highest velocity and may therefore cause more extensive injury than the part of the object closer to the fulcrum.[20,59] Additionally, the pattern formed depends on the weight and speed with which the object impacts the skin, as seen when comparing the bruising caused by a slap versus that caused by a punch. When Randeberg et al[20] studied high-speed, light-weight impacts (comparable to a slap) on domestic pigs, they found through recordings by high speed cameras that these impacts produced intense oscillations in the skin surrounding the impact sites. When they observed low-speed, blunt force impacts (comparable to a punch), they found that the low-speed objects stayed in contact with the skin longer than the high-speed, light objects, thereby diminishing the development of the tissue oscillations. It is possible that the intense tissue oscillations caused by high-speed, light impacts are at least partially responsible for the outline appearance formed by slap marks (Figure 29-5), in contrast to the bruising directly under the contact point caused by low-speed, blunt impacts such as punches. Clearly, inspection for patterns must be thorough and meticulous.

It is not clear how often patterned injuries are observed among abused populations. McMahon et al[4] observed patterned injuries in only 8% of the 371 children they examined who were suspected victims of abuse. Dunstan,[47] however, noted that 57% (of 133 total, ages 1-14 years) of the abused children he studied had injuries with at least one identifiable shape; less than 2% of his control group (189 children) had injuries with identifiable shape. Specifically, identifiable hand prints were seen in 30% of the abused children but none of the controls.[51]

Some bruises have a *pattern formed by the lines of stress* caused by an impact, instead of from the shape of the impacting object. Feldman reported on nine children who had received transverse blows to the buttocks that resulted in vertical bruises along the gluteal cleft.[61] He postulated that this appearance might be caused by either a crimping of the skin along the gluteal crease with impact or from shearing vascular rupture at the junction between compressed vessels on the buttock and the protected vessels within the gluteal crease. Additionally, he reported on four children with petechial bruising along the top of one or both pinnae. He postulated that when the pinna is folded by a forceful impact, the capillaries along this line of folding are injured and result in a rim of petechial bruising.

Table 29-6	Injury Patterns
Method of Injury/ Implement	**Pattern Observed**
Grip/grab	Relatively round marks that correspond with fingertips and/or thumb
Closed-fist punch	Series of round bruises that correspond with the knuckles of the hand
Slap	Parallel, linear bruises (usually petechial) separated by areas of central sparing (Figure 29-5)
Belt/electrical cord	Loop marks or parallel lines of petechiae (the width of the belt/ cord) with central sparing; may see triangular marks from the end of the belt, small circular lesions caused by the holes in the tongue of the belt, and/or a buckle pattern
Rope	Areas of bruising interspersed with areas of abrasion
Other objects/ household implements	Injury in shape of object/implement (e.g., rods, switches, and wires cause linear bruising)
Human bite	Two arches forming a circular or oval shape, may cause bruising and/or abrasion
Strangulation	Petechiae of the head and/or neck, including mucous membranes; may see subconjunctival hemorrhages
Binding/ ligature	Marks around the wrists, ankles, or neck (Figure 29-6); sometimes accompanied by petechiae or edema distal to the ligature mark Marks adjacent to the mouth if the child has been gagged
Excessive hincar (punishment by kneeling on salt or other rough substance)	Abrasions/burns, especially to knees
Hair pulling	Traumatic alopecia; may see petechiae on underlying scalp, or swelling or tenderness of the scalp (due to subgaleal hematoma)
Tattooing or intentional scarring	Abusive cases have been described,[60] but can also be a cultural phenomenon (e.g., Maori body ornamentation)

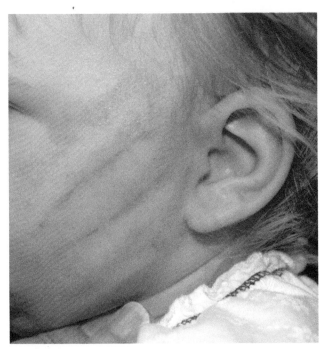

FIGURE 29-5 Slap mark on the cheek of a child.

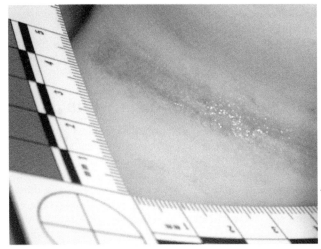

FIGURE 29-6 Ligature marks on the neck of a child.

OTHER CONSIDERATIONS

When evaluating bruises and other skin injuries for possible child abuse, it is important to exclude other causes. If the child only has bruising, with or without other manifestations of bleeding (e.g., subdural hematoma, retinal hemorrhage), evaluation for inherited or acquired coagulopathy is indicated. Children with coagulopathies are sometimes initially misdiagnosed as having been abused,[62,63] which can have obvious, devastating consequences. Approach to coagulopathy evaluation is beyond the scope of this chapter, but there have been several very helpful reviews written.[64-67] Additionally, there are several conditions which predispose the skin to injure easily, including genetic conditions such as Ehlers-Danlos syndrome, and acquired conditions such as corticosteroid atrophy. Conditions which mimic child abuse will be discussed in the next chapter.

COMPLICATIONS OF SOFT TISSUE INJURY

Though the majority of skin and soft tissue injuries are minor, some complications can be life-threatening. Injury with extensive involvement of the muscle tissue can result in rhabdomyolysis.[68-71] Dark or discolored urine can be the initial sign. A urine dipstick can be used as a screening test; rhabdomyolysis will cause a positive result for hemoglobin with an absence of red blood cells. Urine or serum myoglobin levels can confirm the diagnosis. Muscle cell damage causes a proportionate increase in creatinine phosphokinase. Hyperkalemia can result from damage to muscle cells and resulting renal compromise. Because acute renal failure can occur and require dialysis, early recognition is important. Peebles[68] found that 9 of 14 children with rhabdomyolysis caused by physical abuse had resultant renal failure, but none of the cases he reviewed required dialysis. Of those cases, 13 of 14 had injuries to their buttocks or legs.

Skin injuries, especially when not presented for appropriate medical care, can develop infection or heal poorly. Enlarged lymph nodes can be an indication of the chronicity of a skin injury.[7] For example, severe diaper rash accompanied by enlarged inguinal lymph nodes would raise concern for either inadequate immunological function or a chronically neglected dermatitis. Finally, if the diagnosis of child abuse is missed, the child with skin injury may go on to suffer further, sometimes fatal, abuse.

FUTURE RESEARCH DIRECTIONS

Further research is needed around skin injury. One clear deficit in the literature regards bruising in nonwhite children. Many of the landmark papers on bruising either include only white children,[19,26] or the vast majority of subjects are white children.[16,30] Since there may be some differences in the skin's response to trauma among different ethnicities,[15] it will be important to study these groups. Accidental bruising patterns might also be different in children with disabilities or special needs. One small study of accidental bruising supported this conclusion and recommended further study.[72]

Although it has become accepted medical knowledge that we cannot accurately estimate the age of bruises, most of the studies done to date rely on the patient or parent to recall when the injury was sustained. Future studies using subjects having a bruise of verifiable age may yield additional information that will assist in dating bruises.

Additionally, further research is needed into alternative methods of detecting bruises and documenting bruises not visible to the naked eye. The utility of spectrophotometry and alternate light sources requires further investigation. Recent research with animal models suggests that blunt forces might cause hemorrhage deep within the muscular layer that is not visible externally.[20] Establishment of a sensitive and specific way to detect such injury would be very helpful in determining the presence and extent of inflicted injuries.

References

1. Goldsmith LA: My organ is bigger than your organ. *Arch Dermatol* 1990;126:301-302.
2. Johnson CF: Inflicted injury versus accidental injury. *Pediatr Clin North Am* 1990;37:791-814.
3. O'Neill JA Jr, Meacham WF, Griffin JP, et al: Patterns of injury in the battered child syndrome. *J Trauma* 1973;13:332-339.
4. McMahon P, Grossman W, Gaffney M, et al: Soft-tissue injury as an indication of child abuse. *J Bone Joint Surg Am* 1995;77:1179-1183.
5. Galleno H, Oppenheim WL: The battered child syndrome revisited. *Clin Orthop Rel Res* 1982;162:11-19.
6. Johnson CF, Showers J: Injury variables in child abuse. *Child Abuse Negl* 1985;9:207-215.
7. Ellerstein NS: The cutaneous manifestations of child abuse and neglect. *Am J Dis Child* 1979;133:906-909.
8. Sussman SJ: Skin manifestations of the battered-child syndrome. *J Pediatr* 1968;72:99.
9. Velangi SS, Rees JL: Why are scars pale? An immunohistochemical study indicating preservation of melanocyte number and function in surgical scars. *Acta Derm Venereol* 2001;81:326-328.
10. Elsner P, Berardesca E, Wilhelm KP, et al (eds): *Bioengineering of the skin: skin biomechanics.* (Dermatology: Clinical and Basic Science Series). CRC Press, Boca Raton, Fla, 2002.
11. Edwards C, Marks R: Evaluation of biomechanical properties of human skin. *Clin Dermatol* 1995;13:375-380.
12. Orkin M, Maibach HI, Dahl MV (eds): *Dermatology*, ed 1, Appleton and Lange, New York, 1991.
13. Elder DE, Elenitsas R, Johnson BL Jr, et al (eds): *Lever's Histopathology of the Skin*, ed 9, Lippincott Williams & Wilkins, Cedar Knolls, NJ, 2005.
14. Trott A: Mechanisms of surface soft tissue trauma. *Ann Emerg Med* 1988;17(12):1279-1283.
15. Wesley NO, Maibach HI: Racial (ethnic) differences in skin properties: the objective data. *Am J Clin Dermatol* 2003;4:843-860.
16. Sugar NF, Taylor JA, Feldman KW: Bruises in infants and toddlers: those who don't cruise rarely bruise. Puget Sound Pediatric Research Network. *Arch Pediatr Adolesc Med* 1999;153:399-403.
17. Hamdy MK, May KN, Powers JJ: Some biochemical and physical changes occurring in experimentally-inflicted poultry bruises. *Proc Soc Exp Biol Med* 1961;108:185-188.
18. Kaczor K, Pierce MC, Makoroff KL, et al: Bruising and physical child abuse. *Clin Pediatr Emerg Med* 2006;7:153-159.
19. Stephenson T, Bialas Y: Estimation of the age of bruising. *Arch Dis Child* 1996;74:53-55.
20. Randeberg LL, Winnem AM, Langlois NE, et al: Skin changes following minor trauma. *Lasers Surg Med* 2007;39:403-413.
21. Hughes VK, Ellis PS, Burt T, et al: The practical application of reflectance spectrophotometry for the demonstration of haemoglobin and its degradation in bruises. *J Clin Pathol* 2004;57:355-359.
22. Wilson EF: Estimation of the age of cutaneous contusions in child abuse. *Pediatrics* 1977;60:750-752.
23. Langlois NE, Gresham GA: The ageing of bruises: a review and study of the colour changes with time. *Forensic Sci Int* 1991;50:227-238.
24. Carpenter RF: The prevalence and distribution of bruising in babies. *Arch Dis Child* 1999;80:363-366.
25. Bariciak ED, Plint AC, Gaboury I, et al: Dating of bruises in children: an assessment of physician accuracy. *Pediatrics* 2003;112:804-807.
26. Munang LA, Leonard PA, Mok JY: Lack of agreement on colour description between clinicians examining childhood bruising. *J Clin Forensic Med* 2002;9:171-174.
27. Hughes VK, Ellis PS, Langlois NEI: The perception of yellow in bruises. *J Clin Forensic Med* 2004;11:257-259.
28. Schwartz AJ, Ricci LR: How accurately can bruises be aged in abused children? Literature review and synthesis. *Pediatrics* 1996;97:254-257.
29. Hughes VK, Ellis PS, Langlois NEI: Alternative light source (Polilight) illumination with digital image analysis does not assist in determining the age of bruises. *Forensic Sci Int* 2006;158:104-107.
30. Labbe J, Caouette G: Recent skin injuries in normal children. *Pediatrics* 2001;108:271-276.
31. Roberton DM, Barbor P, Hull D: Unusual injury? Recent injury in normal children and children with suspected non-accidental injury. *Br Med J (Clin Res Ed)* 1982;285:1399-1401.

32. Mathew MO, Ramamohan N, Bennet GC: Importance of bruising associated with paediatric fractures: prospective observational study. *Br Med J* 1998;317:1117-1118.

33. Peters ML, Starling SP, Barnes-Eley ML, et al: The presence of bruising associated with fractures. *Arch Pediatr Adolesc Med* 2008;162:877-881.

34. DeGraw M, Little M, Lindberg DM: Likelihood of cutaneous injury associated with fractures in children referred for concern of physical abuse (abstract). Helfer Society, Tucson, 2008.

35. Vogeley E, Pierce MC, Bertocci G: Experience with wood lamp illumination and digital photography in the documentation of bruises on human skin. *Arch Pediatr Adolesc Med* 2002;156:265-268.

36. Barsley RE, West MH, Fair JA: Forensic photography. Ultraviolet imaging of wounds on skin. *Am J Forensic Med Pathol* 1990;11:300-308.

37. Horisberger B, Krompecher T: Forensic diaphanoscopy: how to investigate invisible subcutaneous hematomas on living subjects. *Int J Legal Med* 1997;110:73-78.

38. Hight NB, Rogers MK, Zeskind PS: Documenting a skin exam in babies: are we missing physical abuse? E-PAS2007:61245. Pediatric Academic Societies Annual Meeting, Toronto, 2007.

39. Pierce MC, Kaczor K, Acker D, et al: Bruising missed as a prognostic indicator of future fatal and near-fatal physical child abuse. E-PAS2008:634469. Pediatric Academic Societies Annual Meeting, Honolulu, 2008.

40. Vanezis P: Interpreting bruises at necropsy. *J Clin Pathol* 2001;54:348-345.

41. Stephenson T: Bruising in children. *Curr Paediatr* 1995;5:225-229.

42. Pascoe JM, Hildebrandt HM, Tarrier A, et al: Patterns of skin injury in nonaccidental and accidental injury. *Pediatrics* 1979;64:245-247.

43. Holter JC, Friedman SB: Child abuse: early case finding in the emergency department. *Pediatrics* 1968;42:128-138.

44. Nayak K, Spencer N, Shenoy M, et al: How useful is the presence of petechiae in distinguishing non-accidental from accidental injury? *Child Abuse Negl* 2006;30:549-555.

45. Maguire S, Mann MK, Sibert J, et al: Are there patterns of bruising in childhood which are diagnostic or suggestive of abuse? A systematic review. *Arch Dis Child* 2005;90:182-186.

46. Herr S, Pierce MC, Vogeley E, et al: Auricular bruising as a marker of severe abusive trauma. PAS2003:1102. Pediatric Academic Societies Annual Meeting, Seattle, 2003.

47. Dunstan FD, Guildea ZE, Kontos K, et al: A scoring system for bruise patterns: a tool for identifying abuse. *Arch Dis Child* 2002;86:330-333.

48. Wedgwood J: Childhood bruising. *Practitioner* 1990;234:598-601.

49. Mortimer PE, Freeman M: Are facial bruises in babies ever accidental? *Arch Dis Child* 1983;58:75-76.

50. Tush BA: Bruising in healthy 3-year-old children. *Matern Child Nurs J* 1982;11:165-179.

51. Sibert J: Bruising, coagulation disorder, and physical child abuse. *Blood Coagul Fibrinolysis* 2004;15(suppl 1):S33-S39.

52. Atwal GS, Rutty GN, Carter N, et al: Bruising in non-accidental head injured children; a retrospective study of the prevalence, distribution and pathological associations in 24 cases. *Forensic Sci Int* 1998;96:215-230.

53. Cairns AM, Mok JY, Welbury RR: Injuries to the head, face, mouth and neck in physically abused children in a community setting. *Int J Paediatr Dent* 2005;15:310-318.

54. Johnson CF, Kaufman KL, Callendar C: The hand as a target organ in child abuse. *Clin Pediatr* 1990;29:66-72.

55. Keen JH: Normal bruises in pre-school children. *Arch Dis Child* 1981;56:75.

56. Laing SA, Buchan AR: Bilateral injuries in childhood: an alerting sign. *Br Med J* 1976;2:940-941.

57. Laing SA: Bilateral injuries in childhood: an altering sign? *Br Med J* 1977;2:1355.

58. Labbe J: Determining whether a skin injury could be physical abuse. *Contemp Pediatr* 2003;20:27-49.

59. Swerdlin A, Berkowitz C, Craft N: Cutaneous signs of child abuse. *J Am Acad Dermatol* 2007;57:371-392.

60. Johnson CF: Symbolic scarring and tattooing. Unusual manifestations of child abuse. *Clin Pediatr* 1994;33:46-49.

61. Feldman KW: Patterned abusive bruises of the buttocks and the pinnae. *Pediatrics* 1992;90:633-636.

62. Harley JR: Disorders of coagulation misdiagnosed as nonaccidental bruising. *Pediatr Emerg Care* 1997;13:347-349.

63. Taylor GP: Severe bleeding disorders in children with normal coagulation screening tests. *Br Med J (Clin Res Ed)* 1982;284:1851-1852.

64. Acosta M, Edwards R, Jaffe EI, et al: A practical approach to pediatric patients referred with an abnormal coagulation profile. *Arch Pathol Lab Med* 2005;129:1011-1016.

65. Thomas AE: The bleeding child; is it NAI? *Arch Dis Child* 2004;89:1163-1167.

66. Khair K, Liesner R: Bruising and bleeding in infants and children–a practical approach. *Br J Haematol* 2006;133:221-231.

67. Liesner R, Hann I, Khair K: Non-accidental injury and the haematologist: the causes and investigation of easy bruising. *Blood Coagul Fibrinolysis* 2004;15(suppl 1):S41-S48.

68. Peebles J, Losek JD: Child physical abuse and rhabdomyolysis: case report and literature review. *Pediatr Emerg Care* 2007;23:474-477.

69. Schwengel D, Ludwig S: Rhabdomyolysis and myoglobinuria as manifestations of child abuse. *Pediatr Emerg Care* 1985;1:194-197.

70. Mukherji SK, Siegel MJ: Rhabdomyolysis and renal failure in child abuse. *AJR Am J Roentgenol* 1987;148:1203-1204.

71. Leung A, Robson L: Myoglobinuria from child abuse. *Urology* 1987;29:45-46.

72. Barton C, Finlay F: Bruising in preschool children with special needs. *Arch Dis Child* 2005;90:1318.

30

Skin Conditions Confused with Child Abuse

Kathi L. Makoroff, MD, and Megan L. McGraw, MD

INTRODUCTION

A thoughtful and comprehensive differential diagnosis should be part of any evaluation for suspected child abuse. The medical evaluation for any suspected child abuse victim includes a complete medical history, review of systems, family history, physical examination, and appropriate studies to exclude other medical conditions. Inaccurately making a diagnosis of child abuse is not without significant consequences for those involved, including the patient, patient's family, investigative agencies, and alleged perpetrators. This chapter explores some of the common conditions that can mimic child physical abuse.

CONDITIONS CONFUSED WITH BRUISING

Congenital Conditions

Hemangiomas. Hemangiomas are a common congenital vascular anomaly and are often present at birth. They can be confused with child abuse due to their red-purple discoloration mimicking bruising or deep tissue involvement that appears as swelling.[1,2] In addition, if located in the genital area, hemangiomas may be mistaken as sexual abuse injury.[3]

Dermal melanosis. Dermal melanosis (previously called "Mongolian spots") are congenital hyperpigmented lesions that can be mistaken for bruising associated with child abuse.[1,4,5,6] They are more commonly seen with black, Asian, Latino, and Native American infants but can occur on any infant. Dermal melanosis spots vary in size, shape, and color. Homogenous blue-gray or blue-green patches with irregular borders characterize the typical appearance. Although most commonly located on the lumbosacral, back, shoulders, or buttock areas, dermal melanosis can be located anywhere on the body including the scalp.[4,7] Smaller dermal melanosis can be superimposed on larger melanosis spots, creating the appearance of bruises overlying existing Mongolian spots that can be confused with inflicted injury[8] (Figure 30-1). Differentiating dermal melanosis from bruising can be accomplished by observing the lesion over time. In contrast to dermal melanosis ("Mongolian spots"), bruises are often tender to palpation with an associated reddened, inflammatory appearance that fades over the course of weeks.[3,9] Figure 30-2 illustrates a child who has inflicted linear lesions over an area of dermal melanosis.

DERMATOLOGICAL CONDITIONS

Disorders of Pigmentation

Nevus of Ota/nevus of Ito. Nevus of Ota (nevus fuscoceruleus ophthalmomaxillaris) is a blue-gray or brown irregular, often spotted skin discoloration located on the face in the distribution of the first and second branches of the trigeminal nerve (i.e., the forehead, periorbital, temple, and cheek regions). It is usually unilateral but in 5% of cases is bilateral.[10] The sclera on the affected side might also have a bluish discoloration. Nevus of Ito (nevus fuscoceruleus acromiodeltoideus) differs from nevus of Ota in its distribution that is confined to the neck, shoulder, and proximal arm regions. Nevus of Ota and nevus of Ito each can be seen in isolation or together. Nevus of Ota and nevus of Ito persist into adulthood and sometimes darken in appearance. They can be associated with vascular malformations, Sturge-Weber syndrome, and Klippel-Trenaunay syndrome.[10]

Incontinentia pigmenti (IP). Ciarallo et al[11] reported two cases of IP simulating child abuse. IP is a rare multisystem X-linked disorder with dermatological, dental, neurological, and ophthalmological abnormalities. The patterned cutaneous findings can mimic physical abuse. Cutaneous findings include vesicles in a linear configuration with underlying erythema and at times purpuric appearing that later become linear hyperpigmented lesions along the lines of Blaschko. Diagnosis is made by the constellation of clinical findings and family history; skin biopsy, however, confirms the diagnosis.[10] Since patients with IP can also have neurological and ophthalmological manifestations of the disease, IP can also be confused with inflicted head injury. Differences in presentation should help distinguish between the two. The characteristic skin lesions associated with IP typically occur before the ocular and neurological manifestations and are seen in 90% of patients at 2 weeks of life and in 96% by 6 weeks of life.[10] Seizures are the most common neurological manifestation and can also be associated with microvascular hemorrhagic infarcts and developmental delay.[10] Eye findings include retinal revascularization or detachment, strabismus, cataracts, blindness, and optic nerve atrophy.[10]

Urticaria pigmentosa (UP). Mastocytosis is a group of disorders related to mast cell proliferation that can be limited to the skin or have systemic involvement. UP is the most common form of mastocytosis. The rash associated with UP is characterized by small tan-brown macules and papules. The typical distribution of the rash is on the extremities and

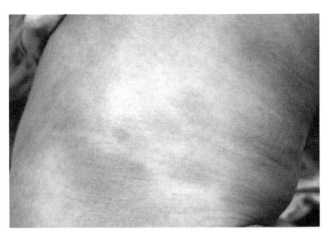

FIGURE 30-1 Mongolian spots on an infant.

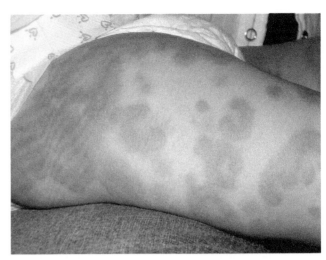

FIGURE 30-3 Classic annular lesions on a child with erythema multiforme.

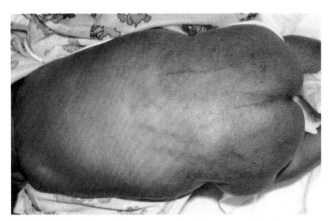

FIGURE 30-2 Inflicted linear pattern bruising on a child with extensive Mongolian spots.

trunk with sparing of the palms and soles. Darier sign (erythema and urticaria with pressure or friction of affected skin) is a common finding in the disorder.[9] The lesions can appear yellow or purple and resemble bruising that can be confused with child abuse.[12,13]

Hypersensitivity Syndromes

Erythema multiforme (EM). EM has previously been confused with child abuse.[14] The initial presentation of EM is the acute onset of symmetric round erythematous plaques that resemble bruises. As the rash evolves, the lesions darken and the annular target type of lesions become apparent (Figure 30-3). EM is a self-limited process thought to be related to infectious agents such as *Mycoplasma* or herpes simplex virus or to a hypersensitivity to medications, particularly penicillins and sulfonamides.[10]

Allergic contact dermatitis. Allergic contact dermatitis is a delayed hypersensitivity reaction resulting from contact with an allergen. Acutely, a well-circumscribed lesion appears that can be erythematous and pruritic. The lesions are typically in the distribution of the allergen; however, due to the patternlike or linear distributions, allergic contact dermatitis can be confused with inflicted injury.

Panniculitis. Panniculitis is a group of skin disorders involving the subcutaneous fat. Cold panniculitis and traumatic fat

necrosis both can resemble bruises. In cold panniculitis erythematous lesions appear hours to days after the exposure to a cold substance and are classically seen on the cheeks of toddlers after eating popsicles. Residual hyperpigmentation can remain for weeks to months after the exposure.[10] Traumatic panniculitis, also known as traumatic fat necrosis, is characterized by hard, inflamed nodules following injury.[10]

Erythema nodosum. Erythema nodosum is a subgroup of the panniculitis type of disorders and is a hypersensitivity reaction distinguished by painful erythematous subcutaneous nodules that as they evolve and darken resemble bruises that can be confused with abusive injury.[2] The lesions typically involve the anterior shins but can be found anywhere on the body containing subcutaneous fat.[10]

Perniosis. Perniosis (chilblains) is described as painful, erythematous, swollen nodules on the fingers or toes occurring 12 to 24 hours after exposure to cold. Localized cyanosis and ulceration can also be present. It is an amplified reaction to cold and is thought to be associated with impaired temperature regulation.[3,10] Because of the erythema and swelling, these lesions can be confused with bruising.

Angioedema. The swelling associated with angioedema can resemble traumatic injury. Thakur et al[15] described an 18-month-old child with recurrent isolated angioedema of the face and scalp without associated urticaria or respiratory compromise. The child had diffuse recurrent noninflammatory scalp swelling and no explanation, which prompted a concern of child abuse.

Vasculitic Disorders

Henoch-Schönlein purpura (HSP). HSP (anaphylactoid purpura) is a small-vessel vasculitis seen in children. The classic clinical manifestations are nonthrombocytopenic palpable purpura, gastrointestinal symptoms, arthritis/arthralgias, and renal disease. The rash is typically symmetric and classically occurs on the bilateral lower extremities and buttocks (dependent areas); however, it can be located anywhere including the face and ears. The initial rash is erythematous macular lesions and urticarial wheals. Over time the rash evolves into a more ecchymotic appearance with petechiae and palpable purpura that has been confused with child abuse.[10,16,17]

Hypersensitivity vasculitis. Palpable purpura and/or petechiae, classically of the lower extremities and dependent areas, characterize the cutaneous findings in hypersensitivity vasculitis. The lesions appear ecchymotic and can be confused with bruising. Waskeritz et al[18] described a child with hypersensitivity vasculitis who had unexplained ecchymotic lesions and purpura initially thought to be abusive injury.

Connective Tissue Disorders

Ehlers-Danlos syndrome (EDS). EDS is an inherited connective tissue disorder characterized by joint hypermobility and skin hyperelasticity. Due to the defects in collagen, patients with EDS can have extensive cutaneous injury with gaping ("fish-mouth") wounds after even mild trauma resulting in the classical reported "cigarette paper" scar.[10] Easy bruising, hematomas, frequent lacerations, poor wound healing, and numerous healed scars often prompt the suspicion of child abuse in these patients.[1,19,20]

Striae distensae. Physiological striae ("stretch marks" or atrophic striae) in adolescents have been confused with linear pattern bruising or scars associated with inflicted injury.[21,22] Striae are common during adolescence and are often related to a recent history of rapid linear growth, obesity, pregnancy, or steroid use. Common sites include the thighs, lower abdomen, breasts, lumbar area, and buttocks. Straie initially appear as thin, pink-red linear marks and have raised inflamed appearing edges. Eventually the lesions fade, becoming flat white atrophic scars.[10]

Hematologic Conditions

Coagulation disorders. Disorders of coagulation can be seen with bruising and/or bleeding. Children with bleeding disorders can have pattern injury from routine care of the child (i.e., fingertip marks from picking up a child). It is important to keep in mind a diagnosis of a bleeding disorder does not exclude child abuse, and these children are at a greater risk for significant bleeding from injury.[23]

Hemophilia. Hemophilia A and hemophilia B are common inherited bleeding disorders that have been previously misdiagnosed as nonaccidental trauma.[2,23-26] Hemophilia A and B are X-linked recessive disorders. Clinical manifestations of hemophilia vary in severity and include excessive bleeding with procedures such as circumcision, bleeding into the joints after trauma, and easy bruising. Patients with hemophilia can have gastrointestinal bleeding, mucosal bleeding, and muscle bleeding after even mild trauma. Laboratory evaluation is significant for a prolonged PTT. Further evaluation demonstrates a decreased factor VIII level (hemophilia A) or factor IX level (hemophilia B).

Platelet disorders. Platelet disorders clinically present as bruises, petechiae, or purpura, all of which are findings that can also be seen in nonaccidental trauma. Platelet disorders can be congenital or acquired and can affect platelet production, destruction, or function. Some medications and viral infections can cause platelet disorders and should be explored in the history. Idiopathic thrombocytopenic purpura (ITP) is an acquired platelet disorder characterized by thrombocytopenia. The most common clinical presentation is petechiae, bruising, bleeding, and/or purpura. Several cases have been published in which children with ITP were initially diagnosed child abuse.[2,24]

Von Willebrand disease (VWD). VWD is the most common inherited bleeding disorder. Symptoms and disease severity can be quite variable, and the condition often goes undiagnosed. Common important clues in the history include history of bleeding with circumcision, easy bruising, nosebleeds, gingival bleeding with routine dental hygiene, excessive menstrual bleeding, and prolonged bleeding after trauma. Due to the predisposition to bleeding and bruising, children with VWD can mistakenly be diagnosed with child abuse.[27]

Vitamin K deficiency. Vitamin K deficiency is seen in several medical conditions and can be associated with a predisposition to bruising and bleeding. Antibiotic use has been related to vitamin K deficiency through alterations in normal intestinal flora and activation in the liver. In addition, vitamin K deficiency can also be related to accidental ingestion of warfarin (i.e., rodenticides).[4] Currently marketed consumer rodenticides contain long-acting anticoagulants that in small amounts are unlikely to cause a coagulopathy. In addition, to protect children from accidental exposures, in 2008 the Environmental Protection Agency (EPA) enacted restrictions for the packaging and distribution of consumer-sized rodenticides, including prohibiting the use of loose bait forms (i.e., pellets) and prohibiting the use of second-generation rodenticides (www.epa.gov). Hemorrhagic disease of the newborn occurs when insufficient amounts of vitamin K are transferred from the mother to the fetus. At birth newborns require supplemental Vitamin K to assist in normal hemostasis and to prevent hemorrhagic disease of the newborn. Infants, particularly those born outside of the hospital, might not have been given prophylactic vitamin K intramuscularly and subsequently have unexplained bleeding, intracranial hemorrhage, and/or bruising.[2,28-30] Coagulation profile abnormalities associated with vitamin K deficiency are a prolongation of both the PT and PTT with a normal platelet count.

Vitamin K deficiency can also be caused by cystic fibrosis (CF). Carpentieri et al[31] presented a case of a child initially diagnosed with neglect, malnutrition, and vitamin K deficiency with associated bruising and petechiae who was found to have cystic fibrosis. CF is associated with pancreatic insufficiency and/or liver disease therefore making patients with CF at risk for fat soluble vitamin deficiencies (vitamins A, D, E, and K). Chronic antibiotic use can also be an additional factor contributing to vitamin K deficiency in this population. Figures 30-4 and 30-5 show an infant who had bruising who was diagnosed with cystic fibrosis.

Hemolytic uremic syndrome (HUS). HUS is characterized by hemolytic anemia, thrombocytopenia, and acute renal compromise. Similar to other disorders of coagulation with thrombocytopenia, HUS can cause easy bruising and petechial rashes.

Other coagulation disorders. Patients with meningitis and associated disseminated intravascular coagulation (DIC) have been reported to be victims of nonaccidental trauma. Kirshner[32] published a case report of two children with meningitis and DIC who were initially diagnosed with head injuries and bruises due to physical abuse. In this same

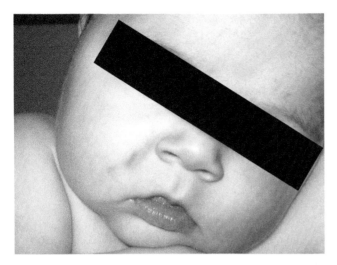

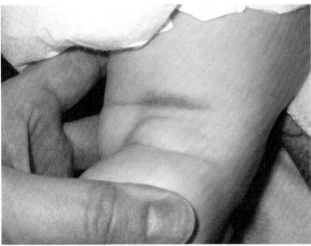

FIGURES 30-4 AND 30–5 Bruising on an infant with cystic fibrosis and associated vitamin K deficiency.

report, Kirshner described a case of purpura fulminans in a child who had severe bruising resembling abusive injury.

Oncological Disorders

Children with undiagnosed oncological conditions can have findings suggestive of nonaccidental injury. For example, children with neuroblastoma can have bilateral eye bruising, classically known as "raccoon eyes." This finding is due to metastasis to the periorbital bones; however, it can be confused with traumatic injury such as basilar skull fractures or direct trauma.[9] Gumus[33] described a case of a 10-month-old female who initially had periorbital swelling and bruising suspected to be child abuse, but when a laboratory investigation revealed significant anemia, hematology was consulted and the diagnosis of neuroblastoma was made. In addition, children with oncological disorders can have cutaneous injury more extensive than expected for the mechanism.[4,34] Bays et al[4] described a case of a child with undiagnosed acute leukemia with extensive buttock bruising after being spanked with a spoon.

Cultural Practices

Coining/spooning. Coining (*cao gio, cheut sah,* "scratch the wind") is a Southeast Asian cultural practice that is performed to improve circulation (get rid of the "bad winds") and to relieve common symptoms including fever, headache, flu, cold symptoms, and seizures.[2] In coining, the affected area is first rubbed with warm medicated oil. A coin is used to scratch the skin's surface in a symmetrical pattern with firm downward linear strokes until ecchymotic lesions appear in the distribution of the skin scratching.[35] Similar to coining, spooning is a cultural practice in which the area is prepped with water and then pinched or massaged. A porcelain spoon is then used to scratch the skin in a linear configuration.[36] The linear petechial or purpuric rashes produced by coining and spooning can be mistaken for physical abuse injury.[2,37-40] The lesions generally resolve in 1 to 2 weeks, but hyperpigmentation can persist.[41] Typically, coining and spooning are not painful and have minimal associated side effects.[42] Transient microscopic hematuria has been described after coining.[43] In addition, cultural practices such as coining or cupping can mask the diagnosis of an underlying bleeding diathesis.[44]

Cupping. Cupping is a technique used by different cultural groups including Russians, Asians, and Mexicans. Cupping is performed to relieve common ailments such as fever, pain, abscesses, and congestion and is believed to increase circulation and release bad toxins.[35,42] Cupping is performed using heated cups to create a vacuum on the skin. An alcohol saturated cotton ball can be used to help create the vacuum while heating the cup. The cup is then immediately placed on the skin in a distribution-related to the symptoms. Two forms of cupping exist: dry and wet. Dry cupping is as described above with the cups being placed on intact skin. In wet cupping, the skin is first prepared by making small cuts on the skin producing bleeding (scarification)[42]. In both types, a vacuum is created as the cup cools, thus producing the characteristic ecchymotic lesions. The circular pattern of bruising and petechiae caused by the cupping has been confused with physical abuse.[43] Less commonly a burn can result and also can be confused with physical abuse.

Other Conditions

Photodermatitis. Phytophotodermatitis is a phototoxic inflammatory skin reaction that occurs when psoralen-containing products (furocoumarin compounds) react with the skin after exposure to UVA light. Psoralen is commonly found in lemon, lime, fig, parsnip, carrot, dill, celery, clover, and buttercup plants.[10] Erythema and blistering can be the initial presentation followed by hyperpigmentation. The unique distribution of the rash, often in a linear configuration or resembling fingerprints/handprints, has been confused with child abuse.[45-48] Berloque dermatitis is another type of photodermatitis and occurs with perfume products containing bergamot (or psoralen). Gruson et al[49] described a case of a 9-year-old female with a blistering linear rash initially diagnosed as child abuse. It was not until further questioning regarding sun exposure and perfume application that the diagnosis was made. It is important to realize that a history to account for the cutaneous findings might be absent until questioned further about plant, perfume, or chemical contact and sun exposure.

Topical application of chemicals. Topical applications of medications or chemicals have caused cutaneous findings mistaken for child abuse. Zurbuchen et al[50] described a case of a child with unexplained skin necrosis after contact with calcium chloride crystals used to melt ice.

Ink/dye staining. Ink, food coloring, dyes, or paint on the skin have been confused with bruising.[2,4,51-53] Clothing dyes are a common cause of bluish discoloration confused with bruising. Children can present for evaluation of bruising with a history of bluish discoloration that persists after bathing. Typically the distribution of the lesions corresponds to contact with clothing.[4] Further questioning frequently reveals a history of the child wearing blue or black denim and/or new or unwashed clothing. Soap and water are often not effective to remove the staining; however, alcohol is usually effective in removing the stains and confirming the diagnosis.[4,54] Povidone iodine stains can also mimic bruises.

Maculae ceruleae. Maculae ceruleae is a skin finding associated with pediculosis pubis infestation. Maculae ceruleae are blue-gray lesions typically found on the thighs or abdomen and are the result of pubic lice bites. When pubic lice bite the skin, they deposit hemosiderin in the deep dermis creating the blue-gray discoloration.[10]

Valsalva effect. Bruising on or around the eyes can be confused with trauma. Mokrohisky et al[55] reported a case of bilateral eye bruising and subconjunctival hemorrhage secondary to the Valsalva effect. The child had a history of urethral stricture and increased straining during voiding before the development of eye bruising and subconjunctival hemorrhage.[55]

CONDITIONS CONFUSED WITH BURNS

Dermatological Conditions

Eczema. Eczema or atopic dermatitis is a chronic inflammatory skin condition that affects infants and children. Eczema in infants has red, scaly, and crusted lesions on the extensor surfaces, cheeks, or scalp. Older children with eczema can have lesions that have serous exudates and crusting. Usually the distribution involves the flexural distribution, especially of the antecubital and popliteal areas, the wrists, ankles, and neck. But, in severe cases any body area can be affected[10] (Figure 30-6).

Epidermolysis bullosa (EB). EB is a disease that manifests as blister or bullae formation occurring with little or no trauma, and in some forms heals with extensive scarring. The bullae can be quite large and quite extensive. The severe forms often start at birth.[10] Although the diagnosis is usually known, there have been several case reports of children with EB who are reported with concerns of severe scalding burns.[4]

Diaper dermatitis from ingested irritants. Irritant diaper dermatitis typically occurs on the areas of the skin that are in direct contact with the diaper and spare the skin not in direct contact with the diaper. Certain diaper irritations have a classic triangular distribution that spares the perianal area. Blistering and skin sloughing can occur but also can be delayed. Since 1997, over-the-counter laxatives contain senna, which is a plant-based cathartic.[56] When ingested senna is held in the diapers over time, severe skin burns can

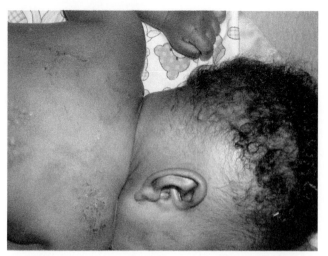

FIGURE 30-6 Eczema on the back and shoulders of an infant.

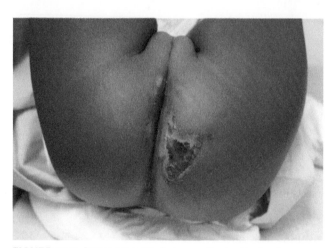

FIGURE 30-7 Diaper dermatitis from over-the-counter laxative use.

occur. The exact mechanism of the severe skin reaction from contact with senna is not known. Other agents in laxatives such as citric acid can also cause irritant diaper dermatitis (Figure 30-7). Because of the often sharp borders (due to the diaper area) and blistering, irritant diaper dermatitis can be confused with inflicted immersion burns.[56]

Contact dermatitis. Allergic or irritant contact dermatitis causes inflammation of the skin as a result of direct contact between a substance and the surface of the skin. The inflammation of the skin can be immediate or delayed. Common irritants in children include nickel and henna tattoos. Since these will leave well-demarcated and patterned lesions that are erythematous and often blistered, it is possible to mistake them for inflicted patterned burns.[9]

Phytophotodermatitis: See Conditions Confused with Bruising section.

Infections

Impetigo. Impetigo is a superficial bacterial infection of the skin that is most commonly caused by strains of staphylococci or streptococci. Nonbullous impetigo consists of papules that progress to pustules that enlarge and break down to form a thick, adherent honey-colored crust.[57]

Nonbullous impetigo lesions can be confused with a cigarette burn, but there are some ways to differentiate the two entities. For example, impetigo involves only the superficial layers of the skin; the lesions have more crusting and heal without scarring. In contrast, cigarette burns involve deeper layers of the skin and heal with scarring. Being able to differentiate the two lesions, however, can be difficult early on.[2,4]

Ecthyma. Ecthyma is an ulcerated skin infection that is most commonly caused by GABHS (group A beta hemolytic streptococcal infections). Similar to impetigo, the lesions can form after minor skin trauma or infected insect bites, but the lesions are deeper than those seen in impetigo. Initially, the lesions resemble pustules with an erythematous base and overlying crusting and are painful. If occurring in groups, ecthyma can be confused with inflicted cigarette burns.[10]

Ringworm. Ringworm or tinea corporis is a dermatophyte infection of the body. Tinea corporis begins as a circular or oval erythematous scaling patch. The border will retain its red color and is usually slightly raised. The result is a lesion-shaped like a ring, hence the name "ringworm.[10]" Because of the scaling patch, the erythema, and the well-demarcated shape of the lesion, these can be confused with a pattern burn.

Cultural Practices

Cupping. See Conditions Confused with Bruising section.

Moxibustion. Moxibustion is another folk remedy used for abdominal pain, colds, fever, and even some behavioral concerns such as temper tantrums. The moxa herb or mugwort herb is ground and then used indirectly with acupuncture needles, or sometimes directly on a patient's skin. There are two types of moxibustion: direct and indirect. In direct moxibustion, a small amount of moxa is placed on top of an acupuncture point and burned. This type of moxibustion can lead to blistering and scarring. The blisters and scars can be mistaken for child abuse.[4]

Complementary and alternative therapies. Herbal therapies are used in some cultures. In the hot-cold balance disease concept, pain is cold therefore should be treated with heat. Garlic is an herbal remedy and is prescribed by naturopathic physicians for a variety of medical purposes. There are a handful of published reports of garlic burns that resulted from applying garlic to the skin.[4] It is important to ask parents and caregivers about the use of any folk remedies, herbal medicines, or other treatments.

Accidental Burns

Car seat burns. Accidental burns from car seat belts and buckles can be confused with abusive burns. The metal and plastic buckles and harnesses can reach high temperatures in a car left in hot climates. As the straps fit snug, infants and small children might not be able to maneuver away from the heat source. The burns can occur on the thighs or torso and can have a patterned appearance[58] (Figure 30-8).

Liquids. Young children can accidentally pull hot liquids off of stove surfaces or countertops and scald themselves. The head/neck, upper torso, and arms tend to be affected in accidental scald burns. Accidental burns tend to have irregular borders and depths, are asymmetric, rarely

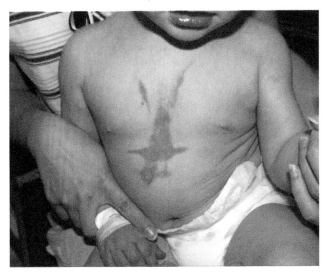

FIGURE 30-8 Car seat pattern burn.

circumferential, and the skin becomes less affected as the liquid flows down the body.[59] Oil or grease burns are usually more severe because the more viscous substance adheres more to the body and holds in the heat.

Contact. Children can accidentally come in contact with hot items in the home. Common items include radiators (particularly steam radiators), clothing irons, and curling irons. Young children can also come in contact with a lit cigarette. Usually, pattern makings are not apparent, but in some cases such as radiators, patterns can be seen. As with all cases, a careful history is important.

Chemical Burns

Hair relaxers and dye. Hair straightening solutions can contain lye or other chemicals. "Lye" relaxers contain sodium hydroxide, which has a pH of 12-14. "No-lye" relaxers are formulated with guanidine hydroxide. Both lye and no-lye relaxers can cause severe burns to the scalp and face when used to straighten hair in children or when children accidently come in contact with them in the household.[60,61] Hair dye has been reported as causing burns in adults. If children accidentally come in contact with hair dye products, burns to the hands face and scalp can occur. A history of product use should be obtained.[60,61]

Other household chemicals. Other chemicals such as over-the-counter analgesic creams can cause burns if applied to a child's skin or if a child accidentally comes in contact with a product.[4] A history of product use or of the presence of such creams and balms in the house should be sought. Also the history of folk practices such as treating "cold" diseases with "hot" remedies should be obtained.

Toxic substances. Millipedes can emit a noxious substance, which consists of a derivative of quinines and can result in skin irritation. The skin appears discolored, but blistering and sloughing of the skin can also occur.[62,63] Because the noxious secretions come from every segment of the millipede, the lesions on the skin are linear or curvilinear (the shape of the insect) and can resemble inflicted burns from an implement such as a hairdryer. These findings have been mistaken for inflicted burns.[63]

CONCLUSION

The number of substantiated cases of physical abuse remains high, and all suspected cases of child abuse must be reported. However, clinicians should also be aware of conditions that can be confused with child abuse. A complete and thorough history and physical examination are necessary. Sometimes laboratory evaluation and consultation with other specialists are needed. Future research should be directed at discerning conditions that can be confused with child abuse.

References

1. Wardinsky TD: Genetic and congenital defect conditions that mimic child abuse. *J Fam Pract* 1995;41:377-383.
2. Wheeler DM, Hobbs CJ: Mistakes in diagnosing non-accidental injury: 10 years' experience. *Br Med J* 1988;396:1233-1236.
3. Jenny C: Cutaneous manifestations of child abuse. *In*: Reece RM, Ludwig S (eds): *Child Abuse Medical Diagnosis and Management*, ed 2, Lippincott Williams & Wilkins, Philadelphia, 2001, pp 23-45.
4. Bays J: Conditions mistaken for child physical abuse. *In*: Reece RM, Ludwig S (eds): *Child Abuse Medical Diagnosis and Management*, ed 2, Lippincott Williams & Wilkins, Philadelphia, 2001, pp 177-206.
5. Asnes RS: Buttock bruises–mongolian spot. *Pediatrics* 1984;74:321.
6. Dungy CI: Mongolian spots, day care centers, and child abuse. *Pediatrics* 1982;69:672.
7. Leung AKC: Extensive mongolian spots with involvement of the scalp. *Pediatr Dermatol* 1999;16:371-372.
8. Leung AKC, Robson WLM: Superimposed mongolian spots. *Pediatr Dermatol* 2008;25:233-235.
9. AlJasser M, Al-Khenaizan S: Cutaneous mimickers of child abuse: a primer for pediatricians. *Eur J Pediatr* 2008;167:1221-1230.
10. Paller AS, Mancini AJ (eds): *Hurwitz clinical pediatric dermatology. A textbook of skin disorders of childhood and adolescence*, ed 3, Elsevier, Philadelphia, 2006.
11. Ciarallo L, Paller AS: Two cases of incontinentia pigmenti simulating child abuse. *Pediatrics* 1997;100:e6.
12. Hannaford R, Rogers M: Presentation of cutaneous mastocytosis in 173 children. *Australas J Dermatol* 2001;42:15-21.
13. Gordon EM, Bernat JR, Ramos-Caro FA: Urticaria pigmentosa mistaken for child abuse. *Pediatr Dermatol* 1998;15:484-485 (letter).
14. Adler R, Kane-Nussen B: Erythema multiforme: confusion with child battering syndrome. *Pediatrics* 1983;72:718-720.
15. Thakur BK, Kaplan AP: Recurrent "unexplained" scalp swelling in an eighteen-month old child: an atypical presentation of angioedema causing confusion with child abuse. *J Pediatr* 1996;129:163-165.
16. Brown J, Melinkovich P: Henoch-Schönlein purpura misdiagnosed as suspected child abuse: a case report and literature review. *JAMA* 1986;256:617-618.
17. Daly KC, Siegel RM: Henoch-Schönlein purpura in a child at risk of abuse. *Arch Pediatr Adolesc Med* 1998;152:96-98.
18. Waskerwitz S, Christoffel KK, Hauger S: Hypersensitivity vasculitis presenting as suspected child abuse: case report and literature review. *Pediatrics* 1981;67:283-284.
19. Owen SM, Durst RD: Ehlers-Danlos syndrome simulating child abuse. *Arch Dermatol* 1984;120:97-101.
20. McNamara JJ, Baler R, Lynch E: Ehlers-Danlos syndrome reported as child abuse. *Clin Pediatr* 1985;24:317.
21. Heller D: Lumbar physiological striae in adolescence suspected to be non-accidental injury. *Br Med J* 1995;311:738.
22. Cohen HA, Matalon A, Mezger A, et al: Striae in adolescents mistaken for physical abuse. *J Fam Pract* 1997;45:84-85.
23. Thomas AE: The bleeding child; is it NAI? *Arch Dis Child* 2004;89:1163-1167.
24. Harley JR: Disorders of coagulation misdiagnosed as nonaccidental bruising. *Pediatr Emerg Care* 1997;13:347-349.
25. Johnson CF, Coury DL: Bruising and hemophilia: accident or child abuse? *Child Abuse Negl* 1988;12:409-415.
26. Pinto FC, Porro FF, Suganuma L, et al: Hemophilia and child abuse as possible causes of epidural hematoma. *Arq Neuropsiquiatr* 2003;61:1023-1025.
27. O'Hare AE, Eden OB: Bleeding disorders and non-accidental injury. *Arch Dis Child* 1987;62:1025-1029.
28. Behrmann BA, Chan W, Finer NN: Resurgency of hemorrhagic disease of the newborn: a report of three cases. *CMAJ* 1985;133:884-886.
29. Brousseau TJ, Kissoon N, McIntosh B: Vitamin K deficiency mimicking child abuse. *J Emerg Med* 2005;29:283-288.
30. Wetzel RC, Slater AJ, Dover GJ: Fatal intramuscular bleeding misdiagnosed as suspected nonaccidental injury. *Pediatrics* 1995;95:771-773.
31. Carpentieri U, Gustavson LP, Haggard ME: Misdiagnosis of neglect in a child with bleeding disorder and cystic fibrosis. *South Med J* 1978;71:854-855.
32. Kirschner RH, Stein RJ: The mistaken diagnosis of child abuse. A form of medical abuse? *Am J Dis Child* 1985;139:873-875.
33. Gumus K: A child with raccoon eyes masquerading as trauma. *Int Ophthalmol* 2007;27:379-381.
34. McClain JL, Clark MA, Sandusky GE: Undiagnosed, untreated acute lymphoblastic leukemia presenting as suspected child abuse. *J Forensic Sci* 1990;35:735-739.
35. Look KM, Look RM: Skin scraping, cupping, and moxibustion that may mimic physical abuse. *J Forensic Sci* 1997;42:103-105.
36. Leung AKC: *Ecchymoses from spoon scratching*, Consultant Live (website): http://www.consultantlive.com/display/article/10162/42529. Accessed April 23, 2009.
37. Gellis SS, Feingold M: Cao-gio (pseudobattering in Vietnamese children). *Am J Dis Child* 1976;130:857-858.
38. Leung AK: Ecchymoses from spoon scratching simulating child abuse. *Clin Pediatr (Phila)* 1986;25:98.
39. Rosenblat H, Hong P: Coin rolling misdiagnosed as child abuse. *CMAJ* 1989;140:417-418.
40. Yeatman GW, Shaw C, Barlow MJ, et al: Pseudobattering in Vietnamese children. *Pediatrics* 1976;58:616-617.
41. Crutchfield CE, Bisig TJ: Coining. *N Engl J Med* 1995;332:1552.
42. Hansen KK, Frasier LD: Child abuse or mimic? *Consult Pediatricians* 2002;99-101.
43. Longmire AW, Broom LA: Vietnamese coin rubbing. *Ann Emerg Med* 1987;16:602.
44. Golden SM, Duster MC: Hazards of misdiagnosis due to Vietnamese folk medicine. *Clin Pediatr* 1977;16:949-950.
45. Coffman K, Boyce WT, Hansen RC: Phytophotodermatitis simulating child abuse. *Am J Dis Child* 1985;139:239-240.
46. Dannaker CJ, Glover RA, Goltz RW: Phytophotodermatitis: a mystery case report. *Clin Pediatr* 1988;27:289-290.
47. Goskowicz MO, Friedlander SF, Eichenfield LF: Endemic "lime" disease: phytophotodermatitis in San Diego county. *Pediatr* 1994;93:828-830.
48. Mehta AJ, Statham BN: Phytophotodermatitis mimicking non-accidental injury or self-harm. *Eur J Pediatr* 2007;166:751-752.
49. Gruson LM, Chang MW: Berloque dermatitis mimicking child abuse. *Arch Pediatr Adolesc Med* 2002;156:1091-1093.
50. Zurbuchen P, Lecoultre C, Calza A, et al: Cutaneous necrosis after contact with calcium chloride: a mistaken diagnosis of child abuse. *Pediatrics* 1996;97:257-258.
51. Lanter RR, Ros SP: Blue jean thighs. *Pediatrics* 1999;88:417.
52. Leiferman KM, Gleich GJ: The case of the blue boy. *Pediatr Dermatol* 1991;8:354.
53. Hansen KK: Folk remedies and child abuse: a review with emphasis on caida de mollera and its relationship to shaken baby syndrome. *Child Abuse Negl* 1998;2:117-127.
54. Harris CR, Mariano C: Blue jean hands syndrome. *Ann Emerg Med* 1984;13:67.
55. Mokrohisky ST, Kesselman NE: Valsalva effect may mimic child abuse. *Pediatrics* 1991;88:420.
56. Leventhal JM, Griffin D, Duncan KO, et al: Laxative-induced dermatitis of the buttocks incorrectly suspected to be abusive burns. *Pediatrics* 2001;107:178-179.
57. Darmstadt GL, Lane AT: Impetigo: an overview. *Pediatr Dermatol* 1994;11:293.
58. Schmitt BD, Gray JD, Britton HL: Car seat burns in infants: avoiding confusion with inflicted burns. *Pediatrics* 1978;62:607-609.
59. Driego DA: Kitchen scalds and thermal burns in children five years and younger. *Pediatrics* 2005;115:10-16.

60. Boucher J, Raglon B, Valdez S, et al: Possible role of chemical hair care products in 10 patients with face, scalp, ear, back, neck and extremity burns. *Burns* 1990;16:146-147.

61. Rauch DA: Hair relaxer misuse: don't relax. *Pediatrics* 2000;105: 1154-1155.

62. Dar NR, Raza N, Rehman SB: Millipede burn at an unusual site mimicking child abuse in an 8-year-old girl. *Clin Pediatr* 2008; 47:490.

63. Shpall S, Frieden I: Mahogany discoloration of the skin due to the defensive secretion of a millipede. *Pediatr Dermatol* 1991;8:25-27.

31

BONE HEALTH AND DEVELOPMENT

Berkeley L. Bennett, MD, MS, and Mary Clyde Pierce, MD

This chapter will focus on bone health and factors such as poor nutrition, disease states, illnesses, and genetic abnormalities that can adversely affect the ability of bone to resist fracture. A brief overview of bone anatomy, physiology, and imaging techniques for evaluating bone quality are also reviewed.

ANATOMY AND BONE DEVELOPMENT

The skeletal system consists of the supporting tissues of the body and includes bone tissue and cartilage. Cartilage is made of cells (chondrocytes) that produce the intercellular matrix containing collagen fibrils. The fibrils are embedded in ground substance, which consists of protein-polysaccharide compounds. Cartilage covers the ends of bones where joint articulation and cushioning are needed; in children cartilage also comprises the growth plates of long bones and sutures of the flat bones of the skull to allow for growth and development. Cartilage is not vascularized.[1]

Bone tissue consists of bone cells and a mineralized intercellular matrix, which also contains ground substance and collagenous fibers. Bone tissue is formed, maintained, modeled, and remodeled by specific bone cells. Bone tissue not only provides critical structural and mechanical support, but also serves as the major body reservoir for calcium, fulfilling a critical physiological need. Osteoblasts (bone forming cells) produce and secrete both collagenous and noncollagenous proteins, producing an organic matrix that is then mineralized. Bone tissue is maintained by the osteocytes, which also in part control bone modeling and remodeling. Osteoclasts (bone resorbing cells) play a central role in new bone formation, bone growth, and calcium homeostasis. Osteoclasts have hormonal receptors related to calcium regulation.[2]

Two different types of bone tissue exist: cancellous (spongy, trabecular) and cortical (compact, dense) bone. Each has unique structural and material properties and therefore has a unique biomechanical response to force application and loading (see Chapter 35). These differences reflect their specific function in providing structural and physiological support. Cancellous bone tissue is characterized by osteocytes, lacunae (spaces that contain the osteocytes), and a solidified matrix. The microstructure of cancellous bone is arranged into spicules or trabecula, resulting in porous tissue filled with marrow. Cortical bone is composed of structural units identified as Haversian systems or osteons. Haversian systems contain a central blood vessel surrounded by layers of mineralized bone (lamella) and lacunae containing bone cells. These systems are connected by cement lines that are thought to help dissipate injury forces.[3-5]

The bony structure in the developing child differs significantly from the adult skeletal system to allow for growth and development. Long bones in children have a hollow, marrow-filled shaft that is cylindrical. This region is termed the diaphysis and the predominant tissue is cortical bone. The shaft flares as it approaches the articular surfaces and transitions into the metaphyseal regions of bone; the ends of bone are termed the epiphyseal regions. Trabecular bone is predominant in the metaphyseal and epiphyseal regions of long bones at the flared ends, next to cartilage. It is trabecular bone that serves as a calcium reservoir for meeting physiological needs.[6] In the developing child, a growth plate is present between the epiphyseal and metaphyseal regions and is termed the physis. This is the site of ossification and allows for cell hypertrophy and growth, and transformation of cartilage to bone (primary spongiosa).

Primary spongiosa is transformed into secondary spongiosa as the bone matrix is laid down and matures;[5] and the biomechanical properties change accordingly. Primary spongiosa has better energy absorbing capacity than the mineralized secondary spongiosa, which is stiffer and more resistant to fatigue failure. The flat bones of the skull are composed of trabecular bone between an inner and outer layer of cortical bone. In children these bones are connected by fibrous sutures that allow for growth and development. They can also serve to dissipate and absorb energy during traumatic events.

A complex and not fully elucidated process occurs at the cellular level to allow for calcium regulation and bone growth and maintenance. Key factors to bone development, bone health, and calcium homeostasis are discussed in separate sections later and include hormonal regulation, calcium and phosphorus regulation, and vitamin D metabolism. In addition to the developmental stage of the child, other factors and conditions also play a key role in bone status and health, such as genetic disorders that affect collagen production, mineral and electrolyte regulation, prenatal and birth history, chronic illness, neuromuscular disorders, exposure to environmental toxins such as lead, nutritional status, diet, and amount of activity and exercise. Specific conditions that can lead to decreased bone strength and ability to resist fracture are discussed later in this chapter.

FACTORS AFFECTING BONE STRENGTH

Fracture patterns in infants and children are a reflection of each child's unique and specific tissue characteristics and stage of development, and loading condition. Important determinants of bone strength and the ability to resist fracture are bone geometry and material properties. Specifically, it is both bone size and bone mineral distribution that affect the ability of a bone to resist fracture.[7] Bone mineral content is an important factor affecting the material properties of bone. Both macro and micro bone structure are also a key factor in ultimate bone strength. The overall structure is related to gestational age and developmental maturation. The microstructure is influenced by the degree of mineralization and whether bone matrix is laid down in a normal progression.

The absence or disruption of the normal mineralization process leads to thinner trabeculae and a thinned cortex, which ultimately affects the ability of bone to resist fracture. Both the structural and material properties are affected by poor mineralization. Mineralization can be adversely affected by poor nutrition, poor stores, prematurity, and vitamin D stores or use abnormalities. In cases where mineralization cannot occur due to matrix abnormalities, osteomalacia occurs, resulting in softer than normal bones.[7]

NONINVASIVE MEASURES OF BONE STRENGTH

Several modalities currently exist for evaluating bone mass and quality but important limitations still exist in correlating data to fracture risk and defining a fracture threshold in children. This is due in part to the difficulty in accurately measuring bone mass in the growing child and the influence of other factors in determining bone strength that are not measured through standard imaging techniques.[7] The most common modalities used for bone mineral assessments are dual-energy x-ray absorptiometry (DXA), quantitative ultrasound (QUS), and quantitative computed tomography (QTC).

The most accepted and widely used modality for evaluating bone mineral content is DXA. DXA uses very low dose x-rays and relies on the differential absorption to distinguish mineralized and soft tissue components.[7,8] From this data, bone mineral content (BMC) is quantified in grams. The demarcated regions of interest are the bone area being evaluated, and are measured in units of cm[2]. To arrive at the bone mineral density (BMD), the attenuation of each pixel in a region of interest or bone area (BA) is compared with a reference standard resulting in units of grams/cm[2]. This value is multiplied by the pixel's area. The bone mineral density is derived through the equation BMD = BMC/BA. Thus DXA values reflect real rather than volumetric densities.[7,8] The resulting values reflect the sum of both trabecular and cortical bone.[7]

Additionally patient positioning can greatly affect the measured results and precision due to the fact that DXA is a two-dimension rather than three-dimensional measurement. Normal controls are required for the correct interpretation of DXA results; this has proven problematic for children due to rapid growth and variability between individuals, and without careful consideration of the data and patient-specific factors, incorrect diagnoses and conclusions can be drawn.[8] The strengths of DXA are that it is low-dose radiation, and results have been shown to predict fracture risk in the elderly. Much work is still needed to establish the role DXA plays in evaluating bone quality and fracture risk in the developing human. An excellent review of pediatric DXA is provided by Binkovitz et al,[8] which highlights both strengths and current limitations of DXA in the pediatric patient.

The second most widely used diagnostic imaging modality for bone mineral assessments is quantitative ultrasound (QUS). Ultrasound uses no ionizing radiation and is a mechanical wave with frequencies that measures bone speed of sound.[7,9] The energy transmitted through bone and the attenuation of the sound waves can be quantified and allows a method for potentially identifying children at higher risk for fracture.[7,9] QUS can evaluate qualitative factors known to be associated with bone strength, including bone elasticity, microarchitecture, and cortical thickness. These are properties important in determining bone strength that are not evaluated by DXA. There remains controversy as to whether QUS results truly correlate with actual bone strength measures. QUS remains a promising modality for assessing bone parameters in the developing child; additional research in children is required to establish its role in understanding actual bone strength and fracture risk.[10,11]

Quantitative computed tomography (QTC) provides key information regarding structural properties that contribute to ultimate bone strength, in addition to BMD measurements; however the high-dose radiation exposure and expense result in a tool that is prohibitive despite its provision of data superior to that obtained from DXA.[7,11] The development of imaging techniques that allow patient-specific bone quality assessments that are highly correlated with bone strength and fracture risk are still needed; continued efforts will one day afford this component to be integrated into critical thinking about fractures and the plausibility of injury.

BONE PHYSIOLOGY AND DISEASE PROCESSES

Calcium Homeostasis and Parathyroid Hormone

Calcium is used by almost every cell in the body and is critical to bone health. Approximately 50% of total circulating calcium is protein bound to albumin; the other 50% is ionized and represents the active fraction.[12] Calcium provides the foundation and mechanical strength of bone, and bone serves as the major reservoir of calcium in the body. Serum calcium levels are tightly regulated by parathyroid hormone (PTH) and 1,25-dihydroxyvitamin D (the active vitamin D metabolite). PTH is secreted by the parathyroid glands. It increases resorption of calcium from the renal distal tubule and mobilizes calcium from bone to maintain appropriate serum levels of calcium. PTH also stimulates proximal renal tubule conversion of 25-hydroxyvitamin D to the active metabolite 1,25-dihydroxyvitamin D, which maximizes calcium availability from the diet by enhancing calcium absorption from the small intestine. Rising serum levels of calcium decrease secretion of PTH and complete the feedback loop.[12] Parathyroid hormone (PTH) is the main hormone responsible for regulation of serum calcium concentration; the production of PTH is controlled by the level of calcium in serum, allowing for tight control within a narrow physiological range.[13] Bone formation is stimulated by PTH, which serves to link new bone formation to bone resorption.[13]

Nutritional Factors that Influence Calcium Balance

Calcium balance is influenced by dietary intake of sodium, protein, and vegetable nutrients. Increased sodium and protein intake increases calcium loss in the urine. Vegetable nutrients, and specifically fiber, can decrease the intestinal absorption of calcium. For this reason, the calcium in milk is approximately twice as available as the calcium in beans and the calcium in some vegetable products may not be bioavailable at all.[13]

Parathyroid Hormone

Serum ionized calcium binds to the surface of parathyroid cells and tightly regulates the secretion of PTH. A fluctuation in ionized calcium of 0.1 mg/dL (0.025 mmol/L) results in a change in serum PTH concentration within minutes.[14] PTH secretion is decreased by 1,25-dihydroxyvitamin D and by increasing levels of serum phosphate.

Hypoparathyroidism

Several genetic mutations have been found to cause decreased PTH production. Autosomal recessive mutations have been shown to effect PTH precursors and parathyroid gland development. Males with X-linked recessive hypoparathyroidism have abnormal parathyroid gland development and have seizures secondary to hypocalcemia.[15,16] An autosomal dominant form of hypoparathyroidism is associated with sensorineural deafness and renal dysplasia. In this form, mutations in the transcription factor GATA3 cause alterations in the embryonic development of the parathyroid glands, kidneys, inner ears, thymus, and central nervous system.[15,16] Mutations in the calcium-sensing receptor are inherited in an autosomal dominant pattern. The effect is that PTH is not secreted appropriately in response to hypocalcemia. These patients often have seizures and tetany.[15]

Patients with DiGeorge syndrome have hypoparathyroidism from parathyroid dysplasia or hypoplasia secondary to an abnormal development of the third and fourth branchial pouches.[15] The constellation of findings include hypoparathyroidism, immunodeficiency, congenital heart defects, and deformities of the ears, nose, and mouth.[16]

The Sanjad-Sakati syndrome includes hypoparathyroidism, mental retardation, facial dysmorphism, and severe growth failure.[15]

Mitochondrial disorders associated with hypoparathyroidism include Kearns Sayre syndrome, MELAS disorder (mitochondrial myopathy, encephalopathy, lactic acidosis, and stroke), and mitochondrial trifunctional protein deficiency syndrome (MTPDS).[15,16]

Pseudohypoparathyroidism

Pseudohypoparathyroidism refers to a group of disorders with signs of hypocalcemia, hyperphosphatemia, and elevated PTH concentrations secondary to PTH resistance rather than defciency.[15,16] The Mutations in GNAS-1 cause an inability of PTH to activate adenyl cyclase upon bonding to kidney or bone receptors. The clinical manifestations vary with maternal or paternal inheritance of the GNAS-1 gene.[15]

Hypomagnesemia

Magnesium is required for PTH release and is important for PTH interactions with kidney and bone. Therefore, hypomagnesemia can cause hypocalcemia via decreased PTH secretion, impaired end organ response to PTH, or decreased production of 1,25-dihydroxyvitamin D. These patients can have prolonged QT and PR intervals, carpopedal spasm, tetany, seizures, muscle weakness, or hypokalemia.[15] Primary hypomagnesemia can be the result of an autosomal recessive mutation in TRPM6, which encodes for a protein kinase and cation permeable channels. Secondary hypomagnesemia occurs from decreased intake or increased urinary losses of magnesium. Children can develop secondary hypomagnesemia from chronic diarrhea or malabsorption and renal tubule disorders and diuretic use.[15]

Phosphate Homeostasis

Phosphate is an important component of bone mineralization, strength, and health. Eighty to ninety percent of phosphate is stored in bone as hydroxyapatite. The remaining phosphate is found in tissues, extracellular fluid, and erythrocytes. Plasma concentrations of phosphate are regulated by PTH. Phosphate homeostasis reflects a balance between intestinal absorption combined with soft tissue and bone stores.[17]

Dietary sources of phosphate include fish, eggs, meat, milk, cheese, bread, fruit, and vegetables. The abundance of bioavailable phosphate in a variety of foods makes dietary deficiencies rare. Antacids containing aluminum or magnesium bind to ingested and secreted phosphate, causing an overall net phosphate loss from the body. Prolonged therapy with these medications can lead to osteomalacia.[18]

Renal regulation of phosphate is the major contributor to maintaining phosphate balance in the body. Phosphate reabsorption from the kidney is modulated by the serum phosphate concentration, parathyroid hormone, and fibroblast growth factor 23.[18] Vitamin D deficiency can induce hypophosphatemia by causing decreased intestinal phosphate absorption and increased PTH in response to hypocalcemia, which then increases renal phosphate excretion.[18]

Hypophosphatemia secondary to renal phosphate wasting is seen in the following disorders:[18]

X-linked Hypophosphatemic Rickets (XLH, also known as vitamin D-resistant rickets). XLH results from a defect in proximal tubular phosphate transport.[17] Hypophosphatemia is often apparent at birth. Other clinical manifestations include lower limb deformities, short stature, radiographic signs of rickets, predisposition to dental abscesses, calcification of tendons and joint capsules, cardiac defects, and hearing loss.[19]

Autosomal Dominant Hypophosphatemic Rickets. This condition results from mutations in fibroblast growth factor 23. Clinical signs are similar to XLH, with variable penetrance.

Hereditary hypophosphatemic rickets and hypercalciuria occurs secondary to dysfunction of renal sodium-phosphate transporters. These patients typically have bone pain and muscle weakness along with signs of rickets and osteomalacia.[19]

Fanconi Syndrome. In Fanconi syndrome there is urinary wasting of compounds that are normally reabsorbed in the proximal tubule. This results in hypophosphatemia, glucosuria, aminoaciduria, and type 2 renal tubular acidosis.[18]

Oncogenic Hypophosphatemic Osteomalacia. This is more common in adults but may be seen at any age. Pediatric patients typically have renal phosphate-wasting rickets, significant bone pain and muscle weakness without growth failure.[17] Very low levels of 1,25-dihydroxyvitamin D combined with hypophosphatemia suggest this diagnosis.[19]

Vitamin D

Vitamin D is an important regulator of calcium and phosphorous metabolism and appropriate levels are critical to bone health.

Vitamin D metabolism. The most common metabolic pathway for vitamin D occurs when 7-dehydrocholesterol is photoisomerized to cholecalciferol (vitamin D_3) in the skin. Vitamin D can also be obtained from dietary sources in the form of ergocalciferol (vitamin D_2). Cholecalciferol and ergocalciferol are transported to the liver for conversion to calcidiol (25-hydroxyvitamin D), which is the major circulating form of vitamin D and is used to determine an individual's vitamin D status. 25-hydroxyvitamin D is biologically inactive and requires conversion by the kidneys to 1,25-dihydroxyvitamin D. Renal production of 1,25-dihydroxyvitamin D is regulated by a negative feedback mechanism and is affected by serum phosphorous and calcium levels. 1,25-dihydroxyvitamin D enhances calcium absorption from the small intestine, increases PTH-mediated bone resorption, and decreases renal calcium and phosphate excretion.[20,21]

Sources of Vitamin D. Approximately 80% of the vitamin D requirement can be produced endogenously from exposure to ultraviolet B radiation from the sun.[21,22] A person's ability to produce adequate amounts of vitamin D in the skin is influenced by pollution, latitude, season, and number of hours of sunshine per day.[22] Synthesis of vitamin D in the skin is dramatically decreased in the winter months at northern latitudes.[22-24] Additional factors contributing to vitamin D formation in the skin include the amount of skin exposed, duration of exposure, use of sunscreen, degree of melanin production, and the age of the individual.[22,25]

Melanin absorbs UV-B photons and reduces the cutaneous production of vitamin D. The synthesis of vitamin D in fair skinned individuals has been shown to be fivefold to tenfold more efficient than in those with highly pigmented skin.[25] Despite the benefits of vitamin D synthesis in the skin, the risk of skin cancer from sunlight exposure creates a challenge for optimizing vitamin D production.[26] One study suggests that minimal sun exposure for infants might be adequate. Infant vitamin D levels could be maintained in the summer months at latitude of 39° with exposure for 30 minutes per week wearing only a diaper, or 2 hours per week if clothed but not wearing a hat.[27] The duration of ultraviolet radiation that is optimal for maintaining vitamin D sufficiency with respect to pigmentation and climate variables is yet to be determined.

The remainder of Vitamin D must be obtained through dietary sources such as fish, eggs, fortified milk, and dietary supplements.[21,28] Current recommendations suggest an intake of 200 IU of vitamin D per day to prevent deficiency.[26] Young infants rely on the vitamin D content of breast milk or formula to supplement vitamin D that is produced in their skin. The vitamin D content of breast milk is low and typically contains less than 25 IU/L.[26] Therefore, the recommended intake of vitamin D cannot be met by breastfeeding alone and supplementation that begins during the first 2 moths of life is advised.[28] All infant formulas sold in the United States have 400 IU/L of vitamin D, providing adequate amounts of this nutrient if the infant consumes at least 500 mL of formula per day.[26] A careful dietary history in addition to consideration of sun exposure and the effects of skin pigmentation is important for determining which infants might be at risk for vitamin D deficiency.

Vitamin D Deficiency. A recent review of published literature on hypovitaminosis D estimated the prevalence to be between 1% and 78% of children and adolescents.[29] This variation is based on individual and environmental factors as described above. Vitamin D status is determined by serum levels of 25-hydroxyvitamin D, and in adults, normal range is between 30 and 90 ng/mL.[21] Currently there is no consensus on optimal hydroxyvitamin D levels in children and what constitutes clinically significant deficiency. Previous authors, however, have defined serum 25-hydroxyvitamin D concentrations of less than 10 ng/mL as overt deficiency, 11 to 20 ng/mL as deficiency, and 21 to 30 ng/mL as vitamin D insufficiency.[30,31]

Vitamin D deficiency is the primary cause of rickets. Rickets is a clinical syndrome that is associated with insufficient endochondral calcification of the growth plates of long bones resulting in deformation and impaired growth. It is also associated with osteomalacia, which is failed mineralization of trabecular and cortical bone. Children can have both rickets and osteomalacia because the growth plates are still forming. Adults with vitamin D deficiency sometimes only have features of osteomalacia.[22]

Young infants of mothers with normal vitamin D status are protected from developing rickets secondary to the transfer of vitamin D metabolites across the placenta in utero.[22] At 3 months of age this protection wanes and their susceptibility to rickets depends upon their exposure to sunlight and vitamin D supplementation. Fractures that occur during this time frame require consideration of bone health issues. Prematurely born infants are more susceptible to vitamin D deficiency. This is because they have had less time to accumulate vitamin D stores and because they have higher vitamin D requirements compared with term infants.[28]

Since the majority of vitamin is produced in the skin, pigmentation and latitude can greatly affect an individual's vitamin D status. In northern locations such as Boston (42.5° north), vitamin D cannot be produced for 4 to 5 months during the winter. Therefore symptoms related to vitamin D deficiency often present during the spring. Optimal vitamin D production during the summer months cannot prevent deficiency that develops secondary to lack of ultraviolet light in the winter, making dietary supplementation necessary for individuals in northern climates regardless of skin pigmentation. Dark skinned individuals living in southern climates can be susceptible to vitamin D efficiency despite optimal latitude for ultraviolet light exposure.[28]

Clinical Manifestations of Vitamin D Deficiency. The clinical presentation of rickets depends on the age of the child and the severity of vitamin D deficiency.[32] Hypocalcemia is seen initially and transiently before the development of hyperparathyroidism. Symptoms related to hypocalcemia are often seen in infants younger than 6 months of age who can have seizures, tetany, stridor, or apneic episodes. Adolescents can also have hypocalcemic symptoms because as hypocalcemia tends to correlate with developmental periods of rapid growth.[33] PTH induces calcium mobilization from bone resulting in demineralization of bones but improved serum calcium levels.[28] As serum calcium levels normalize in response to PTH, skeletal changes associated with rickets can be observed.[22] These findings vary depending upon the developmental stage of the child because infants might show bowing of the forearms whereas toddlers have exaggerated bowing of the legs. The initial bony changes are most prominent at the ends of the long bones. Visible and palpable enlargement of the distal radius and ulna is a common initial finding. Other skeletal changes include: delayed closure of the fontanelles, frontal and parietal bossing, soft skull bones (craniotables), flattening of the posterior skull, enlarged ends of the ribs at the costochondral junction, which appears as visible beading ("rachitic rosary"), and Harrison grooves resulting from muscular pull of the diaphragmatic attachments to the lower ribs.[32] Children born to mothers who are vitamin D deficient can show signs of enamel hypoplasia and delayed eruption of primary dentition.[22] Because a vitamin D receptor is present in skeletal muscle, deficiency can result in proximal muscle weakness with increased frequency of falling.[31] Delayed gross motor milestones can occur as a result of muscle weakness and bone pain that inhibits ambulation. Chest wall deformities and muscle weakness is often associated with frequent pulmonary infections, increased work of breathing, and excessive sweating.[22,34] Dilated cardiomyopathy also has been reported as a complication of rickets.[35] The variable presentation and range of severity illustrates that clinicians should have a low threshold for screening for vitamin D deficiency.

Diagnosis of Rickets. The diagnosis of rickets is determined by clinical features and the presence of radiographic and laboratory findings. Initial radiographic signs include osteopenia and loss of the provisional zone of calcification.

This is followed by widening of the growth plate and metaphyseal cupping and fraying. Hypocalcemia might be present depending upon the stage of rickets and the influence of PTH. Additional laboratory abnormalities may include hypophosphatemia and increased alkaline phosphatase. Levels of 25-hydroxyvitamin D are almost invariably low and can confirm the diagnosis, but might not be necessary if clinical and radiographic features are present.[28]

Screening for vitamin D deficiency should be considered in the following circumstances:

- Dark skinned infants living at northern latitudes[28]
- Infants and children with unexplained poor growth, delay in motor milestones, or excessive irritability[28]
- Children on chronic anticonvulsants or glucocorticoids[28]
- Children with frequent fractures and osteopenia[28]

Alkaline phosphatase can be used as an initial screening test. Additional laboratory evaluation should include serum 25-hydroxyvitamin D, calcium, phosphorous, and PTH. Radiographs of the radius and ulna (anteriorposterior view of the wrists) or tibia and femur (anteriorposterior view of the knees) should also be obtained to evaluate for radiographic signs of rickets.[28]

Metabolic Causes of Rickets. Pseudovitamin D deficiency occurs when there is impaired conversion from 25-hydroxyvitamin D to the active metabolite 1,25-dihydroxyvitamin D. The clinical manifestations of this rare enzyme disorder mimic hypocalcemic rickets. A similar clinic picture occurs with a defect in the vitamin D receptor, which leads to vitamin D resistance.[32]

Biochemical Changes in Rickets. Whether rickets is due to vitamin D deficiency or lack of dietary calcium, the basic defect is an inability to maintain calcium homeostasis. Initial hypocalcemia induces hyperparathyroidism, which causes renal tubular loss of phosphate and hypophosphatemia. Parathyroid hormone also acts on the renal tubules to decrease urinary calcium loss.[22] Alkaline phosphatase is a measure of bone turnover and is usually elevated.[22]

Treatment of Rickets. Treatment of rickets includes vitamin D therapy with ergocalciferol at doses of 2000 to 10,000 IU (40 IU = 1 μg) per day until alkaline phosphatase and skeletal abnormalities return to normal. An alternate approach, called "stosstherapy," consists of a large single oral or intramuscular dose between 150,000 to 600,000 IU.[36] This therapy has been shown to be effective in clearing radiological findings in 2 to 4 weeks.[35] It is important to maintain calcium intake at 1000 mg/day to avoid the "hungry bone" syndrome, which manifests as worsening hypocalcemia after the initiation of vitamin D therapy.[36]

Vitamin D Deficiency and Fractures. The relationship between vitamin D deficiency and risk of fracture is not well understood, but review of the literature illustrates the frequency of fractures associated with nutritional rickets. Bulloch et al[37] reviewed all infants less than 12 months-of-age with rib fractures within a 29 month period at two institutions. Only 1 of 39 infants had rib fractures associated with rickets; this infant also had radiographic and laboratory findings consistent with rickets. In Australia, 232 children younger than 17 years old were evaluated for vitamin deficiency rickets; 87% had vitamin D insufficiency or deficiency and none of these children had clinical symptoms of rickets. While signs of rickets were noted in 42% of children in which radiographs were obtained, no fractures were reported.[24] In Turkey, 42 infants younger than 3 months of age with nutritional rickets were described, none of which were reported to have fractures.[38] DeLucia et al[39] described 43 young children with clinical, biochemical, and radiographic evidence of rickets without associated fractures.[39] An 11-year review in Sydney revealed that 5 of 126 children with nutritional rickets had fractures.[40] Koo et al[41] followed 78 infants with birth weights less than 1500 grams and found that 25% had radiographic findings of fractures and rickets.[41] In Wisconsin, 10% of children with rickets had fractures.[42] These studies illustrate that fractures are a possible but relatively uncommon complication of rickets, compared with other signs and symptoms. In all reports, the children with fractures also had other radiographic or laboratory signs of rickets. It is important to remember that laboratory and radiographic signs of vitamin D deficiency do not exclude the possibility of nonaccidental trauma. Children with vitamin D deficiency can also be victims of abuse. When concerns for inflicted trauma exist, a full evaluation for nonaccidental injury should still be pursued.

Copper Deficiency

Copper deficiency has been argued as a medical cause for fractures in cases of suspected nonaccidental trauma. Predisposing factors for copper deficiency include low birth weight (lower body stores of copper) and dietary deficiency (total parenteral nutrition or cows milk without fortification). Risk for copper deficiency is enhanced by antecedent malnutrition. Psychomotor retardation, hypotonia, hypopigmentation, prominent scalp veins, anemia, and neutropenia have been described.[43,44] Radiographic changes include osteoporosis, blurring and cupping of metaphyses, sickle-shaped metaphyseal spur formation, subperiosteal new bone formation, increased density of the zone of provisional calcification and fractures.[44,45] The skeletal manifestations of copper deficiency are secondary to impaired collagen and elastin cross-linking, which ultimately result in fragile bones with increased risk of fracture.[43]

Features common to copper deficiency can help distinguish this disease from nonaccidental trauma. While radiologic changes are most evident at the ends of metaphyses, copper deficiency affects the entire skeleton. Full-term infants with fractures secondary to copper deficiency have presented between 6 and 60 months of age; fractures in low birth weight infants have occurred between 2 and 7 months of age. Skull fractures have never been reported as sequelae of copper deficiency and rib fractures have never been reported in full-term infants with copper deficiency. All children with fractures have other obvious radiologic abnormalities.[44] These guidelines can be helpful in determining if copper deficiency should be considered in the differential diagnosis. A plasma copper level less than 40 μg/dL and plasma ceruloplasmin level less than 13 mg/dL would be consistent with copper deficiency.[43]

Menkes syndrome is an X-linked recessive disorder that only affects males and causes defective gastrointestinal absorption of copper.[44] These infants have similar findings as in dietary copper deficiency except anemia and neutropenia is absent and intracranial hemorrhage is common.[43] Metaphyseal lesions similar to those found in nonaccidental trauma can be present.[44] Poor prognosis including hypothermia, convulsions, and rapid deterioration can help distinguish Menkes from other causes.[43] Menkes can be distinguished from nonaccidental trauma by the presence of thin, coarse, hypopigmented hair and laboratory confirmation with decreased copper and ceruloplasmin levels.[44]

Vitamin C Deficiency

Ascorbic acid is a necessary cofactor in collagen biosynthesis. The ascorbic acid content of food can be altered by storing and handling practices.[46] Studies have found that bottle systems for storing milk can contribute to decreased ascorbic acid concentration, which could cause risk for vitamin C deficiency in exclusively milk fed infants.[46] Additionally, infants fed evaporated or boiled milk (heat destroys ascorbic acid) or children with significant dietary insufficiencies are at risk for vitamin C deficiency and scurvy. Symptoms are usually apparent 1 to 3 months after inadequate intake, and the onset is usually after the age of 6 months.[44,47] Manifestations of scurvy include rashes, gingival disease, anemia, skeletal muscle degeneration, cardiac hypertrophy, impaired adrenal and bone marrow function, psychiatric symptoms, and arthritis. Insufficient vitamin C intake results in disordered bone structure and function secondary to defects in osteoid matrix and collagen resorption. Associated radiologic changes are due to the suppression of normal cellular activity and a tendency for hemorrhage because of deficiencies within the capillary endothelium.[44] Fractures around growth plates occur and subperiosteal hemorrhages lead to bone pain.[47] Large amounts of calcification can be seen covering the shafts of affected long bones. Metaphyseal findings with scurvy are similar to nonaccidental trauma, but can be distinguished by specific features. A sclerotic zone of provisional calcification (ZPC) combined with a dense ring around the epiphyseal bone and thin cortices, and osteopenia adjacent to the ZPC are consistent findings associated with scurvy.[44] Reduced serum levels of vitamin C can confirm the diagnosis. Full recovery occurs after appropriate therapy.[47]

Vitamin A Intoxication

Hypervitaminosis A initially is seen with nonspecific findings such as anorexia, irritability, and itching. After several weeks or months, hard and tender areas of swelling are noted on the extremities. Subperiosteal new bone formation is found on radiographs and has been described as undulating. There is no metaphyseal involvement and no tendency for fractures.[44]

Caffey Disease

Infantile cortical hyperostosis affects young infants with painful subperiosteal new bone formation and cortical thickening found on multiple bones. Diagnosis is usually during the first 6 months of life and the mandible is involved in 75% of cases. The clavicle and ulna are also commonly affected. There can be a similar history in family members, although the exact cause of Caffey disease is not known. There are no associated fractures or metaphyseal irregularities. The absence of these findings helps distinguish infantile cortical hyperostosis from nonaccidental trauma.[44]

Hypophosphatasia

Hypophosphatasia is an inherited disorder of bone metabolism. Clinical characteristics include rachitic changes in childhood and osteomalacia in adulthood. Premature loss of teeth occurs secondary to the lack of dental cementum.[48] Alkaline phosphatase activity is decreased because of impaired bone and liver contribution to serum alkaline phosphatase activity. Diagnosis is based on clinical symptoms, decreased serum alkaline phosphatase activity, and increased serum pyridoxal-5′-phosphate levels. The severity of disease is inversely related to age at presentation.[49]

Markedly impaired bone mineralization occurs in utero in the perinatal form of hypophosphatasia. Polyhydramnios and still births are not uncommon. The ribs are thin and malformed, which often contributes to lung hypoplasia. Radiological findings such as sclerotic patches in tubular bones and bone spurs on the ulna and fibula are diagnostic. Neonates can have a high-pitched cry, anemia, and seizures.[48]

In the infantile form of hypophosphatasia, neonates appear normal but rachitic disease and failure to thrive is evident by 6 months of age. Premature cranial synostosis is not uncommon. Chest deformities predispose these infants to frequent pulmonary infections. Hypercalcemia causes irritability, poor feeding, vomiting, hypotonia, polydipsia, polyuria, dehydration and constipation. Unexplained episodes of fever and bone pain occur. Radiographs show diffuse demineralization and rachitic signs in the metaphyses.[48]

Hypophosphatasia with onset in childhood is a milder form of the disease, which is seen with bowing of the lower extremities. Focal bony changes at the end of long bones are often diagnostic. Intracranial hypertension, failure to thrive, and craniosynostosis are not uncommon. Spontaneous remission can occur in adolescence but symptoms of the disease often recur in adulthood.[48]

The adult form of hypophosphatasia is usually mild and occurs with osteomalacia, pseudofractures, and increased susceptibility to true fractures.[48]

Osteoporosis

Osteopenia is defined as a reduction in bone mass for age. It is a precursor to osteoporosis, which is characterized as low bone mass with deterioration of bone tissue causing fragility and susceptibility to fractures.[50] It is helpful to distinguish between primary osteoporosis, which results from a bone defect, and secondary osteoporosis, which is the result of nonskeletal disease or side effects of medications.

Primary Osteoporosis. These disorders have in common a genetic defect that affects bone development. They can be further subdivided into heritable disorders of connective tissue and idiopathic juvenile osteoporosis.

Osteogenesis imperfecta (OI) is a well-known inherited disorder of connective tissue and is discussed in detail elsewhere. Patients with Ehlers-Danlos syndrome (EDS) are

similar to patients with OI in that they have joint hypermobility and laxity and easy bruising. Other signs of EDS include recurrent joint dislocations, scoliosis, kyphosis, thoracic lordosis, subluxation of sternoclavicular joints, chest wall deformity, radio-ulnar synostosis, congenital hip dislocation, and club foot. Overall, bone strength is abnormal and leads to increased risk of fractures.[50] One series of 16 patients with ages ranging from 13 months to 36 years found a history of frequent bone fractures in 19%. All of these patients had physical examinations findings consistent with EDS.[51]

Marfan syndrome (MFS) is an autosomal dominant condition with variable skeletal, ocular, and cardiovascular manifestations.[50,52] Osteoporosis is common in adults with this syndrome and approximately 30% of patients with MFS have fractures, although the true susceptibility to fractures in the absence of trauma is not known.[50]

Homocystinuria is an autosomal recessive connective tissue disorder that is associated with cognitive impairments, ectopic lentis, marfanoid body habitus, and early onset thrombotic vascular disease.[50] Skeletal manifestations include scoliosis, arachnodactyly, enlarged carpal bones, pectus deformities, bowing limb deformities, joint contractures, and pes cavus. Osteoporosis is a common feature in young patients but responds to therapy.[50]

Idiopathic juvenile osteoporosis (IJO) presents in previously healthy children most often in the years preceding puberty, although IJO in children as young as 3 years of age has been described. There does not appear to be an inheritance pattern. Symptoms include gradual onset of pain in the back, hips, knees, and feet that can be severe enough to compromise walking. Vertebral compression fractures are common. Metaphyseal fractures and kyphosis, scoliosis, and pectus carinatum can be present.[50] Radiographs can show evidence of new, abnormal bone that appears as a radiolucent, submetaphyseal band. Vertebrae can appear biconcave or wedge-shaped. Maximizing calcium and vitamin D intake has been shown to be beneficial. Many patients experience spontaneous remission over 2 to 5 years.[50]

Secondary Osteoporosis. Secondary osteoporosis results from an underlying disorder or treatment of a medical condition. Broad categories of secondary osteoporosis include prematurity (discussed elsewhere), neuromuscular disease, chronic illness, and endocrine and reproductive disorders.[50] In children with chronic diseases, bone strength and resistance to fracture can be severely compromised resulting in easy fracturability. Additionally, cognitive deficits associated with some chronic diseases can hinder a child's ability to express pain or discomfort, which will make identification of an injury more difficult.

Neuromuscular Disease

Mechanical challenges are critical to optimal bone strength. Children with neuromuscular disorders lack the influence of muscular strength on developing bone. Secondary osteoporosis from this mechanism is a major problem for children with cerebral palsy, Duchenne muscular dystrophy, polio, immobilization, and limb disuse.

Cerebral palsy is a nonprogressive disorder with motor and postural dysfunction that results from a single insult to the brain.[50,53,54] Complications of CP can include mental retardation, epilepsy, visual disorders, speech impairment, and orthopedic disorders.[53] Scoliosis, joint subluxation and dislocation, and progressive hip dysplasia are common skeletal abnormalities.[50,53] Osteopenia results from a decreased rate of bone growth.[53] Fractures occur in 5% to 30 % of children with CP as a result of stiffness due to contractures of major joints, low bone mass secondary to muscle disuse, and vitamin D deficiency secondary to suboptimal sunlight exposure.[50,55] Bone strength can be further hindered by chronic anticonvulsant therapy.[50]

Duchenne muscular dystrophy is an X-linked recessive disorder due to mutations in the gene that codes for the dystrophin protein.[50,56] Dystrophin stabilizes a glycoprotein complex on the plasma membrane of muscle fibers. If dystrophin function is altered by mutation, muscle fibers are more susceptible to degradation by proteases.[56] The most distinctive characteristic is progressive proximal muscle weakness that affects the lower extremities before the upper extremities.[50,56] The onset of symptoms is usually before the age of 3. Affected children have difficulty running, jumping, and walking up steps and are usually wheel chair dependent by age 12. The loss of muscle function causes increased susceptibility to fractures, especially in the lower extremities.[50] An investigation of the fracture prevalence in Duchenne muscular dystrophy revealed that fractures occurred most often in independently mobile children as a result of falling. Forty percent of fractures occurred in the 8 to 11-year-old age group; 8.8% of fractures were in children less than 3 years of age.[57]

Immobilization and limb disuse causes dramatic decreases in bone mass and mineral density. Bone loss begins immediately following an injury or paralysis and the rate of bone loss decreases over time.[50] Patients with immobilization, especially those who do not regain function, are at high risk for pathological fractures.

Chronic Illness

Children with leukemia, rheumatologic disorders, inflammatory bowel disorders, cystic fibrosis, and anorexia nervosa are especially susceptible to bone morbidity.[50] Bone pain is a presenting sign in approximately 20% to 30% of patients with leukemia.[50,58] This can be secondary to leukemic involvement of the periosteum or aseptic necrosis because of bone marrow accumulation of leukemic cells. Thus any child with bone pain and abnormalities on blood peripheral smear should be evaluated by a bone marrow biopsy.[58] In addition to bone pain, children with acute lymphoblastic leukemia (ALL) can have gait abnormalities and are more susceptible to fractures. Findings on radiographs include metaphyseal lucencies, sclerotic lesions, and periosteal reaction.[58] Therapy for ALL can have detrimental effects on the skeleton with the most significant decrease in bone mass occurring during the first 6 months of therapy. Fracture risk is especially high during this time with approximately 30% of patients experiencing fractures.[50,59]

Children with rheumatologic conditions are especially at risk for bone morbidity. Impaired bone metabolism results in decreased bone mass and increased fracture risk. The effects on bone mineral density correlate with the extent of disease and improve during periods of disease inactivity.[50]

Skeletal abnormalities in anorexia nervosa are caused by poor nutrition and manifest as reduced bone mass and increased fracture risk that can persist throughout life.[50]

Reproductive and Endocrine Disorders

A significant portion of bone mass is accrued during puberty and is secondary to the influence of sex steroids. These hormonal changes also are necessary for skeletal growth and completion of epiphyseal maturation.[50] Many women with Turner syndrome have no pubertal development,[60] and thus have associated short stature and increased fracture risk.[50]

Growth hormone (GH) is necessary for bone growth and accumulation of muscle mass. Patients with growth hormone deficiency have decreased bone mineral density because they lack the skeletal benefits of GH and muscle stimulus for bone development.[50] Normal bone mass can be achieved with appropriate therapy.[61]

Thyroid hormone stimulates bone resorption. This process increases serum levels of calcium and phosphorous and suppresses PTH and 1,25-dihydroxyvitamin D, which subsequently reduces gastrointestinal absorption of calcium and phosphate. Therefore hyperthyroidism causes increased porosity of bone and reduced volume of trabecular bone, ultimately resulting in osteoporosis.[50,62] The severity of bone deficits correlates with the duration of hyperthyroidism, and patients with chronic disease are at increased fracture risk.[62] The lifetime risk of fracture for individuals with hyperthyroidism is unknown.[63] Untreated congenital hyperthyroidism is most often associated with growth arrest, delayed bone age, and short stature.[63]

Iatrogenic Agents Associated with Pediatric Osteoporosis

The detrimental effect of glucocorticoid therapy on bone health has been well established.[64,65] Glucocorticoids inhibit bone formation through inhibition of replication, migration, differentiation, and longevity of osteoblasts.[66] Bone loss is dose dependent and is greatest after therapy is initiated and continues at a slower but steady rate thereafter.[50] Children who receive more than four courses of corticosteroids (average of 6 days of therapy for each course) are at greater risk of fracture; the risk of a humerus fracture has been shown to be doubled.[67] The confounding effect of the underlying disease also contributes to suboptimal bone health.

Antiepileptic drugs (AED) are associated with osteoporosis.[50] Phenytoin, phenobarbital, and carbamazepine induce the CYP450 enzyme system, which causes increased clearance of vitamin D. This results in an increase in PTH, which stimulates bone turnover and causes osteomalacia. Nonenzymatic AEDs have negative skeletal effects as well. Children on valproate have a 10% reduction in bone mineral density. The severity of this effect is illustrated by correlating it with adult data; a 7% decrease in bone mineral density is associated with a 50% increase in osteoporotic fractures.[68] A pediatric case series described multiple fractures in children taking valproate who had normal serum levels of parathyroid hormone, calcium, vitamin D, and alkaline phosphatase.[55,69] Falls and tonic clonic movements associated with seizure activity also contribute to the increased risk of

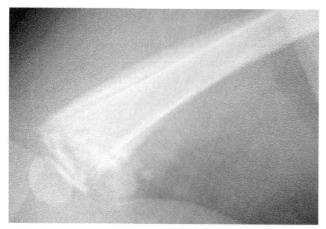

FIGURE 31-1 Ten-week-old with syphilis osteomyelitis with lucent defects in the metaphyseal region of the distal femur and periosteal reaction. *(Image provided by Marguerite Caré, Cincinnati Children's Hospital Medical Center, Cincinnati, Ohio.)*

skeletal injuries. Treatment with vitamin D can be helpful for treatment of osteomalacia.

Infections That Affect Bone Health

Infants with congenital syphilis can have a myriad of manifestations, including hepatosplenomegaly, snuffles, lymphadenopathy, mucocutaneous lesions, pseudoparalysis, edema, rash, hemolytic anemia, and thrombocytopenia.[70] Skeletal abnormalities such as growth arrest lines, metaphyseal destruction, periostitis, and osteitis can be seen on radiographs.[71] Metaphyseal abnormalities can be seen in 90% of infants with symptomatic syphilis and 20% of asymptomatic newborns with positive serological tests (Figure 31-1).[45] Destructive changes of osteomyelitis are seen in the long bones between 1 and 6 months of life. Delayed ossification of the proximal tibial epiphysis can occur in 30% of newborns. Delayed ossification of distal femoral and proximal tibial ossification centers occurs in 10% of newborns with congenital syphilis. Pathological metaphyseal fractures can mimic findings seen in nonaccidental trauma.[45] Serological tests for syphilis are necessary to confirm the diagnosis.

Osteomyelitis affects newborn infants, children, and adolescents (Figure 31-2). Infection is introduced into the bone via hematogenous delivery, direct inoculation, or local invasion from a contiguous infection. Hematogenous delivery is the most common mode of infection in children. Symptoms of osteomyelitis include fever, localized pain, and decreased motility of the affected area. Physical examinations often reveals erythema and swelling. There might be a history of antecedent trauma. Leukocytosis occurs in approximately 30% of patients and serum inflammatory markers are elevated in more than 90% of cases.[72] In infants, osteomyelitis can cause multifocal metaphyseal lesions with subperiosteal new bone formation. Other classic findings of osteomyelitis might not be present. These metaphyseal lucencies are not as well defined compared with metaphyseal changes associated with nonaccidental trauma. Fractures through the physis can result as a complication of metaphyseal osteomyelitis and can be difficult to distinguish from fractures secondary to trauma. Over time callus formation from fracture

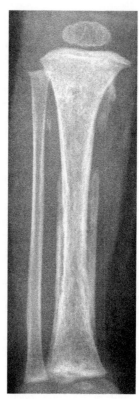

FIGURE 31-2 Ten-month-old with staphylococcal osteomyelitis and prominent tibial periosteal reaction. *(Image provided by Marguerite Caré, Cincinnati Children's Hospital Medical Center, Cincinnati, Ohio.)*

remodeling versus bone destruction from osteomyelitis can be helpful in making the distinction.[44]

Prematurity

Bone health can be adversely affected due to premature birth and/or illnesses occurring during the perinatal and neonatal period. Maximum bone accrual occurs during the third trimester of pregnancy. Nearly 80% of fetal bone becomes mineralized after 26 weeks gestation with peaks at 27 weeks and 34 weeks.[9,73-75] Thus prematurity alone is a significant risk factor for decreased bone strength and ability to resist fracture due to decreased bone density.[73,74,76] Although studies suggest catch up mineralization does occur, and that increased fracture risk does not persist past early childhood,[9,77] it is unclear how soon normal bone mineralization and presumed bone strength occurs. This answer is especially difficult since other illnesses associated with prematurity often require treatment with medications that can adversely affect bone health and mineralization status, such as diuretics (especially furosemide) or steroids. Additionally, many preterm infants require parenteral nutrition, which is also associated with decreased bone density.[9]

Infants born prematurely are at increased risk for fracture if inadequate bone accrual did not occur in utero, and/or if postnatal care required prolonged treatment with medications or parenteral nutrition. Fractures were diagnosed in 1.2% of sick preterm infants requiring prolonged neonatal intensive care treatment. And in very-low-birth-weight (VLBW) infants (weighing <1500 g), the incidence of fractures was 2.1%.[78] Of interest, all but one infant had more than one fracture, all occurring at different times. In this study, four risk factors were identified with bone loss and rickets: (1) cholestatic jaundice; (2) prolonged total parental nutrition (TPN); (3) bronchopulmonary dysplasia; and, (4) prolonged diuretic therapy with furosemide (>2 weeks).[78] Infants born extremely early with very low birth weights (<1000 g) are at markedly increased risk for fractures, with 50% of these infants developing osteopenia with a subsequent fracture rate of 70%.[9,79] The risk for fracture and abnormal bone density does not appear to persist into early childhood however.[9,77] When an infant is diagnosed with a fracture in the outpatient setting, key questions regarding birth history and postnatal course are helpful for identifying factors associated with increased risk of fracture.

Because preterm infants are also at greater risk for abuse, the preterm infant determined to have a fracture must be carefully evaluated for bone disease; the possibility of the trauma being inflicted must also be considered, regardless of bone health status. The presence of osteopenia does not determine whether the trauma causing the fracture was inflicted or accidental in nature. Because prolonged hospitalization of the infant could have interfered with normal bonding and preterm infants also may have increased needs, requiring extra parenting time and skills, added emotional and financial stresses on the parents and family structure can occur. These added stresses can be associated with physical abuse.[9,80] Therefore special consideration must be given to the premature infant with a fracture. A comprehensive and simultaneous evaluation for bone pathology that might lead to increased fracture risk should be done in concert with an evaluation for family social stressors and pathology that might lead to increased risk of violence. Both conditions must be considered, and the appropriate treatment and intervention provided to allow for the best possible outcome for the child.

Preterm infants are known to sustain pathological fractures from simple procedures such as IV placement[81] or hyperflexion positioning for an LP.[82] Rib fractures have been reported rarely from cardiopulmonary resuscitation in a VLBW infant. Prematurity alone, however, is not an adequate explanation for posterior rib fractures.[83] In a study evaluating for the incidence and location of rib fractures in ELBW infants (birth 22-33 weeks gestation), 5 of 72 had rib fracture detected; 3 of 5 had undergone CPR; all 5 infants died before discharge from the NICU; and none of the fractures were posterior. The authors concluded that rib fractures are rare even in ELBW infants, and that none were posterior in location. "The possibility of NAT must be considered irrespective of neonatal history" when a rib fracture is identified.[83]

Osteogenesis Imperfecta

Osteogenesis imperfecta (OI) is a connective tissue disorder with varying presentations, although the hallmark of this disorder is brittle bones. The most severe forms of this disease are lethal at birth; mildly affected individuals sometimes only have symptoms of premature osteoporosis.

The incidence of OI is 1 per 20,000 births, although misdiagnosis is common because of the heterogeneity of presentation.[84,85] More than 200 gene mutations have been associated with OI. The most common mutation is in two genes that code for proteins in Type I collagen; approximately 90% of patients with OI have a mutation in the COL1A1 or COL1A2 gene.[84,86] Type I collagen consists of a triple helix molecule made of two α_1 and one α_2 polypeptide chains. Glycine residues are located at the center of each helical turn and mutations in these amino acids can result in structural abnormalities that impair collagen function.[86] Patients with OI have decreased bone formation and increased bone turnover.[87] Histologically, patients with OI have a disorganized appearance to the bone that varies with the severity of the underlying disease.[84] There is also decreases in cortical width, cancellous bone volume, and number of trabeculas.[84] Collectively, these changes result in a loss of bone strength and decreased resistance to fracture.

The clinical manifestations vary significantly, but the most common features of OI include: excessive number of fractures or fractures resulting from minimal trauma, short stature, scoliosis, blue sclera, hearing loss, fragile teeth (dentinogenesis imperfecta), increased laxity of ligaments and skin, wormian bones, and easy bruisability.[84] More specific clinical manifestations are seen within the different types of OI.

Type I. Type I OI is the most common. These individuals have a minimal amount of bone fragility and stature is often normal. Fractures may occur after they begin ambulating and most frequently involve the long bones of the extremities, the ribs, and the small bones of the hands and feet. Fractures heal at a normal rate.[88] Blue sclera is typical in this phenotype but dentinogenesis imperfecta is uncommon. Vertebral compression fractures can occur during periods of rapid growth such as puberty.[86] Adults with Type I OI may have premature osteoporosis or accelerated osteoporosis after menopause. Hearing loss is found in adulthood and affects approximately 50% of patients.[84]

Type II. Type II is associated with death occurring in utero or early infancy (Figure 31-3). Prenatal determination of lethal versus severe OI is often not possible.[89] These infants often have blue or gray sclera and short, broad bones with decreased density. Mortality is usually secondary to respiratory insufficiency as a result of multiple rib fractures.[86] Other causes of death are CNS malformations and hemorrhages.[89]

Type III. This is the most severe survivable form of OI. Prenatal diagnosis might be possible via ultrasonography.[89] Many infants with type III OI have long bone deformities and multiple fractures at birth (Figure 31-4). Blue sclera, dentinogenesis imperfecta, triangular facies (secondary to underdevelopment of facial bones and a relatively large head), and short stature are also typical manifestations. Children with this type of OI suffer from multiple fractures and usually require the use of a wheel chair before adulthood. Respiratory compromise is a leading cause of death for these patients.[3]

Type IV. The manifestations of this type of OI are extremely diverse ranging from mild disease to wheel chair dependence. Classic signs of OI are often absent; blue sclera is uncommon. It is possible for radiographs to be otherwise normal at the time of the first fractures, but the frequency of this phenomenon is not known.[88] Lucent teeth are often the only associated abnormality and the diagnosis can be difficult to make before tooth eruption.[90] Spontaneous

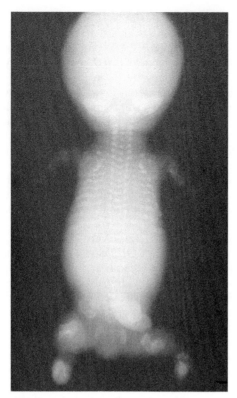

FIGURE 31-3 A newborn with the most severe form of osteogenesis imperfecta, Type II, died shortly after birth.

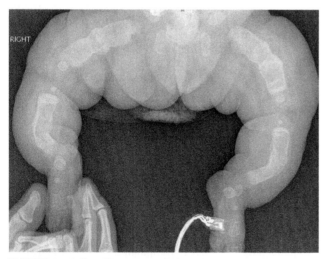

FIGURE 31-4 Type III osteogenesis imperfecta, the most severe survivable form of OI. The newborn had long bone fractures and deformities in utero.

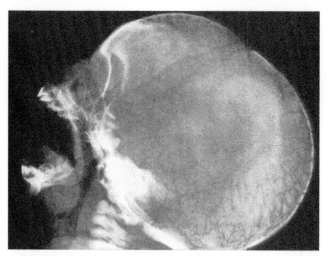

FIGURE 31-5 Wormian bones of the skull in a child with osteogenesis imperfecta.

mutations are common in this manifestation of OI and therefore a family history of bone fragility can be absent. Because of the lack of family history and associated symptoms, type IV OI is sometimes difficult to distinguish from nonaccidental trauma.

Type V. The inheritance pattern for this noncollagen variant is autosomal dominant; although the exact genetic defect is unknown. DNA and protein screening of collagen type I is negative. Disrupted lamellar organization is distinct from OI types I and IV. Blue sclera and dentinogenesis imperfecta is not common. The hallmark of this type of OI is hypertrophic callus formation. These patients often have firm, warm swelling over the bones that is often initially thought to be secondary to inflammation or malignancy.[89] Early calcification of the interosseous membrane between the radius and ulna causes these patients to have limitation of pronation and supination and an increased incidence of radial head subluxation.[86]

Type VI. Patients with this autosomal recessive form of OI have moderate to severe bone deformity and fragility. They do not have blue sclera or dentinogenesis imperfecta. This type of OI can only be diagnosed via bone biopsy, which reveals a mineralization defect within the bone matrix.[89] Histologically the bone lamellas have a fish scale-like appearance. There is also excessive osteoid accumulation despite normal calcium and phosphate metabolism.[86] Radiographs do not show signs of growth plate involvement.[89] These patients do not respond as well to bisphosphonate therapy compared with other types of OI. Similar to type V, DNA and protein screening of type I collagen is negative.[86]

Type VII. This type of OI has moderate to severe bone deformities and often presents in infancy as rhizomelia and coxa vara. OI type VII results from a reduction in expression of cartilage-associated protein (CRTAP) and has an autosomal recessive mode of inheritance.[86]

Laboratory Findings. Biochemical markers of bone and mineral metabolism are usually normal. This helps in distinguishing OI from other skeletal diseases such as rickets. Hypercalciuria is common in OI and correlates with the severity of skeletal disease. Patients with type VI OI can have elevated levels of serum alkaline phosphatase.[84]

Diagnosis. The diagnosis of OI is based on signs and symptoms although the variability of manifestations can make a clinical diagnosis challenging. During the first year of life, radiographs in patients with OI might not have any abnormalities in addition to fractures.[88,91] Wormian bones (Figure 31-5) are frequent but not universal for this disease.[91] A family history with features of skeletal dysplasia raise the suspicion of a bone fragility disorder but the absence of such history does not exclude the diagnosis. There is no definitive lab test for OI but some studies, in combination with clinical suspicion, can direct the diagnosis. Culture of fibroblasts obtained from a skin biopsy can be analyzed to determine if procollagen synthesis is appropriate. Approximately 87% of patients with clinical features of OI will have abnormal collagen production identified by this method.[92] DNA testing of white blood cells for mutations in *COL1A1* and *COL1A2* can detect almost 90% of collagen type I mutations.[84]

DIFFERENTIAL DIAGNOSIS

The differential diagnosis for a child who has one or more fractures should include hypophosphatasia, osteoporosis with renal tubular acidosis, rickets, and nonaccidental trauma.[93] Each of these entities on the differential diagnosis have distinguishing characteristics that allow for differentiation. Specific syndromes that resemble OI include the following.

Cole-Carpenter syndrome is associated with development of metaphyseal fractures within the first year of life, decreased bone density, craniosynostosis, hydrocephalus, ocular proptosis, and facial dysmorphism. Hypercalciuria has also been described. The genetic cause has yet to be defined.[89]

Patients with Bruck syndrome are observed to have brittle bones at birth. The inheritance pattern is recessive. Bone fragility in these patients leads to multiple fractures, joint contractures, and pterygia.[89]

Osteoporosis pseudoglioma syndrome has a recessive inheritance pattern and is associated with mild to moderate OI. Patients with this syndrome also have blindness secondary to hyperplasia of the vitreous, corneal opacity, and secondary glaucoma.[89]

Osteogenesis Imperfecta Versus Nonaccidental Trauma

The physical findings associated with OI can be helpful in distinguishing this disease from nonaccidental trauma.[94] The skeletal deformities of type II and type III can be readily recognized on x-rays. The presence of wormian bones larger than normal (6 × 4 mm) or excessive in number (10 or greater) can indicate OI or another bone fragility condition (Figure 31-5).[95] Type I is almost always associated with blue sclera and this finding can also be seen in family members.[88] The presence of family members with hypermobility of joints, deafness, or dentinogenesis imperfecta can be an indication of an inherited bone fragility disorder.[94] Radiographs of patients with OI often reveal generalized osteoporosis of the axial and appendicular skeleton. The diaphyses are sometimes thinner than normal and the cortices can be thinned as well.[95] Fractures in OI are typically seen in the diaphyses of long bones. The most common presentation is transverse fractures that appear as pathological fractures of osteopenic bones.[95] Classic metaphyseal lesions commonly seen in nonaccidental trauma are not seen in OI without an obvious mineralization defects.[92] When metaphyseal fractures do exist, there is usually additional findings of bone disease on radiographs.[88] Rib fractures are unusual manifestations of OI but when they do occur from minor trauma, other findings (osteopenia and thinning of the ribs) are usually present. Additionally, rib fractures associated with

bone fragility are not usually paired or in different stages of healing.[95]

Challenging cases for child abuse pediatricians occur when an infant has more than one fracture, but no physical findings associated with osteogenesis imperfecta and no family history of blue sclera, dentinogenesis imperfecta, joint hypermobility, or frequent fractures. Sporadic cases of type IV can yield this presentation, but the rate of occurrence is rare. A population study described in an article by Taitz[96] shows that only 5% of cases of OI would not have blue sclera or progressive deformity, and that only an additional 0.6% would not have any family history. Thus if the overall prevalence of OI is 1 in 20,000, the occurrence of this disease in the absence of blue sclera, progressive deformity, or family history would be 1 in 3 million births.[94]

In summary, children with unexplained fractures or fractures that are typical of nonaccidental trauma are unlikely to have OI unless additional features of OI are present. As always, it also is important to note that no one disease state is "protective" against abuse; the two can coexist. A careful and thoughtful assessment can often help distinguish a medical disease process where abuse is also occurring.

Temporary Brittle Bone Disease

Temporary brittle bone disease (TBBD) has generated much discussion in the literature. Patterson et al[97-99] described 39 children with fractures during the first year of life and a retrospective diagnosis of this disease. The underlying pathology is asserted to be a temporary collagen defect due to copper deficiency or another metalloenzyme deficiency,

Table 31-1	Findings Concerning for Child Abuse in Children with Fractures

Metaphyseal corner fractures
Posterior rib fractures
Scapular, acromial, or sternal fractures
Spiral or oblique fractures of long bones without adequate trauma mechanism
Unexplained fractures with normal bone mineralization
Lack of further fracturing while in protective environment
Head injury and retinal findings consistent with inflicted head trauma
Other unexplained injuries

Table 31-2	Features of Osteogenesis Imperfecta in a Child or Family Members

Bone fragility, fractures without significant trauma mechanism
Osteoporosis at a relatively young age
Fragile or translucent teeth
Excessive wormian bones
Poor bone mineralization on radiographs
Deafness or hearing impairment
Ligamentous laxity or hypermobility of joints
Easy bruising
Short stature
Fractures that continue while in a protective environment

Table 31-3 Conditions and Features of Bone Health Abnormalities

Historical Factors	Deficiency or Defect	Age at which Fracture Susceptibility Is Affected	Are Other Clinical Features Present or Do Fractures Occur in Isolation?
Exclusively fed evaporated or boiled milk Rashes, gingival disease, anemia, arthritis	Vitamin C deficiency	>6 months of age	Other clinical features present
Joint hypermobility and laxity Easy bruising 　Joint subluxation 　Spine curvature	Ehlers-Danlos syndrome	Infant	Other clinical features present
Pain in back, hips, knees	Idiopathic juvenile osteoporosis	Toddler	Other clinical features present
Mental retardation Epilepsy Orthopedic disorders	Cerebral palsy	Toddler	Other clinical features present
Proximal muscle weakness	Duchenne muscular dystrophy	Young child	Other clinical features present
Bone pain	Leukemia	Infant	Laboratory signs or other clinical features present
Hepatosplenomegaly 　Snuffles 　Lymphadenopathy 　Mucocutaneous lesions Pseudoparalysis 　Edema 　Rash 　Hemolytic anemia 　Thrombocytopenia Positive serologic testing for syphilis	Congenital syphilis	Neonate	Laboratory signs or other clinical features present
Minimal sunlight exposure Dark skin pigmentation Exclusively breast fed infant without vitamin supplementation Chronic anticonvulsant or glucocorticoid therapy Frequent fractures and osteopenia	Vitamin D deficiency	Young infant	Other radiographic signs present
Low birth weight Total parenteral nutrition Exclusively fed cow's milk without supplementation Malnutrition	Copper deficiency	Full term infants: 6-60 months of age Low birth weight: 2-7 months of age	Other clinical features and radiographic signs present
Male Coarse, hypopigmented hair	Menkes	Young infant	Other clinical and radiographic features usually present
Fever 　Localized bone pain Decreased mobility	Osteomyelitis	Young infant	Metaphyseal lucencies and fractures through the physis may be the only findings

but scientific evidence to support this is lacking.[100] The features described in TBBD have some overlap with fractures associated with nonaccidental trauma and normal variants: fractures in the first year of life, predominance of rib and metaphyseal fractures, fractures found as incidental findings on radiographs, often symmetrical periosteal reaction without associated fracture, delay in bone age, osteopenia, expanded costochondral junctions, vomiting, diarrhea, apnea, hepatomegaly, anemia, and neutropenia.[100] Because of the overlap with nonaccidental injury and lack of scientific evidence, TBBD remains a controversial issue and is generally considered a nonexistent condition.[101]

SUMMARY

Many factors should be considered when evaluating the young child or infant with a fracture(s). Table 31-1 lists common findings in cases of child abuse. Table 31-2 details the features of OI in children and/or family members, and Table 31-3 outlines conditions that lead to bone

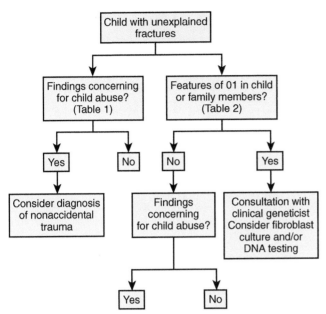

FIGURE 31-6 Flow diagram illustrating the approach to the evaluation of a child with a fracture.

abnormalities and commonly associated features. Figure 31-6 is a flow diagram illustrating the approach to the evaluation of a child with a fracture. Future research is needed to better identify bone health issues and how bone health affects the child's ability to resist fracture. Additionally, work is needed to better identify the abused child regardless of bone health condition or other medical diagnoses, as ill health is not protective against abuse, and might, in fact, increase the risk for abusive injury.

References

1. Reith JR, Ross MH: *Atlas of descriptive histology*, ed 3, Harper & Row, New York, 1977.
2. Aubin JE, Heersche JNM: Bone cell biology. *In*: Glorieux FH, Pettifor JM, Juppner H (eds): *Pediatric Bone, Biology and Diseases.* Elsevier Science, San Diego, 2003, pp 43-75.
3. Gomez MA, Nahum AM: Biomechanics of bone. *In*: Nahum AM, Melvin JW (eds): *Accidental Injury.* Springer-Verlag, New York, 2002, pp 206-227.
4. Summerlee AJS: Bone formation and development. *In*: Summer-Smith G (ed): *Bone in Clinical Orthopedics*, ed 2, Thieme, New York, 2002, pp 1-22.
5. Webster SSJ: Integrated bone tissue physiology: anatomy and physiology. *In*: Cowin SC (ed): *Bone Mechanics Handbook.* CRC Press, Boca Raton Fla, 2001, pp 1-1-1-68.
6. Boskey AL: Bone mineralization. *In*: Cowin SC (ed): *Bone Mechanics Handbook.* CRC Press, Boca Raton Fla, 2001, pp 5-1-5-31.
7. Mora S, Bachrach L, Gilsanz V: Noninvasive techniques for bone mass measurement. *In*: Glorieux FH, Pettifor JM, Juppner H (eds): *Pediatric Bone, Biology and Diseases.* Elsevier Science, San Diego, 2003, pp 303-324.
8. Binkovitz LA, Henwood MJ, Sparke P: Pediatric DXA: technique, interpretation, and clinical applications. *Pediatr Radiol* 2008;38: S227-S239.
9. Carroll DM, Doria AS, Paul BS: Clinical-radiological features of fractures in premature infants—a review. *J Perinat Med* 2007; 35:366-375.
10. Baroncelli GI: Quantitative ultrasound methods to assess bone mineral status in children: technical characteristics, performance, and clinical application. *Pediatr Res* 2008;63(3):220-228.
11. Binkley TL, Berry R, Specker BL: Methods for measurement of pediatric bone. *Rev Endocr Metab Disord* 2008;9:95-106.
12. Ardeshirpour L, Cole DEC, Carpenter TO: Evaluation of bone and mineral disorders. *Pediatr Endocrinol Rev* 2007;5:584-598.
13. Strewler GJ: Parathyroid and calcium homeostasis. *In*: Glorieux FH, Pettifor JM, Juppner H (eds): *Pediatric Bone, Biology and Diseases.* Elsevier Science, San Diego, 2003, pp 135-172.
14. Fuleihan GEH: Parathyroid hormone secretion and action. UpToDate, Waltham, Mass, May 2008.
15. Jeha GS, Kirkland JL: Etiology of hypocalcemia in infants and children. UpToDate, Waltham, Mass, May 2008.
16. Bastepe M, Juppner H, Thakkar RV: Parathyroid disorders. *In*: Glorieux FH, Pettifor JM, Juppner H (eds): *Pediatric Bone, Biology and Disease.* Elsevier, San Diego, 2003, pp 485-508.
17. Caverzasio J, Murer H, Tenenhouse HS: Phosphate homeostasis regulatory mechanisms. *In*: Glorieux FH, Pettifor JM, Juppner H (eds): *Pediatric Bone, Biology and Diseases.* Elsevier, San Diego, 2003, pp 173-192.
18. Agus ZS: Causes of hypophosphatemia. *UpToDate*, Waltham, Mass, Jan 2009.
19. Ward LM: Renal phosphate-wasting disorders in childhood. *Pediatr Endocrinol Rev* 2005;2:342-350.
20. Pazirandeh S, Burns DL: Overview of vitamin D. UpToDate, Waltham, Mass, April 2008.
21. Holick MF: Vitamin D deficiency. *N Engl J Med* 2007;357: 266-281.
22. St Arnaud R, Demay MB: Vitamn D biology. *In*: Glorieux FH, Pettifor JM, Juppner H (eds): *Pediatric Bone, Biology and Diseases.* Elsevier Science, San Diego, 2003, pp 193-209.
23. Ziegler EE, Hollis BW, Nelson SE, et al: Vitamin D deficiency in breastfed infants in Iowa. *Pediatrics* 2006;118:603-610.
24. McGillivray G, Skull SA, Davie G, et al: High prevalence of asymptomatic vitamin D and iron deficiency in East African immigrant children and adolescents living in a temperate climate. *Arch Dis Child* 2007;92:1088-1093.
25. Chen TC, Chimeh F, Lu Z, et al: Factors that influence the cutaneous synthesis and dietary sources of vitamin D. *Arch Biochem Biophys* 2007;460:213-217.
26. Gartner LM, Greer FR: Prevention of rickets and vitamin D deficiency: new guidelines for vitamin D intake. *Pediatrics* 2003;111: 908-910.
27. Specker BL, Valanis B, Hertzberg V, et al: Sunshine exposure and serum 25-hydroxyvitamin D concentrations in exclusively breast fed infants. *J Pediatr* 1985;107:372-376.
28. Misra M, Pacaud D, Petryk A, et al: Vitamin D deficiency in children and its management: review of current knowledge and recommendations. *Pediatrics* 2008;122:398-417.
29. Rovner AJ, O'Brien KO: Hypovitaminosis D among healthy children in the United States: a review of the current evidence. *Arch Pediatr Adolesc Med* 2008;162:513-519.
30. Bowden SA, Robinson RF, Carr R, et al: Prevalence of vitamin D deficiency and insufficiency in children with osteopenia or osteoporosis referred to a pediatric metabolic bone clinic. *Pediatrics* 2007;121:2007-2111.
31. Holick MF, Chen TC: Vitamin D deficiency: a worldwide problem with health consequences. *Am J Clin Nutr* 2008;87:1080S-1086S.
32. Rauch F: Overview of rickets in children. UpToDate, Waltham, Mass, Jan 2007.
33. Ladhani S, Srinivasan L, Buchanan C, et al: Presentation of vitamin D deficiency. *Arch Dis Child* 2004;89:781-784.
34. Joiner TA, Foster C, Shope T: The many faces of vitamin D deficiency rickets. *Pediatr Rev* 2000;21:296-302.
35. Balasubramanian S, Ganesh R: Vitamin D deficiency in exclusively breast fed infants. *Indian J Med Res* 2008;127:250-255.
36. Rauch F: Etiology and treatment of hypocalcemic rickets in children. *UpToDate*, Waltham, Mass, Dec 2008.
37. Bulloch B, Schubert CJ, Brophy PD, et al: Cause and clinical characteristics of rib fractures in infants. *Pediatrics* 2000;105:e48.
38. Hatun S, Ozkan B, Orbak Z, et al: Vitamin D deficiency in early infancy. *J Nutr* 2005;135:279-282.
39. DeLucia MC, Mitnick ME, Carpenter TO: Nutritional rickets with normal circulating 25-hydroxyvitamin D: a call for reexamining the role of dietary calcium intake in North American infants. *J Clin Endocrinol Metab* 2003;88:3539-3545.
40. Robinson PD, Högler W, Craig ME, et al: The re-emerging burden of rickets: a decade of experience from Sydney. *Arch Dis Child* 2004;91:564-568.

41. Koo WWK, Sherman R, Succop P, et al: Fractures and rickets in very low birth weight infants: conservative management and outcome. *J Pediatr Orthop* 1989;9:326-330.
42. Mylott BM, Kump T, Bolton ML, et al: Rickets in the dairy state. *WMJ* 2004;103:84-87.
43. Shaw JCL: Copper deficiency and non-accidental injury. *Arch Dis Child* 1988;63:448-455.
44. Brill PW, Winchester P, Kleinmman PK: Differential diagnosis I: diseases simulating abuse. *In*: Kleinman PK (ed): *Diagnostic Imaging of Child Abuse*, ed 2, Mosby, St Louis, 1998, pp 178-196.
45. Chapman S: Child abuse or copper deficiency? A radiological view. *Br Med J* 1987;294:1370.
46. Francis J, Rogers K, Brewer P, et al: Comparative analysis of ascorbic acid in human milk and infant formula using varied milk delivery systems. *Int Breastfeed J* 2008;3:19-24.
47. Weinstein M, Babyn P, Zlottkin S: An orange a day keeps the doctor away: scurvy in the year 2000. *Pediatrics* 2001;108:e55.
48. Cole DC: Hypophosphatasia. *In*: Glorieux FH, Pettifor JM, Juppner H (eds): *Pediatric Bone, Biology and Diseases*. Elsevier Science, San Diego, 2003, pp 651-678.
49. Cahill RA, Wenkert D, Perlman SA, et al: Infantile hypophosphatasia: transplantation therapy trial using bone fragments and cultured osteoblasts. *J Clin Endocrinol Metab* 2007;92:2923-2930.
50. Ward LM, Glorieux FH: The spectrum of pediatric osteoporosis. *In*: Glorieux FH, Pettifor JM, Juppner H (eds): *Pediatric Bone, Biology and Diseases*. Elsevier Science, San Diego, 2003, pp 401-442.
51. Jui-Lung Y, Shuan-Pei L, Ming-Ren C, et al: Clinical features of Ehlers-Danlos syndrome. *J Formos Med Assoc* 2006;105:475-480.
52. Wright MJ, Connolly HM: The Marfan syndrome. *UpToDate*, Waltham, Mass, 2008.
53. Miller G: Clinical features and diagnosis of cerebral palsy. *UpToDate*, Waltham, Mass, May 2007.
54. Miller G: Epidemiology and etiology of cerebral palsy. *UpToDate*, Waltham, Mass, Dec 2008.
55. Sheth RD: Bone health and pediatric epilepsy. *Epilepsy Behav* 2003;5:S30-S35.
56. Darras BT: Clinical features and diagnosis of Duchenne and Becker muscular dystrophy. *UpToDate*, Waltham, Mass, Jan 2009.
57. McDonald DG, Kinaldi M, Gallagher AC, et al: Fracture prevalence in Duchenne muscular dystrophy. *Dev Med Child Neurol* 2002;44:695-698.
58. Horton TM, Steuber CP: Overview of the presentation and classification of acute lymphoblastic leukemia in children. *UpToDate*, Waltham, Mass, Feb 2008.
59. Halton JM, Atkinson SA, Fraher L, et al: Altered mineral metabolism and bone mass in children during treatment for acute lymphoblastic leukemia. *J Bone Miner Res* 1996;11:1774-1783.
60. Saenger P: Clinical manifestations and diagnosis of Turner syndrome. *UpToDate*, Waltham, Mass, Feb 2002.
61. Rogol AD: Treatment of growth hormone deficiency in children. *UpToDate*, Waltham, Mass, April 2008.
62. LaFranchi S: Clinical manifestations and diagnosis of hyperthyroidism in children and adolescents. *UpToDate*, Waltham, Mass, April 2007.
63. Murphy E, Williams GR: The thyroid and the skeleton. *Clin Endocrinol* 2004;61:285-298.
64. Kelly HW, Van Natta ML, Covar RA, et al: Effect of long-term corticosteroid use on bone mineral density in children: a prospective longitudinal assessment in the childhood asthma management program (CAMP) study. *Pediatrics* 2008;132:e53-e61.
65. Leonard MB: Glucocorticoid induced osteoporosis in children: impact of the underlying disease. *Pediatrics* 2007;119:S166-S174.
66. Raisz LG: Pathogenesis of osteoporosis. *UpToDate*, Waltham, Mass, Sep 2008.
67. van Staa TP, Cooper C, Leufkens HG, et al: Children and the risk of fracture caused by oral corticosteroids. *J Bone Miner Res* 2003;18:913-918.
68. Samaniego EA, Sheth RD: Bone consequences of epilepsy and anti-epileptic medications. *Semin Pediatr Neurol* 2007;14:196-200.
69. Pavlakis SG, Chusid RL, Roye DP, et al: Valproate therapy: predisposition to bone fracture. *Pediatr Neurol* 1998;19:143-144.
70. American Academy of Pediatrics: Syphilis. *In*: Pickering LK, Baker CJ, Long SS, et al (eds): *Red Book: 2006 Report of the Committee on Infectious Diseases*, ed 27, American Academy of Pediatrics, Elk Grove Village Ill, 2006, pp 631-644.
71. Moyer VA, Schneider V, Yetman R, et al: Contribution of long-bone radiographs to the management of congenital syphilis in newborn infants. *Arch Pediatr Adolesc Med* 1998;152:353-357.
72. Krogstad P: Clinical features of hematogenous osteomyelitis in children. *UpToDate*, Waltham, Mass, July 2008.
73. Prentice A: Pregnancy and lactation. *In*: Glorieux FH, Pettifor JM, Juppner H (eds): *Pediatric Bone, Biology and Diseases*. Elsevier Science, San Diego, 2003, pp 249-269.
74. Kovacs CS: Fetal mineral homeostasis. *In*: Glorieux FH, Pettifor JM, Juppner H (eds): *Pediatric Bone, Biology and Diseases*. Elsevier Science, San Diego, 2003, pp 271-302.
75. Backstrom MC, Kuusela AL, Maki R: Metabolic bone disease of prematurity. *Ann Med* 1996;28:275-282.
76. Beyers N, Alheit B, Taljaard JF, et al: High turnover osteopenia in preterm babies. *Bone* 1994;15:5-13.
77. Dahlenburg SL, Bishop NJ, Lucas A: Are preterm infants at risk for subsequent fractures? *Arch Dis Child* 1989;64:1384-1385.
78. Amir J, Katz K, Grunebaum M, et al: Fractures in premature infants. *J Pediatr Orthop* 1988;8:41-44.
79. Moyer-Mileur L, Luetkemeier M, Boomer L, et al: Effect of physical activity on bone mineralization in premature infants. *J Pediatr* 1995;127:620-625.
80. Strathearn L, Gray PH, O'Callaghan MJ, et al: Childhood neglect and cognitive development in extremely low birth weight infants: a prospective study. *Pediatrics* 2001;108:142-151.
81. Phillips RR, Stephen HL: Fractures of long bones occurring in neonatal intensive therapy units. *Br Med J* 1990;301:225-226.
82. Habert J, Haller JO: Iatrogenic vertebral body compression fractures in a premature infant caused by extreme flexion during positioning for a lumbar puncture. *Pediatr Radiol* 2000;30:410-411.
83. Smurthwaite D, Wright N, Russell S, et al: How common are rib fractures in extremely low birth weight preterm infants? *Arch Dis Child Fetal Neonatal Ed* 2009;94:F138-F139.
84. Beary JF, Chines AA: Clinical features and diagnosis of osteogenesis imperfecta. *UpToDate*, Waltham, Mass, 2008.
85. Plotkin H, Primorac D, Rowe D: Osteogenesis imperfecta. *In*: Glorieux FH, Pettifor JM, Juppner H (eds): *Pediatric Bone, Biology and Diseases*. Elsevier Science, San Diego, 2003, pp 443-471.
86. Cheung MS, Glorieux FH: Osteogenesis imperfecta: update on presentation and management. *Rev Endocr Metab Disord* 2008;9:153-160.
87. Chavassieux P, Seeman E, Delmas PD: Insights into material and structural basis of bone fragility from diseases associated with fractures: how determinants of the biomechanical properties of bone are compromised by disease. *Endocr Rev* 2007;28:151-164.
88. Ablin DS, Greenspan A, Reinhart M, et al: Differentiation of child abuse from osteogenesis imperfecta. *AJR Am J Roentgenol* 1989;154:1035-1046.
89. Plotkin H: Syndromes with congenital brittle bones. *BMC Pediatr* 2004;4:16.
90. Augarten A, Laufer J, Szeinberg A, et al: Child abuse, osteogenesis imperfecta and the grey zone between them. *J Med* 1993;24:171-175.
91. Smith R: Osteogenesis imperfecta, non-accidental injury, and temporary brittle bone disease. *Arch Dis Child* 1995;72:169-176.
92. Jenny C, Committee on Child Abuse and Neglect: Evaluating infants and young children with multiple fractures. *Pediatrics* 2006;118:1299-1303.
93. Byers PH, Krakow D, Nunes ME, et al: Genetic evaluation of suspected osteogenesis imperfecta. *Genet Med* 2006;8:383-388.
94. Taitz LS: Child abuse and osteogenesis imperfecta. *Br Med J* 1987;295:1082-1083.
95. Lachman RS, Krakow D, Kleinman PK: Differential diagnosis II: osteogenesis imperfecta. *In*: Kleinman PK (ed): *Diagnostic Imaging of Child Abuse*, ed 2, Mosby, St Louis, 1987, pp 197-213.
96. Sillence DO, Senn A, Danks DM: Genetic heterogeneity in osteogenesis imperfecta. *J Med Genet* 1976;16:101-116.
97. Paterson CR: Osteogenesis imperfecta and other bone disorders in the differential diagnosis of unexplained fractures. *J R Soc Med* 1990;83:72-74.
98. Paterson CR, Burns J, McAllion SJ: Reply to Dr. Bawle: temporary brittle bone disease. *Am J Med Genet* 1994;49:131-132.
99. Paterson CR, McAllion SJ: Osteogenesis imperfecta in the differential diagnosis of child abuse. *Br Med J* 1989;299:1451-1454.
100. Chapman S, Hall CM: Non-accidental injury or brittle bones. *Pediatr Radiol* 1996;27:106-110.
101. Ablin DS, Sane SM: Non-accidental injury: confusion with temporary brittle bone disease and mild osteogenesis imperfecta. *Pediatr Radiol* 1997;27:111-113.

32

Abusive Fractures

Kim Kaczor, MS, and Mary Clyde Pierce, MD

A fracture is an incomplete or complete break in the continuity of bone resulting from excessive stress and/or an abnormal weakness in the bone structure.[1,2] The likelihood of fracture and the amount of energy required to produce a fracture is dependent on intrinsic and extrinsic variables, including the age and bone health of the child, direction and rate of loading, and the tension in the surrounding muscle. Different energy levels and loading characteristics create distinctly different failure patterns or fracture characteristics. The stage of healing also contributes to the characteristics of the fracture. Collectively, these fracture characteristics are known as the fracture morphology and include:

- The specific fracture location along the bone (e.g., epiphyseal, diaphyseal, metaphyseal)
- The fracture type (e.g., transverse, oblique, spiral, buckle, CML)
- Whether there is displacement, separation, or comminution of the fracture
- Whether the fracture is open or closed
- Whether there is more than one fracture along the bone
- The extent of callus formation, if present

Knowledge of how bone structure and material properties affect bone strength and how bone responds to load is essential to understanding fractures in children and discerning the validity of the stated cause of injury and the resultant fracture (see chapters 31 and 35). The goal of this chapter is to provide an evidence-based framework to evaluate fractures in children by applying logical reasoning to the determination of injury plausibility.

Fractures account for 10% to 25% of childhood injuries,[3] with 125.5 total fracture cases per 100,000 children ages 0 to 35 months. One quarter of fractures in children less than 12 months of age are attributable to abuse. This proportion decreases to 2.9% in children 24 to 35 months of age.[4] Some fracture types are highly specific for abuse, but no fracture type is inherently diagnostic or pathognomonic of abusive or accidental trauma (Table 32-1).[5] Therefore, when a child is diagnosed with a fracture, a determination of injury plausibility must be made.

FRACTURE ASSESSMENT AND INJURY PLAUSIBILITY

"Possible" is not the same as "plausible." Although it might be possible for a fracture to occur from a given history, possibility alone does not constitute plausibility. The evaluation of injury plausibility is a multiple-step process requiring a careful and directed history, physical, and psychosocial examination. The history obtained by the medical care provider helps determine whether the particular type and magnitude of loading required to result in the fracture was likely generated from the described cause. In addition to injury and history compatibility, plausibility also includes: how the cause of injury is described by the caregiver; whether the cause of injury is described in a consistent and credible way; whether signs and symptoms are consistent with the details of the history provided; and whether other injuries are present. If more than one fracture or injury is identified, the same rigorous assessment must be applied for each additional injury.

For example, it might be possible for an ambulating child to sustain a femur fracture from falling down the stairs, but if the fracture is severe and there is a delay in seeking care, and/or the child is described as behaving normally and walking after the fall, and/or other serious injuries are identified, then the specific story is not credible and the specific injuries and fracture type are inconsistent with the historical account. The injury is not a plausible accident.

THE PROVIDED VERSUS THE OBTAINED HISTORY

It is important to note that the provided history of injury does not always differentiate between abusive and accidental injuries in children. The "provided" history, however, plays a critical role in guiding the "obtained" history. The "provided" history is information volunteered by the child or caregiver regarding the injury event. The "obtained" history is information solicited by the health care provider pertinent to assessing the injury and history compatibility. The provided history influences the type of questions that are asked to obtain specific details about the injury event.

The caregiver might be cognizant of pertinent details but unaware of their importance for injury reconstruction, so it is up to the interviewer to obtain those details through directed questions. If the history is inconsistent, implausible, or changing, the concern for abusive injury increases. For example, when a child has a complete and overlapping transverse fracture of the femur, it is structurally impossible for the child to walk. If the caregiver states that a child walked normally after the injury, the history is fabricated. In contrast, some fracture types allow a degree of load bearing, but with pain or tenderness. In those cases, history that the

Table 32-1	**Specificity of Radiologic Findings as Indicators of Abuse**

High Specificity

Classic metaphyseal lesions
Rib fractures, especially posterior
Scapular fractures
Sternal fractures

Moderate Specificity

Multiple fractures, especially bilateral
Fractures of different ages
Epiphyseal separations
Vertebral body fractures and subluxations
Digital fractures
Complex skull fractures

Common, but Low Specificity

Subperiosteal new bone formation
Clavicle fractures
Long bone fractures
Linear skull fractures

Adapted from Kleinman PKK (ed): *Diagnostic imaging of child abuse*, ed 2, Mosby, Chicago, 1998, p 9.

child limped with pain after the injury is plausible. Table 32-2 provides a framework for obtaining a detailed and directed history.

Examples of radiographs and illustrations of injury events with the corresponding biodynamics are shown in Figures 32-1 to 32-10. Table 32-3 summarizes the types of loading required to obtain specific fracture morphologies. Table 32-4 provides a summary of the key elements to assess, concepts to consider, and questions or actions that will help evaluate injury plausibility.

BONY INJURIES

Overview of Fracture Incidence

Leventhal et al[4] evaluated the incidence and proportion of fractures attributable to abuse in infants and young children (up to 36 months) in the United States by bone injured and age of the child (Table 32-5). Their findings represent the 2003 data of 3438 hospitals in 36 states, accounting for more than 85% of the U.S. population.

Fractures in Different Stages of Healing

A single unexplained healing fracture or multiple fractures in different stages of healing are highly suspicious for abuse.[6-8] O'Neill et al[9] performed a retrospective review of 110 children evaluated for child abuse; 28 infants and children had skeletal injuries, of which 20 were found to have old fractures in various stages of healing.[9] Fractures of different ages indicate that the child sustained traumatic forces multiple times.

Subperiosteal New Bone Formation

Subperiosteal new bone formation (SPNBF) is a sign of increased metabolic activity in the underlying bone. When shear or torsion loads are applied to bones, the periosteum can separate from the bone, leading to subperiosteal hemorrhage. Radiographically, SPNBF appears as a thin or hazy layer of cortical bone separated from the bone by a thin dark line.[5] The presence of SPNBF is often an indication that the child's bone has been injured. Caretakers of infants with SPNBF have confessed to shaking children or grabbing, twisting, or yanking the involved extremities.[2] SPNBF that is symmetrical can be a normal finding in young infants.

Multiple Fractures

When a child is diagnosed with multiple fractures, the extent of the skeletal injuries is rarely explained by the history. A greater proportion of children with abusive trauma have multiple fractures as compared with children with accidental trauma. As the number of fractures increases, the likelihood of abuse also increases.[4,9-12] King et al[10] analyzed 189 cases of child abuse (ages <1 month to 13 years) and found 429 fractures; 50% of the children had 1 fracture, 21% had 2 fractures; 12% had 3 fractures; and 17% had 4 to 15 fractures. O'Neill et al[9] conducted a retrospective review of 110 children ages 3 weeks to 11 years who were evaluated for child abuse. In nearly one third, fractures were identified, and of those with fractures, 83% (n = 29) had multiple fractures.[9] Akbarnia et al[13] reviewed the records of children admitted with "battered child syndrome," and 74 children were found to have a total of 264 fractures. The children averaged 3.6 fractures per child (range 1-15 fractures). Another study reported a fourfold to sixfold increase in the likelihood of abuse in children less than 36 months of age with three or more fractures compared with children with an isolated fracture (Table 32-6).[4]

Worlock et al[11] compared fractures resulting from abuse to accidental fractures in children less than 60 months of age (Table 32-7). More than half of the children (54%) in the abuse group had three or more fractures compared with none of the children with accidental trauma. In addition, 71% of the abused children had significant bruising, compared with 0.8% of the children in the accident group.[11] In comparison, Sawyer et al[14] analyzed the fracture patterns in children and young adults who fell from significant heights of 10 feet (Table 32-8). Despite significant fall heights (10-40 feet), the average fracture rate was less than two fractures per patient.

While bone diseases can result in more than one fracture, the fracture rate in children with bone abnormalities is still lower than that typically observed in the abused population.[14] Although metabolic disorders should be considered when multiple fractures are identified, the presence of a metabolic disorder does not exclude the possibility of abuse.[15] The diagnostic workup for abuse should occur concomitantly with diagnostic tests for bone disease.[16]

Table 32-2 A Framework to Obtain a Detailed and Directed History

Trauma Chief Complaint with Concern of Injury	Abnormal Sign or Symptom Chief Complaint with Absence of Trauma
Prior to Injury Event	*Prior to Noticing Abnormality*
What was the initial position of the child?	What was the child doing?
Was the child in motion (e.g., running, walking)?	Was anyone else around the child?
	When was the last time the child was free of the abnormality?
During the Injury Event	*At the Time of Noticing Abnormality*
What were the dynamics?	What is the abnormality (e.g., limp, swelling, disuse)?
What was the distance of the fall?	When did you first notice the abnormality?
Were any objects impacted (e.g., coffee table)?	What was the child doing?
What body part landed first?	Was anyone else present?
Did the child fall alone or with a person or object (e.g., car seat, walker)?	
Environmental Factors	*Environmental Factors*
What was the landing surface type (e.g., carpet, wood)?	Where was the child when the abnormality was first noticed (e.g., crib, couch, day care)?
Was the surface wet or slippery?	What is the environment like where the child was first noticed to have the abnormality (e.g., type of crib, presence of bumper pads, rail up/down)?
For stair falls, how many steps did the child fall down? What is the surface type of the stairs and the landing?	Possible injurious surface types in the child's vicinity (e.g., radiator, fireplace, stairs)?
After the Injury Event	*After Noticing Abnormality*
How much time elapsed before seeking medical attention?	How much time elapsed before seeking medical attention?
What was the final landing position of the child?	What were the actions of the child (e.g., get up, walk, remain still)?
What were the actions of the child (e.g., get up, walk, remain still)?	What were the behaviors of the child (e.g., cry, irritable, fussy, no change)?
What were the behaviors of the child (e.g., cry, irritable, fussy, no change)?	What was the behavior of the child during normal child care activities (e.g., dressing, diaper changes, strapping in car seat)?
What was the behavior of the child during normal child care activities (e.g., dressing, diaper changes, strapping in car seat)?	Was there any specific action that seemed to cause the child pain?

Fractures with a High Specificity for Abuse

Classic Metaphyseal Lesions (CML). The CML is a very concerning injury with "... a high predictive value for abuse in infants (<1 year of age).[17]" CMLs occur most often in infants less than 6 months of age.[18] The CML is not the most common fracture encountered in child abuse, but is the fracture type most often found in fatal abuse cases.[17] Diaphyseal fractures occur four times more commonly than metaphyseal fractures, but the CML has a greater specificity for abuse.[5,19]

The histopathology of the CML shows "...a subepiphyseal planar series of microfractures through the most immature portion of metaphyseal bone.[20]" The fracture involves disruption of the primary spongiosa and calcified cartilage core at the metaphysis of long bones, the site where maximum bone growth and turnover is occurring.

Radiographically, the CML often appears as a "corner" or "bucket handle" fracture (Figure 32-11). This variance in the radiographic appearance results from many factors including: (1) the shape of the metaphysis involved; (2) the age of the lesion; (3) the plane of the x-ray beam with regard to the fracture plane; (4) whether the fracture is complete or incomplete; (5) the severity of the trabecular disruption and extent of fracture displacement; and (6) the quality of the radiographs.[20] The disruption and displacement of individual trabeculae allow the bony injury to become visible on radiographs. Once enough disruption occurs and or healing begins, the bony injury becomes radiographically apparent. Of note, microscopic trabecular injury without radiographic evidence has been described by Kleinman et al.[20]

The proximal tibia, distal femur, and proximal humerus are the most common sites for occurrence of CMLs in the abused infant, often occurring bilaterally.[17,21] More than 50% of CMLs were found to involve the knees. Of interest, CML injuries of the distal femur always involved the medial margins, which underscore the importance of an especially careful inspection of this area, including high-quality radiographic imaging in all cases of suspected infant abuse.[22]

The mechanistic failure of bone when loaded under shear or tension is typically transverse or planar. Both intrinsic and extrinsic factors create the unique fracture morphology of the CML. First, the metaphysis of the developing bone has microanatomical and physiological features that result in vulnerability to tensile or shearing forces. As new bone is laid down and older bone is resorbed to allow for growth and remolding, cartilaginous cores are mineralized, forming immature trabeculae. As older trabeculae are removed by osteoclasts to allow for growth and expansion, many holes are created in the region of maximum growth. Just distal to this area of maximum growth is the actual growth plate (epiphysis), which is surrounded by a fibrous terminal extension of the periosteum, termed the subperiosteal collar.[23] This collar surrounds the epiphysis and provides increased biomechanical strength to the growth plate, but also leaves the region of maximum growth just proximal to the collar more susceptible to injury. Under normal circumstances and everyday activity of the nonambulating infant, this region remains healthy and highly functional. Shearing or tensile loads, however, lead to microfailure of trabeculae through the susceptible primary spongiosa. Trabecular bone separates immediately at the point of fracture as a result of a tensile load because it does not contain Haversian systems in its architecture.[24] Tensile loadings could be generated during violent shaking of a child by an adult if the extremities

	Types of Loading Required to Obtain Specific Fracture Morphologies and Biodynamic Examples
Table 32-3	
Biomechanical Conditions	**Fracture Types**
Torsional loading (Figures 32-1, A and B)	Spiral/long oblique
Bending load (Figures 32-2, A and B)	Transverse/short oblique
Compressive loading (Figures 32-3, A and B)	Buckle/impaction
Tension and/or shear loading (Figure 32-11)	Classic metaphyseal lesion
High-energy event (Figure 32-12)	Open and/or comminuted

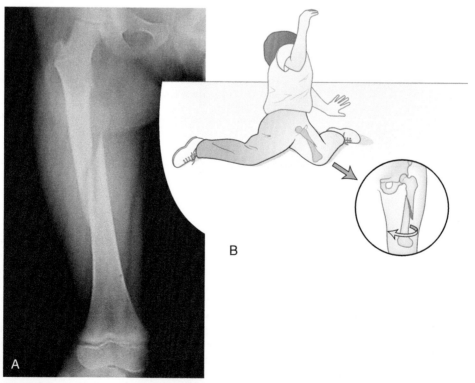

FIGURE 32-1 A, AP view spiral femur fracture. **B,** Example of a history with biodynamics that account for torsional loading: twisting (or rotation) of the leg as the child slips and the leg folds underneath the body.

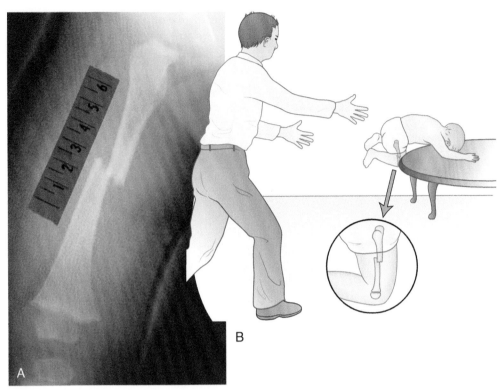

FIGURE 32-2 A, AP view of transverse femur fracture. **B,** Example of a history with biodynamics that account for bending load. Perpendicular impact of the leg.

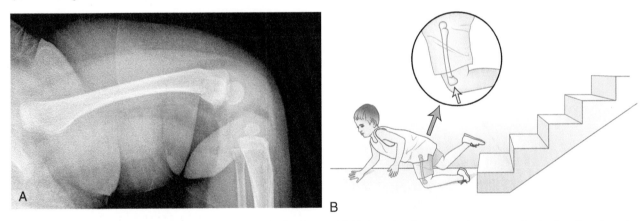

FIGURE 32-3 A, Lateral view of buckle fracture. **B,** Example of a history with biodynamics that account for compressive loading. Knee impacts along the longitudinal axis of the femur as child falls down the stairs.

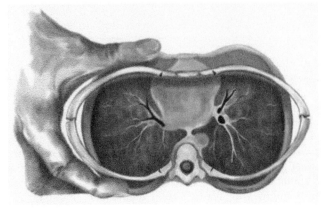

FIGURE 32-4 Common mechanism of infant rib fractures. *(Adapted from Lonergan GF, Baker AM, Morey MK, et al: Child abuse radiologic-pathologic correlation.* Radiographics *2003;23:812.)*

were flailing during the assault. The metaphysis is also exposed to tensile loading by the caregiver grabbing and forcefully yanking a child by the extremity or twisting the extremity to the point of fracture.[2,23,24]

CML injuries caused by tensile and torsional loading from accidental trauma also have been reported.[25,26] Accidental CMLs have occurred during difficult breech deliveries and by manipulations required for club foot repair, where combined loadings of torsion and tension are applied to the bone. These accidental injury scenarios provide insight into the types of loads experienced by abused infants with CMLs.

Rib fractures. Rib fractures account for 5% to 51% of all fractures in studies of abused children.[27] In comparison, in children with accidental trauma, rib fractures account for less than 1% of all fractures.[28] Motor vehicle collisions and pedestrians hit by cars are two events that can result in

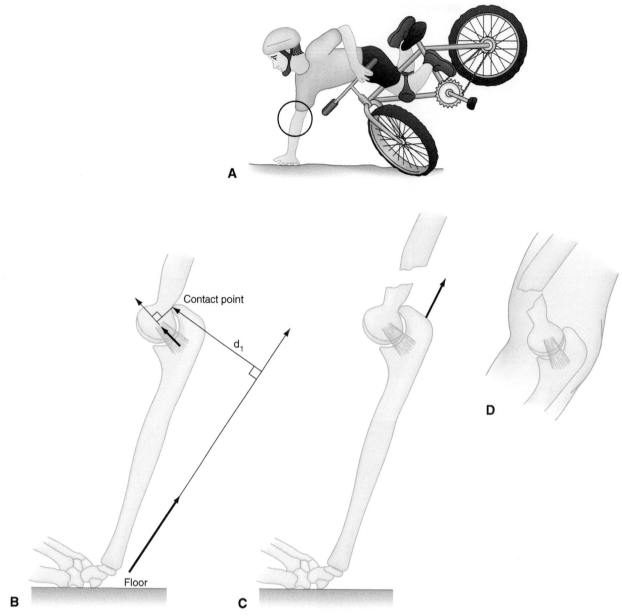

FIGURE 32-5 Mechanism of injury of supracondylar fracture. **A,** Fall on an outstretched arm produces hyperextension of elbow. **B,** Ulna levers against distal humerus. **C,** Humerus fails, triceps exerts unopposed force. **D,** Distal fragment displaces. *(Adapted from Geiderman JM: Humerus and elbow. In: Marx JA [ed]: Rosen's Emergency Medicine: Concepts and Clinical Practice, ed 6, Mosby, Philadelphia, 2006.)*

accident-related rib fractures. In young children, however, rib fractures from accidental causes are uncommon.[11,29] In one study of accidental fractures, only one of 826 children had rib fractures, which resulted from a severe blunt chest trauma during a traffic accident.[11]

The majority of the infants diagnosed with rib fractures resulting from abuse do not have a history of trauma. They often have nonspecific respiratory complaints, a history of fever, irritability, GI complaints, seizures, or changes in mental status attributable to an accompanying intracranial injury.[28] Most rib fractures are clinically unsuspected and detected on a skeletal survey or bone scan.[19] Occasionally,

caregivers report hearing or feeling a "popping" on the chest wall. When infants are irritable due to rib fractures, efforts to comfort them such as picking them up, patting, or rocking often do not console them and result in paradoxical crying.

When unsuspected rib fractures are found in infants, birth trauma and resuscitation efforts are explanations sometimes given by caretakers.[30-34] Rib fractures due to birth trauma, however, rarely occur.[35-36] Bhat et al[35] screened for birth injuries in nearly 35,000 infants and found no rib fractures. Other investigators have reported five cases of infants with rib fractures from birth trauma—all involving infants with large birth weight for gestational age or histories

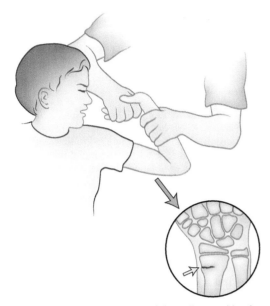

FIGURE 32-6 Compression fracture of the radius resulting from intentional bending of the forearm in order to cause pain.

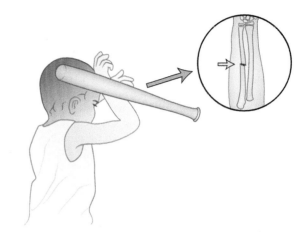

FIGURE 32-8 Protective positioning of the arm resulting in a transverse fracture of the ulna.

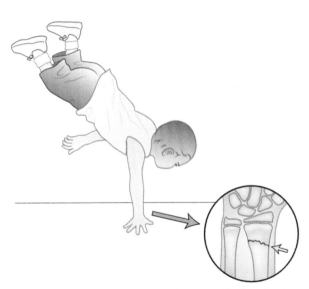

FIGURE 32-7 Fall onto an outstretched arm resulting in a distal forearm fracture.

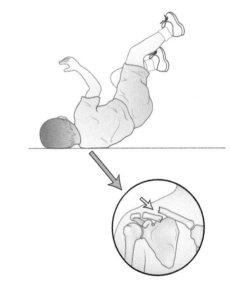

FIGURE 32-9 Clavicle fracture resulting from a fall onto the shoulder.

of difficult deliveries, including shoulder dystocia and forceps/vacuum-assisted extraction.[37-40] Information about the type of delivery and physical examination findings at birth are helpful in determining the plausibility of birth trauma as the cause of the rib fracture. An experienced radiologist can apply dating criteria for rib fractures to help assess whether birth trauma could have been the cause.[41]

Rib fractures from cardiopulmonary resuscitation are uncommonly reported.[32,33] Hoke and Chamberlain[42] compiled all the published skeletal injuries secondary to cardiopulmonary resuscitation (CPR) in children. They found five studies involving a total of 770 children that matched their criteria.[30-34] From this cohort of children, only three cases of rib fractures in infants and children were attributed to CPR. Betz and Leibhardt[30] also investigated whether rib fractures in children can be caused by resuscitation efforts. Out of the

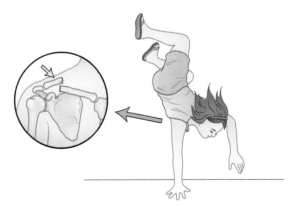

FIGURE 32-10 Clavicle fracture resulting from a fall onto an outstretched arm.

94 resuscitated natural death victims, two had bilateral rib fractures localized in the midclavicular line. The consensus of the current evidence-based literature is that rib fractures from CPR are exceedingly rare.[30,31,33,34,43] One recent study, however, found very subtle anteriolateral rib fractures in 11% of 70 infants who died of natural causes and had been unsuccessfully resuscitated.[44] The fractures were not recognized until the parietal pleura was stripped and the ribs carefully examined. In seven cases there were multiple fractures, and bilateral fractures were found in five cases.

In infants less than 1 year of age, 69.4% of rib fractures are attributable to abuse (Table 32-5). Most abuse-related rib fractures (65%-87%) are found in children under 2 years of age.[4,19] Barsness et al[28] conducted a retrospective study of children 3 weeks to 15 years of age to quantify the association of rib fractures with child abuse. They evaluated more than 3700 children with trauma and identified 78 with rib fractures, of which 51 (65%) were victims of abuse. In children younger than 3 years, the presence of a rib fracture had a positive predictive value for physical abuse of 95%.

The location of the rib fracture helps to discern compatibility between the reported history and the resultant injury. The injury mechanism for rib fractures in the posterior or lateral positions involves anterior-posterior compression. Kleinman and Schlesinger[45] describe the biomechanics of the fractures as follows:

"The posterior ribs and their vertebral articulation act as a lever mechanism. A lever is a rigid bar free to pivot on a fixed point or fulcrum. ... The effort is applied to the ventral portion of the rib, which results in levering of the posterior rib on the transverse process, loading the costovertebral articulation. Assuming that the costovertebral ligaments are stronger than the rib, mechanical failure will occur in the portion of the rib near the fulcrum (fixed point), resulting in fracture near the costotransverse process articulation.[45]"

Figure 32-4 demonstrates this concept.

Rib fractures due to physical child abuse are often located posteriorly and are commonly bilateral. Bulloch et al[40] analyzed rib fractures in infants less than 12 months old.

Table 32-4	**Elements to Assess When Evaluating Injury Plausibility and Fracture Cases in Children**	
Key Elements	**Concepts to Consider**	**Questions or Actions to Help Evaluate Key Elements**
Injury compatibility—Is the fracture morphology accounted for in described injury mechanism?	• Type of loading • Direction and magnitude of force • High or low energy event	The fracture reflects the magnitudes and direction of the applied loads. • What loading failure is reflected by the fracture? • Is the fracture type reflective of high or low energy? Conversely, the described mechanism implies the magnitudes and directions of the loading. • What is the direction and magnitude of the load that can be extrapolated from the described mechanism? • Did the described mechanism provide the required level of energy and type of loading needed to produce the fracture?
History quality—Is the provided history consistent? Is the obtained history detailed?	• The "provided history" is information volunteered by the child or caregiver regarding the injury event. • The "obtained history" is information solicited by the physician pertinent to assessing the injury and history compatibility.	• Is the story consistent from the same caregiver and among different caregivers? • Is the story absent, vague, expanding, or changing in order to explain the injuries or the severity of injury? • Is the caregiver able to respond to directed questions with relevant details?
Developmental compatibility—Are the developmental capabilities of the parties involved congruent with the history?	• Each child's capabilities are unique and must be evaluated individually in order to assess the feasibility of the provided information.	• What is the developmental stage of the child? • What is the child capable of doing?
Postinjury compatibility—Are the described actions and demeanor of the child after the injury consistent with the physical limitations produced by the injury?	• Specific injuries alter anatomy and physiology thereby altering function. • Descriptions of a child's behavior after injury should be consistent with the functionality changes from the injury.	• How did the child act immediately after the injury? • What did the child do?

Table 32–4 Elements to Assess When Evaluating Injury Plausibility and Fracture Cases in Children—cont'd

Key Elements	Concepts to Consider	Questions or Actions to Help Evaluate Key Elements
Timing—Is there a delay in seeking care or a delay in the development of signs/ symptoms?	Inappropriate reasons for a delay in seeking care: • The perpetrator does not want to be discovered and therefore avoids seeking medical attention. • The injury and the child's pain are perceived as minimal or unimportant and reflected in the caregiver's lack of action. • The needs of the caregiver supersede the well-being of the child. • Illicit actions, intoxication, or mental illness of the caregiver adversely affect judgment. • The child is objectified, devoid of importance, or perceived as "property" by the caregiver. Consequently, the child's injury has minimal priority and efforts to seek care occur on caregiver's terms. • A third party arrives at the scene and decides to seek care. Delay in development of signs or symptoms: • Some types of injuries require time to develop the inflammation needed for the injury to become apparent. A delay in seeking care in these circumstances reflects a delay in the development of signs or symptoms; not necessarily indicative of willful neglect.	• When did the caregiver notice something was wrong? • Is the timing of the stated observation consistent with the anatomy, physiology, and functional change caused by the injury? • Is there oxymoronic behavior? Caregivers words and actions are incongruent. • What lead to medical attention being sought? • Did the person taking care of the child at the time of the injury try to dissuade others from seeking care for the child? • Does the lack of action reflect a devoid of caring?
Presence of other injuries— Visual inspection and palpation	• The presence of an injury indicates that the injury threshold has been exceeded. • If multiple injuries are present, the described mechanism must account for the energy and loading required to produce each injury. • Injury to the skin is a visible and easily recognizable form of trauma only requiring a careful and detailed examination. • Palpation can help identify injuries that might otherwise be occult.	• What injuries are discovered through multiple means of investigation? • What is the summary of all of the child's injuries, present and past?
Diagnostic tests Review of prior records	• The exact location of each injury is critical in the injury reconstruction process • Diagnostic imaging and laboratory studies allow the detection of injuries that may not be readily apparent. • Review of prior records allows the detection of injuries that are no longer present but may indicate a pattern of recurrent or escalating injury indicative of the battered child syndrome.	• Head and abdominal imaging • Skeletal imaging • Laboratory studies to evaluate for abdominal organ and muscle injury • Review all records for evidence of any prior injuries including bruises and histories of falls. • Review records for prior medical diagnoses for possible missed trauma (ALTE, seizures, vomiting without diarrhea, irritability, colic).
Social history—Are there concerning social risk factors?	• Many abusers are not forthright about prior social service involvement, domestic violence, and criminal activity, all of which are important when assessing the circumstances surrounding the child's injury. • Trained social workers are highly skilled at obtaining additional information that can help identify otherwise occult risk of injury.	• Are hospital social services available to assist with risk assessment? • Will state social service involvement provide critical information inaccessible to hospital personnel? • Do the factors of the case reach the level required for mandated reporting of child abuse?

Table 32-5	Weighted Proportions of Abusive Fractures Attributable to Abuse, According to Age and Bone, in the 2003 KID

	0-11 mo			12-23 mo			24-35 mo			0-35 mo		
	No.	Proportion from Abuse		No.	Proportion from Abuse		No.	Proportion from Abuse		No.	Proportion from Abuse	
		%	No.		%	No.		%	No.		%	No.
Ribs	809	69.4	561	96	28.5	27	96	27.6	26	1001	61.4	615
Radius/ulna	261	62.1	162	103	19.8	20	293	4.7	14	657	29.8	196
Tibia/fibula	493	58	286	192	16.1	31	384	4.7	18	1069	31.1	332
Humerus	518	43.1	223	545	6.8	37	2108	1.6	34	3172	9.3	295
Femur	1257	30.5	383	761	4.8	36	3008	2.5	75	4026	11.7	471
Clavicle	227	28.1	64	65	16.7	11	95	6	6	388	20.7	80
Skull	3363	17.1	575	948	8.6	81	1575	3.7	58	5886	12.1	712

Adapted from Leventhal JM, Martin KD, Asnes AG: Incidence of fractures attributable to abuse in young hospitalized children: results from analysis of a United States database. *Pediatrics* 2008;122:602.

Table 32-6	Weighted Proportions of Abusive Fractures and Numbers of Fractures in the 2003 KID

	1 Fracture		2 Fractures		≥3 Fractures	
Age (mo)	No.	Proportion from Abuse, %	No.	Proportion from Abuse, %	No.	Proportion from Abuse, %
0-11	5076	18.5	477	55.1	298	85.4
12-23	2489	5.7	149	26.1	39	30.8
24-35	6306	2.6	248	6.2	62	17.6
Total	13,870	9	873	36.3	399	69.5

Adapted from Leventhal JM, Martin KD, Asnes AG: Incidence of Fractures Attributable to Abuse in Young Hospitalized Children: Results From Analysis of a United States Database. *Pediatrics* 2008;122:602.

Table 32-7	Number of Children with Multiple Fractures Due to Abusive and Accidental Trauma

	Number of Fractures		
	1	2	3+
Abuse (n = 35)	9	7	19
Accident (n = 116)	97	19	0

Table generated from the data of Worlock P, Stower M, Barbor PM, et al: Patterns of fractures in accidental and non-accidental injury in children: a comparative study. *Br Med J* 1986;293:100-102.

Thirty-two out of 39 (82%) infants had rib fractures due to abuse, and 20 of the 32 (63%) had fractures located posteriorly. The 32 infants had a total of 119 fractures; 112 of the 119 (94%) fractures were located posteriorly or laterally.

Smurthwaite et al[46] studied rib fractures in extremely low birth weight infants in an intensive care unit and found that 7% had anterior or lateral rib fractures, but no infant had posterior rib fractures, which are most commonly observed in cases of physical abuse.

In addition to the location of the fracture along the rib, the specific rib fractured can serve as an indicator of abuse. Strouse and Owings[47] noted the rarity of fractures of the first rib and determined that most are found in abused children.[48]

Multiple rib fractures also have been found to be more common in abused children. Barsness et al[28] found an average of 5.9 rib fractures in a series of abuse victims while

Table 32-8	Fracture Patterns in Children and Young Adults Who Fall from Significant Heights			
	Age	**# of Patients**	**# of Fractures**	**Average Fractures/Patient**
Infant/toddlers	0-2 years	25	19	0.76
Children	3-10 years	55	55	1
Adolescents/young adults	11-21 years	30	56	1.9

Table generated from the data of Sawyer JR, Flynn JM, Dormans JP, et al: Fracture patterns in children and young adults who fall from significant heights. *J Pediatr Orthop* 2000;20:197-202.

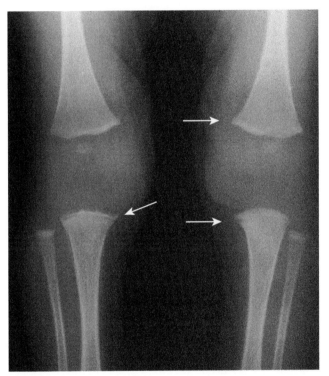

FIGURE 32-11 Radiograph of classic metaphyseal lesions (CML), at arrows.

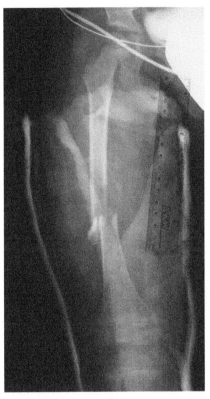

FIGURE 32-12 A comminuted femur fracture resulting from a "high energy event."

children with accidental trauma averaged 1.2 fractures. Worlock et al[11] found fractures of the ribs to be the most common injury in children who had been abused. Additionally, no abused child in their study had only a rib fracture; all had other manifestations of abuse. Therefore, when rib fractures are present, appropriate evaluation for other injuries should be performed. An evaluation for intraabdominal trauma should be considered, especially when lower rib fractures are identified.

Garcia et al[48] analyzed trauma registry data of 2080 children aged up to 14 years with blunt or penetrating trauma to assess the importance of rib fractures as a marker of severe injury in children. Thirty-three of the 2080 children sustained rib fractures, all from blunt trauma. Children with rib fractures were found to be more severely injured than children with blunt or penetrating trauma but without rib fractures. Rib fractures were associated with a high risk of death, with the risk of mortality increasing with the number of ribs fractured. Victims of child abuse (n = 7) had a mean of 4.6

ribs fractured compared with a mean of 4.7 ribs fractured for crash occupants (n = 7) and a mean of 1.3 ribs fractured for children with fall injuries (n = 3). In this study closed head injury was one of the most common injuries associated with rib fractures. Children with concomitant head and thoracic injuries had a 100% increase in mortality over children with thoracic injury alone.

Although rib fractures are commonly associated with other skeletal or head injuries, rib fractures were not associated frequently with nearby bruising. In a retrospective review of 192 children with inflicted fractures, 317 rib fractures were identified and only 29 (9.1%) were found to have a nearby bruise.[49]

Scapular Fractures. Scapular fractures are rare, and currently there is a paucity of evidence-based literature with respect to scapular fractures and the pediatric population. The available literature is about adults or includes few children. Additionally, pediatric literature that is generally focused on fractures, fracture patterns, or incidence of fractures in young children makes no mention of scapular fractures, probably because of their low incidence. The protective nature of the surrounding anatomy (rib cage and soft tissue) and the mobility of the scapula have been suggested as two primary reasons for the rarity of scapular fractures.[50]

Scapular fractures are most commonly seen in young and middle aged males.[51] They require high-energy trauma and occur from motor vehicle collisions, falls from heights, convulsive seizures, or direct trauma.[50-52] Child abuse also can result in scapular fractures, although again, they are uncommonly found.[53]

Associated injuries are found in 80% to 95% of patients with scapular fractures.[51] The injuries can be multiple in number and life threatening.[50] Thompson et al[54] report that patients with scapular fractures have an average of 3.9 other major injuries. Injuries found with scapular fractures include upper extremity and thoracic injuries, such as pneumothorax or lung injuries and fractures of the rib, clavicle, humerus, spine and/or pelvis.[55] In a review of 9453 patients with scapular fractures and 2728 randomly selected controls from a national trauma database (trauma patients with no scapular fractures), rib fractures were identified in 52.9% of patients with scapular fractures and 9.9% of controls, lung injury was identified in 47.1% of patients with scapular fractures versus 12.3% of controls, spinal fractures were identified in 29.1% of patients with scapular fractures versus 11.6% of controls, and clavicle fractures were identified in 25.2% of patients with scapular fractures versus 2.8% of controls.[55]

Due to the multiplicity and severity of the commonly associated injuries, the diagnosis of a scapular fracture is often delayed.[51,52] Tadros et al[52] studied the causes of a delayed diagnosis (>24 hr after hospital admission) of scapular fracture in blunt trauma patients aged 8 to 60 years. Eight cases of missed scapular fractures were compared with 56 cases with a timely diagnosis. They concluded that delayed diagnosis can be because of extensive chest injuries overshadowing the scapula on chest radiographs or by use of chest CT technique that did not cover the entire scapula. Three of the eight cases in the missed fracture group were visualized on plain radiography whereas seven of the eight cases were seen on CT. In this study, CT was a more effective imaging modality for the diagnosis of scapular fracture.

The index of suspicion for a scapular fracture should be heightened in cases where there is severe thoracic injury or blunt trauma to the chest.[52,56] Additionally, if a scapular fracture is identified and a history of high-energy or direct blunt trauma is absent, physical abuse must be suspected.

Sternal and Pelvic Fractures. Sternal and pelvic fractures are injuries that are uncommonly observed secondary to abuse. Pelvic fractures have a prevalence of 0.2% among children up to 16 years.[57] Mok[53] found that the pelvis is among the less commonly fractured bones in her review of abusive injury in children. In both accidental and abusive trauma, fractures to the sternum and pelvis most often result from direct blunt force.[27,58] They are caused by high-energy events. In abusive trauma, a sternal or pelvic fracture might indicate the child has been stomped upon. In contrast, in accident-related traumatic events, traffic accidents and falls are the most common causes of sternal and pelvic fractures.

Von Garrel et al[59] analyzed 200 cases of sternal fractures in patients 9 to 96 years of age. They found that 83% resulted from traffic accidents, 13% from falls, and 4% from other (unspecified) events. Of the traffic accidents, 97% were motor vehicle crashes and 92% of those injured were restrained. Additionally, 63.5% of the patients with sternal fractures had concomitant injuries. Rib fractures, pulmonary injuries, and cardiac injuries, respectively, were the most common. Due to the proportion of sternal fracture patients with other injuries, studies such as troponin levels should be considered to rule out injuries such as cardiac contusions. In the case of pelvic fractures, commonly associated injuries include fractures of the proximal femur, soft tissues injuries, and genitourinary injuries.[60] Any child with a pelvic fracture should be screened for additional injuries. If no history of a high-energy, blunt force trauma event is provided, physical abuse should be suspected in a child with a sternal or pelvic fracture.

Vertebral Fractures. Fractures of the vertebral bodies or spinous processes are uncommon sequelae of physical child abuse. According to Kleinman,[61] two thirds of spinal injuries occur in children less than 3 years of age and one half occur in children less than 1 year of age. The average child's age at which spinal fractures are recognized is 22 months (range: 2 months to 10 years). The specific type of spinal injury sustained is influenced by the age and developmental stage of the child. For example, toddlers are more susceptible to injury from direct blows or sudden deceleration while infants are more likely to be shaken.[62]

Most commonly, spine injuries involve compression of the vertebral bodies. Such injuries are observed along a continuum of severity demonstrating imperceptible to diffuse height loss. These injuries can result from axial loading and/or excessive hyperflexion.[61] When a compression fracture is identified, careful observation of the physical findings is critical to understanding the injury mechanism. For example, evidence of scalp swelling associated with a compression fracture could indicate that the child was forcibly slammed down on his/her head.

Kleinman and Marks[63] described the postmortem radiologic and histopathologic findings in four victims of physical abuse with vertebral body fractures. For each of the children, aged 7 to 36 months, compression deformity was evident on ante mortem radiographs obtained during hospitalization. The four children had a total of 10 fractures with a range of 1 to 6 fractures per child. The following fracture patterns were identified: pure compression (n = 3), superior end plate (n = 2), and mixed pattern (n = 5). None of the fractures involved the posterior elements, no epidural blood or spinal cord abnormalities were identified, and no patient had associated extremity injury. Additionally, none of the fractures were suspected based on history, clinical findings, or gross inspection. These cases demonstrate that vertebral fractures can easily be missed when children present for other reasons given that such fractures are commonly asymptomatic. Alternatively, when vertebral fractures are identified, they can be incidental findings on imaging studies for abdominal or other trauma.[61] Vertebral fractures are most common at the thoracolumbar junction, although they can occur at any level.

Hangman fracture is defined as bilateral fractures of the pedicles of C2, and are characterized as "a traumatic spondylolysis of the axis.[61,64,] This is a rare fracture type associated with hyperextension. Only three cases of hangman fracture have been reported secondary to abuse.[64] McGrory and Fenichel[65] describe the case of a 4-month-old with a hangman fracture where the mother reported forcibly shaking the infant by the shoulders. In cases of accidental trauma involving older children and adults, hyperextension because of a motor vehicle collision or fall can result in hangman fractures.[61,64] A hangman fracture is not always associated with neurological deficits. When other injuries typical of abusive trauma are present, these additional findings should help to differentiate a hangman fracture from a primary spondylolysis.[61]

Spinous process fractures appear to result from avulsion of cartilage and/or bone at the interspinous ligamentous attachments. They usually occur in the middle or lower thoracic region or upper lumbar region, and they can be solitary or multiple in number.[61] Kleinman and Zito[62] reviewed the skeletal surveys and clinical records of 19 infants less than 5 months of age. Injuries of the spinous processes were identified in three infants. In addition, each of the infants also had multiple skeletal fractures typical of abuse.[62]

Spinous process injury can result from blunt force trauma or from violent shaking with hyperextension and hyperflexion of the spine. Kleinman[62] points to associated compression fracture to support the role of hyperflexion in such injuries.

Hand Fractures. Only one paper to date focuses on fractures of the hands in abuse victims. Nimkin et al[66] examined the imaging findings of 11 abused infants ranging in age from 2 months to 2 years with fractures of the hands and feet. Six infants had hand fractures. Although there is limited information on hand fractures and abuse, any infant or young child with a hand fracture or any child with bilateral hand fractures should raise the index of suspicion for abuse. Merten et al[19] note that, although uncommon, such fractures are found sufficiently often to include views of the hands and feet in the skeletal survey.

In general, hand fractures in children most commonly result from household- and sports- related injuries.[67-69] Their cause differs with age and developmental stage. Eighty-three percent of toddlers (up to 2 years) and 87% of preschool (2-5 years) aged children sustain hand fractures at home. In comparison, hand fractures at sporting events are more common in younger (5-10 years) and older (10-16 years) school children, occurring in 41% and 34%, respectively.[67] Other investigators have found "punching" to be the most common fracture causation in children 13 to 16 years of age.[69]

Hand fractures are rare in infancy and early childhood.[67-69] The projected incidence of skeletal hand injury in toddlers according to a prospective clinical study conducted by Vadivelu et al[67] is 34 per 100,000 children per year. Mahabir et al[69] studied 242 hand fractures in children under 16 years old; the incidence of hand fracture rose sharply after age 9 and peaked at age 12. Children ages 11 to 16 years had 64% of all hand fractures observed. Worlock and Stower[68] reviewed 137 hand fractures in 136 children less than 12 years old and found a similar pattern in which the incidence of fracture rose sharply after age 8.

Rennie et al[57] studied the epidemiology of fractures in children, and found that fractures of the finger phalanges were among the five most common fractures in the following age groups: 2 to 4, 5 to 11, and 12 to 16 years. However, the incidence increased with age. Metacarpal fractures also are also among the five most common fractures in children in the 5 to 11 and 12 to 16 year age groups. Vadivelu et al[67] report that toddlers predominantly sustain soft tissue injury to the hand (86%); they are most vulnerable to crush injuries and lacerations. Preschoolers have a slightly increased tendency toward bony injury, and older children most commonly sustain bony injuries (77%). In general, the most commonly fractured digit in children is the little finger followed by the thumb.[67-69]

Of the abuse victims with hand fractures in Nimkin et al's study,[66] 7 of the 11 had three or more additional fractures involving the long bones of the upper and lower extremities, and 7 had additional fractures of the ipsilateral extremity. Based on these observations, they concluded that one of the important aspects of a hand (or foot) fracture is that such fractures can serve as potential indicators of more serious injuries. In their study, only one infant had evidence of bruising or swelling. This is supported by the findings of Peters et al,[49] who found bruising associated with fractures in 192 child abuse victims. A total of three metacarpal fractures were identified. None had a bruise near the fracture site.

Foot Fractures. As with hand fractures, only one study has examined abusive foot fractures. Nimkin et al[66] examined the imaging findings of 11 abused infants ranging in age from 2 months to 2 years, with fractures of the hands and feet; five children had a total of seven fractures of the feet. Six of the fractures were metatarsal fractures. Three were healing and three were acute. Four of the six involved the first metatarsal. The seventh fracture was a proximal phalangeal fracture.

Worlock et al[29] compared the fracture patterns of 35 children with physical abuse to 826 controls who had a fracture to the accident department of a university hospital. A total of 923 fractures were observed, including 71 foot fractures in the control population; 11 were identified in toddlers (10-60 months) and 60 were identified in school-age children (> 60 months). The foot was found to have the third highest rate of fracture (7.7%). No foot fractures were observed in the abuse population.[11,29]

Rennie et al[57] found that fractures of the metatarsus are among the five most common fractures in the children 12 to 16 years of age (4.8%). Fractures of the toe phalanges, calcaneus, and midfoot have lower frequencies, but when present, they are most commonly found in children in the 9- to 11-year age range.

Peters et al[49] identified two metatarsal fractures out of 192 fracture cases. Neither had a bruise near the fracture site.

Fractures Common in Both Abusive and Accidental Trauma (Not Specific for Abuse)

Femur Fractures. Femur fractures account for approximately 1.6% of all bony injuries in children.[70] The incidence of femoral fractures has a trimodal distribution with peaks in early infancy, early childhood, and adolescence.[71-73] The high fracture incidence observed in early infancy and early childhood is largely due to abuse and immature bone strength, respectively. The femur is the largest bone in the body, and consequently it is often thought that high energy mechanisms are required to produce a femur fracture. Although, the exact amount of force required to fracture the femur remains unknown, both high and low energy mechanisms are capable of producing such fractures in young children.[71,74,75] In adolescence, once the bone is fully developed, high velocity trauma is required for fracture.[70] Common causes of femur fractures in children include motor vehicle collisions, motor vehicle-pedestrian accidents, falls, and child abuse.[72,76-81]

As developmental capabilities progress, normal play activities, such as a fall while running or a trip with a twist (or rotation) of the leg, can cause torsional load to be applied to the femur, resulting in a spiral fracture. When a spiral fracture is caused by accidental trauma, other injuries are absent and unusual bruising is uncommon.

Blakemore et al[74] analyzed 42 children with isolated femoral shaft fractures and found that children ages 1 to 5 years can sustain femoral shaft fractures from relatively low-energy injuries, such as a fall from a low height or fall while running. Pierce et al[81] studied 29 children less than 3 years of age with femur fractures resulting from reported stair falls. In 25 children ages 6 to 29 months, the history was determined to be plausible, and 4 fractures in children 2 to 36 months were determined to be suspicious for abuse. In each case specific historical details elucidating the biodynamics of the injury event were essential in determining compatibility between the resultant fracture type and the biomechanical conditions, and ultimately, determining the plausibility of the stated cause of injury.

The primary injury mechanisms for femoral fracture are age dependent. Most femur fractures caused by abusive trauma occur in children less than 2 years of age,[73,76,79] and the vast majority of children with abusive femoral fractures are less than 1 year of age.[71,77,78,82] In children younger than walking age, 60% to 70% of femoral fractures are caused by abuse;[75,77,78] and in children less than 4 years of age up to 30% of femoral fractures could be due to abuse.[71]

Beals and Tufts[71] studied 80 femoral fractures in children under 4 years of age and found abused children were younger (average age 9.6 months) compared with nonabused children (average age 22.6 months). Loder et al[77] analyzed nearly 10,000 femur fractures and concluded that femur fractures resulting from abuse occurred almost exclusively in children less than 2 years of age. Nork et al[77] evaluated 21 children younger than 2 years with a fractured femur and identified child abuse as the mechanism of injury in 67% of children younger than 1year of age and 11% of children between 1 and 2 years of age.

Children in early childhood aged 2 to 4 years are also at risk for abuse. Factors such as parental skills, level of support, and developmental issues such as toilet training can add to the stress that sometimes leads to abusive trauma. Fractures in children 2 to 4 years of age can be associated with disciplinary actions that turn violent. This is likely due to unrealistic expectations regarding the child's developmental stage and the resulting frustrations. When evaluating a young child with a fracture, questions directed at toileting issues are sometimes helpful in determining if an inciting event preceded the injury. For example, it may be helpful to ask: "When did the child last soil himself or herself? How is the toilet training progressing? What methods are being used to help the child learn to use the toilet?" In older children, the injury mechanisms are more commonly accidental in nature and include falls for children less than 6 years, motor vehicle-pedestrian accidents for children 6 to 9 years, and motor vehicle collisions for teenagers.[73,76]

Considering all children 18 years of age and younger, most femur fractures occur in the shaft (70%), with 12% occurring proximally and 18% distally.[76] In children less than 4 years of age, 65% of fractures occur in the middiaphysis, 9% proximally, and 25% distally.[8]

Injury type and severity is influenced by the amount of energy that is available in a given injury event. The most common fracture type and location when a child is struck by a fast moving object, or falls from a significant distance, such as from a second story window, is a transverse or short oblique fracture of the middiaphysis (Figure 32-2). Falls from shorter distances that involve impact to the knee most often produce a buckle fracture at the distal one third of the femur at the junction of the diaphyseal-metaphyseal regions (Figure 32-3). Normal play activities, such as a fall while running or a trip with a twist (or rotation) of the leg, can cause torsional load to be applied to the femur and result in a spiral fracture (Figure 32-1). It is a common belief that spiral fractures are highly suspicious for abuse and that the presence of a spiral fracture signifies that the child's leg was twisted and the injury is abusive in nature. Although this is one possible cause of a spiral fracture, other causes exist and the presence of a spiral fracture in itself is *not* diagnostic of abuse or accident. A spiral femur fracture simply indicates that the bone failed under torsional load. The bone structure of the femur is such that the bone is stronger under axial loading than torsional loading. These biomechanical properties of the femur lead to a lower injury threshold for torsional loading. This lower threshold, in combination with the torque that is produced when the foot is caught during a fall while running or a trip with a twist (or rotation) of the leg, yields a set of circumstances that allow the bone to fail without an associated "high-impact" or "high-energy" mechanism. An infant that is nonambulatory cannot autonomously generate this torsional load, and therefore, spiral fractures (of any long bone) in the very young and developmentally immature population are highly suspicious for abuse.

Studies found no differences in fracture characteristics when comparing abused and nonabused children.[71,74,80,82] Scherl et al[80] performed a review of 207 patients younger than 6 years of age with accidental and abusive femoral shaft fractures, of which 76 patients were investigated for possible abuse. The average age was 2.73 years. Mechanisms of injury included pedestrians struck by motor vehicles, falls, motor vehicle crashes, and child abuse. No one fracture type was exclusively associated with accidental or abusive trauma (Table 32-9). Of the 207 patients studied, 76 were investigated for possible child abuse. The average age of the abused children was 0.89 years. Spiral fractures were less common than transverse fractures overall, and no more common in the abused children, but they were overrepresented in cases that were *investigated* for abuse, probably because of the common misconception that spiral fractures are caused by abuse.[80] Pierce et al[81] analyzed femur fractures resulting from stair falls among children 2 to 36 months of age. They found that fracture type alone was not diagnostic or

Table 32-9	Fracture Characteristics of Abused and Nonabused Children		
Fracture Type	Overall	Investigated for Abuse	Positive for Abuse
Transverse	38%	27%	36%
Spiral	27%	39%	36%
Oblique	17%	15%	7%
Unknown	14%	15%	21%
Greenstick, buckle, or butterfly fragment	4%	4%	0%

Table generated from the results of Scherl SA, Miller L, Lively N, et al: Accidental and nonaccidental femur fractures in children. *Clin Orthop Relat Res* 2000;376:99-105.

predictive of abusive or accidental trauma. Stair falls resulted in transverse, spiral, oblique, or buckle fractures, depending on the fall dynamics. In all of the cases of accidental injury, the loading extrapolated from the historical account was consistent with the resultant fracture type. Conversely, when the stated cause of injury or fall dynamics were fabricated, the historical elements and loading type did not correspond to the resultant fracture type.[81] This study underscores the need to obtain a detailed history of the dynamics of the injury event, and emphasizes the importance of not reflexively concluding that the cause of a fracture is abuse or accident based on fracture type alone.

In 65% to 72% of cases, the femoral fracture is an isolated finding.[79,83] When associated injuries are discovered, the mechanism of injury must have a sufficient quantity of energy available and provide the trauma exposure necessary to account for the additional injuries. Three studies of femoral fractures involving a total of 1500 children found associated injuries in 28% to 35% of cases.[79,83,84] The injury mechanisms that led to femur fractures with associated injuries differed significantly from those with isolated femur fractures.[83] Taylor et al[84] found that the majority of associated injuries were present in patients injured in high energy impacts. Anderson[79] found associated injuries in 41 of 117 patients admitted with femoral fractures. Of the 41, 17 were motor vehicle-pedestrian accidents, 9 were motor vehicle-passenger accidents, and 8 were abuse victims.[79] Rewers et al[83] studied 1139 children ages 0 to 17 years with femoral fractures. Associated injuries were present in 28.6% of cases, more often in older children. In children less than 2 years of age with abusive trauma and associated injuries, the affected body regions include, in order of decreasing frequency, extremities, head and neck, chest, abdomen and pelvis, and face. Children who were abused, hit by a car, or involved in a motor vehicle crash (MVC) were 16 to 20 times more likely to have associated injuries than those with a femur fracture as a result of a fall. Falls lead to associated injuries in only 6.2% of cases, compared with 70% of MVC

cases, and 55% of autopedestrian accidents, and 55% of cases with abusive trauma.[83]

These studies speak to the extremely aggressive nature of an assault causing a femur fracture and the degree of violence to which children in abusive environments are subjected. When a child is diagnosed with a femur fracture and abuse is considered among the possible causes, it is imperative that the child undergo a thorough evaluation for other injuries. Equally, when a femur fracture is diagnosed and associated injuries are identified, the historical information must be carefully scrutinized and should account for the multiplicity of injuries.[15]

According to Peters et al,[49] bruising is infrequently identified in extremity fractures of suspected child abuse victims. In their study, only 5 of 60 femur fractures had an associated bruise.

Tibia/Fibula Fractures. Tibial and fibular fractures are the third most common pediatric long bone fracture; 50% to 70% of tibial fractures occur in the distal one third and the least commonly affected portion of the tibia is the proximal one third. In child abuse, however, the proximal tibia is one of the most common sites for the CML.[21] The proportion of tibial fractures due to abuse in infants exceeds 50%.[4] King et al[10] reported in their study of battered children that the tibia was injured in 26% of all abused children with a fracture.

Tibial and fibular fractures are relatively common skeletal injures once the child begins to ambulate. The classic "toddler fracture" occurs from seemingly innocuous trauma. The toddler fracture is most often a subtle spiral or oblique nondisplaced fracture of the mid or distal tibia. The child can have only a history of a limp and no known traumatic event or a minor event such as a trip or misstep. If the child has a fracture of tibia or fibula but is not yet ambulating, the fracture is highly concerning, and, by definition, cannot be diagnosed as a "toddler" fracture. Spiral or nondisplaced oblique fractures of the tibia can be caused by both accidents and abuse. An abusive fracture can occur when an infant or young child is grabbed or yanked up by the leg or when the lower leg is twisted with the intent to injure or cause pain.

Humerus Fractures. Accidental humeral shaft fractures are not common in children; however, the humerus is one of the most common bones to be fractured from child abuse. The prevalence of abuse in young children with humeral fractures ranges from 8% to 78%.[85] King et al[10] report that the humerus is the bone most commonly injured in children with abusive fractures. In infants less than 12 months of age, the proportion of humeral fractures attributable to abuse is 43.1%. This percentage declines to 6.8% for children 12 to 23 months of age and 1.6% for children 24 to 35 months of age.[4]

Falls are the most common cause of accidental humeral factures, including falls from heights, household objects, and playground equipment.[86] Waltzman et al[87] report that fractures from monkey bars and jungle gym falls involve the upper extremity 90% of the time, of which 40% are supracondylar fractures of the distal humerus. The patients studied ranged in age from 20 months to 12 years with a mean age of 6.2 years. Farnsworth et al[86] analyzed a total of 391 supracondylar humerus fractures. In 70% of cases the mechanism of injury was a fall from a height. Children 3 years old tended to fall off of household objects (beds, couches, other furniture). Overall, they reported that 29% of supracondylar fractures occur on playgrounds. The incidence of supracondylar fractures was found to increase at age 4 years.[86] Shaw et al[88] reviewed 34 cases of humeral shaft fractures, of which, approximately one third resulted from a fall. The mechanism of injury of a supracondylar humerus fracture is typically a fall onto an outstretched arm or, less frequently, a fall onto a flexed elbow. Farnsworth et al[86] determined that children are more likely to fracture their nondominant arm. They proposed the following playground scenario: child slips from the playground apparatus/monkey bars, attempts to hold on with the dominant hand, and lands on the ground with the nondominant arm outstretched, where the elbow is tightly interlocked, concentrating bending forces in the distal humerus (Figure 32-5).[86,89-91] When this fracture type is encountered it is critical not to reflexively assume either an abusive or accidental cause, but rather evaluate all historical, physical, and social factors to best determine the cause of the injury.[92]

While Shaw's study revealed that a history of a fall was common in cases of accidental humeral fracture, a history of a fall was also provided in numerous cases that were deemed abusive in nature.[88] Likewise, Strait et al[85] found that half of the humeral fracture cases with an abusive cause had a history of a fall. Children with abuse-related humerus fractures present commonly with unknown mechanisms of injury, histories that change, and mechanisms of injury that include medical causes or limb disuse.[53,85,88,93]

Williamson and Lowdon[94] analyzed 277 humerus fractures in patients under 16 years of age. The peak incidence of fractures in this study was from 6 to 13 years of age, with lower prevalence in those under 5 years of age. The authors concluded that fractures of the arm in the younger age groups should alert the physician to the possibility of abusive injury. Strait et al[85] studied 124 patients with a total of 124 acute humeral fractures. All children with a humerus fracture that resulted from abuse were less than 2 years of age and 90% were less than 15 months. Abuse was diagnosed in 36% of children less than 15 months old with a humerus fracture and in 1% of children ages 15 months to 3 years.

The humeral shaft is fractured less frequently in children than in adults, accounting for 2% to 5% of all fractures in children.[95] Fractures involving the proximal humeral growth plate represent approximately 0.45% of all childhood fractures. Distal humeral supracondylar fractures account for approximately 30% of limb fractures in children less than 7 years but are uncommon before the age of 2 years.[96]

Shaw et al[88] reviewed 34 cases of humeral shaft fractures in children less than 3 years of age and found that fracture type was not pathognomonic for abuse. Some fracture types, however, are more concerning for abuse than others. Almost 60% of spiral/oblique fractures that occurred in the group less than 15 months of age were from abuse.[85] Worlock et al[11] compared the fracture patterns of 35 children who had been abused to 826 children with accidental injuries. Spiral fractures of the humeral shaft were significantly more common in the abuse group and indicated failure under torsional load. No child under age 5 in the accident group sustained a spiral humerus fracture. This is in contrast to the young child with a spiral femur fracture. The load bearing nature of the leg provides the opportunity to sustain a spiral femur fracture during ambulation. Spiral humerus fractures

of accidental cause are observed at later stages of development because the arms are not typically used for load bearing in infants. When the child attains more advanced developmental capabilities, the arms assume load bearing functions during normal play activities. The developmentally immature infant cannot autonomously generate a torsional load to the humerus. The presence of a spiral humerus fracture in a developmentally immature infant or young child indicates that the torsional load has been applied and might be due to an abusive cause. Each case necessitates careful consideration of the physical and historical findings. Hymel and Jenny[97] reported two young preambulatory infants who sustained midshaft spiral humerus fractures from videotaped and reenacted accidental injury events. Both infants had their arms extended outward from their bodies and were rolled from the prone to the supine position, while their trunks were not lifted from the surface. These two cases are examples in which the torsional load to the humerus was applied by the sibling and caregiver, accidentally causing spiral fractures.

Worlock et al,[11] Leventhal et al,[4] and Thomas et al[75] found that all nonsupracondylar fractures were likely due to abuse, especially in children less than 1 year of age. Strait et al[85] found a higher prevalence of supracondylar humerus fractures because of abuse than previously reported in the literature. In their series, supracondylar fractures accounted for 30% of the fractures resulting from abuse.

Radius/Ulna Fractures. Forearm fractures are common injuries in childhood and account for 40% to 45% of all fractures. Eighty-one percent occur in children age 5 and older.[98,99] Forearm fractures are less common in toddlers and young children, and rare in infants because of the loading conditions required to sustain a forearm fracture. Forearm fractures do not occur in infants as a result of normal activities because infants are nonambulatory and lack the parachute reflex until late infancy.[100,101] Any infant or toddler who has a forearm fracture without an obvious cause requires careful assessment for abuse. Inflicted forearm fractures can be caused by a caregiver grabbing or yanking the infant or young child by the arm. This results in the application of a bending force to the arm and can produce a fracture. Confessions have also included descriptions of angry or malicious caregivers intentionally bending back the forearm to the point of fracture to "teach a lesson" or cause pain (Figure 32-6).

Forearm fractures result most often from an axial load during a fall onto an outstretched arm (Figure 32-7) or a direct lateral impact to the forearm. If the arms are lifted up to the face to protect against a trajectory or a strike with an object, a fracture can result (Figure 32-8). The latter is sometimes referred to as a "nightstick" injury.[91] Consequently, a transverse fracture of the ulna must raise the question of whether the injury is a "defensive wound" from protective positioning when a child is struck with an object.

Skull Fractures. Table 32-10 describes common terms used to describe skull fractures. The prevalence of skull fractures in cases of abuse is estimated at 10% to 13%.[102] Skull fractures are the most common fracture in children less than 2 years of age. The proportion due to abuse is low at 17.1%, yet the number of fractures attributable to abuse is still substantial because of the large number of skull fractures overall. Consequently, skull fractures are the second most common fracture attributable to abuse (Table 32-5).[4]

Table 32-10	Terms Used to Describe Skull Fractures
Fracture Type	**Definition**
Single linear	A fracture consisting of an unbranched line; configurations can be straight, zig zagged, or angular in nature
Multiple or complex	Two or more distinct fractures of any type or a single fracture with multiple components, including branched linear fractures
Basilar	Fracture at the base of the skull
Diastatic	Fracture that occurs along the suture lines of the skull; seen more often in newborns and infants
Depressed	Fracture where the skull has an inward displacement of the bone; normal curvature is disrupted
Stellate	Fracture in which the break lines radiate from a central point
Ping-pong	Type of depressed skull fracture usually seen in young children, resembling the indentation that can be produced with the finger in a ping-pong ball; when elevated it resumes and retains its normal position
Maximum fracture width	The widest point of separation of a linear fracture as measured on radiograph
Growing	An enlarged linear fracture

Adapted, in part, from Hobbs CJ: Skull fracture and the diagnosis of abuse. *Arch Dis Child* 1984;59:246-252.

Accidental skull fractures most commonly result from falls from moderate heights, typically 3 to 6 feet.[103] Such falls include baby chairs, bouncy seats, and car seats placed on tables and countertops, and falls from the arms of a standing caregiver.[103,104] Other accidental injury mechanisms include: falling televisions/heavy furniture, motor vehicle collisions, and falls from windows at heights of one or more stories.[103,104]

Clinical and laboratory research has been conducted to determine whether bed or couch falls could lead to skull fractures and clinically significant injuries in young children. The consensus findings of the clinical studies investigating nearly 600 children indicate bed and couch falls result in a very low incidence of fracture and no serious head injuries.[105,108] These findings are supported by the biomechanical laboratory investigation conducted by Bertocci et al[109] in which an instrumented 3-year-old test dummy and bed fall mock-up were used to test the risk of head and lower extremity injury from bed falls initiated from a side-lying posture. They found such falls present a low risk of head and lower extremity injury. Coats and Margulies[110] studied the mate-

rial properties of the pediatric suture and skull at rates of impact similar to those seen in low height falls. Using human infant cranial suture and bone, they found that the pediatric cranial bone was 35 times stiffer than a pediatric cranial suture. The pediatric cranial suture deformed 30 times more before failure. The strains observed in the bone and suture indicate that the skull can "… undergo dramatic shape changes before fracture, potentially causing substantial deformation in the brain. The sizeable difference between pediatric bone and suture material properties underscores the crucial role that sutures play in the unique response of the pediatric head to impact in low height falls.[110]" Donor infant age was found to have the greatest effect on the elastic modulus and ultimate stress of the cranial bone.

A few publications highlight cases of skull fracture from bed falls or short-distance falls (<3 feet).[103,111,112] The commonality among the cases presented is that each child contacted the edge of a hard surface during the fall: radiator, toy, or table corner. In each case, the fall against the edged surface concentrated the impact to a specific area of the skull and depressed or ping-pong fractures typically were the resultant fracture type.[103,112,113] In short distance falls against flat contact surfaces, the impact forces are dissipated over the surface area of the skull, reducing the likelihood for skull fracture.[112] Consequently, impact surface is an important element of the history that must be obtained to assess injury plausibility. It is important to ask whether the child impacted an object and to obtain a thorough description of the impact surface. Coats and Margulies[114] recently produced the three-dimensional (3D) angular acceleration and impact force data for head impact in infants from low-height falls. They used an instrumented anthropometric infant surrogate and concluded that fall height had little effect on angular motion when the fall was from 1.5 meters or less onto a foam or innerspring crib mattress. In contrast, a fall onto a carpet pad was nearly indistinguishable from concrete with respect to the biomechanical measures of peak acceleration and change in peak-to-peak angular velocity. The goal of this line of research is to determine injury risk and, ultimately, aid clinicians in their differential diagnoses of children with a history of a fall. At this point, however, there is no pediatric injury threshold data available to relate to the biomechanical data obtained from the infant surrogate to traumatic brain injury.[114]

In cases in which a skull fracture results from physical child abuse, the infants and children most often present for medical attention because of a sign or symptom, such as swelling on the head or vomiting. A history of trauma is often absent. When a history is provided, commonly stated causes include: an injury event related to a baby bottle or car seat, bed fall, and/or a vague statement of a sibling causing the injury. In many cases, the caregiver attempts to construct or "remember" a history of trauma after a fracture is identified. In addition, multiple and sometimes life-threatening injuries are often present. To fully assess the compatibility of the injury and history, it is important to solicit a detailed history, as outlined in Table 32-2. When evaluating the history, keep in mind that toddlers who pull to a standing position and then fall to the floor can sustain linear parietal skull fractures. Sometimes the fall goes unnoticed or the toddler cries briefly, and the parent only discovers a "lump" on the head at a later time. The absence of a history is not diagnostic of abuse, especially in a child with a linear fracture and no brain injury.

In children less than 2 years of age sustaining a head injury, skull fracture rates of 8.6% to 43% have been reported, with higher rates in infants.[115] Duhaime et al[113] assert, "Head injury in the youngest age group is distinct from that occurring in older children because of differences in mechanisms, injury thresholds, and the frequency with which the question of child abuse is encountered."

When the skull is impacted, the resultant fracture type is dependent on the injury mechanism and the type and magnitude of force applied. The predominant fracture type and location observed in infants and young children is a simple linear fracture of the parietal bone. Such fractures most commonly result from short distance falls. Hobbs[103] conducted a study of 60 children admitted to the hospital with skull fractures. Only four (6.6%) children had fractures involving nonparietal bones. Shane and Fuchs[115] analyzed 102 cases of acute skull fracture of which 91% had a history of a fall and 90% had a linear fracture. Children with nonparietal fractures were largely those who fell down stairs in a walker.

Duhaime et al[113] compiled a table of the expected injury types associated with accidental mechanisms in young children (Table 32-11). Most commonly, skull fractures resulting from short distance falls in young children are simple linear fractures without any associated intracranial hemorrhage or neurological deficit,[116] or other associated serious or life-threatening injuries. Linear skull fractures are as likely to occur from falls less than 4 feet as from falls greater than 4 feet, stair falls, or falls down stairs in a walker. Complex skull

fractures are associated with higher falls because of the greater biomechanical impact forces generated.[113] Depressed skull fractures occur from falls greater than 4 feet, stair falls, falls onto an edged surface, and impact from a moving object.[103,112,113] "Ping-pong fractures" occur from short falls against a pointed object.[112] Basilar or bilateral fractures without intracranial hemorrhage occurred from stair falls and falls greater than 4 feet.[113]

Cavarial, linear, depressed, and ping-pong fractures commonly occur from falls in young children, as skull deformation can occur with relatively low impact force in this age group. Greater biomechanical forces produce more extensive injuries and skull fractures, but the type of force determines the particular fracture type.[113] Translational or linear forces of greater magnitudes produce more extensive skull fractures. Multiple and complex fractures are often concerning for abuse. Table 32-12 highlights the fracture types observed in accident and abuse cases and their relative frequencies.[103]

Hobbs[103] advises that the following features should raise the suspicion for abuse in children under 2 years old with a skull fracture and a history of minor trauma:

- Multiple or complex fracture
- Depressed fracture
- Diastatic fracture (maximum fracture width greater than 3.0 mm)
- Growing fracture
- Involvement of more than one cranial bone
- Nonparietal fracture
- Associated intracranial injury

The number of cranial bones involved in the fracture is a measure of the extent and severity of the injury. Hobbs[103] found that fractures resulting from accident-related trauma rarely involved more than one cranial bone or crossed the suture line. In comparison, abuse-related trauma commonly involved two or more cranial bones. Hobbs noted that the most severe fractures were from abusive events, and the only equivalent injuries observed in cases of accidental trauma were in children run over by motor vehicles. This

Table 32-11	Expected Injury Types Associated with Accidental Mechanisms in Very Young Children
Mechanism	**Injury Types**
Fall < 4 ft	Concussion/soft tissue injury Linear fracture Epidural hematoma Ping-pong fracture Depressed fracture*
Fall > 4 ft	Injuries listed above plus the following: Depressed fracture Basilar fracture Multiple fractures Subarachnoid hemorrhage Contusion Subdural hematoma* Stellate fracture*
Motor vehicle accident	Injuries listed above plus the following: Subdural hematoma Diffuse axonal injury

Adapted from Duhaime AC, Alario AJ, Lewander WJ, et al: Head injury in very young children: mechanisms, injury types, and ophthalmologic findings in 100 hospitalized patients younger than 2 years of age. *Pediatrics* 1992;90:179-185.
*Uncommonly associated with given mechanism

Table 32-12	Fracture Types Observed in Accident and Abuse Cases and the Relative Frequencies	
Skull Fracture	**Accident (n = 60)**	**Abuse (n = 29)**
Single linear	55	6
Multiple complex	3	23
Depressed	3	12
Maximum width at presentation >3.0 mm	4	10 (of 13)*
Growing	2	6

Adapted from Hobbs CJ. Skull fracture and the diagnosis of abuse. *Arch Dis Child* 1984;59:246-252.
*Only 13 of 29 children received measurements.

observation speaks to the extremely violent nature of physical abuse and the significant force used in these attacks.

Peters et al[49] identified bruising or subgaleal hematoma at the site of skull fracture in 43.3% of patients with skull fractures and suspected abuse.

Clavicle Fractures. Clavicle fractures account for 5% to 15% of childhood fractures, and are the most common type of fracture in children.[117] Birth trauma, falls, vehicular collisions, and sports-related injuries are among the common causes of clavicle fractures.[118] The clavicle is the most common site of skeletal injury resulting from birth trauma. Oppenheim et al[119] reviewed nearly 22,000 live births; 57 newborns had 58 clavicle fractures for an overall incidence of 2.7 clavicle fractures per 1000 live births. McBride et al[120] conducted a prospective screening of 9106 newborns and observed 4.7 fractures per 1000 live births for an overall incidence of 0.5%. Factors that are associated with clavicle fractures at birth include: high birth weight, shoulder dystocia, prolonged gestational age, and forceps or vacuum assisted delivery.[119,120] The diagnosis of a clavicle fracture from birth can be delayed. The fracture might not be detected on imaging until callous formation occurs, or an injury might not be recognized until a palpable mass on the clavicle is discovered.[119]

Stanley et al[121] studied the mechanism of clavicular fracture in a consecutive series of 150 patients presenting to hospitals. In their study, 94% of the patients sustained a clavicle fracture because of a direct injury to the shoulder by falling onto the shoulder (Figure 32-9) or sustaining a direct blow, 6% sustained a clavicle fracture by falling on an outstretched arm (Figure 32-10). They note that fracture is more likely when impact energy is absorbed quickly than when it is dissipated more slowly.

Clavicle fractures also result from abusive trauma. Forces sufficient for fracture can be inflicted by a direct blow to the shoulder or, alternatively, if the child is thrown or pushed and subsequently falls onto his or her shoulder (Figure 32-9). When these children present for medical care, the caregiver often relates that the child is not using his or her arm and there is no history of trauma.[122] There are few publications that discuss pediatric clavicle fractures as a result of abusive trauma. An early publication by Merten et al[19] report that clavicle fractures are unusual in child abuse—detected in only 7 % of abused children. More recently, Leventhal et al[4] studied fractures in hospitalized children less than 3 years old and found that 20.7% of clavicle fractures were due to abuse. The incidence of clavicle fractures attributable to abuse decreased with increasing age of the child. In infants up to 11 months, 28.1% of clavicle fractures were from abuse, in children 12 to 23 months, 16.7%, and in children 24 to 35 months 6.0% were attributed to abuse.

Calder et al[117] analyzed fracture location along the clavicle, and Postacchini et al[123] conducted an epidemiological study of clavicle fractures. In both studies the overwhelming majority of clavicle fractures were located in the middle third of the clavicle. This region is the thinnest portion of the bone and it lacks ligamentous and muscular attachments, so it fractures most easily.

A clavicle fracture is most often a benign injury. An exception is a posteriorly displaced medial clavicular fracture, which requires immediate evaluation for concomitant mediastinal and/or vascular injuries and pneumothora-

ces.[124] In newborns, the injury most commonly associated with a clavicle fracture is a brachial plexus injury. Oppenheim et al[119] found that 1 of every 19 clavicle fractures was associated with a brachial plexus injury.[119] Stanley et al[121] found that 10% of patients sustaining direct injury to the shoulder also had "skin grazing over the point of the shoulder." This study, however, contained both adult and child participants, and it is not noted what ages are included among the 10%. Peters et al[49] identified seven clavicle fractures in abused children and none had a bruise near the fracture site.

SUMMARY

The evaluation of injury plausibility is a multiple-step process requiring a careful and directed history, physical, and psychosocial examination. If more than one fracture or injury is identified, the same rigorous assessment must be applied for each additional injury. Knowledge of how bone structure and material properties affect bone strength and how bone responds to load is essential to understanding fractures in children and discerning the validity of the stated mechanism compared with the resultant fracture. All of the following factors contribute to injury plausibility.

- The history provided by the caregiver
- Between the type of fracture and the described behavior of the child after the fracture
- The developmental capabilities of the child and the described actions leading up to the fracture event
- Between the fracture biomechanics and history of injury
- Between all injuries sustained and the injury potential of the described cause

Further research on children and infants in the following key areas will enhance our understanding of fractures and improve our ability to assess injury plausibility: bone strength and response to loading, injury thresholds, and the biomechanical analysis of common injury events. Additionally, research related to the pertinent intrinsic and extrinsic variables (e.g., bone health, landing surface, and recurring trauma) affecting each of these factors is critical is to the development of a comprehensive understanding of fractures and childhood injuries. Further validation and testing of injury plausibility models are also required. Our investigations and conclusions currently are limited by the biofidelity of our child anatomic testing devices. The improvement of these surrogates is another area of critical need.

References

1. Levine RS: Injury to the extremities. *In*: Nahum AM, Melvin JW (eds): *Accidental Injury Biomechanics and Prevention.* Springer-Verlag, New York, 2002, pp 491-522.
2. Pierce MC, Bertocci G, Vogeley E, et al: Evaluating long bone fractures in children: a biomechanical approach with illustrative cases. *Child Abuse Negl* 2004;28:505-524.
3. Landin LA: Epidemiology of children's fractures. *J Pediatr Orthop B* 1997;6:79-83.
4. Leventhal JM, Martin KD, Asnes AG: Incidence of fractures attributable to abuse in young hospitalized children: results from analysis of a United States database. *Pediatrics* 2008;122:599-604.
5. Kleinman PK: Skeletal trauma: general considerations. *In*: Kleinman PK (ed): *Diagnostic Imaging of Child Abuse*, ed 2, Mosby, Chicago, 1998, pp 8-25.

6. Kogutt MS, Swischuk LE, Fagan CJ: Patterns of injury and significance of uncommon fractures in the battered child syndrome. *Am J Roentgenol Radium Ther Nucl Med* 1974;121:143-149.

7. Kocher MS, Kasser JR: Orthopaedic aspects of child abuse. *J Am Acad Orthop Surg* 2000;8:10-20.

8. Krishnan J, Barbour PJ, Foster BK: Patterns of osseous injuries and psychosocial factors affecting victims of child abuse. *Aust N Z J Surg* 1990;60:447-450.

9. O'Neill JA, Meacham WF, Griffin PP, et al: Patterns of injury in the battered child syndrome. *J Trauma* 1973;13:332-339.

10. King J, Diefendorf D, Apthorp J, et al: Analysis of 429 fractures in 189 battered children. *J Pediatr Orthop* 1988;8:585-589.

11. Worlock P, Stower M, Barbor P: Patterns of fractures in accidental and non-accidental injury in children: a comparative study. *Br Med J* 1986;293:100-102.

12. McClelland CQ, Heiple KG: Fracture in the first year of life: a diagnostic dilemma. *Am J Dis Child* 1982;136:26-29.

13. Akbarnia B, Torg JS, Kirkpatrick J, et al: Manifestations of the battered-child syndrome. *J Bone Joint Surg Am* 1974;56:1159-1166.

14. Sawyer JR, Flynn JM, Dormans JP, et al: Fracture patterns in children and young adults who fall from significant heights. *J Pediatr Orthop* 2000;20:197-202.

15. Jenny C, Committee on Child Abuse and Neglect: Evaluating infants and young children with multiple fractures. *Pediatrics* 2006;118:1299-1303.

16. Pierce MC, Smith S, Kaczor K: Bruising in infants: those with a bruise may be abused. *Pediatr Emerg Care* 2009;25:845-847.

17. Kleinman PK: Problems in the diagnosis of metaphyseal fractures. *Pediatr Radiol* 2008;38:S388-S394.

18. Merten DF, Radkowski MA, Leonidas JC: The abused child: a radiological reappraisal. *Radiology* 1983;146:377-381.

19. Kleinman PK, Marks SC, Richmond JM, et al: Inflicted skeletal injury: A postmortem radiologic-histopathologic study in 31 infants. *AJR Am J Roentgenol* 1995;165:647-650.

20. Kleinman PK: Diagnostic imaging in infant abuse. *AJR Am J Roentgenol* 1990;155:703-712.

21. Kleinman PK, Marks SC, Blackboume B: The metaphyseal lesion in abused infants: A radiologic-histopathologic study. *AJR Am J Roentgenol* 1986;146:895-905.

22. Kleinman PK, Marks SC: A regional approach to the classic metaphyseal lesion in abused infants: the distal femur. *AJR Am J Roentgenol* 1998;170:43-47.

23. Kleinman PK, Marks S: Relationship of the subperiosteal bone collar to metaphyseal lesions in abused infants. *J Bone Joint Surg Am* 1995;77:1471-1476.

24. Gomez MA, Nahum AM: Biomechanics of bone. *In*: Nahum AM, Melvin JW (eds): *Accidental Injury Biomechanics and Prevention*. Springer-Verlag, New York, 2002, pp 206-227.

25. Grayev AM, Boal DK, Wallach DM, et al: Metaphyseal fractures mimicking abuse during treatment for clubfoot. *Pediatr Radiol* 2001;31:559-563.

26. Snedecor ST, Wilson HB: Some obstetric injuries to the long bones. *J Bone Joint Surg Am* 1949;31:378-384.

27. Kleinman PK: Bony thoracic trauma. *In*: Kleinman PK (ed): *Diagnostic Imaging of Child Abuse*, ed 2, Mosby, Chicago, 1998, pp 110-148.

28. Barsness KA, Cha ES, Bensard D, et al: The positive predictive value of rib fractures as an indicator of nonaccidental trauma in children. *J Trauma* 2003;54:1107-1110.

29. Worlock P, Stower M: Fracture patterns in Nottingham children. *J Pediatr Orthop* 1986;6:656-660.

30. Betz P, Liebhardt E: Rib fractures in children: resuscitation or child abuse? *Int J Legal Med* 1994;106:215-218.

31. Price EA, Rush LR, Perper JA, et al: Cardiopulmonary resuscitation-related injuries and homicidal blunt abdominal trauma in children. *Am J Forensic Med Pathol* 2000;21:307-310.

32. Spevak MR, Kleinman PK, Belanger PL, et al: Cardiopulmonary resuscitation and rib fractures in infants: a postmortem radiologic-pathologic study. *JAMA* 1994;272:617-618.

33. Feldman KW, Brewer DK: Child abuse, cardiopulmonary resuscitation, and rib fractures. *Pediatrics* 1984;73:339-342.

34. Bush CM, Jones JS, Cohle SD, et al: Pediatric injuries from cardiopulmonary resuscitation. *Ann Emerg Med* 1996;28:40-44.

35. Bhat BV, Kumar A, Oumachigui A: Bone injuries during delivery. *Indian J Pediatr* 1994;61:401-405.

36. Cumming WA: Neonatal skeletal fractures. Birth trauma or child abuse? *J Can Assoc Radiol* 1979;30:30-33.

37. Rizzolo PJ, Coleman PR: Neonatal rib fracture: birth trauma or child abuse? *J Fam Pract* 1989;29:561-563.

38. Hartmann RW Jr: Radiological case of the month. Rib fractures produced by birth trauma. *Arch Pediatr Adolesc Med* 1997;151:947-948.

39. Barry PW, Hocking MD: Infant rib fracture - birth trauma or non-accidental injury. *Arch Dis Child* 1993;68:250.

40. Bulloch B, Schuber CJ, Brophy PD, et al: Cause and clinical characteristics of rib fractures in infants. *Pediatrics* 2000;105:e48-e51.

41. O'Connor JF, Cohen J: Dating fractures. *In*: Kleinman PK (ed): *Diagnostic Imaging of Child Abuse*, ed 2, Mosby, Chicago, 1998, pp 168-177.

42. Hoke RS, Chamberlain D: Skeletal chest injuries secondary to cardiopulmonary resuscitation. *Resuscitation* 2004;63:327-338.

43. Sewell RD, Steinberg MA: Chest compressions in an infant with osteogenesis imperfecta type II: no new rib fractures. *Pediatrics* 2000;106:e71-e72.

44. Dolinak D: Rib fractures in infants due to cardiopulmonary resuscitation efforts. *Am J Forensic Med Pathol* 2007;28:107-110.

45. Kleinman PK, Schlesinger AE: Mechanical factors associated with posterior rib fractures: laboratory and case studies. *Pediatr Radiol* 1997;27:87-91.

46. Smurthwaite D, Wright N, Russell S, et al: How common are rib fractures in extremely low birth weight preterm infants? *Arch Dis Child Fetal Neonatal Ed* 2009;94:F138-F139.

47. Strouse PJ, Owings CL: Fractures of the first rib in child abuse. *Radiology* 1995;197:763-765.

48. Garcia VF, Gotschall CS, Eichelberger MR, et al: Rib fractures in children: a marker of severe trauma. *J Trauma* 1990;30(6):695-700.

49. Peters ML, Starling SP, Barnes-Eley ML, et al: The presence of bruising associated with fractures. *Arch Pediatr Adolesc Med* 2008;162:877-881.

50. Goss TP: Scapular fractures and dislocations: diagnosis and treatment. *J Am Acad Orthop Surg* 1995;3:22-33.

51. Lapner PC, Uhthoff HK, Papp S: Scapula fractures. *Orthop Clin North Am* 2008;39:459-474.

52. Tadros AMA, Lunsjo K, Czechowski J, et al: Causes of delayed diagnosis of scapular fractures. *Injury* 2008;39:314-318.

53. Mok JYQ: Non-accidental injury in children-an update. *Injury* 2008;39:978-985.

54. Thompson DA, Flynn TC, Miller PW, et al: The significance of scapular fractures. *J Trauma* 1985;25:974-977.

55. Baldwin KD, Ohman-Strickland P, Mehta S, et al: Scapula fractures: a marker for concomitant injury? A retrospective review of data in the national trauma database. *J Trauma* 2008;65:430-435.

56. Harris RD, Harris JH Jr: The prevalence and significance of missed scapular fractures in blunt chest trauma. *AJR Am J Roentgenol* 1988;151:747-750.

57. Rennie L, Court-Brown CM, Mok JYQ, et al: The epidemiology of fractures in children. *Injury* 2007;38:913-922.

58. Canale ST, Beaty JH: Fractures of the pelvis. *In*: Beaty JH, Kasser JR (eds): *Rockwood and Wilkins Fractures in Children*, ed 5, Lippincott, Williams & Wilkins, New York, 2001, pp 883-911.

59. von Garrel T, Ince A, Junge A, et al: The sternal fracture: radiographic analysis of 200 fractures with special reference to concomitant injuries. *J Trauma* 2004;57:837-844.

60. Kleinman PK: Lower extremity. *In*: Kleinman PK (ed): *Diagnostic Imaging of Child Abuse*, ed 2, Mosby, Chicago, 1998, pp 26-71.

61. Kleinman PK: Spinal trauma. *In*: Kleinman PK (ed): *Diagnostic Imaging of Child Abuse*, ed 2, Mosby, Chicago, 1998, pp 149-167.

62. Kleinman PK, Zito JL: Avulsion of the spinous processes caused by infant abuse. *Radiology* 1984;151:389-391.

63. Kleinman PK, Marks SC: Vertebral body fractures in child abuse. Radiologic-histopathologic correlates. *Invest Radiol* 1992;27:715-722.

64. Kleinman PK, Shelton YA: Hangman's fracture in an abused infant: imaging features. *Pediatr Radiol* 1997;27:776-777.

65. McGory BR, Fenichel GM: Hangman's fracture subsequent to shaking in an infant. *Ann Neurol* 1977;2:82.

66. Nimkin K, Spevak MR, Kleinman PK: Fractures of the hands and feet in child abuse: imaging and pathologic features. *Radiology* 1997;203:233-236.

67. Vadivelu R, Dias JJ, Burke FD, et al: Hand injuries in children: a prospective study. *J Pediatr Orthop* 2006;26:29-35.

68. Worlock PH, Stower MJ: The incidence and pattern of hand fractures in children. *J Hand Surg Br* 1986;11(2):198-200.

69. Mahabir RC, Kazemi AR, Cannon WG, et al: Pediatric hand fractures: a review. *Pediatr Emerg Care* 2001;17:153-156.

70. Kasser JR, Beaty JH: Femoral shaft fractures. *In*: Beaty JH, Kasser JR (eds): *Rockwood and Wilkins Fractures in Children*, ed 5, Lippincott, Williams & Wilkins, New York, 2001, pp 941-980.

71. Beals RK, Tufts E: Fractured femur in infancy: the role of child abuse. *J Pediatr Orthop* 1983;3:583-586.

72. Hedlund R, Lindgren U: The incidence of femoral shaft fractures in children and adolescents. *J Pediatr Orthop* 1986;6:47-50.

73. Hinton RY, Lincoln A, Crockett MM, et al: Fractures of the femoral shaft in children. Incidence, mechanisms, and sociodemographic risk factors. *J Bone Joint Surg Am* 1999;81:500-509.

74. Blakemore LC, Loder RT, Hensinger RN: Role of intentional abuse in children 1 to 5 years old with isolated femoral shaft fractures. *J Pediatr Orthop* 1996;16:585-588.

75. Thomas SA, Rosenfield NS, Leventhal JM, et al: Long-bone fractures in young children: distinguishing accidental injuries from child abuse. *Pediatrics* 1991;88:471-476.

76. Loder RT, O'Donnell PW, Feinberg JR: Epidemiology and mechanisms of femur fractures in children. *J Pediatr Orthop* 2006;26:561-566.

77. Nork SE, Bellig GJ, Woll JP, et al: Overgrowth and outcome after femoral shaft fracture in children younger than 2 years. *Clin Orthop Relat Res* 1998;357:186-191.

78. Gross RH, Stranger M: Causative factors responsible for femoral fractures in infants and young children. *J Pediatr Orthop* 1983;3:341-343.

79. Anderson WA: The significance of femoral fractures in children. *Ann Emerg Med* 1982;11:174-177.

80. Scherl SA, Miller L, Lively N, et al: Accidental and nonaccidental femur fractures in children. *Clin Orthop Relat Res* 2000;376:99-105.

81. Pierce MC, Bertocci GE, Janosky JE, et al: Femur fractures resulting from stair falls among children: an injury plausibility model. *Pediatrics* 2005;115:1712-1722.

82. Rex C, Kay PR: Features of femoral fractures in nonaccidental injury. *J Pediatr Orthop* 2000;20:411-413.

83. Rewers A, Hedegaard H, Lezotte D, et al: Childhood femur fractures, associated injuries, and sociodemographic risk factors: a population-based study. *Pediatrics* 2005;115:e543-e552.

84. Taylor MT, Banerjee B, Alpar EK: Injuries associated with a fractured shaft of the femur. *Injury* 1994;25:185-187.

85. Strait RT, Siegel RM, Shapiro RA: Humeral fractures without obvious etiologies in children less than 3 years of age: when is it abuse? *Pediatrics* 1995;96:667-671.

86. Farnsworth CL, Silva MS, Mubarak SJ: Etiology of supracondylar humerus fractures. *J Pediatr Orthop* 1998;18:38-42.

87. Waltzman ML, Shannon M, Bowen AP, et al: Monkeybar injuries: complications of play. *Pediatrics* 1999;103:e58-e61.

88. Shaw BA, Murphy KM, Shaw A, et al: Humerus shaft fractures in young children: accident or abuse? *J Pediatr Orthop* 1997;17:293-297.

89. John SD, Wherry K, Swischuk LE, et al: Improving detection of pediatric elbow fractures by understanding their mechanics. *Radiographics* 1996;16:1443-1460.

90. Kasser JR, Beaty JH: Supracondylar fractures of the distal humerus. *In*: Beaty JH, Kasser JR (eds): *Rockwood and Wilkins Fractures in Children*, ed 5, Lippincott, Williams & Wilkins, New York, 2001, pp 577-624.

91. Minkowitz B, Busch MT: Supracondylar humerus fractures. Current trends and controversies. *Orthop Clin North Am* 1994;25:581-594.

92. Kleinman PK: The upper extremity. *In*: Kleinman PK (ed): *Diagnostic Imaging of Child Abuse*, ed 2, Mosby, Chicago, 1998, pp 72-109.

93. Taitz J, Moran K, O'Meara M: Long bone fractures in children under 3 years of age: is abuse being missed in emergency department presentations? *J Paediatr Child Health* 2004;40:170-174.

94. Williamson DM, Lowdon IMR: Why do children break their arms? *Injury* 1988;19:9-10.

95. Webb LX, Mooney JF: Fractures and dislocations about the shoulder. *In*: Green NE, Swiontkowski MF (eds): *Skeletal Trauma in Children*, vol 3, Saunders, Philadelphia, 2003, pp 322-343.

96. Green NE: Fractures and dislocations about the elbow. *In*: Green NE, Swiontkowski MF (eds): *Skeletal Trauma in Children*, vol 3, Saunders, Philadelphia, 2003, pp 257-321.

97. Hymel KP, Jenny C: Abusive spiral fractures of the humerus: a videotaped exception. *Arch Pediatr Adolesc Med* 1996;150:226-228.

98. Armstrong PF, Joughin VE, Clarke HM, et al: Fractures of the forearm, wrist, and hand. *In*: Green NE, Swiontkowski MF (eds): *Skeletal Trauma in Children*, vol 3, Saunders, Philadelphia, 2003, pp 166-255.

99. Waters PM: Distal radius and ulna fractures. *In*: Beaty JH, Kasser JR (eds): *Rockwood and Wilkins Fractures in Children*, ed 5, Lippincott, Williams & Wilkins, New York, 2001, pp 381-442.

100. Haslam RHA: The nervous system. *In*: Nelson WE (ed): *Nelson Textbook of Pediatrics*, ed 15, WB Saunders, Philadelphia, 1996, pp 1667-1738.

101. Edelson G, Kelly I, Vigder F, et al: A three-dimensional classification for fractures of the proximal humerus. *J Bone Joint Surg Br* 2004;86:413-425.

102. Kleinman PK, Barnes PD: Head trauma. *In*: Kleinman PK (ed): *Diagnostic Imaging of Child Abuse*, ed 2, Mosby, Chicago, 1998, pp 285-342.

103. Hobbs CJ: Skull fracture and the diagnosis of abuse. *Arch Dis Child* 1984;59:246-252.

104. Billmire ME, Myers PA: Serious head injury in infants: accident or abuse? *Pediatrics* 1985;75:340-342.

105. Helfer R, Slovis T, Black M: Injuries resulting when small children fall out of bed. *Pediatrics* 1977;60:533-535.

106. Lyons TJ, Oates RK: Falling out of bed: a relatively benign occurrence. *Pediatrics* 1993;92:125-127.

107. Nimityongskul P, Anderson L: The likelihood of injuries when children fall out of bed. *J Pediatr Orthop* 1987;7:184-186.

108. Selbst SM, Baker MD, Shames M: Bunk bed injuries. *Am J Dis Child* 1990;144:721-723.

109. Bertocci GE, Pierce MC, Deemer E, et al: Using test dummy experiments to investigate pediatric injury risk in simulated short-distance falls. *Arch Pediatr Adolesc Med* 2003;157:480-486.

110. Coats B, Margulies SS: Material properties of human infant skull and suture at high rates. *J Neurotrauma* 2006;23:1222-1232.

111. Johnson K, Fischer T, Chapman S, et al: Accidental head injuries in children under 5 years of age. *Clin Radiol* 2005;60:464-468.

112. Wheeler S, Shope TR: Depressed skull fracture in a 7-month old who fell from bed. *Pediatrics* 1997;100:1033-1034.

113. Duhaime AC, Alario AJ, Lewander WJ, et al: Head injury in very young children: mechanisms, injury types, and ophthalmologic findings in 100 hospitalized patients younger than 2 years of age. *Pediatrics* 1992;90:179-185.

114. Coats B, Margulies SS: Potential for head injuries in infants from low-height falls: laboratory investigation. *J Neurosurg Pediatr* 2008;2:321-330.

115. Shane SA, Fuchs SM: Skull fractures in infants and predictors of associated intracranial injury. *Pediatr Emerg Care* 1997;13:198-203.

116. Case ME: Accidental traumatic head injury in infants and young children. *Brain Pathol* 2008;18:583-589.

117. Calder JDF, Solan M, Gidwani S, et al: Management of paediatric clavicle fractures - is follow-up necessary? An audit of 346 cases. *Ann R Coll Surg Engl* 2002;84:331-333.

118. Ogden JA: Distal clavicular physeal injury. *Clin Orthop Relat Res* 1984;188:68-73.

119. Oppenheim WL, Davis A, Growdon WA, et al: Clavicle fractures in the newborn. *Clin Orthop Relat Res* 1990;250:176-180.

120. McBride MT, Hennrikus WL, Mologne TS: Newborn clavicle fractures. *Orthopedics* 1998;21:317-319.

121. Stanley D, Trowbridge EA, Norris SH: The mechanism of clavicular fracture. *J Bone Joint Surg* 1988;70:461-464.

122. Neviaser JS: Injuries of the clavicle and its articulations. *Orthop Clin North Am* 1980;11:233-237.

123. Postacchini F, Gumina S, De Santis P, et al: Epidemiology of clavicle fractures. *J Shoulder Elbow Surg* 2002;11:452-456.

124. Kwon Y, Sarwark JF: Proximal humerus, scapula, and clavicle. *In*: Beaty JH, Kasser JR (eds): *Rockwood and Wilkins Fractures in Children*, ed 5, Lippincott, Williams & Wilkins, New York, 2001, pp 741-806.

33

Imaging of Skeletal Trauma in Abused Children

Vesna Martich Kriss, MD

INTRODUCTION

Bony fractures are a common part of childhood. In fact, more than 40% of all American males will sustain a fractured bone by the age of 15 years.[1] Fractures occurring from common accidental childhood injuries usually have a characteristic appearance such as a Salter Harris growth plate injury, greenstick fracture, or torus/buckle fracture (Figures 33-1 and 33-2). Inflicted injuries, however, also can fracture bones. Because some inflicted injuries also have a distinct radiographic appearance, it is sometimes possible to characterize a bony injury as likely nonaccidental versus accidental in nature, particularly in infants. Hence, skeletal imaging is a crucial component in the workup for child abuse. Radiographic skeletal surveys and nuclear medicine bone scintigraphy are the main modalities used in the skeletal imaging workup of child abuse.

SKELETAL SURVEY

The primary radiographic tool in the workup of potential abusive skeletal injury is the skeletal survey.[2,3] A skeletal survey provides a radiographic look at all of the child's bones (Table 33-1).

If suspicious areas are seen on the skeletal survey, repeat multiplanar views should be done such as lateral or oblique views to better visualize potential abusive injuries. Sometimes bony injury may remain occult and not visible on the initial radiographic views. If clinical suspicion remains high, repeat skeletal survey can be done 2 weeks later to look for periosteal reaction (healing callus formation), thereby increasing the diagnostic yield of abusive injuries.[4]

In children less than 1 year of age suspected to be abused, skeletal survey yielded unsuspected injuries in 47%.[5] The number dropped to 28% for children from 1 to 2 years of age and was 22% for children 2 to 5 years of age. In children older than 5 years of age, the radiographic yield of unsuspected injuries via skeletal survey was only 9%, rendering this group more amenable to selective radiographic evaluation based on clinical suspicion rather than a full skeletal survey.[5]

Although the number of radiographs in a skeletal survey is large, with proper collimation and positioning the actual radiation dose to each visualized body part is about 0.1 to 0.2 mSv (similar single dose as a routine chest x-ray). In comparison, consider the radiation dose of an abdomen/pelvis CT scan (8-14 mSv) or nuclear medicine bone scintigraphy (2-3 mSv).[6]

NUCLEAR MEDICINE (BONE SCINTIGRAPHY)

Bone scintigraphy (nuclear medicine scan) is another option that can be done to rapidly elucidate the presence of an occult skeletal injury, especially if a high clinical suspicion remains despite an initial negative radiographic skeletal survey. Nuclear medicine bone scans are certainly more sensitive than radiographic skeletal surveys (100% vs. 88%) with fewer false positives (0.8%-12.3%).[7,8] A bone scan also is more cumbersome to perform and is not always available at all hours. For a bone scan, a radiopharmaceutical that is sensitive to areas of increased bony metabolic activity is injected intravenously. If trauma, infection, or tumor is present, the scan will "light up" or show increased uptake of the radiopharmaceutical in the affected areas of bone. In the case of abuse, the injury will be visualized immediately after the event. With radiographs, some lesions are not obvious until healing bone is visualized 2 weeks later (Figure 33-3).

Bone scintigraphy has limitations as well; skull and metaphyseal injuries (that are near metabolically active normal growth plates) can be missed. On the other hand, occult soft tissue injuries are better appreciated with nuclear medicine. In general, radiographic skeletal survey is still considered the first line of imaging for an abusive injury with a bone scan used as a complementary imaging modality when a high index of suspicion still remains after a normal radiographic skeletal survey.[7,8]

RADIOGRAPHIC "RED FLAGS"

Specific radiographic appearances of skeletal trauma in abused children (so-called radiographic "red flags") can help the physician, social worker, and/or law enforcement personnel diagnose bony injuries suspicious for abuse as opposed to those caused by accidents. This chapter will demonstrate six radiographic "red flags" of skeletal trauma that are highly suggestive of inflicted injury:

1. Nonambulatory children with long bone fractures
2. Characteristic fracture lines such as spiral fractures (especially in infants)
3. Multiple injuries of differing ages
4. Metaphyseal "corner" fractures
5. Rib fractures (especially posterior)
6. Skull fractures (especially occipital or "egg-shell")

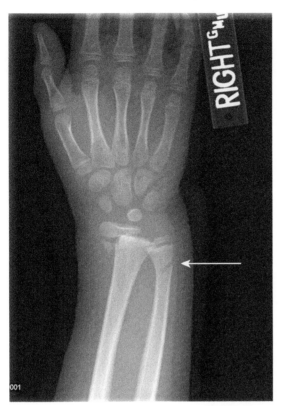

FIGURE 33-1 Fracture involving the radial growth plate known as a Salter-Harris fracture, a common accidental injury. Incidentally noted is a greenstick fracture or incomplete fracture of the distal ulna *(arrow)*.

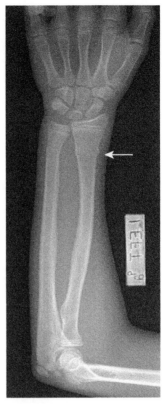

FIGURE 33-2 Another common accidental injury in children is the torus or buckle fracture, often caused by a fall onto an outstretched arm. Note the cortical disruption with adjacent "buckle" of the bony cortex *(arrow)*.

Red Flag No. 1: Nonambulatory Children with Long Bone Fractures

Long bone fractures are a common element in abusive injuries, appearing in 76% of all abusive skeletal injuries in one series of 189 documented abuse cases.[9] Long bone fractures in the nonambulatory infant, however, are particularly worrisome. Walking is one of the early milestones of life, occurring at about 1 year of age. Once a child learns to walk, they are capable of creating true self-imposed accidental injuries such as the common toddler fracture (Figure 33-4). On the other hand, nonambulatory infants are much less likely to experience accidental long bone fractures. The lack of purposeful ambulation stipulates that a young infant's long bone fracture cannot be self-inflicted. Hence, the diagnosis of a long bone fracture of any type in an infant automatically merits investigation to determine a plausible explanation for the injury (Figure 33-5).

In cases of infant abuse, often the only initial reason given for imaging is a "swollen extremity" or "not moving the extremity." In these cases, once the radiographic diagnosis of long bone fracture is made, one should be skeptical of the subsequent appearance of a "new" history of accidental fall or dropping of an infant in an attempt to explain the newly discovered skeletal injury (Figure 33-6).

Even once walking commences, certain types of long bone fractures can still be ominous. For instance, the common accidental toddler fracture mentioned earlier (Figure 33-4) is often seen as just a subtle cortical crack in the otherwise intact distal tibia. Contrast this with the com-

Table 33-1	Complete Skeletal Survey Table

Appendicular Skeleton

Humeri (AP)
Forearms (AP)
Hands (PA)
Femurs (AP)
Lower legs (AP)
Feet (PA) or (AP)

Axial Skeleton

Thorax (AP and lateral), to include ribs, thoracic and upper lumbar spine
Pelvis (AP), to include the mid lumbar spine
Lumbosacral spine (lateral)
Cervical spine (AP and lateral)
Skull (frontal and lateral)

plete separation of the bony shaft of a much larger, stronger bone such as the humerus or femur (Figure 33-7). The force required for the latter is far greater, and in some cases are beyond the force that can occur in true household accidents. In fact, in studies of femoral fractures under age 4, abuse was still the cause in 30% to 79% of cases.[10-12] Multiple studies of childhood falls of less than 3 feet revealed a less than 2% incidence of bony fractures, none of which were the femur.[13-15] The absence of ambulation clearly makes long

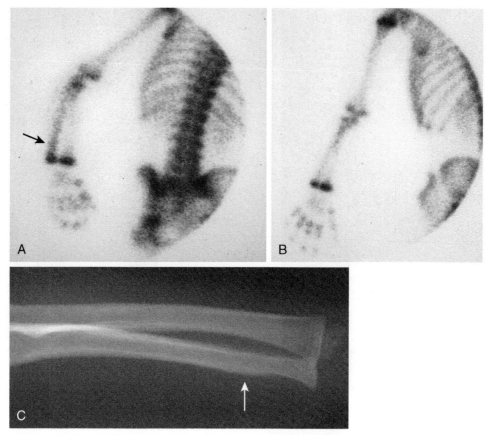

FIGURE 33-3 A, Nuclear medicine scan of a child with a suspected arm injury. Initial radiographs revealed no discernable bony injury. Bone scintigraphy showed increased uptake in the distal ulna *(arrow)*, worrisome for injury. **B,** For comparison, this image is of a *normal* ulnar scintigraphic image of the same region. Note the generalized increased uptake of all the normal growth plates. **C,** Follow-up radiograph of the lower arm of the child seen in **A,** taken 2 weeks later. Distal ulnar periosteal reaction associated with a healing injury is noted *(arrow)*.

bone injuries in young infants more suspicious for an abusive injury.

Red Flag No. 2: Characteristic Fracture Line

There are four descriptive patterns to describe a fracture line: transverse, oblique, spiral, or comminuted, any of which can conceivably occur with abuse. The type of fracture line seen corresponds to the direction and amount of force applied to the bone (see Chapter 36). For instance, comminuted fractures imply great force (such as motor vehicle accidents, gunshot wounds, etc.) because the bone fracture line is fragmented into smaller pieces. Such a fracture is usually accompanied by an appropriate accidental scenario and is rarely seen in young children.

Transverse fractures lines running horizontal to the bony axis are commonly seen with direct blows to the bone (Figure 33-8). Although usually accidental, such an injury can be associated with abuse. For instance, a transverse fracture can result from using a forearm to shield the head or upper body from a direct blow, the so-called "nightstick fracture." Indirect bending of an extremity can also result in a transverse fracture and can be seen in both accidental (planted foot that absorbs a direct blow to one side or falls from great heights) and nonaccidental (holding a leg while swinging/throwing a child) events.

In children, an incomplete transverse fracture is called a "greenstick" fracture line (Figure 33-1), a common accidental injury. Similarly, indirect bending can also result in plastic or bowing fractures as the force applied to the growing bone is enough to bend but not break the cortical margin (Figure 33-9). Although seen with abuse as well, transverse fractures are more commonly seen with accidental injury.

Oblique fracture lines are at any angle other than horizontal to the bony axis (Figure 33-10). Much attention has been given to the presence of a spiral fracture. A spiral fracture is an oblique fracture that winds around a long bone (Figure 33-11). It has a longer fracture length than a simple oblique fracture (often encompassing a third or more of the length of the entire bony shaft) and requires multiple radiographic views to see the entire course of the fracture. The accurate designation of a spiral versus a simple oblique fracture line can be unreliable since it depends on the radiographic views obtained. Still, it is important to attempt to determine the difference between the two fracture lines since the mechanism of injury causing these fractures differs, and hence can be a crucial component in matching an injury to the given clinical history.

Spiral fractures imply torsional forces applied to the long bone. Since many inflicted injuries to the long bones in children involve twisting of extremities, such a fracture line has been linked with abuse, although they are not limited to

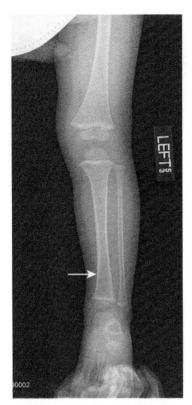

FIGURE 33-4 Common toddler fracture. Note the subtle lucent (black) line through the distal tibial metaphysis in this child who sustained a minor fall *(arrow)*.

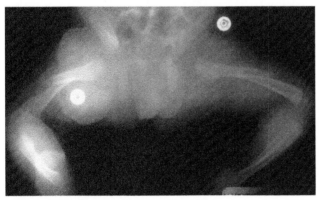

FIGURE 33-5 A 1-month-old infant with bilateral femur fractures.

abuse.[9,16,17-19] In infants, however, spiral fractures are more likely to be abusive than they are in ambulatory children.

Red Flag No. 3: Multiple Injuries of Differing Ages

Abusive injury can often be difficult to prove. The temporal relationship between the visualized radiographic injury and the proffered story are often a vital part of any child abuse workup. Discrepancies in the time frame of the injury as documented by clinical history and radiographic findings are certainly a strong indicator of a suspicious injury. The ability to determine the radiographic age of a fracture depends on the presence or absence of a periosteal reaction

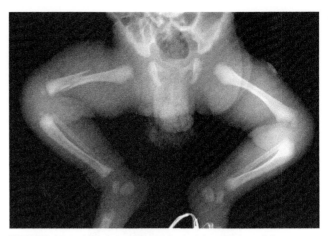

FIGURE 33-6 A 2-week-old infant imaged for a history of "not moving an extremity" that was swollen on clinical examination. Following radiographic confirmation of a right spiral femur fracture, the caretakers then offered a "new story" of dropping the infant.

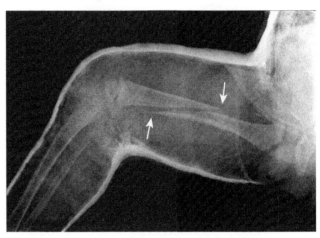

FIGURE 33-7 Long bone spiral fracture. Note the complete separation of fracture fragments and the length of the fracture line *(arrows)*.

(healing new bone formation, also known as callus). This periosteal reaction, however, is not specific to trauma; it can also be seen with any insult to bone including infection or tumor. Usually, the latter two entities are easily ruled out.

Callus is first seen approximately 10 to 14 days after the injury, and even earlier in infants (as early as 8 days postinjury).[20-22] Subperiosteal new bone formation manifests as a thin white (sclerotic) line coursing around the fracture margins of the long bones (Figure 33-10). Blurring of the distinct, sharp fracture line is another early sign of healing as the callus bridges the injury site.[23]

With time (weeks to months), the fracture site remodels with loss of definition of the original injury, usually correcting any previous deformities. Restoration of the original architecture of bone (intact cortex and medullary cavity) then occurs. The time span for a solidly united fracture of an immobilized limb in an adult is close to 3 months, but much earlier in children. An infant can unite a femur fracture in 3 weeks, and an 8-year-old child by 8 weeks (Figure 33-12).[24] Unlike adults, children can undergo extensive bony remodeling with eventual complete restoration of normal

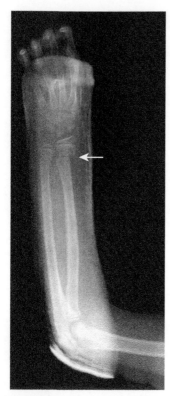

FIGURE 33-8 A transverse fracture is a fracture line that runs horizontal to the bone long axis *(arrow)*.

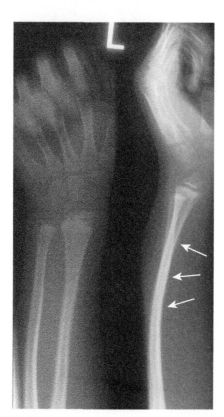

FIGURE 33-9 The bowing or "plastic" fracture occurs when the force on the bone is enough to bend but not break the long bone. As a result, no distinct fracture line is seen, but an obvious deformity is present on the lateral view *(arrows)*.

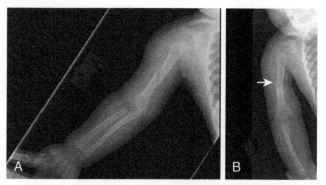

FIGURE 33-10 Oblique fracture. **A,** Note the visualization of the entire fracture course on one view and the shorter overall length of the fracture as compared with a spiral fracture. **B,** With time (3-4 weeks), one can seen the healing oblique fracture of the humerus with associated callus formation bridging the fracture site *(arrow)*.

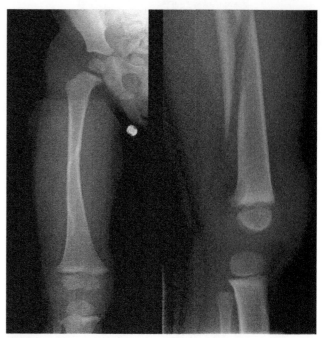

FIGURE 33-11 A, AP view of a spiral fracture. **B,** Lateral view of the same fracture. Note the length of the fracture line and the inability to see the entire fracture length on any one view. In fact, this large fracture is barely visible on the frontal view **(A)**.

bony appearance in a year or two (earlier in infants) even despite original wide displacement or angulation of bony fragments.[25]

The extent and appearance of periosteal reaction can change due to a number of factors. Inadequate diet, particularly with deficiency of vitamin D or calcium, can delay new bone formation.[25] Alternatively, periosteal reaction can magnify if motion remains at the fracture site due to repetitive injuries and/or lack of immobilization of the fracture site. The resulting subperiosteal hemorrhage can be extensive and exuberant (Figure 33-13). This latter finding can also be seen with avulsion of the periosteal membrane from the bone from an abusive twisting of a limb that strips the sensitive membrane from the bone, causing periosteal reaction but paradoxically, not fracture of the underlying bone (Figure 33-14).[26]

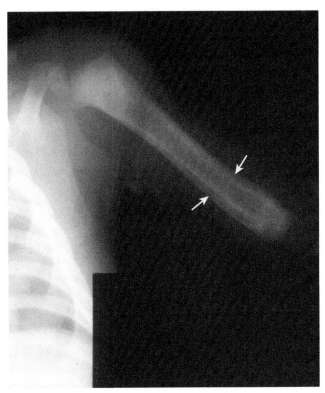

FIGURE 33-12 Remodeling of a distal humeral fracture. The original fracture line is no longer visualized as the callus has virtually repaired the damages *(arrows)*.

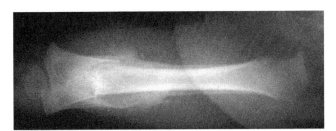

FIGURE 33-13 Exuberant periosteal reaction due to lack of immobilization of this healing fracture.

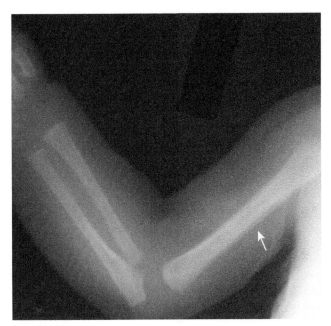

FIGURE 33-14 Periosteal reaction is clearly seen along the shaft of this humerus *(arrow)*, indicative of periosteal injury, yet no visible fracture line is ever seen.

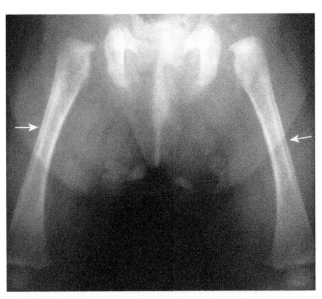

FIGURE 33-15 Physiological periosteal reaction can be seen symmetrically along only a single cortex of the femurs bilaterally *(arrows)*.

Adjacent soft tissue injury/soft tissue swelling is another helpful sign. Normal sharp muscle/fat interface can easily be seen on radiographs. Disruption of this area by hematoma or edema (swelling) signifies a recent injury of less than a week. Restoration of fat planes radiographically can be seen within 3 to 7 days following an injury, longer with an associated bony injury.[25]

Periosteal reaction can also be a normal finding in infants under 6 months of age. Physiologic periosteal new bone formation is commonly seen along the shafts of the long bones (femur, humerus, tibia, and less commonly the radius and ulna). Reported studies document that nearly half of all infants will develop this finding on serial radiographs.[27,28] The hallmark of physiological periosteal reaction is symmetry (same exact finding on bilateral long bones) with appearance of periosteal reaction on only one side of the cortex (Figure 33-15). The presence of periosteal reaction on a long bone that differs from one side of the body to another

or that encompasses both sides of the cortex of a long bone is worrisome for inflicted injury (Figure 33-16).

Care must also be taken with fractures discovered near birth. Birth trauma can result in initially occult fractures, especially fractures of the midsection of the clavicle. Incidence of clavicular birth injuries has been reported at up to 7 per 1000 deliveries (Figure 33-17).[29] However, because healing callus formation in infants is so rapid, it is possible to assert that the lack of callus with a clavicle fracture beyond 11 days after birth effectively excludes birth trauma as a cause. Also, fractures of the proximal and distal ends of the clavicle merit investigation (regardless of the callus timing)

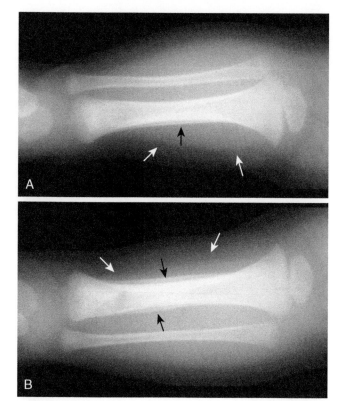

FIGURE 33-16 A, Note the normal physiological periosteal reaction seen only along one side of the cortex *(black arrow)* and intact fat planes on the unaffected tibia *(white arrows).* **B,** The opposite tibia is injured, with double cortical periosteal reaction *(black arrows)* and disrupted fat/muscle interface on the injured side *(white arrows).*

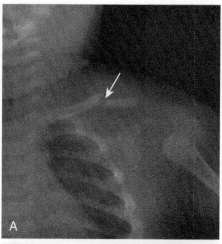

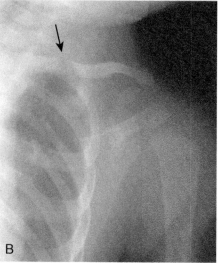

FIGURE 33-17 A, A common midclavicular fracture *(arrow)* in a 1-day-old infant attributed to birth trauma. Note the lack of callus. **B,** An abusive proximal clavicular fracture *(arrow)* in a 1-month-old. Note the lack of callus that this time rules out birth trauma as the cause due to the age of the child.

because these locations are highly unlikely to have been caused by a birth injury.[30]

The presence of fractures of differing ages (as documented radiographically by fractures in various stages of healing) can be a powerful tool in the workup of child abuse (Figures 33-18 to 33-20).

Red Flag No. 4: Metaphyseal "Corner" Fracture (The Classic Metaphyseal Lesion [CML])

Of all the injuries documented in child abuse, the classic metaphyseal lesion, or CML, (commonly referred to as the metaphyseal corner fracture) is probably the most highly specific injury associated with abuse. This injury is usually induced by "human hands" and does not occur with falls or blunt trauma. As described initially by Caffey,[26] and then more extensively by Kleinman,[31] the mechanism involves torsional and shearing strains of the metaphysis (end of the visualized mineralized bone) near the physis by pulling or twisting of the infant extremity, or by shaking the infant. The result is planar microfractures through the primary spongiosa seen at the metaphyseal/physeal interface.[26,31] Common sites include the distal femur, proximal and distal tibia, and proximal humeri. This is an injury seen exclusively in very young children. In abused children under 2 years of age, 39% to 50% have CMLs identified.[32,33]

The actual radiographic appearance of the metaphyseal corner fracture will depend on the projection of the image. From certain angles, this fracture can appear as a curvilinear structure emanating from the metaphysis, hence the common name "bucket-handle" fracture (Figure 33-21). Alternatively, the fracture can be visualized as a tiny bony piece projecting from the corner of the metaphysis or as an irregularity of the metaphyseal margin (Figure 33-22).

Red Flag No. 5: Rib Fractures, Especially Posterior Fractures

Like the CML, rib fractures have a very high specificity for inflicted injury and are commonly seen in abused infants. One study documents that 51% of 31 infants who died from abuse had thoracic cage fractures.[32] Conversely, rib fractures in infants and young children are exceedingly rare in true accidents due to the inherent plasticity, which allows for extreme deformability of the infant rib cage instead of overt fracture in the face of applied forces. As a result, rib fractures

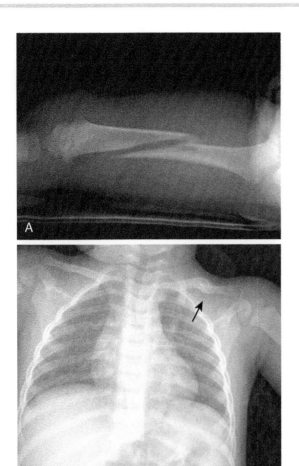

FIGURE 33-18 Two-year-old child who sustained a "fall" that resulted in a spiral femur fracture. Note the absence of callus dating this femur fracture as acute (less than 10-14 days). Subsequent skeletal survey revealed a healing clavicular fracture *(arrow)*, clearly of a different age than the femur injury.

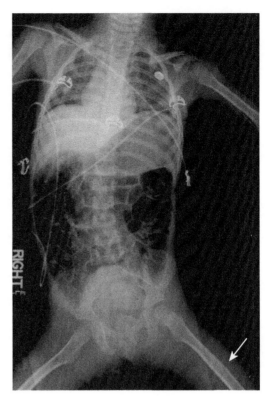

FIGURE 33-19 Radiograph of an obtunded child with a severe head injury following a "fall." Recurrent abuse was substantiated with discovery of a subtle old, remodeled fracture of her left mid femur *(arrow)*.

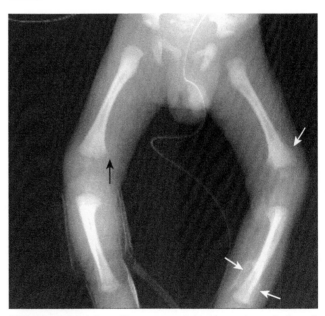

FIGURE 33-20 Infant with an acute subdural hemorrhage. Periosteal reaction can be seen involving the distal left femur and tibia *(white arrow)*, demonstrating injuries of differing ages. Also note the more acute metaphyseal corner fracture involving her distal right femur *(black arrow)* that does not have any callus formation.

in children are a documented marker of severe trauma to the chest.[34]

A clear mechanism, however, explains the pattern of rib fractures seen with abuse. Squeezing of the infant chest by human hands can generate impressive anteroposterior compressive forces that result in fractures preferentially at three sites: the posterior rib at the costo-vertebral junction, the lateral margin of the rib, and the anterior rib. Because of the infant's small thoracic cage in relation to a perpetrator's hands, it is common to see fractures in multiple adjacent ribs.[35]

Initially, fractures of infant ribs (seen as lucent lines across a rib margin) can be difficult to visualize radiographically. It is only with the appearance of healing callus that these fractures become obvious. This callus appears as a rounded white "bulbous" area centered over the fracture site, commonly seen at the posterior costovertebral junction and lateral rib margins (Figure 33-23). Because of the difficulties identifying acute rib fractures, follow-up radiographs or scintigraphy have been recommended for improved detection.[7,36,37] Oblique films of the rib cage can also be helpful to better visualize rib fractures, especially those along the lateral margins (Figure 33-24).[35]

"Handedness" may also play a role in the location of rib fractures. While holding an infant's chest (with the infant looking at the caretaker), the perpetrator's right hand would encircle the infant's left chest. Anecdotally, right-sided infant rib fractures are less common than left-sided rib fractures, possibly related to the fact that most people are right handed

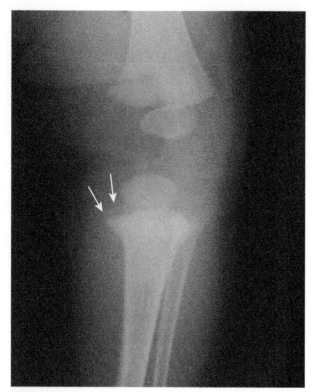

FIGURE 33-21 Curvilinear density projecting off the proximal tibial margin *(arrows)* consistent with a "bucket-handle" appearance of a classical metaphyseal lesion.

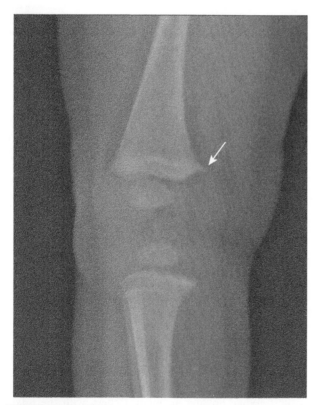

FIGURE 33-22 Metaphyseal corner fracture shows avulsion of a tiny piece of the distal cortical margin *(arrow)* from the distal femur in an infant.

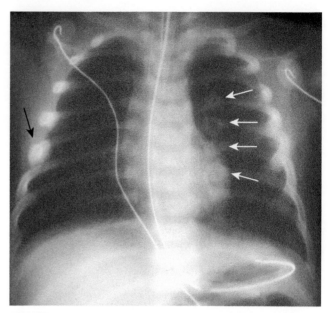

FIGURE 33-23 Classic posterior rib fractures with bulbous callus formation at the costovertebral junction at multiple adjacent levels *(white arrows)*. Lateral margin rib fracture with callus on the right is also present *(black arrow)*.

and therefore stronger on that side. The presence of the less commonly seen right-sided infant rib fractures, then, might help identify a left-handed perpetrator.

Red Flag No. 6: Skull Fractures

Unlike CML and rib fractures, skull fractures are much less definitively associated with abuse. Skull fractures result from blunt contact and can be seen with childhood falls and accidents. Luckily, the infant skull (with its open sutures) has plasticity and is usually able to resist accidental fracture; only 1% to 3% of short household accidental falls in children will result in a skull fracture.[38,39] Yet in abused children, skull fractures accounted for up to 13% of fractures, a number that rose to 29% to 33% in children less than 2 years of age, and to more than 40% in children who subsequently died from abusive injuries.[9,32,35]

Accidental skull fractures tend to have a characteristic radiographic appearance. They carry the label of "simple" skull fracture and appear as a thin, lucent (black) line, often located in the temporal/parietal area (Figure 33-25). Much more worrisome are "complex" skull fractures, which imply increased blunt force contact. These include skull fractures that have more than one fracture line (often with branching points), sometimes described as stellate or "egg-shell" fractures. Fractures that cross suture lines, that are comminuted (multiple pieces), or that are depressed also raise the index of suspicion. Widened fracture margins (greater than 3 mm) and fractures originating from the occipital area are also concerning (Figures 33-26).[40-42]

Skull radiographs are still the best method to image a potential skull fracture, and along with the spine, are the only films of the skeletal survey that always require two views (AP and lateral). CT can be used for potential associated intracranial injury. Due to the projection of the axial images, CT can miss concomitant skull fractures, particularly fractures that run parallel to the axial section plane.[35,43]

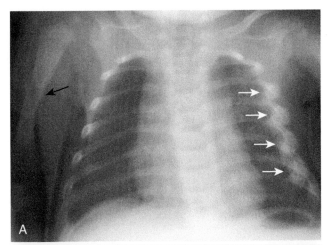

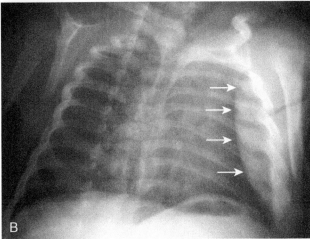

FIGURE 33-24 A, Six-month-old infant with a right oblique humeral fracture *(black arrow)* after being "dropped from her mother's arms." Skeletal survey revealed extensive callus involving multiple right ribs *(white arrows).* **B,** The more characteristic bulbous callus is better seen in the oblique films *(white arrows).*

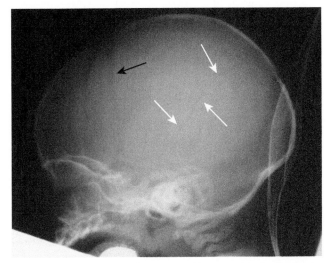

FIGURE 33-25 Simple skull fracture *(white arrows)* in the temporal-parietal area from a documented accidental fall. Note how thin the black fracture line is. Normal coronal sutures are also seen *(black arrows).*

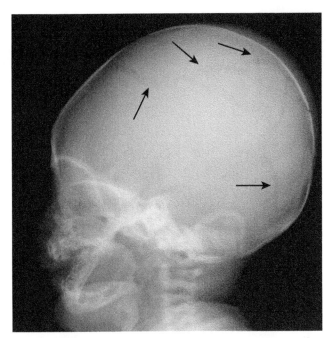

FIGURE 33-26 Complex skull fracture in an abused infant with wide fracture margins and multiple branch points, or "egg-shell" fracture *(arrows).*

Dating a skull fracture is problematic and at best, can only be a gross approximation. The presence of a soft tissue "knot" or swelling adjacent to the bony head injury can help define the fracture as "new" (an acute injury of less than 3 to 7 days), but is not definitive.[44] In addition, the presence of a sharp, well-defined fracture line is associated with a more acute injury. Conversely, a blurring of the skull fracture line that loses clear, sharp definition is seen as a more subacute or chronic injury (Figure 33-27).[25]

Suture widening, as seen on skull radiographs, is potentially a very ominous finding since it can be a harbinger of associated increased intracranial pressure. The presence of expanding cerebral edema/swelling or intracranial hematoma will result in a diffuse widening of all cranial sutures, often best seen involving the coronal sutures on the lateral film (Figure 33-28). Further imaging with CT or MR is warranted in these cases to determine the extent of intracranial involvement. Care must be taken not to mistake sutural widening from increased intracranial pressure with sutural diastasis (splitting) from adjacent fracture extension into a suture.

STRENGTH OF MEDICAL EVIDENCE

The literature strongly supports the imaging findings indicative of skeletal abuse in children. Numerous studies outlined previously have compared accidental to abusive skeletal imaging findings, defining their unique features with clear correlation of data and strong statistical support. Certainly the evidence supporting the abusive cause of most classic metaphyseal lesions and posterior rib fractures in infants is overwhelming. Extensive work on timing of callus formation has resulted in more definitive timetables, a crucial component in the temporal facts of skeletal healing. Recent work more clearly defines the timing of initial periosteal reaction in young infants.[22]

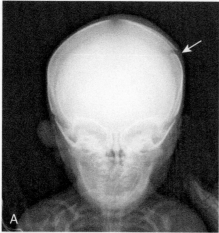

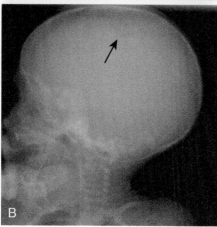

FIGURE 33-27 A, A "new" skull fracture (less than a week old) with soft tissue swelling and a sharp fracture line *(arrows).* **B,** A more subacute, indistinct fracture line *(arrow)* without any adjacent soft tissue swelling.

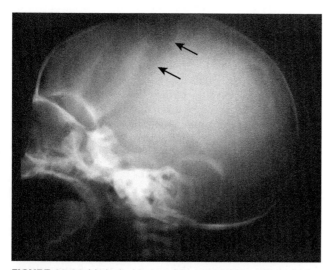

FIGURE 33-28 Marked widening of the cranial sutures *(arrows)* in an abused infant with increased intracranial pressure from subdural hematomas.

FUTURE RESEARCH

Biomechanical modeling of skeletal injuries is ongoing, with the goal of determining the amount of force needed to break juvenile bones. The correlation between heights of falls and types of fractures requires biomechanical modeling as well. Application of new technologies such as digital imaging and its use in the diagnosis of abusive injuries should also be pursued.

References

1. Landin LA: Fracture patterns in children. Analysis of 8,682 fractures with special reference to incidence, etiology and secular changes in a Swedish urban population 1950-1979. *Acta Orthop Scand Suppl* 1983;202:1-109.
2. Faerber EN, Applegate KE, Allen WR Jr, et al: ACR practice guideline for skeletal surveys in children, American College of Radiology (website): http://www.acr.org/SecondaryMainMenuCategories/quality_safety/guidelines/pediatric/skeletal_surveys.aspx. Accessed May 3, 2009.
3. American Academy of Pediatrics Section on Radiology: Diagnostic imaging of child abuse. *Pediatrics* 2009;123:1430-1435.
4. Kleinman PK, Nimkin K, Spevak MR, et al: Follow-up skeletal surveys in suspected child abuse. *AJR Am J Roentgenol* 1996;167:893-896.
5. Merten DF, Radkowski MA, Leonidas JC: The abused child: a radiological reappraisal. *Radiology* 1983;146:377-381.
6. Wolbarst A: *Physics of radiology,* ed 2, Medical Physics, Madison, Wis, 2005.
7. Sty JR, Starshak RJ: The role of bone scintigraphy in the evaluation of the suspected abused child. *Radiology* 1983;146:369-375.
8. Conway JJ, Collins M, Tanz RR: The role of bone scintigraphy in detecting child abuse. *Semin Nucl Med* 1993;23:321-333.
9. King J, Diefendorf D, Apthorp J, et al: Analysis of 429 fractures in 189 battered children. *J Pediatr Orthop* 1988;8:585-589.
10. Beals RK, Tufts E: Fractured femur: the role of child abuse. *J Pediatr Orthop* 1983;3:583-586.
11. Anderson WA: The significance of femoral fractures in children. *Ann Emerg Med* 1982;11:174-177.
12. Gross RH, Stranger M: Causative factors responsible for femoral fractures in infants and young children. *J Pediatr Orthop* 1983;3:341-343.
13. Helfer RE, Slovis TL, Black M: Injuries resulting when small children fall out of bed. *Pediatrics* 1977;60:533-535.
14. Nimityongskul A, Anderson LD: The likelihood of injury when children fall out of bed. *J Pediatr Orthop* 1987;7:184-186.
15. Lyons TJ, Oates RK: Falling out of bed: a relatively benign occurrence. *Pediatrics* 1993;92:125-127.
16. Loder RT, Bookout C: Fracture patterns in battered children. *J Orthop Trauma* 1991;5:428-433.
17. Stewart G, Meert K, Rosenberg N: Trauma in infants less than three months of age. *Pediatr Emerg Care* 1993;9:199-201.
18. Thomas SA, Rosenfield NS, Levanthal JM, et al: Long bone fractures in young children: distinguishing accidental injuries from child abuse. *Pediatrics* 1991;88:471-476.
19. Gross RH, Davidson R, Sullivan JA, et al: Cast brace management of the femoral shaft fracture in children and young adults. *J Pediatr Orthop* 1983;3:572-582.
20. Prosser I, Maguire S, Harrison SK, et al: How old is this fracture? Radiologic dating of fractures in children: a systematic review. *AJR Am J Roentgenol* 2005;184:1282-1286.
21. Islam O, Sobelski D, Symons S, et al: Development and duration of radiographic signs of bone healing in children. *AJR Am J Roentgenol* 2000;175:75-78.
22. Halliday K, Broderick N, Hawkes R, et al: Dating infants' fractures. *Pediatr Radiol* 2008;38(suppl 3):S534.
23. Chapman S: Radiologic dating of injuries. *Arch Dis Child* 1992;67:1063-1065.
24. Salter RB: Special features of fracture and dislocation in children. *In*: Heppenstall RB (ed): *Fracture Treatment and Healing.* WB Saunders, Philadelphia, 1980.
25. O'Connor JF, Cohen J: Dating fractures. *In*: Kleinman PK (ed): *Diagnostic Imaging of Child Abuse.* Mosby, St Louis, 1998.

26. Caffey J: Some traumatic lesions in growing bones other than fractures and dislocations: clinical and radiographic features. *Br J Radiol* 1957;3:225-238.

27. Glaser K: Double contour on roentgenograms of long bones of infants. *AJR Am J Roentgenol* 1949;61:482-492.

28. Shopfner CE: Periosteal bone growth in normal infants. A preliminary report. *AJR Am J Roentgenol* 1966;97:154-163.

29. Cohen AW, Otto SR: Obstetric clavicular fractures. A three year analysis. *J Reprod Med* 1980;25:119-122.

30. Cunming WA: Neonatal skeletal fractures: birth trauma or child abuse? *J Can Assoc Radiol* 1979;30:30-33.

31. Kleinman PK, Marks SC, Blackborne B: The metaphyseal lesion in abused infants: a radiologic histopathologic study. *AJR Am J Roentgenol* 1986;146:895-905.

32. Kleinman PK, Marks SC, Richmond JM, et al: Inflicted skeletal injury: a post mortem radiologic-histopathologic study in 31 infants. *AJR Am J Roentgenol* 1995;165:647-650.

33. Worlock P, Stower M, Barbor P: Patterns of fractures in accidental and non-accidental injury in children: a comparative study. *Br Med J* 1986;293:100-102.

34. Garcia VF, Gotschall CS, Eichelberger MR, et al: Rib fractures in children: a marker of severe trauma. *J Trauma* 1990;30:695-700.

35. Lonergan GJ, Baker AM, Morey MK, et al: Child abuse: radiologic-pathologic correlation. *Radiographics* 2003;23:811-845.

36. Kleinman PK, Nimkin K, Spevak MR, et al: Follow-up skeletal surveys in suspected child abuse. *AJR Am J Roentgenol* 1996;167:893-896.

37. Smith FW, Gilday DL, Ash JM, et al: Unsuspected costo-vertebral fractures demonstrated by bone scanning in the child abuse syndrome. *Pediatr Radiol* 1980;10:103-106.

38. Williams RA: Injuries in infants and small children resulting from witnessed and corroborated free falls. *J Trauma* 1991;31:1350-1352.

39. Tarantino CA, Dowd MD, Murdock TC: Short vertical falls in infants. *Pediatr Emerg Care* 1999;15:5-8.

40. Billmire ME, Myers PA: Serious head injury in infants: accident or abuse? *Pediatrics* 1985;75:340-342.

41. Meservy CJ, Towbin R, McLaurin RL, et al: Radiographic characteristics of skull fractures resulting from child abuse. *AJR Am J Roentgenol* 1987;149:173-175.

42. Hobbs CJ: Skull fracture and the diagnosis of abuse. *Arch Dis Child* 1984;59:246-252.

43. Saulsbury FT, Alford BA: Intracranial bleeding from child abuse: the value of skull radiographs. *Pediatr Radiol* 1982;12:175-178.

44. Kleinman PK, Spevak MR: Soft tissue swelling and acute skull fractures. *J Pediatr* 1992;121:737-739.

34

THE ROLE OF CROSS-SECTIONAL IMAGING IN EVALUATING PEDIATRIC SKELETAL TRAUMA

Peter T. Evangelista, MD, and Kathleen M. McCarten, MD, FACR

INTRODUCTION

Imaging studies are often critical in the assessment of infants and young children with evidence of physical injury, despite the fact that when considering all cases of child abuse and neglect, the incidence of physical injury documented by diagnostic imaging examinations is relatively small.[1] The role of imaging in suspected nonaccidental trauma (NAT) is twofold, first to document the extent of physical injury and second to elucidate all imaging findings that could potentially suggest alternative diagnoses.[2,3] The modalities available for imaging include radiography, scintigraphy, and cross-sectional imaging, which consists of ultrasound, computed tomography (CT), and magnetic resonance (MR) imaging.

Radiography remains the unanimous starting point in the overall imaging workup of skeletal injury. In keeping with this guideline, the radiographic bone survey (RBS) is the accepted standard in the imaging evaluation of suspected NAT and is mandatory in children under the age of 2.[4,5] Certain fractures, including posterior rib fractures, spiral fracture in a nonambulatory child, vertebral fracture, scapular fracture, classic metaphyseal lesion (CML), and fractures of different ages, are highly suggestive of NAT.[3,6,7] Despite a high-quality technique as outlined by the American College of Radiology (ACR) and the Section on Radiology of the American Academy of Pediatrics,[1,8] several factors limit the effectiveness of radiography. First, acute, incomplete, and nondisplaced rib fractures can be difficult to identify,[9] particularly in the young infant. Although oblique rib radiographs can improve detection,[10] they are not routinely performed at most institutions.[11] Second, radiographs are insensitive for evaluating nonosseous injury. Third, there is great variation in imaging protocols among pediatric health care facilities with a little less than half reporting acquisition practices approximating those recommended by the ACR.[11] Bone scintigraphy demonstrates increased activity at sites of healing fractures and has been shown to complement the RBS and to improve the detection of rib fractures and fractures of the spine, pelvis, and acromion.[12] On the other hand, it has poor sensitivity (35%) in detection of CML, largely because the metaphysis is a site of normal intense metabolic activity in young children. Only 4.7% of health care facilities in the Unites States reported routine performance of both RBS and bone scintigraphy in a survey by Kleinman in 2004.[11]

This chapter will explore the current role of cross-sectional imaging (ultrasound, CT, and MRI) in the workup of general skeletal trauma in children, and particularly in the imaging workup of suspected NAT.

ULTRASONOGRAPHY

Diagnostic ultrasonography is a convenient, practical, and cost-effective method for primarily evaluating a variety of musculoskeletal disorders in the pediatric population. It is well suited for use in children because of the increased ratio of cartilage to bone in the immature skeleton.[13,14] Using a transducer, high frequency sound waves (above the frequency range of human hearing) are generated in pulsed packets and sent into the patient. The sound waves are then echoed back to the transducer and processed to form an anatomic image largely based on the reflecting properties of the internal and surface architecture of different tissues. The stronger the reflector, the higher the echo strength and the corresponding brightness on the image. Bone, and in particular its cortical surface, is a very strong reflector and thus makes ultrasonography of structures deep in it impractical. High-quality musculoskeletal ultrasonography is typically performed with a linear array transducer in the range of 5.0 to 10.0 Mhz.[15] As transducer frequency increases, axial resolution increases but the depth of the imaging field decreases.[16] Therefore, for every circumstance, the highest transducer frequency is selected that effectively balances this trade-off. When combined with color Doppler technique, ultrasonography is a uniquely powerful tool for assessing a variety of conditions involving the musculoskeletal system in the pediatric patient.[13] The major benefits of ultrasonography are its lack of ionizing radiation and the rare need for sedation.

The most common use of ultrasonography in general musculoskeletal pediatric clinical practice is for developmental dysplasia of the hip.[17,18] Other common clinical applications include the imaging evaluation of the painful hip,[19] joint effusions,[20] soft tissue infection and osteomyelitis,[21,22] inflammatory arthropathies,[23,24] paraskeletal soft tissue masses,[25] foreign body identification,[26] congenital foot deformities,[27,28] proximal focal femoral deficiency,[29] and image guidance for interventional procedures.[30]

With regard to skeletal trauma, ultrasonography has been demonstrated to be effective in the evaluation of tendon, ligament, and muscle injuries in the general population. However, in children the growth plates are generally weaker and more vulnerable to trauma than tendons and ligaments, so ultrasonography is more commonly used in children to

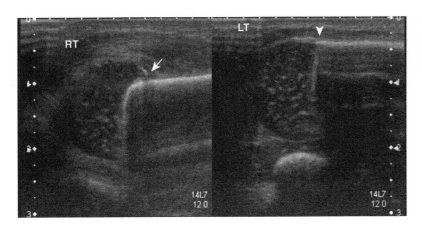

FIGURE 34-1 Newborn infant with decreased right arm movement and suspected birth injury. Ultrasound of affected right and normal left shoulder demonstrates slipped proximal humeral epiphysis (*arrow*) and normal relationship on the left (*arrowhead*).

evaluate epiphyseal-apophyseal detachment rather than injury to the ligament itself.[13] In the adolescent, ultrasonography can be used to evaluate Osgood-Schlatter lesions, which demonstrate fragmentation of the tibial tuberosity and surrounding hypoechoic soft tissue edema related to micro-avulsion from repeat traction injury on the developing tibial tuberosity ossification center.[31] In children under the age of 5, ultrasonography has demonstrated a role in identifying traumatic avulsions of the nonossified medial epicondyle.[32,33] In the newborn, ultrasound assessment of the shoulder can be used to distinguish posterior humeral head displacement in Erb palsy from slipped proximal humeral epiphysis related to birth injury (Figure 34-1).[34,35] Distal humeral physeal separation or fracture separation of the distal humeral epiphysis is difficult to diagnosis radiographically, especially if nondisplaced, because of the nonossified cartilaginous epiphysis. When displaced it manifests radiographically by the abnormal medial and posterior displacement of the ulnar shaft and capitellum relative to the humeral shaft (Figure 34-2). Although an unusual injury, it accounts for a significant number of elbow fractures in children under the age of 3 and indicates the possibility of unsuspected NAT.[36,37] Children can present clinically with swelling of the elbow, disuse of the extremity, or reported/perceived pain.[37] Ziv et al[38] reported a case of distal humeral epiphyseal separation in a neonate easily diagnosed using ultrasonography.

Proximal femoral physeal injuries or proximal femoral epiphysiolysis occur infrequently in infants but are highly correlated with NAT (Figure 34-3).[6,39] The injury should be suspected in any infant having an apparently shortened limb held in the flexed, abducted, and externally rotated position.[40] In infants under 4 months of age, the diagnosis is difficult radiographically due to lack of ossification of the femoral head. In these cases, ultrasonography has been demonstrated to be of value in documenting injuries.[41]

Although using ultrasonography is not advocated as a screening examination for global fracture detection, it has been demonstrated to be effective in cases where there is a clinically indistinct location of pain in children with trauma,[42] or where radiographs are suspicious but not diagnostic.[20] Ultrasonography demonstrates well the displacement or disruption of the perichondral ring diagnostic of a CML that might not be readily apparent by radiographs.[43] Healing fractures are often better appreciated by ultrasonography because a healing callus is visualized sooner by ultrasound than by conventional radiographs.[44] Moreover, ultrasound

has been used to detect occult rib fractures in adults[45,46] and costochondral dislocation of a lower rib in an abused infant of 9 months.[47]

In summary, ultrasonography is not the primary modality in the evaluation of trauma or suspected NAT. However, ultrasound does play an important role as an adjunct study and is of particular benefit in the evaluation of injury to cartilaginous structures such as chondrocostal injury and physeal/epiphyseal injury of the shoulders, elbows, hips, and knees in abused infants. It may also be of benefit in select cases to diagnose radiographically occult long bone fractures.

COMPUTED TOMOGRAPHY

Computed tomography (CT) and, in particular, multidetector CT (MDCT) offers several advantages in the workup of skeletal trauma. First, the fast acquisition time obviates the need for sedation in most cases, and second, the ability to reformat and evaluate images in multiple planes reduces the need to manipulate the patient to achieve optimal imaging of the area of interest.[48] MDCT has been proven superior to conventional radiography in the evaluation of fractures involving complex anatomical regions in the general population, such as of the face, pelvis, and spine.[49-51] It offers superb spatial resolution and is often relied upon for preoperative planning in complex skeletal trauma. The major disadvantage of CT is its significant dose of ionizing radiation as compared with conventional radiography. This is especially true for imaging of the more radiosensitive structures of the axial skeleton and is less of an issue in the least radiosensitive structures of the peripheral appendicular skeleton. Given the fact that children are more radiosensitive than adults and given the potential risk of CT-induced malignancy, it is important that principles guiding the use of ionizing radiation referred to as "ALARA" (as low as reasonably achievable) are always followed.[52-56]

For pediatric skeletal trauma, CT has demonstrated increased sensitivity in the evaluation of radiographic occult fractures, especially in older children. CT has been found to detect occult injuries in 52% of children with joint effusion but otherwise normal radiographs.[48] In evaluation of triplane fractures, which typically occur in older children and account for 6% to 10% of epiphyseal injuries, CT most accurately delineated and analyzed these fractures and concluded that CT is the method of choice for both preoperative

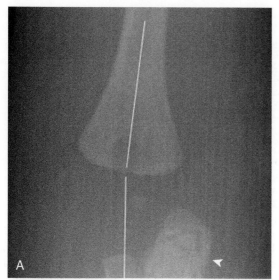

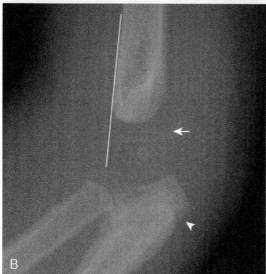

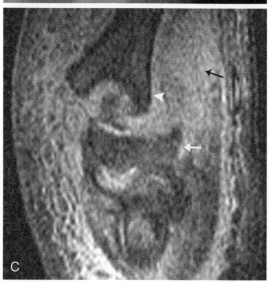

FIGURE 34-2 Ten-month-old girl with suspected NAT and distal humeral physeal separation. Initial humeral AP **(A)** and lateral **(B)** radiographs demonstrate medial translation of the ulna relative to the humerus (ulnar shaft should be in line with humeral shaft, white lines **(A)**. Healing olecranon fracture *(arrowheads)* also noted **(A, B)**. Note posterior displacement of capitellum and ulna *(white line)* **(B)** drawn along the anterior cortex should intersect capitellum) and posteriorly displaced metaphyseal fragment *(arrow)*. Coronal STIR MR image **(C)** better demonstrates medial translation of epiphyseal fragment *(arrow)* relative to the metaphysis *(arrowhead)* with marked surrounding edema *(black thin arrow)*.

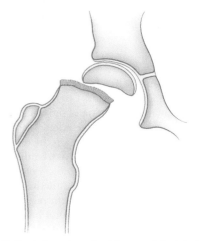

FIGURE 34-3 Illustration of proximal femur epiphysiolysis.

and postoperative evaluation of these injuries.[56] (Note that triplane fractures are not a typical manifestation of child abuse.)

MDCT has largely replaced radiography as the modality of choice for the imaging of major pediatric maxillofacial trauma because it provides the best depiction of facial fractures; radiographs should be reserved for initial evaluation in those patients with low-energy trauma.[57] Although facial fractures occur in only 2.3% of abused children,[58] a level of suspicion for NAT should always be present. Infant mandibular fractures, in particular, should raise suspicion for abuse as a newborn's cranial-to-facial proportion is approximately 8:1, as compared with the adult's 2:1 proportion. In infants, this craniofacial disproportion generally protects the maxilla and mandible.[59]

Rib fractures in infants are the result of NAT in more than 80% of cases,[60-63] and are the most common skeletal injury in child abuse.[64-65] CT has been found to be highly sensitive in adults in detecting radiographically occult rib fractures,[66] and recently was found to be significantly more sensitive than initial chest radiographs in the early detection of rib fractures in abused infants under the age of one.[67] Still, the addition of oblique radiographs to the initial RBS, follow-up radiographs several weeks postinjury, or complementary use of bone scintigraphy are more widely accepted alternatives.[10,12,68,69]

Spinal trauma in the setting of NAT is unusual, with spinal fractures compromising only 3% of abuse-related fractures.[70] Thoracolumbar fracture with listhesis is a rare fracture first described by Swischuk,[71] and one which should prompt suspicion for NAT (Figure 34-4). The injury is most

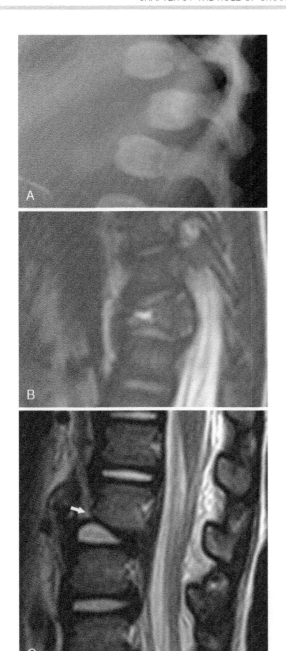

FIGURE 34-4 A 2-year-old boy with back pain, upper lumbar point tenderness, and suspected NAT. Lateral radiograph **(A)** and sagittal CT reconstruction **(B)** demonstrate retrolisthesis of L2 on L3 *(arrow)* with mild anterior L2 compression and widened facet joints *(arrowhead in* **A**). Sagittal T2 weighted image **(C)** demonstrates Salter-type fracture through the inferior endplate apophysis and L2 retrolisthesis.

common at the L1/L2 level, and radiographic findings can be quite subtle and misinterpreted as nontraumatic in etiology.[72] The radiographic findings include subtle listhesis to complete dislocation of one vertebra on another with or without varying compression deformities of the affected vertebra. More chronic injuries can demonstrate paravertebral calcifications. In terms of cause, there is substantial evidence supporting a mechanism of hyperflexion and axial spinal loading.[73,74] A high level of awareness is needed to identify this injury on conventional radiography and it is essential that lateral radiographs of the spine be included

as part of the routine RBS.[74] Cross-sectional imaging studies such as CT or MRI should be obtained in cases of documented spinal pathology. CT and MRI can demonstrate the typical fracture through the neurocentral synchondrosis and the Salter type of fracture through the endplate apophysis.[73]

Numerous studies have documented the utility of performing high-quality postmortem radiography for not only documenting the extent and chronicity of NAT, but potentially to demonstrate normal findings, which can contribute to the accurate classification of death.* Several studies have explored the use of CT as a virtual autopsy.[77,78] Post mortem CT (PMCT) has been shown in deceased infants and children to detect the cause of death when combined with medical history and laboratory data.[79] CT and particularly whole body MDCT might ultimately have a more prominent role in the post-mortem evaluation of NAT.

In summary, CT is not the primary modality for evaluation of skeletal trauma in children and is rarely required in cases of suspected NAT. CT has been shown superior to radiographs in evaluating complex intraarticular and physeal fractures in older children, but is of limited value in the younger children with higher cartilage to bone ratio. In children with suspected NAT, CT should be reserved to the evaluation of complex anatomical regions such as the face in the setting of high clinical suspicion or for further delineation of suspected spinal fractures. It is an important selective tool in evaluation of infants where there is a high suspicion for osseous thoracic NAT and in whom there is the possibility of associated intrathoracic or intraabdominal injury.[67] Lastly it might play a more prominent role in the future in the virtual autopsies of children with suspected NAT.

MAGNETIC RESONANCE IMAGING

Magnetic resonance (MR) imaging offers several advantages over conventional radiography in the evaluation of skeletal trauma. Its main advantages include its high contrast and spatial resolution, and its lack of ionizing radiation. Its main disadvantage in the pediatric population is the relative long examination times, which often require the administration of sedation. With that said, it is the imaging modality of choice in the evaluation of traumatic lesions of cartilage, ligaments, myotendinous units, and soft tissues.[80-84]

Numerous studies have demonstrated the superiority of MR imaging compared with conventional radiographs for the detection of occult bony injury. This is especially true for developing bones, which are largely composed of radiolucent structures.[84-91] For example, stress fractures which occur most commonly in the tibia, fibula, metatarsals, cuboid, calcaneus, and femur in children,[92] demonstrate a sensitivity of as low as 15% on initial radiographs. Further, delayed radiographs only reveal findings in 50% of patients.[93] In these cases, MRI using fat suppressed T2 weighted imaging is extremely sensitive to high signal marrow edema and often subperiosteal edema associated with stress reactions.[93] The presence of a low signal intensity line with high signal marrow edema confirms the presence of a stress fracture.[84]

---

*References 6, 7, 64, 65, 75, 76.

Approximately 15% of all pediatric fractures involve the physis, with the peak age in early adolescence.[94] Although conventional radiography remains the primary means of evaluating these injuries, MR imaging is sometimes used to delineate acute physeal fractures in very young children with unossified epiphyses.[84] Fifteen percent of all physeal fractures lead to growth arrest with the formation of a bone bridge across the physis, which can cause limb shortening or angular deformity.[95] Although the distal radius is the most common site of physeal fracture, the distal femur and distal tibia have disproportionately high incidences of posttraumatic premature physeal fusion.[96] MR imaging (particularly fat suppressed three-dimensional spoiled gradient echo sequences) is the modality of choice in evaluating physeal growth arrest.[97-99] The goal of imaging is to accurately depict the size and location of bone bridges relative to the remainder of the physis to guide surgical management.[84] Optimal surgical correction results when 2 years of expected longitudinal growth remains and when the physeal bridge involves less than 50% of the growth plate area.[100,101]

MR imaging can be used to evaluate epiphyseal injuries in infants, such as those occurring at the proximal/distal humerus and at the proximal femur. Although these are most often the result of birth trauma, in this age group they also can be nonaccidental in nature. Currently ultrasonography is the preferred imaging modality because it can rapidly establish the diagnosis without the need for sedation.[102] MR imaging is more frequently used in the evaluation of elbow trauma in children beyond infancy.[84] MR imaging is a valuable adjunct in evaluating the previously discussed entity of distal humeral physeal separation, which has been associated with NAT (Figure 34-2). MR imaging is of particular value in cases where the fracture is nondisplaced or where there is uncertainty with regard to the diagnosis.[36,37]

Regarding global MR imaging in the evaluation of NAT, there is very little data in the literature to support its use. There is only a single case report espousing MR imaging for the evaluation of NAT in children.[103] MR imaging was performed in this case report employing the short-tau inversion recovery sequence, which is highly sensitive to extracellular water in both bone marrow and soft tissues, and when used to image the entire body enables a survey of the entire musculoskeletal system and multiple organ systems in a single imaging test. There are numerous references supporting the usefulness of the whole-body, short-tau inversion recovery (WB-STIR) sequence for the staging of malignant disease in adults and children.[104-106] Mentzel et al[107] in 2004 concluded that WB-STIR was more sensitive than bone scintigraphy for the detection of multifocal skeletal metastasis in children.

Preliminary unpublished data from our institution demonstrates that coronal WB-STIR MR imaging complements but does not replace the initial RBS for the investigation of NAT in children. Although MR imaging can demonstrate acute osseous injuries that are missed on the initial bone survey (Figures 34-5 and 34-6), it performed poorly in the detection of chronic fractures and in the identification of classic metaphyseal lesions [CMLs] (Figure 34-7). Furthermore, WB-STIR might have an important forensic role in assessing the age of a fracture since most of the chronic fractures were not associated with marrow or periosteal edema. There are two possible reasons why WB-STIR MR imaging performed poorly in detection of CMLs. First these fractures are thought to represent shear type injuries through the primary spongiosa.[108] This mechanism might generate only minimal edema in a manner similar to distraction type fractures described by Palmer.[109] Secondly, suffering similar limitations of bone scintigraphy, the physeal region is normally high in signal on WB-STIR MR imaging and therefore makes edema less conspicuous.

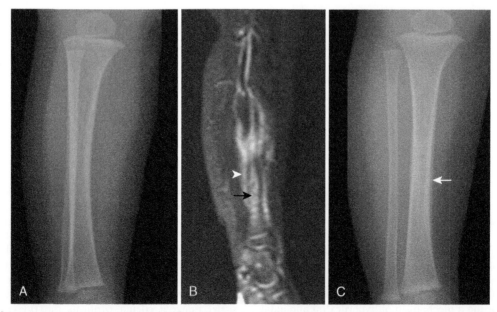

FIGURE 34-5 Seven-month-old boy with suspected NAT. **A,** No fracture was diagnosed on the initial RBS of the right tibia. **B,** Coronal WB-STIR obtained 1 day later shows marrow edema *(arrow)* and perosseous edema *(arrowhead)* suspicious for acute nondisplaced fracture. **C,** Follow-up RBS 29 days later demonstrates periosteal reaction *(arrow)* compatible with healing nondisplaced fracture. A fracture line is not discretely visualized.

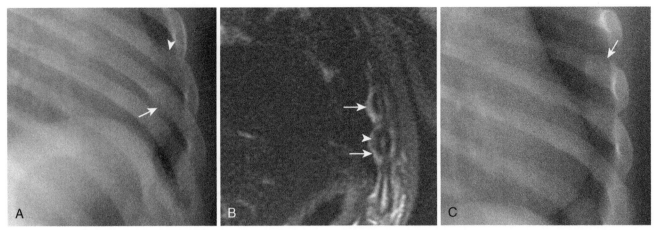

FIGURE 34-6 Four-month-old boy with suspected NAT. **A,** Initial RBS demonstrates subacute sixth rib fracture *(arrow).* Early subacute fifth rib fracture is only evident by subtle periosteal reaction *(arrowhead),* which was missed prospectively. **B,** WB-STIR demonstrates subperiosteal edema *(arrows)* around subacute fifth and sixth rib fractures. Sixth rib fracture demonstrates intermediate signal callus *(arrowhead).* **C,** Follow-up RBS obtained 20 days later demonstrates interval callus formation *(arrow)* at the fifth rib fracture.

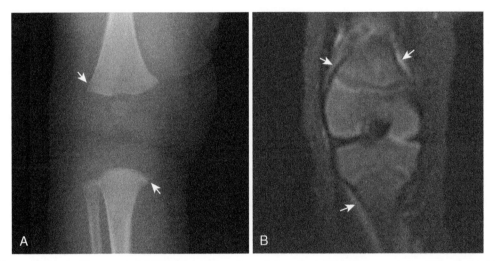

FIGURE 34-7 Six-week-old boy with suspected NAT. **A,** Extremity radiograph from the initial RBS demonstrates CMLs *(arrows)* of the distal femur and proximal tibia. **B,** Coronal WB-STIR 3 days later demonstrates subperiosteal edema *(arrows)* extending to the physis of the distal femur and proximal tibia. The CMLs are not discretely visualized.

As expected, coronal WB-STIR can also identify a variety of superficial and deep soft tissue injuries (Figure 34-8), some of which are primary traumatic lesions. The identification of these soft tissue abnormalities can be of great value in documenting the nature and extent of soft tissue injuries that one routinely detects on the RBS.

Given the additional expense and the sedation requirement, the role of WB-STIR in the workup of NAT is yet to be determined. We currently are only using coronal WB-STIR MR imaging in children referred for brain MR imaging by the hospital's Child Protection Program for suspected abusive head injury.

In summary, MRI is the modality of choice for evaluating nonosseous traumatic lesions in the pediatric population and for the evaluation of radiographically occult osseous injury. It plays a crucial role in the evaluation of physeal injury, although conventional radiography remains the initial examination of choice. With regard to suspected NAT, MR imaging is a useful adjunct study in the evaluation of physeal and epiphyseal injuries in the young child, although ultrasonography is often preferred since it can be performed without sedation. MR imaging and particularly coronal WB-STIR MR imaging maintain great promise as a complementary screening tool in the imaging workup of NAT.

SUMMARY

Conventional radiography remains the unanimous starting point in the overall imaging workup of skeletal injury. In keeping with this guideline, the RBS is the accepted standard in the imaging evaluation of suspected NAT.

Ultrasonography is an important adjunct study in the evaluation of trauma and suspected NAT. It is of particular benefit in the evaluation of injury to cartilaginous structures such as chondrocostal injury and physeal/epiphyseal injury of the shoulders, elbows, hips, and knees in abused infants. It can also be of benefit in select cases to diagnose radiographically occult long bone fractures.

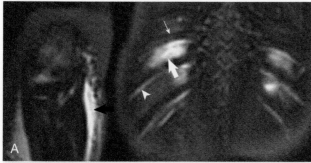

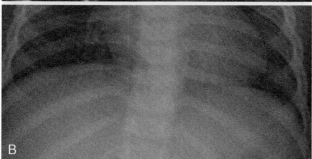

FIGURE 34-8 Seventeen-month-old boy with suspected NAT. **A,** Coronal WB-STIR of posterior chest wall and right elbow demonstrates edema of intercostal muscles *(large arrow)* but no fracture of adjacent ribs *(thin arrow)*. Note normal hyperintense subcostal neurovascular bundle *(arrowhead)*. There is diffuse subcutaneous edema of right antecubital fossa *(black arrow)* related to failed angiocatheter placement. **B,** Corresponding RBS corroborates absence of rib fractures.

CT plays an important adjunct role in the workup of skeletal trauma in children but is of limited utility in suspected NAT. In children with suspected NAT, CT should be reserved for the evaluation of complex anatomical regions such as the face in the setting of high clinical suspicion or for further delineation of suspected spinal fractures. For the latter, however, MR imaging is the favored modality. It has a selective role in the evaluation of infants with a high suspicion for occult osseous thoracic injury and in which there is suspected internal injury. Future research is needed into the utility of postmortem CT and MR imaging, also known as virtual autopsy, in children who die from suspected NAT.

In young children with suspected NAT, MR imaging is a useful adjunct study in the evaluation of physeal and epiphyseal injuries, although ultrasonography is often preferred, especially in infants, since sedation is not needed for ultrasound. It also is of value in further evaluating young children with traumatic spinal pathology. The current use of MR imaging as a whole body screening tool in the imaging workup of NAT is anecdotal and case specific. Future research is needed to determine the optimal role of whole body MR imaging in the imaging workup of NAT.

The strength of the medical evidence is moderate for ultrasonography and computed tomography, and weak to moderate for magnetic resonance imaging with regard to the use of these cross-sectional imaging modalities in the workup of NAT.

References

1. American Academy of Pediatrics Section on Radiology: Diagnostic imaging of child abuse. *Pediatrics* 2009;123:1430-1435.
2. Ablin DS, Sane SM: Nonaccidental injury: confusion with brittle bone disease and mild osteogenesis imperfecta. *Pediatr Radiol* 1997;27:111-113.
3. Merten DF, Radkowski MA, Leonidas JC: The abused child: a radiological reappraisal. *Radiology* 1983;146:377-381.
4. American College of Radiology: Imaging the child with suspected physical abuse. ACR appropriateness criteria. *Radiology* 2000;215(suppl):805-809.
5. Kemp AM, Butler A, Morris S, et al: Which radiological investigations should be performed to identify fractures in suspected child abuse? *Clin Radiol* 2006;61:723-736.
6. Kleinman PK: *Diagnostic Imaging of Child Abuse.* Mosby-Year Book, St Louis, 1998.
7. Kleinman PK, Blackbourne BD, Marks SC, et al: Radiologic contributions to the investigation and prosecution of cases of fatal infant abuse. *N Engl J Med* 1989;320:507-511.
8. Faerber EN, Applegate KE, Allen WR Jr, et al: *ACR practice guideline for skeletal surveys in children,* American College of Radiology (website): http://www.acr.org/SecondaryMainMenuCategories/quality_safety/guidelines/pediatric/skeletal_surveys.aspx. Accessed May 3, 2009.
9. Lonergan GJ, Baker AM, Morey MK, et al: Child abuse: radiologic-pathologic correlation. *Radiographics* 2003;23:811-845.
10. Ingram JD, Connell J, Hay TC, et al: Oblique radiographs of the chest in nonaccidental trauma. *Emerg Radiol* 2000;7:42-46.
11. Kleinman PL, Kleinman PK, Savageau JA: Suspected infant abuse: radiographic skeletal survey practices in pediatric health care facilities. *Radiology* 2004;233:477-485.
12. Mandelstam SA, Cook D, Fitzgerald M, et al: Complementary use of radiological skeletal survey and bone scintigraphy in detection of bony injuries in suspected child abuse. *Arch Dis Child* 2003;88:387-390.
13. Bellah R: Ultrasound in pediatric musculoskeletal disease: techniques and applications. *Radiol Clin North Am* 2001;39:597-618.
14. Harcke HT: Musculoskeletal ultrasound in pediatrics. *Semin Musculoskelet Radiol* 1998;2:321-330.
15. Roberts CS, Beck Jr DJ, Heinsen J, et al: Diagnostic ultrasonography: applications in orthopaedic surgery. *Clin Orthop Relat Res* 2002;401:248-264.
16. van Holsbeeck MT, Introcaso JH: Sonography of ligaments. *In*: Bralow L (ed): *Musculoskeletal Ultrasound,* ed 2, Mosby Year-Book, St Louis, 2000, pp 171-192.
17. Harcke HT: Screening newborns for developmental dysplasia of the hip: the role of sonography. *AJR Am J Roentgenol* 1994;162:395-397.
18. Graf R, Schuler P: *Guide to sonography of the infant hip.* Thieme Medical, New York, 1987.
19. Dorr U, Ziegler M, Hauke H: Ultrasonography of the painful hip: prospective studies in 204 patients. *Pediatr Radiol* 1987;17:233-237.
20. Keller MS: Musculoskeletal sonography in the neonate and infant. *Pediatr Radiol* 2005;35:1167-1173.
21. Wright NB, Abbott GT, Carty HM: Ultrasound in children with osteomyelitis. *Clin Radiol* 1995;50:623-627.
22. Riebel TW, Nasir R, Nazarenko O: The value of sonography in the detection of osteomyelitis. *Pediatr Radiol* 1996;26:291-297.
23. Lamer S, Sebag G: MR imaging and ultrasound in children with juvenile chronic arthritis. *Eur J Radiol* 2000;33:85-93.
24. Cellerini M, Salti S, Trapani S, et al: Correlation between clinical and ultrasound assessment of the knee in children with mono-articular or pauci-articular juvenile rheumatoid arthritis. *Pediatr Radiol* 1999;29:117-123.
25. Abiezzi SS, Miller LS: The use of ultrasound to the diagnosis of soft tissue masses in children. *J Pediatr Orthop* 1995;15:566-673.
26. Gilbert FJ, Campbell RSD, Bayliss AP: The role of ultrasound in the detection of non-radiopaque foreign bodies. *Clin Radiol* 1990;41:109-112.
27. Gigante C, Talenti E, Turra S: Sonographic assessment of clubfoot. *J Clin Ultrasound* 2004;32:235-242.
28. Aurell Y, Johansson A, Hansson G, et al: Ultrasound anatomy in the normal neonatal and infant foot: an anatomic introduction to ultrasound assessment of foot deformities. *Eur Radiol* 2002;12:2306-2312.
29. Gillespie R, Torode IP: Classification and management of congenital abnormality of the femur. *J Bone Joint Surg Br* 1983;65:557-568.

30. Shin HJ, Amaral JG, Armstrong D, et al: Image-guided percutaneous biopsy of musculoskeletal lesions in children. *Pediatr Radiol* 2007;37: 362-369.

31. Lanning P, Heikkinen E: Ultrasound features of the Osgood-Schlatter lesion. *J Pediatr Orthop* 1991;11:538-540.

32. Davidson RS, Markowitz RI, Dormans J, et al: Ultrasonographic evaluation of the elbow in infants and children after suspected trauma. *J Bone Joint Surg Am* 1994;76:1804-1813.

33. May DA, Dilser DG, Jones EA, et al: Using sonography to diagnose an unossified medial epicondyle avulsion in a child. *AJR Am J Roentgenol* 2000;174:1115-1117.

34. Hunter JD, Franklin K, Hughes PM: The ultrasound diagnosis of posterior shoulder dislocation associated with Erb's palsy. *Pediatr Radiol* 1998;28:510-511.

35. Ziegler M, Dorr U, Schultz R: Sonography of slipped humeral epiphysis due to birth injury. *Pediatr Radiol* 1987;17:425-426.

36. Gilbert SR, Conklin MJ: Presentation of distal humeral physeal separation. *Pediatr Emerg Care* 2007;23:816-819.

37. Nimkin N, Kleinman P, Teeger S, et al: Distal humeral physeal injuries in child abuse: MR imaging and ultrasonography findings. *Pediatr Radiol* 1995;25:562-565.

38. Ziv N, Litwin A, Katz K, et al: Definitive diagnosis of fracture-separation of the distal humeral epiphysis in neonates by ultrasonography. *Pediatr Radiol* 1996;26:493-496.

39. Ogden JA, Lee KE, Rudicel SA, et al: Proximal femoral epiphysiolysis in the neonate. *J Pediatr Orthop* 1984;4:285-292.

40. Canale SF, Tolo VT: Fractures of the femur in children. *Instr Course Lect* 1995;44:255-273.

41. Jones JCW, Feldman KW, Bruckner JD: Child abuse in infants with proximal physeal injuries of the femur. *Pediatr Emerg Care* 2004;20: 157-161.

42. Moritz JD, Berthold LD, Soenksen SF, et al: Ultrasound in diagnosis of fractures in children: unnecessary harassment or useful addition to x-ray? *Ultraschall Med* 2008;29:267-274.

43. Markowitz RI, Hubbard AM, Harty MP, et al: Sonography of the knee in normal and abused infants. *Pediatr Radiol* 1993;23: 264-267.

44. Allen GM, Wilson DJ: Ultrasound and the diagnosis of orthopaedic disorders. *J Bone Joint Surg Br* 1993;81:944-951.

45. Mariacher-Gehler SM, Michel BA: Sonography: a simple way to visualize rib fractures. *AJR Am J Roentgenol* 1994;163:1268.

46. Kara M, Dikmen E, Erdal HH, et al: Disclosure of unnoticed rib fractures with the use of ultrasonography in minor blunt chest trauma. *Eur J Cardiothorac Surg* 2003;24:608-613.

47. Smeets AJ, Robben SGF, Meradji M: Sonographically detected costochondral dislocation in an abused child: a new sonographic sign to the radiological spectrum of child abuse. *Pediatr Radiol* 1990;20: 556-567.

48. Chapman V, Grottkau B, Albright M, et al: MDCT of the elbow in pediatric patients with posttraumatic elbow effusions. *AJR Am J Roentgenol* 2006;187:812-817.

49. Rhea J, Rao P, Novelline R: Helical CT and three-dimensional CT of facial and orbital injury. *Radiol Clin North Am* 1999;37:489-513.

50. Sheridan R, Peralta R, Rhea J, et al: Reformatted visceral protocol helical computed tomographic scanning allows conventional radiographs of the thoracic and lumbar spine to be eliminated in the evaluation of blunt trauma patients. *J Trauma* 2003;55:665-669.

51. Guillamondegui O, Pryor J, Gracias V, et al: Pelvic radiography in blunt trauma resuscitation: a diminishing role. *J Trauma* 2002;53: 1043-1047.

52. Frush DP: Pediatric CT: practical approach to diminish the radiation dose. *Pediatr Radiol* 2002;32:714-717.

53. Brenner D, Elliston C, Hall E, et al: Estimated risks of radiation-induced fatal cancer from pediatric CT. *AJR Am J Roentgenol* 2001; 176:289-296.

54. Beir V: *Health effects of exposure to low levels of ionizing radiation*, National Academies Press (website): http://www.nap.edu/openbook.php?isbn =0309039959. Accessed May 4, 2009.

55. Frush DP, Donnelly LF, Rosen NS: Computed tomography and radiation risks: what pediatric health care providers should know. *Pediatrics* 2003;112:971-972.

56. Shah NM, Platt ST: ALARA: is there a cause for alarm? Reducing radiation risk from computed tomography scanning in children. *Curr Opin Pediatr* 2008;20:243-247.

57. Feldman F, Singson RD, Rosenberg ZS, et al: Distal tibial triplane fractures: diagnosis with CT. *Radiology* 1987;164:429-435.

58. Alcala-Galiano A, Arribas-Garcia IJ, Martin-Perez MA, et al: Pediatric facial fractures: children are not just small adults. *Radiographics* 2008;28:441-461.

59. Zimmerman CE, Troulis MJ, Kaban LB: Pediatric facial fractures: recent advances in prevention, diagnosis and management. *Int J Oral Maxillofac Surg* 2006;35:2-13.

60. Schlievert R: Infant mandibular fractures: are you considering abuse? *Pediatr Emerg Care* 2006;22:181-183.

61. Barsness KA, Cha ES, Bensard DD, et al: The positive predictive value of rib fractures as an indicator of nonaccidental trauma in children. *J Trauma* 2003;54:1107-1110.

62. Bulloch B, Schubert CJ, Brophy PD, et al: Cause and clinical characteristics of rib fractures in infants. *Pediatrics* 2000;105:e48-e52.

63. Cadzow SP, Armstrong KL: Rib fractures in infants: red alert! *J Paediatr Child Health* 2000;36:322-326.

64. Kleinman PK, Marks SC, Nimkin K, et al: Rib fractures in 31 abused infants: postmortem radiologic-histopathologic study. *Radiology* 1996; 200:807-810.

65. Kleinman PK, Marks SC, Richmond JM, et al: Inflicted skeletal injury: a postmortem radiologic-histopathologic study in 31 infants. *AJR Am J Roentgenol* 1995;165:647-650.

66. Niitsu M, Takeda T: Solitary hot spots in the ribs on bone scan: value of thin-section reformatted computed tomography to exclude radiography-negative fractures. *J Comput Assist Tomogr* 2003;27: 469-474.

67. Wootton-Gorges SL, Stein-Wexler R, Walton JW, et al: Comparison of computed tomography and chest radiography in the detection of rib fractures in abused infants. *Child Abuse Negl* 2008;32:659-663.

68. Kleinman PK, Nimkin K, Spevak MR, et al: Follow-up skeletal surveys in suspected child abuse. *AJR Am J Roentgenol* 1996;167: 893-896.

69. Zimmerman S, Makoroff K, Care M, et al: Utility of follow-up skeletal surveys in suspected child physical abuse evaluations. *Child Abuse Negl* 2005;10:1075-1083.

70. Carrion WV, Dormans JP, Drummon DS, et al: Circumferential growth plate fracture of the thoracolumbar spine from child abuse. *J Pediatr Orthop* 1996;16:210-214.

71. Swischuk LE: Spine and spinal cord trauma in the battered child syndrome. *Radiology* 1969;92:733-738.

72. Levin TL, Berdon WE, Cassell I, et al: Thoracolumbar fracture with listhesis-an uncommon manifestation of child abuse. *Pediatr Radiol* 2003;33:305-310.

73. Gabos PG, Tuten HR, Leet A, et al: Fracture-dislocation of the lumbar spine in an abused child. *Pediatrics* 1998;101:473-477.

74. Tran B, Silvera M, Newton A, et al: Inflicted T12 fracture-dislocation: CT/MRI correlation and mechanistic implications. *Pediatr Radiol* 2007;37:1171-1173.

75. McGraw EP, Pless JE, Pennington DJ: Postmortem radiography after unexpected death in neonates, infants, and children: should imaging be routine? *AJR Am J Roentgenol* 2002;178:1517-1521.

76. Thomsen TK, Elle B, Thomsen JL: Post-mortem radiological examination in infants: evidence of child abuse? *Forensic Sci Int* 1997;90: 223-230.

77. Thali MJ, Yen K, Schweizer W, et al: Virtopsy, a new imaging horizon in forensic pathology: virtual autopsy by postmortem multi-slice computed tomography (MSCT) and magnetic resonance imaging (MRI)—a feasibility study. *J Forensic Sci* 2003;48:386-403.

78. Ezawa H, Yoneyama R, Kandatsu S, et al: Introduction of autopsy imaging (AI) redefines the concept of autopsy: 30 cases of clinical experience. *Pathol Int* 2003;53:865-873.

79. Oyake Y, Takeshi A, Shiotani S, et al: Postmortem computed tomography for detecting causes of sudden death in infants and children: retrospective review of cases. *Radiat Med* 2006;24:493-502.

80. Lee K, Siegel MJ, Lau DM, et al: Anterior cruciate ligament tears: MR imaging-based diagnosis in a pediatric population. *Radiology* 1999;213:697-704.

81. Bates DG, Hresko MT, Jaramillo D: Patellar sleeve fracture: demonstration with MR imaging. *Radiology* 1994;193:825-827.

82. Bencardino J, Rosenberg Z, Brown R, et al: Traumatic musculotendinous injuries of the knee: diagnosis with MR imaging. *Radiographics* 2000;20:S103-S120.

83. Palmer W, Kuong S, Elmadbouh H: MR imaging of myotendinous strain. *AJR Am J Roentgenol* 1999;173:703-709.

84. Ecklund K: Magnetic resonance imaging of pediatric musculoskeletal trauma. *Top Magn Reson Imaging* 2002;13:203-218.

85. Naranja RJ Jr, Gregg JR, Dormans JP, et al: Pediatric fracture without radiographic abnormality. *Clin Orthop Relat Res* 1997;342: 141-146.

86. Berger P, Ofstein R, Jackson D, et al: MRI demonstration of radiographically occult fractures: what have we been missing? *Radiographics* 1989;9:407-436.

87. Lee J, Yao L: Occult intraosseous fracture: magnetic resonance appearance versus age of injury. *Am J Sports Med* 1989;17:620-623.

88. Haramati N, Staron R, Barax C, et al: Magnetic resonance imaging of occult fractures of the proximal femur. *Skeletal Radiol* 1994;23: 19-22.

89. Yao L, Lee J: Occult intraosseous fracture: detection with MR imaging. *Radiology* 1988;167:749-751.

90. Rizzo P, Gould E, Lyden J, et al: Diagnosis of occult fractures about the hip: magnetic resonance imaging compared with bone scanning. *J Bone Joint Surg Am* 1993;75:395-401.

91. Griffith JF, Roebuck DJ, Cheng JCY, et al: Acute elbow trauma in children: spectrum of injury revealed by MR imaging not apparent on radiographs. *AJR Am J Roentgenol* 2001;176:53-60.

92. Ogden J: Fractures associated with pediatric disease. In Ogden J (ed): *Skeletal Injury in the Child*. WB Saunders, Philadelphia, 1990, pp 299-303.

93. Anderson MW, Greenspan A: Stress fractures. *Radiology* 1996;199: 1-12.

94. Mizuta T, Benson WM, Foster BK, et al: Statistical analysis of the incidence of physeal injuries. *J Pediatr Orthop* 1987;7:518-523.

95. Peterson HA: Physeal and apophyseal injuries. In Rockwood CA, Wilkins KE, Beaty JH (eds): *Fractures in Children*, ed 3, Lippincott-Raven, Philadelphia, 1996, pp 103-165.

96. Peterson HA, Madhok R, Benson JT, et al: Physeal fractures: part I. Epidemiology in Olmsted County, Minnesota. 1979-1988. *J Pediatr Orthop* 1994;14:423-430.

97. Rogers LF, Poznanski AK: Imaging of epiphyseal injuries. *Radiology* 1994;191:297-308.

98. Eucklund K, Jaramillo D: Patterns of premature physeal arrest: MR imaging of 111 children. *AJR Am J Roentgenol* 2002;178:967-972.

99. Sailhan F, Chotel F, Guibal AL: Three-dimensional MR imaging in the assessment of physeal growth arrest. *Eur Radiol* 2004;14:1600-1608.

100. Langenskiöld A: Surgical treatment of partial closure of the growth plate. *J Pediatr Orthop* 1981;1:3-11.

101. Peterson HA: Partial growth arrest and its treatment. *J Pediatr Orthop* 1984;4:246-258.

102. Broker FH, Burbach T: Ultrasonic diagnosis of separation of the proximal humeral epiphysis in the newborn. *J Bone Joint Surg Am* 1990;72:187-191.

103. Stranzinger E, Kellenberger CJ, Braunschweig S, et al: Whole-body STIR MR imaging in suspected child abuse: an alternative to skeletal survey radiography? *Eur J Radiol Extra* 2007;63:43-47.

104. Kavanagh E, Smith C, Eustace S: Whole-body turbo STIR MR imaging: controversies and avenues for development. *Eur Radiol* 2003;13(9):2196-2205.

105. Kellenberger CJ, Epelman M, Miller SF, et al: Fast STIR whole-body MR imaging in children. *Radiographics* 2004;24:1317-1330.

106. Mazumdar A, Siegel MJ, Narra V, et al: Whole-body fast inversion recovery MR imaging of small cell neoplasms in pediatric patients: a pilot study. *AJR Am J Roentgenol* 2002;179:1261-1266.

107. Mentzel HJ, Kentouche K, Sauner D, et al: Comparison of whole-body STIR-MRI and ^{99m}Tc-methylene-diphosphonate scintigraphy in children with suspected multifocal bone lesions. *Eur Radiol* 2004; 14:2297-2302.

108. Kleinman PK: Problems in the diagnosis of metaphyseal fractures. *Pediatr Radiol* 2008;38(suppl 3):S388-S394.

109. Palmer WE, Levine SM, Dupuy DE: Knee and shoulder fractures: association of fracture detection and marrow edema on MR images with mechanism of injury. *Radiology* 1997;204:395-401.

35

LONG BONE FRACTURE BIOMECHANICS

Gina Bertocci, PhD, PE

INTRODUCTION

Fractures in children can occur as a result of either accident or abuse. Clinicians are often asked to determine whether a fracture could have resulted from a stated cause such as a fall from a sofa or bed. To determine whether a stated cause is compatible with a presenting fracture, a basic understanding of biomechanics as it relates to fractures can be useful. Biomechanics relies upon the use of engineering or physics principles to study the response of biological tissue to physical phenomena such as force, acceleration, or pressure. Biomechanical principles can provide an improved understanding of how a bone will respond to the application of a force and its likelihood to fracture under certain conditions.

The objectives of this chapter are:

1. To describe characteristics of bone tissue anatomy that are related to bone strength and biomechanical response to loading
2. To describe fundamental biomechanical concepts important to fracture prediction
3. To describe biomechanical factors that affect the likelihood of bone fracture

OVERVIEW OF LONG BONE ANATOMY

Long bones, such as the femur, tibia, and humerus, consist of the shaft, or diaphyseal region, which consists of compact or cortical bone (Figure 35-1). The segments on either end of the diaphysis consist of cancellous or trabecular bone, and are called the metaphyseal region. A connective tissue layer, periosteum, covers the outer surface of long bones.

Cortical bone tissue is dense, and is composed of haversian microsystems, which include concentric rings of lamellas constructed of mineralized collagen fibers and lacunae. The lacunae contain bone cells, or osteocytes. The number, size, and distribution of the lacunae affect the cortical bone's response to loading.[2]

Cancellous bone tissue is made up of a network of rods and plates that resemble a honeycomb structure. The plates are mineralized and their thickness and direction of alignment affects load-bearing capacity. The honeycomb structure of cancellous bone tissue is made up of microstructure units referred to as trabeculas. Cancellous bone is less dense than cortical bone and is porous in nature with a high surface area.

These differences in cancellous and cortical bone microstructure lead to differences in the transmission of forces through the bone tissue and their load carrying capacity. Each type of bone has unique biomechanical properties and therefore has a unique response to the application of force. These differences reflect their specific function in the human body. Cortical bone is primarily responsible for the supportive load-bearing function of the skeleton, while cancellous bone provides cushioning to skeletal structures during loading.

A more detailed description of bone anatomy is provided in Chapter 31.

BIOMECHANICAL CONCEPTS IMPORTANT TO UNDERSTANDING FRACTURES

To determine whether a bone is likely to fracture under a given loading condition, key biomechanical terms and concepts must first be understood. Table 35-1 lists biomechanical terms and definitions.

Force

The application of a force tends to cause a body or object with mass to accelerate, change position, or change shape. *Force* can be defined as the mass of an object times its acceleration. Figure 35-2 illustrates the response of a spring to a compressive force and tensile (pulling) force. A combination of multiple forces along with their direction of application can be defined as the *loading condition*.

Moment

A moment is the tendency to produce an object's rotation when applied at a perpendicular distance (moment arm) from the axis of rotation.[3] A moment can be defined as the force applied times the moment arm. The concepts related to a moment can be illustrated by the action of a seesaw (Figure 35-3). When two individuals of equal mass are sitting on the seesaw, it is balanced, the moments on each side are equal, and no movement occurs. However, when an individual of larger mass (delivering a greater downward force to the seesaw) sits on one side of the seesaw this will generate a larger moment, which serves to offset the balance of the seesaw creating its downward motion on the side of the individual with greater mass. This downward movement tends to rotate the seesaw about is axis of rotation.

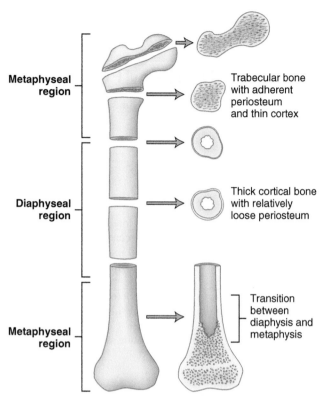

FIGURE 35-1 Illustration of bone architecture. *(From Pierce MC, Bertocci GE, Vogeley E, et al: Evaluating long bone fractures in children: a biomechanical approach with illustrative cases. Child Abuse Negl 2004;28:505-524.)*

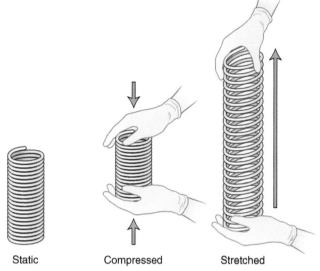

FIGURE 35-2 Response of spring to compression *(center)* and tension *(right)*. Application of these forces alters the shape of the spring.

BIOMECHANICAL MATERIAL PROPERTIES

Properties inherent to a specific biological material that influence how it will respond when exposed to physical phenomena (e.g., force, acceleration) are referred to as *biomechanical material properties*. These properties characterize biological tissues and are *not* dependent on the size or shape (geometry) of the material. An example of a biomechanical material property is elasticity.

Elasticity

A material is said to be *elastic* if it deforms under external force, but returns to its original shape when the force is removed. A biomechanical material property that describes the elastic nature of a material is *elasticity*. Elasticity can be thought of as defining the stiffness of a material, and it is often described through a parameter known as the *elastic modulus* (abbreviated as E_1). The elastic modulus, E, of a material can be derived for a material by knowing the ratio of stress to strain. E is independent of the size and shape of a material. The elastic modulus is a commonly reported material property in engineering handbooks for biological materials and for common materials such as metals, wood, plastics, etc. Often engineers will perform an experiment that entails applying a force or stress to a material, while measuring the corresponding deformation or strain. These quantities are then plotted against each other and the slope of the line formed by the plot can be determined to yield the elastic modulus (Figure 35-7). A material with a low elastic modulus (E_2 in Figure 35-7) would have greater deformation (greater strain) under a given load (or stress) as compared with a material with a high elastic modulus (E_2 in Figure 35-7).

Stress

Force normalized over the area to which it is applied is referred to as *stress*. Stress can be determined by dividing the force by the cross-sectional area of force application. Therefore, for a given force, as the cross-sectional area decreases, stress increases. That is, a force applied to a small cross-sectional area will yield a higher stress than when that same force is applied to a large cross-sectional area (Figure 35-4). The stress that develops within a bone under force application is an important factor in determining how the bone will respond and whether the bone will fracture. Stress also can be described based upon the direction or type force that is applied to an object. Terms that define specific types of stress depend upon the characteristics of force application; these include compression, tension, bending, torsion, and shear (Table 35-1). Figure 35-5 demonstrates graphical depictions of stress applications.

Strain

The change in length of an object (e.g., bone) normalized to its original length is referred to as *strain*. Strain can be determined by dividing the change in length of an object by its original length (Figure 35-6). Strain is also an important factor in determining whether or not a bone fractures under certain loading conditions.

Yield Strength

From a stress:strain curve, additional material properties can be defined and are important to predicting a bone's

Table 35-1	Biomechanical Terms and Definitions
Term	**Definition**
Anisotropy	Material that displays different material properties and responds differently to loading in different directions. Long bones are typically strongest in compression and weakest in shear loading.
Bending stress	Occurs when a force is applied perpendicular to the long axis of a structure or object causing tension on one side and compression on the other.
Biomechanical material properties	Characterizes a material and defines how a material will respond to exposure to physical phenomena (e.g., force, acceleration). Modulus of elasticity is an example of a material property.
Biomechanics	Study of response of biological tissue to physical phenomena such as force, acceleration, pressure, etc.
Compression	Stress created by compressing or "squeezing" an object or structure.
Deformation	Change in size or shape of an object due to application of force. Deformation can be elastic or permanent.
Elasticity	Material is said to be elastic if it deforms under stress (e.g., external forces), but then returns to its original shape when the stress is removed. Often described through modulus of elasticity, E, which is the ratio of stress to strain and can be thought of as defining the stiffness of a material.
Force	Application of which tends to cause a body or object with mass to accelerate, change position, or child shape. (Force = Mass × Acceleration)
Fracture	Failure of structure such that it is unable to support or withstand the applied load.
Fracture threshold	Level of force or stress above which a fracture will occur.
Load	Describes the application of forces or moments to a body or object.
Moment	The tendency of a force to produce body or object rotation when applied at a perpendicular distance (moment arm) from the axis of rotation.[3] (Moment = Force × Moment Arm)
Shear stress	Stress produced when force application is aligned with the surface of a body or object.
Strain	Change in length normalized to the original length of a body or object.[3] (Strain = Change in Length/Original Length)
Stress	Force normalized to the area over which it is applied.[3] The same force applied to a smaller cross section will yield a higher stress. (Stress = Force/Cross-Sectional Area)
Tension	Stress created by extending or "pulling" an object or structure.
Torsional stress	Results from twisting an object or structure about its longitudinal axis.
Ultimate strength	Stress beyond which an object or structures will fail or fracture.
Viscoelasticity	Material is said to exhibit viscoelastic behavior if its response is dependent upon rate of strain application. A viscoelastic material will appear stiffer at higher rates of strain application.
Yield strength	Also known as *elastic limit*. Stress beyond which an object or structure will undergo permanent deformation. Material responds elastically below the yield strength.

response to loading. The *yield strength* of a material can be defined as the stress beyond which an object or structure will undergo permanent or *plastic* deformation. (*Note: Although the term "plastic" is often used clinically to indicate a reversible situation, in contrast the terminology "plastic" behavior or deformation in reference to material response indicates a permanent or irreversible response.*) In other words, a material responds elastically below the yield strength (material returns to its original shape when the load

is removed) and deformation is reversible in this region. In contrast, stresses greater than the yield strength will lead to plastic, irreversible, deformation. Figure 35-8 illustrates the point on the stress:strain curve that identifies a material's yield strength. The stress:strain curve illustrates key properties related to a material's response to loading. The material will respond elastically at stresses below the yield strength, and plastically when stresses exceed the yield strength.

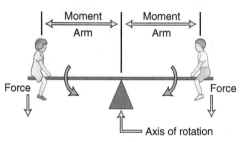
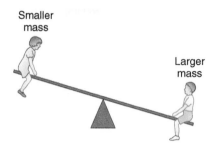

FIGURE 35-3 Individuals with equal mass balance the seesaw creating equal moments *(left)*. The individual with greater mass generates a larger moment causing the seesaw to rotate *(right)*.

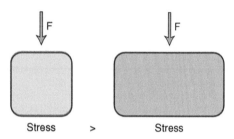

FIGURE 35-4 A force applied to a smaller cross-sectional area generates a higher level of stress as compared to when this same force is applied to a larger cross-sectional area.

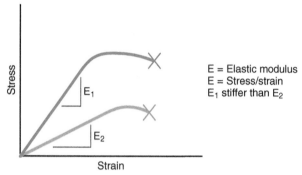

FIGURE 35-7 *Elastic modulus* is the slope of the stress:strain curve. It is often referred to as the stiffness of a material. In this diagram, the material defined by E_1 is stiffer than the material defined by E_2.

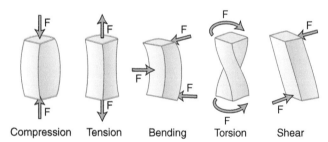

FIGURE 35-5 Type of stress depends upon the characteristics of force application.

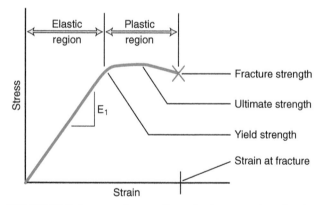

FIGURE 35-8 Stress:strain curve illustrating key properties related to a material's response to loading. The material will respond elastically at stresses below the yield strength, and plastically when stresses exceed the yield strength.

Ultimate Strength

The *ultimate strength* of a material is the stress at which a material or structure will fail. In the case of bone tissue, failure would be defined as fracture.

Anisotropy

Some materials respond differently when loading is applied from different directions. These materials are defined as *anisotropic*. Materials responding similarly under loading

FIGURE 35-6 Force applied to an object can stretch or deform the object. The change in length as compared with an object's original length is defined as *strain*.

conditions applied from varying directions are referred to as *isotropic*. The material will respond elastically at stresses below the yield strength, and plastically when stresses exceed the yield strength.

FACTORS AFFECTING LIKELIHOOD OF FRACTURE

The likelihood of a fracture occurring in a specific bone is dependent upon a number of factors that can be categorized as *extrinsic* or *intrinsic* factors. Models capable of predicting fractures are dependent upon accurate representation of both intrinsic and extrinsic factors. Whether or not a fracture occurs depends upon the internal stresses developed within the bone, and whether these internal stresses exceed the fracture threshold.

Intrinsic Factors

The response of bone to loading is dependent upon intrinsic factors that include both material and structural or geometric characteristics of the bone.

Bone Material Properties

Elastic Modulus. Table 35-2 provides elastic moduli for cortical bone and trabecular bone in comparison with other common materials. Table 35-2 illustrates that cortical bone is stiffer than trabecular bone ($E_{cortical} > E_{trabecular}$). Therefore, for a given loading condition (below the yield strength), trabecular bone will undergo greater deformation as compared with cortical bone. Trabecular bone tissue found at the epiphysis and metaphysis of long bones has a high level of porosity, providing the ability to deform without failure. The openings in trabecular bone tissue are filled with marrow and fat, which help to provide a degree of energy absorption under loading.[4,5]

Anisotropy and Strength. As previously stated, bone tissue is considered an *anisotropic* material, responding differently under varying directions of loading. For example, Table 35-3 shows that femoral cortical bone tissue loaded longitudinally (parallel to the long axis of the bone) in tension has a higher ultimate strength (133 MPa) as compared to when the same tissue is loaded in a transverse direction (perpendicular to the long axis of the bone) under tension (51 MPa).[6]

Long bones also typically have increased strength under compressive loading conditions, and exhibit the lowest strength under application of shear loading. Table 35-3 also illustrates this concept for femoral cortical bone tissue.[6] When the femur is loaded longitudinally (parallel to the long axis of the bone) under compression, the ultimate strength is 193 MPa, whereas when it is loaded longitudinally in tension, the ultimate strength decreases to 133 MPa. This difference in strength is also seen when the comparing compression and tension loading in the transverse direction.

Table 35-2	Elastic Moduli for Bone Tissue and Other Materials[3]
Material	**E (GPa)***
Cortical bone	12-24[†]
Trabecular bone	0.005-1.5[†]
Stainless steel	190
Polyethylene[‡] (UHMWPE)	1.2

*Gigapascal = 10^9 pascal.
[†]Depends upon density and direction of loading.
[‡]Ultra high molecular weight polyethylene, used in joint replacements.

Table 35-3	Ultimate Strength and Elastic Modules for Femoral Cortical Bone Under Varying Loading Conditions and Directions				
	Type of Bone	**Direction**	**Loading Condition**	**Ultimate Strength**	**Elastic Modulus**
	Cortical bone, femur	Longitudinal	Tension	133 MPa	17.0 GPa
	Cortical bone, femur	Longitudinal	Compression	193 MPa*	17.0 GPa
	Cortical bone, femur	Transverse	Tension	51 MPa	11.5 GPa
	Cortical bone, femur	Transverse	Compression	133 MPa	11.5 GPa

*Strength of femoral cortical bone tissue varies depending upon loading direction and characteristics of the load. The red box designates the conditions under which the femoral cortical bone has the greatest strength.[7] (The specimens evaluated in this study were harvested from cadavers ranging in age from 19-80 years.)
MPa, Millipascal; *GPa*, gigapascal.

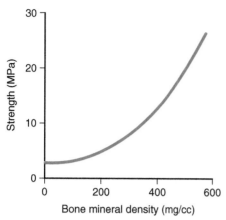

FIGURE 35-9 Compressive strength of femoral trabecular bone tissue increases with increasing bone mineral density.[8]

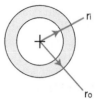

FIGURE 35-10 Approximation of long bone cross-sectional geometry (r_i = inner radius; r_o = outer radius).

Table 35-4	Femoral Geometric Characteristics and Moment of Inertia for Newborn vs. 6-Month-Old Child		
Age	**Moment of Inertia**	**Outer Diameter**	**Cortical Thickness**
Newborn	63 mm^4	6.0 mm	2.15 mm
6 months	291 mm^4	9.0 mm	2.0 mm

Density and Strength. Bone tissue strength is also dependent upon bone mineral density.[7] In general, the strength of bone tissue increases with increasing bone mineral density as illustrated in Figure 35-9. Trabecular bone mineral density ranges from 0.1 to 1.0 g/cc, whereas cortical bone tissue density is approximately 1.8 g/cc. Since bone mineral density is directly related to strength, it is important when assessing the likelihood of fracture to consider those conditions that can alter bone mineral density (see Chapter 31).

Bone Geometric Characteristics. The geometric characteristics of the bone structure will also affect its response to loading. Depending on whether the bone is subjected to bending, axial loading or torsion determines which aspects of the bone geometry relates to its resistance to fracture. Important geometric characteristics can include the inner and outer diaphysis radii, along with the cross-sectional area, or cortical wall thickness, of the bone structure.

The Importance of Intrinsic Factors Related to Pediatric Bone Tissue

Curry[8] compared age-related bone tissue from younger children to adults. Bone tissue from younger children dissipated more energy before fracture. With larger haversian canals, a child's bone is more porous and thus tolerates a greater level of strain as compared with adult bones prior to fracture.

Extrinsic Factors

Bone tissue response to loading is also dependent upon *extrinsic factors* such as loading characteristics.

Types and Characteristics of Loads

The characteristics of the loading applied to a bone are key to understanding its resistance to fracture. The magnitude, distribution, and direction of loading are important to whether or not a bone will fracture. Various combinations of geometric characteristics (*intrinsic factors*) are key to a bone's ability to resist fracture depending upon the characteristics of loading. Two common loading conditions, bending and torsion, are discussed in greater detail next.

Bending. When a bending load, or moment, is applied to a bone, the maximum *internal stress* (σ) developed within that bone is dependent upon the magnitude of the applied *moment* and the geometric characteristics of the bone. The internal stress is directly related to the bending *moment* applied and indirectly related to the *moment of inertia* (described later).

In a simplified representation of a long bone cross-sectional geometry as a hollow tube, the inner radius (ri, center of bone to medullary canal wall) and outer radius (r_o, center of bone to outer cortical wall) affect the level of stress developed within the bone (Figure 35-10). When a bending load is applied, the structure is in tension on the side of load application, and in compression on the opposite side. The ability of a bone to resist bending stress is dependent upon its moment of inertia, I. When a long bone is approximated as a hollow tube, the *moment of inertia* can be defined as;

$$I = \Pi/4\left(r_o^4 - r_i^4\right)$$
$$\text{Where } \Pi = 3.14159265.$$

As an example, Table 35-4 compares geometric characteristics that are used to determine the moment of inertia for the femur of a newborn and 6 month-old-infant to illustrate this concept. As shown, the 6-month-old child has a moment of inertia, which is 4.6 times that of a newborn.

The maximum internal stress, σ, associated with a application of a bending *moment*, M, can then be estimated as;

$$\sigma = My/I,$$

where y = distance from the neutral axis, or ro when estimating the maximum internal stress.

Using the previous comparison of the newborn and 6-month-old child's femur geometry and moment of inertia, it can be shown that for a given bending moment application, the internal femoral stress, σ, experienced by the 6-month-old is one third of that experienced by the newborn.

Once the maximum internal bending stress, σ, has been estimated, this value is then compared with the ultimate strength of the bone tissue to determine the response of the bone. If σ exceeds the ultimate bending strength of the bone tissue, then the bone will fail or fracture.

Torsion. A similar type of analysis can be undertaken as it relates to torsional loading conditions applied to a long bone. In torsional loading, internal bone stress is directly related to the torque (force times moment arm) or twisting applied to the bone. The bone's ability to resist fracture under these conditions is dependent upon the *polar moment of inertia,* J. Assuming again that the cross-section of a long bone can be approximated as a hollow tube (Figure 35-10), the polar moment of inertia, J, can be defined as;

$$J = \Pi/2\left(r_o^4 - r_i^4\right)$$

Table 35-5 compares the femoral geometric characteristics and polar moment of inertia of a newborn and 6-month-old child. Table 35-5 shows that the 6-month-old child has a femoral polar moment of inertia that is 4.6 times that of a newborn. This difference is important because it relates to the bone's ability to resist fracture.

When torque is applied to a bone, the associated maximum internal torsional stress, τ, can be determined using the following equation:

$$\tau = Tr/J$$

where *r* represents the radius of the bone, T represents the torque applied, and J represents the polar moment of inertia. Using the geometric data provided and polar moment of inertia determined (Table 35-5) for the newborn and 6-month-old child, the maximum internal torsional stress for a given applied torque can be expressed as:

$$T_{6mo} = T(4.5)/582 \quad T_{newborn} = T(3)/126$$

$$\boxed{T_{6mo} : T_{newborn} = 0.33}$$

Therefore, it can be shown that for a given torque application to the femur, the internal torsional stress experienced by the 6-month-old child would be one third of that experienced by a newborn.

Again, once the maximum internal torsional stress has been determined, this value can be compared with the ultimate torsional strength of the bone tissue to determine whether or not a fracture would occur. Internal stress values that exceed the strength of the bone will lead to failure or fracture of the bone.

Response to Rate (Speed) of Loading Application

Bone tissue response is also dependent upon the rate at which the loading is applied. Materials that are time- or rate-dependent are referred to as *viscoelastic*. Figure 35-11 illustrates the influence of strain rate (rate of deformation) on cortical bone ultimate strength and elastic modulus.[9] This figure shows that the ultimate strength and elastic modulus increase with rapid loading or deformation. The ultimate strength increases by roughly a factor of 3, while the elastic modulus increases by a factor of approximately 2 over the strain rate range. (Note that normal activities typically occur at a strain rate of <0.01/sec.)

Combining Intrinsic and Extrinsic Factors

The process by which one determines whether a fracture occurs in a laboratory setting is obviously somewhat different than that which can be used in a clinical setting. Nonetheless, it is of value to understand the idealized steps that one would take assuming that all information relevant to an incident, the associated loading conditions, and the child's bone structure and properties could be obtained. Figure 35-12 provides an overview of the idealized conceptual process that would be used to determine whether a fracture would occur for a given incident.

In this idealized approach, the loading characteristics (direction of application, location of application, and magnitude) associated with an incident are extracted or determined through close examination of the event. These loading characteristics are used to estimate the internal stress developed within the bone structure. The internal stress developed within the bone is then compared with the strength of the bone tissue to determine the resultant response.

Although the approach presented in Figure 35-12 provides an "ideal" method for assessing fractures, many unknowns usually exist, preventing clinical application of this approach. Unknowns might include complex loading

Table 35-5	Femoral Geometric Characteristics and Polar Moment of Inertia for a Newborn *vs.* 6-Month-Old Child		
Age	Polar Moment of Inertia	Outer Diameter	Cortical Thickness
Newborn	126 mm⁴	6.0 mm	2.15 mm
6 Months	582 mm	9.0 mm	2.0 mm

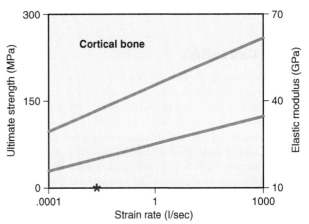

FIGURE 35-11 Ultimate cortical bone strength and elastic modulus in tension versus strain rate. Both properties increase with increasing strain rate.

* = Strain rate of typical normal activities.

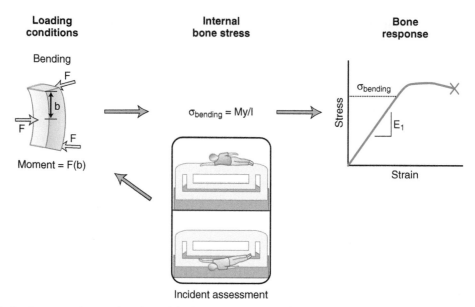

FIGURE 35-12 Idealized conceptual approach to determining bone response to loading for a given incident.

conditions that consist of a combination of loading types, unknown magnitude and direction of the loading, and unknown biomechanical properties of the specific child's bone tissue. Because such a quantitative approach often falls short in a clinical setting, a qualitative, modified approach to fracture assessment (described below), which is based in principle upon the idealized quantitative approach, can usually be implemented.

QUALITATIVE FRACTURE ASSESSMENT MODEL

In the absence of quantitative data regarding the specific event and the child's bone tissue properties, the determination of whether a fracture is biomechanically compatible with a stated cause can be aided by using the components described in Figure 35-13. The proposed qualitative Fracture Assessment Model attempts to convey the interrelationship of injury causation, injury mechanism, and fracture type. The components of this model can be defined as follows.

Injury Causation

Injury causation is a detailed description of the event that leads to a specific fracture or injury. Often the stated cause of the injury is presented by the caregiver. The description should include as many details as possible, such as the child's initial position and posture, dynamics during the fall, landing position, and surface upon which the child fell. An example of injury causation is a child rolling from an 18 inch high bed from a horizontal posture onto a carpeted floor landing onto an outstretched arm.

Injury Mechanism

The injury mechanism describes how forces or accelerations associated with the injury causation (i.e., event) can be

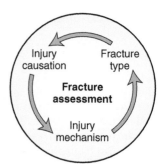

FIGURE 35-13 Fracture Assessment Model. A model to assess fractures and their biomechanical compatibility with a stated cause is dependent upon three components: injury causation, injury mechanism, and fracture type. There should be continuity between these three components.

transmitted to the bone structure (or region of the body) where a fracture is present. The description should include the direction of force(s), the planes of the body where the force(s) are applied, and an evaluation of the transmission of these forces to the bone. An example of an injury mechanism is a torsional load applied to the tibia when a toddler's foot becomes entangled with a toy or carpet while running or walking in the forward direction. A typical resulting fracture from this type of torsional load application would be a non-displaced spiral fracture of the tibia.

Fracture Type

The fracture type is the morphological description of the resulting fracture pattern and its location on the bone. An example of fracture type is a spiral fracture to the midshaft of the tibia. Pierce et al[1] provides a detailed overview of fracture types associated with various loading conditions. Loading conditions and resulting fracture types are covered in Chapter 32.

This model should be applied in a stepwise progression starting with the *injury causation* moving through the *injury mechanism* and finally onto the resulting *fracture type*. There should be continuity of flow from one component of the model to the next. Evaluating each component of this model will help the clinician to qualitatively "reconstruct" the event and evaluate the compatibility of the fracture and the stated cause. That is, the *injury causation* must be capable of generating specific forces of a magnitude and direction that can lead to an *injury mechanism* that is capable of generating a specific *fracture type*. If the *injury causation* can lead to fall dynamics that are capable of generating a loading pattern that can create a specific *fracture type*, then the clinician has an improved level of confidence that the stated cause could have resulted in the fracture. (This same assessment model can also be used for other types of injuries.) The simplified examples provided below will help to illustrate application of the Qualitative Fracture Assessment Model.

Fracture Assessment Case 1: Skiing Incident

Stated Cause: 5-year-old child involved in skiing incident.
Injury Causation: Child was downhill skiing and the tip of her ski caught on a tree trunk. The child continued to move forward down the slope, abruptly falling to the ground, facing supine with her leg folded beneath her. The child was subsequently unable to bear weight on one lower extremity.
Injury Mechanism: The tree trunk retained the tip of the ski such that the ski rotated relative to the child's lower extremity, introducing a torsional (twisting) load on the tibia.
Fracture Type: Spiral fracture to the diaphysis of the tibia.
Fracture Assessment: In this case the injury causation can lead to an injury mechanism that can cause the presenting fracture. As previously stated, torsional loading will lead to spiral fractures and given the injury causation in this case, it is reasonable that torsional type loading will be present. The assessment of this case is that the stated cause is compatible with and supports the resulting fracture.

Fracture Assessment Case 2: Sofa Fall

Stated Cause: 6-month-old child fell from sofa.
Injury Causation: The caregiver stated that the child was lying on a sofa 18 inches above a padded carpeted floor and then rolled off the sofa. The caregiver also stated that the child fell free to the floor, did not impact any object during the fall, and no limbs were retained by the sofa.
Injury Mechanism: When evaluating the fracture type (spiral comminuted), one would evaluate the injury causation to determine if torsional loading (necessary to generate a spiral fracture) could result. Given that the fall was a free fall to the floor, however, and no limbs were impinged within the sofa, it is difficult to envision how a torsional load could be introduced during this event. The most likely loading pattern resulting from a free fall from a sofa is a bending or compression pattern. Also of interest in this case, the presence of bone fragments suggests a high level of energy was imparted to the child's femur. A fall from a sofa onto a carpeted floor would not be classified as a high-energy event.

Fracture Type: Comminuted spiral fracture of the femur.
Fracture Assessment: In this case the injury mechanism necessary to create a comminuted spiral femur fracture cannot be ascertained from the injury causation. A comminuted spiral fracture of the femur would require exposure to high level of torsional loading. Therefore the continuity of flow from one component of the model to the next is broken, and it can be concluded that the stated cause of injury and presenting fracture are biomechanically incompatible.

KEY POINTS IN FRACTURE ASSESSMENT

- Knowledge of biomechanics is important when attempting to determine whether a bone will fracture under given loading conditions.
- Both intrinsic and extrinsic factors must be considered when attempting to determine whether a bone will fracture under given loading conditions.
  - Intrinsic factors important to determining likelihood of fracture:
    - Bone biomechanical or material properties (elastic modulus, yield strength, ultimate strength, etc.)
    - Bone geometry (cortical wall thickness, inner and outer radii)
  - Extrinsic factors important to determining likelihood of fracture:
    - Characteristics of loading (type, direction and rate of application)
- Internal bone stress is dependent upon loading conditions and geometrical characteristics of the bone.
- Bone tissue response to loading is dependent upon internal bone stress as well as the material or biomechanical properties of the bone.
- When assessing fractures, injury causation, injury mechanism and fracture morphology must be considered.
- Fracture morphology must be compatible with a specific injury mechanism which can be derived from a specific injury causation. There must be continuity between injury causation, injury mechanism and fracture type.

References

1. Pierce MC, Bertocci GE, Vogeley E, et al: Evaluating long bone fractures in children: a biomechanical approach with illustrative cases. *Child Abuse Negl* 2004;28:505-524.
2. Mullender MG, Huiskes R, Versleyen H, et al: Osteocyte density and histomorphometric parameters in cancellous bone of the proximal femur in five mammalian species. *J Orthop Res* 1996;14:972-979.
3. Lucas GL, Francis CW, Friis EA: *A primer of biomechanics.* Springer, New York, 1999.
4. Hall SJ: *Basic biomechanics,* ed 3, WCB McGraw-Hill, Boston, 1999.
5. Gomez MA, Nahum AM: Biomechanics of bone. *In:* Nahum A, Melvin J (eds): *Accidental Injury: Biomechanics and Prevention,* ed 2, Springer-Verlag, New York, 2002, pp 206-227.
6. Reilly DT, Burstein AH: The elastic and ultimate properties of compact bone tissue. *J Biomech* 1975;8:393-405.
7. Lotz JC, Gerhart TN, Hayes WC: Mechanical properties of trabecular bone for the proximal femur: a quantitative QCT study. *J Comput Assist Tomogr* 1990;14:107-114.
8. Currey JD, Butler G: The mechanical properties of bone tissue in children. *J Bone Joint Surg* 1975;57:810-814.
9. Wright TM, Hayes WC: Tensile testing of bone over a wide range of strain rates: effects of strain rate, microstructure and density. *Med Biol Eng Comput* 1976;14:671-680.

36

ABDOMINAL AND CHEST INJURIES IN ABUSED CHILDREN

Sandra M. Herr, MD

INTRODUCTION

Abdominal trauma is the second most common cause of death resulting from abuse (after head injury), with a mortality rate as high as 40% to 50%.[1-3] It is often listed as a "rare" but lethal form of child abuse and is significantly less common than cutaneous, skeletal, and intracranial injuries in abused children, with rates as low as 2%.[4-7] This low rate likely represents underrecognition of the true incidence of intraabdominal injuries in child abuse cases. Traditionally, laboratory and/or radiographic evaluations for abdominal injuries were only carried out in those patients with signs and symptoms of abdominal pathology including abdominal pain or tenderness, bruising of the abdominal wall, or abdominal distension. These findings are frequently absent in child abuse victims; young age, delay in presentation, concomitant severe head or skeletal injuries, and the lack of underlying bony structures all play a role in diminishing the signs and symptoms of abusive trauma to the thoracic and abdominal regions. Coant et al[8] performed screening liver enzyme levels in suspected abuse patients *without* clinical signs of abdominal trauma, and found that 4 of 49 (8.2%) had abnormal levels, with three of these patients having liver lacerations on computed tomography (CT) scan. Improved identification of less severe cases with more liberal laboratory and radiological screening would likely both increase the reported incidence and decrease the reported mortality rate of abdominal injuries in child abuse cases.

Significant intrathoracic trauma is unusual in abuse cases, most likely because of the plasticity of the thoracic skeletal structures. Except for rib fractures, abuse-related thoracic injuries are most often discovered incidentally in the evaluation for other injuries, and are rarely the sole finding.

EPIDEMIOLOGY

Although abdominal trauma related to abuse is seen in all age groups, the peak incidence of severe and fatal abusive abdominal injuries is in toddlers.[1,9] Both sexes are affected, with a slight male predominance, and there are no significant racial differences. As stated previously, the exact incidence of abusive thoracoabdominal injuries is unclear. Various sources have found rates ranging from 2% to 3% of all abuse cases to as high as 20%. In the study by Sivit et al,[10] the authors looked at 69 cases of child abuse evaluated by the trauma team over a 3-year period and identified 14 of 69 children (20.3%) with "abdominal or lower thoracic visceral injury." Even with this high rate, the investigators only performed abdominal CT or abdominal exploration on those patients with clinical evidence of abdominal pathology; it is unclear what percentage of the remaining children might have had subclinical abdominal injuries. They found that 74% of those patients with signs and symptoms of abdominal injury had nonskeletal thoracic or abdominal injuries on CT or at autopsy. In one study of fatal abuse cases, 14% had intraabdominal injuries.[11] Gaines et al[12] found duodenal injuries in 2.8% of their child abuse admissions; the rate of all intra-abdominal injuries was not presented but was likely much higher.[12] In the absence of a large, prospective evaluation of known and suspected child abuse cases with screening laboratory and/or radiological tests for abdominal trauma, the true incidence of this important injury complex will remain unknown.

PATHOPHYSIOLOGY

Mechanisms of Injury

The absence of a clear and truthful history in the majority of child abuse cases makes determination of the exact mechanism of injury difficult. Information gleaned from confessions, witnessed assaults, and experimental data as well as similar injury complexes resulting from known accidental trauma have all been used to attempt to determine the mechanisms of injury in abusive abdominal trauma cases. The most commonly injured structures include small bowel (especially duodenum and proximal jejunum), the left lobe of the liver, and pancreas; these structures are often injured together in the same patient. This spectrum of injuries is similar to that seen in bicycle handlebar injuries, suggesting a focal intrusion type of mechanism, such as a punch or kick to the upper abdomen. Suggested mechanisms for the common injuries include direct compression of the underlying structures against the spinal column, increased intraluminal pressure in bowel and blood vessels, or shearing forces caused by differential mobility around points of fixation. It is likely that a combination of these factors is involved. Structures that are "fixed" in position are most vulnerable, including the liver and pancreas, and the portions of duodenum and jejunum on either side of the ligament of Treitz.

Spectrum of Injuries

Any thoracic or abdominal tissue or organ can be injured by significant blunt trauma to the area. Multiple studies and case series have delineated the injuries most commonly seen in abusive abdominal trauma, with solid organ injuries predominating in most series but hollow viscus injuries being significantly more common than with accidental blunt abdominal trauma.[3,13,14] Bowel injuries are more common in abusive abdominal trauma than accidental blunt abdominal trauma resulting from motor vehicle crashes; in addition, small bowel injuries predominate in child abuse whereas colonic injuries are more common in accidental trauma.[15]

A significant percentage of the bowel injuries from accidental trauma results from motor vehicle crashes with seatbelt-related abdominal trauma, which might account for the higher proportion of colonic injuries. The higher proportion of small bowel injuries from child abuse could be the result of upward kicks or punches to the abdomen, similar to the intrusion-type mechanism seen with handlebar injuries. The study by Wood et al[3] demonstrated that 39% of the abused patients had *both* hollow viscus and solid organ injury, compared with none of the accidentally injured patients.

Intraabdominal Solid Organ Injury

Liver lacerations are the most common solid organ injuries in most series of inflicted abdominal trauma. In contrast to accidental hepatic injuries, the left lobe is most commonly involved in abusive injuries. This is thought to be due to the more central impact point of a kick or punch to the abdomen versus more lateral impact in accidental blunt abdominal trauma. Injuries to the liver can vary from simple contusion or laceration to massive laceration with hemoperitoneum and shock. Pancreatic contusions or lacerations occur less commonly, and frequently occur in conjunction with duodenal and hepatic injuries. The more protected position of the pancreas, with bowel overlying and surrounding the majority of the gland, most likely accounts for this lower incidence relative to the superficial and anteriorly positioned liver. Lacerations of the pancreas can be complicated by pseudocyst formation. Adrenal hemorrhage can result from direct blunt trauma to the adrenal gland, from shearing of perforating vessels as they enter the gland, or from increased venous pressure associated with abdominal trauma; unilateral hemorrhage into the medullary portion of the right adrenal gland is most commonly described.[16] Adrenal injury is most commonly discovered incidentally on abdominal CT or autopsy, and is usually associated with major thoracic, abdominal, and other abusive injuries; ipsilateral rib fractures and abdominal visceral injuries are particularly common. Isolated splenic and renal injuries are less commonly seen in abusive abdominal trauma, most likely caused by their more protected positions within the abdominal cavity. These injuries are most often seen in massive abdominal injury in conjunction with other intraabdominal injuries such as bowel and liver lacerations (Figures 36-1, 36-2, and 36-3).

Intraabdominal Hollow Viscus Injury

Hollow viscus injury is more common in abusive abdominal trauma than accidental trauma. Although the injuries can

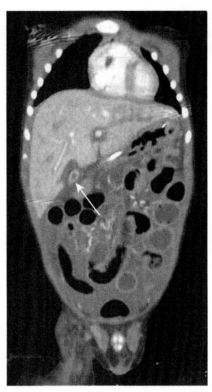

FIGURE 36-1 Axial CT image of a 2-year-old male who presented in full arrest with no history of trauma. CT demonstrates liver lacerations, hemoperitoneum, and fluid surrounding the gall bladder *(arrow).*

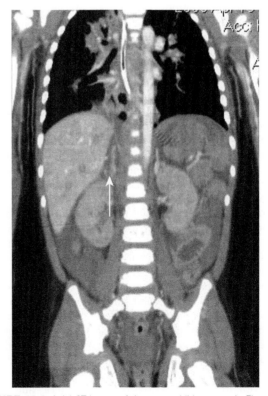

FIGURE 36-2 Axial CT image of the same child as seen in Figure 37-1. The *arrow* demonstrates a right adrenal hematoma; comparison can be made to the normal left adrenal gland. Autopsy revealed a partially avulsed gallbladder, hepatic and splenic lacerations, multiple bowel perforations and hematomas, and the right adrenal hematoma.

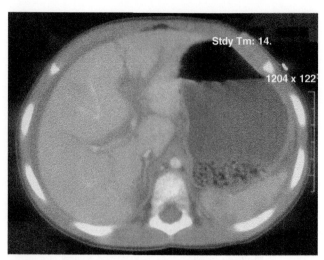

FIGURE 36-3 Abdominal CT image of a 3-year-old girl who presented with a syncopal event; there was no history of trauma. Lacerations to the liver and spleen are seen, along with hemoperitoneum. The stomach is fluid filled and dilated as a result of duodenal hematoma and perforation.

vary from localized hematoma to perforation, intramural hematoma is the most frequently encountered injury. Bowel injuries typically occur at points of fixation and most commonly involve the small bowel. The most common location is the duodenum (especially the junction of the third and fourth parts) and proximal jejunum.[17-19] This location is particularly susceptible because of the underlying vertebral column and the fixation of the bowel at the ligament of Treitz, allowing compression and shearing of the bowel in that area. The third part of the duodenum is also located between the superior mesenteric vessels anteriorly and the aorta and spinal column posteriorly. Injuries to the duodenum vary from localized bowel wall hematoma, to focal perforation, to partial or complete transaction. Perforation is particularly common in the posterior, retroperitoneal region of the fourth part of the duodenum. The study by Ledbetter et al[15] found that bowel injury was much more common in abusive (65%) than non-abusive abdominal trauma (8%), and that the injuries were more commonly small bowel in inflicted and colonic in accidental cases. This study also demonstrated that the small bowel perforations and other hollow viscus injuries in abused patients are associated with a higher mortality rate than similar injuries in accidental cases. This increased mortality is most likely related to the common delay in presentation, the number and severity of associated injuries and co-morbidities (malnutrition), and delays in diagnosis caused by an incomplete or absent history. Mesenteric tears and contusions are also fairly common in abusive abdominal trauma, often in association with bowel injury. Disruption of the vascular supply to the adjacent bowel occurs with severe mesenteric tears, resulting in bowel ischemia and the potential for delayed necrosis and perforation. Fossum and Descheneaux[20] described a group of patients with autopsy findings consistent with long-standing, repetitive mesenteric and small bowel trauma, resulting in mesenteric and bowel wall scarring. The authors theorized that the dense, fibrotic mass fixed the adjacent bowel in place, making it more susceptible to repetitive trauma with resultant bowel rupture. CT can

also demonstrate bowel abnormalities related to generalized hypoperfusion, or "shock bowel." This is commonly seen in those patients with hemorrhagic shock after arrest or prolonged apnea. Other rare hollow viscus injuries described in cases of inflicted abdominal trauma include gastric rupture and bladder tears or rupture.

Miscellaneous Abdominal Injuries

Vascular and biliary tree injuries are rare intraabdominal injuries seen in abusive trauma. As with hollow viscus injuries, stretch, compression, and/or differential mobility at points of fixation are theorized to contribute to these injuries. Intimal tears, pseudoaneurysm formation, and partial or total disruption of both major and minor blood vessels and the biliary tree have all been described in child abuse victims. Forceful blows to the abdomen, flank, or back were the suspected mechanisms of injury in these cases. Unexplained or worsening peritonitis, anemia from ongoing blood loss, and radiographic (portal venous gas) or laboratory evidence of biliary system injury led to the diagnosis.[21] Biliary structures, including the hepatic artery, common bile duct, and portal vein, course together within the hepatoduodenal ligament from the liver to the duodenum; case series and reports have described injuries to one or more of these structures from major abusive abdominal trauma.[22] All of these cases had severe or fatal injuries. Cases of aortic injury, including complete transection of the abdominal aorta, have been described with absent or diminished lower extremity pulses, lower extremity paralysis, and severe anemia and acidosis.[23] As with accidental blunt abdominal trauma, these injuries are rare but should be suspected in patients with abnormal lower extremity neurovascular examination findings.

Thoracic Injuries

Major thoracic injuries, other than rib fractures, are uncommon in abusive trauma. In general these injuries are discovered incidentally during the evaluation of other abusive trauma on skeletal survey or abdominal CT. Injuries such as pulmonary contusion, parenchymal tears, hemothorax, pneumothorax, cardiac contusion or rupture, pericardial effusion, or vascular injuries are most often seen in conjunction with multiple rib fractures. Chylothorax can result from disruption of the intrathoracic lymphatic system. These injuries, like the rib fractures with which they are usually associated, typically result from violent blows to or compression of the chest. Vascular or lymphatic injuries can also result from rapid deceleration when a child is thrown into a stationary object. Cardiac injuries resulting from abuse are rare, but severe blunt chest or upper abdominal trauma can cause contusions or tears to any of the layers of the heart. Intimal tears of the right atrium have been described in association with increased intraabdominal pressure caused by blunt abdominal trauma.[24] Myocardial injury involving the conducting system can result in cardiac arrhythmias, and commotio cordis has been described.

Associated Injuries

As with all abusive injuries, abusive abdominal trauma is rarely an isolated finding. Isolated inflicted abdominal trauma is more common in older abuse victims; infants are more likely to have multiple injuries. The most frequently associated injuries are bruises (60%-95%), followed by fractures and head injuries.

DIAGNOSTIC EVALUATION

History

The majority of patients with inflicted thoracoabdominal injuries present with no history of trauma, but rather with complaints related to their underlying injuries. As with other abusive injuries, patients with inflicted abdominal injuries often present with a history of a short-distance fall: off a bed or couch, from a crib, from a standing position, from a caretaker's arms, or down stairs. Huntimer et al[25] conducted a literature review of small bowel perforations and stair falls, and found that none of the 312 small bowel perforations in the literature resulted from a stair fall, and none of 677 stair falls resulted in intraabdominal injuries.[25] Any significant intraabdominal injury allegedly resulting from a short-distance fall should raise concern for inflicted injury.

Delay in presenting for care is a common feature of all inflicted injuries; the subtle and nonspecific signs and symptoms of abdominal injuries, along with delayed onset of symptoms in some specific injury complexes, augment this delay in abusive abdominal trauma. Those patients with isolated small bowel perforations, particularly involving retroperitoneal segments of bowel, often have delays of several days prior to presentation. The bowel contents and resulting inflammatory response are initially "walled off" or contained within the retroperitoneum, and it may take several days for diffuse peritonitis and the associated symptoms to develop. Bowel wall hematomas also take hours to days to become symptomatic, depending on the level of bowel involved and degree of lumen obstruction. Progressively worsening abdominal pain and vomiting (usually bilious) are typical, with varying degrees of distension depending on the level of the obstruction. Some inflicted abdominal injuries, including bowel wall hematomas and small contusions or lacerations to the liver or other solid organ, are self limited and resolve without treatment. Abused patients sometimes present for evaluation of other injuries or illnesses, or even well child care, at a time when their abdominal injuries are already resolved or resolving.

The presenting complaints of patients suffering abusive abdominal trauma are frequently related to their other injuries. If the patient has associated injuries, particularly head trauma, the presenting symptoms can be related to the head injury rather than the abdominal injuries. As with accidental trauma victims, patients with significant extremity or rib fractures or head injury have "distracting" injuries that can mask the signs and symptoms of abdominal trauma. In addition, the signs and symptoms of the common intraabdominal injuries are vague and non-specific: nausea and vomiting, abdominal pain or distension, non-specific crying or pain in infants and young children. Respiratory distress resulting from associated rib fractures or the presence of subdiaphragmatic blood from a lacerated or ruptured spleen or liver is another potential presentation. Referred shoulder pain related to diaphragmatic irritation from a ruptured liver or

spleen can be a presenting complaint. Pallor related to blood loss might also be noted.

Common thoracic abusive injuries, such as rib fractures, pneumothorax or hemothorax, and pulmonary contusion, can appear with respiratory distress or tachypnea, but often produce few symptoms severe enough to bring the patient to medical attention. As stated previously, these injuries are usually discovered during the evaluation of other abusive injuries. Major vessel and cardiac injuries are rare, but when they occur, they appear with syncope, sudden arrest, or significant cardiorespiratory compromise.

Physical Examination

Abdominal wall bruising is the examination finding that most often leads to an investigation for intraabdominal injuries, but it is absent in a significant proportion of patients. Some series have found that less than 20% of patients with abusive abdominal trauma have any bruising on examination. Ledbetter et al,[15] in a 7-year review of abusive blunt abdominal trauma, found that 2 of 17 patients (11.8%) with intraabdominal injuries had any bruising of the abdominal wall at the time of presentation. Several factors likely play a role in the absence of abdominal wall bruising in these patients. First, the common delay in presentation allows subtle bruising to resolve. Second, there is no bone directly under the abdominal wall soft tissues; the forces associated with a blow to the abdominal wall are therefore transmitted to the intraabdominal contents without resultant bruising or damage to the skin and subcutaneous tissues. Finally, some thoracoabdominal injuries result from blows to the chest wall or back/flank or from deceleration as the child is thrown, making bruising to the abdominal wall unlikely. When abdominal wall bruises are present, they are often subtle and small, belying the often significant underlying intraabdominal injuries (Figure 36-4).

Findings on physical examination can include localized or diffuse tenderness, distension, peritoneal signs, or diminished bowel sounds. Systemic findings suggesting intrathoracic or intraabdominal pathology include unexplained tachycardia, hypotension, or fever related to peritonitis. Shock related to occult hemorrhage results in altered mental status, pallor, and poor perfusion. Respiratory distress and tachypnea are sometimes noted, particularly in those patients with shock and those with significant hemoperitoneum.

Examination findings suggesting thoracic injuries include tachypnea and respiratory distress, hypoxia, tachycardia, and hypotension. Significant hemothorax or pneumothorax will result in diminished breath sounds on the involved side. Crepitus or localized tenderness can be present if there are overlying acute rib fractures. Diminished heart tones, hypotension, and poor pulses can indicate cardiac tamponade.

Laboratory Evaluation

The use of screening "trauma labs" is well established in the evaluation of significant accidental blunt abdominal trauma.[26] These screening tests commonly include hepatic and pancreatic enzyme levels, a complete blood count, and a urine dip or urinalysis. Exact cutoff levels for "significant"

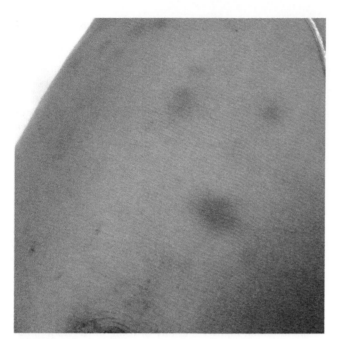

FIGURE 36-4 Rounded bruises on the abdominal wall of the 3-year-old whose CT images are shown in Figure 36-3. The child presented in hemorrhagic shock and required massive fluid and blood resuscitation and emergent laparotomy to repair bowel perforations and to control intraabdominal hemorrhaging.

abnormalities vary, but these levels are then used to determine which patients should undergo radiological evaluation. These data are not easily extrapolated to inflicted abdominal trauma because the time frame for presentation is significantly different and frequently unknown, and the exact mechanism of injury is also unclear, fabricated, or unknown. In the Coant study,[8] two of the three patients with unsuspected liver lacerations had levels significantly below those typically used in accidental trauma cases to indicate the need for radiological evaluation. The authors suggest the use of screening liver enzymes in all suspected abuse cases, and the use of CT for *any* level outside of the normal range. There are little data on the use of amylase/lipase levels or urinalysis in suspected abuse cases. Given that pancreatic, renal, and bladder injuries do occur in abusive abdominal trauma, application of similar screening "trauma labs" to these patients with more liberal criteria for radiological testing than used in accidental cases is warranted. Discovery of any elevation of hepatic or pancreatic enzymes, hematuria, or unexplained anemia warrants further investigation.

Radiographic Evaluation

CT is the imaging modality most commonly used for evaluation of blunt abdominal trauma.[24,27] As discussed previously, CT should be performed in any case of known or suspected child abuse with abnormal screening laboratory values. In addition, CT should be performed in those patients with abnormal examination findings, including abdominal wall bruising, abdominal distension, tenderness, or peritoneal signs. It is critical to remember that these patients often present many hours, days, or even weeks after

their abdominal injuries occurred, and both laboratory and examination findings might have improved or resolved. Those abused patients with neurological compromise or hemodynamic instability might also warrant evaluation with CT (or surgical evaluation with diagnostic peritoneal lavage or laparotomy). Intravenous contrast should be used to improve identification and delineation of solid organ, bladder, and vascular injuries. Oral contrast improves the ability to identify hollow viscus injuries (especially bowel wall hematoma) but is difficult to administer in cases with significant nausea and vomiting and might delay the imaging study. Upper gastrointestinal series (UGI) is helpful in identifying bowel wall hematomas, strictures, or other partial obstructions. UGI is the best study to demonstrate these lesions, particularly with small or resolving intramural hematomas. UGI should be performed in any suspected abuse case with abdominal signs or symptoms and a normal CT. Ultrasound is being used more frequently as a screening tool in accidental abdominal trauma cases; identification of abnormal intraabdominal fluid is an indication for further imaging with CT. There is little information on the use of screening abdominal ultrasound in abuse cases. Ultrasound can be used to identify and delineate bowel wall hematomas and pancreatic injuries including pseudocysts.

Thoracic injuries resulting from child abuse are most often discovered during the evaluation of other injuries. Chest and thoracic spine radiographs are included in the skeletal survey and may reveal rib or spinal fractures as well as pneumothorax or hemothorax and pulmonary contusion. Abdominal CT routinely includes the lower lung fields, heart, and portions of the great vessels, and it can again reveal lower thoracic injuries. CT of the chest or angiography to evaluate the great vessels are rarely necessary in abusive trauma, but should be considered in patients with evidence of severe thoracic trauma with hemodynamic instability or those with abdominal CT or chest x-ray findings suggesting cardiac or great vessel injury. Although CT may allow better identification of rib fractures than plain radiography, the risk of additional radiation exposure outweighs this benefit in patients with no evidence of significant pulmonary or vascular injury.

A critical issue in discussing the laboratory and radiological evaluation of abusive abdominal trauma cases is what can be considered a "significant" injury. In the setting of accidental trauma, the diagnosis of a grade I liver laceration or pancreatic contusion is not going to change the patient's management in any significant way; the levels of screening laboratory abnormalities that warrant CT or other radiological evaluation are set based on this fact. The goal is to identify those injuries that require either surgery or a change in the management of the patient in order to ensure a good outcome. In the setting of abusive trauma, however, it is an issue of *forensic significance*. In addition to the question of whether the patient requires surgery or another intervention, the question arises of whether there are any injuries, how many there are, and the timing of the various injuries. Each identified injury, no matter how small or surgically "insignificant," provides another piece of information in the question of whether the injuries are the result of abuse, how severe/repetitive was the abuse, when/where/how did it occur, and most importantly, where will this patient (and any siblings) be safe after discharge.

OUTCOMES

The mortality of abusive thoracoabdominal trauma is typically stated to be 40% to 50%. With increased awareness of these injuries and the increased use of screening laboratory and radiological evaluation, more recent data suggest a significantly lower mortality rate, particularly in patients with isolated abdominal injuries.[9,12,28] In a study by Canty et al,[28] a 12-year review of gastrointestinal injuries resulting from blunt trauma demonstrated that 19% of the injuries were caused by inflicted injury, but half of the deaths occurred in victims of child abuse. The mortality rate for the abuse victims was 20% (3/15) versus 4.7% (3/64) in the accidental blunt abdominal trauma cases. In most series, the majority of the mortality was due to the head and other associated injuries rather than the abdominal injuries. Long-term morbidity related to bowel injuries with secondary strictures or adhesions is seen in patients with complicated bowel perforations requiring extensive or repeated surgeries. The majority of solid organ and vascular injuries are treated conservatively, and those patients who survive the initial injury are unlikely to suffer long-term morbidity related to their thoracic and abdominal injuries.[28]

STRENGTH OF THE MEDICAL EVIDENCE

As stated previously, the literature on this topic has been limited by the use of screening laboratory and radiological tests on patients identified by historical or physical examination indicators of abdominal injuries. Although the literature clearly delineates the spectrum of thoracoabdominal abusive injuries, the true incidence and mortality rate remain unclear. In addition, little information regarding exact mechanisms of injury exists in the current literature.

SUGGESTED DIRECTIONS FOR FUTURE RESEARCH

Future research regarding inflicted thoracoabdominal injuries should include clinical and animal and/or experimental models to clarify mechanisms of injury, and large, prospective evaluation of known and suspected abuse cases using broad screening for abdominal injuries to better clarify the true incidence and mortality of these important injuries. Biochemical markers of injury have been used for decades to identify cardiac injury and are used in abdominal trauma to identify liver or pancreatic injury; more recently, biochemical markers have been used to identify those patients with brain injury. Future research should attempt to identify biochemical markers for bowel injury that are sensitive and specific enough to help guide the radiological evaluation and management of these patients.

References

1. Cooper A, Floyd T, Barlow B, et al: Major blunt abdominal trauma due to child abuse. *J Trauma* 1988;28:1483-1486.

2. Ellis PSJ: The pathology of fatal child abuse. *Pathology* 1997;29:113-121.

3. Wood J, Rubin DM, Nance ML, et al: Distinguishing inflicted versus accidental abdominal injuries in young children. *J Trauma* 2005;59:1203-1208.

4. Hobbs CJ: Abdominal injury due to child abuse. *Lancet* 2005;366:187-188.

5. Merten DF, Carpenter BLM: Radiologic imaging of inflicted injury in the child abuse syndrome. *Pediatr Clin North Am* 1990;37:815-837.

6. DiGiacomo JC, Frankel H, Haskell RM, et al: Unsuspected child abuse revealed by delayed presentation of periportal tracking and myoglobinuria. *J Trauma* 2000;49:348-350.

7. Davis HW, Carrasco MM: Child abuse and neglect. *In:* Zitelli BJ, Davis HW (eds): *Atlas of Pediatric Physical Diagnosis*, ed 5. Mosby, Philadelphia, 2007, pp 161-240.

8. Coant PN, Kornberg AE, Brody AS, et al: Markers for occult liver injury in cases of physical abuse in children. *Pediatrics* 1992;89:274-278.

9. Trokel M, Discala C, Terrin NC, et al: Patient and injury characteristics in abusive abdominal injuries. *Pediatr Emerg Care* 2006;22:700-704.

10. Sivit CJ, Taylor GA, Eichelberger MR: Visceral injury in battered children: a changing perspective. *Radiology* 1989;173:659-661.

11. Pollanen MS, Smith CR, Chiasson DA, et al: Fatal child abuse-maltreatment syndrome: a retrospective study in Ontario, Canada, 1990-1995. *Forensic Sci Int* 2002;126:101-104.

12. Gaines BA, Shultz BS, Morrison K, et al: Duodenal injuries in children: beware of child abuse. *J Pediatr Surg* 2004;39:600-602.

13. Barnes PM, Norton CM, Dunstan FD, et al: Abdominal injury due to child abuse. *Lancet* 2005;366:234-235.

14. Roaten JB, Partrick DA, Nydam TL, et al: Nonaccidental trauma is a major cause of morbidity and mortality among patients at a regional level 1 pediatric trauma center. *J Pediatr Surg* 2006;41:2013-2015.

15. Ledbetter DJ, Hatch EI, Feldman KW, et al: Diagnostic and surgical implications of child abuse. *Arch Surg* 1988;123:1101-1104.

16. Nimkin K, Teeger S, Wallach MT, et al: Adrenal hemorrhage in abused children: imaging and postmortem findings. *Am J Roentgenol* 1994;162:661-663.

17. Tracy T, O'Connor TP, Weber TR: Battered children with duodenal avulsion and transection. *Am Surg* 1993;6:342-345.

18. Champion MP, Richards CA, Boddy SA, et al: Duodenal perforation: a diagnostic pitfall in non-accidental injury. *Arch Dis Child* 2002;87:432-433.

19. Bowkett B, Kolbe A: Traumatic duodenal perforations in children: child abuse a frequent cause. *Aust N Z J Surg* 1998;68:380-382.

20. Fossum RM, Descheneaux KA: Blunt trauma of the abdomen in children. *J Forensic Sci* 1991;36:47-50.

21. Wu JW, Chen MYM, Auringer ST: Portal venous gas: an unusual finding in child abuse. *J Emerg Med* 2000;18:105-107.

22. deRoux SJ, Prendergast NC: Lacerations of the hepatoduodenal ligament, pancreas and duodenum in a child due to blunt impact. *J Forensic Sci* 1998;43:222-224.

23. Fox JT, Huang YC, Barcia PJ, et al: Blunt abdominal aortic transection in a child: case report. *J Trauma* 1996;41:1051-1053.

24. Kleinman PK: Visceral trauma. *In:* Kleinman PK (ed): *Diagnostic Imaging of Child Abuse*, ed 2. Mosby, Chicago, 1998, pp 248-284.

25. Huntimer CM, Muret-Wagstaff S, Leland NL: Can falls on stairs result in small intestine perforations? *Pediatrics* 2000;106:301-305.

26. Hennes HM, Smith DS, Schneider K, et al: Elevated liver transaminase levels in children with blunt abdominal trauma: a predictor of liver injury. *Pediatrics* 1990;86:87-90.

27. Boal DKB: Child abuse. *In:* Kuhn JP, Slovis TL, Haller JO (eds): *Caffey's Pediatric Diagnostic Imaging*, ed 10. Elsevier, Philadelphia, 2004, pp 2304-2318.

28. Canty TG Sr, Canty TG Jr, Brown C: Injuries of the gastrointestinal tract from blunt trauma in children: a 12-year experience at a designated pediatric trauma center. *J Trauma* 1999;46:234-239.

37

EAR, NOSE, AND THROAT INJURIES IN ABUSED CHILDREN

Philip V. Scribano, DO, MSCE, and Russell A. Faust, PhD, MD, FAAP

INTRODUCTION

Children who sustain injuries from abuse often experience trauma to the face, mouth, and neck regions. An estimated 50% to 75% of abused children have injuries in these locations,[1-5] with a higher prevalence in the younger child or infant. In a large case series of over 1248 children evaluated for all types of abuse and neglect, 37.5% included injuries to the head, face, mouth, or neck. The prevalence increased to 75.5% when the investigators evaluated only those children who became involved with the child protective services system for suspected physical abuse.[2]

The high prevalence of injuries to the face and neck supports the concept that the relative easy accessibility to that part of the body as well as the psychological importance of these areas predisposes them as frequent targets for the offender trying to silence a crying child.[2,6-8]

Despite the frequency of face and neck injuries, there is a relatively low prevalence of injuries to the mouth (2%).[2,6,9] This could be due to medical providers' unfamiliarity with examining the oral cavity. In addition, given the rapid healing potential of mucus membranes, oral injuries might resolve before being identified by a medical provider. While some abusive injuries can be severe and life threatening, most face, mouth, or neck injuries reported in the literature are less serious. Nevertheless, these findings can be harbingers of significant risk for more severe and repeated trauma if not detected as such.[1,3,10-12] Therefore, it is paramount that abuse-related injuries are promptly recognized. Table 37-1 lists common otolaryngological injuries caused by abuse.

FACIAL INJURIES

The face is the most frequently injured area of the body from physical abuse. Abrasions and bruises comprise most (87%) of the injuries, whereas lacerations account for 6% to 7%.[4] Abusive facial injuries are most often caused by a hand punching or slapping the oro-facial region or by an object impacting the face. The most common sign of open-hand blows to the face is multiple parallel marks representing the fingers (Figure 37-1). Bruising to the cheeks or anterior neck region (Figure 37-2) is suspicious for abuse, since this soft tissue does not overlie any bony prominence and therefore requires significant impact for ecchymoses to occur. The risk of *accidental* injury to the face is similar to that for the head and scalp, with the greatest risk existing for young children who are learning to crawl and walk.

Facial fractures in children are rare and should prompt a high index of suspicion for abuse unless the circumstances of the trauma are sufficiently credibile.[13,14] Facial fractures are known to result from motor vehicle accidents, from falls of significant heights, and from traumatic deliveries of newborns.[15] Mandible fractures are quite rare in infants and would not be expected to occur after a short household fall.[16] Given this fact, any infant presenting with a fractured mandible should be evaluated for possible child abuse if a major accident has not been confirmed.

EAR INJURIES

Ear injuries prompting suspicion of abuse include any lacerations of the external auditory meatus or hematomas, ecchymoses, or bruises of the auricle. Bruising to the pinna, which includes anterior as well as posterior injury, is highly suggestive of pinching or grabbing of the ear (Figure 37-3). Evidence of tympanic membrane perforation or ossicular discontinuity is especially suspicious; this can result from a forcible slap to the external ear with an open hand. Ultimately, chronic, recurring trauma can result in deformation of auricles[17,18] as well as sensorineural hearing loss.[3] Penetrating trauma can cause injury to the external auditory meatus, tympanic membrane, and middle ear.[1] The classic triad of unilateral ear bruising, retinal hemorrhages, and ipsilateral cerebral edema with obliteration of the basilar cisterns and associated subdural hemorrhage describes the tin ear syndrome.[19] In the original case report, three children under 3 years of age had similar bruises of the antitragus, the helix, and the triangular fossa, and in the interior folds of the ear without other bruises or lacerations of the head, external auditory meatus, or tympanic membranes. The three children died as a result of their abusive head trauma which included uncal herniation. On autopsy, ipsilateral subdural hemorrhage with absence of coup or contra coup injury was noted. The postulated mechanism was blunt trauma to the side of the head impacting at the point of the ear, which resulted in significant rotational acceleration of the head. These injuries point out the importance of ear bruises in children as a sign of possible associated injuries. Another type of ear injury, recurrent auricular hematomas ("cauliflower ear") is common in boxers, but unusual in other sports and extremely rare in accidental trauma.

Table 37-1	Otolaryngological Injuries Suspicious for Abuse

Ear

- Auricular hematoma/ecchymoses
- Laceration of external auditory canal
- Tympanic membrane perforation
- Ossicular discontinuity
- Total hearing loss associated with vertigo
- Facial nerve paresis
- Cerebral spinal fluid otorrhea
- Persistent otitis media with effusion

Nose

- Recurrent epistaxis
- Septal deviation/perforation
- Columella destruction
- Impaired naso-maxillary development
- Foreign body insertion with internal nasal trauma
- Cerebral spinal fluid rhinorrhea

Oropharynx

- Bruising of the palate or fauces
- Lacerations or evidence of foreign body trauma
- Dental avulsion/subluxation
- Burns to lips or oral mucosa
- Abrasions or scars at the lip, commissures
- Labial frena tear
- Vocal cord paralysis

Other Injuries/ Conditions

- Facial/mandibular fractures
- Retropharyngeal soft tissue neck trauma
- Functional hearing loss
- Vocal cord nodules
- Lesions consistent with sexually transmitted diseases

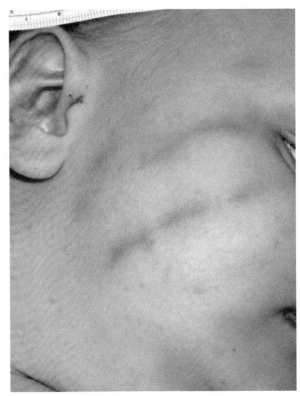

FIGURE 37-1 A 3-year-old boy with characteristic, hand slap bruise over the right cheek.

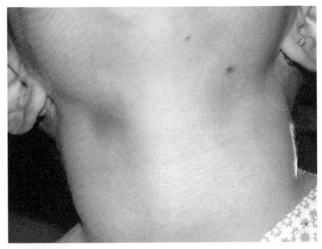

FIGURE 37-2 An 8-year-old who reported being choked by an adult while being sexually abused. Patterned finger marks support the history of choking.

Of particular concern is any injury associated with total hearing or balance loss, facial nerve paralysis, or cerebrospinal fluid (CSF) otorrhea (or CSF rhinorrhea). These injuries should prompt additional evaluation to determine the circumstances of injury, since accidental injuries of the ear and associated neurological structures are uncommon.[3] It can be challenging to distinguish perforation of the tympanic membrane caused by infection and rupture from the perforation caused by trauma; the presence of hemotympanum in the absence of purulence should prompt greater scrutiny and consideration of an abusive episode. Facial nerve paresis combined with any other evidence of trauma warrants a computerized tomography (CT) scan of the temporal bone to rule out fracture. Similarly, cerebrospinal fluid otorrhea, even as an isolated finding, is cause for suspicion. It can reflect a blow of significant force, resulting in either temporal bone fracture or rupture of the membranous inner ear.

It is important to recognize that falsification of symptoms of ear disease has been described.[20] One case involved a mother who reported that her 8-month-old infant had recurrent, at times, bloody discharge from his external auditory meatus. An analysis of the fluid from the ear identified a high level of salivary amylase, proving the "ear discharge" to be saliva. Clinicians were able to recognize this as a case of factitious illness, but only after multiple evaluations, surgical intervention (myringotomy), and hospital admissions. An astute nurse recognized that the "symptom" only occurred with the mother was alone with the child. Other otolaryngological manifestations of factitious illness have been reported, such as persistent cerebrospinal fluid otorrhea, sinusitis, hearing loss, and apnea caused by suffocation.[21-25]

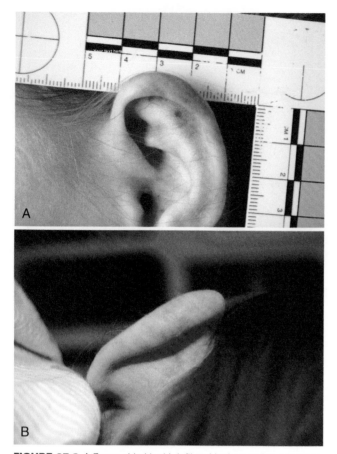

FIGURE 37-3 A 7-year-old girl with inflicted bruises on her left pinna. **A,** Anterior view. **B,** Posterior view.

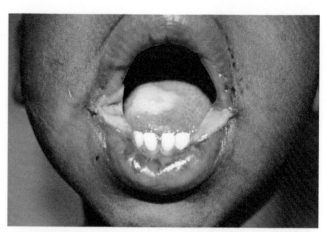

FIGURE 37-4 A 4-year-old boy who reported being burned with a kitchen spoon. He sustained intra-oral and commissure burns; the posterior pharynx was spared.

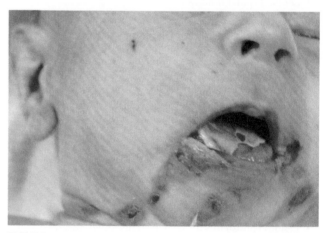

FIGURE 37-5 A 6-week-old infant who was admitted with burns to the face and oral mucosa after being fed a bottle of milk overheated in a microwave.

NASAL INJURIES

Accidental injuries to the nose are not uncommon. Intranasal injuries, however, should prompt suspicion, since these injuries require significant force. In addition, although children commonly insert foreign bodies into their noses, associated injury to intranasal structures is rare and when encountered, abuse should be considered.[26] Examination findings such as recurrent epistaxis, blood clots, or deviation of the nasal septum are not diagnostic of abuse, but the history should include a reasonable mechanism of injury. Blunt force trauma to the nose with nasal cartilage fracture and resulting septal hematoma will lead to resorption of the cartilage with perforation and possible nasal deformity if not managed acutely. The findings of septal perforation or columella destruction can be sequelae of old, untreated injuries. Hematoma and abscess of the nasal septum resulting in nasal deformity and other complications have been described as resulting from child abuse.[27] In general, the nose does not bruise without direct impact or pinching. Nasal tip or columella bruising is highly suspicious for intentional injury from pinching these structures.

ORAL INJURIES

Signs of abuse in the oral cavity can be subtle and difficult to recognize if the clinician is not conducting a thorough examination. A comprehensive examination should include inspection of the hard and soft palates, labial and lingual frena, gingiva, tongue, buccal mucosa, posterior pharynx, and teeth if present. Injury to the lips is the most common abusive injury to the mouth.[13] Repeated trauma can leave scars over the lips. Localized abrasions or bruises to the commissures suggest injury from a mouth gag. Burns to the mouth and commissure can be caused by application of heated implements to the mouth, such as a heated spoon (Figure 37-4). Burns to the mouth and lips also can be due to unintentional events (Figure 37-5). A torn labial frenum has been regarded as pathognomonic of abuse in non-ambulatory children.[2,6,8,28,29] A frustrated caregiver trying to silence a crying infant using a hand or other object such as a bottle can result in these lesions (Figure 37-6). Oral (buccal) lacerations or bruising of the palate in a young, pre-ambulatory child is highly suspicious for abuse and can result from the forcible insertion of an object into the mouth or from a direct blow to the mouth. The oral cavity is also a site for identifying sexual abuse trauma. Lesions can result from sexually transmitted infections. Petechiae and bruising at the junction of the soft and hard palates or on the floor of the mouth can be caused by forced fellatio.[6,13] Injuries to the tongue have

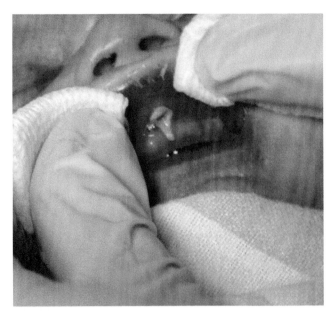

FIGURE 37-6 A 7-week-old with an upper labial frenum laceration. *(Courtesy of Jonathan Thackeray, MD, Columbus, Ohio.)*

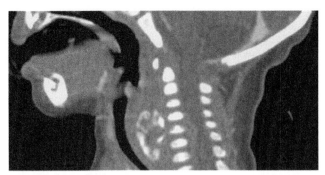

FIGURE 37-7 CT scan of the neck of a 2½-month-old with bilateral femur fractures. Skeletal survey revealed a calcification on lateral neck x-rays. The CT scan identified a resolving retropharyngeal calcified hematoma adjacent to a C5 compression fracture and epidural hematoma. This prior injury was correlated with a period of respiratory difficulty approximately 3 weeks before the study.

resulted from an adult biting an infant's tongue. The arc of the bite (the concave surface of the mark) in the direction toward the lips instead of toward the posterior pharynx suggests the injury is the result of non-accidental trauma rather than self-inflicted injury.[30] Because of the healing characteristics and excellent blood supply of the mucus membranes, oral lacerations rarely require surgical repair.

Teeth can be injured and result in fracture, avulsion, luxation, or displacement. Although fractures are more likely to be the result of accidental trauma, it is important to obtain a detailed history to understand the cause of these injuries. Tooth avulsions caused by abuse (direct force apical to the crown of the tooth, resulting in expulsion of the tooth) are almost exclusively limited to the anterior teeth because of their single root structure, where a sufficient blow to the alveolar ridge of the mouth can result in this trauma.[8] Forced dental extraction by parents as a form of child abuse has been reported where intact teeth were forcibly removed from a child's mouth while the child was restrained.[31] Luxation, or disruption of the tooth causing injury to the periodontal ligament supporting the tooth in the alveolar ridge, can present as a loose tooth and can be displaced lingually (more likely in abusive events) or labially because of an object or hand strike to the mouth and teeth.

NECK/PHARYNGEAL INJURIES

Pharyngeal/hypopharyngeal injuries, which should prompt further evaluation for possible non-accidental trauma, include hypopharyngeal laceration, esophageal perforation, and retropharyngeal hematoma with associated cervical spine and cervical cord trauma (Figure 37-7).[10,11,32,33] These injuries result from forcible insertion of foreign objects and/or hyperextension/hyperflexion of the neck, and characteristically present with an inconsistent or absent history to explain the injuries. Often, there has been a delay in seeking care. Symptoms include hemoptysis, noisy breathing, difficulty feeding, drooling, stridor, or subcutaneous emphy-

sema.[34] Evidence of enlargement of the retropharyngeal space, retropharyngeal air, or pneumomediastinum is sometimes found on imaging studies.

Vocal cord paralysis (unilateral or bilateral) can be caused by strangulation or can result from a severe head injury. Patients present with respiratory distress, stridor, choking spells, or frank apnea.[33] In one report, a 13-month-old child was co-sleeping with her mother. The mother had very long hair, and the child was strangled accidentally by her mother's hair.[35] Specific indicators of possible strangulation include laryngeal edema, hyoid bone fracture, petechiae of the neck and face, and ligature marks on the neck. At autopsy, findings of fat necrosis with subsequent calcification in the soft tissues of the neck (necklace calcification), Tardieu's spots (subpleural ecchymoses following death from strangulation), and subintimal hemorrhage of the carotid artery, have been described after strangulation, and they should warrant high suspicion for non-accidental injury.[36-38] In some cases, strangulation abuse leaves no identifiable injury pattern.

STRENGTH OF THE MEDICAL EVIDENCE

The medical evidence with regard to otolaryngologic injuries in abused children consists of multiple case reports and case series that demonstrate characteristic injury patterns in maltreated children. As such, it provides a growing evidence of certain injuries commonly occurring in abused children. There is little literature, however, comparing inflicted and accidental injuries. Such studies would facilitate greater diagnostic accuracy in determining the causes of injuries to the face, nose, ears, mouth and pharynx.

SUGGESTED DIRECTIONS FOR FUTURE RESEARCH

Future research efforts should focus on distinguishing characteristics that assist the clinician in determining the mechanism of injuries. There is a need for greater clinical and diagnostic injury identification, especially in the oropharynx and neck. Also, research on methods to improve the detection of occult injuries would improve clinical care.

References

1. Manning SC, Casselbrant M, Lammers D: Otolaryngologic manifestations of child abuse. *Int J Pediatr Otorhinolaryngol* 1990;20:7-16.
2. da Fonseca MA, Feigal RJ, ten Bensel RW: Dental aspects of 1248 cases of child maltreatment on file at a major county hospital. *Pediatr Dent* 1992;14:152-157.
3. Crouse CD, Faust RA: Child abuse and the otolaryngologist: part II. *Otolaryngol Head Neck Surg* 2003;128:311-317.
4. Cairns AM, Mok JYQ, Welbury RR: Injuries to the head, face, mouth and neck in physically abused children in a community setting. *Int J Paediatr Dent* 2005;15:310-318.
5. Becker DB, Needleman HL, Kotelchuck M: Child abuse and dentistry: oro-facial trauma and its recognition by dentists. *J Am Dent Assoc* 1978;97:24-28.
6. Jessee SA: Orofacial manifestations of child abuse and neglect. *Am Fam Physician* 1995;52:1829-1834.
7. Fabian AA, Bender L: Head injury in children: predisposing factors. *Am J Orthopsychiatry* 1947;17:68-79.
8. Mouden L, Kenney J: Oral injuries. *In:* Giardino AP, Alexander R (eds): *Child Maltreatment: A Clinical Guide and Reference*, ed 3. GW Medical Publishing, St Louis, 2005, pp 91-102.
9. Willging JP, Bower CM, Cotton RT: Physical abuse of children—a retrospective review and an otolaryngology perspective. *Arch Otolaryngol Head Neck Surg* 1992;118:584-590.
10. Pramuk LA, Sirotnak A, Friedman NR. Esophageal perforation preceding fatal closed head injury in a child abuse case. *Int J Pediatr Otorhinolaryngol* 2004;68:831-835.
11. Ng CS, Hall CM, Shaw DG: The range of visceral manifestations of non-accidental injury. *Arch Dis Child* 1997;77:167-174.
12. Maguire SA, Hunter B, Hunter LM, et al: Diagnosing abuse: a systematic review of torn frenum and intra-oral injuries. *Arch Dis Child* 2007;92:1113-1117.
13. Tanaka N, Uchide N, Suzuki K, et al: Maxillofacial fractures in children. *J Craniomaxillofac Surg* 1993;21:289-293.
14. Siegel MB, Wetmore RF, Potsic WP, et al: Mandibular fractures in the pediatric patient. *Arch Otolaryngol Head Neck Surg* 1991;117:533-536.
15. Lustmann J, Milhem I: Mandibular fractures in infants: review of the literature and report of seven cases. *J Oral Maxillofac Surg* 1994;52:240-245.
16. Schlievert R: Infant mandibular fractures: are you considering child abuse? *Pediatr Emerg Care* 2006;22:181-183.
17. Leavitt EB, Pincus RL, Bukachevsky R: Otolaryngologic manifestations of child abuse. *Arch Otolaryngol Head Neck Surg* 1992;118:629-631.
18. Willner A, Ledereich PS, deVries EJ: Auricular injury as a presentation of child abuse. *Arch Otolaryngol Head Neck Surg* 1992;118:634-637.
19. Hanigan WC, Peterson RA, Njus G: Tin ear syndrome: rotational acceleration in pediatric head injuries. *Pediatrics* 1987;80:618-622.
20. Bennett AM, Bennett SM, Prinsley PR, et al: Spitting in the ear: a falsified disease using video evidence. *J Laryngol Otol* 2005;119:926-927.
21. Mra Z, MacCormick JA, Poje CP: Persistent cerebrospinal fluid otorrhea: a case of Munchausen's syndrome by proxy. *Int J Pediatr Otorhinolaryngol* 1997;41:59-63.
22. Samuels MP, McClaughlin W, Jacobson RR, et al: Fourteen cases of imposed upper airway obstruction. *Arch Dis Child* 1992;67:162-170.
23. Southall DP, Stebbens VA, Rees SV, et al: Apnoeic episodes induced by smothering: two cases identified by covert video surveillance. *Br Med J* 1987;294:1637-1641.
24. Southall DP, Plunkett MC, Banks MW, et al: Covert video recordings of life-threatening child abuse: lessons for child protection. *Pediatrics* 1997;100:735-760.
25. Feldman KW, Stout JW, Inglis AF Jr: Asthma, allergy, and sinopulmonary disease in pediatric condition falsification. *Child Maltreat* 2002;7:125-131.
26. Fischer H, Allasio D: Nasal destruction due to child abuse. *Clin Pediatr* 1996;35:165-166.
27. Canty PA, Berkowitz RG: Hematoma and abscess of the nasal septum in children. *Arch Otolaryngol Head Neck Surg* 1996;122:1373-1376.
28. Thackeray JD: Frena tears and abusive head injury: a cautionary tale. *Pediatr Emerg Care* 2007;23:735-737.
29. Sirotnak AP, Grigsby T, Krugman RD: Physical abuse of children. *Pediatr Rev* 2004;25:264-277.
30. Lee, LY, Mulvey IJ: Human biting of children and oral manifestations of abuse. A case report and literature review. *ASDC J Dent Child* 2002;69:92-95.
31. Carrotte PV: An unusual case of child abuse. *Br Dent J* 1990;168:444-445.
32. Myer CM, Fitton CM: Vocal cord paralysis following child abuse. *Int J Pediatr Otorhinolaryngol* 1988;15:217-220.
33. Tostevin PMJ, Hollis LJ, Bailey CM: Pharyngeal trauma in children—accidental and otherwise. *J Laryngol Otol* 1995;109:1168-1175.
34. Ramnarayan P, Qayyum A, Tolley N, et al: Subcutaneous emphysema of the neck in infancy: under-recognized presentation of child abuse. *J Laryngol Otol* 2004;118:468-470.
35. Milkovich SM, Owens J, Stool D, et al: Accidental childhood strangulation by human hair. *Int J Pediatr Otorhinolaryngol* 2005;69:1621-1628.
36. Carty H. Case report: child abuse- necklace calcification- a sign of strangulation. *Br J Radiol* 1993;66:1186-1188.
37. Jain V, Ray M, Singhi S: Strangulation injury, a fatal form of child abuse. *Indian J Pediatr* 2001;68:571-572.
38. Bird CR, McMahan JR, Gilles FH, et al: Strangulation in child abuse: CT diagnosis. *Radiology* 1987;163:373-375.

SUDDEN INFANT DEATH SYNDROME OR ASPHYXIA?

Henry F. Krous, MD, and Roger W. Byard, MD

INTRODUCTION

There are many causes of infant death that result from natural diseases, accidents, or inflicted injuries. Some of these become quite apparent after review of the medical history, careful scene investigation, and/or thorough autopsy with ancillary radiographic and laboratory studies.[1] If a specific cause is not ascertained, however, a diagnosis of sudden infant death syndrome (SIDS) is often made.[2,3]

One of the most perplexing and pressing dilemmas currently facing those involved in the field is the differentiation of SIDS from asphyxia, whether accidental or inflicted. This is particularly true for those cases without diagnostic physical findings at autopsy. In such cases, careful and repeated questioning of the caretakers, thorough scene evaluations and reconstructions where the infants were found lifeless, and reviews of the circumstances of death are mandatory given the extraordinarily divergent consequences that will follow if the manner of death is certified as natural, accident, or homicide.[4]

This chapter provides a brief review of SIDS and asphyxia, focuses on approaches that have been undertaken to differentiate these two conditions, and discusses controversial areas in their differentiation.

SUDDEN INFANT DEATH SYNDROME

Definition and Epidemiology

SIDS is currently defined as the sudden and unexpected death of an infant under 1 year of age, with onset of the lethal episode apparently occurring during sleep, which remains unexplained after a thorough investigation including performance of a complete autopsy and review of the circumstances of death and the clinical history.[3] This general "San Diego" definition was then stratified to accommodate the differing levels of certainty of making a SIDS diagnosis and to facilitate research.[3] In addition, another category, unclassified sudden infant death (USID) was created for "deaths not meeting the criteria for Category 1 or II SIDS, but where alternative diagnoses of natural or unnatural conditions are equivocal."[3] This includes cases where autopsies have not been performed. It should also be noted that this new scheme also allows cases that have undergone cardiopulmonary resuscitation to be classified as SIDS.

The "Back to Sleep" campaign in the United States and equivalent public educational programs designed to modify infant care practices in other countries led to dramatic declines in SIDS rates in all developed countries. For example, the SIDS rate in the United States in 2004 was 0.54/1000 live births compared with rates two to three times that before the early 1990s.[5] In 2005, the rate was 0.41 in England and Wales.[6] Nevertheless, SIDS is still the most common cause of postneonatal infant death accounting for approximately 23% of all postneonatal infant deaths; six SIDS deaths occur each day in the United States.

Recent data have suggested that the decline in SIDS rates in the United States is a result of a shift in death classification and reporting. The overall postneonatal mortality rate between 1991 and 1996 declined 21.9% compared with a reduction in the SIDS rate of 38.9%.[7] The same study also found that the proportion of the postneonatal mortality contributed by SIDS declined from 37.1% in 1991 to 28.8% in 1996 whereas rates for deaths ascribed to asphyxia in a bed or cradle significantly increased, suggesting that only a very small number of SIDS deaths were reclassified as asphyxia. Similar data are available from Australia.[8]

Risk Factors

SIDS occurs primarily between 1 and 5 months of age, with 90% of cases occurring by the sixth postnatal month. In most studies, males generally predominate over females by a ratio of 2:1. Premature birth, low birth weight, lower socioeconomic class, young maternal age, and short inter-gestational interval place an infant at increased risk of SIDS. African American, Native American, Alaskan native, Australian aboriginal, and Maori ethnicity have also been cited as risk factors. Exposure to prenatal, gestational, and/or postnatal cigarette smoke is an important and modifiable risk factor.[9-13]

Several other risk factors for SIDS must be carefully evaluated when considering the possibility that asphyxia caused the death of an infant in whom there are no significant post-mortem findings. These include prone sleep position, especially for unaccustomed or first-time prone sleepers; soft bedding; soft objects in the bed; and the infant being found with his or her head covered by blankets.[14-18] Although the precise role of prone sleep position in SIDS is unknown, external airway obstruction has been considered. In this regard, an analysis of intrathoracic petechiae, a likely marker of terminal upper airway obstruction, found no differences in SIDS cases found with their face directly into the sleep surface compared with those found with their faces to the side or up, thereby suggesting a role for rebreathing or hyperthermia.[19]

Head covering deserves additional comment since it raises the possibility of suffocation. A recent review of population-based age-matched controlled studies addressing the significance of head covering and the risk of SIDS found that the pooled prevalence of head covering in SIDS victims was 24.6% compared with 3.2% among the controls.[20] Although the risk varied in strength across all studies, the pooled adjusted odds ratio from studies mainly conducted after the fall in the SIDS rate was 16.9. These findings suggest that avoidance of head covering might lead to a 25% reduction in SIDS deaths. Another study concluded that head covering was not an agonal event since these SIDS cases were often sweaty, suggesting that it preceded, and could have been causally related to, the death.[21]

Bed sharing is another important SIDS risk factor. Without careful scene investigation and reconstruction, especially in the absence of a witness, the certifying pathologist is faced with the dilemma of differentiating SIDS from overlaying. To date, there are no studies that show a protective effect of bed sharing against SIDS.[22-25] This risk is particularly important during the first 4 months of age and remains after controlling for cigarette smoke exposure and is not affected by breastfeeding.[25]

Autopsy Findings

Routine autopsy examinations and ancillary studies do not identify a specific cause of death in SIDS despite the frequent presence of often minor pathologic findings. Intrathoracic petechiae are the most common gross autopsy finding, but their presence is neither pathognomonic nor does their absence exclude a diagnosis of SIDS.[19,26,27] Their unique distribution, however, suggests their pathogenesis is related to breathing against an obstructed upper airway or deep gasping, rather than being the result of external airway obstruction with oronasal compression.[19,26-28]

Minor inflammatory infiltrates are not uncommonly identified microscopically in the airways and lungs, but are not evident to the naked eye.[29,30] However, we found that SIDS cases were no different than accidental or inflicted suffocation control cases with respect to the type and severity of inflammation within the lungs, results of postmortem cultures, or a history of upper respiratory infection.[31] On the other hand, another study found that *Staphylococcus aureus* or *Escherichia coli* were isolated significantly more often from postmortem cultures taken from infants whose deaths were unexplained than did those from infants whose deaths were of non-infective causes, suggesting that these bacteria might be important in the mechanism of death.[6]

Sophisticated studies of the central nervous system have identified subtle abnormalities that appear critical to increasing the vulnerability of an infant to sudden unexpected death during sleep. Absence or severe hypoplasia of the arcuate nuclei has been shown in a small percentage of SIDS cases.[32,33] Abnormalities in brainstem neurotransmitter receptors affect a much larger proportion of cases.[34-38]

Triple Risk Hypothesis

Although suggested in some form by others before them,[39] Filiano and Kinney[40] proposed the "triple risk" hypothesis for SIDS that has captured increasing recognition and acceptance by those working in the field. They stated, "According to this model, sudden death in SIDS results from the intersection of three overlapping factors: (1) a vulnerable infant; (2) a critical developmental period in homeostatic control; and, (3) an exogenous stressor(s). An infant will die of SIDS only if he/she possesses all three factors; the infant's vulnerability lies latent until he/she enters the critical period and is subject to an exogenous stressor."[40] This hypothesis continues to be refined with expanding recognition and understanding of the contribution of risk factors, pathologic findings, and developmental physiology of the young infant. For example, the medullary serotonergic defect hypothesis has been advanced to account for a significant proportion of SIDS deaths. This hypothesis proposes that SIDS, or a subset of SIDS, is due to a developmental abnormality in a medullary network of serotonergic neurons, including the arcuate nucleus, that results in a failure of protective responses to life-threatening stressors (e.g., asphyxia, hypoxia, and hypercapnia) during sleep as the infant passes through a critical period in homeostatic control.[36]

Disorders Mimicking Sudden Infant Death Syndrome

There are a number of disorders that can cause sudden unexpected infant death and therefore mimic SIDS. Fortunately many of these disorders can be identified through comprehensive evaluation of the circumstances of death and postmortem examination, including ancillary studies for which there are standardized protocols to assist in this approach (http://www.cdc.gov/SIDS/PDF/SUIDIforms.pdf).[41-43]

Cardiac sodium and potassium ion channel mutations leading to prolongation of the QT interval cause 2% to 5% of sudden unexpected infant deaths.[44-48] A large Italian study brought particular attention to this relationship.[49] To date, mutational analyses have revealed about 103 distinct mutations in the sodium channel gene SCN5A.[50] Confirmation of the diagnosis requires either characteristic findings on an antemortem electrocardiogram, which is rarely available, or molecular testing of fresh tissues taken at autopsy. Electrocardiographic demonstration of long QT intervals in either parent may be helpful, but negative results do not exclude the diagnosis in the infant since approximately half of the cases of long QT interval are the result of a new mutation.

Metabolic disorders disrupting energy metabolism and glucose homeostasis are another cause of sudden infant death.[51] Among these disorders, those characterized by disordered fatty acid oxidation are the most frequently encountered. Medium chain acyl-CoA dehydrogenase (MCAD) deficiency is the most common, although other fatty acid oxidation disorders including very long chain acyl-CoA dehydrogenase deficiency, long chain acyl-CoA dehydrogenase deficiency, and short chain acyl-CoA dehydrogenase have also been implicated. Other diseases that can cause sudden infant death are defects in carnitine uptake and glutaric acidemia type 2.[52] It is now estimated that approximately 5% of sudden infant deaths are a result of metabolic disorders.[52] In contrast to earlier times, tandem mass spectrometric testing of blood obtained either from the newborn or at the time of autopsy is a very comprehensive and rather inexpensive method to establish these diagnoses.[53,54] It should be noted that amino acidemias and organic acidemias are rarely associated with sudden unexpected death; rather, death is typically preceded by varying periods of clinically evident deterioration.

Other causes of sudden infant death include, but are not limited to congenital malformations, especially obstructive lesions of the left heart, as well as neoplasms, myocarditis, and sepsis.[1,55-57]

ASPHYXIA

Generally the term *asphyxia* is used when an animal or human is exposed to insufficient oxygen levels to sustain normal metabolic processes. Complete deprivation of oxygen results in anoxia and partial deprivation causes hypoxia. Although asphyxia originally meant a lack of pulse (from the Greek *asphuxia*: a—not; *sphuxis*—pulse), asphyxia nowadays is limited to situations in which an individual is not receiving adequate amounts of oxygen. A variety of situations and mechanisms reduces the availability of oxygen at the cellular level.[58] Before examining the difficulties that occur in attempting to differentiate SIDS from various asphyxial deaths, it is appropriate to review definitions, classifications, and mechanisms of asphyxial deaths.

Historical Developments

Originally asphyxia denoted cessation of respiration or apnea, usually as a result of strangulation, hanging, or suffocation. Understanding of the underlying processes was variable, with some authors considering that terminal mechanisms involved only the lungs and airways whereas others acknowledged that more complex interactions occurred.[59-62] For example, Taylor[62] in the mid-nineteenth century noted that the airway was not necessarily obstructed in hanging, and that compression of blood vessels in the neck was an important part of the lethal process involving (as he put it) "… apoplexy of the congestive kind."[62]

Although the diagnosis of an asphyxial death was based on the finding of a congested face, frothing at the mouth, dilatation of the right side of the heart and fluid, dark blood,[59,60] it is now recognized that these findings are entirely nonspecific.[63]

Pathophysiology

One of the difficulties with understanding asphyxial processes has been the tendency to classify cases according to the circumstances of death rather than the underlying pathophysiological mechanisms. Although there is no doubt that it is practically very useful to categorize infant and early childhood deaths based on the death scene and autopsy findings into groups such as hanging, wedging, and smothering, cases can also be separated into four main groups based on the different mechanisms that have impeded oxygenation. These consist of (1) insufficient oxygen in the surrounding atmosphere, (2) reduced transfer of oxygen from the atmosphere to the blood, (3) impaired oxygen transport in the circulating blood, and (4) interference with oxygen uptake at the cellular level.[63] In addition, combinations of these four mechanisms can occur together.

Since the range of activities for infants and the very young is limited, the most common types of asphyxial deaths involve feeding/eating and sleeping accidents that result in deaths caused by lethally low oxygenation of the circulating blood and reduced oxygen transport (Categories 2 and 3).

Categories

(1) Insufficient Oxygen in the Surrounding Atmosphere

(a) Displacement of Oxygen. This rarely occurs when infants or children are exposed to environments in which oxygen has been displaced by inert gases such as carbon dioxide or methane, or in drowning.[64,65] Loss of consciousness can occur within seconds if the oxygen concentration in inspired air is reduced to below 25% of normal, followed by death within minutes.[66]

(b) Consumption of Oxygen. If toddlers are accidentally or deliberately confined in airtight spaces such as refrigerators or become entrapped in plastic bags, the limited amount of oxygen present might not be sufficient to sustain life.[67]

(2) Reduced Transfer of Oxygen from the Atmosphere to the Blood

(a) External Airway Obstruction (Smothering). Blockage of the mouth and nostrils is deliberate in homicides where pillows are held over infants' faces, or inadvertent in cases where infants lie face down on soft bedding or wrap themselves in plastic sheeting or bags.[67] Wetting of sheets or blankets with vomitus or saliva also increases resistance to airflow and assists in molding of material around the mouth and nose, thus increasing the possibility of asphyxia. Certain types of beds and bedding predispose to smothering. Infants who slip down between the arms of U-shaped pillows or who slip into a space between a crib side and a mattress can die from external airway obstruction. Portable mesh-sided and inflatable cribs are also potentially dangerous if infants move into a position where their faces are pressed against the plastic sides or base.[68-70] On occasion, the mechanism involved can be quite complex. An example of this concerns overhead-suspended rocking cradles where infants slip into a position in which they are unable to lift their faces off the mattress and bedding. A feature common to many of these potentially lethal situations is the presence of a trough or depression into which an infant has slipped. Infants and children with underlying conditions such as cerebral palsy can be at increased risk of asphyxia deaths.[71,72] We have also reported examples of infants who died while breastfeeding, suggesting that maternal distraction can be a contributory factor.[73,74]

(b) Internal Airway Obstruction. Infants and toddlers can occlude their upper airways from organic conditions such as intraluminal hemangiomas, lingual thyroglossal duct cysts, and acute epiglottitis.[75] Inhalation of foreign bodies is also a danger in the young, most commonly parts of toys or incompletely masticated solid food. A problem with infants and toddlers is that the incisor teeth develop before the molars, so it is possible to bite off chunks of food before it is possible to chew properly. Large fragments of food can then be inhaled, resulting in critical airway narrowing or

occlusion.[76,77] If resuscitation has been attempted, obstructive foreign material might have been removed from the upper airways, so it is important to obtain statements from attending medical personnel and to obtain the aspirated material for measurement and evaluation. Hanging can also cause tracheal obstruction in the young, particularly given the pliability of the tracheal cartilaginous rings.

(c) Extrinsic Compromise of Thoracic Cage Function. Infants who become wedged between a mattress and a crib side or wall can have their respiratory excursion critically limited, preventing the respiratory muscles from expanding the chest cage and filling the lungs with air. This represents mechanical/positional asphyxia. If there is pressure on the chest, for example, when a toddler becomes trapped under a piece of furniture, death can result from crush asphyxia.[78]

(d) Intrinsic Compromise of Thoracic Cage Function. This can occur in vehicle accidents if an infant suffers multiple rib fractures or a pneumothorax. The adverse effects are similar at all ages with compromise of the bellows function of the chest cage and diaphragm.

(3) Impaired Oxygen Transport in the Circulating Blood

(a) Reduced Oxygen-Binding Capacity. The most common scenario involves exposure to carbon monoxide, a tasteless, odorless non-irritating gas that is derived from burning organic materials when there is an inadequate supply of oxygen for complete combustion. Inhalation of carbon monoxide can be lethal as it has up to 250 to 300 times the binding affinity for hemoglobin compared with oxygen. Thus, even quite small amounts of carbon monoxide can displace oxygen from hemoglobin and significantly deplete the amount of circulating oxygen within the blood. Carbon monoxide also acts at the cellular level and impairs mitochondrial respiration.[66]

Carbon monoxide toxicity should be suspected in cases in which there are multiple unexpected infant deaths, either at the same time or sequentially in the same room or house, since environmental contamination from faulty heaters might have occurred. Lethal carbon monoxide toxicity in early life is also not uncommon in cases of familial murder-suicide.[79] House fires are another situation in which lethal levels of carbon monoxide can be encountered. Although infants succumb to lower levels of carboxyhemoglobin than older individuals, it is also important to test for other substances such as cyanide from burning plastic materials. Cherry-pink discoloration of the skin often provides the first indication of possible lethal carbon monoxide exposure.

(b) Local Vascular Compression. Infants and toddlers who hang themselves can significantly slow venous return from the head or stop arterial blood flow, without occluding their airways. This leads to a critical reduction in cerebral oxygenation with fatal consequences.

(4) Interference with Oxygen Uptake at the Cellular Level

(a) Chemical Asphyxia. This refers to poisoning at the cellular level where substances such as cyanide directly impair use of oxygen because of deleterious effects on enzyme systems.

(5) Combinations of Mechanisms that Impede Oxygenation

Many lethal asphyxial circumstances involve more than one of the previously mentioned mechanisms.[80] For example, wedging can cause death because of a combination of smothering and mechanical asphyxia casused by covering of the face and splinting of the chest.[81] Hanging involves vascular and airway occlusion, the latter caused by direct pressure on the trachea as well as to lifting of the tongue and parapharyngeal soft tissues. In addition, vagal inhibition can play a role in terminal mechanisms.[82] Infants are at risk of hanging if they slip down in strollers and become suspended from webbing, and toddlers can hang themselves from curtain cords or get their clothing caught on projections such as bolts and nuts found inside old, repaired, or homemade cots.[83,84] Head entrapment is also a problem that is encountered in exploratory toddlers when they manage to insert their heads into narrow spaces but are then unable to successfully extricate themselves.[85]

The death of an infant while sleeping in bed with an adult has been referred to as overlaying based on the time-honored concept that these infants have been asphyxiated when the adult has lain across them. This has evoked passionate debate with opponents of the idea claiming that it is virtually impossible for an adult not to realize that an infant is under them. For this reason the deaths of infants when sharing sofas with an adult have been classified as "SIDS" without consideration of the likelihood of an accidental manner of death. It would seem reasonable to accept, however, that any infant who is asleep in proximity to an adult is at risk of asphyxia from a variety of mechanisms. These include obstruction of the nose and mouth and chest compression.[83,84,86] Strangulation from a mother's long hair has rarely been reported.[87] Certain factors increase the risk of asphyxiation, such as soft, abundant bedding; young age of the infant; large body mass index of the adult(s); and intoxication, sedation, or fatigue.[88,89] It has also been noted that certain infants are predisposed to respiratory arrest after relatively short periods of airway obstruction.[90] Underlying diseases and conditions such as bronchopulmonary dysplasia and anemia may increase an infant's susceptibility to asphyxia by reducing baseline levels of oxygenation.

Although drowning is associated with exposure to reduced environmental oxygen levels, the mechanisms of death are quite complex, involving not only asphyxia from oxygen displacement, but also possible airway obstruction from laryngospasm, electrolyte disturbances from hemodilution, and sometimes vagal inhibition from cold ambient temperatures.[91,92]

Inflicted suffocation involves placing a pillow or plastic bag over an infant's head and/or lying over the victim, thus introducing an element of positional/crush asphyxia.

Pathological Features

Establishing the diagnosis of asphyxia can be extremely difficult at autopsy since there are often no morphological markers present to suggest the diagnosis and acute hypoxia has no specific histologic features. For this reason, there has been considerable energy expended in recent years to ensure that all unexpected infant and toddler deaths undergo comprehensive death scene evaluation by trained examiners. Published protocols are available to provide guidelines for this.[92] Whereas entrapment or exposure to suffocating gases is readily identified at the scene, wedging deaths and possible overlaying are less easy to prove, particularly if the scene is disturbed with removal of the body. Hanging is usually diagnosable given the characteristic scene features and parental histories, although on occasion care givers might alter the scene findings to reduce their feelings of guilt, as was the case with a mother whose young son had hung himself from a cord that she had left hanging from a cupboard door handle.[1]

Careful external examination should be conducted along with a full skeletal survey to check for occult bone trauma. Patterned abrasions or parchmented areas of skin can indicate injury associated with entrapment or wedging. Similarly, patterns of lividity and pressure blanching should correspond to the known or reported position of the infant when found. Circumferential parchmented ligature marks around the neck will usually indicate hanging or possible ligature strangulation. Manual strangulation can cause oval fingertip bruises of the neck and underlying strap muscles—the latter demonstrated by careful layer dissection of the neck. Fractures of the hyoid bone and thyroid cartilage are rare in infants given the pliable nature of these cartilaginous structures in the young. In cases of crush asphyxia there will sometimes be markings on the skin corresponding to the object under which the child was allegedly found.

Despite the citing of petechial hemorrhages, fluidity of the blood, cyanosis, and congestion, edema, and engorgement of the right heart as so-called "classical" signs of asphyxia, these are not reliable and are found in a range of other situations. While survival for some time can lead to changes of hypoxic-ischemic encephalopathy with neuronal nuclear pyknosis and cytoplasmic eosinophilia,[93] no consistent histological, histochemical or biochemical markers for acute hypoxia have been found. This is perhaps not surprising given the variety of mechanisms that contribute to asphyxial deaths.

Petechiae

Petechial hemorrhages are pinpoint collections of blood found in certain circumstances in the skin, sclera, and conjunctivae, and under serous surfaces such as the pleura and pericardium. They vary in size from approximately 0.1 to 2 mm and are caused when an acute rise in venous pressure results in rupture of thin-walled peripheral venules. The reason for their preferential appearance in tissues such as the eyelid and serous membranes is thought to be due to the reduced amounts of perivascular supporting tissue. It has been estimated that it requires at least 15 to 30 seconds for petechiae to develop.[94]

One of the difficulties in the interpretation of petechiae in the very young is the paucity of studies in infancy and childhood,[95] and the fact that facial petechiae appear to occur less often in infants than in adults.[96] The distribution and number of petechiae in adults have also been influenced by the position and mass of bodies and the extent of dependent lividity.[94,97] Given the debate that has occurred regarding the potential significance and pathogenesis of petechiae, it is perhaps worthwhile briefly reviewing the literature, with

the caveat that studies have focused on adult populations and not on children or infants.

In a study of 5000 consecutive autopsy reports, petechial hemorrhages of the conjunctivae were recorded in 227 (4.5%) of cases.[98] Although this has the likelihood for under-reporting, it does show the lack of sensitivity and specificity of petechiae as markers of asphyxia (i.e., not all of the deaths attributed to asphyxia had conjunctival petechiae and they were also present in cases of natural death, mostly resulting from cardiovascular disease). The authors suggested that conjunctival petechiae were caused by several mechanisms including hypoxia and an acute rise in local vascular pressure caused by either acute right heart failure or mechanical vascular obstruction. They postulated that direct endothelial injury was required with or without an associated coagulopathy.[98]

The concept of capillary wall injury being necessary for the development of petechiae has been challenged, however, with suggestions that these small hemorrhages result purely from elevations in intravascular pressure unrelated to hypoxia.[99] Thus the likelihood of petechiae appearing is reduced by lowered arterial pressure and enhanced by elevated venous pressure. This is exemplified by the capillary fragility test in which petechiae are created in the skin when a tourniquet around the upper arm occludes venous but not arterial flow. The lack of petechiae in cases of smothering by plastic bags in which there has been no increase in intravascular pressures is also supportive of this concept.[100]

Infants and young children who have been crushed often demonstrate similar features as adults under the same circumstances with numerous confluent petechiae of the face, head, and upper body, with intense facial congestion.[77,78] Given that these individuals have suffered generalized hypoxia, the presence of petechiae in congested areas and the absence elsewhere further support raised intravascular pressures as being essential to their etiology. Of interest, the absence of petechiae under tight supportive clothing indicates that compression of vessels preventing an increase in intravascular pressures will inhibit petechiae despite hypoxic conditions.[101]

When petechial hemorrhages are caused by factors other than venous engorgement, such as circulating toxins in sepsis and coagulopathies in hematological disorders,[27,102] the distribution should be generalized and not geographic. Care must be taken in assessing the distribution of petechiae in infants with dark skin as they might only be visible in the conjunctivae. Thus a dark-skinned infant with petechiae resulting from meningococcal sepsis could only have visible hemorrhages in the eyes.

Oronasal Blood. Oronasal blood is an important finding in cases of acute life-threatening events (ALTEs) and sudden infant death. It is relatively common in cases of attempted, but unsuccessful, inflicted suffocation, being observed in 11 of 38 patients with an ALTE undergoing covert video surveillance but none of 46 controls.[103] On the other hand, it is rarely described by caretakers who have discovered an infant lifeless or by emergency medical technicians called upon to resuscitate them or by scene investigators from a medical examiner's office. As opposed to serous, mucus, and/or pink secretions, oronasal blood was described in 28 of 406 cases (7%) of unexpected infant deaths in the San Diego SIDS Research Project database.[104] In the same study, oronasal blood could not be attributed to resuscitation attempts among 14 of the 28 cases with oronasal blood present. Only 10 of 300 SIDS cases (3%), 2 of 14 accidental suffocation cases (14%), and 2 of 13 undetermined cases (15%) had oronasal blood reported. Oronasal blood in the absence of, or prior to, CPR was observed in only 1 of 300 SIDS cases (0.3%) found both supine and alone in a safe crib. Conversely, the lack of a safe sleep environment is reflected by the fact that 8 of 10 SIDS cases in which oronasal blood was present were bedsharing; 5 of these were with both parents, and in 2 cases, the infant was between the parents, suggesting the possibility of overlaying.

Whether in a living or dead infant, oronasal blood observed before CPR is probably of oronasal skin or mucous membrane origin and is a suspicious sign of accidental or inflicted suffocation. Therefore, use of an otoscope to establish the origin of oronasal blood is recommended in cases of sudden infant death.

Pulmonary Intraalveolar Siderophages

The presence of pulmonary intraalveolar siderophages has been proposed as a morphologic marker to aid in distinguishing SIDS from "soft" asphyxia.[105-111] Despite the absence of any or appropriate controls, some have suggested that SIDS is an inappropriate diagnosis when siderophages are present in large numbers.[105,109,112] We were unable to confirm this view after retrospective assessment of siderophages in iron-stained lung sections in 91 SIDS cases and 29 cases of death caused by asphyxia (27 accidents and 2 homicides) from the San Diego SIDS/SUDC Research Project (SDSSRP) database.[113] Given that the number of pulmonary siderophages varied widely in the SIDS and suffocation control cases, they cannot be used as an independent variable to ascertain past attempts at asphyxia.[113] Interstitial hemosiderin is also found in a significant number of otherwise unremarkable SIDS cases.[114]

Pulmonary Intra-Alveolar Hemorrhage. Similarly, the presence of pulmonary intra-alveolar hemorrhage has been suggested as a morphologic marker to possibly aid in distinguishing SIDS from "soft" suffocation.[106,107] Again, we were unable to confirm this proposal in our study that compared the severity of pulmonary hemorrhage in 34 SIDS cases that were found supine, alone, and in a safe sleep environment, with 40 cases of suffocation that was either accidental (37 cases) or inflicted asphyxia (3 cases).[115] Age and the duration of cardiopulmonary resuscitation and postmortem interval had no effect on the severity of pulmonary intraalveolar hemorrhage in SIDS.

Other Findings. Other features of asphyxia such as congestion and swelling of the face and lips may occur with crush asphyxia, hanging, and strangulation, but they are quite variable. Although low suspension hanging can lead to facial and conjunctival petechiae, full suspension with compression of the carotid arteries often results in a pallid face. Lifting of the tongue can result in protrusion of the tip of the tongue from the mouth with artefactual drying. Casper[116] quite elegantly summarized the situation: "How often do we read in purely theoretical authors of the violet, bluish-red, swollen countenance of those strangled! Nothing, however is so erroneous as to suppose that everyone hanged has such an appearance."

Pulmonary and cerebral edema can be present in asphyxial deaths, in part due to an increase in venous pressure, but are quite nonspecific and are found in deaths from many other causes. Similarly, congestion and edema of other tissues and organs are of no use in establishing or refuting the diagnosis. Engorgement of the right side of the heart with the left side of the heart being empty, and fluid blood are also completely unreliable.

The significance of large amounts of gastric contents within the airways is debatable and does not necessarily indicate asphyxial death from aspiration. Again, studies have concentrated on adult populations, but as many as 20% to 25% of individuals may aspirate food agonally, unrelated to the precise cause of death. Postmortem transport and movement of bodies have been shown to move gastric contents into the airways.[117]

The clinical significance of aspiration of gastric contents into the airways and lungs of previously well infants has had limited attention in cases of sudden infant death. In one study, it was not considered to be a significant factor in the deaths of previously well infants.[118] Not all previous studies, however, have addressed the potential role of attempts at cardiopulmonary resuscitation of infants that could artifactually force gastric contents into the distal lung. In a study of SIDS cases who had not undergone cardiopulmonary resuscitation, 10 of 69 cases (14%) of SIDS infants revealed microscopic evidence of gastric aspiration into the distal lung; this group was not otherwise clinically or pathologically different from cases of SIDS infants without aspiration.[119] Thus gastric aspiration can be a terminal event that some infants in a subset of SIDS cases cannot overcome.

DIFFERENTIATION FROM SIDS

Although the lack of pathognomonic pathologic features at autopsy sometimes makes the diagnosis of asphyxia difficult in adults, it is even more difficult in infants.[120] Infants' small size and lack of strength means that they can be asphyxiated either deliberately or accidentally without significant struggling, thus leaving no bruises or abrasions to assist in determining the circumstances surrounding the lethal episode. Pressure on the nose and mouth can also be sufficient to occlude the airways without leaving any markings on the skin. Guidelines for scene and autopsy features that assist in making the diagnosis of asphyxia have been recently published;[63] both asphyxial deaths in the young and SIDS, however, can have identical autopsy findings.[121]

Although scene examination is essential in all cases of unexpected infant death, the scene usually has been altered by parents or care givers in their attempts to revive the infants. The scene can be further altered by ambulance officers who transported the moribund or dead child to the hospital. If resuscitation is attempted and the oropharynx is suctioned, foreign material responsible for choking can be removed, resulting in an essentially negative autopsy. Important items such as cords or bedding that assist in differentiating an asphyxial death from one caused by SIDS also might have been removed, and parents often clean the room where the infant died.

Pressure blanching can be found on the body that corresponds to objects such as crib sides that have pressed against the head of a potentially wedged infant. Therefore it is important for the pathologist to examine the crib and sleeping arrangement if asphyxia is suspected. Unusual markings should not be present in SIDS deaths. Similarly, parchmented ligature marks around the neck should suggest a diagnosis of hanging or ligature strangulation. A doll can be used to demonstrate the position in which the infant was found.

Facial and conjunctival petechiae are not found in SIDS infants, and are also found less often in infants who have asphyxiated than in older individuals,[96,122,123] although it has been suggested that the combination of conjunctival petechiae and acute pulmonary emphysema indicates asphyxia in the young.[124] If florid petechiae are found in the skin of the face and drainage area of the superior vena cava, the possibility of chest and/or neck compression should be strongly considered.[125,126] Profuse petechial hemorrhaging of the face has been termed *masque ecchymotique* and precludes a diagnosis of SIDS.[63,126] Neck dissections should always be performed in cases of unexpected infant deaths; bruises, however, are not always found in cases of hanging or strangulation, and the pliability of the laryngeal cartilages and hyoid bone makes fractures rare.

A good example of the lack of findings at autopsy in infants who are known to have died of asphyxia was a 1-month-old girl who was found in cardiac arrest beneath her unconscious mother in a public washroom. Her mother had succumbed to an overdose of self-administered opiates and had fallen on the child.[89] Despite resuscitation, the girl died a day later in hospital of hypoxic-ischemic encephalopathy. The infant had been carefully examined in hospital and at autopsy by attending pediatricians and the pathologist specifically for evidence of asphyxia but showed no abnormal skin markings, external petechiae, or other findings of note. In fact, the autopsy findings were identical to those normally found in SIDS. Thus, in a case of undisputed death caused by a combination of suffocation and crush asphyxia, determination of the events initiating lethal hypoxic-ischemic encephalopathy relied entirely on scene information. This case clearly illustrates that physical findings in suffocation and SIDS can be indistinguishable.[120,127] and that determining whether an infant has been accidentally or deliberately suffocated, or has died of SIDS, is not always possible at autopsy. It is now recognized that there are a number of cases in which multiple deaths of infants in the same family that were incorrectly attributed to SIDS were due to inflicted asphyxia.[128-132]

CONCLUSION

Because SIDS is by definition a diagnosis of exclusion, significant problems arise in trying to differentiate it from asphyxia in infancy when there are no specific autopsy findings. Determining whether asphyxia or SIDS has occurred, therefore, requires careful evaluation of all aspects of the history, scene, and autopsy, as well as the exclusion of other possibilities. For these reasons the diagnosis of both asphyxiation and SIDS in infancy must be approached with circumspection and with consideration of a range of possibilities, some of which may remain unclear even after extensive investigation. Unfortunately, even after full investigations have been performed according to standard protocols, a definitive diagnosis is not always possible and a number of issues concerning possible lethal terminal mechanisms remain unresolved.

References

1. Byard RW: *Sudden Death in Infancy, Childhood and Adolescence*, ed 2. Cambridge University Press, Cambridge, 2004.
2. Willinger M, James LS, Catz C: Defining the sudden infant death syndrome (SIDS): deliberations of an expert panel convened by the National Institute of Child Health and Human Development. *Pediatr Pathol* 1991;11:677-684.
3. Krous HF, Beckwith JB, Byard RW, et al: Sudden infant death syndrome and unclassified sudden infant deaths: a definitional and diagnostic approach. *Pediatrics* 2004;114:234-238.
4. Byard RW: Unexpected infant death: lessons from the Sally Clark case. *Med J Aust* 2004;181:52-54.
5. Mathews TJ, MacDorman MF: Infant mortality statistics from the 2004 period linked birth/infant death data set. *Natl Vital Stat Rep* 2007;55:1-32.
6. Weber M, Klein N, Hartley J, et al: Infection and sudden unexpected death in infancy: a systematic retrospective case review. *Lancet* 2008;371:1848-1853.
7. Malloy MH: Trends in postneonatal aspiration deaths and reclassification of sudden infant death syndrome: impact of the "Back to Sleep" program. *Pediatrics* 2002;109:661-665.
8. Tursan d'Espaignet E, Bulsara M, Wolfenden L, et al: Trends in sudden infant death syndrome in Australia from 1980-2002. *Forensic Sci Med Pathol* 2008;4:83-90.
9. Mitchell EA, Milerad J: Smoking and the sudden infant death syndrome. *Rev Environ Health* 2006;21:81-103.
10. Shah T, Sullivan K, Carter J: Sudden infant death syndrome and reported maternal smoking during pregnancy. *Am J Public Health* 2006;96:1757-1759.
11. Fleming P, Blair PS: Sudden Infant Death Syndrome and parental smoking. *Early Hum Dev* 2007;83:721-725.
12. Moon RY, Horne RS, Hauck FR: Sudden infant death syndrome. *Lancet* 2007;370:1578-1587.
13. Blair PS, Fleming PJ, Bensley D, et al: Smoking and the sudden infant death syndrome: results from 1993-5 case-control study for confidential inquiry into stillbirths and deaths in infancy. Confidential Enquiry into Stillbirths and Deaths Regional Coordinators and Researchers. *Br Med J* 1996;313:195-198.
14. Mitchell EA, Ford RP, Taylor BJ, et al: Further evidence supporting a causal relationship between prone sleeping position and SIDS. *J Paediatr Child Health* 1992;28 (Suppl 1):S9-S12.
15. Mitchell EA, Tuohy PG, Brunt JM, et al: Risk factors for sudden infant death syndrome following the prevention campaign in New Zealand: a prospective study. *Pediatrics* 1997;100:835-840.
16. Taylor JA, Krieger JW, Reay DT, et al: Prone sleep position and the sudden infant death syndrome in King County, Washington: a case-control study. *J Pediatr* 1996;128:626-630.
17. Mitchell EA, Thach BT, Thompson JM, et al: Changing infants' sleep position increases risk of sudden infant death syndrome. New Zealand Cot Death Study. *Arch Pediatr Adolesc Med* 1999;153:1136-1141.
18. Hauck FR, Herman SM, Donovan M, et al: Sleep environment and the risk of sudden infant death syndrome in an urban population: the Chicago Infant Mortality Study. *Pediatrics* 2003;111:1207-1214.
19. Krous HF, Nadeau JM, Silva PD, et al: Intrathoracic petechiae in sudden infant death syndrome: relationship to face position when found. *Pediatr Dev Pathol* 2001;4:160-166.
20. Blair PS, Mitchell EA, Heckstall-Smith EM, et al: Head covering—a major modifiable risk factor for sudden infant death syndrome: a systematic review. *Arch Dis Child* 2008;93:778-783.
21. Mitchell EA, Thompson JM, Becroft DM, et al: Head covering and the risk for SIDS: findings from the New Zealand and German SIDS case-control studies. *Pediatrics* 2008;121:e1478-e1483.
22. Mitchell EA: Recommendations for sudden infant death syndrome prevention: a discussion document. *Arch Dis Child* 2007;92:155-159.
23. Horsley T, Clifford T, Barrowman N, et al: Benefits and harms associated with the practice of bed sharing: a systematic review. *Arch Pediatr Adolesc Med* 2007;161:237-245.
24. Carpenter RG: The hazards of bed sharing. *Paediatr Child Health* 2006;11(Suppl A):24A-28A.

25. Ruys JH, de Jonge GA, Brand R, et al: Bed-sharing in the first four months of life: a risk factor for sudden infant death. *Acta Paediatr* 2007;96:1399-1403.

26. Krous HF: The microscopic distribution of intrathoracic petechiae in sudden infant death syndrome. *Arch Pathol Lab Med* 1984;108:77-79.

27. Krous HF, Jordan J: A necropsy study of distribution of petechiae in non-sudden infant death syndrome. *Arch Pathol Lab Med* 1984;108:75-76.

28. Poets CF, Meny RG, Chobanian MR, et al: Gasping and other cardiorespiratory patterns during sudden infant deaths. *Pediatr Res* 1999;45:350-354.

29. Beckwith JB: The sudden infant death syndrome. *Curr Probl Pediatr* 1973;3:1-36.

30. Krous HF: The pathology of sudden infant death syndrome: an overview. *In:* Culbertson JL, Krous HF, Bendell RD (eds): *Sudden Infant Death Syndrome. Medical Aspects and Psychological Management.* The John Hopkins University Press, Baltimore, 1988, pp 18-47.

31. Krous HF, Nadeau JM, Silva PD, et al: A comparison of respiratory symptoms and inflammation in sudden infant death syndrome and in accidental or inflicted infant death. *Am J Forensic Med Pathol* 2003;24:1-8.

32. Filiano JJ, Kinney HC: Arcuate nucleus hypoplasia in the sudden infant death syndrome. *J Neuropathol Exp Neurol* 1992;51:394-403.

33. Matturri L, Biondo B, Suarez-Mier MP, et al: Brain stem lesions in the sudden infant death syndrome: variability in the hypoplasia of the arcuate nucleus. *Acta Neuropathol (Berl)* 2002;104:12-20.

34. Kinney HC, Filiano JJ, Sleeper LA, et al: Decreased muscarinic receptor binding in the arcuate nucleus in sudden infant death syndrome. *Science* 1995;269:1446-1450.

35. Panigrahy A, Filiano JJ, Sleeper LA, et al: Decreased kainate receptor binding in the arcuate nucleus of the sudden infant death syndrome. *J Neuropathol Exp Neurol* 1997;56:1253-1261.

36. Kinney HC, Filiano JJ, White WF: Medullary serotonergic network deficiency in the sudden infant death syndrome: review of a 15-year study of a single dataset. *J Neuropathol Exp Neurol* 2001;60:228-247.

37. Kinney HC, Randall LL, Sleeper LA, et al: Serotonergic brainstem abnormalities in Northern Plains Indians with the sudden infant death syndrome. *J Neuropathol Exp Neurol* 2003;62:1178-1191.

38. Paterson DS, Trachtenberg FL, Thompson EG, et al: Multiple serotonergic brainstem abnormalities in sudden infant death syndrome. *JAMA* 2006;296:2124-2132.

39. Guntheroth WG, Spiers PS: The triple risk hypotheses in sudden infant death syndrome. *Pediatrics* 2002;110:e64.

40. Filiano JJ, Kinney HC: A perspective on neuropathologic findings in victims of the sudden infant death syndrome: the triple-risk model. *Biol Neonate* 1994;65:194-197.

41. Matturri L, Ottaviani G, Lavezzi AM: Guidelines for neuropathologic diagnostics of perinatal unexpected loss and sudden infant death syndrome (SIDS): a technical protocol. *Virchows Arch* 2008;452:19-25.

42. Krous HF, Byard RW: International standardized autopsy protocol for sudden unexpected infant death. Appendix I. *In:* Byard RW, Krous HF (eds): *Sudden Infant Death Syndrome: Problems, Progress and Possibilities.* Arnold, London, 2001, pp 319-333.

43. Iyasu S, Rowley D, Hanzlick R: Guidelines for death scene investigation of sudden, unexplained infant deaths: Recommendations of the Interagency Panel on Sudden Infant Death Syndrome. *MMWR Morb Mortal Wkly Rep* 1996;45:1-6. Available at http://www.cdc.gov/mmwr/preview/mmwrhtml/00042657.htm. Accessed May 6, 2009.

44. Tester DJ, Ackerman MJ: Sudden infant death syndrome: how significant are the cardiac channelopathies? *Cardiovasc Res* 2005;67:388-396.

45. Ackerman MJ, Siu BL, Sturner WQ, et al: Postmortem molecular analysis of SCN5A defects in sudden infant death syndrome. *JAMA* 2001;286:2264-2269.

46. Ackerman MJ, Anson BD, Tester DJ, et al: Molecular autopsy of HERG defects in sudden infant death syndrome. *J Am Coll Cardiol* 2002;39:111A-112A.

47. Schwartz PJ, Priori SG, Bloise R, et al: Molecular diagnosis in a child with sudden infant death syndrome. *Lancet* 2001;358:1342-1343.

48. Wedekind H, Smits JP, Schulze-Bahr E, et al: De novo mutation in the SCN5A gene associated with early onset of sudden infant death. *Circulation* 2001;104:1158-1164.

49. Schwartz PJ, Stramba-Badiale M, Segantini A, et al: Prolongation of the QT interval and the sudden infant death syndrome. *N Engl J Med* 1998;338:1709-1714.

50. Moric E, Herbert E, Trusz-Gluza M, et al: The implications of genetic mutations in the sodium channel gene (SCN5A). *Europace* 2003;5:325-334.

51. Bonham JR, Downing M: Metabolic deficiencies and SIDS. *J Clin Pathol* 1992;45:33-38.

52. Boles RG, Buck EA, Blitzer MG, et al: Retrospective biochemical screening of fatty acid oxidation disorders in postmortem livers of 418 cases of sudden death in the first year of life. *J Pediatr* 1998;132:924-933.

53. Rinaldo P, Matern D: Disorders of fatty acid transport and mitochondrial oxidation: challenges and dilemmas of metabolic evaluation. *Genet Med* 2000;2:338-344.

54. Bennett MJ, Rinaldo P: The metabolic autopsy comes of age. *Clin Chem* 2001;47:1145-1146.

55. Valdes-Dapena M, Gilbert-Barness E: Cardiovascular causes for sudden infant death. *Pediatr Pathol Mol Med* 2002;21:195-211.

56. Dettmeyer RB, Padosch SA, Madea B: Lethal enterovirus-induced myocarditis and pancreatitis in a 4-month-old boy. *Forensic Sci Int* 2006;156:51-54.

57. Krous HF, Chadwick AE, Isaacs H Jr: Tumors associated with sudden infant and childhood death. *Pediatr Dev Pathol* 2005;8:20-25.

58. Byard RW, Cains G: Lethal asphyxia—pathology and problems. *Minerva Med* 2007;127:273-282.

59. Mann JD: *Forensic Medicine and Toxicology,* ed 3. Charles Griffin & Co., London, 1902.

60. Reese JJ: *Text-book of Medical Jurisprudence and Toxicology,* ed 7. P. Blakiston's Son & Co, Philadelphia, 1906.

61. Giffen GH: *Students' Manual of Medical Jurisprudence and Public Health,* ed 2. William Bryce. Edinburgh, 1906.

62. Taylor AS: *The Principles and Practice of Medical Jurisprudence.* John Churchill & Sons, London, 1865.

63. Byard RW, Jensen LL: Fatal asphyxial episodes in the very young: classification and diagnostic issues. *Forensic Sci Med Pathol* 2007;3:177-181.

64. Byard RW, Wilson GW: Death scene gas analysis in suspected methane asphyxia. *Am J Forensic Med Pathol* 1992;133:69-71.

65. Byard RW, Cains G, Simpson E, et al: Drowning, haemodilution, haemolysis and staining of the intima of the aortic root—preliminary observations. *J Clin Forensic Med* 2006;13:121-124.

66. DiMaio VJ, DiMaio D: *Forensic Pathology,* ed 2. CRC Press, Boca Raton, 2001.

67. Byard RW, Simpson E, Gilbert JD: Temporal trends over the past two decades in asphyxial deaths in South Australia involving plastic bags or wrapping. *J Clin Forensic Med* 2006;13:9-14.

68. Byard RW, Beal SM: V-shaped pillows and unsafe infant sleeping. *J Paediatr Child Health* 1997;33:171-173.

69. Byard RW: Inflatable beds and accidental asphyxia in infants. *Scand J Forensic Sci* 2006;12:22-24.

70. Byard RW, Bourne AJ, Beal SM: Mesh-sided cots—yet another potentially dangerous infant sleeping environment. *Forensic Sci Int* 1996;83:105-109.

71. Amanuel B, Byard RW: Accidental asphyxia in bed in severely disabled children. *J Paediatr Child Health* 2000;36:66-68.

72. Brogan T, Fligner CL, McLaughlin JF, et al: Positional asphyxia in individuals with severe cerebral palsy. *Dev Med Child Neurol* 1992;34:169-173.

73. Byard RW: Is breast feeding in bed always a safe practice? *J Paediatr Child Health* 1998;34:418-419.

74. Krous HF, Chadwick AE, Stanley C: Delayed infant death following catastrophic deterioration during breast-feeding. *J Paediatr Child Health* 2005;41:215-217.

75. Byard RW: Mechanisms of unexpected death in infants and young children following foreign body ingestion. *J Forensic Sci* 1996;41:438-441.

76. Wick R, Gilbert JD, Byard RW: Cafe coronary syndrome-fatal choking on food: an autopsy approach. *J Clin Forensic Med* 2008;13:135-138.

77. Byard RW: Unexpected death due to acute airway obstruction in daycare centers. *Pediatrics* 1994;94:113-114.

78. Byard RW, Hanson KA, James RA: Fatal unintentional traumatic asphyxia in childhood. *J Paediatr Child Health* 2003;39:31-32.

79. Byard RW, Knight D, James RA, et al: Murder-suicides involving children: a 29-year study. *Am J Forensic Med Pathol* 1999;20:323-327.

80. Byard RW, Tsokos M: Infant and early childhood asphyxial deaths—diagnostic issues. *In:* Tsokos M (ed): *Forensic Pathology Reviews,* Vol 2. Humana Press, Totowa, NJ, 2005, pp 101-123.

81. Collins KA: Death by overlaying and wedging: a 15-year retrospective study. *Am J Forensic Med Pathol* 2001;22:155-159.

82. Green H, James RA, Gilbert JD, et al: Fractures of the hyoid bone and laryngeal cartilages in suicidal hanging. *J Clin Forensic Med* 2000;7:123-126.

83. Byard RW, Beal S, Bourne AJ: Potentially dangerous sleeping environments and accidental asphyxia in infancy and early childhood. *Arch Dis Child* 1994;71:497-500.

84. Byard RW: Hazardous infant and early childhood sleeping environments and death scene examination. *J Clin Forensic Med* 1996;3:115-122.

85. Jensen L, Charlwood C, Byard RW: Shopping cart injuries, entrapment and childhood fatality. *J Forensic Sci* 2008;53:1178-1180.

86. Byard RW, Beal S, Blackbourne B, et al: Specific dangers associated with infants sleeping on sofas. *J Paediatr Child Health* 2001;37:476-478.

87. Milkovich SM, Owens J, Stool D, et al: Accidental childhood strangulation by human hair. *Int J Pediatr Otorhinolaryngol* 2005;69:1621-1628.

88. Byard RW, Hilton J: Overlaying, accidental suffocation and sudden infant death. *J SIDS Infant Mort* 1997;2:161-165.

89. Mitchell E, Krous HF, Byard RW: Pathological findings in overlaying. *J Clin Forensic Med* 2002;9:133-135.

90. Byard RW, Burnell RH: Apparent life threatening events and infant holding practices. *Arch Dis Child* 1995;73:502-504.

91. Byard RW, Houldsworth G, James RA, et al: Characteristic features of suicidal drownings: a 20-year study. *Am J Forensic Med Pathol* 2001;22:134-138.

92. Byard RW, Krous HF (eds): *Sudden Infant Death Syndrome. Problems, Progress & Possibilities.* Arnold, London, 2001.

93. Byard R, Blumbergs P, Rutty G, et al: Lack of evidence for a causal relationship between hypoxic-ischemic encephalopathy and subdural hemorrhage in fetal life, infancy and early childhood. *Pediatr Dev Pathol* 2007;10:500-501.

94. Saukko P, Knight B: *Knight's Forensic Pathology*, ed 3. Arnold, London, 2004, pp 352-367.

95. Byard RW, Krous HF: Petechial hemorrhages and unexpected infant death. *Leg Med (Tokyo)* 1999;1:193-197.

96. Moore L, Byard RW: Pathological findings in hanging and wedging deaths in infants and young children. *Am J Forensic Med Pathol* 1993;14:296-302.

97. Bockholdt B, Maxeiner H, Hegenbarth W: Factors and circumstances influencing the development of hemorrhages in livor mortis. *Forensic Sci Int* 2005;149:133-137.

98. Rao N, Smith RE, Choi JH, et al: Autopsy findings in the eyes of fourteen fatally abused children. *Forensic Sci Int* 1988;39:293-299.

99. Ely SF, Hirsch CS: Asphyxial deaths and petechiae: a review. *J Forensic Sci* 2000;45:1274-1277.

100. Haddix TL, Harruff RC, Reay DT, et al: Asphyxial suicides using plastic bags. *Am J Forensic Med Pathol* 1996;17:308-311.

101. Byard RW: The brassiere "sign"—a distinctive marker in crush asphyxia. *J Clin Forensic Med* 2005;12:316-319.

102. Byard RW, Krous HF: Petechial hemorrhage and unexpected infant deaths. *Legal Med* 1999;1:193-197.

103. Southall DP, Plunkett MC, Banks MW, et al: Covert video recordings of life-threatening child abuse: lessons for child protection. *Pediatrics* 1997;100:735-760.

104. Krous HF, Nadeau JM, Byard RW, et al: Oronasal blood in sudden infant death. *Am J Forensic Med Pathol* 2001;22:346-351.

105. Becroft DM, Lockett BK: Intra-alveolar pulmonary siderophages in sudden infant death: a marker for previous imposed suffocation. *Pathology* 1997;29:60-63.

106. Potter S, Berry PJ, Fleming P: Pulmonary haemorrhage in sudden unexpected death in infancy. *Pediatr Dev Pathol* 1999;2:394-395.

107. Yukawa N, Carter N, Rutty G, et al: Intra-alveolar haemorrhage in sudden infant death syndrome: a cause for concern? *J Clin Pathol* 1999;52:581-587.

108. Becroft DM, Thompson JM, Mitchell EA: Nasal and intrapulmonary haemorrhage in sudden infant death syndrome. *Arch Dis Child* 2001;85:116-120.

109. Hanzlick R, Delaney K: Pulmonary hemosiderin in deceased infants: baseline data for further study of infant mortality. *Am J Forensic Med Pathol* 2000;21:319-322.

110. Hanzlick R: Pulmonary hemorrhage in deceased infants: baseline data for further study of infant mortality. *Am J Forensic Med Pathol* 2001;22:188-192.

111. Schluckebier DA, Cool CD, Henry TE, et al: Pulmonary siderophages and unexpected infant death. *Am J Forensic Med Pathol* 2002;23:360-363.

112. Jackson CM, Gilliland MG: Frequency of pulmonary hemosiderosis in Eastern North Carolina. *Am J Forensic Med Pathol* 2000;21:36-38.

113. Krous HF, Wixom C, Chadwick AE, et al: Pulmonary intra-alveolar siderophages in SIDS and suffocation: a San Diego SIDS/SUDC Research Project report. *Pediatr Dev Pathol* 2006;9:103-114.

114. Byard RW, Stewart WA, Telfer S, et al: Assessment of pulmonary and intrathymic hemosiderin deposition in sudden infant death syndrome. *Pediatr Pathol Lab Med* 1997;17:275-282.

115. Krous HF, Haas EA, Masoumi H, et al: A comparison of pulmonary intra-alveolar hemorrhage in cases of sudden infant death due to SIDS in a safe sleep environment or to suffocation. *Forensic Sci Int* 2007;172:56-62.

116. Casper JL: A Handbook of the Practice of Forensic Medicine Based Upon Personal Experience. Vol II. The New Sydenham Society, London, 1862.

117. Knight BH. The significance of the postmortem discovery of gastric contents in the air passages. *Forensic Sci* 1975;6:229-234.

118. Byard RW, Beal SM: Gastric aspiration and sleeping position in infancy and early childhood. *J Paediatr Child Health* 2000;36:403-405.

119. Krous HF, Masoumi H, Haas EA, et al: Aspiration of gastric contents in sudden infant death syndrome without cardiopulmonary resuscitation. *J Pediatr* 2007;150:241-246.

120. Banaschak S, Schmidt P, Madea B: Smothering of children older than 1 year of age-diagnostic significance of morphological findings. *Forensic Sci Int* 2003;134:163-168.

121. Byard RW: Inaccurate classification of infant deaths in Australia: a persistent and pervasive problem. *Med J Aust* 2001;175:5-7.

122. Byard RW: Possible mechanisms responsible for the sudden infant death syndrome. *J Paediatr Child Health* 1991;27:147-157.

123. Matsumura F, Ito Y: Petechial hemorrhage of the conjunctiva and histological findings of the lung and pancreas in infantile asphyxia—evaluation of 85 cases. *Kurume Med J* 1996;43:259-266.

124. Betz P, Hausmann R, Eisenmenger W: A contribution to a possible differentiation between SIDS and asphyxiation. *Forensic Sci Int* 1998;91:147-152.

125. Oehmichen M, Gerling I, Meissner C: Petechiae of the baby's skin as differentiation symptom of infanticide versus SIDS. *J Forensic Sci* 2000;45:602-607.

126. Perrot LJ: Masque ecchymotique. Specific or nonspecific indicator for abuse. *Am J Forensic Med Pathol* 1989;10:95-97.

127. Kleemann WJ, Wiechern V, Schuck M, et al: Intrathoracic and subconjunctival petechiae in sudden infant death syndrome (SIDS). *Forensic Sci Int* 1995;72:49-54.

128. Meadow R: Munchausen syndrome by proxy. The hinterland of child abuse. *Lancet* 1977;2:343-345.

129. Meadow R: Munchausen syndrome by proxy. *Arch Dis Child* 1982;57:92-98.

130. Byard RW, Beal SM: Munchausen syndrome by proxy: repetitive infantile apnoea and homicide. *J Paediatr Child Health* 1993;29:77-79.

131. Byard RW, Burnell RH: Covert surveillance in Munchausen syndrome by proxy. Ethical compromise or essential technique? *Med J Aust* 1994;160:352-356.

132. Byard RW, Sawaguchi T: Sudden infant death syndrome or murder? *Scand J Forensic Sci* 2008;14:14-16.

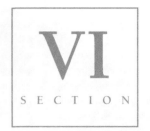

ABUSIVE HEAD TRAUMA

Deborah E. Lowen, MD

39

ABUSIVE HEAD TRAUMA

Kent P. Hymel, MD, and Katherine P. Deye, MD

Abusive pediatric head trauma begins with intense frustration and anger. In its aftermath, lives, relationships, families, and futures can be changed forever. Violent acts that result in traumatic brain injuries lead irrevocably to powerful, stressful experiences for involved family members and for many of the professionals who respond to treat, support, consult, investigate, protect, testify, prosecute, defend, and/or judge.

INCIDENCE AND EPIDEMIOLOGY

The incidence of inflicted head trauma during the first 1 or 2 years of life has been estimated in various studies to range from 16.1 to 33.8 cases per 100,000 infants per year.[1-5] A preponderance of evidence supports a conclusion that male infants are at greater risk.[1,5-7] Infants living in families experiencing socioeconomic or other acute stress are also at increased risk.[4,8] Race and ethnicity have not been found to be a significant predictor of inflicted pediatric neurotrauma.[9] Abusive head trauma appears to be the leading cause of infant homicide in the United States.[10]

HISTORICAL CONTEXT

The number and quality of published, peer-reviewed research studies regarding abusive head trauma have increased dramatically in recent years. Interpreting this expanding body of work is an ongoing challenge that requires an understanding of the historical context. Some individuals have played prominent roles by raising public awareness about abusive head trauma, by questioning widely held assumptions, or by redirecting our clinical or research priorities.

In 1946, Dr. John Caffey[11] published a landmark paper titled, "Multiple fractures in the long bones of infants suffering from chronic subdural hematoma." In this paper, he described six children with subdural hematomas and multiple fractures. Caffey was the first to suggest that trauma explained this combination of findings. He advised physicians to look for fractures in children with subdural hematomas, and vice versa.

On November 14, 1956, Virginia Jaspars was sentenced to 10 to 22 years in prison. Investigations revealed evidence supporting a conclusion that, between 1948 and 1956, Ms. Jaspars killed or injured at least 15 infants left in her care. New Haven, Connecticut physicians Drs. Paul Goldstein, Steve Downing, Michael Kashgarian, and (most importantly) Robert Salinger uncovered vital clues that ultimately revealed the nature of Ms. Jaspars' abusive actions. When Ms. Jaspars confessed to the death of Jennifer Malkan, she reported that she was irritated by the child's persistent crying and therefore, "... shook the child to cause her head to bob back and forth." She added, "The baby lost her breath and her eyes were funny in her head."[12]

In 1971, Dr. Norman Guthkelch, the first pediatric neurosurgeon in Great Britain, published an article in the *British Medical Journal* titled "Infantile subdural haematoma and its relationship to whiplash injuries."[13] He described multiple infants with subdural hematomas whose caregivers described violently shaking the children. Dr. Guthkelch's manuscript represents the first clear reference to shaking as a mechanism for intracranial injuries in infants and young children.

In 1987, pediatric neurosurgeon Dr. Ann-Christine Duhaime and colleagues published a landmark paper in the *Journal of Neurosurgery*.[14] Their retrospective analysis of 48 cases of shaken baby syndrome led Duhaime and her colleagues to conduct a series of biomechanical experiments. They concluded, "... severe head injuries commonly diagnosed as shaking injuries require impact to occur," and, "... shaking alone in an otherwise normal baby is unlikely to cause the shaken baby syndrome."

Recently, some professionals have opined that the shaken baby syndrome is an unproven myth. Widely held theories of shaking-whiplash injury are now directly challenged.[15,16] On the other hand, a considerable body of literature supports a conclusion that isolated shaking can injure or kill babies.[13,17-20] The debate continues—in the medical literature, in the lay press, and in courtrooms. Chapter 41, "The Case for Shaking," provides a more detailed overview of this topic.

NOMENCLATURE

In response to this ongoing debate, clinicians and researchers have assigned a variety of labels to the constellation of clinical signs and cranial injuries that they have interpreted to be the result of abusive actions. These labels have included shaken baby syndrome, whiplash-shaken infant syndrome, shaking-impact injury, shaking-slam injury, abusive head trauma, inflicted head trauma, inflicted pediatric neurotrauma, and inflicted traumatic brain injury. In recent years, more and more clinicians and researchers are choosing to use more inclusive and less specific labels (e.g., "abusive head trauma" or "inflicted head trauma") when referring to these cases, avoiding labels that imply unrealistic certainty regarding the specific injury mechanisms (e.g., "shaken baby syndrome"). In 2009, the American Academy of Pediatrics Committee on Child Abuse and Neglect recommended use of the phrase "abusive head trauma" when describing an inflicted injury to the head and its contents.[21]

RESPONSIBILITIES OF THE CHILD ABUSE MEDICAL SPECIALIST

Child abuse medical specialists who play a role in these real-life dramas are expected to do all of the following competently and consistently:

- To recognize cases of abusive head trauma masquerading as accidental trauma
- To recognize cases of accidental head trauma misinterpreted as abusive
- To direct an appropriately thorough child abuse diagnostic evaluation
- To assemble and integrate the relevant historical, clinical, laboratory and radiological information
- To actively consider, confirm, and/or exclude *nontraumatic* etiologies for the child's clinical presentation, physical examination findings, and radiological findings
- To formulate objective, forensic impressions of reasonable medical certainty regarding the nature, extent, severity, mechanisms, and timing of the child's traumatic injuries, and
- To communicate those impressions clearly, consistently, and without bias—to family members, to other health care providers, to child protection case workers, to police investigators, and later, to attorneys, judges, and/or juries.

In this chapter, we summarize an approach to accomplish these tasks reliably.

THE CLINICAL SPECTRUM

A majority of infant victims of inflicted head trauma present with recent, sudden onset of clear and persistent clinical signs, attributed to an accidental cranial impact (e.g., a fall). A few will present initially for medical treatment with acute and severe *but delayed* clinical deterioration following an earlier, unrecognized, or unreported head injury event. Only rare cases of inflicted pediatric neurotrauma will present with a thorough caregiver accounting of his or her abusive acts that preceded the victim's acute clinical deterioration.

Abusive acts can involve isolated contact injury mechanism(s), isolated inertial injury mechanism(s), or combined contact and inertial injury mechanisms. The resulting primary and secondary traumatic cranial injuries can be closed or penetrating, superficial or deep, and focal or diffuse. The associated clinical manifestations can be mild, moderate, life-threatening or fatal; acute, delayed, or late; and recognized or missed. The caregiver's specific explanation for the child's traumatic cranial injuries and clinical presentation can be complete, incomplete, or absent; consistent or inconsistent (with repetition over time); adequate or inadequate (to explain the child's clinical, laboratory, and/or radiological findings); and truthful, partially truthful, or fabricated.

In recognition of this extraordinary clinical variability and the potential for historical inconsistencies, researchers have used a wide variety of definitional criteria to categorize and to compare cases of accidental versus inflicted pediatric head trauma. In hindsight, it appears that some of the earliest definitional criteria used by researchers to categorize cases as accidental or inflicted were fundamentally flawed with inherent biases or by circular reasoning. Despite these limitations, our child maltreatment medical literature provides overwhelming evidence that adults' abusive actions can cause devastating or fatal traumatic brain injuries in infants and young children.[22-31]

Abusive acts have been linked to subdural, subarachnoid, and retinal hemorrhages;[7,22,32-35] localized axonal injury in the region of the craniocervical junction; acute respiratory compromise or arrest; loss of consciousness; hypotension;[36-40] and secondary, diffuse, hypoxic-ischemic brain injury with swelling.[23,39,41-42] Young victims of inflicted head trauma frequently present with associated cutaneous injuries[32,43] and fractures of the skull,[22,44,45] ribs, or extremities.[11,46] At the time of initial neuroimaging, many young victims of abusive head trauma reveal radiological evidence of prior (and therefore repetitive) traumatic, intracranial injuries.[24]

Acute clinical signs (appearing within seconds, minutes, or hours) can include craniofacial soft tissue injuries, inconsolability, loss of appetite, vomiting, altered sleep patterns, seizures, alteration or loss of consciousness, and cardiorespiratory compromise and/or arrest. *Delayed* clinical signs (appearing later, but within hours, days, or weeks) can include inconsolability, recurrent vomiting, loss of appetite, altered sleep patterns, seizures, alteration or loss of consciousness, and cardiorespiratory compromise or arrest. *Late* clinical signs (appearing weeks, months, or years after injury) can include feeding difficulties, sensory deficits, motor impairments, macrocephaly, microcephaly, behavioral dysfunctions, developmental delays, intellectual deficits, attention deficits, and educational dysfunctions. For a more complete discussion of outcomes, see Chapter 48, "Outcome of Abusive Head Trauma."

MISSED CASES

Considered in isolation, each of these clinical manifestations of traumatic brain injury is nonspecific. Each can result from inflicted head trauma, from noninflicted head trauma, or from other nontraumatic etiologies. Young victims of abusive head trauma who present for medical evaluation and treatment with isolated, less severe, nonspecific clinical signs (e.g., irritability, lethargy, recurrent vomiting, loss of appetite, and/or altered sleep patterns) are frequently misdiagnosed. In their 1999 analysis, Jenny and colleagues[47] reported that physicians recognized less than one in five cases of inflicted pediatric head trauma if the victim presented with normal respirations, no seizures, and no facial or scalp soft tissue injuries, and if the victim came from a Caucasian family with two adult caregivers.

A high index of suspicion is warranted. Without a high index of suspicion, cases will be missed, victims will be returned to their abusive environment, and children will be reinjured. In their 1999 study, Jenny and colleagues[47] reported that 27.8% of victims of inflicted head trauma were reinjured after a missed diagnosis.

REPORTING SUSPECTED ABUSE

Medical providers are not trained or mandated to investigate a crime scene or to assess psychosocial risk of child abuse or neglect. We *are* mandated by law in all 50 states to report any *suspicion* of abuse. Defining precisely what constitutes a reasonable suspicion of abusive head trauma is difficult, if not impossible. Yet, experienced clinicians have come to recognize numerous specific examples of clinical presentations (involving an infant or young child) that create a reasonable suspicion of abusive head trauma and prompt a report of suspected abuse to child protective services. These examples include the following:

- Unexplained loss of consciousness, lethargy, hypotonia, seizures, coma, respiratory distress, apnea, persistent irritability, recurrent vomiting, and/or poor feeding when infectious, metabolic, or toxic causes have been excluded
- Clear and persistent clinical signs that prompt diagnostic evaluation revealing evidence of traumatic brain injury, nonfocal subdural or subarachnoid hemorrhage and/or extensive, dense, multilayered retinal hemorrhages—unexplained by traumatic childbirth, a motor vehicle accident, a complex accidental fall (e.g., down stairs in an infant walker or in the arms of a falling adult), a fall from an elevated height (usually greater than 6 feet) or other equivalent accidental trauma
- Facial or scalp soft tissue injuries not overlying bony prominences, involving the external ears or associated with intraoral trauma or bleeding (e.g., torn frenulum or gingival laceration)
- Facial or scalp soft tissue injuries or skull fractures in a preambulatory infant, or
- Skull fractures that are multiple, complex, or diastatic—attributed to a short-distance fall (usually less than 6 feet).

THE RELEVANT FORENSIC ISSUES

In cases of suspected inflicted head trauma, the relevant forensic issues to be addressed by the child abuse medical consultant include the following:

- Have *nontraumatic* etiologies for the child's clinical, laboratory, and radiological findings been reasonably excluded?
- Does the caretaker's account or explanation of the child's head injury event adequately explain the child's clinical presentation and traumatic cranial injuries?
- What is the best estimate of the timing of the child's head injury event?

THE DIFFERENTIAL DIAGNOSIS

To identify inflicted injuries masquerading as accidental trauma, a high index of suspicion for inflicted pediatric head trauma is essential. To identify accidental injuries misinterpreted as abusive, and to identify nontraumatic etiologies for the child's clinical, laboratory, and/or radiological findings, *objectivity* is equally important. Birth trauma, accidental head trauma, and other nontraumatic explanations for intracra-

nial bleeding and/or brain injury must be *actively* considered. These differential diagnostic considerations fall into the following general categories:

- Nonabusive trauma (e.g., forceps delivery, vacuum extraction, breech delivery, motor vehicle crash, a complex accidental fall, a fall from an elevated height)
- Congenital or metabolic condition or variation of normal (e.g., aneurysm, arteriovenous malformation, benign expansion of the extra-axial spaces, glutaric acidemia)
- Neoplastic diseases (e.g., brain tumor, acute leukemia)
- Bleeding diathesis (e.g., hemorrhagic disease of the newborn, hemophilia, idiopathic thrombocytopenic purpura, von Willebrand's disease)
- Acquired causes (e.g., meningitis, superior sagittal sinus thrombosis, obstructive hydrocephalus), and
- Connective tissue disease (e.g., osteogenesis imperfecta, Ehlers-Danlos syndrome)

For a more complete discussion of conditions confused with abusive head trauma, see Chapter 47, "Conditions Confused with Head Trauma."

INJURY MECHANISMS

Does the account or explanation of the child's head injury event adequately explain the child's clinical presentation and traumatic cranial injuries? To answer this question, a biomechanics-based approach is recommended.[48] Work backwards, from injury to history: (1) What are the child's primary cranial injuries? (2) What mechanisms of injury (i.e., contact and/or inertial) are required to explain each of these primary cranial injuries? and (3) Are these specific, required mechanisms of injury evident in the history provided by the caregiver? If not, child abuse must be considered.

Primary traumatic cranial injuries are those that occur at the moment of injury and result from mechanical distortions and strains. All primary traumatic cranial injuries derive from one of two mechanisms of injury: contact or inertial. A *contact* cranial injury results solely from skull deformation and requires cranial impact. Examples of contact cranial injuries include the following: (1) craniofacial bruising, abrasions, lacerations, or soft tissue swelling, (2) subgaleal hemorrhage or cephalohematoma, (3) skull fractures, and, (4) any associated epidural, subarachnoid, or subdural hemorrhage; brain contusions;or brain lacerations resulting solely from skull deformation. Contact cranial injuries can be viewed as those injuries that result from cranial impact if/when the head is fixed and prevented from accelerating (or decelerating) as a consequence of that impact.

An *inertial* cranial injury results solely from whole-head cranial acceleration or deceleration. Because the head is tethered to the body by the neck, cranial acceleration (or deceleration) is usually rotational rather than straight-line. Inertial cranial injuries can be induced in two ways: (1) impulsively, via forces transmitted through the neck (e.g., a whiplash injury), or (2) by cranial impact, if the impact causes cranial acceleration (or deceleration). Examples of inertial cranial injuries include the following: (1) acute concussion, (2) diffuse traumatic axonal injury, (3) nonfocal, acute subdural hematoma that results from tearing of one or more bridging veins, and (4) any associated subarachnoid hemorrhage, brain contusions, or brain lacerations resulting solely from rotational cranial acceleration. Inertial mechanisms of cranial injury have been linked to worse outcomes.[30]

Because inertial cranial injuries can result from cranial impact, victims of inflicted pediatric head trauma can reveal a combination of contact and inertial primary injuries. However, some cranial impacts that produce clinically significant inertial cranial injuries do *not* produce visible, external, soft tissue injuries at the site of impact. In fatal cases of pediatric neurotrauma, scalp reflection at the time of autopsy might reveal evidence of cranial impact that did not produce visible, external, soft tissue injuries.[14] It follows that in living children with isolated inertial cranial injuries, impact can never be definitively excluded (or shaking confirmed) as the mechanism of that child's inertial cranial injuries. For a more complete discussion of head injury biomechanics, see Chapter 40, "Biomechanics of Head Trauma in Infants and Young Children."

TIMING OF INJURY

Child protective services and police investigators—not medical providers—investigate child abuse. On the other hand, when a medical provider can reasonably identify the *timing* of a victim's inflicted head injury event, the victims' caregiver at that time will appropriately become the subject of a child abuse investigation. Under ideal circumstances, this investigation will lead to court actions that protect an abused child from re-injury. For these reasons, accurate assessment of the timing of abusive head trauma is an essential skill of the child abuse medical specialist.

Serial cranial imaging studies that reveal an expected progression of posttraumatic findings (e.g., the evolution and resolution of brain or scalp swelling, the degradation of posttraumatic subdural collections, or the evolution of posttraumatic encephalopathic changes) facilitate only very broad estimates of the timing of a child's head injury event. The vast majority of young victims of moderate to severe (accidental or inflicted) pediatric neurotrauma become rapidly, clearly, and persistently ill.[49-54] It follows that precise documentation of the timing of onset of the victim's most severe and persistent clinical signs (of traumatic brain injury) facilitates an estimation of the timing of the child's head injury event. Stated more simply, to estimate the timing of head injury, answer this question: When did the child first become clearly and persistently ill with clinical signs linked to his or her traumatic cranial injuries?[49]

Severe *and delayed* acute clinical deterioration is possible after accidental or inflicted childhood neurotrauma.[50,51,55-60] The published literature regarding this phenomenon suggests that delayed clinical deterioration will occur if and when a child with focal intracranial injuries (e.g., epidural hematoma) experiences secondary systemic hypoxemia and/or ischemia, brain swelling, increased intracranial pressure, herniation, and/or brainstem compression. The vast majority of children who experience delayed and severe clinical deterioration after closed head trauma are not completely asymptomatic before their subsequent clinical deterioration, but manifest persistent or recurrent, less severe, nonspecific clinical signs of their initial head injury (e.g., recurrent vomiting, persistent irritability, prolonged loss of appetite, abnormal sleep patterns, seizures, accelerating head growth).

THE DIAGNOSTIC EVALUATION

In the absence of visible craniofacial soft tissue injuries, alteration or loss of consciousness, seizures, or cardiorespiratory compromise, abusive head trauma is frequently missed, misdiagnosed, or not even considered.[47] Diagnostic uncertainty increases if/when the caretaker of the head-injured child delays seeking medical care and/or denies any history of closed head trauma to explain the child's acute clinical signs. Victims of closed head trauma sometimes fail to reveal visible, external signs of their accidental or abusive cranial impacts.[14] Some infants with traumatic intracranial injuries will have a normal neurological examination.[61-67] Vigilance and a high index of suspicion are required. To *diagnose* inflicted head trauma, we must first *consider* the diagnosis.[47]

In a majority of cases, a diagnosis of abusive head trauma will be challenged, appropriately, by other medical providers, by family members, and/or later in a courtroom. To avoid over- and/or under-diagnosis of abusive head trauma, objectivity is essential. To ensure objectivity, a *consistently thorough* diagnostic evaluation is warranted. This evaluation must include a comprehensive history; meticulous physical examination; and specific laboratory testing, imaging studies, and/or consultations by medical specialists that facilitate *active* consideration of inflicted head trauma *and* alternate diagnoses. In some cases, and in some jurisdictions, you will find it necessary to order tests specifically to "rule out" an alternate diagnosis.

History

Obtain an independent *history of the present illness* from any and all potential caretakers, ideally in isolation from all other potential perpetrators of inflicted trauma (Table 39-1). How, when, and where did the child first became clearly and persistently ill? Document verbatim any and all statements made by caregiver(s) to explain the child's presenting clinical signs. Meticulously document the specific circumstances of any alleged, accidental, head injury event *and* the subsequent, acute clinical consequences of that event. If the infant or child suffered an accidental cranial impact but did not become clearly and persistently symptomatic thereafter, the injury event was likely inconsequential. Use direct quotations whenever possible. Document when and to whom the statements are made. A thorough medical history will allow you to ascertain the nature and the clinical severity of the child's injury or condition and may capture information that will prove to be forensically significant.

Obtain a *past medical history, family medical history* and a *review of systems* that are sufficiently comprehensive to allow you to reasonably exclude (or to elucidate) alternate potential explanations for the child's presenting clinical signs, laboratory, and/or radiological findings (Tables 39-2, 39-3, and 39-4). *Actively* seek information regarding alternative diagnoses, including congenital brain defects, variations, neoplasia, or acquired conditions; a bleeding diathesis; connective tissue disease; birth asphyxiation or trauma; and previous, clinically significant, traumatic, or hypoxic-ischemic brain injuries. Take a thorough *social history* to

| Table 39-1 | History of Present Illness |

- When was the last time that your child was acting, eating, and interacting in a completely normal way?
- When did your child first become clearly and persistently ill or symptomatic?
- What was the very first thing that you noticed about your child that concerned you?
- What did you observe next?
- What other clinical signs appeared thereafter?
- How long did these clinical signs last?
- Did your child have an alteration or a loss of consciousness?
- Was he ever completely limp like a rag doll?
- Could you awaken him?
- Did you try to awaken him?
- What did you try to do to awaken him?
- Did he stop breathing?
- Did he have difficulty breathing?
- What were his respiratory efforts like?
- Did he turn blue?
- Did he stiffen his entire body?
- Did his eyes roll backwards?
- Did he have a seizure?
- Did his arms or legs jerk repeatedly?
- What did these arm or leg movements look like?
- Were his eyes or his gaze deviated to one side?
- Which adult(s) first observed your child's abnormal behaviors?
- When, where, and how did this adult discover or first observe these abnormal behaviors?
- What happened?
- Did your child fall?
- Who witnessed this fall?
- How far did he fall?
- Onto what kind of surface?
- Precisely how did your child land when he fell?
- What part of his body impacted first?
- What part of his body impacted next?
- How did he act immediately after the fall?
- How did he act over the next several minutes (and hours) after the fall?

identify past and current stressors and risk factors for abuse (Table 39-5). Supplement your medical history by reviewing the child's birth and outpatient medical records thoroughly (Table 39-6).

Physical Examination

Practitioners should follow these guidelines during physical examination:

Supplement your understanding of the child's acute clinical condition and course by reviewing his or her EMT and emergency department records. Then perform a meticulous initial physical examination. Carefully measure and plot growth parameters for potential evidence of acute or chronic malnutrition, macrocephaly (e.g., potentially related to a chronic subdural collection, posttraumatic hydrocephalus, or acute brain swelling) or microcephaly (e.g., potentially related to posttraumatic cerebral atrophy). Assess vital signs, skin color and perfusion, respirations, and overall respon-

siveness for evidence of diffuse or deep brain injury associated with respiratory insufficiency and/or compensated shock. Look for asymmetrical movements and functional deficits.

Visually inspect the child's entire body. Accidental bruising of the knees, shins, elbows, and forehead are common in cruising or ambulatory children, but very uncommon in infants who are not yet cruising.[68] Some bruises are easily overlooked (e.g., in the scalp or involving the external ears). A majority of pediatric victims of blunt abdominal trauma will not reveal abdominal wall bruising. Document, measure, and describe all traumatic skin injuries in the medical record.

Carefully palpate the head and scalp, extremities, and ribs for tenderness, swelling, induration, deformity or crepitus—signs that might indicate an underlying fracture. Palpate the sutures and fontanels for signs of increased intracranial pressure. Carefully inspect the external ears, tympanic membranes, nose, mouth, and hypopharynx. Inflicted traumatic injuries are common in these locations. Inspect the child's retina bilaterally in a darkened room. Be patient, because the examination requires time. Consider a short-acting mydriatic to improve retinal visualization. For a more complete discussion of eye injuries in child abuse, see Chapter 44, "Eye Injuries in Child Abuse."

Compare and contrast respiratory movements, effort, and breath sounds to help confirm or exclude clinically significant traumatic thoracic injuries. Examine the abdomen for signs of tenderness, rigidity, rebound, guarding, or loss of bowel sounds. Inspect the genitalia and anus for bleeding or other potential signs of penetrating trauma.

Perform a careful neurological examination. Objectively document the child's mental status, responsiveness, clinical injury severity, and coma scores. Compare your observations to similar assessments made at the scene of injury, during transport, and/or in the emergency department. Remember that intracranial injuries can be clinically subtle or silent.[69]

Re-examine the child serially. Some bruises evolve over time or appear only after treatment for shock. Serial physical examinations can reveal evolution of patterned bruises, delayed soft-tissue swelling, signs of an acute abdomen, bony deformities, evolving losses of function and/or evolving neurological deficits. Serial photo documentation of traumatic soft tissue injuries is strongly recommended.

Neuroimaging

In an infant or young child with *acute*, unexplained neurological signs or symptoms and suspected child abuse, obtain an initial, unenhanced cranial CT scan (with brain and bone window settings) and a standard radiographic (four-view) skull series. If the initial cranial CT scan is positive (or if the initial CT scan is negative but suspicion of child abuse remains high), obtain cranial MRI with T1- and T2-weighted conventional or fast spin echo imaging, different susceptibility-weighted sequences (such as gradient echo and diffusion-weighted), and FLAIR sequences. Consider magnetic resonance angiography (MRA) and venography (MRV) to help confirm or exclude vascular lesions, especially if/when parenchymal lesions are discovered.

In an infant or young child with *chronic* neurological signs and suspected child abuse, obtain cranial MRI with T1- and

Table 39-2 Past Medical History

- Did you (mother) experience complications during your pregnancy?
- What complications did you experience?
- Did you (mother) experience post-partum hemorrhage?
- Was your child born prematurely?
- How prematurely?
- Do you know *why* your child was born prematurely?
- How was your child delivered? Vaginally? By caesarean section?
- Did the doctor have to use forceps or a vacuum machine to help deliver your baby?
- Did your child have to be delivered urgently or emergently?
- Do you know *why* he had to be delivered urgently or emergently?
- During labor, did your child's heart rate drop too low prior to his/her birth?
- In the delivery room, immediately after his birth ...
  - ... did your child cry vigorously right away?
  - ... did his/her body become pink quickly?
  - ... did your child quickly begin to move his/her arms and legs actively?
  - ... did his/her body turn blue after his birth?
  - ... for how long did he/she look blue?
  - ... was he/she ever limp and floppy like a rag doll?
  - ... for how long was he/she limp and floppy like a rag doll?
  - ... did somehow have to help your child to start breathing?
  - ... what interventions were required to help your child start breathing?
  - ... did someone perform chest compressions?
- During his/her stay in the newborn nursery, did your child ...
  - ... ever have a seizure?
  - ... become lethargic, limp, or unresponsive?
  - ... receive treatment with intravenous antibiotics?
  - ... receive treatment with oxygen?
  - ... receive rescue breathing?
  - ... require a breathing tube?
  - ... require a ventilator?
  - ... require chest compressions?
  - ... undergo circumcision?
  - ... experience prolonged bleeding from his circumcision site?
- How long did your baby stay in the hospital after birth?
- Since your child's discharge from the newborn nursery, has he/she ever ...
  - ... been hospitalized?
  - ... had surgery?
  - ... had a broken bone?
  - ... had a seizure?
  - ... suffered a concussion?
  - ... become unconscious?
  - ... become completely limp like a rag doll?
  - ... become lethargic?
  - ... become completely unresponsive?
  - ... stopped breathing?
  - ... turned blue?
  - ... received treatment with oxygen?
  - ... required rescue breathing?
  - ... required a breathing tube?
  - ... required a ventilator?
  - ... required chest compressions?
  - ... been inconsolable?
  - ... experienced prolonged, recurrent vomiting?
  - ... required treatment for a head injury?
  - ... experienced frequent or prolonged nasal or oral bleeding?
  - ... manifested frequent or easy bruising, especially in "unusual" places?
  - ... passed blood in his urine or stools?
  - ... experienced prolonged, post-operative bleeding?
  - ... had oozing, prolonged bleeding, or hematoma formation at the site of immunizations?

Table 39-3	Family Medical History

Is there a family medical history of ...
- ... easy bruising?
- ... a blood clotting or bleeding disorder?
- ... menorrhagia?
- ... prolonged post-operative bleeding?
- ... severe or recurrent nosebleeds?
- ... excessive bleeding with dental procedures?
- ... mental retardation?
- ... cerebral palsy?
- ... seizures?
- ... developmental delays?
- ... hearing loss?
- ... blindness?
- ... frequent fractures?
- ... dental problems?
- ... brittle bone disease or osteogenesis imperfecta?
- ... any other connective tissue or bone disease?
- ... sudden, unexpected infant death or crib death?
- ... kidney disease?
- ... mental illness?
- ... any other genetic or hereditary condition affecting young children?

Table 39-4	Review of Systems

"Has your child ever ..."
- ... experienced unexplained weight loss?
- ... become very lethargic or very hard to wake up?
- ... become completely floppy like a rag doll?
- ... been completely unresponsive?
- ... had problems with vision or hearing?
- ... experienced bleeding from the nose, ears, or mouth?
- ... experienced shortness of breath?
- ... stopped breathing?
- ... turned blue or appeared dusky around the lips?
- ... experienced recurrent vomiting?
- ... demonstrated prolonged loss of appetite?
- ... had blood in the urine or stools?
- ... had unexplained bruises, abrasions, or cuts?
- ... had a seizure?
- ... seemed continually irritable or inconsolable?
- ... had very swollen lymph glands?
- ... had a fracture or broken bone?
- ... appeared to not be using one extremity like the one on the opposite side?

T2-weighted conventional or fast spin echo imaging, along with gradient echo and FLAIR sequences to exclude (or to confirm) older injuries. For a more complete discussion of imaging of abusive head trauma, see Chapter 42.

Laboratory Studies, Medical Consultations and Secondary Diagnostic Evaluations

Young victims of moderate or severe closed head trauma deserve broad laboratory screening and additional medical

Table 39-5	Social History

- What are the names and ages of the biological parents?
- How long have they known each other?
- Are they currently married to each other?
- If so, for how long?
- If not, were they ever married to each other?
- For how long?
- When did they separate or divorce?
- Why did they separate or divorce?
- Is either biological parent now remarried?
- Was the pregnancy for this child planned?
- Who now lives in the home with this child?
- Has this child (or any other child living in this home) ever been the subject of a previous report to child protective services?
- Which of the adults who live with this child provides primary care for this child?
- Do these adults also work outside the home?
- Have these adults had to deal with issues of poverty or unemployment?
- Domestic violence?
- Alcohol abuse?
- Drug abuse?
- Incarceration?
- Depression?
- Other mental health problems?
- What other adults also provide child care for this child?
- Does the child attend day care?
- How often?

Table 39-6	Review of Birth and Outpatient Records

- Do the child's birth records document ...
  - ... prolonged late decelerations?
  - ... cord around the neck?
  - ... a premature delivery?
  - ... a spontaneous vaginal delivery?
  - ... forceps extraction?
  - ... vacuum-assisted delivery?
  - ... neonatal asphyxiation?
  - ... neonatal resuscitation?
  - ... prolonged bleeding with circumcision?
  - ... vitamin K prophylaxis?
  - ... neonatal seizures?
  - ... neonatal lethargy?
  - ... neonatal sepsis?
- Do the child's outpatient medical records document ...
  - ... immunization status?
  - ... current medications?
  - ... current allergies?
  - ... normal growth and development?
  - ... developmental delays?
  - ... macrocephaly or microcephaly?
  - ... excessive bruising?
  - ... bruising before cruising?
  - ... bruising in unexpected places?
  - ... patterned bruising?
  - ... sensory deficits?
  - ... apparent life-threatening events?
  - ... prior fractures?
  - ... prior seizures?
  - ... other unexplained trauma?
  - ... failure to thrive?

consultations as required to help confirm or exclude occult trauma and its potential complications (e.g., hypovolemic shock, peritonitis associated with an occult ruptured hollow viscous, acquired consumptive coagulopathy). At a minimum, in cases of suspected physical abuse involving a child less than 2 years of age, the diagnostic evaluation should include the following: (1) CBC with platelet count, (2) coagulation screening tests, (3) serum chemistries, liver, and pancreatic function tests, (4) urinalysis, (5) pediatric ophthalmology evaluation, and (6) an initial radiographic skeletal survey. Definitive confirmation (or exclusion) of specific diagnoses may require serial laboratory testing, additional screening (or definitive) laboratory testing, additional medical specialty consultations, and/or ancillary radiographic studies (Table 39-7).

Table 39-7	**Laboratory Studies, Medical Consultations, and Secondary Diagnostic Evaluations**

- Obtain CBC with platelet count
- Obtain screening coagulation tests
- Obtain serum chemistry panel, liver and pancreatic function tests
- Obtain urinalysis
- Obtain an initial radiographic skeletal survey
- Obtain pediatric ophthalmology consultation
- In the presence of shock or possible internal traumatic injuries, obtain trauma services consultation
- In the presence of possible or probable seizures, obtain pediatric neurology consultation
- In a child with abnormal coagulation screening tests, an abnormal bleeding history, or an abnormal initial cranial imaging study:
  - Obtain initial and serial PT, PTT, CBC with platelet count, thrombin time, fibrinogen level, fibrin split products and D-dimer to exclude (or to confirm) an acquired consumptive coagulopathy (e.g., DIC)
  - Consider von Willebrand's screening tests
  - Consider pediatric hematology consultation
- In a child with an unexplained alteration in mental status:
  - Consider urine and serum toxicology screening
  - Consider pediatric neurology consultation
- In the presence of cranial imaging results compatible with glutaric academia (type 1), obtain serum amino acid and urine organic acid testing
- When connective tissue, metabolic, or nutritional bone disease is a diagnostic consideration:
  - Obtain serum calcium, phosphorus, and alkaline phosphatase
  - Consider testing for 1,25-OH vitamin D and its precursors
  - Consider skin biopsy or genetic testing to confirm (or to exclude) connective tissue disease
  - Consider metabolic disease consultation
- After stabilization and/or before hospital discharge:
  - Consider nuclear medicine bone scan
  - Consider physical therapy consultation
  - Consider audiological evaluation
  - Consider speech therapy consultation
  - Consider occupational therapy consultation
  - Plan a neurodevelopmental evaluation
  - Order a follow-up radiographic skeletal survey

DIAGNOSTIC OBJECTIVITY

To ensure objectivity, a *consistently thorough* diagnostic approach is essential. A comprehensive medical history, meticulous physical examination(s), and the appropriate use of laboratory tests, imaging studies, and medical specialty consultations—coupled with *active* consideration of alternate diagnoses—will frequently (although not inevitably) lead to a reasonable degree of medical certainty regarding the nature, extent, severity, mechanisms, and timing of pediatric neurotrauma. In many cases of suspected pediatric abusive head trauma, it is the discovery of associated *noncranial* traumatic injuries suspicious for abuse (e.g., patterned bruises, bruises in a pre-ambulatory infant, rib fractures) that provides the most compelling evidence that an infant's *cranial* injuries were also inflicted.

COMMUNICATION

Communicating your diagnostic impressions—clearly and effectively; orally and in writing; in a hospital room or in a courtroom; to parents, investigators, attorneys, judges, and jurors—can be extraordinarily challenging. Communication failures can lead to failures to protect children at risk. When testifying, keep it simple. Make eye contact when speaking. Maintain a professional demeanor. Remember that jurors tend to remember what they hear first and last. Experience helps.

STRENGTH OF THE MEDICAL EVIDENCE

Abusive head trauma is a well-recognized clinical entity. Our substantial (and growing) collective clinical experience—summarized in our published, peer-reviewed, medical literature regarding this subject—leads us to one incontrovertible conclusion: abusive actions directed toward an infant or young child can cause devastating traumatic intracranial injuries. This conclusion derives largely from Class 3 scientific evidence (i.e., retrospective case reports and clinical series). Higher (Class 1 or 2) scientific evidence is virtually nonexistent, since direct testing of hypotheses (e.g., is shaking dangerous?) is impossible in humans.

Current controversies regarding abusive head trauma derive almost exclusively from the inevitable requirement to interpret specific historical, clinical, laboratory, and/or radiological findings in a *forensic* context. Does the caregiver's account of the child's head injury event reasonably explain the child's clinical, physical, laboratory, and radiological findings? If not, why not? Have nontraumatic etiologies been reasonably excluded? Can we reasonably conclude that the child was abused?

Preliminary studies of our initial *forensic* impressions regarding hypothetical cases of pediatric head trauma reveal significant variations that require further analysis.[70] In many cases, reasonable doubt arises if/when a clinical, physical, laboratory, or radiological finding is considered in isolation, rather than within the context of the child's entire presentation. What is the best unifying explanation for the child's clinical, physical, laboratory, and radiological findings?

Prospective, multicentered, comparative studies of clinical presentations, mechanisms, injuries, and outcomes following accidental versus inflicted pediatric head trauma are limited in number. Meta-analyses of these studies are difficult, because researchers have used highly variable definitional criteria to categorize cases as accidental versus inflicted. Prospective, *long-term* outcome studies following abusive head trauma are nonexistent.

The practice recommendations that appear in this chapter (e.g., active consideration of alternate diagnoses) derive from our own past professional experiences or "lessons learned."

SUGGESTED DIRECTIONS FOR FUTURE RESEARCH

We need objective, widely accepted, definitional criteria for categorizing cases of pediatric head trauma as accidental versus inflicted. We need to use these definitional criteria uniformly in future, multicentered, prospective, comparative studies of clinical presentations, injuries, mechanisms, and outcomes following (accidental versus inflicted) pediatric head trauma. We need research studies that clarify how—and why—medical professionals reach specific *forensic* conclusions. Finally, and perhaps most urgently, because perpetrators rarely disclose their abusive actions and head-injured infants can have normal neurological examinations, we need rapid, noninvasive, sensitive, and specific screening tests that will facilitate detection of subtle, easily missed, traumatic brain injuries in infants and young children. For a more complete discussion of biochemical markers of head trauma in children, see Chapter 46.

CONCLUSION

Medical providers with child abuse expertise enter and exit the real life dramas that surround cases of abusive head trauma at two predictable times—shortly after a head-injured child is admitted to a hospital, and much later, in a courtroom. Both entrances can be highly emotionally charged. To function effectively, a child abuse medical specialist must listen carefully, remain objective, execute a thorough diagnostic evaluation, actively consider alternate potential explanations, and communicate results and forensic impressions clearly. If you can accomplish these tasks consistently, you will speak with conviction. More importantly, you will help to protect children from repetitive abusive trauma.

References

1. Keenan HT, Runyan DK, Marshall SW, et al: A population-based study of inflicted traumatic brain injury in young children. *JAMA* 2003;290:2542-2543.
2. Sills MR, Libby AM, Orton HD: Prehospital and in-hospital mortality: a comparison of intentional and unintentional traumatic brain injuries in Colorado children. *Arch Pediatr Adolesc Med* 2005;159:665-670.
3. Ellingson KD, Leventhal JM, Weiss HB: Using hospital data to track inflicted traumatic brain injury. *Am J Prev Med* 2008;34:S157-162.
4. Minns RA, Jones PA, Mok JY: Annual incidence of shaken impact syndrome in young children. *Am J Prev Med* 2008;34:S126-133.
5. Barlow KM, Minns RA: Annual incidence of shaken impact syndrome in young children. *Lancet* 2000;356:1571-1572.
6. Jayawant S, Rawlinson A, Gibbon F, et al: Subdural hemorrhages in infants: population based study. *Br Med J* 1998;317:1558-1561.
7. Feldman KW, Bethel R, Shugerman RP, et al: The cause of infant and toddler subdural hemorrhage: a prospective study. *Pediatrics* 2001;108:636-646.
8. Keenan HT, Marshall SW, Nocera MA, et al: Increased incidence of inflicted traumatic brain injury in children after a natural disaster. *Am J Prev Med* 2004;26:189-193.
9. Sinal SH, Petree AR, Herman-Giddens M, et al: Is race or ethnicity a predictive factor in shaken baby syndrome? *Child Abuse Negl* 2000;24:1241-1246.
10. Overpeck MD, Brenner RA, Trumble AC, et al: Risk factors for infant homicide in the United States. *N Engl J Med* 1998;339:1211-1216.
11. Caffey J: Multiple fractures in the long bones of infants suffering from chronic subdural hematoma. *Am J Roentgen* 1946;56:163-173.
12. Jenny C: On the theory and practice of shaking infants: where have we come in the 30 years since shaken baby syndrome was first identified? Oral keynote presentation; Fourth National Conference on Shaken Baby Syndrome, Salt Lake City, Utah; 12 September 2002.
13. Guthkelch AN: Infantile subdural haematoma and its relationship to whiplash injuries. *Br Med J* 1971;2:430-431.
14. Duhaime AC, Gennarelli TA, Thibault LE, et al: The shaken baby syndrome: a clinical, pathological and biomechanical study. *J Neurosurg* 1987;66:409-415.
15. Goldsmith W, Plunkett J: A biomechanical analysis of the causes of traumatic brain injury in infants and children. *Am J Forensic Med Pathol* 2004;25:89-100.
16. Donohoe M: Evidence-based medicine and shaken baby syndrome: part I—literature review, 1966-1998. *Am J Forensic Med Pathol* 2003;24:239-242.
17. Hadley MN, Sonntag VKH, Rekate HL, et al: The infant whiplash-shake injury syndrome: a clinical and pathological study. *Neurosurgery* 2000;24:536-540.
18. Saternus KS, Kernbach-Wighton G, Oehmichen M: The shaking trauma in infants—kinetic chains. *Forensic Sci Int* 2000;109:203-213.
19. Starling SP, Patel S, Burke BL, et al: Analysis of perpetrator admissions to inflicted traumatic brain injury in children. *Arch Pediatr Adolesc Med* 2004;158:454-458.
20. Biron D, Shelton D: Perpetrator accounts in infant abusive head trauma brought about by a shaking event. *Child Abuse Negl* 2005;29:1347-1358.
21. Christian CW, Block R, AAP Committee on Child Abuse and Neglect: Abusive head trauma in infants and children. *Pediatrics* 2009;123:1409-1411.
22. Duhaime AC, Alario AJ, Lewander WJ, et al: Head injury in very young children: mechanisms, injury types, and ophthalmologic findings in 100 hospitalized patients younger than 2 years of age. *Pediatrics* 1992;90:179-185.
23. Duhaime AC, Christian C, Moss E, et al: Long-term outcome in infants with the shaking-impact syndrome. *Pediatr Neurosurg* 1996;24:292-298.
24. Ewing-Cobbs L, Kramer L, Prasad M, et al: Neuroimaging, physical, and developmental findings after inflicted and noninflicted traumatic brain injury in young children. *Pediatrics* 1998;102:300-307.
25. Barlow K, Thompson E, Johnson D, et al: The neurological outcome of non-accidental head injury. *Pediatr Rehabil* 2004;7:195-203.
26. Ewing-Cobbs L, Prasad M, Kramer L, et al: Inflicted traumatic brain injury: relationship of developmental outcome to severity of injury. *Pediatr Neurosurg* 2000;31:251-258.
27. Goldstein B, Kelly MM, Bruton D, et al: Inflicted versus accidental head injury in critically injured children. *Crit Care Med* 1993;21:1328-1332.
28. Haviland J, Russell RI: Outcome after severe non-accidental head injury. *Arch Dis Child* 1997;77:504-507.
29. Prasad MR, Ewing-Cobbs L, Swank PR, et al: Predictors of outcome following traumatic brain injury in young children. *Pediatr Neurosurg* 2002;36:64-74.
30. Hymel KP, Makoroff KL, Laskey AL, et al: Mechanisms, clinical presentations, injuries and outcomes from inflicted versus noninflicted head trauma during infancy: results of a prospective, multicentered, comparative study. *Pediatrics* 2007;119:922-929.
31. Keenan HT, Hooper SR, Wetherington CE, et al: Neurodevelopmental consequences of early traumatic brain injury in 3-year-old children. *Pediatrics* 2007;119:e616-e623.
32. Reece RM, Sege R: Childhood head injuries: accidental or inflicted? *Arch Pediatr Adolesc Med* 2000;154:11-15.

33. Bechtel K, Stoessel K, Leventhal JM, et al: Characteristics that distinguish accidental from abusive injury in hospitalized young children with head trauma. *Pediatrics* 2004;114:165-168.

34. Keenan HT, Runyan DK, Marshall SW, et al: A population-based comparison of clinical and outcome characteristics of young children with serious inflicted and noninflicted traumatic brain injury. *Pediatrics* 2004;114:633-639.

35. Levin AV: Retinal haemorrhage and child abuse. *In:* David TJ (ed): *Recent Advances in Pediatrics.* Churchill Livingstone, London, 2000, pp 151-219.

36. Geddes JF, Whitwell HL, Graham DI: Traumatic axonal injury: practical issues for diagnosis in medicolegal cases. *Neuropathol Appl Neurobiol* 2000;26:105-116.

37. Geddes JF, Vowles GH, Hackshaw AK, et al: Neuropathology of inflicted head injury in children. II. Microscopic brain injury in infants. *Brain* 2001;124:1299-1306.

38. Geddes JF, Hackshaw AK, Vowles GH, et al: Neuropathology of inflicted head injury in children. I. Patterns of brain damage. *Brain* 2001;124:1290-1298.

39. Johnson DL, Boal D, Baule R: Role of apnea in nonaccidental head injury. *Pediatr Neurosurg* 1995;23:305-310.

40. Karandikar S, Coles L, Jayawant S, et al: The neurodevelopmental outcome in infants who have sustained a subdural haemorrhage from non-accidental head trauma. *Child Abuse Rev* 2004;13:178-187.

41. Duhaime AC, Bilaniuk L, Zimmerman R: The "big black brain": radiographic changes after severe inflicted head injury in infancy. *J Neurotrauma* 1993;10:S59.

42. Zimmerman RA, Bilaniuk LT, Bruce D, et al: Computed tomography of craniocerebral injury in the abused child. *Radiology* 1979;130:687-690.

43. Atwal GS, Rutty GN, Carter N, et al: Bruising in non-accidental head injured children: a retrospective study of the prevalence, distribution and pathological associations in 24 cases. *Forensic Sci Int* 1998;96:215-230.

44. Leventhal JM, Thomas SA, Rosenfield NS, et al: Fractures in young children. Distinguishing child abuse from unintentional injuries. *Am J Dis Child* 1993;147:87-92.

45. Merten DF, Radkowski MA, Leonidas JC: The abused child: a radiological reappraisal. *Radiology* 1983;146:377-381.

46. Kleinman PK, Marks SC Jr, Richmond JM, et al: Inflicted skeletal trauma: a postmortem radiologic-histopathologic study in 31 infants. *Am J Roentgenol* 1995;165:647-650.

47. Jenny C, Hymel KP, Ritzen A, et al: Analysis of missed cases of abusive head trauma. *JAMA* 1999;281:621-626.

48. Hymel KP, Bandak FA, Partington ME, et al: Abusive head trauma? A biomechanics-based approach. *Child Maltreat* 1998;3:116-128.

49. Hymel KP: The timing of clinical presentation after inflicted childhood neurotrauma. *In:* Reece RM, Nicholson CE (eds): *Inflicted Childhood Neurotrauma.* American Academy of Pediatrics, Elk Grove Village, IL, 2003, pp 65-68.

50. Wilman KY, Bank DE, Senac M, et al: Restricting the time of injury in fatal inflicted head injuries. *Child Abuse Negl* 1997;21:929-940.

51. Levin HS, Aldrich EF, Saydjari C, et al: Severe head injury in children: experience of the Traumatic Coma Data Bank. *Neurosurgery* 1992;31:435-443.

52. Nachelsky MB, Dix JD: The time interval between lethal infant shaking and onset of symptoms. A review of the shaken baby syndrome literature. *Am J Forensic Med Pathol* 1995;16:154-157.

53. Starling SP, Holden JR, Jenny C: Abusive head trauma: the relationship of perpetrators to their victims. *Pediatrics* 1995;95:259-262.

54. Gilles EE, Nelson MD: Cerebral complications of nonaccidental head injury in childhood. *Pediatr Neurol* 1998;19:119-128.

55. Reilly PL, Graham DI, Adams JH, et al: Patients with head injury who talk and die. *Lancet* 1975;2:375-377.

56. Lobato RD, Rivas JJ, Gomez PA, et al: Head-injured patients who talk and deteriorate into coma. Analysis of 211 cases studied with computerized tomography. *J Neurosurg* 1991;75:256-261.

57. Snoek JW, Minderhoud JM, Wilmink JT: Delayed deterioration following mild head injury in children. *Brain* 1984;107:15-36.

58. Bruce DA, Alavi A, Bilaniuk L, et al: Diffuse cerebral swelling following head injuries in children: the syndrome of "malignant brain edema." *J Neurosurg* 1981;54:170-178.

59. Gilliland MG: Interval duration between injury and severe symptoms in nonaccidental head trauma in infants and young children. *J Forensic Sci* 1998;43:723-725.

60. Arbogast KB, Margulies SS, Christian CW: Initial neurologic presentation in young children sustaining inflicted and unintentional fatal head injuries. *Pediatrics* 2005;116:180-184.

61. Dietrich AM, Bowman MJ, Ginn-Pease ME, et al: Pediatric head injuries: can clinical factors reliably predict an abnormality on computed tomography? *Ann Emerg Med* 1993;22:1535-1540.

62. Lloyd DA, Carty H, Patterson M, et al: Predictive value of skull radiography for intracranial injury in children with blunt head injury. *Lancet* 1997;349:821-824.

63. Quayle KS, Jaffe DM, Kupperman N, et al: Diagnostic testing for acute head injury in children: when are head computed tomography and skull radiographs indicated? *Pediatrics* 1997;99:e11.

64. Gruskin KD, Schutzman SA: Head trauma in children younger than 2 years of age: are there predictors for complications? *Arch Pediatr Adoles Med* 1999;153:15-20.

65. Greenes DS, Schutzman SA: Clinical indicators of intracranial injury in head-injured infants. *Pediatrics* 1999;104:861-867.

66. Rubin DM, Christian CW, Bilaniuk LT, et al: Occult head injury in high-risk abused children. *Pediatrics* 2003;111:1382-1386.

67. Laskey AL, Holsti M, Runyan DK, et al: Occult head trauma in young suspected victims of physical abuse. *J Pediatr* 2004;144:719-722.

68. Sugar NF, Taylor JA, Feldman KW: Bruises in infants and toddlers. *Arch Pediatr Adolesc Med* 1999;153:399-403.

69. Hymel KP: Traumatic intracranial injuries can be clinically silent. *J Pediatrics* 2004;144:701-702.

70. Laskey AL, Sheridan MS, Hymel KP: Physicians' initial forensic impressions of 16 hypothetical cases of pediatric traumatic brain injury. *Child Abuse Negl* 2007;31:329-342.

40

BIOMECHANICS OF HEAD TRAUMA IN INFANTS AND YOUNG CHILDREN

Susan Margulies, PhD, and Brittany Coats, PhD

INTRODUCTION

Traumatic brain injury (TBI) is a leading cause of death and disability among children and young adults in the United States, and it results in over 2500 childhood deaths, 37,000 hospitalizations, and 435,000 emergency department visits *each year*.[1] Head injury in infancy results in higher morbidity and mortality than that seen in older children, and it has become increasingly clear that the significant incidence of inflicted injury in the youngest patients is in large part responsible for this difference.[2-5] Skull fracture, intracranial bleeding, and traumatic axonal injury are the most common findings in serious head injuries in infancy and those associated with non-accidental causes. Determining the biomechanical conditions that cause these injuries and others in infants and older children will yield more effective prevention, diagnosis, and treatment strategies, as well as provide valuable information to help discern between accidental and inflicted injury etiologies.

MECHANICS OF TRAUMATIC BRAIN INJURY

Head injuries often occur with rapid head accelerations or decelerations that produce injurious brain deformations, or head impact that can deform or fracture the skull and produce underlying local brain deformations. Most frequently, both inertial (acceleration-deceleration) and contact mechanisms occur together such as in motor vehicle crashes, falls, and accidental and abusive impacts. Although rapid accelerations can be linear or rotational, high angular acceleration and velocity of the head are often correlated with intracranial hemorrhages and traumatic axonal injury in the brain.[6-12]

The underlying pathology of traumatic diffuse axonal injury (DAI) is the widespread damage to axons in the white matter of the brain, and the level of immediate neurological impairment is correlated with the extent and severity of axonal damage.[13] Biomechanical analyses of primate and porcine inertial models of DAI indicate a link between brain material deformation (tissue strain) and white matter injury.[14,15] Galbraith[16,17] confirmed this finding, showing that uniaxial tensile strain, not stress, caused short- and long-term neural dysfunction in unmyelinated axons. Subdural hematomas (SDHs) are caused by the rupture of the parasagittal bridging veins. In a primate inertial model for SDH,[18] biomechanical analysis revealed strong association of SDH with the elongation of the bridging veins beyond their ultimate or rupture strain as the brain moved relative to the skull during sudden acceleration or deceleration.[11] Taken together, these studies demonstrate that tissue deformation is closely associated with the primary axonal and vascular damage found in DAI and SDH.

Previous studies have attempted to define head injury tolerances for adults and children by determining the maximum load experienced by the head without injury. The most common head injury load tolerance, used extensively in automobile occupant safety research, is the head injury criterion (HIC), which is calculated from the acceleration of a head motion over a certain time interval.[19] Unfortunately, the HIC was derived from impact experiments on adult cadavers, does not differentiate between rotational and translational loads, and is not sensitive to the direction of head movement, making it an ineffective parameter for pediatric head injury.

Traditionally, a biomechanical analysis of head injury in the infant and young child assumes that they respond as miniature adults, with identical tissue properties and injury thresholds.[19-23] Using an engineering approach called *dimensional analysis*, critical inertial loading conditions associated with SDH and DAI can be scaled from the adult to the infant as a function of brain mass.[24,25] These analyses conclude that the lower brain mass of the young child allows the pediatric brain to sustain higher rotational accelerations than its adult counterpart before the onset of injury. However, differences between adults and children in tissue composition, mechanical properties, and brain vulnerability can influence the predictions of injury from scaling. As we describe later in this chapter, studies have shown significant age-related differences in brain and skull properties, indicating that the pediatric head cannot be modeled as a miniature adult head. Unfortunately, the biomechanical data used in most scaling approaches involve adult tissue composition, mechanical properties, and injury thresholds, and so must be interpreted with caution. Pediatric biomechanical models incorporating age-specific data are necessary to accurately mimic the pediatric head response to impact or rotation.

MATERIAL RESPONSE OF PEDIATRIC BRAIN AND SKULL TO LOADS

To date, human,[26] porcine,[26,27] and rodent[28] brain tissue testing studies reveal that when undergoing large deformations, the immature brain is approximately twice as stiff as adult brain. This finding is due, in part, to the presence of unmyelinated axons in the pediatric brain. Biomechanical models have reported that axons, rather than the surrounding matrix of astrocytes and oligodendrocytes, contribute more effectively to the stiffness of brain tissue.[29] Lipids have a low shear modulus,[30] suggesting that the increasing volume of myelin in the brain will decrease the effective shear modulus (stiffness) of brain tissue. Axons in the pediatric brain are undergoing rapid myelination during the first year of life and do not reach adult levels of myelination until approximately 18 months old. Although the pediatric brain is stiffer than adult brain, two studies[31,32] found human pediatric dural tissue to be approximately half as stiff as adult dura,[33] assuming similar thicknesses across age. Because the meninges provide support and protection to the brain during trauma, the pediatric brain might be less protected against loads than the adult brain. Material tests on pia and arachnoid in children and adults, however, is needed before this assertion can be made.

At birth, the skull begins as a single cortical bone layer approximately 1 mm thick, but as the bone continues to develop, the single layer of cortical bone differentiates into three layers: an outer table of cortical bone, middle spongy diploe layer, and an inner table of cortical bone, with a composite thickness of 5 to 6 mm. In a series of studies on fetal cranial bone, McPherson and Kriewall[34,35] report a significant increase in cranial bone stiffness (elastic modulus) with increased fetal development (20-40 weeks' gestation). More recently, Coats and Margulies[36] measured the elastic modulus in infants (36 weeks' gestation to 1 year) and found an increase in stiffness with age, such that the adult modulus is more than 30 times higher than the 1-month-old infant,[37] the 1-year-old is 18 times higher than the infant,[36] and the adult is 1.5 times higher than the 6-year-old.[38] Human infant cranial suture was 35 times lower than pediatric cranial bone, and tolerated significantly larger deformations prior to fracture or rupture, indicating that the infant braincase can withstand large shape distortions prior to fracture, unlike the adult skull.[36]

ANIMAL MODELS OF PEDIATRIC TRAUMATIC BRAIN INJURY

In adult head injury, limits of acceleration associated with concussion have been suggested based on measurements made from instrumented football players[39] and boxers,[40] and those specific for SDH and DAI have been suggested based on scaled rotational accelerations from inertial head injury studies in adult primates.[19,41] In pediatric head injury, there are no human data on load tolerances causing concussion, SDH, or DAI, but pediatric animal models are used to investigate mechanisms of brain injury under controlled impact or inertial conditions. Most pediatric animal models for head injury have evaluated the effect of contusional brain injury on the immature rat brain.[42-44] These models have

been particularly useful in characterizing the focal injuries that often occur with head impact, primarily to the gray matter.[43-48]

Adelson and colleagues[47] have developed a model of diffuse brain injury in 17-day-old rats. However, unlike humans, rodents have lissencephalic brains and little white matter, as well as a very different maturational sequence from humans. With little white matter, DAI is difficult to characterize in the rat.[6,49] Developmentally, the rodent brain has its growth spurt entirely in the postnatal period, whereas humans peak in brain growth at the time of birth,[50] and the small brain size of rodents poses challenging biomechanical constraints when designing a device to create an animal model for inertial injury (widespread axonal injury, SDH). Because biomechanical analysis of mechanisms of pediatric brain injury depends on animal models that include salient differences between human infant and adult brains, such as differential development of the gray and white matter, regional cerebral metabolism and blood flow, changes in receptor density and distribution at different ages, and changes in biomechanical properties, rodent models are limited in their ability to provide data relevant to understanding head injury in human infants and young children.[51]

In contrast, piglets provide many advantages in modeling the immature human brain; the overall shape, gyral pattern, and distribution of gray and white matter is similar in pigs and humans. The growth pattern of the postnatal brain is similar to that of human infants; brain weight nearly doubles between the neonatal and juvenile periods and triples to reach the adult weight.[50,52,53] The response of the piglet to hypoxia and ischemia appears to parallel that in human infants. Cerebral blood flow and metabolism are similar, and the piglet brain matures in a similar manner with respect to myelination and brain electrical activity.[50,54-58] Visual-evoked response remains immature until 2 weeks after birth.[59] Whereas rodent models of TBI have limited their focus to only contusion injury, piglet TBI models have investigated fluid percussion[45] and inertial rotation injuries,[12] in addition to contusion injury,[60-63] that produce distributed white matter and SDH in infant and juvenile pigs.

Some fluid percussion studies report the pediatric brain to be more vulnerable to injury,[44,45] whereas other weight-drop (contusional) studies report no significant differences between the adult and pediatric animals.[64] The applied load in these studies, however, is not precisely scaled across age for infants and adults. In a study with the applied load scaled to age, Duhaime et al[61] produced cortical lesions across three age groups of piglets (5 day "infant," 1 month "toddler," and 4 months "adolescent") and reported that 1 week after injury the infant piglets had the smallest cortical lesion, and the adolescent group had the largest at 1 week after injury, indicating that the younger infant brain was either less vulnerable to acute injury and/or was able to have a quicker recovery than the older pigs. In inertial injury studies in piglets and adult pigs experiencing the same angular velocity and acceleration, Raghupathi and Margulies[12] reported at only 6 hours after injury that the piglets had 3.4 times more injured axons per area than the adults, indicating that the pediatric brain is more vulnerable to acute rotational injury than the adult. A later study by Duhaime and colleagues[65] confirmed age-dependent temporal pattern, such that lesion volume 1 day after cortical impact injury in infant piglets was larger than adolescents, but that lesion volume for the infant pigs was smaller at 7 days and 30 days after injury. Finally, in a subsequent study from the Margulies lab,[66] repeated rapid horizontal head rotation 15 minutes after the initial rotation produced significantly more regions of injured axons than animals experiencing a single rotation, suggesting a cumulative effect of injury.

Interestingly, recent data indicate that there is a directional dependence on pediatric head injury,[67] with sagittal rotations resulting in the worst clinical findings with the greatest loss of consciousness, 100% apnea, and lowest cerebral blood flow, and the best outcomes from coronal rotations. Inertial head injury studies in the adult primate also report significant effects of rotational direction on brain trauma,[7,68] but differences between head and neck orientation in the biped compared with the quadruped make direct comparison difficult. In summary, animal models demonstrate that injury severity depends on developmental age, rotational direction and/or impact location, time after the injury, the number of insults to the brain, and the time between those insults.

Although animal models are useful for determination of injury response and time course, as well as development of new diagnosis and treatment strategies, they cannot be used to determine local tissue deformations that are primarily responsible for acute TBI, or determining minimum accelerations or impact forces necessary to produce concussion, SDH, or DAI. The inability to measure intracranial deformations hinders the extension of these animal model results to other types of loads (faster rates, different directions, distributed rather than focal loads) and to humans.

MECHANISMS OF ABUSIVE HEAD TRAUMA

In infants and toddlers, the majority of serious TBI is due to child abuse,[2] and abused children with brain injury have a worse outcome than those with accidental brain injury.[69] Although contact head trauma is a frequent finding in abusive head trauma,[70] many researchers believe that shaking alone can cause SDH, retinal hemorrhage, and death.[71,72] These authors argue that the lack of evidence of contact injury (skull fracture, cranial bruising, or scalp swelling) is evidence of shaking alone. If the infant's head strikes a padded surface such as a mattress, however, the force of the impact is widely dissipated and might not be associated with evidence of impact, even though the brain decelerates rapidly. The mechanism of injury responsible for SDH, retinal hemorrhage, and skeletal trauma that characterize abusive head trauma has been debated during the past decade. Duhaime et al[21] suggested that impact was necessary for SDH by demonstrating that the magnitude of angular deceleration is 45 times as great when an infant anthropomorphic surrogate model's head is struck as when it is shaken alone, and that the thresholds for concussion, SDH and DAI are exceeded at the moment of impact. Prange and others[73] later confirmed these findings and demonstrated that vigorous shaking produces accelerations that are significantly smaller than the rebound the head experiences from a 1-foot fall onto concrete. Unfortunately, surrogates only yield insight into the accelerations and contact loads experienced during a fall or simulated abusive scenario and cannot predict injuries. Furthermore, the utility of surrogates is compromised when their biofidelity or humanness (e.g., resistance of the neck to flexion/extension, compliance of the head and thorax, mass of the head/torso/limbs) is not considered in the construction of the surrogate. As more data regarding the kinematics and mechanical properties of children become available, the response of surrogates should be validated with human child data to ensure that they mimic children's responses.

COMPUTATIONAL MODELS OF PEDIATRIC HEAD INJURY

To relate the deformation occurring within the brain to a specific applied contact force or acceleration-deceleration of the head, finite element computational models are often used. These computational models are useful in extending the experimental results beyond scenarios tested in the experiments and to develop prevention and protection strategies. Many computational models of brain injury have been developed for the adult, but only a few have been developed for the child.[74-79] Many of these models have idealizations that can limit their validity, such as the use of simplified material properties and geometries. If assigned realistic parameters, computational models are a powerful tool to predict the stress and strain distributions throughout the brain, but are not capable of predicting the incidence of tissue injury. Tissue injury thresholds, or specific mechanical limits of the tissue related to functional or structural failure, must be developed to determine whether a focal tissue distortion predicted by the model would produce a specific injury, such as edema or axonal injury.

ROLE OF BIOMECHANICS IN ABUSIVE HEAD TRAUMA

Biomechanics provides empirical data regarding the global and focal mechanisms of head injury. Each biomechanical tool (animal experiments, human and animal tissue testing, anthropomorphic surrogate studies, and computational models) provides a crucial piece of the puzzle, but the best approach to understanding mechanisms of head injuries in child abuse is to combine the information from each of these tools and compare with data from clinical studies to answer the question: What mechanisms cause what injuries in children of what age? Before a comprehensive answer can be given, however, more research is needed to define tissue injury thresholds and to create biofidelic anthropomorphic surrogates and computational models that mimic the child's responses. Continued research in these areas will open pathways for enhanced traumatic head injury prevention, detection, and treatment strategies specific to infants and toddlers.

References

1. Langlois JA, Rutland-Brown W, Thomas KE: *Traumatic Brain Injury in the United States: Emergency Department Visits, Hospitalizations, and Deaths.*

Centers for Disease Control and Prevention, National Center for Injury Prevention and Control, Atlanta, 2004.

2. Billmire ME, Myers PA: Serious head injury in infants: accident or abuse? *Pediatrics* 1985;75:340-342.

3. Duhaime AC, Alario AJ, Lewander WJ, et al: Head injury in very young children: Mechanisms, injury types, and ophthalmologic findings in 100 hospitalized patients under two years of age. *Pediatrics* 1992;90:179-185.

4. Luerssen TG, Bruce DA, Humphreys RP: Position statement on identifying the infant with nonaccIdental central nervous system injury (the whiplash-shake syndrome). The American Society of Pediatric Neurosurgeons. *Pediatr Neurosurg* 1993;19:170.

5. Luerssen TG, Huang JC, McLone DG, et al: Retinal hemorrhages, seizures, and intracranial hemorhages: relationships and outcomes in children suffering traumatic brain injury. *In:* Marlin AE: *Concepts in Pediatric Neurosurgery,* vol 11. Karger, Basel, Switzerland, 1991, pp 87-94.

6. Gennarelli TA: The spectrum of traumatic axonal injury. *Neuropath Appl Neurobiol* 1996;22:509-513.

7. Gennarelli TA, Thibault LE, Adams JH, et al: Diffuse axonal injury and traumatic coma in the primate. *Ann Neurol* 1982;12:564-574.

8. Gennarelli TL, Thibault LE, Ommaya A: Pathophsiological response to rotational and translational accelerations of the head. *SAE Transactions* 1972;720970:797-803.

9. Gennarelli TA, Thibault LE: Biomechanics of acute subdural hematoma. *J Trauma* 1982;22:680-686.

10. Margulies SS, Meaney DF, Smith D, et al*: A comparison of diffuse brain injury in the newborn and adult pig.* International Research Committee on the Biokinetics of Impact, Barcelona, Spain, 1999.

11. Meaney DF: *Biomechanics of acute subdural hematoma in the subhuman primate and man (PhD Thesis),* University of Pennsylvania, 1991.

12. Raghupathi R, Margulies SS: Traumatic axonal injury after closed head injury in the neonatal pig. *J Neurotrauma* 2002;19:843-853.

13. Gennarelli TA, Thibault LE: Biological models of head injury. *In:* Becker DP, Povlishock JT: *Central Nervous System Trauma Status Report.* National Institutes of Health, National Institute of Neurological & Communicative Disorders & Stroke, 1985, pp 391-404.

14. Margulies SL, Thibault LE, Gennarelli TA: Physical model simulations of brain injury in the primate. *J Biomech* 1990;23:823-836.

15. Miller RT, Margulies SS, Leoni M, et al: Finite element modeling approaches for predicting injury in an experimental model of severe diffuse axonal injury. *In: Proceedings of 42nd Stapp Car Crash Conference.* Society of Automotive Engineers, Tempe, AZ, 1998.

16. Galbraith JA: *The effects of mechanical loading on the electrophysiology of the squid giant axon PhD Thesis.* University of Pennsylvania, 1988.

17. Galbraith JA, Thibault LE, Matteson DR: Mechanical and electrical responses of the squid giant axon to simple elongation. *J Biomech Eng* 1993;115:13-22.

18. Thibault LE, Gennarelli TA: Biomechanics of acute subdural hematoma. *J Trauma* 1982:22:680-686.

19. Margulies SS, Thibault LE: A proposed tolerance criterion for diffuse axonal injury in man. *J Biomech* 1992;25:917-923.

20. Dejeammes, M, Tarriáfre C, Thomas T, et al: Exploration of biomechanical data towards a better evaluation of tolerance for children involved in automotive accidents. *SAE Transactions* 1984;#840530:427-441.

21. Duhaime AC, Gennarelli TA, Thibault LE, et al: The shaken baby syndrome: a clinical, pathological, and biomechanical study. *J Neurosurg* 1987;66:409-415.

22. Mohan D, Bowman BM, Snyder RG, et al: A biomechanical analysis of head impact injuries to children. *J Biomech Eng* 1979;101:250-260.

23. Sturtz G: Biomechanical data of children. *SAE Transactions* #801313 1980:513-559.

24. Ommaya AK, Fisch FJ, Mahone RM, et al: Comparative tolerances for cerebral concussion by head impact and whiplash injury in primates. *SAE transactions* #700401, 1970.

25. Ommaya AK, Yarnell P, Hirsch AE: Scaling of experimental data on cerebral concussion in sub-human primates to concussion threshold for man. *In: Proceedings of 11th Stapp Car Crash Conference.* Society of Automotive Engineers, Los Angeles, 1967.

26. Prange MT: *Comparative tolerances for cerebral concussion by head impact and whiplash injury in primates (PhD thesis).* University of Pennsylvania, Philadelphia, 2002.

27. Prange MT, Margulies SS: Regional, directional, and age-dependent properties of brain undergoing large deformation. *J Biomech Eng* 2002;124:244-252.

28. Gefen A, Genen N, Zhu Q, et al: Age-dependent changes in material properties of the brain and braincase of the rat. *J Neurotrauma* 2003;20:1163-1177.

29. Arbogast KB, Margulies SS: A fiber-reinforced composite model of the viscoelastic behaviour of the brainstem in shear. *J Biomech* 1999;32:865-870.

30. Yamada H: *Strength of Biological Materials.* Williams and Wilkins, Baltimore, 1990.

31. Bylski DI, Kriewall TJ, Akkas N, et al: Mechanical behavior of fetal dura mater under large deformation biaxial tension. *J Biomech* 1986;19:19-26.

32. Kriewall TJ, Akkas N, Bylski DI, et al: Mechanical behavior of fetal dura mater under large axisymmetric inflation. *J Biomech Eng* 1983;105:71-76.

33. Galford JE, McElhaney JH: A viscoelastic study of scalp, brain, and dura. *J Biomech* 1970;3:211-221.

34. Kriewall TJ: Structural, mechanical, and material properties of fetal cranial bone. *Am J Obstet Gynecol* 1982;142:707-714.

35. McPherson GK, Kriewall TJ: The elastic modulus of fetal cranial bone: a first step toward understanding of the biomechanics of fetal head molding. *J Biomech* 1980;13:9-16.

36. Coats B, Margulies SS: Material properties of human infant skull and suture at high rates. *J Neurotrauma* 2006;23:1222-1232.

37. McElhaney JH, Gogle JL, Melvin JW, et al: Mechanical properties of cranial bone. *J Biomech* 1970;3:495-511.

38. Hubbard RP: Flexure of layered cranial none. *J Biomech* 1971;4:251-263.

39. Pellmen EJ, Viano DC, Tucker AM, et al: Concussion in professional football: reconstruction of game impacts and injuries. *Neurosurgery* 2003;53:799-814.

40. Breton F, Fincemaille Y, Tarriere C, et al: Event-related potential assessment of attention and the orienting reaction in boxers before and after a fight. *Biol Psychol* 1991;31:57-71.

41. Gennarelli TA, Abel JM, Adams H, et al: Differential tolerance of frontal and temporal lobes to contusion induced by angular acceleration. *In: Proceedings of the 23rd Stapp Car Crash Conference,* 1979.

42. Bittigau P, Sifringer M, Pohl D, et al: Apoptotic neurodegeneration following trauma is markedly enhanced in the immature brain. *Ann Neurol* 1999;24:724-735.

43. Grundy PD, Biagas KV, Kochanek PM, et al: Early cerebrovascular response to head injury in immature and mature rats. *J Neurotrauma* 1994;11:135-148.

44. Prins ML, Lee SM, Cheng CL, et al: Fluid percussion brain injury in the developing and adult rat: a comparative study of mortality, morphology, intracranial pressure and mean arterial blood pressure. *Brain Res Dev Brain Res* 1996;95:272-282.

45. Armstead WM, Kurth CD: Different cerebral hemodynamic responses following fluid percussion brain injury in the newborn and juvenile pig. *J Neurotrauma* 1994;11:487-497.

46. Giza CC, Griesbach GS, Hovda DA: Experience-dependent behavioral plasticity is disturbed following traumatic injury to the immature brain. *Behav Brain Res* 2005;157:11-22.

47. Adelson PD, Robichaud P, Hamilton RL, et al: A model of diffuse traumatic brain injury in the immature rat. *J Neurosurg* 1996;85:877-884.

48. Bittigau P, Sifinger M, Pohl D, et al: Apoptotic neurodegeneration following trauma is markedly enhanced in the immature brain. *Ann Neurol* 1999;45:724-735.

49. Meaney DF, Lenkinski RE, Alsop DC, et al: Biomechanical analysis of experimental diffuse axonal injury. *J Neurotrauma* 1995;12:689-694.

50. Dickerson JW, Dobbing J: Prenatal and postnatal growth and development of the central nervous system of the pig. *Proc R Soc London* 1966;166:384-395.

51. Gennarelli TA: Animate models of human head injury. *J Neurotrauma* 1994;11:357-368.

52. Coppoletta JM, Wolbach SB: Body length and organ weights of infants and children. *Am J Pathol* 1933;9:55-70.

53. Thomas JM, Beamer JL: Age-weight relationships of selected organs and body weight for miniature swine. *Growth* 1971;35;259-272.

54. Pampiglione G: Some aspects of development of cerebral function in mammals. *Proc R Soc Med* 1971;64:429-435.

55. Wagerle LC, Kumar SP, Delivoria-Papadopoulos M: Effect of sympathetic nerve stimulation on cerebral blood flow in newborn piglets. *Pediatr Res* 1986;20:131-135.

56. Buckley NM: Maturation of circulatory system in three mammalian models of human development. *Comp Biochem Physiol A Comp Physiol* 1986;83:1-7.

57. Aminoff MJ: Electroencephalography, *In:* Berg BO (ed): *Principles of Child Neurology.* McGraw-Hill, New York, 1996, pp 23-38.

58. Sarnat HB: Neuroembryology. *In:* Berg BO (ed): *Principles of Child Neurology.* McGraw-Hill, New York, 1996, pp 607-628.

59. Mattsson JL, Fry WN, Boward CA, et al: Maturation of the visual evoked response in newborn miniature pigs. *Am J Vet Res* 1978;29:1279-1281.

60. Madsen FF, Reske-Nielsen E: A simple mechanical model using a piston to produce localized cerebral contusions in pigs. *Acta Neurochir (Wien)* 1987;88:65-72.

61. Duhaime AC, Margulies SS, Durham SR, et al: Maturation-dependent response of the piglet brain to scaled cortical impact. *J Neurosurg* 2000;93:455-462.

62. Madsen FF: Changes in regional cerebral blood flow after hyperventilation in the pig with an induced focal cerebral contusion. *Acta Neurochir (Wien)* 1990;106:164-169.

63. Madsen FF: Regional cerebral blood flow in the pig after a localized cerebral contusion treated with barbiturates. *Acta Neurochir (Wien)* 1990;106:24-31.

64. Adelson PD, Robichaud P, Hamilton RL, et al: A model of diffuse traumatic brain injury in the immature rat. *J Neurosurg* 1996;85:877-884.

65. Duhaime AC, Hunter JV, Grate LL, et al: Magnetic resonance imaging studies of age-dependent responses to scaled focal brain injury in the piglet. *J Neurosurg* 2003;99:542-548.

66. Raghupathi R, Mehr MF, Helfaer MA, et al: Traumatic axonal injury is exacerbated following repetitive close head injury in the neonatal pig. *J Neurotrauma* 2004;21:307-316.

67. Eucker S: *Regional cerebral blood flow response following brain injury depends on direction of head motion.* Presented at the National Neurotrauma Society, Orlando, FL, 2008.

68. Gennarelli TA, Thibault L, Tomei G, et al: *Directional dependence of axonal brain injury due to centroidal and non-centroidal acceleration.* 31st Stapp Car Crash Conference, 1987.

69. Ewing-Cobbs L, Kramer L, Prasad M, et al: Neuroimaging, physical, and developmental findings after inflicted and noninflicted traumatic brain injury in young children. *Pediatrics* 1998;102:300-307.

70. Gilliland MG, Folberg R: Shaken babies—some have no impact injuries. *J Forensic Sci* 1996;41:114-116.

71. Alexander R, Sato Y, Smith W, et al: Incidence of impact trauma with cranial injuries ascribed to shaking. *Am J Dis Child* 1990;144:724-726.

72. Hadley MN, Sonntag VK, Rekate HL, et al: The infant whiplash-shake injury syndrome: a clinical and pathological study. *Neurosurgery* 1989;24:536-540.

73. Prange MT, Coats B, Duhaime AC, et al: Anthropomorphic simulations of falls, shakes, and inflicted impacts in infants. *J Neurosurg* 2003;99:143-150.

74. Lapeer RJ, Prager RW: Fetal head moulding: finite element analysis of a fetal skull subjected to uterine pressures during the first stage of labour. *J Biomech* 2001;34:1125-1133.

75. Desantis Klinich K, Hulbert GM, Schneider LW: Estimating infant head injury criteria and impact response using crash reconstruction and finite element modeling. *Stapp Car Crash J* 2002;46:165-194.

76. Coats B, Margulies SS, Ji S: Parametric study of head impact in the infant. *Stapp Car Crash J* 2007;51:1-15.

77. Roth S, Raul JS, Ludes B, et al: Finite element analysis of impact and shaking inflicted to a child. *Int J Legal Med* 2007;121:223-228.

78. Roth S, Raul JS, Ludes B, et al: Biofidelic child head FE model to simulate real world trauma. *Comput Methods Programs Biomed* 2008;90:262-274.

79. Coats B, Margulies SS: Potential for head injuries in infants from low-height falls. *J Neurosurg Pediatr* 2008;2:321-330.

41

THE CASE FOR SHAKING

Mark S. Dias, MD, FAAP

INTRODUCTION

A causal link between abusive trauma and subdural hemorrhages (SDHs) during infancy was first proposed by Guthkelch[1] in 1972. Shortly thereafter Caffey[2,3] suggested the term *whiplash shaken infant syndrome* to describe infants with abusive subdural and retinal hemorrhages but without external evidence of physical trauma. The term *shaken baby syndrome* (SBS) has been used subsequently to describe the combination of intracranial injury (brain injury and/or intracranial hemorrhage) and retinal hemorrhages from an abusive mechanism involving a rotational acceleration of the head caused by violent infant shaking. Intracranial injuries include acute and/or chronic SDH, axonal injury (AI), gliding contusions, cortical tears, and intracerebral edema. Retinal hemorrhages are reported in 30% to 100% of cases; averaging several series yields an approximate frequency of about 80%.[4]

In 1987 Duhaime and colleagues[5] in a landmark study reported evidence of impact injury in 63% of cases, and 100% of fatal cases of SBS. Subsequent publications have confirmed evidence of impact (e.g., scalp ecchymosis, soft tissue swelling, and skull fracture) in many infants with abusive head injuries. Duhaime's study also evaluated the accelerational forces generated by both shaking and impact using doll models, comparing these forces with established injury thresholds and suggesting that the forces acting on an infant's head during shaking alone were insufficient to cause SDH or AI. In this study only impact could generate forces sufficient to reach these injury thresholds, leading the authors to suggest that the term *shaken impact syndrome* was a better description of the causal mechanisms involved. The American Academy of Pediatrics has recently recommended that the term *abusive head trauma* (AHT) be used to avoid drawing any conclusions about the underlying mechanistic cause of the injuries.[6]

Over the past several years, the relationship between shaking and intracranial injury has come under intense scrutiny and criticism, with several authors questioning the assertion that shaking alone can achieve established injury thresholds for SDH or brain injury, and therefore, infant shaking, no matter how violent, cannot cause or contribute to the pathophysiology of AHT.[7-10] The logical conclusion is that abusive head trauma cannot be alleged in the absence of physical signs of external injury from impact, leading to widely disparate expert medical opinion in individual court cases about whether or not abuse has occurred. The arguments against shaking reached such a fevered pitch in the

United Kingdom that all such cases were re-reviewed and in three cases sentences were changed based, in part, upon a "new understanding" of the biomechanics of infant shaking.

Unfortunately, nobody has yet marshaled a coherent and comprehensive argument in support of shaking as a causal mechanism for abusive head injury. This chapter reviews the available literature to make such an argument, emphasizing the following key concepts:

1. The biomechanical data regarding various injury thresholds are based upon experimental observations performed in *adult primates*. There is no evidence to support that injury thresholds derived from these studies are applicable to infant brains, and recent evidence suggests that injury thresholds in infant brains are considerably less than in adults.
2. The experimental primate studies used single-cycle rotational injuries with approximately 30-msec cycle times; there is no evidence that the injury thresholds derived from these experiments are applicable to the biomechanical parameters (repetitive 250- to 350-msec cycle times) during violent infant shaking.
3. Recent studies also suggest that secondary metabolic responses of infants to head injuries are both quantitatively and qualitatively different than in older children or adults; moreover, those injuries identified as abusive in nature by clinical criteria seem to engender an even greater secondary metabolic response.
4. These metabolic responses might reflect developmental *critical periods* during which the infant is uniquely susceptible to the effects of head injury and particularly to abusive head injuries. The injury thresholds for initiating these cascades have not been determined.
5. The clinical spectrum (both neurological presentation as well as neuroimaging and pathological findings) that follows *accidental* head injuries in infants and children has been well described in the literature in numerous publications. The extent, character, profile, and pattern of these accidental injuries are overwhelmingly consistent, and are wholly different from both the types and pattern of inflicted injuries.
6. A number of studies have addressed the clinical and pathological features of admitted (or confessed) cases of abusive head injury. Although evidence of blunt force trauma (impact) is reported in 20% to 63% of these cases (even among those cases in which only shaking was admitted), violent infant shaking remains a strikingly

common element in these confessions, with shaking admitted in up to 71%. In addition, a well-documented case of "shaken adult syndrome" having retinal and SDHs and AI has been described,[11] suggesting that shaking can be injurious even beyond infancy.

7. Although it is obvious that some of these confessions are erroneous, *in order to accept the thesis that shaking alone cannot achieve injury thresholds for brain injury or intracranial hemorrhage, every case of admitted shaking would have to involve numerous systematic and consistent lies*, something that defies logic.

BIOMECHANICS

A Brief Primer

A number of elegant biomechanical analyses of infant shaking have already been published. (See references 12 and 13 for examples of contrasting views.) In this text, Margulies provides a more detailed analysis of the biomechanics of AHT. (See Chapter 40, "Biomechanics of Head Trauma in Infants and Young Children.") A brief review, however, will help to better understand the arguments put forth by various authors. A *force* (measured in Newtons), when applied to an object (such as the brain) will result in a deformation, the magnitude of which will depend upon the magnitude and direction of the force, the rate at which the force is applied, the surface area over which the force is applied, and the *intrinsic material properties of the object to which the force is applied*. *Stress* is defined as the force divided by the surface area over which the force is applied (measured in Newtons/m², or Pascals). The application of force to an object results in a *deformation* of the object. The amount of deformation is called *strain*. The *Elastic (or Young's) Modulus* is the ratio of stress to strain and is a constant for any uniform material. The smaller the elastic modulus, the more readily deformation occurs.

An *elastic* deformation is one in which the deformation is proportional to the force applied and is entirely reversible. The brain and skull, however, like many biological substances, are *viscoelastic*, meaning that the elastic properties will vary depending upon the rate of application of a force. For events of short duration in which the force is rapidly applied, the brain is relatively resistant to deformation (i.e., it is relatively "stiff"). In contrast, for events of longer duration during which forces are applied more slowly, deformation is greater (i.e., the brain is "less stiff"). For short duration events, the deformation, or strain, is proportional to force multiplied by the time. Since force is directly proportional to mass times the acceleration (F = ma) and velocity is proportional to acceleration times the time (v = at), then the strain for events of short duration is proportional to mass and velocity; strain is dependent more upon the velocity of an applied load for short duration loads. For events of longer duration, the acceleration of the applied load is the more critical factor.

Studies of the biomechanics of traumatic brain injuries began with Holbourn's studies in 1943,[14] which suggested that brain injury results from shear strains in which tissues deform as they translate past one another in a gliding fashion, rather than by compressive or tensile strains in which the tissues are either compressed or pulled apart. He postulated that *impact loading* (a focal blow) to a stationary head results

in localized deformation of the skull and underlying brain, inducing maximal shearing in the superficial tissues and producing *superficial contusions*. In contrast, *impulse loading*, or accelerational brain injuries, produce higher degrees of diffuse shear strain that is distributed deeper in the brain substance. He suggested that *linear* acceleration produces primarily compressive strains and therefore little deformation (since brain is relatively incompressible), whereas *rotational* acceleration produces higher degrees of shear strain that would be more injurious. He also recognized the importance of viscoelasticity in the generation of brain injuries and proposed that the transition between short-duration (velocity-dependent) events and long-duration (acceleration-dependent) events occurred at 2 to 200 msec. Finally, he concluded that sagittal rotations produced the greatest midline shear and therefore were most likely to injure the bridging parasagittal veins and produce SDH. These strains were reproduced in gelatin brain models that, although lacking some important features (such as the falx and tentorium), nonetheless supported these basic conclusions.

Applicability of Biomechanical Studies to Human Infant Shaking

Experimental verification of Holbourne's theories came during the 1960s with studies by Gennarelli, Thibault, Ommaya, and others at the University of Pennsylvania.[15-19] In these studies, *adult non-human primates* were subjected to rapid single accelerations of increasing magnitude while seated on a sled, with the head either immobilized (producing linear head acceleration) or not (producing angular acceleration). Critical thresholds capable of producing loss of consciousness (concussion), SDH, and AI were established in three different primate species having different brain masses. These results suggested (1) The thresholds for rotational velocity and acceleration were on average 50% higher for whiplash events not associated with impact compared with those events associated with impact, (2) the critical thresholds were inversely proportional to the brain mass (specifically [brain mass]^{2/3}) in the three species examined (Figure 41-1), and (3) SDH was more frequent following short-duration events lasting 5 msec or less, whereas AI more commonly followed longer-duration events lasting >6 msec. It is important to again point out that these injury thresholds were established for *adult non-human primates undergoing single cycle accelerational events*.

In 1987 Duhaime and colleagues[5] attempting to biomechanically model the forces that could be generated by shaking and impact, studied a "biofidelic" doll model having a head filled with wet cotton to approximate the weight distribution of a human infant head. Peak velocities and accelerations generated by either shaking the doll or impacting the doll against either a hard or soft surface were compared against the established injury thresholds derived from the previous experimental primate studies. Duhaime concluded that shaking alone (with cycle times of approximately 100-250 msec) achieved maximum velocities and accelerations well below the identified thresholds for SDH or AI (Figure 41-2). On the other hand, impact injuries against hard or soft surfaces (with cycle times of approximately 30 msec) consistently exceeded these injury thresholds. The authors concluded that shaking *alone* was unlikely to generate

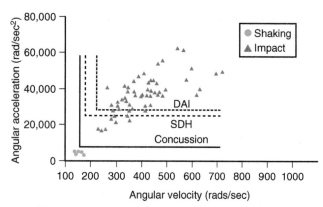

FIGURE 41-1 Illustration of injury thresholds for producing diffuse axonal injury *(DAI)*, subdural hemorrhage and concussion as derived from adult primate data. *(Adapted from Duhaime AC, Gennarelli TA, Thibault LE, et al: The shaken baby syndrome. A clinical, pathological, and biomechanical study. J Neurosurg 1987;66:409-415.)*

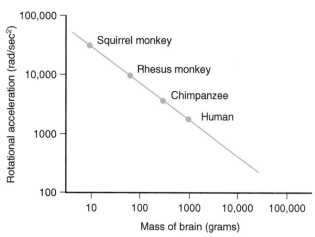

FIGURE 41-2 Relationship between injury thresholds in various species based upon mass scaling. Thresholds were experimentally derived from adult specimens of each of the three primate species studied; theoretical injury thresholds for adult humans are extrapolated from the experimental data on primates assuming the injury threshold is proportional to $1/m^{2/3}$, where m = brain mass. *(Adapted from Ommaya AK, Fisch FJ, Mahone RM, et al. Comparative tolerances for cerebral concussion by head impact and whiplash injury in primates. Warrendale, PA, 1970, Society of Automotive Engineers.)*

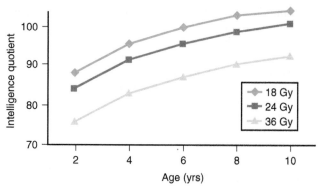

FIGURE 41-3 Effect of age on the effect of external beam whole brain radiation therapy on the intelligence quotient (IQ). For each radiation dose, the IQ declines as the therapy is delivered at progressively younger ages. *(Adapted from Silber JH, Radcliffe J, Peckham V, et al. Whole-brain irradiation and decline in intelligence: The influence of dose and age on IQ score. J Clin Oncol 1992;10:1390-1396.)*

enough force/load to produce SDH and AI described in the SBS and suggested that a *combination of shaking plus impact* was more common, and perhaps even necessary, to achieve the requisite injury thresholds.

The thrust of much of the medical research over the ensuing two decades has focused on proving (or disproving) that shaking alone can (or cannot) achieve the injury thresholds derived from the original experimental primate studies. There are several concerns with both the methodology and underlying assumptions of this line of research. First, the biofidelity of the original Duhaime model, particularly as it relates to the kinetics of neck motion, is in question, and significant differences in peak velocity and acceleration have been achieved simply by varying the parameters of the neck model in various studies.[20-22]

More critical, however, are the difficulties with the underlying assumptions: (1) The differences in thresholds for brain injury (SDH and AI in particular) can be accounted for *solely* by size scaling (smaller brains are less susceptible to injury than are larger brains), (2) brain injury thresholds (after size scaling) are identical for both mature and immature brains, and (3) the injury thresholds for single impulse whiplash injuries as determined in the primate studies are comparable to cyclic impulse loading (shaking). Simply put, *can injury thresholds derived from adult non-human primates undergoing a single acceleration on a sled be reliably extrapolated, using only mass scaling, to a human infant undergoing repetitive shaking?*

An Infant Is not Simply a Small Adult

Although it is intuitively obvious, an infant is not simply a scaled-down adult (and even less, a small adult monkey). A number of physical features of the infant brain are significantly different, including (1) The relative size of the head to the body, (2) the strength of the neck muscles, (3) the water content of the brain, (4) the degree of myelination, and (5) the relative absence of nodes of Ranvier (which in adults form the locus for traumatic AI).

Two well-known examples illustrate the fallibility of using the response to external forces in an adult (or even an older child) to predict the response in an infant. In the first example, the effect of radiation injury to the developing human brain as a function of age, the results are quantitative and predictable—cranial radiation to treat cancer results in a decline in IQ that is dependent upon both the radiation dose and child's age (Figure 41-3). In the second example, the effects of eye patching on vision, the response of the infant is qualitatively different and unexpected compared with the response of the older child or adult. A child >6 years of age undergoing a period of monocular eye patching will sustain no significant lasting visual effects, whereas an infant subjected to the same period of monocular eye patching will suffer a significant and lasting visual loss that is not predicted by the response of the older child.[23]

Experimental evidence from animal models also suggests that the responses of the developing brain to traumatic brain injury (TBI) are significantly different from those of the adult brain. The developing piglet brain is a reasonable model for studying the effects of trauma on developing brain tissue. Experimental evidence has suggested that (1) The developing brain sustains greater injury at a lower threshold than adult brain, and (2) the effects of repetitive impulse loading are cumulative. The elastic shear modulus of the 2- to 3-day piglet brain (corresponding to a 1-month-old human) is significantly lower (that is, the tissue is more readily deformed) than that of the adult porcine brain, suggesting that injury thresholds are significantly lower for infant brains than predicted by simple mass scaling,[24] and no minimum threshold for injury has yet been established for piglet brains. Moreover, piglets subjected to two impulse loads within 15 minutes sustain greater injury at lower peak rotational velocities than do piglets undergoing single impulse loads[25]; the effect of *repetitive cyclic events over seconds* that would be analogous to shaking has not been systematically studied.

Neither has the effect of natural (or harmonic) frequency on brain injury thresholds been examined. The natural frequency is an inherent property of a material that results in a summation of forces that are applied cyclically at the natural frequency. The natural frequency has been estimated at between 5 and 10 Hz (corresponding to cycle times of 100-200 msec) for non-human primate brains, and between 4 and 5 Hz (corresponding to cycle times of 200-250 msec) for human brains.[18,26] The natural frequency for human brain is well within the frequency range for shaking (4-10 Hz) as derived from Duhaime's study.[5] A study by Thibault and Margulies[27] suggests that both adult and infant brains are increasingly susceptible to repetitive (or *oscillatory*) loading at lower frequencies down to 20 Hz, the lowest frequency studied; the effects of lower frequency events have not yet been evaluated.

THE BIOCHEMICAL RESPONSE OF THE DEVELOPING BRAIN TO ABUSIVE HEAD INJURY

Mounting evidence suggests that the biochemical and metabolic responses to head injury are significantly and fundamentally different in the young infant than that of the older child or adult. These biochemical responses are likely developmentally regulated and occur during "critical developmental periods" during which the developing brain is uniquely susceptible to outside forces that at other times would be innocuous. These developmentally regulated critical periods are well known throughout developmental biology and are responsible for the visual loss to monocular eye patching described previously.

The metabolic responses to abusive head injury have been thoroughly reviewed by Kochanek and colleagues,[28-30] and the interested reader is referred to these and other reviews for more complete information. The purpose here is to synthesize and condense the evolving information about this complex topic to explain how the infant response in general, and the response to abusive head injury in particular, differ in important ways from the responses seen in older children and adults. TBI sets in motion a number of metabolic cascades which contribute to *secondary* neuronal injury and death hours or days following injury. These secondary insults can be divided mechanistically into five broad categories: (1) excitotoxicity, (2) ischemia, (3) inflammation, (4) oxidative stress and free radical damage, and (5) apoptosis or programmed cell death. For each, the immature brain has been shown to be more vulnerable than the developed brain and, in many cases, uniquely susceptible to secondary metabolic insults.

Glutamate, an excitatory amino acid, has been implicated as one of the most clinically significant mediators of excitotoxicity both in animal models and in humans. Glutamate exerts its effects through the activation of both *N*-methyl-D-aspartate (NMDA) receptors and non-NMDA receptors. Increased levels of glutamate sufficient to cause neuronal cell death have been described in the cerebrospinal fluid (CSF) of both adults and children after TBI,[31,32] and its effects have been studied extensively. These include the initiation of a calcium-mediated metabolic cascade that leads to activation of intracellular proteases, lipases, and endonucleases; the release of superoxide radicals and nitric oxide; and ultimately, cell death. Ruppel and colleagues[32] demonstrated significantly greater rises in CSF glutamate after TBI both in young children (<4 years of age) and those with abusive injuries. Peak CSF glutamate levels were seven*fold greater* after abusive injuries compared with accidentally injured controls, and the elevations were much more sustained compared with the response to accidental injuries. These studies suggest that TBI in infants can produce a quantitatively different glutamate response, and that abusive injuries appear to be particularly injurious in this regard. Other studies suggest that the metabolic *response* to glutamate is also age dependent. The glutamate NMDA receptor is developmentally regulated with its glutamate-modulated activation producing a greater calcium influx in the immature brain. Intracerebral injection of NMDA produces a much greater degree of damage in immature rat brains than in adults.[33] Finally, developing neurons are more susceptible to this excitotoxic cascade than are mature neurons.

Cerebral ischemia is common in the first 24 hours following TBI and is more common in children than adults.[34] Secondary ischemic injuries play an important role in abusive head injury, particularly in the genesis of the severe global hypodensities or "big black brain" on CT scans commonly seen in abusive head injuries.[35] Diffusion-weighted MRI confirms multifocal and global ischemic abnormalities in these infants without any demonstrated macrovascular (arterial or venous) occlusion on magnetic resonance angiography or venography.[36,37] *In vitro* studies in adult pigs suggest that the brainstem is inherently vulnerable to shear injury compared with the cerebrum,[38] and pathological studies in fatal cases of AHT have found *traumatic* AI at the cervicomedullary junction and upper cervical spinal cord,[12,39-42] with secondary *ischemic* AI at more rostral levels of the neuraxis.[41,42] This has led to the hypothesis that *focal* AI at the lower brainstem, cervicomedullary junction, and/or upper cervical spinal cord can produce transient apnea and/or circulatory changes that lead to global ischemic encephalopathy.[40,41]

Molecular responses to infant TBI might also contribute significantly to ischemic brain injury. Endothelin-1, a peptide with potent vasoconstrictor properties, is significantly increased in the CSF of infants and children with TBI,[43] and in a piglet model of TBI.[44] Endothelin-1 influences cerebral autoregulation in juvenile and particularly newborn piglets, and the response is mitigated by treatment with endothelin-1 antagonists.[44]

Another pair of molecular species, adenosine and vascular endothelial growth factor (VEGF), protects against ischemic injury. Adenosine stimulates the formation of VEGF following TBI. VEGF is vasoactive, angiogenic, and neuroprotective; it increases vascular permeability, stimulates angiogenesis, protects against ischemia, and reduces glutamate-induced excitotoxicity. Although both adenosine and VGEF are increased in CSF following TBI in infants and children, the increase is less following AHT compared with accidental injuries.[45]

Another secondary metabolic injury pathway that is set in motion following TBI results in oxidative cellular damage. Free radicals such as superoxide, hydroxyl radicals, hydrogen peroxide, and oxidative nitrogen species such as peroxynitrite interact with a number of intracellular molecules, causing damage to cell membranes, proteins, and nucleic acids. F2-isoprostane, a marker of lipid peroxidation, is increased in the CSF of children following TBI.[46] In an experimental model of daily shaking in 6-day-old rats, hydroxyl radicals were increased following the third shaking episode; both this oxidative response and intracerebral hemorrhage were diminished by pretreatment with tirilazad, an antioxidant.[47]

A number of inflammatory mediators have been implicated in secondary cellular damage following TBI. Tumor necrosis factor (TNF), interleukin (IL)-1, IL-6, and IL-8 are increased in the CSF of both adults and children following TBI and produce vasomotor paralysis, vasodilation, hyperemia, and tissue edema.[48-50] A number of inflammatory reactants are particularly increased in infants and in victims of abusive head injury including IL-4, IL-6, IL-8, IL-10, IL-12, the soluble intracellular adhesion molecule-1, and quinolinic acid.[51-53] In particular, quinolinic acid rises significantly *earlier* following AHT compared with accidental TBI, which might reflect either prior episodes of head injury or a delay in seeking medical care following AHT.[54,55]

Apoptosis is a developmentally regulated energy-dependent process that results in cell death and is characterized histologically by DNA fragmentation and pyknosis; the resulting DNA fragments are readily identified in immunohistochemical preparations. In contrast, *necrosis* is a cell death resulting from a metabolic failure with swelling and cell lysis. Apoptosis occurs throughout embryogenesis and early childhood and is responsible for a variety of developmentally regulated processes such as remodeling of the digits by elimination of interdigital tissue, and the development of nephrons to form the kidney. Apoptosis in the brain is important for the elimination of neurons and remodeling of intercellular connections during brain and spinal cord development.

Apoptosis is principally regulated by mitochondrial membrane cytochrome *c*, which is increased in the CSF of children and infants with TBI, particularly in victims of abusive head injury and following fatal accidental head injuries.[56,57] In addition, Bcl-2, which regulates cytochrome *c* and is protective against apoptosis, is *higher* in the CSF of children with TBI, but remarkably *lower* (and not significantly different than controls) in the subset of infants with abusive head injury.[57]

Table 41-1 summarizes those CSF markers that are increased to a greater degree in abusive head trauma

Table 41-1	Relative Changes in Cerebrospinal Fluid Markers Following AHT Compared with Accidental Neurotrauma	
Marker	**Physiological Role**	**Change (Compared with Accidental Trauma)**
Glutamate	Neurotoxin	↑↑↑
Quinolinic acid	Neurotoxin	↑↑, more rapid peak in AHT
ICAM-1	Inflammation	↑
Cytokines	Inflammation	↑
Bcl-2	Neuroprotectant	↓
Adenosine	Neuroprotectant	↓
Procalcitonin	Neuroprotectant	↓
S-100 Protein	Neuronal marker	↑
MBP	Myelin marker	↑
NSE	Neuronal marker	↑

compared with accidental trauma in young infants. The net result of these five metabolic cascades (excitotoxicity, ischemia, inflammation, oxidative stress, and apoptosis) is that infants, particularly those suffering AHT, are at particularly greater risk for secondary cellular damage and death. Markers of both glial injury, such as myelin basic protein, and neuronal injury and death such as S-100 protein and neuron-specific enolase, are higher, rise earlier, and are more sustained in younger infants following AHT compared with older children and those with accidental injuries.[58,59] In particular, the sustained rise in neuron-specific enolase suggests that neuronal death is ongoing, likely the result of secondary metabolic destruction. To what degree the activation of these destructive metabolic pathways is dependent on young age as opposed to mechanism of injury is unclear, since most severe *infant* head injuries are also abusive and a multivariate analysis is not yet possible with the small sample sizes studied. *Nonetheless, it is clear that the metabolic response of the immature brain to TBI is both quantitatively and qualitatively different than that of the developed brain, and the thresholds necessary to initiate these metabolic cascades in the developing brain has never been examined properly.*

ACCIDENTAL BRAIN INJURIES—SPECTRUM AND PATTERN OF INJURIES

Research by Prange and colleagues[20] using biofidelic dummies suggested that shaking results in changes in both angular velocity and angular acceleration comparable to a fall from a 1.5-meter height onto concrete. In fact, "short fall defenses" have been used by various expert witnesses to explain the injuries in many court proceedings involving alleged abusive injuries. Plunkett[60] has published "evidence" suggesting that short falls can be fatal. It therefore seems reasonable to contrast the severity and pattern of injuries seen in cases of alleged AHT with those that are commonly seen following short falls as an example of impact injury. A wealth of studies have described the injuries after short falls in young children, including falls at home from sofas, beds, high chairs, or changing tables; falls from cribs while in hospitals; and falls down stairs (with or without walkers). Both the published literature and the author's 17-years experience as a full-time pediatric neurosurgeon are consistent— the spectrum of injuries includes skull fractures and small contact epidural, subdural, or subarachnoid hemorrhages (typically underlying the impact site) or contusions. Among 1815 pediatric short falls (<10 feet) reviewed by Alexander et al,[61] 44 (2.4%) had skull fractures and only 8 (0.04%) had any intracranial injuries. Among 1037 pediatric stairway falls (including 524 in walkers), 34 (3.2%) had skull fractures, 13 (1.2%) had intracranial injuries, and 1 (0.09%) died. A more recent epidemiologic analysis of short falls (<1.5 m) among children in California by Chadwick et al[62] suggested that the odds of death resulting from short falls was less than 0.48 per million children per year. Even the evidence provided by Plunkett,[60] consisting of a review of over 75,000 reports of childhood injuries from playground equipment reported to the U.S. Consumer Product Safety Commission, identified only 18 deaths, an incidence of less than 0.02%; moreover, half of the deaths were caused primarily by either large space-occupying extra-axial (subdural or epidural) hemorrhages or large arterial distribution cerebral infarctions (one with identified post-mortem vertebral artery dissection) that are rarely seen in AHT.

Many comparative studies have confirmed that the nature and pattern of intracranial injuries following accidental falls is distinctly different from that following AHT.[63-70] Summarizing the findings in these studies, AHT differs significantly from accidental injury in the following ways: (1) More frequently causing prolonged coma and lower initial Glasgow Coma Scores, (2) having both more frequent, repeated, and more difficult to control seizures, (3) having more frequent SDHs *and* more extensive or diffuse SDHs yet *less* frequent epidural hemorrhages, (4) having much more frequent retinal hemorrhages (approximately 75%-80% on average) *as well as* more extensive, multilayered retinal hemorrhages, and retinoschisis; and (5) having a significantly higher mortality and worse long-term neurological outcomes. In addition, these injuries—both the pattern and extent—are observed both in cases that lack *any* history of trauma, and among those having other recognized abusive injuries such as bite marks, patterned soft tissue injuries, rib fractures, classic metaphyseal skeletal injuries, and others.

The wealth of evidence suggests that, although there are rare exceptions, inertial (impact) injuries from falls generate a consistent pattern of injury from an impact such as rare skull fractures and even rarer focal intracranial injuries. These injuries are well tolerated, resulting in serious intracranial injury or death in only rare isolated cases. In contrast, infants with AHT consistently present with injuries that are clinically, radiographically, and pathologically distinct from accidental injuries. Perhaps most importantly, clinical studies confirm that although evidence of impact is certainly present in a proportion of cases of AHT, impact is significantly less common in AHT than in accidental injuries.[64] How, then, are we to explain the mechanics of these injuries?

CLINICAL EVIDENCE OF SHAKING— PERPETRATOR CONFESSIONS

Confessed perpetrators in various studies have admitted to shaking alone, shaking with impact, or impact alone. In one study, 46% admitted to shaking only, 29% to impact only, and 25% to a combination of shaking and impact. Combining the first and third groups, 71% of the total admitted to shaking with or without additional impact.[70] There is no disputing the physical evidence of impact in a proportion (35%-63% of cases) of confessed abusive head injury, even among those who confessed to shaking only. Nor is there any argument that impact increases the applied force and, from a strictly biomechanical standpoint, makes the injuries potentially worse. However, if the biomechanical data are accepted at face value, then shaking without impact should *never* achieve sufficient force to produce prolonged traumatic coma, AI, or SDHs. The evidence from perpetrator confessions suggests otherwise.

For example, Starling[71] reviewed 171 cases of AHT, comparing 81 having perpetrator confessions with 90 having none. Of the 81 cases having perpetrator confessions, 69 had additional clinical evidence sufficient to make a reasonable determination regarding the mechanism of abuse (shaking alone, shaking with impact, or impact alone). Among the 32 cases with admitted shaking alone, 4 (13%) had evidence of impact injury, whereas evidence of impact injury was found in 5 of 17 cases (29%) of admitted shaking plus impact, and 12 of 20 (60%) of cases of admitted impact only. Neither the presenting clinical features nor the ultimate outcomes were dependent upon the mechanism described by the perpetrator. The frequency of SDHs was similar in all three groups, and retinal hemorrhages were *more* common in the cases of admitted shaking only. The authors concluded that shaking alone is sufficient to cause both subdural and retinal hemorrhages. A more recent review of perpetrator confessions (excluding the study by Starling above) found legitimate evidence of intracranial injury by shaking alone in 11 of 54 (20%) cases, providing further support for the importance of shaking as a mechanism of injury despite the author's conclusion that there is no "... support for many of the commonly stated aspects of the so-called shaken baby syndrome."[72]

One underlying weakness in all studies of confessed perpetrator admissions is the possibility (perhaps even the likelihood) that the perpetrator is either lying outright about the mechanism of injury, or omitting critical portions of the story. Unfortunately, this inherent weakness will likely not be overcome without the development of an unequivocal lie detector test. It is striking, however, that perpetrators consistently volunteer the same mechanism of injury—shaking the infant—when they are asked to describe what happened. *This common and consistent admission by the perpetrator to shaking the infant (whether or not cranial impact injury is described or discovered by physical examination, radiographic studies, or autopsy) overwhelmingly suggests that shaking is an important component of infant abusive TBI and is, in fact, sufficient to cause the intracranial injuries found in AHT. To suggest otherwise (as required by the biomechanical evidence) would require that every confessed perpetrator has to have been consistently and universally lying about the same phenomenon, something that defies logic and common sense.*

TOWARD A BETTER UNDERSTANDING OF THE MECHANISMS OF SHAKING-INDUCED TRAUMATIC BRAIN INJURY

It is becoming increasingly clear from both neuroimaging studies[36,37,73,74] and post-mortem analyses of fatal cases[40,41] that the widespread cerebral and axonal damage in cases of AHT are, in fact, ischemic rather than directly traumatic in nature. There is also mounting evidence that the primary damage involves a previously unemphasized upper cervical spinal cord or brain stem injury, especially in fatal cases.[39-42] The presence of uncontrolled early seizures, so prevalent during the initial 24 to 72 hours after both AHT[68] and hypoxic-ischemic encephalopathy (HIE),[75,76] but rare following accidental trauma,[68] also strongly supports an ischemic pathophysiological basis for AHT. Whether the cerebral ischemia is primary and due to the apnea so commonly reported in these cases,[71,77] or due to secondary metabolic cascades as discussed above, is uncertain. Acute elevations of glutamate in particular could be a common final pathway for seizures in both AHT and HIE.[76] What is abundantly clear, however, from multiple clinical observations is that shaking, with or without impact, plays an important role in the pathogenesis of infant abusive brain injuries. Unfortunately, we have spent decades trying to determine whether infant shaking can achieve "magical" thresholds for brain injury—thresholds derived from experimental studies on adult primates and applied to human infants based solely upon mass scaling with no recognition of the many unique anatomical, biochemical, and developmental determinants of the developing infant brain. A simple biomechanical approach to injury modeling for AHT is therefore unlikely to get us any closer to the truth since we will never be able to know the specific injury thresholds for initiating these complex metabolic injury cascades in infants.

There are many similarities between the current controversies surrounding infant shaking and those that led to the discovery of the nature of insect flight. For centuries scientists were unable to fully explain insect flight, which seemed to violate known Newtonian principles. The prevailing experimental approach prior to the 1980s was to apply known, steady-state aerodynamic principles (those that govern fixed wing airplane flight) to insect flight, which, unfortunately, failed to fully explain how insects could fly. Insects placed in experimental wind tunnels could generate less than half of the lift required to maintain flight. Eventually, studies elucidated the mechanism: a dynamic leading edge vortex, generated by changes in the wing's position during flight, which spirals air along the wing's leading edge and creates the additional lift required for flight. Nobody would have suggested prior to this discovery that insect flight was impossible because it "lacked a sufficient factual base"—the observations spoke for themselves! However, it took a quantum change in thinking to discover the underlying mechanism.[78]

Similarly, understanding the pathophysiological role of shaking in AHT will likely require a quantum change in our thinking from the classical biomechanical paradigms of the 1970s to a model that takes into account new observations regarding metabolic pathways, the role of brainstem and/or upper cervical spinal cord injury, or other factors yet undiscovered. To those who argue that the contribution of shaking to the pathophysiology of AHT is a hypothesis lacking a sufficient evidentiary base, the consistent and repeated observation that confessed shaking results in stereotypical injuries that are so frequently encountered in AHT—and which are so extraordinarily rare following accidental/impact injuries—*is* the evidentiary basis for shaking. The thrust of current research should be to better understand why this occurs, rather than dismiss these important observations out of hand.

A quote from Richard Feynman[79] seems an appropriate way to end this chapter: "In general we look for a new law by the following process. First we guess it. Then we compare the consequences of the guess to see what would be implied if this law that we guessed is right. Then we compare the result of the computation to *nature*, with experiment or *experience*, compare it directly with *observation*, to see if it works. If it disagrees with experiment it is wrong. In that simple statement is the key to science. It does not make any difference how beautiful your guess is. It does not make any difference how smart you are, who made the guess, or what his name is. If it disagrees with experiment (or experience), … it is wrong."[79]

References

1. Guthkelch AN: Infantile subdural hematoma and its relationship to whiplash injury. *Br Med J* 1972;2:430-431.
2. Caffey J. On the theory and practice of shaking infants. *Am J Dis Child* 1972;124:161-169.
3. Caffey J. The whiplash shaken infant syndrome: manual shaking by the extremities with whiplash-induced intracranial and intraocular bleedings, linked with residual permanent brain damage and mental retardation. *Pediatrics* 1974;54:396-403.
4. Levin AV: Retinal haemorrhages and child abuse. *In*: David TJ (ed): *Recent Advances in Paediatrics.* Churchill Livingstone, Edinburgh, 2000, pp 151-219.
5. Duhaime AC, Gennarelli TA, Thibault LE, et al: The shaken baby syndrome. A clinical, pathological, and biomechanical study. *J Neurosurg* 1987;66:409-415.
6. Christian CW, Block R, Committee of Child Abuse and Neglect, American Academy of Pediatrics: Abusive head trauma in infants and children. *Pediatrics* 2009;123:1409-1411.
7. Uscinski RH: Shaken baby syndrome: an odyssey. *Neurol Med Chir* 2006;46:57-61.
8. Geddes JF, Plunkett J: The evidence base for shaken baby syndrome. We need to question the diagnostic criteria. *Br Med J* 2004;328:720-721.
9. Donohoe M: Evidence-based medicine and shaken baby syndrome: part I—literature review. *Am J Forensic Med Pathol* 2003;24:239-242.
10. Squire W: Shaken baby syndrome: the quest for evidence. *Dev Med Child Neurol* 2008;50:10-14.
11. Pounder DJ: Shaken adult syndrome. *Am J Forensic Med Pathol* 1997;18:321-324.
12. Shannon P, Smith CR, Deck J, et al: Axonal injury and the neuropathology of shaken baby syndrome. *Acta Neuropathol* 1998;95:625-631.
13. Ommaya AK, Goldsmith W, Thibault L: Biomechanics and neuropathology of adult and paediatric head injury. *Br J Neurosurg* 2002;16:220-242.
14. Holbourne AHS: Mechanics of head injuries. *Lancet* 1943;2:438-441.
15. Ommaya AK, Fisch FJ, Corrao P, et al: Comparative tolerances for cerebral concussion by head impact and whiplash injury in primates. *In*: Backaitis SH (ed): *Biomechanics of Impact Injury and Injury Tolerances of*

the Head and Neck Complex. Society of Automotive Engineers, Warrendale, PA, 1993, pp 265-274.

16. Gennarelli TA, Thibault LE: Biomechanics of head injury. *In:* Wilkins RH, Rengachary SS (eds): *Neurosurgery.* McGraw-Hill, New York, 1985, pp 1531-1536.

17. Gennarelli TA, Thibault LE, Ommaya AK: Pathophysiologic responses to rotational and translational accelerations of the head. *In:* Backaitis SH (ed): *Biomechanics of Impact Injury and Injury Tolerances of the Head and Neck Complex.* Society of Automotive Engineers, Warrendale, PA, 1993, pp 411-423.

18. Ommaya AK, Grubb RLJ, Naumann RA: Coup and contre-coup injury: observations on the mechanics of visible brain injuries in the rhesus monkey. *J Neurosurg* 1971;35:503-516.

19. Ommaya AK, Hirsch AE: Tolerances for cerebral concussion from head impact and whiplash in primates. *J Biomechanics* 1971;4:13-21.

20. Prange MT, Coates B, Duhaime A-C, et al: Anthropomorphic simulations of falls, shakes, and inflicted impacts in infants. *J Neurosurg* 2003;93:455-462.

21. Wolfson DR, McNally DS, Clifford MJ, et al: Rigid-body modeling of shaken baby syndrome. *Proc Inst Mech Eng* 2005;219:63-70.

22. Massi M, Jenny C: Biomechanics of the shaken baby: A comparison of the APRICA 2.5 and APRICA 3.4 anthropomorphic test devices. Presented at: Pediatric Abusive Head Trauma: Medical, Forensic, and Scientific Advances and Prevention. Hershey, PA, July, 2007.

23. Keech RV, Kutschke PJ: Upper age limit for the development of amblyopia. *J Pediatr Ophthalmol Strabismus* 1995;32:89-93.

24. Thibault KL, Margulies SS: Age dependent material properties of the porcine cerebrum: effect on pediatric inertial head injury criteria. *J Biomechanics* 1998;31:1119-1126.

25. Raghupathi R, Mehr MF, Helfaer MA, et al: Traumatic axonal injury is exacerbated following repetitive closed head injury in the neonatal pig. *J Neurotrauma* 2004;21:307-316.

26. Ommaya AK, Faas F, Yarnell P: Whiplash injury and brain damage: an experimental study. *JAMA* 1968;204:285-289.

27. Thibault KL, Margulies SS: Age dependent material properties of the porcine cerebrum: effect on pediatric inertial head injury criteria. *J Biomechanics* 2002;31:1119-1126.

28. Ruppel RA, Clark RSB, Bayir H, et al: Critical mechanisms of secondary damage after inflicted head injury in infants and children. *Neurosurg Clin North Am* 2002;13:169-182.

29. Berger RP, Kochanek PM, Pierce MC: Biochemical markers of brain injury: could they be used as diagnostic adjuncts in cases of inflicted traumatic brain injury? *Child Abuse Negl* 2004;28:739-754.

30. Kochanek PM, Clark RSB, Ruppel RA, et al: Biochemical, cellular, and molecular mechanisms in the evolution of secondary damage after severe traumatic brain injury in infants and children: lessons learned from the bedside. *Pediatr Crit Care Med* 2000;1:4-19.

31. Palmer AM, Marion DW, Botscheller ML, et al: Increased neurotransmitter amino acid concentration in human ventricular CSF after brain trauma. *Neuroreport* 1994;6:153-156.

32. Ruppel RA, Kochanek PM, Adelson PD, et al: Excitatory amino acid concentrations in ventricular cerebrospinal fluid after severe traumatic brain injury in infants and children: the role of child abuse. *J Pediatrics* 2001;138:18-25.

33. McDonald JW, Silverstein FS, Johnson MV: Neurotoxicity of N-methyl-D-aspartate is markedly enhanced in developing rat central nervous system. *Brain Res* 1988;459:200-203.

34. Adelson PD, Clyde B, Kochanek PM, et al: Cerebrovascular response in infants and young children following severe traumatic brain injury: a preliminary report. *Pediatr Neurosurg* 1997;26:200-207.

35. Duhaime AC, Durham S: Traumatic brain injury in infants: the phenomenon of subdural hemorrhage with hemispheric hypodensity ("Big Black Brain"). *Prog Brain Res* 2007;161:293-302.

36. Biousse V, Suh DY, Newman NJ, et al: Diffusion-weighted magnetic resonance imaging in shaken baby syndrome. *Am J Ophthalmol* 2002;133:249-255.

37. Ichord RN, Naim M, Pollock AN, et al: Hypoxic-ischemic injury complicates inflicted and accidental traumatic brain injury in young children: the role of diffusion-weighted imaging. *J Neurotrauma* 2007;24:106-118.

38. Arbogast KB, Margulies SS: Material characterization of the brainstem from oscillatory shear tests. *J Biomechanics* 1998;31:801-807.

39. Hadley MN, Sonntag VKH, Rekate HL, Murphy A: The infant whiplash-shake injury syndrome. A clinical and pathological study. *Neurosurgery* 1989;24:536-540.

40. Geddes JF, Hackshaw AK, Vowles GH, et al: Neuropathology of inflicted head injury in children I. Patterns of brain damage. *Brain* 2001;124:1290-1298.

41. Geddes JF, Vowles GH, Hackshaw AK, et al: Neuropathology of inflicted head injury in children II. Microscopic brain injury in infants. *Brain* 2001;124:1299-1306.

42. Brennan LK, Rubin D, Christian CW, et al: Neck injuries in young pediatric homicide victims. *J Neurosurg Pediatr* 2009;3:232-239.

43. Ruppel RA, Kochanek PM, Adelson PD, et al: Endothelin-1 is increased in cerebrospinal fluid following traumatic brain injury in children. *Crit Care Med* 1999;27:A76.

44. Armstead WM: Role of endothelin-1 in age-dependent cerebrovascular hypotensive responses after brain injury. *Am J Physiol* 1999;277:H1884-H1894.

45. Robertson CL, Bell MJ, Kochanek PM, et al: Increased adenosine in cerebrospinal fluid after severe traumatic brain injury in infants and children: association with severity of injury and excitotoxicity. *Crit Care Med* 2001;29:2287-2293.

46. Bayir H, Kagan VE, Tyurina YY, et al: Assessment of antioxidant reserves and oxidative stress in cerebrospinal fluid after severe traumatic brain injury in infants and children. *Pediatr Res* 2002;51:571-578.

47. Smith SL, Andrus PK, Gleason DD, et al: Infant rat model of the shaken baby syndrome: preliminary characterization and evidence for the role of free radicals in cortical hemorrhaging and progressive neuronal degeneration. *J Neurotrauma* 1998;15:693-705.

48. Goodman JC, Robertson CS, Grossman RG, et al: Elevation of tumor necrosis factor in head injury. *J Neuroimmunol* 1990;30:213-217.

49. Kossman T, Hans VHJ, Imhof HG, et al: Intrathecal and serum interleukin-6 and the acute-phase response in patients with severe traumatic brain injuries. *Shock* 1995;4:311-317.

50. McClain CF, Cohen D, Phillips R, et al: Increased plasma and ventricular fluid interleukin-6 levels in patients with head injury. *J Lab Clin Med* 1991;118:225-231.

51. Whalen MJ, Carlos TM, Kochanek PM, et al: Interleukin-8 is increased in cerebrospinal fluid of children with severe head injury. *Crit Care Med* 2000;28:929-934.

52. Whalen MJ, Carlos TM, Kochanek PM, et al: Soluble adhesion molecules in CSF are increase in children with severe head injury. *J Neurotrauma* 1998;15:777-787.

53. Bell MJ, Kochanek PM, Doughty LA, et al: Interleukin-6 and interleukin-10 in cerebrospinal fluid after severe traumatic brain injury in children. *J Neurotrauma* 1997;14:451-457.

54. Sinz EH, Kochanek PM, Heyes MP, et al: Quinolinic acid is increased in CSF and associated with mortality after traumatic brain injury in humans. *J Cereb Blood Flow Metab* 1998;18:610-615.

55. Bell MJ, Kochanek PM, Heyes MP, et al: Quinolinic acid in the cerebrospinal fluid of children after traumatic brain injury. *Crit Care Med* 1999;27:491-497.

56. Janesko KL, Satchell MA, Kochanek PM: IL-1 converting enxyme (ICE), IL-1, and cytochrome *c* in CSF after head injury in infants and children. *J Neurotrauma* 2000;17:956.

57. Clarke RS, Kochanek PM, Adelson PD, et al: Increases in bcl-2 protein in cerebrospinal fluid and evidence for programmed cell death in infants and children after severe traumatic brain injury. *J Pediatrics* 2000;137:197-204.

58. Berger RP, Pierce MC, Wisniewski SR, et al: Neuron-specific enolase and S100B in cerebrospinal fluid after severe traumatic brain injury in infants and children. *Pediatrics* 2002;109:e31.

59. Berger RP, Adelson PD, Pierce MC, et al: Serum neuron-specific enolase, S100B, and myelin basic protein concentrations after inflicted and noninflicted traumatic brain injury in children. *J Neurosurg* 2005;103(1 Suppl):61-68.

60. Plunkett J: Fatal pediatric head injuries caused by short-distance falls. *Am J Forens Med Pathol* 2001;22:1-12.

61. Alexander RC, Levitt CJ, Smith WL: Abusive head trauma. *In:* Reece RM, Ludwig S (eds): *Child Abuse Medical Diagnosis and Management,* ed 2. Lippincott Williams & Wilkins, Philadelphia, 2001, pp 47-80.

62. Chadwick DL, Bertocci G, Castillo E, et al: Annual risk of death resulting from short falls among children: less than 1 in 1 million. *Pediatrics* 2008;121:1213-1224.

63. Hymel KP, Rumack CM, Hay TC, et al: Comparison of intracranial computed tomographic (CT) findings in pediatric abusive and accidental head trauma. *Pediatr Radiol* 1997;27:743-747.

64. Hymel KP, Makaroff KL, Laskey AL, et al: Mechanisms, clinical presentations, injuries, and outcomes from inflicted versus noninflicted head trauma during infancy: results of a prospective, multicentered comparative study. *Pediatrics* 2007;119:922-929.

65. Ewing-Cobbs L, Kramer L, Prasad M, et al: Neuroimaging, physical, and developmental findings after inflicted and noninflicted traumatic brain injury in young children. *Pediatrics* 1998;102:300-307.

66. Goldstein B, Kelly MM, Bruton D, et al: Inflicted versus accidental head injury in critically ill children. *Crit Care Med* 1993;21:1328-1332.

67. Reece RM, Sege R: Childhood head injuries. Accidental or inflicted? *Arch Pediatr Adolesc Med* 2000;154:11-15.

68. Bechtel K, Stoessel K, Leventhal JM, et al: Characteristics that distinguish accidental from abusive injury in hospitalized young children with head trauma. *Pediatrics* 2004;114:165-168.

69. Duhaime AC, Alario AJ, Lewander WJ, et al: Head injury in very young children: Mechanisms, injury types and ophthalmologic findings in 100 hospitalized patients younger than 2 years of age. *Pediatrics* 1992;90:179-185.

70. Arbogast KB, Margulies SS, Christian CW: Initial neurologic presentation in young children sustaining inflicted and unintentional fatal head injuries. *Pediatrics* 2005;116:180-184.

71. Starling SP, Patel S, Burke BL, et al: Analysis of perpetrator admissions to inflicted traumatic brain injury in children. *Arch Pediatr Adolesc Med* 2004;158:454-458.

72. Leetsma JE: Case analysis of brain-injured admittedly shaken infants. 54 cases, 1969-2001. *Am J Forensic Med Pathol* 2005;26:199-212.

73. Chan Y-L, Chu WCW, Wong GWK: Diffusion-weighted MRI in shaken baby syndrome. *Pediatr Radiol* 2003;33:574-577.

74. Parizel PM, Ceulemans B, Laridon A, et al: Cortical hypoxic-ischemic brain damage in shaken baby (shaken impact) syndrome: value of diffusion-weighted MRI. *Pediatr Radiol* 2003;33:868-871.

75. Volpe JJ (ed): *Neurology of the Newborn*, ed 3. WB Saunders, Philadelphia, 1995.

76. Pu Y, Garg A, Corby R, et al: A positive correlation between alpha-glutamate and glutamine on brain 1H-spectroscopy and neonatal seizures in moderate and severe hypoxic-ischemic encephalopathy. *AJNR Am J Neuroradiol* 2008;29:216.

77. Johnson DL, Boal D, Baule R: Role of apnea in nonaccidental head injury. *Pediatr Neurosurg* 1995;23:305-310.

78. Dudley R: *The Biomechanics of Insect Flight: Form, Function, Evolution*. Princeton University Press, Princeton, NJ, 2002.

79. Feynman R: *The Character of Physical Law*. Random House, New York, 1994, p 150.

42

IMAGING OF ABUSIVE HEAD TRAUMA

Glenn A. Tung, MD, FACR

INTRODUCTION

Traumatic head injury is one of the leading causes of death and disability in infants and children.[1] Abusive head trauma (AHT) occurs in 12% of children who are physically abused and is associated with a mortality rate of 12.5% to 40%.[2-5] Neuroimaging has become critical for the timely and accurate diagnosis of traumatic head injury and has three primary objectives. The first objective of neuroimaging is to detect the injury in a child who might not be fully cooperative or, even worse, who is critically ill or unconscious. The second is to evaluate the full extent and severity of head injury. This is particularly important when weighing the need for urgent medical or surgical intervention. The third objective of neuroimaging is to characterize any detected lesions, and to differentiate them from others that might mimic traumatic head injury. In the case of AHT, characterizing the traumatic lesion often also involves an assessment of the time that the injury occurred for forensic purposes.

THE NEUROIMAGING EXAMINATION

Medical clinicians caring for children should have a low threshold for performing neuroimaging to investigate traumatic head injury. Even in the absence of overt neurological symptoms or signs of head injury, young children with physical signs or skeletal injuries that raise the suspicion of inflicted trauma should undergo neuroimaging. Examples of injuries that should raise such suspicion include classic metaphyseal lesions, posterior rib fractures, fractures in a non-ambulatory child, or fractures of different ages. A panel of medical experts has published criteria for the imaging evaluation of AHT based on the age of the child, medical history, and neurological examination.[6] In the majority of cases of suspected AHT, the neuroimaging evaluation will involve either or both computed tomography (CT) and magnetic resonance imaging (MRI).

Computed Tomography

Traditionally, noncontrast head CT is performed first to evaluate the child in whom abusive head injury is suspected. Multidetector, noncontrast CT imaging of the head can be performed on critically ill children, and can be completed in less than 10 seconds of imaging time. It is readily available in most emergency rooms, and can easily accommodate cardiorespiratory monitoring equipment and orthopedic fixation hardware. Noncontrast CT is sensitive for acute intracranial hemorrhage, skull fracture, severe cerebral edema, and mass effect (Figure 42-1). One of the critical imperatives of the initial imaging is to identify head injuries that require immediate medical or neurosurgical intervention. Hematomas, cerebral edema, or depressed skull fractures that cause significant mass effect are all readily detected by noncontrast CT. Compared with MRI, however, CT is less sensitive for small and non-hemorrhagic traumatic brain injuries.

To evaluate the spectrum of traumatic head injury with the highest sensitivity, noncontrast CT examinations of the head should be reviewed in at least two different level-window settings optimized to evaluate injuries of the brain (level, 30-50 Hounsfied units [HU]; window, 80-120 HU) and calvarium (level, 450-500 HU; window, 2000-4000 HU). Some also advocate reviewing CT images with a third setting that is more sensitive for small subdural or epidural hematomas (EDH) (level, 50-100 HU; window, 150-300 HU). Regarding skull fracture, the time-honored diagnostic examination has been the plain film radiograph. Multidetector CT, however, enables the rapid acquisition of a 3-dimensional volume of x-ray attenuation data and facilitates reformatted viewing in the coronal or sagittal plane, or as a 3-dimensional image. In many cases, multidetector CT with 3-dimensional image reformation is superior to skull radiography for the diagnosis and characterization of skull fractures, particularly those in which the plane of the fracture is primarily transverse (Figure 42-2). As such, multidetector CT complements the radiographic bone survey for the detection and description of skull, maxillofacial, and skull base fractures.

Magnetic Resonance Imaging

MRI of the head is recommended in any patient who has sustained a closed head injury when neurological symptoms or signs are not explained sufficiently by findings on noncontrast head CT or if findings on CT need to be characterized with greater specificity. MR imaging of the brain is more sensitive than noncontrast CT for nearly all traumatic head injuries, particularly for those involving the brain parenchyma. Ghahreman and colleagues[7] reviewed 65 consecutive cases of AHT in a single pediatric neurosurgical unit over 7 years. In almost half of the 37 children who underwent MR imaging, additional diagnoses not seen on initial CT were made. These included cases of cerebral ischemia and infarction, shear injury, and small subdural or subarachnoid hemorrhages. The increased sensitivity of MR imaging is attributed to the ability to evaluate a broader spectrum of pathophysiology, such as the magnetic susceptibility of iron in the hemoglobin of blood, decreased water diffusion associated with ischemic cytotoxic edema, and time-dependent changes in the signal intensity of blood products.

Since patient motion can create artifacts that obscure important information, adequate sedation is an important prerequisite to obtaining diagnostic MR images in most infants and children. Sedation should be administered and monitored by a team of personnel who are not only familiar with the pharmacology of the sedatives used, but who can also rapidly identify and treat cardiorespiratory complications, emesis, and hypersalivation. Sedation can be

achieved using a wide range of short-acting agents and can be administered by several routes, including local, transmucosal, oral, rectal, intramuscular, intravenous, and inhalational.[8] The intravenous route is preferred for the deeper level of sedation that is often required in children who are injured or are in pain since it facilitates the rapid onset and reversal of sedation, and the administration of supplemental medication if necessary. In addition, since MRIs occurs in an environment of a strong static magnetic field, it can be unsafe for patients with certain biomedical implants or devices because of movement or dislodgement of objects made from ferromagnetic materials.[9,10] Constant vigilance by health care personnel is necessary to maintain a safe MR imaging environment for patients.

A complete discussion of MRI technology is beyond the scope of this chapter. For the investigation of traumatic head injury, however, a suggested standard MRI protocol on a 1.5-Tesla system includes spin-echo T1-weighted, turbo spin-echo T2-weighted, T2*-weighted gradient-echo, and diffusion-weighted MR imaging, as well as fluid-attenuated inversion recovery (FLAIR) pulse sequences. Using a phased-array head coil and parallel MR imaging techniques, this protocol can be completed in 20 minutes of imaging time. The FLAIR and T2-weighted sequences are sensitive for intracerebral mass lesions, such as brain contusion, intracerebral hematoma, or cerebral edema. The FLAIR sequence is also helpful in detecting and characterizing subdural hematoma (SDH) and subarachnoid hemorrhage. T2*-weighted imaging is both sensitive and specific for brain hemorrhage, whether acute or chronic, and is particularly valuable for detecting small foci of white matter hemorrhage that characterize diffuse axonal injury (DAI). Both T1- and T2-weighted MR images characterize mass lesions detected on the FLAIR sequence, and provide information to estimate the age of intracranial blood.

Diffusion, or Brownian motion, refers to the constant, random thermal motion of molecules. In clinical diffusion-weighted MR imaging, "apparent" water diffusion is investigated and reflects not only thermal water diffusion, but also other sources of water mobility, such as flow along pressure gradients and changes in membrane permeability. Decreased water diffusion in brain tissue that is detected on

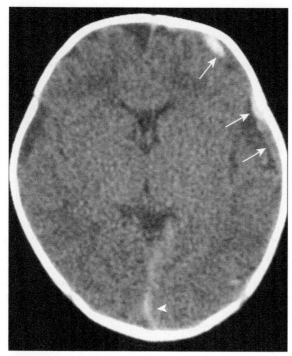

FIGURE 42-1 An 8-month-old girl with acute subdural hematoma from abusive head trauma. Noncontrast CT shows mixed-density left frontal *(arrows)* and hyperdense interhemispheric *(arrowhead)* subdural hematomas.

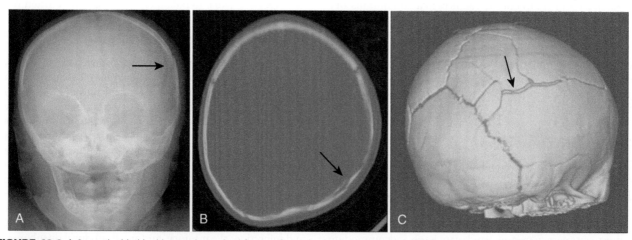

FIGURE 42-2 A 6-month-old girl with complex parietal fracture from abusive head trauma. **A,** Skull radiograph from radiographic bone survey shows left parietal fracture *(arrow)*. **B,** Noncontrast CT with bone window settings confirms impaction *(arrow)* from parietal fracture. **C,** Extent and complexity of fracture is demonstrated on volume-rendered image from multidetector CT.

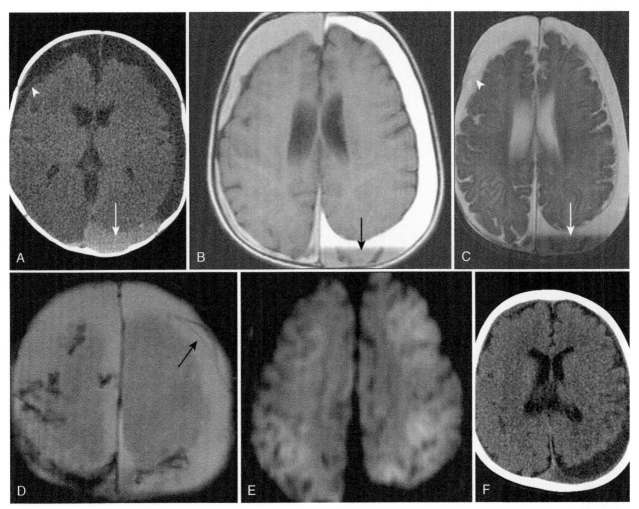

FIGURE 42-3 A 5-month-old girl with acute and chronic subdural hematomas and ischemic infarction from abusive head trauma. **A,** Head CT demonstrates bilateral hypodense chronic subdural hematomas containing linear membrane *(arrowhead)*. Hyperdense clot *(arrow)* forms sediment in acute left subdural hematoma. **B,** Note loss of gray-white matter differentiation in the brain tissue. **C,** Nine days later, hyperintense subdural hematomas, membranes *(arrowhead)*, and hypointense sediment *(arrow)* containing clots are seen on FLAIR **(B)** and T2-weighted **(C)** MR images. **D,** T2*-weighted gradient echo image shows hypointense membrane *(arrow)* in chronic subdural hematoma and bilateral hypointense acute blood clots. **E,** Multifocal cortical hyperintensities in both parietal and left frontal lobes, consistent with cerebral ischemia, are seen on diffusion-weighted image but not on other pulse sequences. **F,** Follow-up CT performed 2 years later shows asymmetrical left parietal and frontal encephalomalacia.

diffusion-weighted imaging (DWI) is believed to reflect both cytotoxic edema, which is associated with acute ischemic or hypoxic brain injury, and intramyelinic edema, which can occur with diffuse axonal brain injury. In contrast, increased water diffusion reflects vasogenic or interstitial edema. In children under the age of 2 years, DWI may be particularly valuable for the diagnosis of acute brain ischemia since both normal unmyelinated cerebral white matter and abnormal brain edema are high in signal intensity on T2-weighted and FLAIR MR imaging (Figure 42-3). Suh and colleagues[11] have reported the value of DWI in infants with suspected AHT. Sixteen (89%) infants had abnormal findings on DWI including lesions that were multifocal in 15 (94%) and global in 4 (25%). In the majority of cases, abnormalities were more apparent and extensive on DWI than on any other MRI sequence. There was a significant relationship between the extent of abnormality on DWI and poor clinical outcome. DWI can be used to show many shear injuries but is less sensitive than T2*-weighted gradient echo MRI for shear injuries associated with small foci of hemorrhage.[12]

Supplementing these standard pulse sequences are MR spectroscopy and MR angiography. MR spectroscopy is used to assess both normal and pathologic biochemical constituents of brain tissue. In pediatric head trauma a significant increase in tissue lactate concentration has been observed in regions of brain contusion and infarction (Figure 42-4).[13] In a study of serial MR spectroscopy performed over 3 weeks in three abused infants, Haseler et al[14] reported that brain metabolites remained normal up to 24 hours after head injury but decreased to 40% of normal within 5 to 12 days, with lactate and lipid levels more than doubling in concentration. MR angiography is used to assess the patency of cerebral arteries and veins. For example, MR arteriography can demonstrate tapered narrowing, occlusion, or pseudoaneurysm that occurs with traumatic arterial dissection.

Total Body MR Imaging

Brain imaging is also included as a part of more comprehensive MR imaging of the entire body. MR imaging of the

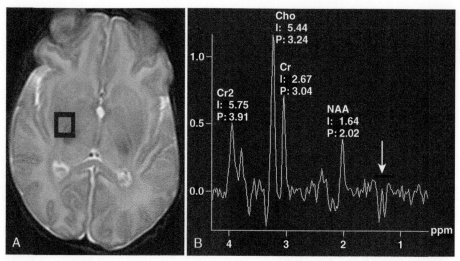

FIGURE 42-4 Hypoxic-ischemic injury in neonate on single-voxel proton MR spectroscopy. **A,** T2-weighted MR image shows symmetric deep grey nuclei. Box indicates volume element for single-voxel spectroscopy. **B,** Intermediate echo time spectrum demonstrates inverted doublet peak *(arrow)* at 1.33 ppm, indicating lactate from anaerobic glycolysis or in response to release of glutamate, an excitatory amino acid neurotransmitter.

entire body in the coronal plane using the short-tau inversion recovery (STIR) sequence can be completed in less than 30 minutes of imaging time and complements the radiographic bone survey in the comprehensive evaluation of suspected abusive injury. Unpublished data from the author's institution suggest that coronal images of the brain from whole-body STIR demonstrates most important traumatic head injuries, such as SDH and cerebral swelling, and can distinguish subarachnoid from subdural fluid. It might not be as sensitive as dedicated brain MR imaging, however, for small SDHs less than 3 mm wide.

SPECIFIC TRAUMATIC HEAD INJURIES

AHT includes those injuries caused by impact to the head (from either a direct blow or by the head striking another object), from shaking, or from some combination of these mechanisms.[15-18] Traumatic head injury is frequently classified by location. In general, traumatic injury of the brain itself (intraaxial injury) has a poorer prognosis than injury involving only the extracerebral soft tissues, calvarium, or dural spaces over the brain (extraaxial spaces). Another classification of traumatic head injury is based on the biomechanical mechanism of blunt head injury.[19,20] In this classification, the *primary injury* results from a direct impacting or rotational force acting on the head, whereas a *secondary injury* results from hemodynamic or metabolic derangements indirectly related to the primary head injury, such as ischemic or hypoxic brain injury. An impact force causes a focal primary injury of the scalp, skull, or brain at and directly below the point of contact, but does not cause diffuse brain injury and concussion.[21] An inertial injury is a primary injury that results from an acceleration-deceleration force that can injure the brain at a distance from a point of contact (e.g., the contre-coup cortical contusion). A diffuse primary injury is associated with a rotational inertial force and is characterized clinically by the sudden loss of consciousness. Violent shaking causes an extreme rotational movement of the brain within the cranial vault that can tear superficial cortical veins and shear brain

tissue at the interface between grey matter and white matter, which differ in density and other mechanical properties.[21] As a result, subdural and subarachnoid hemorrhage, both focal and diffuse axonal brain injury, and retinal hemorrhage and retinoschisis are observed with inertial forces.[17]

Traumatic Injuries of the Brain

A *cortical contusion* results from an impact injury to the cerebral cortex and often extends deeper to adjacent subcortical white matter as well. Since direct impact is implicated in its pathophysiology, scalp hematoma or skull fracture often accompanies the brain contusion. Larger contusions are more common in adults and involve cortical brain tissue that abuts corrugated surfaces of the inner calvarium such as the orbitofrontal, anterior frontal, anteroinferior temporal, and occipital lobes. Furthermore, an impact injury that produces a cortical contusion in an older child or adult is more likely to cause an axonal injury in the immature brain.[18,22] Thus cortical contusions are distinctly unusual in infants and might be very small. On noncontrast CT, an acute brain contusion is as an ill-defined, low-density lesion that can contain small foci of hyperdense petechial hemorrhage. Frequently, small contusions visible on T2-weighted, FLAIR, T2*-weighted, or diffusion-weighted MR imaging sequences are not seen on noncontrast CT (Figure 42-5). A focal region of encephalomalacia at times represents the sequelae of a cortical contusion.

An extreme rotational or acceleration-deceleration force may cause an unequal translation of brain tissues that differ in density; tensile injury to axons and small vessels is also possible. In the adult brain, this *axonal* or *shear injury* is manifested by axonal swelling, focal accumulations of axoplasm (eosinophilic retraction balls), microhemorrhage, and Wallerian degeneration when evaluated at autopsy.[23,24] Immediate loss of consciousness is a clinical manifestation of DAI and the prognosis is related to both the number and location of lesions.[25] The subcortical white matter is disrupted with a lesser inertial force than that which disrupts successively

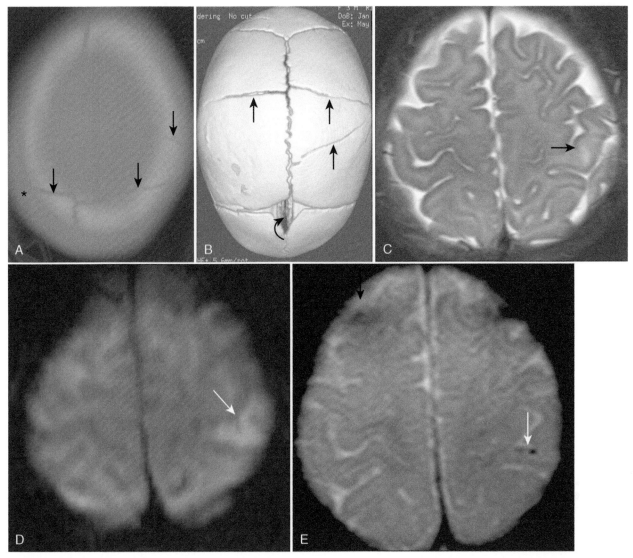

FIGURE 42-5 Bilateral skull fractures, scalp edema, and small cortical contusion from abusive head trauma in a 4-month-old girl. **A,** CT displayed with bone window setting shows linear biparietal skull fractures *(arrows)* and scalp edema (*) but no contusion on brain window settings. **B,** Volume-reconstruction from multidetector CT confirms linear skull fractures *(arrows);* note open anterior fontanelle *(curved arrow).* **C** and **D,** Both T2-weighted **(C)** and diffusion-weighted MR images **(D)** show hyperintense cortical edema *(arrow)* in left postcentral gyrus. **E,** There are also punctate foci of hypointense blood *(arrow)* on T2*-weighted gradient echo image consistent with small brain contusion.

deeper tissues such as the corpus callosum, basal ganglia, and rostral brainstem.[26]

Neuroimaging can detect axonal injury in characteristic sites. On CT, punctate foci of hyperdense hemorrhage with or without surrounding hypodense edema can be seen in frontotemporal subcortical white matter, although in many cases and particularly in children, the CT scan is normal.[27] Small hemorrhages are not commonly seen in young children with axonal brain injury because blood vessels are more elastic and do not shear as readily, even when adjacent axons are torn.[17] Nearly one third of patients with a normal CT scan will have manifestations of axonal injury on MR imaging. Multiple foci of hyperintensity in the subcortical white matter or corpus callosum on FLAIR, T2-weighted, or diffusion-weighted pulse sequences are characteristic of edema associated cerebral shear injury (Figure 42-6). In a study of 25 adults with DAI, Huisman et al[12] reported foci of decreased water diffusion in 64% of cases, reflecting

cytotoxic edema, intramyelinic edema, or both. In 24% of cases, water diffusion was increased, indicating focal vasogenic edema.[12] On T2*-weighted gradient-echo sequence, small foci of marked hypointensity from microhemorrhage is typical, may be the only sign of DAI, and can remain for years (Figure 42-7). More recently, susceptibility-weighted MR imaging, which uses a high spatial resolution, three dimensional–gradient echo sequence with phase post-processing, has been shown to demonstrate even more foci of microhemorrhage than conventional two-dimensional, T2*-weighted gradient echo MR imaging.[28,29]

In infants under the age of 6 months, a violent rotational force may cause a focal, slit-shaped laceration in white matter. This rare macroscopic shear lesion, termed *contusion tear* by Lindenberg,[30] is often accompanied by microscopic markers of DAI as well as subdural and subarachnoid hemorrhage.[17,30,31] On neuroimaging, the contusion tear appears as a well-defined cavity in the subcortical white matter of the

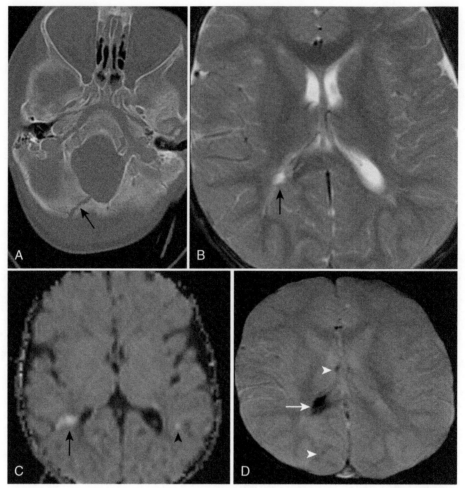

FIGURE 42-6 A 20-month-old boy with diastatic occipital fracture and shear injury from AHT. **A,** Noncontrast CT shows diastatic occipital fracture *(arrow)*. **B-D,** Hyperintense signal in periatrial white matter *(arrow)* on both T2-weighted **(B)** and diffusion-weighted **(C)** MR images corresponds to focus of hemorrhage on T2*-weighted gradient echo image **(D)**. Other, smaller foci of shear injury *(arrowheads)* are shown on both diffusion- and T2*-weighted MR images.

frontal or parietal lobe, sometimes containing a sediment of blood (Figure 42-8).

Brain swelling occurs more often in children than adults after closed head injury and has been reported in as many as 65% of physically abused children.[32-34] Cerebral autoregulation is impaired in these severely injured children and this may lead to hyperemic brain swelling and intracranial hypertension.[35] Cerebral edema is nonspecific and has been reported after a rotational inertial force that causes DAI; with hypoxic brain injury from strangulation, suffocation, posttraumatic apnea, or prolonged seizure; and from ischemic brain injury. Damage to brainstem centers that control cardiac and respiratory function from transtentorial herniation or primary axonal injury are suspected of causing apnea and secondary hypoxemic brain edema in some abused infants.[36-38] The neuroimaging signs of brain swelling include loss of grey-white matter differentiation and mass effect. On noncontrast CT, hypodense edema in the cerebral cortex will reduce image contrast between the cortex and subcortical white matter, resulting in loss of grey-white matter differentiation. When the hypodensity of the cerebral cortex and white matter from edema is profound and extensive on CT, there is often a striking relative increased density of the basal ganglia, cerebellum, and brainstem, the so-called "reversal sign" or "bright cerebellum" sign (Figure 42-9).[39,40] This sign indicates particularly severe and irreversible hypoxic-ischemic brain injury.

In the report by Han and colleagues,[39] any child with this ominous sign who survived had profound neurological deficits and severe developmental delay. On T2-weighted and FLAIR MR imaging, the diagnosis of cerebral edema in infants and young children can be difficult to identify because unmyelinated white matter and brain edema are both hyperintense. In these cases, DWI or MR spectroscopy might demonstrate excessive brain edema or lactate, respectively. If marked, mass effect from cerebral swelling can manifest as compression and effacement of the cerebral sulci, ventricles, or the cisterns at the skull base including the ambient, quadrigeminal, or suprasellar cisterns.

Extraaxial Injury in Abusive Head Trauma

SDH is one of the most characteristic head injuries associated with AHT.[18,41-43] An extreme angular

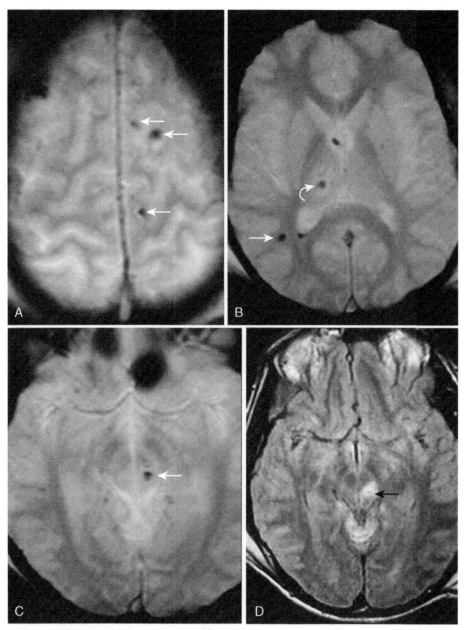

FIGURE 42-7 A 17-year-old boy with shear injury on MR imaging after motorcycle crash. **A-C,** T2*-weighted gradient echo MR images show multiple foci of microhemorrhage at grey-white matter junction (*arrows* in **A**), right thalamus (*curved arrow* in **B**), and dorsolateral upper midbrain (*arrow* in **C**). **D,** On FLAIR, there is hyperintense edema in dorsolateral midbrain (*arrow*).

acceleration-deceleration force, with or without impaction, causes the brain to move at a different speed than the relatively fixed dural venous sinuses and calvarium. As a result hemorrhage can occur in the subdural space and/or the subarachnoid space if there is tearing of superficial cortical veins. Electron microscopy of the subdural part of these bridging veins shows a relatively thin wall and absent mural reinforcement at the arachnoid trabeculae; these factors contribute to relative vascular fragility.[44] Severe accidental head trauma, most often from vehicular crash, can also cause SDH but relatively minor traumatic head injury, such as a fall from a short vertical height of less than 4 feet, would be an uncommon cause of an SDH.[45-48] Dashti and colleagues[41] reported that only 7% of accidental head injuries were associated with SDH and 80% of these were

from motor vehicle collisions. In contrast, 69% of inflicted head injuries were associated with acute SDH. In a retrospective review of 287 children with head injuries, Reece and Sege[43] reported SDH in 46% of children with AHT and in only 10% of those with accidental head trauma. SDH has been reported as a complication of both vaginal and caesarian delivery, after ventricular shunting, and in children with large subarachnoid spaces from volume loss or in those with bleeding diatheses.

On neuroimaging, the subdural hemorrhage is a crescent-shaped hemorrhage between the skull and brain that crosses cranial sutures but is limited by the falx and tentorium. Subdural hemorrhage occurs over the convexity of the brain, next to the falx between the cerebral hemispheres (interhemispheric), or both, and can be quite extensive

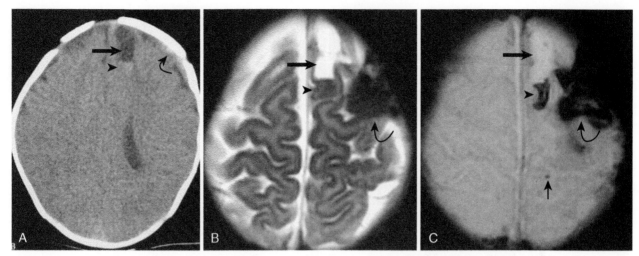

FIGURE 42-8 Contusional tear on CT and MR imaging. **A,** Head CT shows dependent hyperdense blood *(arrowhead)* in hypodense left frontal white matter laceration *(arrow)* and small hyperdense subdural hemorrhage *(curved arrow)*. **B** and **C**, T2-weighted **(B)** and T2*-weighted gradient echo **(C)** MR images show hyperintense white matter laceration *(arrow)* in left superior frontal gyrus with sediment of hypointense acute blood *(arrowhead)* and large extraaxial clot *(curved arrow)*. Note microhemorrhage consistent with shear injury in left postcentral gyrus *(small arrow in* **C**).

(see Figures 42-1 and 42-3). When large, the associated mass effect is manifested by effacement of sulci or cisterns, compression or displacement of the ventricles, and midline shift (subfalcine herniation), and warrants the designation "subdural hematoma." Studies in adults have shown that, as the hemorrhage organizes over the ensuing week to month, neovascularization and collagen production form membranes within subacute and chronic subdural hemorrhages (see Figure 42-3).[49]

Temporal changes in the radiodensity and signal intensity of SDH are discussed in greater depth later in this chapter. Briefly, the acute SDH is hyperdense on noncontrast CT, and becomes first isodense and then hypodense over the next 2 or 3 weeks. On MR imaging, the acute subdural hematoma is hypointense on T2-weighted MR imaging. In the subacute stage, the SDH is hyperintense on T1-weighted imaging and becomes hyperintense on the FLAIR sequence in the subacute and chronic stages (Figure 42-10).

Subarachnoid hemorrhage fills fissures and sulci between the arachnoid and pial leptomeninges, is often focal, and can be adjacent to a skull fracture, cortical contusion, or subdural hematoma. Subarachnoid hemorrhage occurs with over 70% of traumatic subdural hemorrhages since both result from the tearing of small cortical veins. In one study, subarachnoid hemorrhage occurred in 31% of AHT and in only 8% of accidental trauma.[43] Subarachnoid hemorrhage is detected readily on noncontrast CT as hyperdense blood filling the subarachnoid space within cortical sulci or basilar cisterns. In contrast to the hypointensity of normal CSF, subarachnoid blood is hyperintense on FLAIR, and this enables the detection of SAH on MR imaging with a sensitivity that is equal to or greater than noncontrast CT (Figure 42-11).[50,51]

Intraventricular hemorrhage can result from primary rupture of subependymal veins, or either reflux of subarachnoid hemorrhage or dissection of an intracerebral hematoma into the ventricles. On transverse axial CT or MR imaging, small intraventricular hemorrhages are detected as a horizontal fluid-fluid level within the dependent occipital horn in a supine patient. This fluid-fluid level represents a sedi-

ment of clotted blood below a supernatant of CSF mixed with unclotted blood. Using the FLAIR sequence, intraventricular hemorrhage appears hyperintense compared with CSF when MR imaging is performed during the first 48 hours after injury but varies in signal intensity later (see Figure 42-11).[52]

Epidural hematoma (EDH) is much less common after inflicted injury compared with subdural and subarachnoid hemorrhage.[4,53,54] Of 26 extracerebral fluid collections detected on CT in 47 abused children, Merten and colleagues[53] reported only two EDHs. The mechanism of injury that causes EDH is a linear impact to the calvarium that directly lacerates a vessel or the dura, and so EDH is accompanied by a fracture of the skull in 90% of cases.[55] In infants, a parietal EDH from laceration of the posterior branch of the middle meningeal artery can expand rapidly. A venous EDH following laceration of the superior sagittal or transverse dural sinus might not expand as quickly since it is more likely to undergo tamponade by the brain or dura. On CT, the EDH is a focal biconvex or lentiform hyperdense mass adjacent to the calvarium that is restricted by cranial sutures but crosses the falx or tentorium. The EDH compresses the underlying brain and subarachnoid space. Scalp edema and calvarial fracture often accompany the EDH at the impact site, and there might be a contralateral SDH (Figure 42-12).

After long bones, the skull is the most common site of fracture in abused children and any *calvarial fracture* should trigger a search for an intracranial injury.[56,57] The pediatric skull, softer and thinner than the adult skull, is more susceptible to fracture despite its more pliable nature. A linear parietal fracture is the most common type of skull fracture and usually does not require additional treatment beyond that of closing an associated scalp laceration. Many simple, linear fractures are caused by accidental injury, such as a fall from a height of less than 4 feet, and are not associated with serious intracranial injury.[45-48] Although no pattern of fracture is pathognomonic for inflicted injury, skull fractures that are multiple, bilateral, diastatic, cross sutures, or growing are more prevalent after AHT.[45,53,58-60] In a study of 126 children with skull fractures from abusive head injury, 54% were

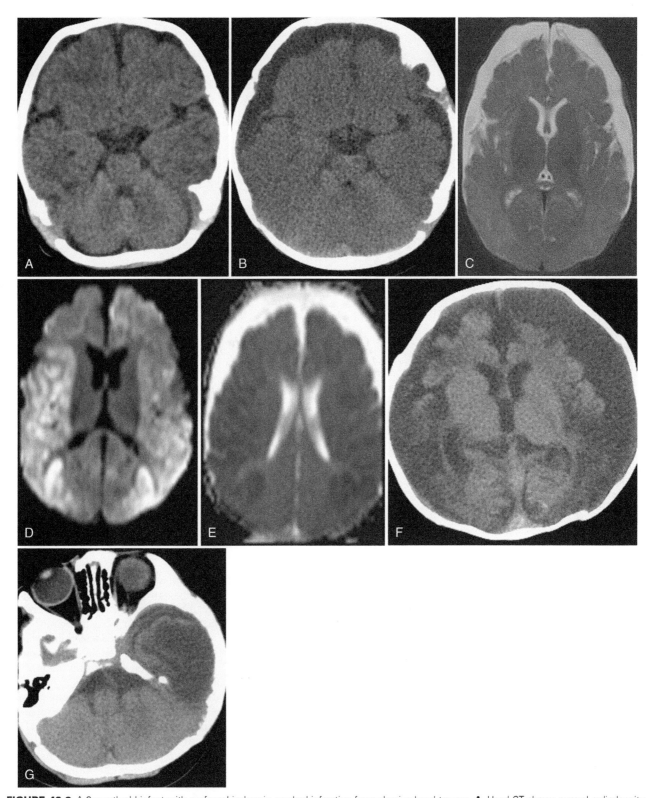

FIGURE 42-9 A 3-month-old infant with profound ischemic cerebral infarction from abusive head trauma. **A,** Head CT shows normal radiodensity of grey and white matter in both cerebrum and cerebellum. **B,** Two months later, head CT shows diffuse hypodensity in cerebral cortex and subdural fluid–containing membranes; attenuation of cerebellum is normal ("CT reversal sign"). **C,** T2-weighted MR image demonstrates hyperintense subdural hematomas, subtle biparietal cortical hyperintensity, and normal basal ganglia. **D** and **E,** Diffusion-weighted **(D)** and apparent diffusion coefficient map images **(E)** show diffuse abnormal signal intensity in cerebral cortex sparing basal ganglia. **F** and **G,** Head CT performed 6 weeks later shows global cerebral encephalomalacia and relatively normal basal ganglia and cerebellum.

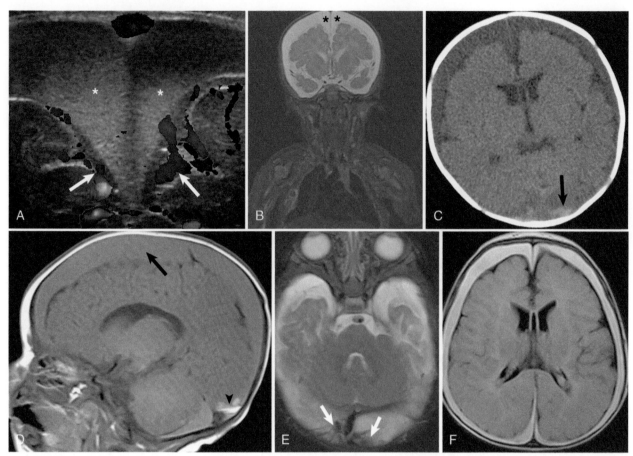

FIGURE 42-10 A 9-week-old infant with acute-on-chronic subdural hematoma. **A** and **B,** Transcranial Doppler sonogram **(A)** and whole-body short-tau inversion recovery (WB-STIR) MR image **(B)** in coronal plane show bihemispheric subdural fluid containing no vessels (*).On ultrasound, compressed superficial cortical vessels in subarachnoid space *(arrows)* lie against surface of brain. **C,** Noncontrast CT demonstrates hypodense subdural hematomas and sediment of hyperdense clot *(arrow).* **D,** Sagittal T1-weighted MR imaging performed 1 day after CT shows slightly hyperintense SDH *(arrow)* and hyperintense clot *(arrowhead).* **E** and **F,** Transverse T2-weighted **(E)** and FLAIR **(F)** images shows hyperintense chronic subdural hematomas and dependent hypointense clot *(arrows).*

wide (>3 mm) and complex, and 33% were multiple.[59] Linear fractures can be missed on CT, particularly when the plane of the fracture is collinear with the plane of imaging. Volume-rendered presentation of multidetector CT information increases the sensitivity for all types of skull, facial, and orbital fractures (see Figure 42-2).[61,62]

Scalp edema and *hematoma* are important signs of an acute head injury and should generate a search for an associated skull fracture or intracranial injury. The converse is not true, however, since significant intracranial injuries can occur with little or no scalp swelling.[18]

DETERMINING THE AGE OF HEAD INJURY

One of the important characteristics of inflicted injury is an inconsistency between the documented injury and its explanation based on expected patterns of injury from biomechanical, epidemiologic, and neurodevelopmental information. In cases of AHT, the age of the injury is important in child protection as well as prosecution issues. Therefore, in addition to documenting the presence, nature, and extent of head injury, another objective of neuroimaging is

to provide a reasonable estimation of the age of that injury. There are several imaging signs that suggest a head injury has occurred recently. These include scalp edema, cerebral edema, subarachnoid hemorrhage, hyperdense hemorrhage on CT, and "acute" blood products (e.g., deoxyhemoglobin) on MR imaging. Other signs suggest that an injury is older. For instance, the presence of an organizing membrane within an SDH on CT or MR imaging, which can be enhanced after contrast material is administered, suggests that the hemorrhage is at least 1 week old.[63,64]

The radiodensity or x-ray attenuation of blood on CT is related to its protein content and hematocrit, and by convention is described relative to the radiodensity of normal brain tissue. Freshly extravasated blood is the same or slightly more radiodense than brain tissue on noncontrast CT, but within several hours becomes more hyperdense because of hemoconcentration and clot formation.[65-67] Hyperdense blood can be seen from the time of injury to as long as 7 to 10 days after the traumatic event.[68,69] During the 1 to 3 weeks after injury, the density of blood decreases by an average of 0.7 to 1.5 Hounsfield units per day because of clot proteolysis (Figure 42-13).[70,71] Thus at some time in its resolution, hemorrhage will be the same density as adjacent brain tissue, rendering it more difficult to detect.[64,72,73] After

3 weeks, blood will be predominately hypodense on CT and appears grossly like crank-case oil when examined at surgery or autopsy.[64]

This temporal pattern of hemorrhage regression on CT is a generalization, and exceptions should be considered. For instance, within the first day after head injury, an SDH can be of mixed density with both hyperdense and hypodense components, or rarely, predominately hypodense.[68,69,74-76] Wells and Sty[76] reported that the first appearance of low-attenuation fluid in SDH was during the first week after the traumatic event in 80% of 55 children and that mixed-density subdural fluid could occur after a single traumatic insult. In an acute SDH, blood that is lower in radiodensity reflects unclotted blood (because of active bleeding or coagulopathy), separation of serum from a sediment of clotted blood, or admixture with CSF from a co-existent tear in the arachnoid membrane.[77]

Blood also undergoes a change in signal intensity over time on MR imaging. This temporal change has been confirmed largely from empirical investigations of adult subjects with intraparenchymal bleeding.[78,79] The pathophysiology of the changes in the signal intensity of blood on MR imaging is influenced by both biological factors, such as the oxygenation of hemoglobin, oxidation of iron in hemoglobin, and the integrity of the red blood cell (RBC) membrane, as well as technical factors relating to MR imaging, such as pulse sequence selection and the magnetic field strength of the scanner.[78-80] By convention, the temporal changes in the signal intensity of intracerebral hematoma and SDH on MR imaging have been divided into four stages, which is illustrated in Figure 42-13 and summarized in Table 42-1. Intracerebral hematomas are classified as "acute" (between several hours and 3 days after bleeding into the brain parenchyma), "early subacute" (approximately 3 days to 1 week), "late subacute" (1 week to 1 month), or "chronic" (over 1 month). In the acute stage, blood has begun to clot and contains deoxyhemoglobin within intact RBCs. On T1-weighted MR images, acute blood is the same signal intensity (isointense) or slightly hypointense compared with normal brain tissue, and on T2-weighted images, blood containing deoxyhemoglobin is hypointense. In the early subacute stage, clot retraction occurs and deoxyhemoglobin is oxidized to methemoglobin. Since the RBCs are still intact at this stage, methemoglobin is in the intracellular compartment. On T1-weighted images, early subacute blood is

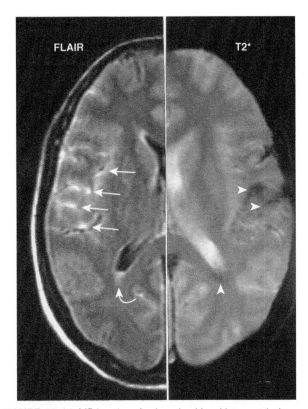

FIGURE 42-11 MR imaging of subarachnoid and intraventricular hemorrhage. Composite image of FLAIR (left side of image) and T2*-weighted gradient echo images (right side) shows hyperintense Sylvian subarachnoid *(arrows)* and intraventricular *(curved arrow)* hemorrhage on FLAIR. Hemorrhage *(arrowheads)* is hypointense on T2*-weighted gradient echo image.

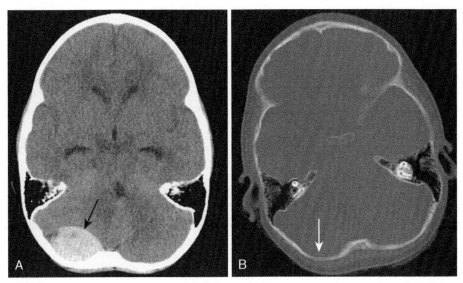

FIGURE 42-12 Venous epidural hematoma in a 2-year-old child after a fall. **A,** CT scan viewed with brain window shows biconvex hyperdense hematoma *(arrow)* in posterior fossa. **B,** CT viewed with bone window shows linear right occipital skull fracture next to right lateral dural venous sinus.

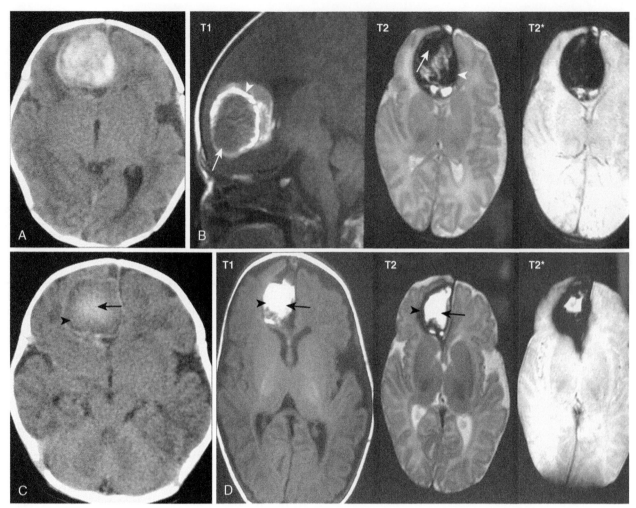

FIGURE 42-13 CT and MR imaging of intracerebral hematoma in acute and subacute stages in a 1-year-old child. **A,** Noncontrast CT shows hyperdense hematoma in right frontal lobe 4 hours following blunt traumatic head injury. **B,** Montage of MR images performed 48 hours after injury shows center of hematoma *(arrow)* is isointense relative to white matter on sagittal T1-weighted image *(left image)* consistent with deoxyhemoglobin. Peripheral rim *(arrowhead)* of hematoma is hyperintense, consistent with intracellular methemoglobin. On T2-weighted *(middle)* and T2*-weighted gradient echo *(right)* images, hematoma is markedly hypointense. **C,** CT scan performed 7 days after injury shows rim of hematoma *(arrowhead)* is isodense but center *(arrow)* is hyperdense. **D,** Montage of MR imaging performed 12 days after injury shows that hematoma *(arrow)* is hyperintense on T1-weighted *(left)* and T2-weighted *(middle)* images consistent with extracellular methemoglobin. Hemosiderin-containing rim *(arrowhead)* is hypointense on T2-weighted and T2*-weighted gradient echo *(right)* images.

hyperintense because of the methemoglobin. On T2-weighted images, early subacute blood is hypointense compared with normal brain tissue. After about 1 week, RBCs begin to lyse and methemoglobin becomes extracellular; this defines the late subacute stage. On both T1- and T2-weighted MR imaging, extracellular methemoglobin is hyperintense. After about 1 month from the time of initial brain hemorrhage, iron from catabolized hemoglobin becomes stored as water-soluble ferritin or water-insoluble hemosiderin in glial cells that surround the contracting blood clot. Both ferritin and hemosiderin are markedly hypointense on T2-weighted MR imaging and are isointense on T1-weighted MR images.

There have been far fewer published investigations of the temporal regression of SDH than parenchymal hemorrhage on MR imaging. In general, the changes in signal intensity of SDH over time are similar to those of intracerebral hematoma but differences have been reported (see Figure 42-1).[75,81-83] In one of the earliest studies, Fobben and colleagues[82] reported that the signal intensity of blood products

in four acute, four early subacute, and four late-subacute subdural hematomas were similar to those of intracerebral hematoma of the same age. Unlike the brain hematoma, however, only 1 in 13 chronic SDHs contained T2-hypointense hemosiderin, and the authors suggested that the absence of a blood–brain barrier in the subdural space enabled hemosiderin resorption to occur.[82] More recently, Vinchon and colleagues[75] studied posttraumatic SDH of known age on both noncontrast CT and MR imaging in 20 children. After a single traumatic event, acute hematomas that were heterogeneous in signal intensity could be found on MR imaging. T1-hyperintense sediment was seen as early as 3 days after trauma and in most SDHs between 3 and 14 days after trauma. An investigation of traumatic SDH in adults by Duhem and colleagues[81] also reported heterogeneous signal intensity in the temporal evolution of SDH and concluded that this was not a sign of repetitive head trauma. They found that the temporal changes in SDH differed from intracerebral hematoma in 83% of 18 patients (see Table 42-1).[81]

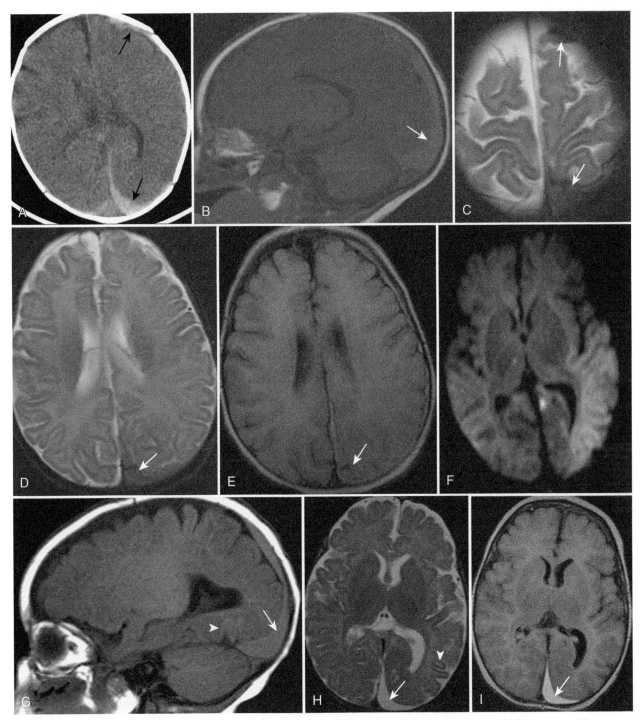

FIGURE 42-14 A 10-week-old with subdural hematoma (SDH) and ischemic infarction from abusive head trauma. **A,** Noncontrast CT shows acute, hyperdense left occipitoparietal and frontal SDHs *(arrows)*. **B,** Sagittal T1-weighted MR imaging performed 2 days later shows increased signal intensity in acute SDH *(arrow)*. **C** and **D,** Transverse axial T2-weighted images show decreased signal intensity *(arrows)* in acute SDH. **E,** FLAIR shows isointense signal intensity in acute SDH *(arrow)*. **F,** Diffusion-weighted image demonstrates left temporoparietal hyperintensity that was not seen on other pulse sequences or on CT. **G,** Sagittal T1-weighted MR imaging performed 16 days after CT shows hyperintense signal in dependent, late subacute SDH *(arrow)* and faint laminar hyperintensity in temporal cortex *(arrowhead)*. **H** and **I,** Late subacute hematoma *(arrow)* is hyperintense on both transverse T2-weighted **(H)** and FLAIR **(I)** MR imaging. Also note enlargement of left lateral ventricle and slight parietal atrophy *(arrowhead)* consistent with focal encephalomalacia.

Table 42-1	Temporal Changes in Signal Intensity of Blood on 1.5-Tesla MR Imaging		ICH		SDH*	
Stage	**Time**	**Hemoglobin**	**T1**	**T2**	**T1**	**T2**
Acute	Hours-3 days	Deoxyhemoglobin	↓/=	↓	=	↓
Early subacute	3-10 days	Methemoglobin (IC)	↑	↓	↑	=/↑
Late subacute	<3 wk	Methemoglobin (EC)	↑	↑	↑	↑
Chronic	>3 wk	Hemosiderin	=	↓	↓	↑

↑, Hyperintense compared to normal brain tissue; =, isointense; ↓, hypointense; *EC*, extracellular; *IC*, intracellular; *ICH*, intracerebral hematoma; *SDH*, subdural hematoma; *T1*, T1-weighted MR imaging; *T2*, T2-weighted MR imaging.
*Data from the investigation of Duhem R, Vinchon M, Tonnelle V, et al: [Main temporal aspects of the MRI signal of subdural hematomas and practical contribution to dating head injury]. *Neurochirurgie* 2006;52:93-104.

DIFFERENTIAL DIAGNOSIS

Chapter 47 ("Conditions Confused with Head Trauma") presents a thorough discussion of the differential diagnoses to be considered when evaluating a child with possible AHT. Knowledge of the radiological characteristics of these conditions is imperative.

Benign Extraaxial Fluid of Infancy (BEAF)

This condition, alternatively called *benign enlargement of the subarachnoid space* or *expanded arachnoid collections of infancy*, is characterized by enlargement of the subarachnoid space over and between the cerebral hemispheres in children with normal neurological development and no signs of intracranial hypertension. It is usually diagnosed within the first year of life, resolves without treatment by the age of 2 years, and is often familial.[84] Many of these children present for neuroimaging because of an increasing head circumference that exceeds the 95th percentile by the age of 6 months. Neuroimaging reveals symmetrical enlargement of the subarachnoid spaces around and between the frontal lobes and within the Sylvian fissures but without mass effect. The lateral and third ventricles are sometimes slightly enlarged. MR imaging as well as color Doppler sonography performed through the acoustical window of an open anterior fontanel can differentiate BEAF from chronic SDH.[85,86] The subarachnoid space normally contains numerous superficial cortical veins, whereas blood within the subdural space does not. Furthermore, CSF in the enlarged subarachnoid spaces should be the same density and signal intensity as that in the lateral ventricles. On Doppler ultrasound, the visualization of color-encoded veins in anechoic extracerebral spaces over the convexity of the frontal lobes is consistent with BEAF (Figure 42-15). With abnormal subdural fluid collection, these same cortical veins are displaced inward and appear to be compressed along the surface of the brain by subdural fluid of variable echogenicity (see Figure 42-10).[85] A membrane might also be seen if the subdural fluid is a subacute or chronic subdural hemorrhage.

The importance of BEAF is not only that it might be confused with chronic SDH on neuroimaging, but also that some believe that it predisposes to the development of SDH (see Figure 42-15).[86,87] Biomechanical models suggest that when the width of the subarachnoid space increases to 6 mm from a normal size of about 3 mm, excessive brain translation may cause superficial cortical veins to tear.[88] Yet a recent finite element model study has yielded the exact opposite conclusion, where increased extraaxial fluid actually *stabilized* bridging vessels, decreasing bridging vein strain resulting from rotational acceleration of the head.[89] Theoretically, BEAF might increase the likelihood of a small localized SDH with impact, but it should not account for the severe encephalopathy often associated with AHT.

Accidental Head Trauma

Differentiating accidental from AHT on the basis of neuroradiology alone is difficult if not impossible. The history provided must be compared with the clinical signs and symptoms as well as the neuroimaging findings to ultimately determine the etiology. Nonetheless, some features deserve mention. The disproportionately higher prevalence of SDH and diffuse cerebral edema in AHT speaks to differences between accidental and inflicted head trauma.[41,43,90,91] Cortical contusion, DAI, and EDH seem to be more prevalent in accidental head injury, particularly those from motor vehicle crashes.[90,92] SDH that occurs after an accident is more often unilateral and adjacent to a direct contact injury, such as skull fracture or scalp hematoma. Mixed-density SDH has been shown to be significantly more prevalent in AHT but can be observed in cases of head injury from accidental trauma as well, and interhemispheric SDH, once thought to be a defining injury of abuse, might be as likely to occur after accidental head trauma, particularly if SDH from birth are categorized as "accidental" injueries.[68] Datta and colleagues[92] reported findings in 49 cases of inflicted head injury, 3 cases of accidental traumatic brain injury, and 11 cases of SDH that resulted from miscellaneous causes (meningitis, postsurgery, hemorrhagic disease of newborn, and benign effusion). SDHs of different density or signal intensity were seen in 26 (53%) cases of

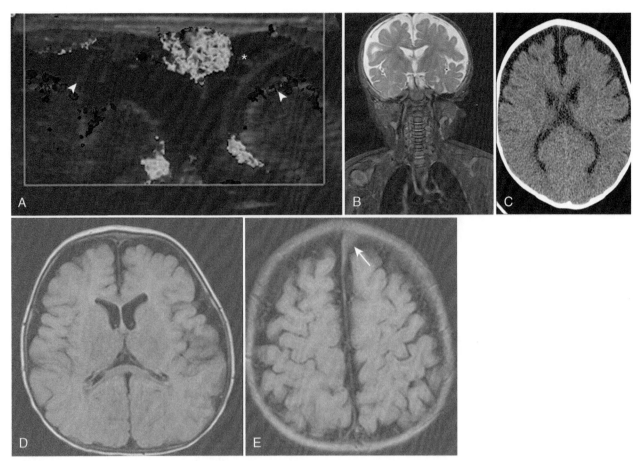

FIGURE 42-15 Asymptomatic 7-month-old boy referred for large head circumference with expanded arachnoid collections of infancy and small left subdural hematoma (SDH). **A,** Coronal transcranial Doppler sonogram demonstrates vessels coursing in right frontal subarachnoid space *(arrowheads)* and small, vessel-free left extraaxial space (*). **B,** Coronal whole-body short-tau inversion recovery shows vessels coursing through large bifrontal subarachnoid spaces. **C,** Noncontrast CT demonstrates large bifrontal and interhemispheric extraaxial spaces that are isodense compared with ventricular CSF. **D** and **E,** FLAIR images show large bifrontal subarachnoid spaces that are isointense compared with ventricular CSF as well as small left frontal SDH *(arrow)* that is higher in signal intensity compared with CSF.

AHT but in none of the SDH from the other causes. Focal or diffuse cerebral edema was seen in 12 (24%) cases of AHT and generalized edema associated with SDH was only seen with inflicted head injury.[92]

Parturitional Head Trauma

The prevalence of asymptomatic SDH ranges from 8% to 46% after uncomplicated vaginal or cesarean delivery.[83,93,94] Rooks and colleagues[83] reported SDH in 46% of 101 asymptomatic term infants who underwent cranial MRI 72 hours after delivery. All were supratentorial and in the posterior half of the cranium, 43% were also infratentorial, and nearly all were 3 mm or smaller (Figure 42-16). Several studies have reported that these small, birth-related subdural hematomas resolve within a few months after discovery.[83,94]

Infectious and Inflammatory Disease

Bacterial and viral infections uncommonly produce neuroimaging findings that are similar to those of AHT. A well-described complication of *Haemophilus influenzae* and *Neisseria meningitidis* meningitis in infants is a subdural collection that may contain clear, xanthochromic, hemorrhagic, or purulent

fluid.[95] A protein-rich subdural effusion or empyema could mimic chronic SDH on CT but the clinical presentation and CSF profile should be distinctive (Figure 42-17). Some neuroimaging signs of herpes encephalitis and AHT are somewhat similar. In some cases of herpes encephalitis, MR imaging demonstrates cortical hemorrhage, but SDH would not be expected.[96] Since early diagnosis is important, infants with an unidentified encephalopathy should undergo neuroimaging and have CSF evaluated for herpes infection.

Coagulopathy

Spontaneous or traumatic intracranial hemorrhage can occur with inherited coagulopathy or acquired bleeding diatheses caused by systemic diseases or their treatment. Hemorrhagic disease of the newborn, hemophilia A and B, and von Willebrand disease are inherited coagulopathies that might rarely cause intracranial hemorrhage.[97-101] SDH and other intracranial hemorrhages in children have been reported with leukemia, as a complication of anticoagulation therapy or bone marrow transplantation, and from acquired coagulopathies, such as drug-induced or idiopathic immune-thrombocytopenic purpura and consumption coagulopathy.[102-106]

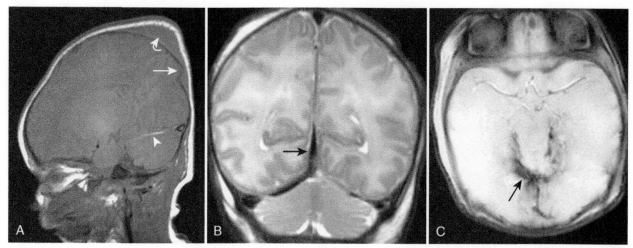

FIGURE 42-16 SDH in neonate with mild hypotonia 5 days after vaginal delivery. **A,** Sagittal T1-weighted MR image shows overriding calvarial bones *(arrow)*, scalp hematoma *(curved arrow)*, and small, linear hyperintense subtentorial hemorrhage *(arrowhead)*. **B,** Coronal T2-weighted image demonstrates hypointense posterior interhemispheric *(arrow)* and subtentorial hemorrhage. **C,** Markedly hypointense subtentorial *(arrow)* and posterior subdural hemorrhage is confirmed on transverse axial T2*-weighted gradient echo MR image.

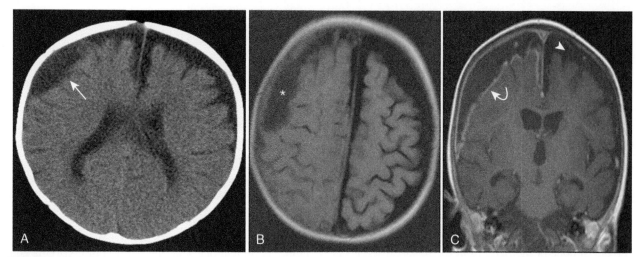

FIGURE 42-17 Subdural empyema resulting from meningitis. **A,** CT shows excessive bifrontal extraaxial fluid with mass effect on right frontal lobe *(arrow)*. **B,** Fluid in right subdural space (*) is higher in signal intensity than left subarachnoid fluid on transverse axial T1-weighted MR image. **C,** There is contrast enhancement of both thickened dura and along deep margin *(curved arrow)* of right subdural empyema on coronal T1-weighted image. Vessels course through fluid in enlarged nonenhancing left subarachnoid space *(arrowhead)* that is isointense with cerebrospinal fluid in lateral ventricles. *(Case courtesy of Kathleen McCarten, MD, Hasbro Children's Hospital, Providence, RI.)*

Metabolic Disease

Glutaric aciduria type 1 (GA1) can be associated with SDH. Since retinal hemorrhages are also infrequently reported with this rare metabolic disease, GA1 may mimic AHT.[107-109] Findings on neuroimaging that suggest GA1 include widening of the Sylvian fissures and expansion of the CSF spaces anterior to the temporal lobe from temporal lobe hypoplasia. Abnormal hyperintense signal in the putamen, either in isolation or with the caudate nucleus, is a result of depletion of neurons or of proliferation of astrocytes.[110]

FUTURE DIRECTIONS FOR RESEARCH

One of the most important directions for future research regarding neuroimaging of head trauma involves the use of advanced MR imaging techniques to investigate traumatic brain injury in infants and young children. The detection and accurate characterization of cerebral injury may enable earlier and more specific intervention to prevent potentially devastating long-term morbidity of traumatic brain injury. Whole-body STIR could be a useful adjunct to conventional brain MR imaging for distinguishing subarachnoid effusion from SDH in infants, and for the detection of traumatic skull and scalp injuries. Other neuroimaging techniques have shown that brain tissue that appears normal on CT and conventional MR imaging techniques can be structurally or functionally impaired. Newer gradient-echo MR imaging techniques, such as susceptibility-weighted imaging, increase the sensitivity of MR imaging for superparamagnetic blood products. In a study of seven children, Tong and colleagues[29] showed that the number of hemorrhagic shear injuries was six times greater and the volume was twice as large on susceptibility-weighted MR imaging compared with conventional T2*-weighted gradient echo MR imaging. Proton MR spectroscopy enables the *in vivo* analysis of key biochemical constituents of brain tissue. In 14 subjects with mild traumatic brain injury, decreased concentrations of *N*-acetylaspartate, an amino acid marker of neuronal function, and increased levels of choline, a marker of cell membrane repair, were detected in cerebral tissue that was normal on conventional MR imaging.[111] Another study found a strong correlation between elevated brain lactate levels and poor clinical outcome in children who had suffered AHT.[112]

Diffusion-tensor imaging (DTI) evaluates the integrity of white matter and has been used to create exquisite maps of white matter tracts (diffusion-tensor tractography). Huisman and colleagues[113] reported that abnormal diffusion tensor measurements in the internal capsule and callosal splenium reflect damage to axonal microstructure and correlate better with clinical assessments of brain injury than conventional DWI. Others have found that DTI detects damage to areas of the brain remote from direct brain injury, suggesting that it might be a useful technique to study distal axonal and transsynaptic effects of brain injury.[114] These seminal investigations of newer MR imaging techniques need to be confirmed and extended before promulgation of whole-body STIR, susceptibility-weighted MR imaging, proton MR spectroscopy, and diffusion tensor imaging can be recommended for the routine evaluation of AHT.

References

1. Kraus JF, Fife D, Conroy C: Pediatric brain injuries: the nature, clinical course, and early outcomes in a defined United States' population. *Pediatrics* 1987;79:501-507.
2. Bruce DA, Zimmerman RA: Shaken impact syndrome. *Pediatr Ann* 1989;18:482-484, 486-489, 492-484.
3. Conway EE Jr: Nonaccidental head injury in infants: "the shaken baby syndrome revisited." *Pediatr Ann* 1998;27:677-690.
4. Duhaime AC, Alario AJ, Lewander WJ, et al: Head injury in very young children: mechanisms, injury types, and ophthalmologic findings in 100 hospitalized patients younger than 2 years of age. *Pediatrics* 1992;90:179-185.
5. Duhaime AC, Christian C, Moss E, et al: Long-term outcome in infants with the shaking-impact syndrome. *Pediatr Neurosurg* 1996;24:292-298.
6. American College of Radiology: *ACR Appropropriateness Criteria*, 2005. Available at http://www.acr.org/SecondaryMainMenuCategories/quality_safety/app_criteria/pdf/ExpertPanelonPediatricImaging/SuspectedPhysicalAbuseChildDoc9.aspx. Accessed July 4, 2009.
7. Ghahreman A, Bhasin V, Chaseling R, et al: Nonaccidental head injuries in children: a Sydney experience. *J Neurosurg* 2005;103:213-218.
8. Krauss B, Green SM: Sedation and analgesia for procedures in children. *N Engl J Med* 2000;342:938-945.
9. Shellock FG: Magnetic resonance safety update 2002: implants and devices. *J Magn Reson Imaging* 2002;16:485-496.
10. Shellock FG, Spinazzi A: MRI safety update 2008: part 2, screening patients for MRI. *AJR Am J Roentgenol* 2008;191:1140-1149.
11. Suh DY, Davis PC, Hopkins KL, et al: Nonaccidental pediatric head injury: diffusion-weighted imaging findings. *Neurosurgery* 2001;49:309-318.
12. Huisman TA, Sorensen AG, Hergan K, et al: Diffusion-weighted imaging for the evaluation of diffuse axonal injury in closed head injury. *J Comput Assist Tomogr* 2003;27:5-11.
13. Holshouser BA, Ashwal S, Luh GY, et al: Proton MR spectroscopy after acute central nervous system injury: outcome prediction in neonates, infants, and children. *Radiology* 1997;202:487-496.
14. Haseler LJ, Arcinue E, Danielsen ER, et al: Evidence from proton magnetic resonance spectroscopy for a metabolic cascade of neuronal damage in shaken baby syndrome. *Pediatrics* 1997;99:4-14.
15. Caffey J: On the theory and practice of shaking infants. Its potential residual effects of permanent brain damage and mental retardation. *Am J Dis Child* 1972;124:161-169.
16. Caffey J: The whiplash shaken infant syndrome: manual shaking by the extremities with whiplash-induced intracranial and intraocular bleedings, linked with residual permanent brain damage and mental retardation. *Pediatrics* 1974;54:396-403.
17. Case ME, Graham MA, Handy TC, et al: Position paper on fatal abusive head injuries in infants and young children. *Am J Forensic Med Pathol* 2001;22:112-122.
18. Duhaime AC, Gennarelli TA, Thibault LE, et al: The shaken baby syndrome. A clinical, pathological, and biomechanical study. *J Neurosurg* 1987;66:409-415.
19. Bandak FA: On the mechanics of impact neurotrauma: a review and critical synthesis. *J Neurotrauma* 1995;12:635-649.
20. Ommaya AK: Head injury mechanisms and the concept of preventive management: a review and critical synthesis. *J Neurotrauma* 1995;12:527-546.
21. Gennarelli TA: Mechanisms of brain injury. *J Emerg Med* 1993;11 (Suppl 1):5-11.
22. Kriel RL, Krach LE, Sheehan M: Pediatric closed head injury: outcome following prolonged unconsciousness. *Arch Phys Med Rehabil* 1988;69:678-681.
23. Adams JH, Graham DI, Gennarelli TA, et al: Diffuse axonal injury in non-missile head injury. *J Neurol Neurosurg Psychiatry* 1991;54:481-483.
24. Adams JH, Graham DI, Murray LS, et al: Diffuse axonal injury due to nonmissile head injury in humans: an analysis of 45 cases. *Ann Neurol* 1982;12:557-563.
25. Ommaya AK, Gennarelli TA: Cerebral concussion and traumatic unconsciousness.Correlation of experimental and clinical observations of blunt head injuries. *Brain* 1974;97:633-654.
26. Adams JH, Doyle D, Ford I, et al: Diffuse axonal injury in head injury: definition, diagnosis and grading. *Histopathology* 1989;15:49-59.
27. Mittl RL, Grossman RI, Hiehle JF, et al: Prevalence of MR evidence of diffuse axonal injury in patients with mild head injury and normal head CT findings. *AJNR Am J Neuroradiol* 1994;15:1583-1589.
28. Sigmund GA, Tong KA, Nickerson JP, et al: Multimodality comparison of neuroimaging in pediatric traumatic brain injury. *Pediatr Neurol* 2007;36:217-226.
29. Tong KA, Ashwal S, Holshouser BA, et al: Hemorrhagic shearing lesions in children and adolescents with posttraumatic diffuse axonal injury: improved detection and initial results. *Radiology* 2003;227:332-339.
30. Lindenberg R, Freytag E: Morphology of brain lesions from blunt trauma in early infancy. *Arch Pathol Lab Med* 1969;87:298-305.
31. Calder I, Hill I, Scholtz C: Primary brain trauma in non-accidental injury. *J Clin Pathol* 1984;37:1095-1100.
32. Bruce DA, Alavi A, Bilaniuk L, et al: Diffuse cerebral swelling following head injuries in children: the syndrome of "malignant brain edema." *J Neurosurg* 1981;54:170-178.
33. Cohen RA, Kaufman RA, Myers PA, et al: Cranial computed tomography in the abused child with head injury. *AJR Am J Roentgenol* 1986;146:97-102.
34. Zimmerman RA, Bilaniuk LT, Bruce D, et al: Computed tomography of pediatric head trauma: acute general cerebral swelling. *Radiology* 1978;126:403-408.
35. Sharples PM, Matthews DS, Eyre JA: Cerebral blood flow and metabolism in children with severe head injuries. Part 2: Cerebrovascular resistance and its determinants. *J Neurol Neurosurg Psychiatry* 1995;58:153-159.
36. Geddes JF, Hackshaw AK, Vowles GH, et al: Neuropathology of inflicted head injury in children. I. Patterns of brain damage. *Brain* 2001;124:1290-1298.
37. Geddes JF, Vowles GH, Hackshaw AK, et al: Neuropathology of inflicted head injury in children. II. Microscopic brain injury in infants. *Brain* 2001;124:1299-1306.
38. Punt J, Bonshek RE, Jaspan T, et al: The "unified hypothesis" of Geddes et al. is not supported by the data. *Pediatr Rehabil* 2004;7:173-184.
39. Han BK, Towbin RB, De Courten-Myers G, et al: Reversal sign on CT: effect of anoxic/ischemic cerebral injury in children. *AJNR Am J Neuroradiol* 1989;10:1191-1198.
40. Harwood-Nash DC: Abuse to the pediatric central nervous system. *AJNR Am J Neuroradiol* 1992;13:569-575.

41. Dashti SR, Decker DD, Razzaq A, et al: Current patterns of inflicted head injury in children. *Pediatr Neurosurg* 1999;31:302-306.

42. Gilles EE, Nelson MD Jr: Cerebral complications of nonaccidental head injury in childhood. *Pediatr Neurol* 1998;19:119-128.

43. Reece RM, Sege R: Childhood head injuries: accidental or inflicted? *Arch Pediatr Adolesc Med* 2000;154:11-15.

44. Yamashima T, Friede RL: Why do bridging veins rupture into the virtual subdural space? *J Neurol Neurosurg Psychiatry* 1984;47:121-127.

45. Hobbs CJ: Skull fracture and the diagnosis of abuse. *Arch Dis Child* 1984;59:246-252.

46. Nimityongskul P, Anderson LD: The likelihood of injuries when children fall out of bed. *J Pediatr Orthop* 1987;7:184-186.

47. Tarantino CA, Dowd MD, Murdock TC: Short vertical falls in infants. *Pediatr Emerg Care* 1999;15:5-8.

48. Williams RA: Injuries in infants and small children resulting from witnessed and corroborated free falls. *J Trauma* 1991;31:1350-1352.

49. Friede RL, Schachenmayr W: The origin of subdural neomembranes. II. Fine structural of neomembranes. *Am J Pathol* 1978;92:69-84.

50. Campbell BG, Zimmerman RD: Emergency magnetic resonance of the brain. *Top Magn Reson Imaging* 1998;9:208-227.

51. Noguchi K, Seto H, Kamisaki Y, et al: Comparison of fluid-attenuated inversion-recovery MR imaging with CT in a simulated model of acute subarachnoid hemorrhage. *AJNR Am J Neuroradiol* 2000;21:923-927.

52. Bakshi R, Kamran S, Kinkel PR, et al: MRI in cerebral intraventricular hemorrhage: analysis of 50 consecutive cases. *Neuroradiology* 1999;41:401-409.

53. Merten DF, Osborne DR, Radkowski MA, et al: Craniocerebral trauma in the child abuse syndrome: radiological observations. *Pediatr Radiol* 1984;14:272-277.

54. Shugerman RP, Paez A, Grossman DC, et al: Epidural hemorrhage: is it abuse? *Pediatrics* 1996;97:664-668.

55. Leggate JR, Lopez-Ramos N, Genitori L, et al: Extradural haematoma in infants. *Br J Neurosurg* 1989;3:533-539.

56. Loder RT, Bookout C: Fracture patterns in battered children. *J Orthop Trauma* 1991;5:428-433.

57. Skellern CY, Wood DO, Murphy A, et al: Non-accidental fractures in infants: risk of further abuse. *J Paediatr Child Health* 2000;36:590-592.

58. Billmire ME, Myers PA: Serious head injury in infants: accident or abuse? *Pediatrics* 1985;75:340-342.

59. Carty H, Pierce A: Non-accidental injury: a retrospective analysis of a large cohort. *Eur Radiol* 2002;12:2919-2925.

60. Meservy CJ, Towbin R, McLaurin RL, et al: Radiographic characteristics of skull fractures resulting from child abuse. *AJR Am J Roentgenol* 1987;149:173-175.

61. Lee HJ, Jilani M, Frohman L, et al: CT of orbital trauma. *Emerg Radiol* 2004;10:168-172.

62. Medina LS: Three-dimensional CT maximum intensity projections of the calvaria: a new approach for diagnosis of craniosynostosis and fractures. *AJNR Am J Neuroradiol* 2000;21:1951-1954.

63. Firsching R, Frowein RA, Thun F: Encapsulated subdural hematoma. *Neurosurg Rev* 1989;12(Suppl 1):207-214.

64. Scotti G, Terbrugge K, Melançon D, et al: Evaluation of the age of subdural hematomas by computerized tomography. *J Neurosurg* 1977;47:311-315.

65. New PF, Aronow S: Attenuation measurements of whole blood and blood fractions in computed tomography. *Radiology* 1976;121:635-640.

66. Norman D, Price D, Boyd D, et al: Quantitative aspects of computed tomography of the blood and cerebrospinal fluid. *Radiology* 1977;123:335-338.

67. Kaufman HH, Singer JM, Sadhu VK, et al: Isodense acute subdural hematoma. *J Comput Assist Tomogr* 1980;4:557-559.

68. Tung GA, Kumar M, Richardson RC, et al: Comparison of accidental and nonaccidental traumatic head injury in children on noncontrast computed tomography. *Pediatrics* 2006;118:626-633.

69. Vinchon M, Noizet O, Defoort-Dhellemmes S, et al: Infantile subdural hematomas due to traffic accidents. *Pediatr Neurosurg* 2002;37:245-253.

70. Dolinskas CA, Bilaniuk LT, Zimmerman RA, et al: Computed tomography of intracerebral hematomas. I. Transmission CT observations on hematoma resolution. *AJR Am J Roentgenol* 1977;129:681-688.

71. Dolinskas CA, Bilaniuk LT, Zimmerman RA, et al: Computed tomography of intracerebral hematomas. II. Radionuclide and transmission CT studies of the perihematoma region. *AJR Am J Roentgenol* 1977;129:689-692.

72. Bergstrom M, Ericson K, Levander B, et al: Computed tomography of cranial subdural and epidural hematomas: variation of attenuation related to time and clinical events such as rebleeding. *J Comput Assist Tomogr* 1977;1:449-455.

73. Moller A, Ericson K: Computed tomography of isoattenuating subdural hematomas. *Radiology* 1979;130:149-152.

74. Dias MS, Backstrom J, Falk M, et al: Serial radiography in the infant shaken impact syndrome. *Pediatr Neurosurg* 1998;29:77-85.

75. Vinchon M, Noule N, Tchofo PJ, et al: Imaging of head injuries in infants: temporal correlates and forensic implications for the diagnosis of child abuse. *J Neurosurg (Pediatrics 2)* 2004;101:44-52.

76. Wells RG, Sty JR: Traumatic low attenuation subdural fluid collections in children younger than 3 years. *Arch Pediatr Adolesc Med* 2003;157:1005-1010.

77. Zouros A, Bhargava R, Hoskinson M, et al: Further characterization of traumatic subdural collections of infancy. Report of five cases. *J Neurosurg* 2004;100:512-518.

78. Bradley WG Jr: MR appearance of hemorrhage in the brain. *Radiology* 1993;189:15-26.

79. Gomori JM, Grossman RI, Yu-Ip C, et al: NMR relaxation times of blood: dependence on field strength, oxidation state, and cell integrity. *J Comput Assist Tomogr* 1987;11:684-690.

80. Parizel PM, Van Goethem JW, Ozsarlak O, et al: New developments in the neuroradiological diagnosis of craniocerebral trauma. *Eur Radiol* 2005;15:569-581.

81. Duhem R, Vinchon M, Tonnelle V, et al: [Main temporal aspects of the MRI signal of subdural hematomas and practical contribution to dating head injury]. *Neurochirurgie* 2006;52:93-104.

82. Fobben ES, Grossman RI, Atlas SW, et al: MR characteristics of subdural hematomas and hygromas at 1.5 T. *AJR Am J Roentgenol* 1989;153:589-595.

83. Rooks VJ, Eaton JP, Ruess L, et al: Prevalence and evolution of intracranial hemorrhage in asymptomatic term infants. *AJNR Am J Neuroradiol* 2008;29:1082-1089.

84. Hellbusch LC: Benign extracerebral fluid collections in infancy: clinical presentation and long-term follow-up. *J Neurosurg* 2007;107:119-125.

85. Chen CY, Chou TY, Zimmerman RA, et al: Pericerebral fluid collection: differentiation of enlarged subarachnoid spaces from subdural collections with color Doppler US. *Radiology* 1996;201:389-392.

86. Wilms G, Vanderschueren G, Demaerel PH, et al: CT and MR in infants with pericerebral collections and macrocephaly: benign enlargement of the subarachnoid spaces versus subdural collections. *AJNR Am J Neuroradiol* 1993;14:855-860.

87. McNeely PD, Atkinson JD, Saigal G, et al: Subdural hematomas in infants with benign enlargement of the subarachnoid spaces are not pathognomonic for child abuse. *AJNR Am J Neuroradiol* 2006;27:1725-1728.

88. Papasian NC, Frim DM: A theoretical model of benign external hydrocephalus that predicts a predisposition towards extra-axial hemorrhage after minor head trauma. *Pediatr Neurosurg* 2000;33:188-193.

89. Raul JS, Roth S, Ludes B, et al: Influence of the benign enlargement of the subarachnoid space on the bridging veins strain during a shaking event: a finite element study. *Int J Legal Med* 2008;122:337-340.

90. Ewing-Cobbs L, Prasad M, Kramer L, et al: Acute neuroradiologic findings in young children with inflicted or noninflicted traumatic brain injury. *Childs Nerv Syst* 2000;16:25-33.

91. Hymel KP, Rumack CM, Hay TC, et al: Comparison of intracranial computed tomographic (CT) findings in pediatric abusive and accidental head trauma. *Pediatr Radiol* 1997;27:743-747.

92. Datta S, Stoodley N, Jayawant S, et al: Neuroradiological aspects of subdural haemorrhages. *Arch Dis Child* 2005;90:947-951.

93. Looney CB, Smith JK, Merck LH, et al: Intracranial hemorrhage in asymptomatic neonates: prevalence on MR images and relationship to obstetric and neonatal risk factors. *Radiology* 2007;242:535-541.

94. Whitby EH, Griffiths PD, Rutter S, et al: Frequency and natural history of subdural haemorrhages in babies and relation to obstetric factors. *Lancet* 2004;363:846-851.

95. Vinchon M, Joriot S, Jissendi-Tchofo P, et al: Postmeningitis subdural fluid collection in infants: changing pattern and indications for surgery. *J Neurosurg* 2006;104:383-387.

96. Kurtz J, Anslow P. Infantile herpes simplex encephalitis: diagnostic features and differentiation from non-accidental injury. *J Infect* 2003;46:12-16.

97. Balak N, Silav G, Kilic Y, et al: Successful surgical treatment of a hemophiliac infant with nontraumatic acute subdural hematoma. *Surg Neurol* 2007;68:537-540.

98. Dietrich AM, James CD, King DR, et al: Head trauma in children with congenital coagulation disorders. *J Pediatr Surg* 1994;29:28-32.

99. Myles LM, Massicotte P, Drake J: Intracranial hemorrhage in neonates with unrecognized hemophilia A: a persisting problem. *Pediatr Neurosurg* 2001;34:94-97.

100. Rutty GN, Smith CM, Malia RG: Late-form hemorrhagic disease of the newborn: a fatal case report with illustration of investigations that may assist in avoiding the mistaken diagnosis of child abuse. *Am J Forensic Med Pathol* 1999;20:48-51.

101. Ziv O, Ragni MV: Bleeding manifestations in males with von Willebrand disease. *Haemophilia* 2004;10:162-168.

102. Colosimo M, McCarthy N, Jayasinghe R, et al: Diagnosis and management of subdural haematoma complicating bone marrow transplantation. *Bone Marrow Transplant* 2000;25:549-552.

103. Kolluri VR, Reddy DR, Reddy PK, et al: Subdural hematoma secondary to immune thrombocytopenic purpura: case report. *Neurosurgery* 1986;19:635-636.

104. Lin CH, Hung GY, Chang CY, et al: Subdural hemorrhage in a child with acute promyelocytic leukemia presenting as subtle headache. *J Chin Med Assoc* 2005;68:437-440.

105. Seckin H, Kazanci A, Yigitkanli K, et al: Chronic subdural hematoma in patients with idiopathic thrombocytopenic purpura: A case report and review of the literature. *Surg Neurol* 2006;66:411-414; discussion 414.

106. Streif W, Andrew M, Marzinotto V, et al: Analysis of warfarin therapy in pediatric patients: A prospective cohort study of 319 patients. *Blood* 1999;94:3007-3014.

107. Bishop FS, Liu JK, McCall TD, et al: Glutaric aciduria type 1 presenting as bilateral subdural hematomas mimicking nonaccidental trauma. Case report and review of the literature. *J Neurosurg* 2007;106:222-226.

108. Gago LC, Wegner RK, Capone A Jr, et al: Intraretinal hemorrhages and chronic subdural effusions: glutaric aciduria type 1 can be mistaken for shaken baby syndrome. *Retina* 2003;23:724-726.

109. Osaka H, Kimura S, Nezu A, et al: Chronic subdural hematoma, as an initial manifestation of glutaric aciduria type-1. *Brain Dev* 1993;15:125-127.

110. Twomey EL, Naughten ER, Donoghue VB, et al: Neuroimaging findings in glutaric aciduria type 1. *Pediatr Radiol* 2003;33:823-830.

111. Govindaraju V, Gauger GE, Manley GT, et al: Volumetric proton spectroscopic imaging of mild traumatic brain injury. *AJNR Am J Neuroradiol* 2004;25:730-737.

112. Ashwal S, Holshouser BA, Shu SK, et al: Predictive value of proton magnetic resonance spectroscopy in pediatric closed head injury. *Pediatr Neurol* 2000;23:114-125.

113. Huisman TA, Schwamm LH, Schaefer PW, et al: Diffusion tensor imaging as potential biomarker of white matter injury in diffuse axonal injury. *AJNR Am J Neuroradiol* 2004;25:370-376.

114. Ptak T, Sheridan RL, Rhea JT, et al: Cerebral fractional anisotropy score in trauma patients: a new indicator of white matter injury after trauma. *AJR Am J Roentgenol* 2003;181:1401-1407.

43

NECK AND SPINAL CORD INJURIES IN CHILD ABUSE

Stephen C. Boos, MD, FAAP, and Kenneth Feldman, MD

INTRODUCTION

Despite the relatively small size of the neck compared with the rest of the body, it has numerous vital structures, many of which are shared with or connected in some fashion to other regions of the body. Injury to neck structures caused by child abuse is not rare but is frequently unrecognized. Willging et al[1] described a series of abused children seen in an emergency department. Of 4342 children referred for possible abuse, 105 (2.4%) had injury to structures of the neck. Naidoo[2] described 389 injuries in 300 abused children. Twenty-four of the injuries (6.2%) involved the neck, and 41 (10%) involved the mouth. The structures of the neck can be injured via access through the mouth because of sustained force against the neck such as during strangulation, by a blow to the neck, or by transmitted forces during violent motion of the head or body. This chapter discusses injury of the neck's many structures, organized by mechanism of injury (Table 43-1). Abusive injuries are described, including their presentation, recognition or documentation, and differentiation from similar nonabusive injuries. The relationship between cervical injury and abusive head trauma merits special consideration and is discussed in detail.

INJURY VIA ACCESS THROUGH THE MOUTH

Many structures of the anterior neck, including the hypopharynx, larynx, trachea, and esophagus, are extensions of the mouth. As such, many injuries to these structures occur via oral access. Forceful introduction of a finger, penis, or foreign object or material can mechanically damage these structures. Foreign objects can remain behind and irritants can cause inflammation, obstructing the airway and causing suffocation. Ingestion or administration of caustic agents can chemically injure anatomic structures. Evidence of injury can be quite varied. Some presentations are immediately apparent as trauma. In other cases recognition of traumatic injury might only occur during in-depth investigations because of other problems such as airway inflammation or difficulty swallowing. Radiological imaging or direct visualization through endoscopy is often critical for making the diagnosis.

Hypopharyngeal Laceration

Hypopharyngeal injury is perhaps the best example of orally induced trauma. Thevasagayam and colleagues[3] described a case of hypopharyngeal injury and reviewed reports of 24 additional cases. The presentation of hypopharyngeal injury was quite varied. Case reports described symptoms such as oral bleeding, drooling, breathing difficulties, trouble swallowing, fever, sepsis, subcutaneous emphysema, stiffness of the neck, a mass in the neck or superior chest, or swelling of the neck, face, and chest. Oral blood and subcutaneous emphysema were more likely to suggest trauma. The occurrence of visible traumatic oral lesions, particularly laceration of the labial frenula, tonsilar pillars, palate, or posterior pharyngeal wall, led to consideration of trauma in other cases. Recognition of injuries outside the neck and mouth prompted consideration of trauma and abuse in a few cases. Many cases, however, were treated supportively without a clear diagnosis until the case failed to resolve in the anticipated time period, recurred, or worsened.

Hypopharyngeal injury is documented by three principle means. The presence of a mass in the retropharyngeal space, parapharyngeal tissues, or mediastinum is often noted on plain radiography or computed tomography (CT). The lateral neck film, taken during inspiration with the neck somewhat extended, is the standard initial evaluation. A retropharyngeal space greater than half the width of the adjacent vertebral body or the presence of air in the tissues identifies the abnormality. Contrast-enhanced conventional radiography, CT, or magnetic resonance imaging (MRI) will elucidate soft tissue masses and air in the soft tissues. In addition, entry of the contrast medium into the laceration and retention of the contrast in the soft tissues can demonstrate the originating traumatic laceration (Figure 43-1). Some authors suggest that barium is more effective than water-soluble contrast for this purpose.

Direct endoscopic visualization was performed in many reported cases, and it allows diagnosis, photo documentation, and access for further exploration and treatment. In some cases, involvement of the carotid sheath has been identified, illustrating the added seriousness of neck injury. Intraoral injury or foreign body can also cause elevated salivary amylase levels.

Hypopharyngeal injury that occurs outside the medical setting should always prompt concern for child abuse. Only 5 of the 25 cases described by Thevasagayam[3] were clearly not inflicted. Falling with a long object, such as a knitting needle or toothbrush, in the mouth caused three of these injuries. Eating a sharp object or having one propelled into the mouth explained other cases. The *abusive* hypopharyngeal injuries in this case series were identified based on an

Table 43-1	Injuries to Neck Structures, by Mechanism of Injury	
Mechanism of Injury	**Described Abusive Injuries**	
Oral access	Hypopharyngeal laceration	
	Subcutaneous emphysema	
	Foreign body ingestion/aspiration	
	Particulate (pepper) concretions	
	Caustic agent ingestion/aspiration	
Direct trauma to the neck (strangulation)	Bruises, abrasions, and lacerations of the neck	
	Petechiae of the face	
	Fractures of cartilage and hyoid	
	Cartilage, joint, and muscle hemorrhages	
	Cervical vertebral fracture	
	Vocal cord paralysis	
	Airway, vein, and artery obstruction	
	Brain infarction	
Direct trauma to the neck (blunt force)	Bruises and abrasions	
Indirect forces from relative motion of head and torso	Hangman's fracture (pars interarticularis fracture of C2 with subluxation on C3)	
	Other vertebral fracture	
	Disc rupture	
	Ligamentous injury of the spine	
	Vertebral and carotid artery injury	
	Subarachnoid, subdural, and epidural hemorrhage of the spine	
	Contusion, swelling, and infarction of the spinal cord	
	Axonal injury of the spine and spinal nerve roots	
	Hemorrhage in cervical musculature	

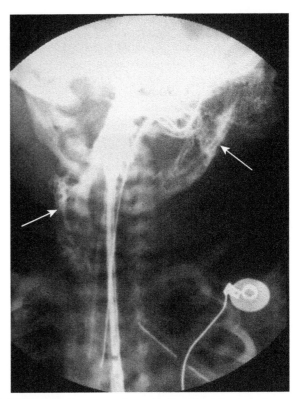

FIGURE 43-1 A contrast-enhanced radiograph of the neck of a 4-week-old. The infant had the epiglottis pulled on by a hand, ripping it from the surrounding soft tissues. The arrows mark contrast material that has seeped into the surrounding soft tissues.

absent, inconsistent, or changing history, or because other abuse injuries were discovered.

Medical instrumentation can also cause pharyngeal, hypopharyngeal, laryngeal injury, and injury to the strap muscles of the neck, which must be distinguished from pre-existing injury.[4]

Introduction of a Foreign Body

Several reports have described the effects of the abusive introduction of objects through a child's mouth.[5-7] These objects included coins, other metallic objects, broken glass, a small rubber ball, and baby wipes. Presentation depends on the nature of the object and where and how the object lodges. Sharp objects that enter the pharynx or esophagus can cause perforation, as discussed previously. Objects that fill the pharynx, cover the larynx, or enter the trachea can obstruct the airway, resulting in acute respiratory distress or apnea. Foreign bodies that produce a partial obstruction are sometimes more difficult to diagnose, presenting with chronic cough or intermittent wheeze. Objects that lodge in the esophagus can produce pain, drooling, dysphagia, or respiratory complaints. In one unusual case, repeated abusive feeding of coins to an infant was associated with an unexplained death.[5]

When no history of aspiration of a foreign body is reported, it can be difficult to recognize the diagnosis. Unreported foreign bodies can be found during attempts to establish an airway, on imaging studies, or during endoscopy for persistent symptoms. Foreign body ingestion and aspiration are well-known accidental injuries in childhood, and distinguishing abuse from accidents is sometimes challenging.[8-11] Inflicted foreign body aspiration was suspected in case reports in part because of the very young ages of the children (3-6 months). When the child's reported or implied behaviors are inconsistent with his or her developmental level, the medical history suggests abuse.

The frequency of laceration or abrasion of the hypopharynx accompanied by injuries to other parts of the body has been found to be higher in inflicted incidents than in accidental ones. Even "accidental" ingestion or aspiration in young children can be due to supervisory neglect. Careful assessment by extensive history, physical examination, and appropriate imaging studies should be performed in cases of foreign body ingestion or aspiration.

Introduction of Caustic or Irritating Agents

Injury caused by oral introduction of caustic and irritating substances has been reported from intentional abuse, supervisional neglect of children, and unsafe storage of these materials. Two series of children who were injured by ingestion of caustic materials have been reported. In one,[12] the caustic materials were household chemicals that were improperly stored or inadequately monitored. In the other,[13] the materials were being used in the manufacture of methamphetamine. In each of these reports, the children themselves ingested or inhaled the agent and the cases were considered neglectful.

Cohle et al[14] summarized the histories of eight children who died from inhaled and ingested black pepper. In seven of the eight, the pepper was administered by an adult as a form of punishment. In some cases, pepper concretions and soft tissue edema resulted in airway obstruction. These cases were considered abusive and labeled as homicides. In nonlethal cases, children presented with symptoms from irritation, burning, and swelling of the pharynx, larynx, and esophagus. Stridor and dysphagia were recognized and respiratory distress often led to intubation. Burns, injuries, or inflammation was evident in the oropharynx and sometimes on the face. In the cases of neglect, the history included ingestion or aspiration of the pepper. In the fatal cases, a false history of the children themselves ingesting pepper was often given.

In the fatal pepper ingestions, more than half of the children had historical and physical findings indicating prior physical abuse. The volume of pepper found in the pharynx, larynx, esophagus, and sometimes the stomach was quite large, and therefore inconsistent with the history of the child ingesting it. Scene investigations were often vital in pointing out the falsehoods of the given histories. Cohle et al[14] also gathered reports of nonfatal pepper exposures from local poison control centers. These reports were nearly always limited to mild irritation of the mouth, throat, or eyes. A careful history, physical examination, and scene investigation is needed to distinguish between neglectful, abusive, and nonabusive causes of these injuries.

DIRECT EXTERNAL TRAUMA TO THE NECK (STRANGULATION)

Both the external surface and internal structures of the neck can be injured by direct contact. Manual or ligature strangulation is the most commonly reported cause of external neck injury. Strangulation causes injuries through focal or circumferential compression of the airway and vascular structures. Visible signs include indentations (Figure 43-2), bruises, or abrasions on the skin of the neck where a hand, object, or ligature made contact. Petechiae of the neck and face above the level of vascular obstruction are common with neck compression that produces *venous* but not *arterial* obstruction.[15] Petechiae are *not* present after complete suspension that compromises arterial blood supply to the head.

Sometimes vertically oriented abrasions are found on the neck that are caused by the victims' fingernails when they attempt to grab the strangling object to relieve the obstruction. Many strangulation victims are dead at presentation. Survivors can manifest hypoxic-ischemic injuries of the brain, pulmonary congestion, and swelling within the injured airway.[16,17]

Fractures of the boney and cartilaginous structures of the throat, fractures of the vertebrae, and spinal cord injuries have been reported, but they are rarer in children than in

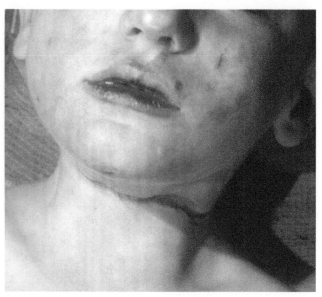

FIGURE 43-2 Indentation of the neck after hanging.

adults.[16,18] Maxeiner,[19] however, reports that these injuries are often missed at autopsy because of dissection technique. Verma[20] described 28 strangulation deaths in children less than 18 years old. Five had fractures of the thyroid horns and two had fractures of the hyoid bone. Fractures were more common in older children, perhaps because of their increased bony calcification. In living patients, CT scan has been used to identify bony and cartilaginous injury of the larynx. MRI scan has been found to be a very sensitive way to detect soft tissue injuries related to strangulation in adults.[21] Vocal cord paralysis from injury to the recurrent laryngeal nerve has been reported.[22]

Relatively small amounts of direct pressure above the hyoid bone will result in obstruction of the airway.[23] The necessary pressure varies with age and individual characteristics, but on average, 1.6 lb of force will obstruct the airway of a small child and 5 lb of force will obstruct the airways of all children under 6 years of age.[24] Airway obstruction alone can produce hypoxic injury of various organs, notably the brain, but airway compromise is not required for strangulation. For example, death has occurred in subjects with a tracheostomy below the site of their neck constriction.[25] Some authors emphasize, whereas others minimize, the effect of carotid stimulation during strangulation. In theory, this might result in bradycardia, dysrhythmias, or even cardiac arrest, adding ischemia to the hypoxic challenge. Ischemic injury of the brain also results from vascular compression and obstruction.[16] A child's lower blood pressure should indicate that less compression is needed in a child to obstruct arterial blood flow to the head.

In most cases of strangulation, the circumstances in which the child was found or the injuries on the body will indicate the cause of the injury. A few reports suggest that strangulation injuries can be occult and require special attention or study. Carty[26] reported a 3½-month-old girl with recurrent apnea and severe hypoxic ischemic brain injury. Bilateral supraclavicular subcutaneous calcium deposits described as "necklace calcifications" were attributed to fatty necrosis from direct trauma during strangulation. Bird et al[27] suggested that three children with unilateral brain swelling and subdural hemorrhage had been strangled by being grasped around the neck during shaking. One child had intramural hemorrhages of the carotid artery at autopsy, but there was no direct evidence of vascular injury in the necks of the other two. Unilateral swelling with traumatic brain injury has been more widely recognized since this report, and Bird's presumptions of strangulation have not been widely accepted as its cause.[28]

Injury to laryngeal structures from strangulation must be distinguished from the results of resuscitative efforts. Bush et al[29] reported 211 deceased children under age 12 who had received cardiopulmonary resuscitation. Fifteen had neck injuries attributed to resuscitation efforts, but no laryngeal injuries were reported. Using laryngeal findings alone to identify strangulation following attempted resuscitation appears to be difficult, at best.[30]

The reported frequency of abusive strangulation injuries varies. Feldman and Simms[16] found only 1 of 233 strangulation cases was attributed to inflicted injury. Consumer Product Safety Commission reports were the source of 195 of these cases (which by definition would exclude recognized inflicted cases), leaving an abuse rate of 2.6% in the remaining cases. Another report of a series of 13 children with strangulation injury found one surviving child who was repeatedly strangled (7.7%).[17] Yet in Verma's series of 28 strangulation deaths from India,[20] 93% were attributed to homicide. None of the authors describe how inflicted strangulation was determined, but Verma also reported an assortment of other bodily injuries, including bites, evidence of sexual assault, and injuries that were "defensive in nature." Maxeiner and Bockholdt[31] compared 63 homicides with 19 suicides by ligature strangulation. More severe injury by the ligature itself, scene characteristics such as ligature marks but no ligature found, and other evidence of assault on the body were cited in homicidal cases. Twelve of the homicide victims were children; none had fractures of laryngeal bones and cartilages.

Strangulation by hair has been reported in both homicides and accidents.[32] Accidental strangulation of infants and toddlers by long hair has been reported twice.[33,34] The second report demonstrated the strength of a strand of hair as a strangling ligature. Although this did not establish the truth of the reported incident, it led the court to drop charges against the family.

NONSTRANGULATION BLUNT TRAUMA

Cutaneous injuries to the neck from mechanisms other than strangulation represent the majority of neck injuries seen in abused children. Because of the neck's small and relatively protected surface, patterned injuries on the neck from objects are not often seen. Because it is a natural grab or catch point, grip marks, bruises, abrasions, and streaks of petechiae from grabbing are much more common, sometimes associated with other intracranial injuries. Willging et al[35] reported 70 ecchymoses, 32 abrasions, 5 lacerations, and 5 burns in their series of 105 children with abusive neck injuries. Only two of his cases involved noncutaneous structures.

Blunt trauma of the larynx is a well-known form of injury in both adults and children. Contusion and swelling of the airway, fracture of laryngeal bones and cartilages, and even traumatic rupture of the airway have been reported. These injuries occur in motor vehicle and bicycle crashes, from direct blows, from falls, or from the classical "clothesline" mechanism. Injuries to the carotid or vertebral arteries have been reported following "clothesline" injuries, from contact with a shoulder belt during motor vehicle crashes, or accompanying contusions to the neck from other trauma.[36] Rarely, blunt trauma to the neck will injure the thyroid, which can result in significant bleeding and thyrotoxicosis.[37] Blunt traumatic injury of the parathyroid is even rarer, but can result in calcium dysregulation.

INDIRECT APPLICATION OF FORCES TO THE NECK

The neck is a small, light-weight structure connecting the heavy head with the much heavier body. Any motion or acceleration that is not imparted equally to both the head and the body will impart motion and force to the structures of the neck. This is the most difficult form of neck injury to understand and has generated the greatest controversy. Before proceeding, an understanding of neck anatomy and biomechanics is important.

Anatomy of the Neck

The spinal column of the neck is composed of seven vertebrae, from the highest vertebra of the thorax to occipital condyles of the skull. The lower five cervical vertebrae are similar to one another. These vertebrae are each composed of a cylindrical body, an arch surrounding a canal containing the spinal cord, and lateral and posterior projections, or processes. The lateral processes of the cervical vertebrae contain ostia, which provide two canals that contain the vertebral arteries. Each of these vertebrae is connected to adjacent vertebra above and below by three joints and a variety of ligaments. The main joint bridges vertebral body to vertebral body. A gel-filled disc and a surrounding joint capsule provide cushioning and connection. Facet joints form a bridge between adjacent arches, posterior-laterally. The facet joints are lubricated by fluid and enclosed by a joint capsule. Longitudinal ligaments reinforce the intervertebral connections anterior to the vertebral body, posterior to the vertebral body, inside the dorsum of the spinal canal, and between the lateral and posterior spinous processes.

With a tripod of connecting joints and so much reinforcement, the neck would be quite stiff if each connecting element did not allow for distraction, compression, lateral motion, and rotatory motion. The neck of a young child is highly flexible because of great elasticity in all of the joints and ligaments. Certain features of the child's spine make the immature neck more flexible than the neck of adults. In adults, the facet joints are tipped into the vertical plane, giving greater protection against one vertebra slipping forward over the inferior vertebra. Children's facet joints are much more horizontal, allowing for greater relative motion between vertebrae. Adult cervical vertebrae also possess a lateral hook, the uncinate process, which protects one vertebra from slipping laterally or spinning over the inferior vertebra. This is absent in children, again providing for greater mobility.

The first and second vertebrae are very different. Inferiorly, the second vertebra, or axis, is much like the lower five, articulating through its body, posterior facet joints, and ligaments. Superiorly, however, the body projects upward as the dens, an anterior toothlike extension. The first vertebra, or atlas, has no vertebral body and forms a complete ring surrounding the dens and the spinal canal. Its "facets" form larger joints, articulating below with the modified facets of the axis and above with the occipital condyles of the skull. Additional ligaments connect the dens to the anterior arch of the atlas and the atlas to the base of the skull. This arrangement allows for significantly greater movement, particularly rotation, of the skull-C1-C2 system.

SPINE BIOMECHANICS

Spinal injuries caused by obstetrical care focused attention on the biomechanical properties of the spinal column and cord as early as the nineteenth century. In 1874, Duncan[38] measured tensile forces that caused spinal column and neck failure in intact fetal cadavers. The spinal column gave way with sustained application of 400 to 654 Newtons (90-147 lb force) and decapitation occurred at 404 to 725 Newtons (91-163 lb force). The neck will tolerate much greater forces when they are rapidly and briefly applied,[39] an effect that increases significantly with falling age. Because of this effect, measurements applicable to static loading during obstetrical maneuvers cannot be directly applied to dynamic situations of trauma. In 1922 Crothers[40] observed tensile properties of the infant spine in cadavers. These observations showed that the spinal column can vary in length up to 2 inches from full compression to full extension. However, during full extension, the cord stretched one quarter inch less than the bony spinal column. As a result the cervical cord and attached brainstem moved downward in the spinal column. This effect helped explain cervical cord injuries that resulted from difficult breech extraction.

In the modern era, animal models and mathematical models have been used to further understand the behavior of the pediatric spinal column. This work has demonstrated the effect of age and anatomy on the spinal resistance to and range of motion throughout childhood. Pediatric spines from children age 2 through 12 years old have been tested, in tension, to the point of failure.[41] In one study, isolated spinal columns began to fail at between 490 and 920 Newtons, at which point they were stretched 13.8 to 23.6 mm. Age was associated with but was not completely predictive of how the spines performed. Again, in this study loading was relatively slow, occurring over 3 to 5 seconds, not the milliseconds typical of traumatic injury. Thus, the applicability of this study to understanding clinical events is still quite limited.

It has been noted that infants and young children tend to suffer injury to the upper cervical spine, whereas older children and adolescents, like adults, tend to suffer injury of the lower cervical and upper thoracic spine. The predilection for upper cervical injury is attributed to geometric changes, rather than vertebral strength. Testing of animal spinal segments suggests that upper spinal vertebrae are sometimes stronger than lower vertebrae.[42] However, the fulcrum during flexion is higher in young children versus older children. This results in injury at C2-3, instead of C5-6.

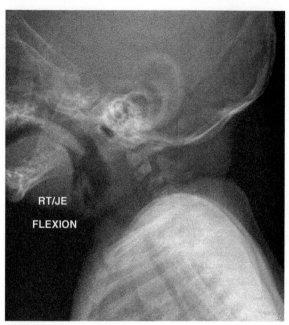

FIGURE 43-3 A "hangman's fracture" (pars interarticularis fracture of C2 with subluxation on C3) on a lateral neck radiograph.

NECK AND CERVICAL SPINE INJURIES REPORT IN CHILD ABUSE CASES

Injury of the Bony Spine and Surrounding Ligaments

The most radiographically evident form of spinal injury involves the vertebrae and the tissues that maintain their alignment. A number of case reports describe children with abusive injury to these structures. "Hangman's fractures" (fractures of the pedicles connecting the bony arch surrounding the spinal canal to the vertebral body of C2), have been describe in four cases (Figure 43-3).[43-46] Other spine injuries described include cervical dislocation and spontaneous reduction,[47] fracture of C2,[48] compression of the body of C5 with anterior subluxation of C4,[49] fracture-dislocation of C5 on C6,[49] and anterior rupture of an intervertebral disk.[50] One infant was reported to have ligamentous injury of the atlanto-occipital junction, atlanto-axial subluxation, rupture of the transverse ligament of the atlas, and fracture of C1.[51] Another child had an avulsion fracture of the odontoid process of C2 and subluxation of C1 on C2.[52]

Injury to Vascular Structures of the Neck

Case reports also demonstrate the varying presentation of cervical vascular injuries resulting from child abuse, including periadventitial hemorrhage with vertebral artery compression and cerebellomedullary infarction,[53] dissection of the vertebral arteries,[48,54] and vascular territory infarcts caused by thrombosis downstream from an internal carotid artery dissection.[48]

Extraaxial Hemorrhage of the Spine

Subarachnoid, subdural, and epidural hemorrhage of the cervical spinal cord have been identified, principally at

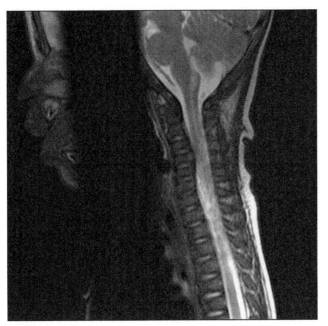

FIGURE 43-4 T2 MRI image of a posterior profusion of the body of C-4 with associated central spinal cord hemorrhage, extending up into the pons.

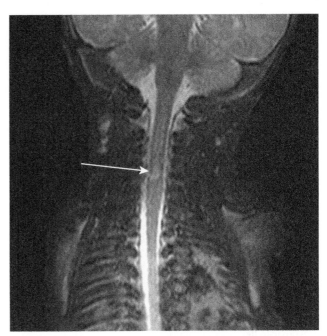

FIGURE 43-5 A short tau inverse recovery (STIR) MRI of the spinal cord in an abused infant showing swelling of the cervical cord *(arrow)* causing "central cord syndrome" and posterior protrusion of C4 vertebral body.

autopsy in abuse cases, but also radiographically.[48-50,53-57] Oemichen and colleagues[58] compared a group of children believed to be shaken with a group dying from other causes including SIDS, nontraumatic illnesses, or trauma not involving the head. Four of eleven "shaken" children had spinal epidural hemorrhage at the cervicothoracic junction, whereas none of nine "control" children had this finding. Feldman et al[59] evaluated 12 children with abusive head trauma using cervical MRI (T1 and T2 sequences). Although MRI did not identify any injury, one autopsied child had subdural hemorrhage around the cervical spine and three had subarachnoid hemorrhage of the cervical spine.

Injuries of the Spinal Cord

Spinal cord injuries have been reported after abuse in many case studies and series (Figures 43-4 and 43-5). Injuries include spinal cord swelling[47,60] contusions,[55,56] lacerations,[56] axonal injury in the cervical spine and nerve roots,[58,61,62] and "spinal cord injury without radiologic abnormality" (SCIWORA).[62-65] In the SCIWORA cases, the diagnosis of spinal cord injury was often delayed because of co-existing brain injury.[65]

Using β-amyloid precursor protein (β-APP) stains, Shannon et al[61] showed staining of nerve roots and white matter tracts in the cervical spine in 7 of 11 cases where the infant was considered to have been shaken, and in none of 7 children dying from brain hypoxia/ischemia.

Injury of Other Cervical Structures

Injury of the muscles and soft tissues of the neck resulting from indirectly applied forces during abuse have been reported, including hemorrhage into the interspinous musculature and the sternocleidomastoid.[50,58]

Presenting Symptoms in and Associated Injuries in Cases of Spinal Injuries in Abused Children

Table 43-2 lists the presenting symptoms and associated injuries in infants and young children presenting with spinal injuries after abuse.[47-54,60,62,65] Some of the symptoms were consistent with spinal cord injury, and some were likely caused or potentiated by associated injuries.

In many of the cases reported, shaking was the mechanism of injury (either confessed to by a perpetrator, or presumed by the evidence, whereas in others, no mechanism was established.[44,48,50,51,53,55,56,58,60,65] A recent study from Philadelphia examined cervical findings in all homicide victims under 3 years of age from 1995 to 2003.[66] Of the 52 victims, 41 (79%) died of abusive head trauma. Of the 41, 29 (79%) had cervical cord injuries; 21 had parenchymal injuries, 24 meningeal hemorrhages, and 16 nerve root avulsions or dorsal root ganglion hemorrhages. None had spinal fractures. Six of the 29 (21%) had soft tissue injury to the neck, and 14 (48%) had brainstem injuries. Six of the children with abusive head trauma had no evidence of an impact to the head, and all six had primary cervical spinal cord injury. Cervical spinal injury was not significantly associated with hypoxic-ischemic injury, herniation, or brain infarction.

Recognizing Cervical Injuries in Abused Children

In studies of cervical injuries in abused children, diagnosis was often delayed or only discovered on autopsy because of the child's clinical status. Two subgroups emerge from these many case reports and series. The first group consists of those patients with head injuries. The evaluation of the neck in patients with head injury is problematic in both abused

Table 43-2	Presenting Signs, Symptoms, and Associated Injuries in Children with Cervical Spine Injuries Caused by Abuse[43-54,62]

Neurological Symptoms

Coma
Seizures
Lethargy
Neck rigidity
Limp, hypotonic extremities
Leg pain on flexion
Central cord syndrome

Systemic Symptoms

Cardiopulmonary arrest
Bradycardia
Respiratory difficulties
Irritability

Associated Injuries

Hypoxic-ischemic brain injury
Cranial subdural, epidural and subarachnoid hemorrhage
Cerebral edema
Retinal hemorrhages
Facial bruising
Liver laceration
History of hypopharyngeal perforation
Pneumomediastinum
Pulmonary contusion
Multiple fractures
Hip dislocation
Metaphyseal fractures
Torticollis
Healing burns
Cerebral infarcts
Toxic ingestion

and nonabused children. High-risk criteria designed to guide radiological evaluation of the neck in trauma patients were developed for the National Emergency X-radiography Utilization Study (NEXUS).[67] This very large study included only 30 children under age 18 with positive radiograph studies. All were identified by the NEXUS criteria of cervical tenderness, additional injuries distracting attention from the neck, altered level of consciousness, neurological findings, or intoxication. Garton and Hammer[68] published a series of 190 children with documented cervical spine injuries. NEXUS criteria identified 94% of the neck-injured children less than 8 years old and 100% of neck-injured children over age 8 years old. Head-injured abused children, however, are frequently considerably younger than 8 years old, and many have attention-distracting injuries or an altered level of consciousness. Few can accurately report on neck or neurological symptoms. Therefore, a larger proportion of these children require neck imaging and needs to have their neck protected until they can be cleared. Plain radiographs do not appear to be adequate to do this. A review of 75,172 children in the National Pediatric Trauma Registry identified 1098 children with cervical spine injury, of whom 385 (35%)

had spinal cord injury without radiographic abnormality (SCIWORA).[69] In Garton and Hammer's study,[68] plain films identified 75% of neck injuries in children under age 8 and 93% in children over age 8. CT scans, flexion-extension views and occasionally MRI demonstrated the injuries in the other patients. These authors recommended adding CT scans of the occiput through C3 to the evaluation of young children.

Some have suggested that MRI is a diagnostically superior and cost-effective way of evaluating the spine in children who lack a reliable neurological examination.[70] Others have suggested that the MRI will overestimate the degree of injury compared with intraoperative findings.[71] At this time a single protocol cannot be recommended.

The second group, which overlaps significantly with the first, is deceased patients. The recognition of cervical injuries at autopsy requires special dissection techniques to preserve the integrity of the cervicomedullary junction, which is severed during the traditional autopsy approach.[72] Some of the findings cited previously required special staining techniques as well, notably immunohistochemical staining for β-APP.

Practitioners evaluating children with abusive and nonabusive head/neck injuries must avoid misdiagnosing normal cervical variants as trauma.[73,74] The problem of distinguishing hangman's fracture from congenital abnormalities of the C2 pedicles deserves special note. Van Rijn et al[75] reported an abused child with congenital ossification defects that were initially suspected to be pedicle fractures.

DIFFERENTIATING ABUSIVE FROM NONABUSIVE CERVICAL INJURIES

The previous case reports and series do not define particular neck injures that distinguish abuse from nonabusive trauma. The case-control series of Oemichen et al[58] and Shannon et al[61] compared abused children to nontraumatic controls and did not define features that differentiate abusive from nonabusive trauma. Instead, the child's full constellation of injuries and accompanying history defined these children as abused. In many of these cases, the authors believed these findings indicated that the child was shaken. The relationship between shaking and neck injuries has become a particular focus of interest.

Neck Injury and Shaking

Early theories on the pathogenesis of the shaken baby syndrome attributed brain injury to mechanical strains throughout the brain during rotational movements of the head leading to traumatic diffuse axonal injury (tDAI). Subsequently, a hypothesis was put forth that these brain injuries were a secondary effect of hypoxic ischemic stresses brought about by apnea and bradycardia.[56] Because the nuclei that regulate heart rate and respiration extend from the low brainstem into the upper cervical cord, it was thought that mechanical strain in this region during shaking would lead to apnea and bradycardia. In an interesting report, Koch et al[76] described the outcome of 199 infants receiving "the gentle impulse the chiropractor can administer by manipulation" of the atlantooccipital region. One half demonstrated some form of "vegetative reaction" and 22% were said to have become apneic. Although this study has been cited as verification of cervical strain-induced apnea, the authors describe these events as less than 10 seconds long and terminated by blowing into the child's face, events that sound more like pain or surprise than centrally induced apnea. The theory received considerable acceptance after Geddes et al[62] published her series of 53 victims of nonaccidental head injury. In babies who died from inflicted head injuries, the authors attributed their commonly observed histologic findings to hypoxic-ischemic injury. Geddes's hypoxia theory remains unsubstantiated.[77] Cerebral axonal injury, when it was found, rarely demonstrated a pattern the authors felt was the result of a traumatic cause. Only three children had true tDAI, but eight had focal traumatic axonal injury in the brainstem and three had focal traumatic axonal injury in cervical cord roots.

Biomechanical arguments regarding the sufficiency of shaking have also focused interest on cervical injury. Prange et al[78] indicated that kinematic measurements of head motion when anthropomorphic dummies were shaken predicted forces that "... fell within the range of estimated infant cranio-cervical tolerance." They explained that this result predicted cervical injury in some, but not all, cases when infants were shaken as the dummies had been. Bandak[79] performed a similar analysis, which predicted major structural failure of the spine in virtually all cases. In a letter to the editor, Margulies,[80] Rangarajan,[81] and others, repeated Bandak's calculations and found parameters were at least 10 times lower than those reported by Bandak. They suggested, again, that cervical injury might possibly occur during severe shaking without impact. These conclusions, however, have been based on available static neck tolerances noted previously, not on dynamic tolerances of infant tissue.

Much is yet to be learned about the biomechanics of the cervicocranial system. Recently, an animal model was developed to study the relationship between head trauma and axonal injury in the cervical spinal cord.[82] Impact with acceleration of the head provoked axonal injury in the spinal cord of rats. This effect was greatest at the craniocervical junction and decreased with distance along the spinal cord. Zhu et al[83] showed that motions of the neck result in displacement of the brain in the skull case in an *in vivo* human model. These results could not be specifically related to injury. By contrast, Feipel and colleagues[84] did not demonstrate strain on the dura mater during motions of the neck in a cadaver model. The links among traumatic events, primary injuries, secondary effects, and secondary injuries during shaking and head impact remain a fertile area for investigation.

Strength of the Evidence

Nearly all the evidence on abusive injury of the neck comes from individual cases, small series of abuse cases, or small numbers of abused children within large series of nonabusively injured children. As such, the evidence is descriptive. A few case-control studies assist in separating neuropathological findings of abusive head and neck trauma from nontraumatic causes of death; none of this evidence develops patterns that separate abusive from nonabusive cervical trauma. Cervical injuries must currently be judged by the history that accompanies them, associated findings of abuse, and circumstantial evidence.

Biomechanical arguments regarding the neck have rested on both excellent biomechanical and anatomical data and on very old data with questionable research methodology. In some cases, the original meaning of very old cadaver data has been distorted through citation and sub-citation. There is a growing body of high-quality animal and cadaver research–based biomechanical data on the behavior of the neck. Both physical and mathematical models of neck behavior will hopefully become available to predict injuries and evaluate the sufficiency of explanations of injury in the future. Currently published biomechanical modeling results range from the preliminary, but informative, to irreproducible and misleading.

The data on the relationship between cervical injury, apnea, and hypoxic-ischemic brain injury are still developing. However, the possibility of hypoxia being a cause of cranial subdural hemorrhage has been refuted.[76,77,85] Optimization and standardization of dissection and histological technique at autopsy are likely to significantly impact future results. Data on appropriate imaging of the neck in traumatized children are also still developing. The meaning of the term *SCIWORA* is likely to change as CT, MRI, and other techniques become standard practice when evaluating these children.

AREAS FOR NEW RESEARCH

Because cervical injury is an uncommon finding in abuse cases, only a very large multicentered database of abused and accidentally injured children, containing great detail, is likely to have the power to identify findings that discriminate abusive from nonabusive cervical trauma. Such a database would benefit many areas of child abuse medicine and conceivably other areas of trauma medicine, such as radiographic assessment of the spine in traumatized children.

The ability to judge the sufficiency of a given history, using biomechanical data, requires significant development. The behavior of the spine in intact living children, under many different traumatic conditions, remains to be modeled successfully. The tolerances of multiple cervical tissues have yet to be determined for various ages and trauma scenarios. Only when this work has significantly advanced can injury predictions be made reliably, based on a clinical history.

Finally, basic research on the pathophysiology of brain injury will need to evaluate the growing focus on hypoxia and ischemia and secondary neurological events such as seizures and cerebral blood flow. Increasingly, this effort will need to consider injury to the cervical cord, cervical blood vessels, and the cervical spine.

References

1. Willging JP, Bower CM, Cotton RT: Physical abuse of children, a retrospective review and an otolaryngology perspective. *Arch Otolaryngol Head Neck Surg* 1992;118:584-590.
2. Naidoo S: A profile of the oro-facial injuries in child physical abuse at a children's hospital. *Child Abuse Negl* 2000;24:521-534.
3. Thevasagayam MS, Siemers MD, Debelle GD, et al: Paediatric hypopharyngeal perforation: child abuse until proved otherwise? *Int J Pediatr Otorhinolaryngol* 2007;71:665-670.
4. Raven KP; Reay DT; Harruff RC: Artifactual injuries of the larynx produced by resuscitative intubation. *Am J Forens MedPath* 1999; 20:31-36.

5. Nolte KB: Esophageal foreign bodies as child abuse: potential fatal mechanisms. *Am J Forens Med Path* 1993;14:323-326.

6. Weintraub B: A case of airway obstruction: A rubber ball in a baby's throat didn't get there on its own. Is it abuse. *Am J Nurs* 2006;106:35-38.

7. Krugman SD, Lantz PE, Sinal S, et al: Forced suffocation of infants with baby wipes: a previously undescribed form of child abuse. *Child Abuse Negl* 2007;31:615-621.

8. Center for Disease Control and Prevention: Nonfatal choking-related episodes among children–United States, 2001. *MMWR Morb Mort Wkly Rep* 2002;51:945-948.

9. Ngo A, Ng KC, Sim TP: Otorhinolaryngeal foreign bodies in children presenting to the emergency department. *Singapore Med J* 2005;46:172-178.

10. Tomaske M, Gerber AC, Stocker S, et al: Tracheobronchial foreign body aspiration in children–diagnostic value of symptoms and signs. *Swiss Med Wkly* 2006;136:533-539.

11. Gregori D, Salerni L, Scarinzi C, et al: Foreign bodies in the upper airways causing complications and requiring hospitalization in children aged 0-14 years: results from the ESFBI study. *Eur Arch Otorhinolaryngol* 2008;265:971-978.

12. Friedman EM: Caustic ingestions and foreign body aspirations: an overlooked form of child abuse. *Ann Otol Rhinol Laryngol* 1987;96:709-712.

13. Farst K, Duncan JM, Moss M, et al: Methamphetamine exposure presenting as caustic ingestion in children. *Ann Emerg Med* 2007;49:341-343.

14. Cohle SD, Trestrail JD, Graham MA, et al: Fatal pepper aspiration. *Am J Dis Child* 1988;142:633-636.

15. Luke JL, Reay DT, Eisele JW, et al: Correlation of circumstances with pathological findings in asphyxial deaths by hanging: a prospective study of 61 cases from Seattle. *J Forensic Sci* 1985;30:1140-1147.

16. Feldman KW, Simms RJ: Strangulation in childhood: epidemiology and clinical course. *Pediatrics* 1980;65:1079-1085.

17. Sabo RA, Hanigan WC, Flessner K, et al: Strangulation injuries in children. Part 1. Clinical analysis. *J Trauma* 1996;40:68-72.

18. Sep D, Theis KC: Strangulation injuries in children. *Resuscitation* 2007;74:386-391.

19. Maxeiner H: "Hidden" laryngeal injuries in homicidal strangulation: how to detect and interpret these findings. *J Forensic Sci* 1998;43:784-791.

20. Verma SK: Pediatric and adolescent strangulation deaths. *J Forens Legal Med* 2007;14:61-64.

21. Yen K, Vock P, Christe A, et al: Clinical forensic radiology in strangulation victims: forensic expertise based on magnetic resonance imaging (MRI) findings. *Int J Legal Med* 2007;121:115-123.

22. Myer CM, Fitton CM: Vocal cord paralysis following child abuse. *Int J Pediatr Otorhinolaryngol* 1988;15:217-220.

23. Stevens RR, Lane GA, Milkovik SM, et al: Prevention of accidental childhood strangulation, a clinical study. *Ann Otol Rhinol Laryngol* 2000;109:797-802.

24. Brouardel, PCH: *La pendaison, la strangulation, la suffocation, la submersion*. Librairie J.B. Baillière et fils, Paris, 1897. Available at http://books.google.com. Accessed May 10, 2009.

25. Spitz WU, Fisher RS: *Medicolegal Investigation of Death*. Charles C Thomas, Springfield, 1965, pp 278-374.

26. Carty H: Case report: child abuse–necklace calcification–a sign of strangulation. *Br J Radiol* 1993;66:1186-1188.

27. Bird CR, McMahan JR, Gilles FH, et al: Strangulation in child abuse: CT diagnosis. *Radiology* 1987;163:373-375.

28. Duhaime AC, Durham S: Traumatic brain injury in infants: the phenomenon of subdural hemorrhage with hemispheric hypodensity ("Big Black Brain"). *Prog Brain Res* 2007;161:293-302.

29. Bush CM, Jones JS, Cohle SD, et al: Pediatric injuries from cardiopulmonary resuscitation. *Ann Emerg Med* 1996;28:40-44.

30. Raven KP, Reay DT, Harruff RC: Artifactual injuries of the larynx produced by resuscitative intubation. *Am J Forens Med Pathol* 1999;20:31-36.

31. Maxeiner H, Bockholdt B: Homicidal and suicidal ligature strangulation—a comparison of the postmortem findings. *Forens Sci Int* 2003;137:60-66.

32. Ruszkiewicz AR, Lee KA, Landgren AJ: Homicidal strangulation by victim's own hair presenting as natural death. *Am J Forens Med Pathol* 1994;15:340-343.

33. Chegwidden HJ, Poirier MP: Near strangulation as a result of hair tourniquet syndrome. *Clin Pediatr* 2005;44:359-361.

34. Milkovich SM, Owens J, Stool D, et al: Accidental childhood strangulation by human hair. *Int J Pedatr Otorhinolaryngol* 2005;69:1621-1628.

35. Willging JP, Bower CM, Cotton RT: Physical abuse of children, a retrospective review and an otolaryngology perspective. *Arch Otolaryngol Head Neck Surg* 1992;118:584-590.

36. Sliker CW, Shanmuganathan K, Mirvis SE: Diagnosis of blunt cerebrovascular injuries with 16-MDCT: accuracy of whole-body MDCT compared with neck MDCT angiography. *AJR Am J Roentgenol* 2008;190:790-799.

37. Delikoukos S, Mantzos F: Thyroid storm induced by blunt thyroid gland trauma. *Am Surg* 2007;73:1247-1249.

38. Duncan JM: Laboratory note: on the tensile strength of the fresh adult foetus. *Br Med J* 1874;2:763-764.

39. Pintar FA, Yoganandan N, Voo L: Effect of age and loading rate on human cervical spine injury threshold. *Spine* 1998;23:1957-1962.

40. Crothers B: The effect of breech extraction upon the central nervous system of the fetus. *Med Clin North Am* 1922;5:1287-1304.

41. Ouyang J, Zhu Q, Weidong Z, et al: Biomechanical assessment of the pediatric cervical spine under bending and tensile loading. *Spine* 2005;30:E716-E723.

42. Nuckley DJ, Ching RP: Developmental biomechanics of the cervical spine: tension and compression. *J Biomech* 2006;39:3045-3054.

43. Curphey TJ, Kade H, Noguchi TT, et al: The battered child syndrome. Responsibilities of the pathologist. *Calif Med* 1965;102:102-104.

44. McGrory BE, Fenichel GM: Hangman's fracture subsequent to shaking in an infant. *Ann Neurol* 1977;2:82.

45. Kleinman PK, Shelton YA: Hangman's fracture in an abused infant: imaging features. *Pediatr Radiol* 1997;27:776-777.

46. Ranjith RK, Mullett JH, Burke TE: Hangman's fracture caused by suspected child abuse. A case report. *J Pediatr Orthop B* 2002;11:329-332.

47. Swischuk L: Spine and spinal cord trauma in the battered child syndrome. *Radiology* 1969;92:733-738.

48. Agner C, Weig SG: Arterial dissection and stroke following child abuse: case report and review of the literature. *Childs Nerv Syst* 2005;21:416-420.

49. Rooks VJ, Sisler C, Burton B: Cervical spine injury in child abuse: report of two cases. *Pediatr Radiol* 1998;28:193-195.

50. Saternus KS, Kernbach-Wighton G, Oemichen M: The shaking trauma in infants – kinetic chains. *Forensic Sci Int* 2000;109:203-213.

51. Ghattan S, Ellenbogen RG: Pediatric spine and spinal cord injury after inflicted trauma. *Neurosurg Clin North Am* 2002;13:227-233.

52. Oral R, Rahhal R, Elshershari H, et al: Intentional avulsion fracture of the second cervical vertebra in a hypotonic child. *Pediatr Emerg Care* 2006;22:352-354.

53. Gleckman AM, Kessler SC, Smith TW: Periadventitial extracranial vertebral artery hemorrhage in a case of shaken baby syndrome. *J Forensic Sci* 2000;45:1151-1153.

54. Nguyen PH, Burrowes DM, Ali S, et al: Intracranial vertebral artery dissection with subarachnoid hemorrhage following child abuse. *Pediatr Radiol* 2007;37:600-602.

55. Hadley MN, Sonntag VKH, Rekate HL, et al: The infant whiplash-shake injury syndrome: a clinical and pathological study. *Neurosurgery* 1989;24:536-540.

56. Johnson D, Boal D, Baule R: Role of apnea in nonaccidental head injury. *Pediatr Neurosurg* 1995;23:305-310.

57. Sun PP, Poffenbarger GJ, Durham S, et al: Spectrum of occipitoatlantoaxial injury in young children. *J Neurosurg* 2000;93(1 Suppl):28-39.

58. Oemichen M, Schleiss D, Pedal I, et al: Shaken baby syndrome: re-examination of diffuse axonal injury as cause of death. *Acta Neuropathol* 2008;116:317-329.

59. Feldman KW, Weinberger E, Milstein JM, et al: Cervical spine MRI in abused infants. *Child Abuse Negl* 1997;21:199-205.

60. Piatt JH, Steinberg M: Isolated spinal cord injury as a presentation of child abuse. *Pediatrics* 1995;96:780-782.

61. Shannon P, Smith CR, Deck J, et al: Axonal injury and the neuropathology of shaken baby syndrome. *Acta Neuropathol* 1998;95:625-631.

62. Geddes JF, Hackshaw AK, Vowles GH, et al: Neuropathology of inflicted head injury in children I. Patterns of brain damage. *Brain* 2001;124:1290-1298.

63. Feldman KW, Avellino AM, Sugar NF, et al: Cervical spinal cord injury in abused children. *Pediatr Emerg Care* 2008;24:222-227.

64. Pang D: Spinal cord injury without radiographic abnormality in children, 2 decades later. *Neurosurgery* 2004;55:1325-1343.

65. Brown RL, Brunn MA, Garcia VF: Cervical spine injuries in children: a review of 103 patients treated consecutively at a level 1 pediatric trauma center. *J Pediatr Surg* 2001;36:1107-1114.

66. Brennan LK, Rubin D, Christian CW, et al: Neck injuries in young pediatric homicide victims. *J Neurosurg Pediatr* 2009;3:232-239.

67. Viccellio P, Simon H, Pressman BD, et al: A prospective multicenter study of cervical spine injury in children. *Pediatrics* 2001;108: e20.

68. Garton HJL, Hammer MR: Detection of pediatric cervical spine injury. *Neurosurgery* 2008;62:1-8.

69. Patel JC, Tepas JJ, Mollitt DL, et al: Pediatric cervical spine injuries: defining the disease. *J Pediatr Surg* 2001;36:373-376.

70. Frank JB, Lim CK, Flynn JM, Dormans JP: The efficacy of magnetic resonance imaging in pediatric cervical spine clearance. *Spine* 2002;27:1176-1179.

71. Goradia D, Linnau KF, Cohen WA, et al: Correlation of MR imaging findings with intraoperative findings after cervical spine trauma. *AJNR Am J Neuroradiol* 2007;28:209-215.

72. Judkins AR, Hood IG, Mirchandani HG, et al: Technical communication: rationale and technique for examination of nervous system in suspected infant victims of abuse. *Am J Forensic Med Pathol* 2004;25:29-32.

73. Lustrin ES, Karakas SP, Ortiz AO, et al: Pediatric cervical spine: normal anatomy, variants, and trauma. *Radiographics* 2003;23: 539-560.

74. Khanna G, El-Khoury GY: Imaging of cervical spine injuries. *Skeletal Radiol* 2007;36:477-494.

75. van Rijn RR, Kool DR, deWitt Harner PC, et al: An abused five-month-old girl: hangman's fracture or congenital arch defect? *J Emerg Med* 2005;29:61-65.

76. Koch LE, Biedermann H, Sternus KS. High cervical stress and apnoea. *Forens Sci Int* 1989;97:1-9.

77. Richards PG, Bertocci GE, Bonshek, RE, et al: Shaken baby syndrome. Before the Court of Appeal. *Am J Dis Child* 2008;91:205-206.

78. Prange MT, Meyers BS: Pathobiology and biomechanics of inflicted childhood neurotrauma – reponse. *In:* Reece RM, Nichols CE (eds): *Inflicted Childhood Neurotrauma.* American Academy of Pediatrics Press, Elk Grove Village, IL, 2003.

79. Bandak FA, Shaken baby syndrome: A biomechanics analysis of injury mechanisms. *Forens Sci Int* 2005;151:71-79.

80. Margulies S, Prange M, Meyers BS, et al: Shaken baby syndrome: a flawed biomechanical analysis. *Forens Sci Int* 2006;164:278-279.

81. Rangarajan N, Shams T: Re: shaken baby syndrome: a biomechanics analysis of injury mechanisms. *Forens Sci Int* 2005;151:71-79.

82. Czeiter E, Pal J, Kovesdai E, et al: Traumatic axonal injury in the spinal cord evoked by traumatic brain injury. *J Neurotrauma* 2008;25:205-213.

83. Zhu SJ, Dougherty L, Margulies SS: In vivo measurements of human brain displacement. *Stapp Car Crash J* 2004;48:227-237.

84. Feipel V, Berghe MV, Rooze MA: No effects of cervical spine motion on cranial dura mater strain. *Clin Biomech* 2003;18:389-392.

85. Byard RW, Blumberg P, Rutty G, et al: Lack of evidence for a causal relationship between hypoxic-ischemic encephalopathy and subdural hemorrhage in fetal life, infancy and early childhood. *Pediatr Devel Path* 2007;10:348-350.

44

EYE INJURIES IN CHILD ABUSE

Alex V. Levin, MD, MHSc, FAAP, FAAO, FRCSC

INTRODUCTION

The eye can be injured directly or indirectly as a result of abusive head trauma. Direct trauma to the face can result in a blunt injury to the globe, surrounding bones, or periocular tissues. Blunt impact trauma to the head can result in forces being transmitted via the skull bones to the optic nerve.[1,2] Brain injury can secondarily affect the eye via papilledema in the setting of increased intracranial pressure, injury to the optic chiasm or visual tracts, or cortical visual impairment resulting from parenchymal brain damage. Severe repeated acceleration-deceleration forces (shaken baby syndrome) with or without blunt head impact can result in intraocular bleeding, disruption of the intraocular contents, or optic nerve injury.[3]

The exact incidence of eye injuries in abusive head trauma is unknown. In the setting of shaken baby syndrome, approximately 85% of children will have retinal hemorrhage with fewer numbers having vitreous hemorrhage, optic atrophy, cortical visual impairment, and even less often other damage to the intraocular contents.[3-5] The incidence of retinal hemorrhages decreases if one includes children who suffer single impact head injury,[6] and approaches 100% in fatal cases of abusive head injury.[7] It has been estimated that 4% to 6% of abused children first present to the ophthalmologist.[8] One small study found that approximately 25% of physically abused children had eye involvement.[9]

BLUNT IMPACT INJURIES TO THE EYE

Any injury to the eye as a result of trauma could be caused through abuse as part of a head injury scenario. It is beyond the scope of this chapter to review all eye injuries; rather, the emphasis is on those ocular findings that might lead to a conclusion to a greater or lesser degree of certainty that trauma occurred (Table 44-1), although the etiology could be abusive or accidental. Those ocular signs that are certainly due to trauma do not necessarily imply an abusive act, but if no history of trauma is offered, then the history is most likely false. For those injuries listed as usually caused by trauma, there are uncommon nontraumatic causes for the same findings. For example, hyphema can rarely be due to juvenile xanthogranulomatosis or iris neovascularization. In the former, characteristic skin lesions are usually present and there is most often a solitary yellow-whitish lesion on the iris representing the iris equivalent of the skin lesions. Iris neovascularization is extremely rare in infants and almost always associated with a known preexisting ophthalmic disease such as uveitis.

Although periorbital ecchymosis can be caused by trauma, it can also be the presenting sign of metastatic neuroblastoma to the orbital bones or leukemia. With neuroblastoma, there is often proptosis and/or restricted eye movements. With leukemia a complete blood count is virtually always abnormal. A single blow to the forehead, by abuse or accident, can also result in bilateral periocular ecchymosis and subconjunctival hemorrhage as the blood tracks down in the subgaleal space and subcutaneous tissues. Practitioners must be particularly careful not to date periocular hemorrhage since the loose attachments of this skin allow for excess and sometimes dramatic accumulations of subcutaneous hemorrhage, thus making timing of the injury very unreliable.

Subconjunctival hemorrhage is most often caused by direct blunt trauma to the globe. Unlike adults, spontaneous subconjunctival hemorrhage is extremely uncommon in children, even in the setting of coagulopathy. This is likely because the conjunctival vessels are supported by more robust substantia propria compared with the elderly in whom spontaneous bleeding is common. Birth by any means can be associated with small, often triangular, subconjunctival hemorrhage at the limbus (cornea-sclera junction) that usually resolves in the first 2 weeks of life.[10-12] Pertussis can be associated with severe bilateral subconjunctival hemorrhage as, in addition to the cough, the organism invades the vessel walls making them weaker.

Asphyxiation/strangulation/suffocation can result in strong Valsalva maneuvers as the child attempts to breathe. The resulting subconjunctival hemorrhage might also be associated with petechia of the lids.[13,14] This has been reported as manifestation of medical child abuse (previously called Münchausen syndrome by proxy).[15] Lastly, subconjunctival hemorrhage has also been reported in abusive head injury such as shaken baby syndrome.[16,17] It is unclear whether this reflects a direct impact lesion to the eye as part of the event, increased intrathoracic pressure, or an indirect trauma to conjunctival vessels brought on by the repeated strong acceleration-deceleration forces.

The lesions listed in Table 44-1 as possibly caused by abuse are often caused by other factors such as infection, uveitis, and genetic conditions. The ophthalmologist might be able to discern such nontraumatic causes by examination alone or by history, such as a family history of infantile cataracts, a prior knowledge of a classic herpetic dendritic corneal lesion, associated Stickler syndrome in a child with retinal detachment, a prior craniopharyngioma in a child with optic atrophy, or the systemic features of Marfan syndrome in a child with ectopia lentis. Trauma should be

402

Table 44-1	Likelihood of Trauma as the Cause of Ocular Findings

Certain Evidence of Trauma

Corneal or scleral laceration (e.g., ruptured globe)
Avulsion of optic nerve
Avulsion of vitreous base
Retinal bruise (e.g., commotio, Berlin edema)
Orbital bone fracture

Usually Resulting from Trauma

Hyphema
Periorbital ecchymosis
Subconjunctival hemorrhage

Possibly Resulting from Trauma (Especially If Unilateral)

Cataract
Corneal scar
Ectopia lentis
Retinal detachment
Optic atrophy

expected when no known diagnostic or contributing factors are present. Systemic causes usually (but not always) manifest bilaterally. When these signs are unilateral, trauma should be considered as a possible cause.

INDIRECT OCULAR AND VISUAL INJURY RELATED TO ABUSIVE HEAD INJURY

Abusive head injury can affect the visual system in several ways without direct blunt eye trauma. First, brain injury involving the occipital cortex, or less commonly, the optic chiasm or optic tracts within the white matter of the brain, will result in visual compromise. This is true regardless of whether the injury was abusive or accidental. Cortical visual impairment can rarely be a transient acute phenomenon after severe blunt impact to the head but is more often a chronic condition that can be quite disabling. In shaken baby syndrome, it can result from severe cerebral edema with infarction of the circulation to the occipital cortex, coup or contra-coup parenchymal contusion, or occipital cortical laceration.[3] Long-term low vision or blindness as a result of abusive head injury is well recognized.[18-22]

The second most common cause of visual loss after abusive head injury is optic atrophy.[3] Although this is most commonly associated with repeated acceleration-deceleration (see below), it can also occur infrequently as a result of severe direct blunt trauma to the frontal bone, or less commonly, the temporal or other bones of the orbital rim, whereby forces are transmitted via the bones to the optic foramen, thus injuring the nerve.[1,2] It must be emphasized that this would not be expected after minor trauma such as a short fall and would most likely be accompanied by obvious signs of the blunt impact such as bruising and swelling. Even less common would be the transsynaptic retrograde death of neurons as a result of postsynaptic injury (i.e., posterior to the lateral geniculate body). This would not be seen in minor or acute brain injury.

Fracture of the orbital bones occurs as a result of blunt impact of the orbital rim, particularly when the zygomatic arch or frontal bone is involved. If the eye is impacted directly and caused to translate posteriorly into the orbit, the orbital bony walls, especially the medial and inferior walls, can sustain "blow out" injuries. The source of orbital fracture can thus be differentiated based on history, affected bone, and evidence of periorbital trauma. Rarely, in severe impact trauma, if the fracture extends posteriorly, the optic nerve can be injured. More common complications of fractures relate to interference with the function of the extraocular muscles, with restriction of gaze in one or more directions or displacement of the globe caused by orbital hemorrhage.

Retinal hemorrhages can occur from direct blunt eye trauma or more commonly, as discussed below, from repeated acceleration-deceleration of the head and neck with or without blunt head impact. Retinal hemorrhage rarely results in a long-term effect on vision. Large hemorrhages obscuring the fovea will reduce vision as long as they are present, and if asymmetric between the two eyes, might lead to a preference for visual development in the less impaired eye, thus adding amblyopia on top of the organic obstruction to vision.[4] For this reason, young children (i.e., those in the shaken baby syndrome age range) with hemorrhage in or over the fovea must be followed after injury for months until one can be certain that visual development has been reestablished equally in both eyes. Less commonly, macular scarring can result in chronic effects on vision.[21]

Lastly, this discussion would be incomplete without mention of nonorganic functional visual loss. Children can present with a variety of unusual ocular symptoms such as transient or alleged permanent visual loss, visual obscuration, blinking, photophobia, and eyelid pulling. Any of these symptoms, in the absence of organic explanatory pathology after full ophthalmology consultation, could be indicators of a variety of psychoemotional stressors in a child's life, including covert physical (or sexual) abuse. Although it would be inappropriate to investigate every child with functional ocular symptoms for possible abuse, consideration of abuse or other factors should come into play when symptoms persist beyond 3 months after the eye doctor appointment or are replaced by other functional symptoms.[23]

RETINAL HEMORRHAGE

Incidence

Retinal hemorrhage is a cardinal manifestation of abusive head trauma characterized by repeated acceleration-deceleration with or without blunt impact (shaken baby syndrome). Approximately 85% of victims will have retinal hemorrhage and the incidence does not appear to vary with age or with whether there are signs of blunt impact to the head.[4,5] In papers that include single acceleration-deceleration blunt impact abusive head trauma along with shaking cases, the reported incidence drops significantly because it is the repeated forces that characterize the syndrome of which retinal hemorrhage is a part. When postmortem series are reviewed, the incidence of retinal hemorrhage rises and even approaches 100%, particularly if microscopic hemorrhage is included since such hemorrhage is beyond the resolution of clinically used instrumentation. Rarely, retinal hemorrhage can occur in the absence of radiologically identified brain injury or intracranial hemorrhage.[24,25]

Types and Patterns

Perhaps the most important aspect of understanding and assessing the diagnostic implication of retinal hemorrhage with respect to child abuse is the recognition of the importance of differentiating retinal hemorrhage on the basis of types, number, extent, and patterns of distribution. In order to do so, a basic familiarity with retinal anatomy is essential.

The retina lines the inner surface of the eye and extends from posterior to anterior so that its edge, the ora serrata, is located just behind the iris. The entire retina is approximately the size of a postage stamp. The retina has ten layers, the bottom one of which, the retinal pigmented epithelium (RPE), is more firmly attached to an underlying vascular layer, the choroid. The choroid brings oxygen and nutrition to the deepest layers of the retina via diffusion. It lies between the retina and the outer shell of the eye, the sclera. The other nine layers of the retina form the "neurosensory retina" and it is these layers together that become involved with a full-thickness retinal detachment, thus leaving the RPE behind. At autopsy, it is common for the neurosensory retina to become artifactitiously detached, which can be distinguished from true premortem retinal detachment by the absence of subretinal blood or exudates.

Posteriorly, the optic nerve enters the eye and is seen just nasal to the visual axis as the optic nerve head (also known as the optic disc) (Figure 44-1). The central retinal vein and artery are carried within the center of the optic nerve. Upon entering the eye, these vessels branch into four major arcades on the surface of the retina: superior temporal, superior nasal, inferior temporal, and inferior nasal (see Figure 44-1).

These retinal vessels continue to branch over the retinal surface, extending to the ora. They also send deeper branches into the retina ending approximately two thirds into the retinal thickness. Retinal venous outflow collects in the central retinal vein in the center of the optic nerve, but exits the optic nerve approximately one third of the way back from the eye before the optic nerve exits the apex of the orbit. This vein then connects with a rich network of non-valved orbital and other veins.

Light that flows into the eye is focused by the cornea and lens as it travels through the pupil and comes to lie straight back within the inside of the eye on an area of specialized retina called the fovea. The fovea lies temporal to the optic nerve and appears as a darker area (see Figure 44-1). The fovea is responsible for our central visual acuity. Surrounding the fovea is a variably defined area that roughly encompasses the two temporal arcades and is called the *macula* (see Figure 44-1). The macula, optic nerve, and some peripapillary (i.e., around the optic nerve) retina all together make up the posterior pole of the eye (see Figure 44-1).

Hemorrhage can lie on the surface of the retina (preretinal hemorrhage), within the renal tissue (intraretinal hemorrhage), or under the neurosensory retina (subretinal hemorrhage) (Figure 44-2). Another term for preretinal hemorrhage is *subhyaloid hemorrhage*, meaning that the blood is between the retina and the well-formed pediatric vitreous gel that fills the eye behind the iris and pupil. If the blood extends into that gel, it is referred to as *vitreous hemorrhage*. Hemorrhage within the retinal tissue is classified as *flame* (also know as *splinter*) *hemorrhage*, since it lies in the most superficial retinal layer made up of millions of nerve fibers streaming from the retina to the optic nerve, thus causing the characteristic linear streaking appearance. Hemorrhage deeper in the retina is referred to as *dot* (smaller) or *blot* (larger) *hemorrhage*, which is round or more amorphous in shape (see Figure 44-2). There are no strict guidelines for using the term *dot* versus *blot* with regards to hemorrhage size. Hemorrhages can have white centers for a variety of reasons including septic emboli, central resolution, or a result of the light reflex from the examining instrument. There is no value in commenting on

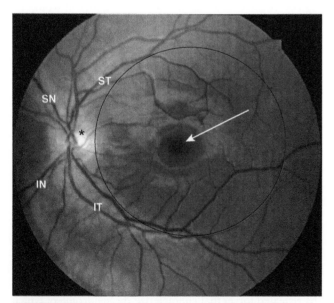

FIGURE 44-1 Normal posterior pole of the left eye. The circle encompasses the macula. *IN*, Inferior nasal arcade; *IT*, inferior temporal arcade; *SN*, superior nasal arcade; *ST*, superior temporal arcade; *arrow*, fovea; * = optic nerve head (optic disc).

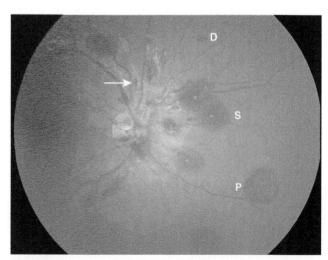

FIGURE 44-2 Types of retinal hemorrhages. *D*, Dot intraretinal hemorrhage; *P*, preretinal hemorrhage; *S*, subretinal hemorrhage; *arrow*, flame (nerve fiber layer, splinter) superficial intraretinal hemorrhage.

the presence or absence of white centers unless there is a specific diagnostic indicator such as obvious leukemic infiltrates.

Retinoschisis refers to the neurosensory retina layers splitting apart. Although there are other forms of retinoschisis that are easily distinguished (e.g., genetic X-linked juvenile retinoschisis), in abusive head trauma a distinct form of retinoschisis occurs wherein blood accumulates in the macula, most often under the most superficial of the retinal layers, the internal limiting membrane (ILM) (Figure 44-3). Blood within a schisis cavity often separates by gravity to create a visible blood-serum level. Sub-ILM blood can also be found over blood vessels (Figure 44-4), where it is a nonspecific finding that can occur with any cause of bleeding resulting from large vessel incompetence or coagulopathy. Rarely in abusive head injury, schisis cavities can occur elsewhere in the retina.[26] Practitioners might find a hemorrhagic or

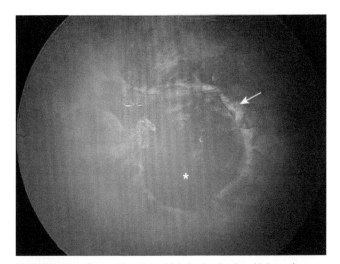

FIGURE 44-3 Traumatic retinoschisis in abusive head injury. *Arrow* indicates perimacular retinal fold; the asterisk indicates blood under the internal limiting membrane within a schisis cavity and extending out into vitreous.

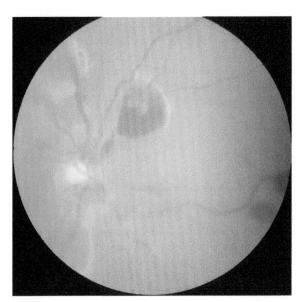

FIGURE 44-4 Subinternal limiting membrane blood (retinoschisis) over a blood vessel. This is a nonspecific finding.

hypopigmented circumlinear demarcation at the edges of a macular schisis lesion. Hypopigmentation arises because of traumatic disruption of the underlying RPE. These lines may or may not be associated with a fold or pleat in the retina, referred to variably and interchangeably in the literature as *perimacular* or *paramacular folds* (see Figure 44-3). After postmortem formalin fixation, the infant retina normally develops multiple folds including a circumferential fold (Lange's fold) at the ora. These normal folds are differentiated by their random multidirectionality, short length, lack of correlation with any anatomical structure, and absence of hemorrhage. The perimacular folds of abusive head trauma form arcs or full circles in the posterior pole. Perimacular folds are usually seen with schisis, but schisis can occur without folds and folds can be seen without schisis.

Both schisis and perimacular folds are often associated with residual vitreous strands, seen on autopsy, attached to the apex of the folds. In infants, the vitreous is firmly attached to the macula, optic nerve, superficial retinal blood vessels, and the area straddling the ora, which includes the last few millimeters of retina before the ora (the peripheral retina). The retina between the periphery and the posterior pole is known as the *midperipheral retina*, which can be relatively spared from hemorrhage in some cases of abusive head trauma.

When describing retinal hemorrhages, practitioners can first describe the number of hemorrhages, ranging from none to "too numerous to count." Several authors have attempted to offer grading schemes for describing retinal hemorrhage but none are in universal use. The types of hemorrhage, particularly the presence of macular retinoschisis and the appearance of lines or folds at the cavity edges, should be noted. Hemorrhage can be bilaterally symmetric, asymmetric, or even unilateral. Specific patterns of hemorrhage can also be recognized. For example, in vasculitis or coagulopathy, hemorrhages are often strictly perivascular (although this pattern does not rule out abuse). In central retinal vein occlusion, a very rare disorder in childhood, the veins are dilated and tortuous, and hemorrhages are too numerous to count, mostly intraretinal, radiating out from the optic nerve centripetally in a very classic and recognizable pattern. Specific retinal disorders, such as capillary hemangioma, can be distinguished on the basis of the retinal appearance, and, for example, associated yellow-white retinal exudates. Likewise, hypertension, which almost never causes retinal hemorrhage in infancy, is associated with a preponderance of exudates compared with hemorrhage. Perhaps most importantly, retinal hemorrhage can be associated with swelling of the optic nerve (papilledema) when caused by increased intracranial pressure. These hemorrhages are found on the optic disc or immediately surrounding the disc and are mostly flame hemorrhages (Figure 44-5). The presence or absence of papilledema should always be noted.

Retinal hemorrhage cannot be dated. It might even be inaccurate to differentiate "new" versus "old" hemorrhage, since hemorrhages sustained at the same time can resolve at variable rates. Although much is known about the resolution of birth hemorrhage (flame hemorrhage is almost always gone by 1 week and usually by 3 days; dot/blot is almost always gone by 4 weeks and usually by 1 week),[3] these intervals cannot be applied for hemorrhage caused by abusive

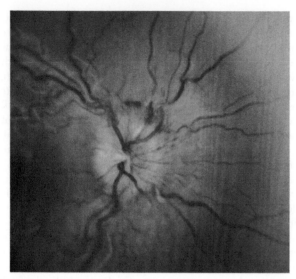

FIGURE 44-5 Papilledema with characteristic peripapillary splinter hemorrhages. Note the blurring of disc margins and loss of visibility of blood vessels on optic nerve head surface.

head trauma because the mechanisms are different and there might be varying tissue injury. The usefulness of the resolution rates for birth hemorrhages comes in identifying whether or not a given type of hemorrhage is due to birth. In abusive head injury, flame and dot/blot hemorrhages sometimes resolve remarkably quickly. Hundreds of small hemorrhages can be gone in 24 hours. But this is not always the case. Preretinal and subretinal hemorrhage take longer to resolve, and blood within a schisis cavity or in the vitreous tends to be slowest to resolve. Although vitreous hemorrhage can occur at the instant of the injury, particularly if there is a retinal tear or detachment, it more often results after a 1- to 3-day delay in which blood spreads from a preretinal location or from within a schisis cavity. There is a correlation between the severity of brain injury and the severity of the hemorrhagic retinopathy, which suggests that the more severe the retinopathy, the more likely that it occurred proximate to the brain injury.

In the "shaken baby" form of abusive head trauma, almost two thirds of victims have too numerous to count, multilayered (preretinal, intraretinal, and subretinal) hemorrhage covering most of the retina (sometimes with midperipheral sparing) and extending to the ora.[5] The absence of retinal hemorrhage, or a small number of hemorrhages confined to the posterior pole, does not rule out abuse. Macular retinoschisis is seen in approximately one third of victims and is frequently unilateral.[5] Asymmetrical and unilateral retinal hemorrhage can also occur.[4,5]

Mechanisms

Several mechanisms have been advanced to explain retinal hemorrhage as seen in abusive head trauma. Although some theories have not been well substantiated by the last 30 years of research in this area, they do identify factors that might modulate the degree of hemorrhagic retinopathy in individual patients. The overwhelming body of research, using clinical, postmortem, animal, mechanical model, and computer model data continuously supports vitreoretinal

traction as the main mechanism of hemorrhage in repeated acceleration-deceleration injury with or without head impact.[3]

One theory that has been presented is that an impairment of venous return out of the eye, in the face of unrestricted arterial supply, could result in rupture of retinal capillaries and venules, with the development of retinal hemorrhage. This impairment was considered possible hypothetically as a result of either increased intrathoracic pressure or increased intracranial pressure. The former is seen in a well-recognized entity called Purtscher retinopathy.[27-30] First described in adults with severe accidental traumatic chest crush injuries, this retinopathy is characterized by polygonal retinal white patches that predominate over the hemorrhages. The pathogenesis of these lesions in incompletely understood and might involve infarction or fat emboli related to long bone fractures, but there clearly is a role for activation of the complement system with microembolization since this entity is also described in no traumatic adult systemic disorders such as pancreatitis.[27,31] Given the incidence of rib fractures in abusive head injury and the frequency of retinal hemorrhages in neonates, this theory was initially given some hypothetical support. But Purtscher retinopathy is rarely seen in abusive head trauma,[29] and the literature offers no suggestion of a correlation between the presence of retinal hemorrhage and rib fractures.[5] In other conditions where there is increased intrathoracic pressure via Valsalva maneuvers, such as coughing,[32] seizures,[33-35] and vomiting,[36] retinal hemorrhage is not seen in children. Multiple studies have shown that the chest compressions of cardiopulmonary resuscitation, which can even be applied too aggressively by caretakers in the field before the arrival of emergency services, rarely cause retinal hemorrhage. When they do, the hemorrhages tend to be very few in number and confined to the posterior pole.[37-41] Valsalva retinopathy itself has a distinct clinical picture with usually a single preretinal hemorrhage or a predominance of preretinal hemorrhages in the posterior pole, which is very different than the hemorrhagic retinopathy of abusive head trauma.[42-44]

The thought that retinal venous outflow impairment can originate from increased intracranial pressure stems from the observation in adults of another well-known entity, Terson syndrome. This condition, which describes the association of intracranial hemorrhage with intraocular hemorrhage, is common in adults with subarachnoid hemorrhage.[45,46] The etiology is poorly understood and might be related to either acutely increased intracranial pressure or blood that tracks down the optic nerve sheath from the intracranial space. We do know from human and animal studies that the optic nerve sheath does dilate in the presence of increased intracranial pressure.[47-50] Excluding the peripapillary hemorrhage characteristic of papilledema described previously, more extensive retinal hemorrhage is not observed. There are reports of intraocular hemorrhage after acute intracranial or optic nerve sheath hemorrhage,[51] but such findings have not been easy to replicate in animal models.[52]

Several lines of evidence indicate that this pathogenic mechanism is not operative in young children. When children with intracranial hemorrhage are studied, Terson syndrome is rarely observed. When it does occur, it appears to cause only a small number of intraretinal and preretinal hemorrhages confined to the posterior pole. One study suggested a maximal incidence of 8%, although empirical experience suggests the number is far lower.[53] The study by Schloff and coworkers did suffer from an older average age of children and a lower incidence of subarachnoid hemorrhage. The rarity of Terson syndrome in children is also supported by the very low number of children who sustain any retinal hemorrhage after accidental head injury (<3%), with most studies indicating incidence closer to zero.[3] If the increased intracranial pressure hypothesis was true, one would expect a much higher incidence of hemorrhage in such studies since many of these children have acutely raised intracranial pressure. Even if one considers fatal car accidents, the incidence of hemorrhage is less than 20%, and few cases of extensive retinal hemorrhage have been reported.[54,55] Studies have also failed to find a correlation between retinal hemorrhage and indicators of increased intracranial pressure in abused children.[5] Finally, the mechanism of venous outflow impairment by any means suffers from the flaw of being inconsistent with the pattern of hemorrhages seen in retinal venous obstruction and the anatomy of the retinal venous drainage as described previously.

Another hypothesis of retinal hemorrhage causation is that hypoxia leads to retinal hemorrhages. The major paper that raised this thought did not examine any eyes at all and the concept was later retracted in court by one of the senior authors.[56,57] Animal models of hypoxia with and without reperfusion do not result in retinal hemorrhage.[58] Other theories have included a possible subclinical vitamin C deficiency, including the idea that routine childhood vaccination raises histamine levels, which induces a temporary decline in vitamin C. These theories are all predicated on the notoriously unreliable and variable serum vitamin C level, which fluctuates widely even in the course of a day and with diet.[59] Lymphocyte vitamin C must be used to study this issue further,[60] but even in frank scurvy few reliable reports of significant intraocular hemorrhage exist.

Victims of abusive head trauma often experience transient mild to moderate coagulopathy as a result of the brain injury.[61] Although this might be responsible for aggravating the appearance of hemorrhage, retinal hemorrhages even in the face of severe coagulopathies such as hemophilia are uncommon,[62] although no systematic study of patients with coagulopathy plus head trauma has been conducted. Other potential modulating factors such as thrombophilia or anemia have not been well studied but in and of themselves are not common causes of extensive retinal hemorrhage in children.

The lines of evidence that support vitreoretinal traction as the primary cause of retinal hemorrhage in abusive head injury are many. Perhaps most striking is the unique presence of macular retinoschisis that, with the exception of the two cases of fatal head crush injury[63,64] and a series of fatal motor vehicle accidents,[54] has not been reported in children less than 5 years old. The presence of perimacular folds and vitreous attachments at histology supports the role of traction. This has most recently been studied using optical coherence tomography.[65] That vitreous traction would result in a unique schisis injury to infants is also consistent with the unique vitreoretinal anatomy of this age group. Why the two cases of head crush injury just cited showed schisis remains unknown.[66] In adults, where the ILM is perhaps more "detachable" than in children, lesions that mimic the

hemorrhagic schisis cavity of abusive head trauma have been described in circumstances of acute severe hemorrhage into the sub-ILM space.[67] Perhaps in fatal crush injury an extraordinary hemorrhage pressure wave is created that is enough to cause this finding or perhaps there is actually vitreoretinal traction induced by compression of the globe.[66] Orbit fracture is a common manifestation of crush injury. Another study that looked at a series of fatal crush injuries did not find severe hemorrhagic retinopathy or schisis.[68] It is interesting that the cases in which schisis and severe hemorrhagic retinopathy was seen after fatal motor vehicle accidents in young children were characterized by repeated acceleration-deceleration forces (i.e, "roll overs").[54] Perhaps it is the very uniqueness of the nature of the injury in abusive head trauma with repeated acceleration-deceleration that allows hemorrhagic retinopathy to occur. Of course, rarely if ever will the situation arise where one would be considering an unknown, unreported fatal crush head injury or motor vehicle accident in the differential diagnosis.

Also supporting the role of vitreoretinal traction is the high incidence of retinal hemorrhage in the peripheral retina, another location where the vitreous is firmly attached. This has been shown to be statistically more likely to indicate abusive head trauma versus accidental head injury.[6] Sparing of the midperiphery is additional evidence, since the vitreous is least attached in this area.

Animal models offer some further insights. In cats, vitreoretinal shear induces altered vascular autoregulation and the vessel walls become patulous and more permeable.[69] This autonomic dysregulation might be the common biochemical pathway by which retinal hemorrhage develops. The orbital finding of hemorrhage within the cranial nerve sheaths[70] is relevant in that the cranial nerves carry the autonomic supply to the eye, which is in part responsible for vascular autoregulation. Recent evidence suggests that one of the primary factors in the development of birth retinal hemorrhage is the effect of prostaglandins, which have a potent effect on vascular autoregulation.[71,72]

Animal models have been less helpful in terms of actually replicating the development of retinal hemorrhage caused by repeated acceleration-deceleration forces. Mouse and rat models of shaking have in some laboratories produced mild hemorrhagic retinopathy, although the details of the hemorrhages have not been well described.[73-75] We have been able to replicate optic nerve sheath hemorrhage but not retinal hemorrhage in a rat model (Levin et al, 2003, unpublished). It appears that the small mass and volume of the rodent eye and the lack of a well-defined orbit make it a poor model, since the amount of force needed to model the infant human scale would be impossible to obtain without causing severe tissue disruption to the animal. Examination of the eyes of kittens and rabbits shaken to death by a dog failed to reveal retinal hemorrhage, likely for the same reason in addition to the mode of shaking (grasping by the posterior neck), which is very different than abusive head trauma.[76] Larger mammals will be needed to develop a better model. An immature pig model using a single acceleration-deceleration of the head without impact is currently under study.[77] An interesting model is the woodpecker, an animal that spends its lifetime submitting itself to repeated acceleration-deceleration with impact.[78] Woodpeckers have no orbital space in which the globe can move, since the bone is closely approximated around the eye. The eye is also held from moving in the orbit by anterior fascial attachments and eyelid closure with each strike. In addition, its vitreous is not attached to the retina. But the woodpecker has the advantage of a superb shock-absorbing skull, small eyes that would require perhaps more force than it can generate to induce ocular injury, an anticipated strike, and a strike that is nearly purely in the anterior-posterior axis every time. All birds have these adaptations, but all birds peck—so perhaps these adaptations are what allowed woodpeckers to evolve such dramatic behaviors.

Several groups have reported computer-based finite element models wherein known tissue properties are used to build a virtual eye, orbit, and orbital contents in the computer that can then be submitted to repeated acceleration-deceleration forces.[79-81] The computer cannot predict tissue injury but it can predict where the retina will experience the greatest stress. Our group and others have shown that the predicted areas of greatest stress on the retina occur at the macula and peripheral retina in keeping with what is observed clinically, again underscoring the importance of vitreoretinal traction.[81,82]

Differential Diagnosis

In addition to the disorders discussed previously, there are many things that can cause retinal hemorrhage (Table 44-2).[3] These diagnoses are almost all readily diagnosed by history, laboratory, eye examination, and/or systemic physical examination. The pattern of hemorrhages seen in these conditions is usually a small number of preretinal and intraretinal hemorrhages confined to the posterior pole of the eye. This nonspecific pattern (Figure 44-6) can also occur in child abuse but does not allow diagnostic comments to be made based on the eye alone. With the exception of birth leukemia, fatal head crush injury, and fatal severe motor vehicle accidents, the extensive multilayered retinal hemorrhages, too numerous to count, extending to the ora seems to have particular specificity for abusive head injury (see Figure 44-3). When considering a differential diagnosis, it is important to avoid "circular reasoning" by which all children with severe hemorrhagic retinopathy are victims of

abuse and therefore the possibility of an alternative diagnosis is not considered. Likewise, there are many areas deserving further research such as the incidence of retinal hemorrhages when multiple factors are combined such as the child who has a severe accidental head injury and then suffers from hypoxia, increased intracranial pressure, anemia, hypotension, and coagulopathy. Although not rigorously studied, we do know that thousands of such children have been examined and clinical experience alone tells us that neither the combination nor the individual factors would cause an extensive hemorrhagic retinopathy. One must be careful of literature that ascribed such retinopathy to nonabusive causes if the eye examinations were not conducted by an ophthalmologist through dilated pupils,[83] or child abuse was not sufficiently evaluated or excluded. Lastly, one must avoid making a diagnosis of abusive head injury based solely on the eye examination without considering other systemic and historical factors.

DOCUMENTATION AND THE ROLE OF THE OPHTHALMOLOGIST

All patients in whom there is a suspicion of abusive head trauma, particularly those under 5 years old, should have a complete eye examination, including pharmacological dilatation of the pupil (unless the pupils are fixed and dilated as a result of neurological injury) and indirect ophthalmoscopy. Preferably, the examination should be conducted by a pediatric ophthalmologist or retinal specialist who is well versed in abusive head injury and in its retinal manifestations as well as in the examination of young children. It is sometimes necessary to insert a lid speculum. When necessary, the eye can be turned and "indented" through a process known as scleral depression, which allows a view of the retina to its periphery. This examination is easily conducted with topical anesthesia alone. Since hemorrhage may increase over the first few days of hospitalization in sick children[84]—presumably caused by the biochemical injury cascade that alters vascular permeability once initial hemorrhage has occurred, brain injury–induced mild coagulopathy, or other factors—it is desirable that the ophthalmology consultation take place in the first 24 hours after admission and certainly no more than 72 hours. If there is an increase in hemorrhages, one would not expect the change to be from a nonspecific "few hemorrhages in the posterior pole" to a more diagnostic

Table 44-2	Some Disorders Associated with Retinal Hemorrhage (Incomplete List)

Coagulopathies
Leukemia
Hyper/hyponatremia
Anemia
Carbon monoxide poisoning
Extracorporeal membrane oxygenation
Increased intracranial pressure
Glutaric aciduria type I
Malaria
Meningitis
Vasculitis
Osteogenesis imperfecta
Accidental head injury
Endocarditis

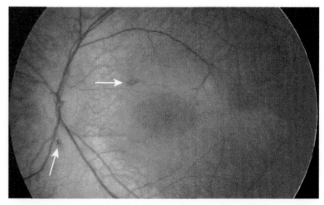

FIGURE 44-6 Mild nonspecific retinal hemorrhages. Arrows indicate small nerve fiber layer (flame) hemorrhages.

severe and extensive hemorrhagic retinopathy. Yet, the earliest documentation is preferred.

It is absolutely acceptable and encouraged for non-ophthalmologists to attempt to view the retina using a direct ophthalmoscope. Such examinations are accurate over 80% of the time with regard to the presence or absence of hemorrhage.[85] False positives and false negatives have been reported,[4,85] and therefore such examinations should never replace the need for a timely formal ophthalmology consult. The non-ophthalmologist examination might, for example, help to raise greater concern of abuse in a differential if hemorrhage is seen, although the absence of observed hemorrhage should also not remove concern of abuse if raised by the presence of non-ophthalmic factors. The direct ophthalmoscope is not capable of seeing beyond the posterior pole, and it is difficult for non-ophthalmologists using this tool to distinguish types or patterns of hemorrhage.[83,85] After performing the eye examination, non-ophthalmologists should document their findings in the chart with the caveat that the note reflects "... preliminary examination pending ophthalmology consultation." Should the non-ophthalmologist find no hemorrhage and the ophthalmologist find some, or even extensive, hemorrhage, the explanation would more likely be a false-negative examination by the non-ophthalmologist than new hemorrhages that occurred in the intervening period between the two examinations.

It is inadvisable for the non-ophthalmologist to instill dilating drops prior to ophthalmology consultation unless an ophthalmology specialist is absolutely unavailable. The ophthalmologist or their designate should check the pupils themselves (rather than preordering dilating drops) when possible, particularly to look for a Marcus Gunn pupil (afferent pupillary defect), which can indicate early optic nerve damage, and to identify any trauma to the anterior segment of the eye (e.g., pupil tear, traumatic mydriasis, hyphema).

There are virtually no other common contraindications, other than known allergy, for pharmacological dilation. There might be times when the attending physician or neurosurgeon caring for an acutely ill child requests that the pupils not be pharmacologically dilated. Although one can debate the evidence to support this practice, the scenario is commonplace. Ophthalmology consultation should still be obtained and several options considered. Shorter-acting agents such as phenylephrine 2.5% and tropicamide 1% can allow for a return of pupillary reactivity usually within 4 to 6 hours, although the size of pupillary dilatation may not be maximal. Another option is to dilate one eye, wait for its pupillary reactivity to return, and then examine the other eye (usually the next day). Lastly, and least preferably, the ophthalmologist can use "small pupil techniques" to examine the retina, usually yielding a limited view of the posterior pole only. If this is the chosen option, the ophthalmologist should be called back to reexamine the child when full pharmacological dilatation of the pupils is considered safe.

Ophthalmologists are encouraged to write detailed descriptions of their observations. This is the standard of care. Although some ophthalmologists have less artistic prowess, drawings are encouraged even if they are "summaries" and not every hemorrhage is drawn, provided that the labeling and descriptions make up for lack of detail in the drawing. The ophthalmology consult should be dated and timed. Since these cases have great medicolegal implications, academic teaching centers should consider embracing a policy requiring staff physicians to write all or part of the consult note. It is important for trainees to examine these children for educational purposes, but if they are to write notes in the chart, they should clearly note their training level and indicate that their findings are "... to be confirmed by attending staff." Staff ophthalmologists should be encouraged to write an assessment that includes a differential diagnosis (if relevant to the case) and indicates appropriate follow-up care. Brain-injured children, even in the absence of retinal hemorrhage, are at risk for strabismus, amblyopia, optic atrophy, and cortical visual loss. If there is no eye injury at all, a follow-up visit in no more than 4 to 6 months to screen for such sequelae is indicated. Shorter follow-up will sometimes be appropriate, particularly when there is hemorrhage in or in front of the fovea, vitreous hemorrhage, or retinoschisis.

In addition to the clinical note, photodocumentation is helpful. This is not an obligatory part of the child's care and in some cases might even hamper the evaluation of the child, either directly, by causing retinal hemorrhage in premature babies, or indirectly, by introducing photos that are of poor quality or have artifacts that can confuse those non-physicians involved in legal proceedings. But when available, photodocumentation is encouraged and can be obtained through a number of retinal cameras now available. Assuming the child is too young or sick to voluntarily sit for the usual upright fundus cameras, there are currently three main options for supine photography. I discuss them from personal experience and, in the case of RetCam, from a prospective study not involving hemorrhage.[86] Further research is needed to clarify the implications of the differences among these tools. Retinal photographs do not replace the need for a skilled ophthalmology consult. Although telemedicine becomes a possibility with digital images, the 3-dimensional view and color accuracy of a live examination remains far superior to photographs.

The Nidek camera (Nidek Co., Ltd., Tokyo, http://www.nidek-intl.com/fundus.html#nm200d) was the first to tout the ability to obtain photographs of the retina without pharmacological dilatation of the pupils. It is relatively easy to use and perhaps the least expensive, but the quality of the photographs is less good than the other two cameras discussed here and it is difficult to view the peripheral retina. The Kowa camera (Kowa Co., Ltd., Tokyo, http://www.kowa.co.jp/e-life/products/fc/genesis_d.htm) offers the best color accuracy (see Figures 44-4 and 44-5) at a moderate cost, but it is technically the most difficult to use compared to the other two cameras. Like the Nidek, its view is of lesser angle. The RetCam camera (Clarity Medical Systems, Inc., Pleasanton, CA, http://www.claritymsi.com/us/contact-clarity.html) is technically the easiest to use and offers the advantage of excellent wide-angle views (see Figures 44-1 to 44-3 and 44-6). It is by far the most expensive and least portable. RetCam photography also can induce artifact at its edges, and retinal hemorrhage can take on a darker appearance, with fainter hemorrhages sometimes appearing faded with less contrast.

Retinal hemorrhage has been documented by magnetic resonance imaging (MRI) and computed tomography (CT), but this is a very inferior means of detection since only raised hemorrhages (e.g., schisis or preretinal hemorrhage) of significant size, retinal detachment, and vitreous hemorrhage can be noted; even then, accurate diagnosis of the radiographic finding is impossible and clinical correlation must be obtained. Ultrasound of the eye (B scan) is very useful in detecting similar findings as MRI but cannot distinguish intraretinal hemorrhage well. It is used when there is an obstruction to the view of the retina (e.g., cataract, vitreous hemorrhage). If vitreous hemorrhage is obstructing the view of the retina, clinical examination should be arranged at periodic intervals of perhaps every 1 to 2 weeks until a retinal view is obtained, understanding that retinal hemorrhages might have resolved in the interim.

POSTMORTEM EXAMINATION AND FINDINGS

When a child dies without a premortem eye examination, postmortem indirect ophthalmoscopy is possible up to 72 hours after death although the progression of corneal cloudiness that obstructs the view will occur faster in some cases. For physicians not familiar with the technique of indirect ophthalmoscopy, monocular means of view are also reported.[87] Such examinations should not replace the need for enucleation with gross and histological examination of the eyes. Postmortem ocular endoscopy has been described[88-90] but also should not replace enucleation. Endoscopy allows some view of the retina but can cause iatrogenic retinal injury such as detachment. For the same reason, vitreous sampling for toxicology and other forensic use is not advisable if abusive head trauma is strongly suspected.

It is beyond the scope of this chapter to discuss all of the postmortem reports regarding eyes of victims of abusive head trauma. These postmortem studies add two important findings. First, there may be hemorrhage, which is not easily visible such as hemorrhage in the choroid, microscopic intraretinal hemorrhage, or small amounts of subretinal hemorrhage.[7,91,92] Hemosiderin detection is not possible without histological section. The value of hemosiderin in general remains unclear and in the retina the timing implications are likely so variable as to limit its forensic utility other than to identify that hemorrhage was present at some point in time.[93,94]

More importantly, autopsy offers the ability to examine the orbital contents including, but not limited to, the optic nerve. Protocols have been established for removal of the eye *en bloc* along with the entire orbital contents using a combined anterior and intracranial approach.[95] This method allows detection of orbital findings such as hemorrhage into the fat, extraocular muscles, optic nerve dura, and optic nerve sheath, as well as intrascleral hemorrhage, which could help to distinguish accidental from nonaccidental injury.[96-100] Since these findings would not be as visible using the routine standard anterior approach enucleation, orbital evisceration is strongly recommended. After the globe and orbital contents are removed, formalin fixation for 72 hours is recommended. The globe should not be sectioned before fixation since the sticky vitreous is more likely to cause retinal detachment. Postmortem documentation of the gross findings is essential and can be achieved through a variety of photographic means.[100,101]

Removal of the eye postmortem, especially when the diagnosis of abuse remains uncertain, may have cultural and societal obstacles. It is paradoxical that such objections are less commonly made to the extensive organ removal and surgical opening that otherwise characterizes routine autopsy. But this is a psychosocial reality of many societies and is likely best dealt with through informed consent, education of professionals, and the establishment of routine protocols for standard of care. Removal of the globe and orbital contents might be considered routine in any case, especially in children less than 5 years old, where the cause of death is unknown, and abuse is possibly in the differential. This would include cases of sudden unexplained infant death with normal physical examination. It is important to note that removal of the globe and orbital contents in no way alters the cosmetic appearance of the corpse after preparation by a funeral home for viewing. Even in cases in which people die without removal of the eyeballs, the lids are shut over plastic shells that cover the eye as well as add fullness to the appearance, since eyes normally become somewhat enophthalmic after death. If the orbital tissues are removed, the orbit can be filled with gauze or other substances to reestablish a normal appearance of the closed lids.

STRENGTH OF THE MEDICAL EVIDENCE

That abusive head trauma, especially when characterized by repeated acceleration-deceleration forces with or without head impact, is associated with retinal hemorrhages is virtually incontrovertible with multiple strong clinical and postmortem studies that demonstrate this. Multiple lines of research continue to converge on the theory that vitreoretinal traction is the major factor in the pathogenesis of retinal hemorrhages. Some authors continue to raise other possible mechanisms, but as discussed previously, there is strong evidence to refute these claims, although the exact role of these other factors in modulating the appearance of the hemorrhages remains unknown.

SUGGESTED DIRECTIONS FOR FUTURE RESEARCH

As in all fields of medicine, there is much research to be done in the field of ocular manifestations of abusive head trauma. First, we must improve on our ability to accurately describe the hemorrhages observed on clinical and postmortem examination by developing a standardized mechanism of description and perhaps scoring. This will be an invaluable tool for all future research. It will also be useful to do serial examinations of large cohorts of children to see if we can develop some precision around dating of these hemorrhages. These studies should also involve carefully controlled development and testing of various photographic systems.

Work should continue in the area of differential diagnosis and pathogenesis. With regard to the former, formal prospective studies should be performed to document accurately the retinal manifestations, if any, of the entire range of potential differential diagnoses such as hypoxia and coagulopathy. We are currently involved in a prospective multicenter examination of children with acutely raised intracranial pressure. Abused children and victims of accidental head injury should also be carefully examined with regards to potential modulating factors such as blood pressure, lymphocyte vitamin C levels, and thrombophilia. For example, if a child is genetically thrombophilic, as are 5% of North American children, would this alter the retinal response to minor accidental head trauma and allow for a hemorrhagic retinopathy that would otherwise not be expected? Studying these potential modulating factors might also give insight into pathogenesis, although animal studies would be particularly useful in this regard if an appropriate model is developed. Non-animal strategies could also involve a study of the biochemical content of vitreous in victims of abuse and accidental head trauma to measure proxy chemicals indicating potential vascular autonomic dysregulation. The concept of autonomic dysregulation can also be explored by continued examination of postmortem orbital specimens and the surgical denervation of animal eyes prior to submitting the animal to repetitive acceleration-deceleration with or without blunt impact.

References

1. Goldenberg-Cohen N, Miller NR, Repka MX: Traumatic optic neuropathy in children and adolescents. *J AAPOS* 2004;8:20-27.
2. Lessell S: Indirect optic nerve trauma. *Arch Ophthalmol* 1989;107:382-386.
3. Levin AV: Retinal haemorrhage and child abuse. *In:* David TJ (ed): *Recent Advances in Paediatrics*, Vol 18. London, Churchill Livingstone, 2000, pp 151-219.
4. Kivlin JD, Simons KB, Lazoritz S, et al: Shaken baby syndrome. *Ophthalmology.* 2000;107:1246-1254.
5. Morad Y, Kim YM, Armstrong DC, et al: Correlation between retinal abnormalities and intracranial abnormalities in the shaken baby syndrome. *Am J Ophthalmol* 2002;134:354-359.
6. Bechtel K, Stoessel K, Leventhal JM, et al: Characteristics that distinguish accidental from abusive injury in hospitalized young children with head trauma. *Pediatrics* 2004;114:165-168.
7. Munger CE, Peiffer RL, Bouldin TW, et al: Ocular and associated neuropathologic observations in suspected whiplash shaken infant syndrome. A retrospective study of 12 cases. *Am J Forensic Med Pathol* 1993;14:193-200.
8. Friendly DS: Ocular manifestations of physical child abuse. *Trans Am Acad Ophthalmol Otolaryngol* 1971;75:318-332.
9. Hendeles S, Barber K, Willshaw HE: The risk of ocular involvement in non-accidental injury. *Child Care Health Dev* 1985;11:345-348.
10. Anteby II, Anteby EY, Chen B, et al: Retinal and intraventricular cerebral hemorrhages in the preterm infant born at or before 30 weeks' gestation. *J AAPOS* 2001;5:90-94.
11. Baum JD, Bulpitt CJ: Retinal and conjunctival haemorrhage in newborn. *Arch Dis Child* 1970;45:344-349.
12. Katzman GH: Pathophysiology of neonatal subconjunctival hemorrhage. *Clin Pediatr (Phila)* 1992;31:149-152.
13. Hawley DA, McClane GE, Strack GB: A review of 300 attempted strangulation cases Part III: injuries in fatal cases. *J Emerg Med* 2001;213:317-322.
14. Ely SF, Hirsch CS: Asphyxial deaths and petechiae: a review. *J Forensic Sci* 2000;45:1274-1277.
15. Levin AV: Ophthalmic manifestations. *In:* Levin AV, Sheridan MS (eds): *Munchausen Syndrome by Proxy; Issues in Diagnosis and Treatment.* New York, Lexington Books, 1995, pp 207-212.
16. Bohnert M, Grosse Perdekamp M, Pollak S: Three subsequent infanticides covered up as SIDS. *Int J Legal Med* 2005;119:31-34.
17. Spitzer SG, Luorno J, Noël LP: Isolated subconjunctival hemorrhages in a nonaccidental trauma. *J AAPOS* 2005;9:53-56.
18. Han DP, Wilkinson WS: Late ophthalmic manifestations of the shaken baby syndrome. *J Pediatr Ophthalmol Strabismus* 1990;27:299-303.
19. Haviland J, Russell RI: Outcome after severe non-accidental head injury. *Arch Dis Child* 1997;77:504-507.
20. Makaroff KL, Putnam FW: Outcomes of infants with inflicted traumatic brain injury. *Dev Med Child Neurol* 2003;45:497-502.
21. McCabe CF, Donahue SP: Prognostic indicators for vision and mortality in shaken baby syndrome. *Arch Ophthalmol* 2000;118:373-377.
22. Case ME: Inflicted traumatic brain injury in infants and young children. *Brain Pathol* 2008;18:571-582.
23. Vrabec TR, Levin AV, Nelson LB: Functional blinking in childhood. *Pediatrics* 1989;83:967-970.
24. Morad Y, Avni I, Benton SA, et al: Normal computerized tomography of brain in children with shaken baby syndrome. *J AAPOS* 2004;8:445-450.
25. Morad Y, Avni I, Capra L, et al: Shaken baby syndrome without intracranial hemorrhage on initial computed tomography. *J AAPOS* 2004;8:521-527.
26. Greenwald MJ, Weiss A, Oesterle CS, et al: Traumatic retinoschisis in battered babies. *Ophthalmology* 1986;93:618-625.
27. Behrens-Baumann W, Scheurer G, Schroer H: Pathogenesis of Purtscher's retinopathy: an experimental study. *Graefes Arch Clin Exp Ophthalmol* 1992;230:286-291.
28. Kelley JS: Purtscher's retinopathy related to chest compression by safety belts. *Am J Ophthalmol* 1972;74(2):278-283.
29. Tomasi LG, Rosman NP: Purtscher retinopathy in the battered child syndrome. *Am J Dis Child* 1975;129:1335-1337.
30. Agrawal A, McKibbin MA: Purtscher's and Purtscher-like retinopathies: a review. *Surv Ophthalmol* 2006;51:129-136.
31. Toshniwal PK, Berman AA, Axelrod AJ: Purtscher's retinopathy secondary to pancreatitis. Aspects of the topography of retinal abnormalities. *J Clin Neuroophthalmol* 1986;6:160-165.
32. Goldman M, Dagan Z, Yair M, et al: Severe cough and retinal hemorrhage in infants and young children. *J Pediatr* 2006;148:835-836.
33. Mei-Zahav M, Uziel Y, Raz J, et al: Convulsions and retinal haemorrhage: should we look further? *Arch Dis Child* 2002;86:334-335.
34. Sandramouli S, Robinson R, Tsaloumas M, et al: Retinal haemorrhages and convulsions. *Arch Dis Child* 1997;76:449-451.
35. Tyagi AK, Scotcher S, Kozeis N, et al: Can convulsions alone cause retinal haemorrhages in infants? *Br J Ophthalmol* 1998;82:659-660.
36. Herr S, Pierce MC, Berger RP, et al: Does Valsalva retinopathy occur in infants? An initial investigation in infants with vomiting caused by pyloric stenosis. *Pediatrics* 2004;113:1658-1661.
37. Fackler JC, Berkowitz ID, Green WR. Retinal hemorrhage in newborn piglets following cardiopulmonary resuscitation. *Am J Dis Child* 1992;146:1294-1296.
38. Gilliland MG, Luckenbach MW: Are retinal hemorrhages found after resuscitation attempts? A study of the eyes of 169 children. *Am J Forens Med Pathol* 1993;14:187-192.
39. Goetting MT, Sowa B: Retinal haemorrhage after cardiopulmonary resuscitation in children: an etiologic evaluation. *Pediatrics* 1990;85:585-588.
40. Kanter RK: Retinal hemorrhage after cardiopulmonary resuscitation or child abuse. *J Pediatr* 1986;180:430-432.
41. Odom A, Christ E, Kerr N, et al: Prevalence of retinal hemorrhages in pediatric patients after in-hospital cardiopulmonary resuscitation: a prospective study. *Pediatrics* 1997;99:E3.
42. Duane TD: Valsalva hemorrhagic retinopathy. *Trans Am Ophthalmol Soc* 1972;70:298-313.
43. Jain AK, Gaynon M: Images in clinical medicine. Macular hemorrhage from bungee jumping. *N Engl J Med* 2007;357:e3.
44. Skorin L Jr, Keith JF. Valsalva retinopathy: examples of classic and secondary occurrences. *Clin Refract Optommol* 2008;19:36-40.
45. Khan SG, Frenkel M: Intravitreal hemorrhage associated with rapid increase in intracranial pressure (Terson's syndrome). *Am J Ophthalmol* 1975;80:37-43.
46. Medele RJ, Stummer W, Mueller AJ, et al: Terson's syndrome in subarachnoid hemorrhage and severe brain injury accompanied by acutely raised intracranial pressure. *J Neurosurg* 1998;88:851-854.
47. Galetta S, Byrne SF, Smith JL: Echographic correlation of optic nerve sheath size and cerebrospinal fluid pressure. *J Clin Neuroophthalmol* 1989;9:79-82.
48. Gangemi M, Cennamo G, Maiuri F, et al: Echographic measurement of the optic nerve in patients with intracranial hypertension. *Neurochirugia (Stuttg)* 1987;30:53-55.
49. Hansen HC, Helmke K: The subarachnoid space surrounding the optic nerves. An ultrasound study of the optic nerve sheath. *Surg Radiol Anat* 1996;18:323-328.
50. Hansen HC, Helmke K: Validation of the optic nerve sheath response to changing cerbrospinal fluid pressure: ultrasound findings during intrathecal infusion tests. *J Neurosurg* 1997;87:34-40.
51. Vanderlinden RG, Chisholm LD: Vitreous hemorrhages and sudden increased intracranial pressure. *J Neurosurg* 1974;41:167-176.

52. Smith DC, Kearns TP, Sayre GP: Preretinal and optic nerve-sheath hemorrhage: pathologic and experimental aspects in subarachnoid hemorrhage. *Trans Am Acad Ophthalmol Otolaryngol* 1957;61:201-211.

53. Schloff S, Mullaney PB, Armstrong DC, et al: Retinal findings in children with intracranial hemorrhage. *Ophthalmology* 2002;109:1472-1476.

54. Kivlin JD, Currie ML, Greenbaum VJ, et al: Retinal hemorrhages in children following fatal motor vehicle crashes: a case series. *Arch Ophthalmol* 2008;126:800-804.

55. Vinchon M, Noizet O, Defoort-Dhellemmes S, et al: Infantile subdural hematomas due to traffic accidents. *Pediatr Neurosurg* 2002;37:245-253.

56. Geddes JF, Tasker RC, Hackshaw AK, et al: Dural haemorrhage in non-traumatic infant deaths: does it explain the bleeding in "shaken baby syndrome"? *Neuropathol Appl Neurobiol* 2003;29:14-22.

57. R. v Harris and Others: Supreme Court of Judicature Court of Appeal (Criminal Division), United Kingdom, 2005.

58. Ozbay D, Ozden S, Müftüoğlu S, et al: Protective effect of ischemic preconditioning on retinal ischemia-reperfusion injury in rats. *Can J Ophthalmol* 2004;39:727-732.

59. Fung EL, Nelson EA: Could vitamin C deficiency have a role in shaken baby syndrome? *Pediatr Int* 2004;46:753-755.

60. Emadi-Konjin P, Verjee Z, Levin AV, et al: Measurement of intracellular vitamin C level in human lymphocytes by reverse phase high performance liquid chromatography (HPLC). *Clin Biochem* 2005;38:450-456.

61. Hymel KP, TC Apshire, DW Luckey, et al: Coagulopathy in pediatric abusive head trauma. *Pediatrics* 1997;99:371-375.

62. Rubenstein RA, Yanoff M, Albert DM: Thrombocytopenia, anemia, and retinal hemorrhage. *Am J Ophthalmol* 1968;65:435-439.

63. Lantz PE, Sinal SH, Stanton CA, et al: Perimacular retinal folds from childhood head trauma. *Br Med J* 2004;328:754-756.

64. Lueder GT, Turner JW, Paschall R: Perimacular retinal folds simulating nonaccidental injury in an infant. *Arch Ophthalmol* 2006;124:1782-1783.

65. Scott AW, Farsiu S, Enyedi LB, et al: Imaging the infant retina with a hand-held spectral-domain optical coherence tomography device. *Am J Ophthalmol* 2009;147:364-373.

66. Levin AV: Retinal hemorrhages of crush head injury: learning from outliers. *Arch Ophthalmol* 2006;124:1773-1774.

67. Sadeh AD, Lazar M, Loewenstein A: Macular ring in a patient with Terson's syndrome. *Acta Ophthalmol Scand* 1999;77:599-600.

68. Gnanaraj L, Gilliland MG, Yahya RR, et al: Ocular manifestations of crush head injury in children. *Eye* 2007;21:5-10.

69. Nagaoka T, Sakamoto T, Mori F, et al: The effect of nitric oxide on retinal blood flow during hypoxia in cats. *Invest Ophthalmol Vis Sci* 2002;43:3037-3044.

70. Wygnanski-Jaffe T, Levin AV, Shafiq A, et al: Postmortem orbital findings in shaken baby syndrome. *Am J Ophthalmol* 2006;142:233-240.

71. Gonzalez Viejo I, Ferrer Novella C, Pueyo Subias M, et al: Hemorrhagic retinopathy in newborns: frequency, form of presentation, associated factors and significance. *Eur J Ophthalmol* 1995;5:247-250.

72. Schoenfeld A, Buckman G, Nissenkorn I, et al: Retinal hemorrhages in the newborn following labor induced by oxytocin or dinoprostone. *Arch Ophthalmol* 1985;103:932-934.

73. Bonnier C, Mesplès B, Carpentier S, et al: Delayed white matter injury in a murine model of shaken baby syndrome. *Brain Pathol* 2002;12:320-328.

74. Smith SL, Andrus PK, Gleason DD, et al: Infant rat model of the shaken baby syndrome: preliminary characterization and evidence for the role of free radicals in cortical hemorrhaging and progressive neuronal degeneration. *J Neurotrauma* 1998;15:693-705.

75. Bonnier C, Mesples B, Gressens P: Animal models of shaken baby syndrome: revisiting the pathophysiology of this devastating injury. *Pediatr Rehabil* 2004;7:165-171.

76. Serbanescu I, Brown SM, Ramsay D, et al: Natural animal shaking: a model for inflicted neurotrauma in children? *Eye* 2008;22:715-717.

77. Binenbaum G, Forbes BJ, Reghupathi R, et al: Animal model to study retinal hemorrhages in a non-impact brain injury. *J AAPOS* 2007;11:84-85.

78. Wygnanski-Jaffe T, Murphy CJ, Smith C, et al: Protective ocular mechanisms in woodpeckers. *Eye* 2007;21:83-89.

79. Cirovic S, Bhola RM, Hose DR, et al: A computational study of the passive mechanisms of eye restraint during head impact trauma. *Comput Methods Biomech Biomed Engin* 2005;8:1-6.

80. Cirovic S, Bhola RM, Hose DR, et al: Mechanistic hypothesis for eye injury in infant shaking: an experimental and computational study. *Forensic Sci Med Pathol* 2005;1:53-59.

81. Bhola RM, Cirovic S, Parson MA, et al: Modeling of the eye and orbit to simulate shaken baby syndrome. *Invest Ophthalmol Vis Sci* 2005;46:E-Abstract 4090.

82. Rangarajan N, Kamalakkannan SB, Hasija H, et al: Finite element model of ocular injury in abusive head trauma. *J AAPOS* 2009;13:364-369.

83. Levin AV: Fatal pediatric head injuries caused by short-distance falls. *Am J Forensic Med Pathol* 2001;22:417-419.

84. Gilles EE, McGregor ML, Levy-Clarke G: Retinal hemorrhage asymmetry in inflicted head injury: a clue to pathogenesis? *J Pediatr* 2003;143:494-499.

85. Morad Y, Kim YM, Mian M, et al: Nonophthalmologist accuracy in diagnosing retinal hemorrhages in the shaken baby syndrome. *J Pediatr* 2003;142:431-434.

86. Erraguntla V, Mackeen LD, Atenafu E, et al: Assessment of change of optic nerve head cupping in pediatric glaucoma using the RetCam 120. *J AAPOS* 2006;10:528-533.

87. Lantz PE, Adams GG: Postmortem monocular indirect ophthalmoscopy. *J Forens Sci* 2005;50:1450-1452.

88. Amberg R, Pollak S: Postmortem endoscopy of the ocular fundus. A valuable tool in forensic postmortem practice. *Forensic Sci Int* 2001;124:157-162.

89. Davis NL, Wetli CV, Shakin JL: The retina in forensic medicine: applications of ophthalmic endoscopy: the first 100 cases. *Am J Forensic Med Pathol* 2006;27:1-10.

90. Tsujinaka M, Bunai Y: Postmortem ophthalmologic examination by endoscopy. *Am J Forensic Med Pathol* 2006;27:287-291.

91. Marshall DH, Brownstein S, Dorey MW, et al: The spectrum of postmortem ocular findings in victims of shaken baby syndrome. *Can J Ophthalmol* 2001;36:377-384.

92. Emerson MV, Jakobs E, Green WR: Ocular autopsy and histopathologic features of child abuse. *Ophthalmology* 2007;114:1384-1394.

93. Elner SJ, Elner VM, Albert DM, et al: The medicolegal implications of detecting hemosiderin in the eyes of children who are suspected of being abused-Reply. *Arch Ophthalmol* 1991;109:322.

94. Gilliland MG, Folberg R, Hayreh SS: Age of retinal hemorrhages by iron detection: an animal model. *Am J Forensic Med Pathol* 2005;26:1-4.

95. Gilliland MG, Levin AV, Enzenauer RW, et al: Guidelines for postmortem protocol for ocular investigation of sudden unexplained infant death and suspected physical child abuse. *Am J Forensic Med Pathol* 2007;28:323-329.

96. Elner SG, Elner VM, Arnall M, et al: Ocular and associated systemic findings in suspected child abuse. A necropsy study. *Arch Ophthalmol* 1990;108:1094-1101.

97. Levin AV: Discussion: the spectrum of postmortem ocular findings in victims of shaken baby syndrome. *Can J Ophthalmol* 2001;36:383-384.

98. Lin K, Glasgow B: Bilateral periopticointrascleral hemorrhages associated with traumatic child abuse. *Am J Ophthalmol* 1999;127:473-475.

99. May K, Parsons MA, Doran R: Hemorrhagic retinopathy of shaking injury: clinical and pathological aspects. *In:* Minns RA, Brown JK (eds): *Shaking and Other Non-accidental Head Injuries in Children.* MacKeith Press, London, 2006, pp 185-207.

100. Gilliland MG, Folberg R: Retinal hemorrhages: replicating the clinician's view of the eye. *Forensic Sci Int* 1992;56:77-80.

101. Nolte KB: Transillumination enhances photographs of retinal hemorrhages. *J Forensic Sci* 1997;42:935-936.

45

NEUROPATHOLOGY OF ABUSIVE HEAD TRAUMA

Lucy B. Rorke-Adams, MD

INTRODUCTION

Injuries from abusive head trauma (AHT) most frequently occur in infants less than 2 years of age.[1-3] Infants beyond 1 month to 2 years of age are most vulnerable. In general, younger infants tend to be injured by shaking and/or blunt trauma.[4] Lethal shaking of a child older than 3 years of age is more difficult, since neck muscles and spinal ligaments are better developed by that time, and the child can more effectively resist the attack. In neonates, when abuse is suspected, intracranial and spinal injuries caused by birth must be distinguished from inflicted trauma.[5-8]

Clinicians and pathologists faced with decisions about whether abuse has occurred have an awesome task, since an affirmative decision has serious legal implications and a profound effect on the future of the putative perpetrator. It is incumbent upon the professionals charged with making the judgment to use all available investigative, clinical, and pathological findings before arriving at a decision.

The pathologist must be privy to all available information regarding circumstances leading to injury, hospitalization, clinical course, and diagnostic studies. Even though there is suspicion that the death was unnatural, he or she should approach the case with objectivity. Pathologists are "friends of the court," in that their primary responsibility is to thoroughly establish the postmortem findings and relate them to the investigative and clinical facts.

Judkins et al[9] published a detailed protocol for examining the central nervous system (CNS) in unexpected child death cases. The forensic pathologist will examine and document all external and internal injuries, separating those findings consequent to treatment.

NEUROPATHOLOGICAL FINDINGS

CNS lesions resulting from accidental and inflicted trauma are basically similar; a decision regarding in which category they belong rests upon the historical and clinical aspects of the case and pattern of lesions. When there is an uncontested history of a serious accident, the decision is generally noncontroversial. In contrast, if events leading to a sudden, life-threatening collapse of an apparently well infant/child are vague or inconsistent with the severity of the injury, a decision regarding accidental versus nonaccidental trauma is a greater challenge. Examination and documentation of findings by the neuropathologist should include a thorough external and internal examination of the face, head, and neck, including soft tissues, bone, meninges, brain, spinal cord and nerves, and eyes.

External Examination

Lethal CNS injury can occur in the absence of recognizable external soft tissue damage,[10] as in infants whose death is ascribed to shaking alone. (This issue of the significance of shaking and impact in AHT is discussed in Chapter 41, "The Case for Shaking," and Chapter 43, "Neck and Spinal Cord Injuries in Child Abuse.")

Soft tissue bruises, contusions, and/or lacerations involving face, eyes, ears, head, back, or indeed any other part of the body in infants who are not yet crawling or walking should arouse suspicion of inflicted trauma. Such injury can occur from burns (e.g., hot water, cigarettes), bites, or patterned lesions produced by objects. Establishing the age of the soft tissue injury is a difficult issue, details of which can be found elsewhere.[11,12]

Internal Soft Tissue Injury

Internal soft tissue injury can be present even when no external injury is apparent. Most commonly, this consists of hemorrhages in the deep layers of the scalp, galea, and periosteum (Figure 45-1). Hemorrhages in temporalis muscles, cervical musculature, or back musculature can be found consequent to blunt trauma; lacerations are characteristic if a sharp object has been used. Periosteal hemorrhage can be present with or without an associated fracture.

Fractures

The majority of skull fractures in children result from accidental falls, are not usually associated with significant clinical symptoms, and do not require treatment.[13] More complex skull fractures occur in serious accidental or inflicted trauma. In the latter instance, they occur when the victim's head is either struck forcefully by a hard object or is itself struck against the hard object. In infants, striking of the head onto an object is a more common mechanism. Fracture frequency varies from 25% to 40% in victims of inflicted trauma.[14-16] A study by Coats and Margulies[17] of the material properties of human infant skull and sutures determined that the infant skull can undergo dramatic shape changes before fracture, hence allowing for substantial deformation of the brain.

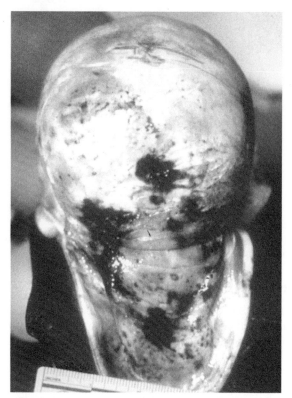

FIGURE 45-1 Galeal and periosteal hemorrhages on paramedian and left parietooccipital skull of a 3-month-old abused infant.

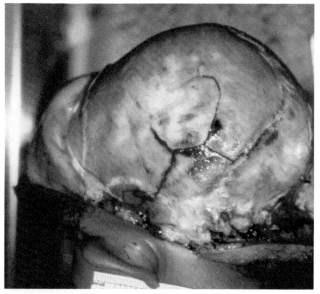

FIGURE 45-2 Left complex parietooccipital fractures in a 4-month-old infant whose head was struck against a bathroom vanity.

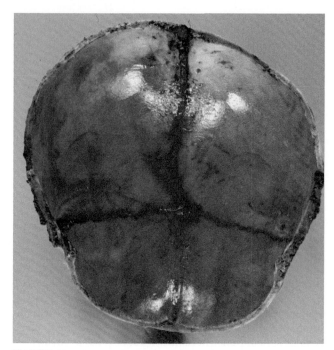

FIGURE 45-3 Inner surface of cranial cap of a 7-month-old abused infant showing sutural diastasis resulting from severe brain swelling and increased intracranial pressure.

Fractures are most commonly located in the parietooccipital bones but can be anywhere. When they extend into the base of the skull, it can be concluded that the force exerted was considerable. The entire thickness of the skull is ordinarily affected, but unless the dura is stripped, a fracture can be missed (Figure 45-2). Sutural diastasis results from massive brain swelling and rarely from blunt trauma, and should be distinguished from fractures (Figure 45-3).

Spinal fractures are rare, even when significant whiplash injury has occurred; however, if present, they are most easily identified by radiological study.[18] In severe shaking there is subluxation rather than fracture of vertebrae, a phenomenon that cannot be identified postmortem.

Intracranial Hemorrhage

The most common pathological finding in infants and children who have sustained inflicted neurotrauma is hemorrhage. It is found in one or more of the spaces or potential spaces surrounding brain and spinal cord or within parenchyma, although these are less frequent. In the majority of cases, the hemorrhages are not in and of themselves life threatening, but rather serve as markers that trauma has occurred. At the same time, the pathogenesis of intracranial hemorrhage might be unrelated to trauma, since it can result from coagulopathies, leukemia, certain metabolic disorders, or even ruptured vascular malformations.[19-24] Under these circumstances, the hemorrhages are most often parenchymal or in an unusual extraparenchymal location.

Epidural Hemorrhage (EDH)

If present, EDH is most commonly found in the posterior fossa in association with fracture of the occipital bone, and around the rostral cervical cord and foramen magnum when the victim has been shaken vigorously or subjected to blunt trauma. Blunt trauma to more caudal levels of the back can also lead to EDH. In addition, spinal EDH is often seen in premature newborns who have cardiopulmonary insufficiency, resulting from back pressure in the venous system. These must not be confused with inflicted injury.

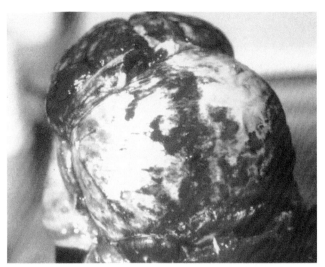

FIGURE 45-4 The brain partially covered by dura (posterior seven eighths of brain) of a 3-month-old abused infant. Note epidural hemorrhage overlying sagittal sinus and spreading laterally posteriorly. Note tension of dura beneath which is a severely swollen brain. This is protruding above the surface of the cut border of the dura anteriorly. The dura on the right has a bluish cast—a characteristic color when there is underlying blood. Note the small amount of subdural blood at anterior dural edge on the left.

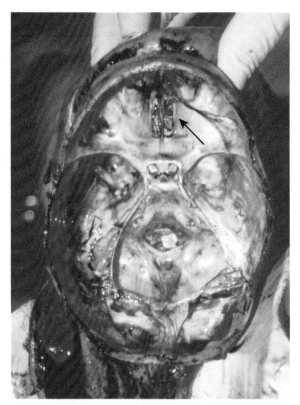

FIGURE 45-6 Skull base of same infant pictured in Figures 45-2 and 45-5. Note pooling of subdural blood along left side of the anterior and middle fossae. Note also acute hemorrhages in olfactory grooves bilaterally *(arrow)*.

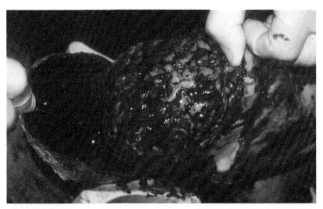

FIGURE 45-5 The brain of the 4-month-old infant with the fractures pictured in Figure 46-2. Note extensive subdural blood pooled in the cranial cap that has been reflected (and patchy subdural blood over the vertex of the brain bilaterally), subarachnoid hemorrhage, and severe brain swelling.

EDH in the supratentorial cavity is most often seen along the sagittal sinus and is usually associated with subdural hemorrhage (Figure 45-4). Elsewhere, it is typically, but not always, associated with temporal bone fracture, a rarity in infants and children.[25] If this occurs, however, it can be concluded that the amount of force applied to the head was extraordinarily strong, since without it, the dura, which is the functional periosteum of the inner table of the skull, would not separate from the bone.

Subdural Hemorrhage (SDH)

The characteristic CNS lesion in victims of AHT is SDH.[14,26-28] This hemorrhage can be unilateral or bilateral, is often paramedian, and most abundant in the posterior interhemispheric fissure (Figure 45-5). Blood can also pool

along the roof of the orbits or floor of the middle fossa (Figure 45-6). The volume of subdural blood generally is not sufficient to require surgical drainage, although in rare cases, it can be a large space-occupying lesion, and if not evacuated promptly, leads to death from increased intracranial pressure. When consequent to a tear of the vein of Galen, the bulk of the blood is located in the region of the quadrigeminal plate/pineal gland, and can extend into the posterior fossa as well.

Subdural blood often surrounds the spinal cord in traumatized individuals, and the issue of its origin can be problematic. If SDH is identified in the supratentorial space, some have assumed that the blood can be transported by gravity to the caudal levels. This assumption is untenable, since it is not possible for the blood to gain access to the posterior fossa or spinal subdural space; the tentorium, brainstem, and cerebellum block exit from the supratentorial space. Instead, subdural blood, which typically originates at the vertex of the brain, can only fall by gravity to the skull base in the anterior and middle fossa, where it is often seen (see Figure 45-6). Still, subdural blood originating in the posterior fossa has easy access to the spinal subdural space if the foramen magnum is not blocked by a swollen brainstem and herniated cerebellar tonsils. Hence, if blood is found around the cord, origin is either local (i.e., from primary trauma to the back) or from trauma affecting the posterior fossa structures (Figure 45-7).

It is the majority opinion among experts involved in diagnosis and treatment of individuals with CNS trauma that SDHs result from tearing of bridging veins that normally

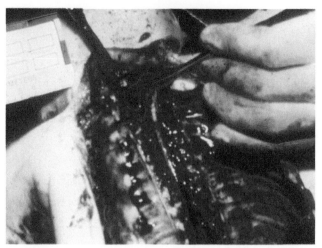

FIGURE 45-7 Posterior view of spinal region of a 7-week-old abused infant showing acute, extensive epidural/subdural hemorrhages.

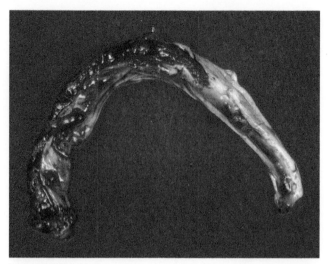

FIGURE 45-9 Falx cerebri of a 3-day-old infant who died consequent to complication of a diaphragmatic hernia. This was an incidental finding.

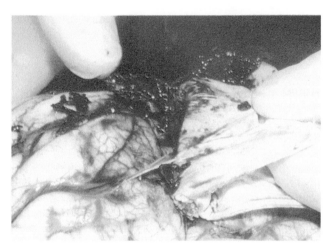

FIGURE 45-8 Vertex of left hemisphere of a severely battered 3-year-old child. The dura has been retracted to show an intact bridging vein entering the sagittal sinus. Subdural clots are located more anteriorly and are located at the vertex of the hemisphere and in the interhemispheric fissure.

leave the subarachnoid space to enter the sinuses (Figure 45-8).[29] Although all bridging veins are vulnerable to tearing, those most commonly affected are located at the vertex of the brain that enter the sagittal sinus. In severe trauma, the sinus itself can be torn.

The leaves of the falx cerebri, which are formed by two apposed sheets of dura, can contain hemorrhage of variable size; the dura, which itself consists of two layers, typically contains hemorrhage within its substance in trauma-induced SDH. Intrafalcine and tentorial hemorrhages are not uncommon in newborns or neonates and are associated with the birth process (Figure 45-9).[7] Some claim that blood in the subdural space originates within the dura or falx and then leaks into the space, a major cause of such hemorrhage being hypoxia, but this novel suggestion by Geddes et al[30] was withdrawn 4 years following publication,[31] and the literature contains no scientific support from other investigators for this hypothesis.

It has also been asserted that a subdural space does not exist.[32] If such were the case, there could be no entity called "subdural hematoma," and the pathologist would always be forced to remove a brain encased in dura. Moreover, if the dura were attached to the arachnoid, that membrane would be torn in the process of separating the dura and brain. This simply never occurs unless earlier inflammation has led to formation of adhesions binding the two.

The anatomical and biomechanical factors that underlie the pathogenesis of subdural hematomas are outlined as follows: (1) the dura is firmly attached to the inner table of the skull, since it is the functional periosteum of the bones, and hence does not move, (2) in certain regions of the skull, two separate leaves of dura come together to form sinuses, of which the most important in this context is the superior sagittal sinus, (3) in order for the cerebral veins to drain into the sinuses, they must leave the protection of the leptomeninges and traverse the space between the arachnoid and the sinus, which is the subdural space, (4) under the normal activities of daily living there is no problem. However, if a force is exerted on the head and the brain is free to move, but the dura containing the sinuses is fixed, then movement of brain places stress on the veins and causes them to tear. The torn veins are sometimes identified during surgery; Maxeiner[33] has outlined a technique that allows postmortem identification.[33,34]

Since subdural blood is most often of venous origin, it is dark red-purple in the fresh state, and the hematoma is often described as a "currant jelly clot." Arterial tears also occur but are uncommon.[33] For an in-depth discussion of the biomechanics of shaking and pathogenesis of subdural bleeding, see Morrison and Minns.[35]

If left undisturbed and the individual survives, the blood is encapsulated by formation of a two-layered membrane. The outer membrane is composed of fibrous granulation tissue and is adjacent to the dura, whereas the denser fibrous tissues comprising the inner membrane is adjacent to, but separate from, the arachnoid. Vasculature in the outer membrane can bleed, but the volume of such hemorrhaging is not often clinically important, even though this mecha-

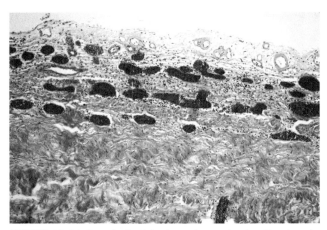

FIGURE 45-10 Organized subdural membrane showing fibrosis and striking neovascularization. The infant was abused at 5 weeks of age and died of pneumonia 11 months later (H&E stain ×100).

nism is all-too-often invoked to explain sudden collapse of an otherwise apparently normal infant (Figure 45-10). In particular, defense experts postulate that infants sustain a primary subdural bleed days or weeks before they present with life-threatening symptoms. The experts claim that the acute event is consequent to a re-bleed from an organized hematoma. Such an argument is unsound because the primary hematoma would have to be quite large in order to produce a membrane with sufficiently abundant vascularity to cause to a re-bleed of large enough volume to result in clinical symptoms. It is unlikely that such a large original hematoma would remain clinically silent and that a secondary bleed would result in catastrophic collapse and/or death. Furthermore, a re-bleed would occur over a period of time, during which symptoms of CNS dysfunction would become apparent. Medical attention would most likely be sought before the complications of increased intracranial pressure became irreversible.

Finally, postmortem examination would reveal the offending membrane and re-bleed, along with evidence of mass effect, unilateral cerebral compression, and the attendant herniation that are the pathological hallmarks of such an event. In reality, such findings are rare in infants with putative AHT.

At the same time, an isolated postmortem finding of a thin subdural membrane or hemosiderin in the dura or leptomeninges should not necessarily excite suspicion of inflicted trauma. Small subdural, intradural, intrafalcine/tentorial, and subarachnoid hemorrhages are common postmortem findings in infants who die of a variety of non-CNS disorders, are most likely associated with the birth process, and are of no clinical significance.[6-8]

Subarachnoid Hemorrhage (SAH)

SAH of various sizes (usually small) and distribution frequently accompany SDH and are the result of bleeding from small arteries in the subarachnoid space; they can be distinguished from subdural blood of venous origin by their bright red color.[26] Because of their small size, they might not be visualized on radiological studies (see Figure 45-5).

SAH of nontraumatic origin can result from venous thromboses, coagulopathies of various types, vasculitides of inflammatory or obscure origin, or rupture of a vascular malformation or aneurysm (giant or mycotic). SAH unaccompanied by SDH or other features suggestive of trauma is most likely a consequence of natural disease.[19-24]

Parenchymal/Intraventricular Hemorrhage

Parenchymal hemorrhages of traumatic origin are typically small and most commonly associated with gliding contusions, callosal tears, and primary brainstem trauma. If isolated or large, their origin is more likely caused by a coagulopathy, venous thrombosis, or rupture of a vascular malformation. Parenchymal hemorrhage arising either in the CNS or elsewhere in the body while the infant/child is under medical surveillance should alert the clinician to the possibility that a natural disease rather than trauma is the likely cause.

If blood is found in the occipital horns and there is no obvious source of hemorrhage in the cerebrum, the possibility that it originated from a vertebral artery tear must be seriously considered and investigated. Under these circumstances, a small amount of blood is usually present around the caudal brainstem and adjacent cervical spinal cord. The blood in these regions and the occipital horn represents anterograde flow from the primary site of injury.

Cerebrospinal Contusions/Lacerations

By definition, contusions/lacerations (C/L) are caused by trauma. Theoretically they can occur at any superficial and/or deep site and can be isolated or numerous. In reality, the majority exhibit a well-recognized distribution pattern that often allows the pathologist to reconstruct the likely events that produced the injury. When superficial, they are easily identifiable, since they typically contain hemorrhages. They extend into underlying cortex and sometimes white matter for a variable distance.

There are three major categories of C/Ls: coup, contrécoup, and intermediate coup. The first two types are generally located superficially, whereas the latter can only be diagnosed after the tissue has been sectioned. Intermediate coup injury is not always accompanied by significant hemorrhage, and microscopic study might be necessary to recognize it. C/Ls occur at the time of the primary trauma.

Localization of the lesions is dependent upon biomechanical factors. Specifically, if the moving head strikes a hard object such as in a simple fall in which the back of the head hits the ground, the coup lesion (involving neural tissue immediately below the impact site of the skull, specifically occipital lobes) will be minimal or absent, whereas the portion of brain in a line opposite the impact site will exhibit contrécoup injury, namely of the orbital surfaces of frontal lobes and temporal poles. On the other hand, if a moving object strikes the stationary head, the coup lesion in the brain below the impact site will be more severe than the contrécoup injury 180 degrees opposite to the primary blow. There may or may not be a fracture in either instance. Intermediate coup lesions can arise consequent to either angular or linear acceleration.

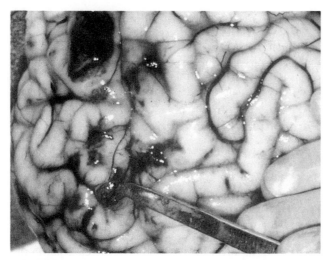

FIGURE 45-11 Acute contusions/lacerations and subarachnoid hemorrhage involving cerebral gyri of 1-month-old abused infant.

Superficial Contusions/Lacerations

Superficial C/Ls in infants/children with AHT most commonly involve the olfactory bulbs and tracts and are typically produced by shaking or other forces producing angular acceleration. If, on the other hand, the head has been subjected to blunt trauma, either by being hit by some object or by being struck against a hard surface, the location of the C/Ls will be related to the specific features of the injury. Repetitive trauma can cause C/Ls of different ages.

Recognition of these lesions is straightforward, since acute lesions are hemorrhagic and display disruption of surface tissue that may or may not be swollen, depending upon survival time after injury (Figure 45-11). In the subacute stage, swelling recedes as there is retraction of tissue and the color of the lesion changes while hemoglobin breaks down into hemosiderin, which is a brownish green-gold (Figures 45-12 and 45-13). Long-standing lesions are typically retracted and more golden than brown, reflecting further transformation into hematoidin.

Deep Contusions/Lacerations

Included in this group are intermediate coup lesions. These are often localized to the temporal and insular cortex in individuals who have sustained trauma to lateral regions of the skull, and tend to occur in pedestrians or bicyclists struck by vehicles or those thrown from vehicles; they are rarely seen in infants or children with AHT. In contrast, the most common deep lesions found after abusive infant head trauma are consequent to shearing forces produced by angular acceleration, and tend to occur in particular sites, such as cerebral white matter, corpus callosum, internal capsule and other fiber tracts at various levels, and in the rostral pons at the level of the locus ceruleus; they are infrequently found in cerebellar white matter. In especially violent trauma the ependyma can tear, allowing fragments of brain tissue to enter the ventricle. These are identifiable on microscopic study, especially in the aqueduct where they become stuck. The majority of the deep C/Ls in infants and children fall into two groups: gliding contusions and axonal injury.

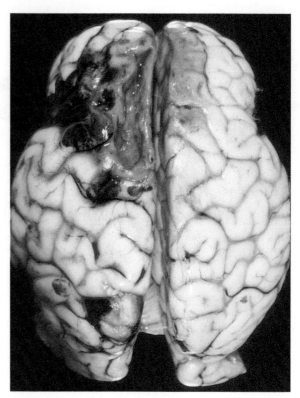

FIGURE 45-12 Vertex view of cerebral hemispheres of an 8-week-old infant who was subjected to repeated blunt trauma to the head. Note organized contusions/lacerations bilaterally (left greater than right) and more recent hemorrhages.

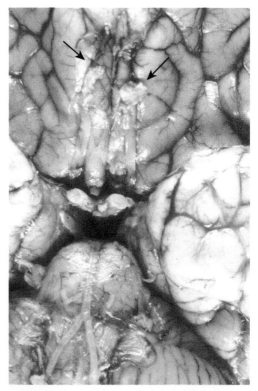

FIGURE 45-13 Base of brain of an 18-month-old infant showing organization of contusions/lacerations of olfactory bulbs (arrows).

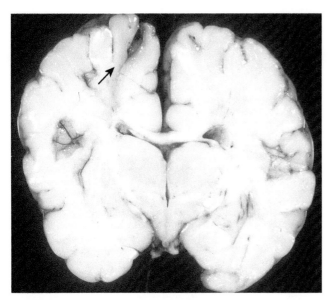

FIGURE 45-14 Coronal section through mid-cerebrum of a 1-year-old female showing gliding contusion on left. This is extending from the surface of the superior frontal convolution into the white matter. Note small residual hemorrhage.

Gliding Contusions/Lacerations. In contrast to those in superficial sites, deep C/Ls are not ordinarily associated with a significant amount of hemorrhage. Gliding contusions consist of dorsoventral slits in paramedian cerebral white matter and are most often found in the frontal lobes, but they can occur at any level if traumatic forces are unusually severe (Figures 45-14 and 45-15). Lesions of this type were described by Lindenberg and Freytag,[36] who suggested that they resulted from shearing forces acting upon the gelatinous, unmyelinated white matter of the infant. White matter of the developing brain, which is unmyelinated for the most part, has a much higher concentration of water than exists in the fully mature brain, and hence is more vulnerable to tears.

Lesions in the same locations are common in older children and adults who sustain closed head injury in bicycle, motorcycle, vehicular, or pedestrian trauma. These lesions have more prominent hemorrhages than those seen in the infant, and frank cavitation of tissue occurs only in exceptional circumstances. Microscopic findings are a function of the age of the injury. In the early stage, the tissue cleft contains some red blood cells along the margin and a few inflammatory cells (see Figure 45-15). After 24 hours, inflammatory cells are more abundant, gitter cells with and without hemosiderin become an important component of the inflammatory reaction, and astrocytic proliferation at the margins becomes apparent. In the chronic stage, a sharply demarcated cavity marks the site of injury (Figure 45-16).

Other white matter lesions, aside from axonal injury (see below) consist of edema associated with acute swelling of oligodendroglia, the nuclei of which are sometimes pyknotic and/or karyorrhectic (Figure 45-17).

Focal and general neuroinflammatory response consequent to diffuse traumatic brain injury includes activation of resident microglia and macrophages recruited from peripheral circulation and can be evaluated by use of immunohistochemical procedures for expression of CD163 or CD68.[37]

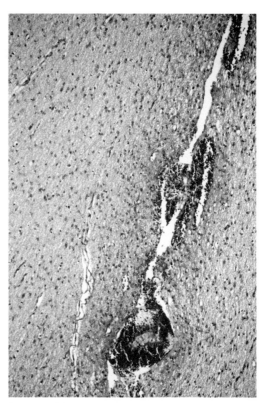

FIGURE 45-15 Photomicrograph of gliding contusion in frontal lobe of a 1-month-old infant. Note split in the tissue and presence of hemorrhage (H&E stain ×100).

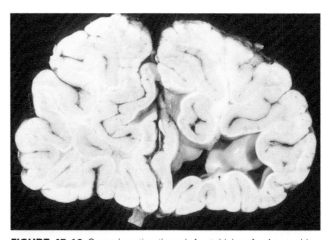

FIGURE 45-16 Coronal section through frontal lobe of a 4-year-old child who was abused at 4 months of age. Note the large, sharply demarcated cavity on the right side. This has replaced most of the white matter on that side.

The more elegant techniques, such as confocal or electron microscopy at the disposal of laboratory investigators, are not feasible in the majority of young victims of AHT because of varying degrees of autolysis consequent to respirator therapy.

Of all CNS fiber tracts, the corpus callosum is the most frequent target of injury, although identification of the lesions is often difficult if the victim has been on life support for more than 24 hours. The lesions are characterized by

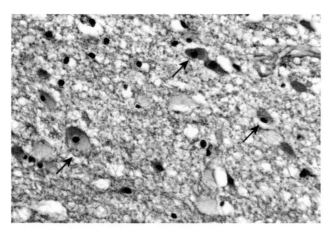

FIGURE 45-17 Acutely swollen oligodendroglia in edematous, damaged white matter *(arrows)* (H&E stain ×100).

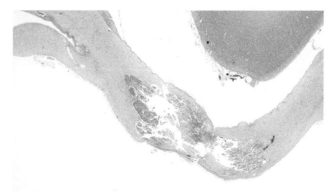

FIGURE 45-19 Photomicrograph of the corpus callosum of an 8-week-old infant who arrived at the hospital dead on arrival. Note tissue fractures and hemorrhage in center of corpus callosum. The cingulate gyrus is just dorsal to the callosum (H&E stain ×10).

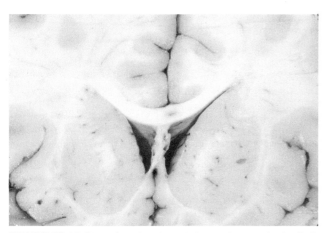

FIGURE 45-18 Coronal section through the cerebrum at the level of the corpus striatum. Note small hemorrhage in corpus callosum just to the right of midline.

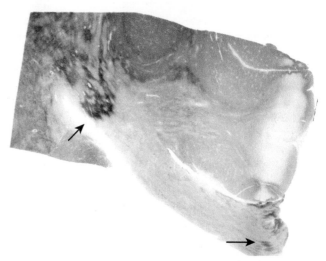

FIGURE 45-20 Hemisection of corpus callosum and cingulate gyrus just above lateral ventricle and caudate nucleus of a 9-month-old infant. Note the dark brown irregular expression of β-amyloid precursor protein (β-APP) at lateral edge of callosal fibers at their junction with the centrum ovale *(arrows)* and torn central fibers of callosum (immunoperoxidase technique for expression of β-APP ×10).

tears and petechial or larger hemorrhage, most commonly in the posterior third of the body and splenium. It is good practice to gently separate the hemispheres while the brain is *in situ* to determine gross evidence of such injury. If autolysis is advanced, identification might be impossible.

Recognition of callosal injury is easier on examination of coronal sections, and varies from total to partial transection with or without injury of the adjacent cingulate gyrus. If partial, it is always localized to the dorsally placed fibers (Figures 45-18 and 45-19). Premortem damage is usually accompanied by hemorrhages along the torn edges. On the other hand, linear, horizontally, or irregularly oriented hemorrhages are sometimes seen unassociated with a gross tear. Occasionally, callosal damage becomes apparent only on microscopic study and can be localized anywhere along the callosum or at its junction with the centrum ovale (Figure 45-20).

A focal contusional-type lesion localized to the ventrolateral brainstem in infants and children whose head has been subjected to violent angular acceleration, consequent to either repeated blunt trauma or shaking, consists of complete, or more often, incomplete subpial necrosis. This is characterized by fragmentation of neuropil, a variable

number of retraction balls (see below), accumulation of lipid-laden macrophages, and acutely swollen, sometimes necrotic, oligodendroglia with or without petechial hemorrhages (Figure 45-21). It rarely occurs in subpial regions of cerebral gyri.

Axonal Injury. Axonal injury consequent to head trauma was first described by Strich[38] over 50 years ago. It results from exertion of powerful forces causing angular acceleration or impact injury; it is not necessarily lethal unless localized within brainstem structures controlling cardiorespiratory functions. At the same time, however, axonal damage in the cerebrum can have a profound effect on psychomotor function if the victim survives.

Axonal injury occurs at the time of the primary trauma, and progresses thereafter.[29] It is not solely caused by trauma but is associated with vascular and metabolic events.[38-44] In the infant, nontraumatic axonal injury is most commonly seen in white matter necrosis as a result of perfusion injury, primarily in prematurely born neonates, a disorder known as *periventricular leukomalacia.*[45] Such lesions have characteristic

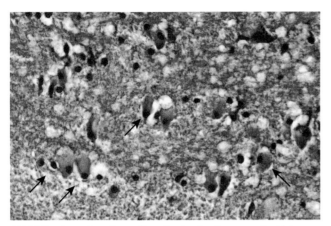

FIGURE 45-21 Acutely swollen oligodendroglia, some of which are pyknotic, in subpial ventral pontine tissue (*arrows*) (H&E stain ×100).

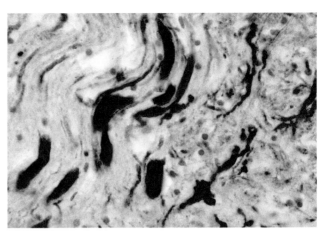

FIGURE 45-23 Swollen, damaged axons in midbrain of a 4-month-old abused infant (immunoperoxidase technique for expression of *Beta* APP ×600).

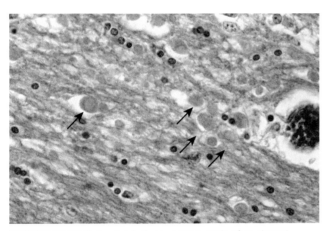

FIGURE 45-22 Retraction balls in centrum ovale of an abused 4-month-old infant (arrows) (H&E stain ×100).

clinical and pathological features that are not likely to be confused with trauma.

When consequent to abusive head injury, axonal damage is most commonly found in corpus callosum and fiber tracts in cerebrum, brainstem, and spinal cord, as well as in cranial and spinal nerve roots. If there is vascular damage, associated hemorrhage is present. Axonal injury in the upper outer quadrant of the pons at the level of the locus ceruleus is typically associated with hemorrhage and parenchymal damage and hence can often be diagnosed on gross examination.

Although it has been noted that axonal injury is almost universal in individuals who die following head injury, it is difficult to diagnose unless survival has been greater than 2 hours, although it may be presumed if there is hemorrhage.[40] In those who survive 18 to 24 hours, the routine H&E-stained sections contain small, eosinophilic, round structures called *retraction balls* (Figure 45-22). It is often possible to recognize axonal swelling, but a more precise assessment of axonal injury can be made if a silver staining technique, such

as Bodian's, is used.[46] Currently it is preferable to use immunohistochemical techniques to look for expression of β-amyloid precursor protein (β-APP); antibodies for neurofilament protein expression in axons can also be used (Figures 45-20 and 45-23).[47,48]

When axonal damage results from ischemia or metabolic disturbances, it can be difficult to distinguish from that induced by trauma, especially if located in cerebral or cerebellar white matter.[43,44] If other features of frank infarction are present, it is not generally problematic, or if it is located in fiber tracts (i.e., corpus callosum, internal capsule, descending tracts in brainstem, spinal cord white matter, or nerve roots) as isolated ischemic necrosis in these regions, it is rare. Tissue autolysis that occurs after cerebral circulation has ceased but the individual is maintained on life support ("respirator brain") does not cause axonal injury. As noted, use of the antibody CD163 for identification of macrophages is helpful in evaluating the parenchymal lesions in all categories.

Brainstem and Spinal Injuries

While there are many ways of inflicting injury to an infant, among the more common is shaking and impact. Shaking usually precedes the impact, which typically involves striking the head against a hard object. On the other hand, postmortem study of some infants reveals no evidence of blunt trauma to scalp or skull, and although it is conceivable that the head was impacted against a soft surface (e.g., mattress or cushions), the possibility that only shaking was involved is likely.[35] Some perpetrators describe what they did (e.g., only "shook the infant"),[49] and it is entirely possible to produce serious injury by shaking alone, the mechanism being that of a whiplash phenomenon.[26,27,50,51]

Every parent knows that the heavy head of the infant must be supported until structures in the neck are sufficiently developed to allow independent head control, usually by about 8 to 12 months of age when the baby is at least able to sit without support.[52] The upper two cervical vertebrae of the infant are particularly mobile because spinal ligaments are not well developed, hence the cervical spinal cord is

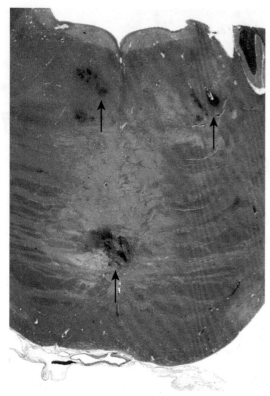

FIGURE 45-24 Section of rostral pons showing multifocal primary hemorrhagic contusions in the tegmentum and basis pontis of a 3-year-old girl subjected to multiple blows to the head *(arrows)* (H&E stain ×5).

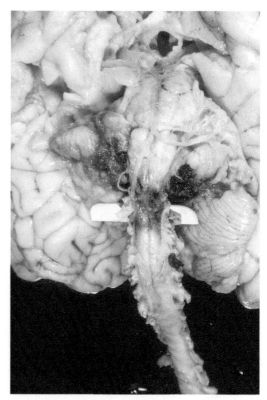

FIGURE 45-25 Primary hemorrhagic contusions/lacerations of cervicomedullary junction of an abused infant.

especially vulnerable to damage if the neck is hyperextended. Such injuries to the cervical cord have, in fact, been documented in complicated deliveries.[53]

In traumatic whiplash—whether accidental or inflicted—brainstem, rostral spinal cord, nerve roots, vertebral arteries, and soft tissues are all potential targets for injury. Fractures are uncommon, since the bony involvement is typically subluxation; soft tissue damage is not often conspicuous. Occasionally the caretaker of an infant in whom there is an allegation of abuse will report that the infant developed breathing difficulty and became limp following shaking. Even without such an admission, it is obvious that this combination of symptoms is characteristic of spinal shock.[54]

Because the whiplash injury typically involves caudal brainstem and rostral cord, it is absolutely necessary to follow the dissection procedure described by Judkins et al.[9] If this is not done, the lesion(s) can be missed. The lesions are typically hemorrhagic and can be found in many different sites, including brainstem, vertebral arteries, meninges, nerve roots and ganglia, and spinal cord (Figures 45-24 and 45-25). Hemorrhages can be epidural, intradural, subdural, or subarachnoid. Axonal damage involving roots and spinal cord is most easily identified when studied for expression of ß-APP. Spinal cord C/Ls typically include partial parenchymal tears or complete transaction (Figures 45-25, 45-26, 45-27, and 45-28). Lesions consisting primarily of acute neuronal necrosis or frank infarction are more likely as a result of cardiorespiratory failure and shock than direct trauma.

It should be understood that any level of spinal cord and/or surrounding structures can be traumatized by mecha-

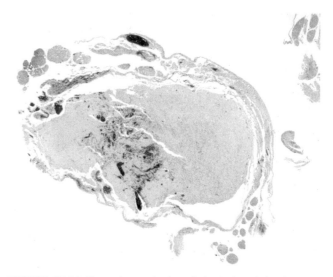

FIGURE 45-26 Photomicrograph of cervical spinal cord showing hemorrhagic contusions/lacerations (H&E stain ×5).

nisms other than whiplash, such as slamming or hitting the victim's back against a hard object, or forceful beating. In rare instances, forceful blows to the top of the head will produce C/L of the central tissue of the spinal cord.

Traumatic Brain Injury/Edema/Swelling

Primary damage to nerve cells and blood vessels occurs consequent to mechanical forces of sufficient magnitude,

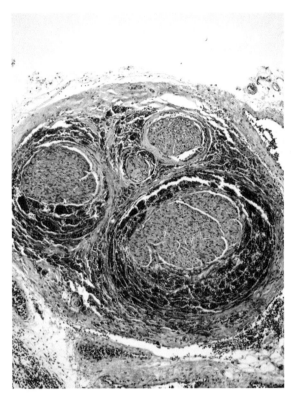

FIGURE 45-27 Photomicrograph of cervical spinal nerve roots surrounded by abundant subdural and intradural hemorrhage from a 1-month-old abused infant (H&E stain ×40).

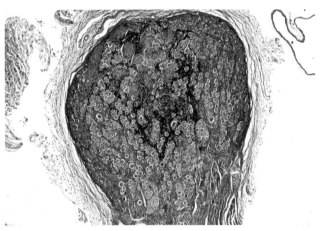

FIGURE 45-28 Acute hemorrhage in dorsal root ganglion in an abused 3-month-old infant (H&E stain ×40).

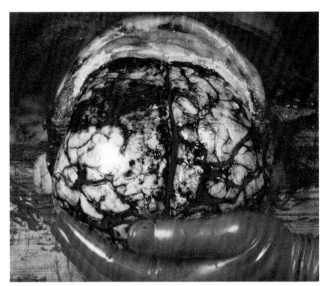

FIGURE 45-29 Cerebrum *(in situ)* of an abused 3-year-old showing severe brain swelling characterized by gyral widening and flattening and sulcal attenuation. Note severe superficial congestion and subarachnoid hemorrhage.

and then as a result of complicated cascades of membranous and biochemical events. Breakdown of cell membranes, endothelial injury, and disturbance of blood–brain barrier all contribute to general brain dysfunction aside from the more obvious C/Ls and axonal injury, and most likely play a major role in pathogenesis of edema and swelling.[29] Edema and swelling of the brain are commonly present if the infant survives for several hours after injury.[55-58] Details of the complex, multifactorial pathogenesis are presented in elegant detail by Blumbergs et al[29] and Minns and Brown.[59]

If the infant dies, the brain swelling is characterized by gyral widening and flattening and sulcal effacement (Figure 45-29). Uncal/parahippocampal grooves are rare in infants because the cranial sutures are still open. On the other hand, the posterior fossa of the infant is a more confined space, since its roof is the tentorium, and the only opening is the foramen magnum, which has a fixed diameter, even in an infant. The tentorial notch is, of course, filled with the brainstem. The brainstem and cerebellum are often swollen, either primarily because of primary injury (brainstem) or as a result of vascular compression. If severe, this often leads to necrosis of cerebellar tonsils, which, when the infant is maintained on a respirator, become autolytic and float into the spinal subdural and/or subarachnoid space. Durét hemorrhages do not occur in infants; hence if brainstem hemorrhages are present, the most likely pathogenesis is trauma.

The *intra vitem* autolysis that occurs after the brain tissue has already died, but the infant is maintained on a respirator hinders, but might not totally obviate, microscopic study.

Anoxic Encephalomyelopathy/ Infarction

At least 75% of abused infants and children exhibit hypoxic-ischemic lesions of brain and/or spinal cord.[58] Gross and microscopic features are generally not difficult to identify, and although pathophysiological features overlap, hypoxic lesions will be discussed separately from those that are ischemic.

Hypoxic Lesions

When the partial pressure of arterial oxygen decreases to a critical level, the phenomenon of cerebral autoregulation is set in motion.[60] Cerebral arteries dilate and capillary beds open to allow for maximal flow as a compensatory mechanism for inadequate oxygen delivery to the tissues. If severe, the cardiac muscle, which is also deprived of oxygen, begins to fail, thereby leading to ischemia. Ensuing neuronal/parenchymal necrosis precipitates brain swelling. This may

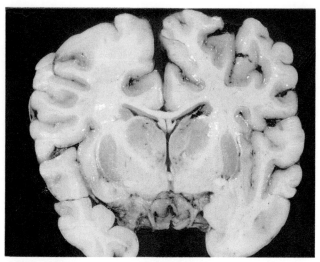

FIGURE 45-30 Coronal section through midcerebrum showing classical dark pink gray matter characteristic of acute anoxic encephalopathy.

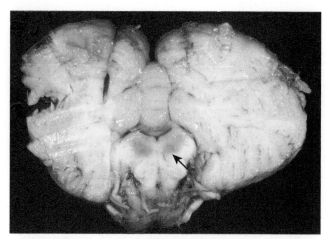

FIGURE 45-31 Transverse section of medulla and cerebellum. Note the striking dusky brown color of the medullary tegmentum *(arrow)* characteristic of hypotensive brainstem necrosis.

be accentuated by traumatic brain injury described previously and is often diagnosed by neuroimaging studies.[61-64]

Pathological features of severe asphyxia from any cause, including accidental or homicidal smothering, are often striking, since dilatation of the vascular bed consequent to autoregulation is prominent, both in subarachnoid and parenchymal vessels. Because the arterial pO_2 is decreased and the pCO_2 is elevated, the usual light pink color of grey matter is transformed into a peach or purple color, depending upon the severity of the asphyctic state, since the pCO_2 in the arteries is more similar to that normally carried by veins (Figure 45-30).

Infants who have been smothered are often regarded as victims of so-called SIDS. Hence, if the pathologist is unaware of the pathophysiology of asphyxia and color changes just described, that error is easily made. In particular, the brain of an individual of any age who dies suddenly does not display the congestion and discoloration of the asphyctic brain with the possible exception of cases of "near-miss SIDS." If the individual dies within a short time, the expected microscopic lesions associated with acute anoxia might not be recognizable.

Ischemic Lesions

Individuals who have a sudden cardiac arrest and/or shock, but who are resuscitated and survive for a variable length of time thereafter, exhibit a unique pathological picture that was described and named "hypotensive brainstem necrosis" by Gilles et al.[65] This circumstance typically causes global necrosis, but the gross pathological features of the brainstem are particularly striking. There is obvious duskiness of inferior colliculi, pontine and medullary tegmentum, and olivary and dentate nuclei produced by vascular dilatation and congestion, consequent to reflow into damaged regions (Figure 45-31). Hypotensive brainstem necrosis may occur at any age and should not be confused with primary brainstem trauma.

Infarction resulting from severe ischemia can occur anywhere in the brain and/or spinal cord, the extent being a function of the length and severity of the insult. Microscopic

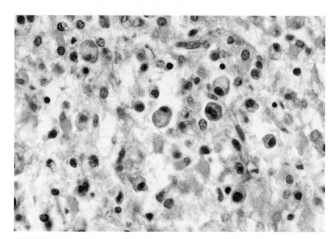

FIGURE 45-32 Photomicrograph of organizing infarction 2 weeks after the ictus in a 2-month-old abused infant (H&E stain ×200).

features of grey matter necrosis in the infant are sometimes more exaggerated than those occurring in adults if the infant survives for a week or more, since the infarcted regions often contain an extraordinary number of fat-laden macrophages (gitter cells), some of which may be multinucleated (Figure 45-32).

Chronic Lesions

All victims of inflicted neurotrauma, even those with severe injury, do not necessarily die immediately. In those who survive for months or years, the separation of traumatic injury from hypoxic-ischemic damage can be challenging (Figure 45-33). Subdural membranes are often present and are recognizable without difficulty. Although severe surface scars and deep gliding contusions are not problematic, retraction balls and damaged axons months or years after the primary event are not ordinarily identified.

Optic Nerve and Retinal Injury

Injuries to the optic nerve and retina are common in infants who are victims of inflicted neurotrauma.[4,10,66-70] At the same

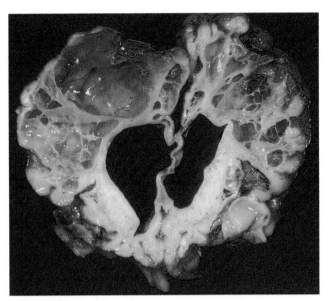

FIGURE 45-33 Coronal section through frontal lobes of infant who was abused at 2 months of age but died 10 months later. Note replacement of normal cortex and white matter by cysts and the golden color of tissue, especially on the left side.

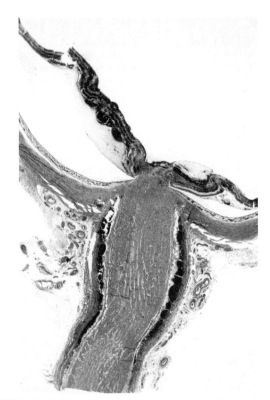

FIGURE 45-35 Photomicrograph of an optic nerve, disc, and posterior portion of retina of a 4-month-old abused infant showing extensive subdural and retinal hemorrhages that occupies all layers (H&E stain ×10).

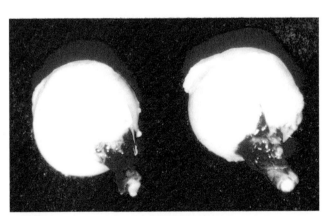

FIGURE 45-34 Globes with attached optic nerves from a 7-week-old abused infant. Note acute hemorrhages extending from the junction of the globe and nerve.

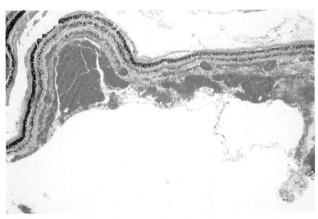

FIGURE 45-36 Photomicrograph of a retina showing extensive retinal, preretinal, and vitreous hemorrhage of a 7-week-old abused infant (H&E stain ×40).

time, pathogenesis of these lesions is a controversial issue. (See Chapter 44, "Eye Injuries in Child Abuse.")

Forensic study of an infant or child who has died of trauma, accidental or inflicted, must include examination of the eyes: globes, optic nerves, surrounding meninges, and soft tissue. The most prominent findings consist of hemorrhage in and beneath the dura surrounding the optic nerve as well as retinal hemorrhage. Optic nerve sheath hemorrhages are typically located at the junction of the nerve and globe and extend toward the brain for a variable distance. Although these are most often found within the dura and subdural space, it is not unusual to identify them in epidural soft tissues and subarachnoid spaces. The optic nerve is ordinarily not damaged directly (Figures 45-34 and 45-35).

In contrast, the retina is a common target for injury, incidence ranging from 50% to 100%, but the most frequent figure is 80%.[10,69,71] Only one or both eyes can be affected.

Retinal hemorrhages extend from the disc, often symmetrically, for a variable distance toward the ora serrata and can involve one or more, sometimes all, layers of the retina (Figure 45-36). When severe, the retina can be thrown into folds or tear, and there can also be vitreous hemorrhage. Folds and tears should be investigated during gross examination since the retina is often separated from the choroid in the process of slide preparation. If the victim survives, organization of the hemorrhages, retinal scarring, and Wallerian degeneration ensue.

MEDICAL EVIDENCE RELATING TO INFLICTED NEUROTRAUMA

Abuse of infants and children has been a grim reality throughout the history of mankind, and the type of abuse has involved a wide spectrum, ranging from culturally approved sacrifices to gods, and runs the gamut of starvation, abandonment, burning, smothering, drowning, shaking, beating, and throwing from buildings, over cliffs, or against objects. Aside from physical means, including widespread sexual abuse, more subtle and difficult to define psychological trauma to children has been, and is, all too common.[72]

In 1942, John Caffey focused attention on a constellation of features that he called "whiplash-shaken baby syndrome." This included traumatic injury of the nervous system, with or without bony injuries, and retinal hemorrhages.[73,74] In the ensuing 62 years an enormous body of literature has become available documenting social, clinical, and pathological features of infants and children alleged to have been victims of abuse. A considerable proportion of this literature consists of case reports ranging from one to many examples of putative inflicted trauma and falls into the category of clinical research. This has been a time-honored method for sharing observations of medical issues with colleagues and has formed the cornerstone of medical knowledge throughout centuries. Indeed, journals devoted to human diseases affecting various organ systems have, do, and will in future publish peer-reviewed papers that fall into the category of clinical research.

In this venue, physicians worldwide have reported their experiences in dealing with clinical problems similar to those described by Caffey, such that there currently exists a mountain of evidence in support of the hypothesis that a recognizable clinical entity does indeed exist produced by severe shaking-battering of an infant. In addition, the forensic literature is replete with reports of postmortem findings of such cases, along with supporting investigative data collected by police.[75]

The current state of knowledge that has accumulated over the years may thus be summarized as follows:

1. An apparently well infant suddenly experiences difficulty breathing, loss of tone, and unconsciousness.
2. The infant is alone with the caretaker.
3. Although emergency medical personnel might succeed in resuscitation, the infant remains unresponsive, remains ventilator dependent, and often requires vasopressor agents.
4. Evidence of soft tissue trauma and/or fractures might or might not be found.
5. Radiologic studies typically identify a small subdural hematoma, usually in a posterior, paramedian location, with or without evidence of profound hypoxic-ischemic injury, the so-called black brain.
6. Unilateral or bilateral retinal hemorrhages are commonly diagnosed by an experienced ophthalmologist.
7. Postmortem examination discloses a constellation of any or all of the following: soft tissue injury, skull fracture, SDH, SAH, brain swelling, C/Ls (superficial or deep, and in various sites, ranging from brain to spinal cord), axonal injury, hypoxic-ischemic damage, and optic nerve and retinal hemorrhages.

This list does not imply that these features are found in every infant or child that is abused, but only summarizes the common findings amongst this group. Naturally each case is unique, but there is no established natural disease for which this combination of features is diagnostic, other than inflicted trauma. To make this diagnosis, it is absolutely necessary to consider *all* aspects of the case, since any one or two features could have a nonsuspicious etiology.

Into this arena has come a small group of physicians and engineers who aggressively challenge the reality of inflicted neurotrauma in infants and children, claiming that the clinical-pathological features most characteristically found in these victims of abuse are actually a consequence of hypoxia-ischemia, increased intracranial pressure, increased intravascular pressure, and excessive coughing.[30,76-78] There is no evidence-based literature to support their point of view, but this does not seem to deter them.

Even though the clinical-pathological features of inflicted neurotrauma in infants and children are firmly established, there remain questions, such as understanding the biomechanics involved in shaking and the pathogenesis of retinal hemorrhages. It is often claimed that this constellation of abnormalities might result from a short fall, but there is currently considerable evidence to the contrary.[59]

Inflicted neurotrauma is a uniquely human affliction and for this reason cannot be studied objectively in the laboratory. The current state of knowledge regarding inflicted neurotrauma is well summarized in publications edited by Minns and Brown[79] and Reece and Nicholson,[80] but it is clear to experts in the field that experimental studies that approximate more closely the human situation must be performed if we are to advance our knowledge of the mechanisms involved in this devastating social, medical, and legal problem.

References

1. Myhre MC, Grøgaard JB, Dyb GA, et al: Traumatic head injury in infants and toddlers. *Acta Paediatr* 2007;96:1159-1163.
2. Duhaime AC, Alario AJ, Lewander WJ, et al: Head injury in very young children: mechanisms, injury types, and ophthalmologic findings in 100 hospitalized patients younger than 2 years of age. *Pediatrics* 1992;90:179-185.
3. Keenan HT, Runyan DK, Marshall SW, et al: A population-based study of inflicted traumatic brain injury in young children. *JAMA* 2003;290:621-626.
4. Budenz DL, Farber MG, Mirchindani HG, et al: Ocular and optic nerve hemorrhages in abused infants with intracranial injuries. *Ophthalmology* 1994;101:559-565.
5. Nelson JS: Developmental and perinatal neuropathology. *In:* Nelson JS, Mena H, Parisi JE, et al (eds): *Principles and Practices of Neuropathology*, ed 2. Oxford University Press, New York, 2003, pp 24-44.
6. Looney CB, Smith JK, Merck LH, et al: Intracranial hemorrhage in asymptomatic neonates: Prevalence on MR images and relationship to obstetric and neonatal risk factors. *Radiology* 2007;242:535-541.
7. Schwartz P: *Birth Injuries of the Newborn*. Hafner Publishing, New York, 1961.
8. Rooks VJ, Eaton JP, Ruess L, et al: Prevalence and evolution of intracranial hemorrhage in asymptomatic term infants. *AJNR Am J Neuroradiol* 2008;29:1082-1089.
9. Judkins AR, Hood IA, Mirchindani HG, et al: Technical communication. Rationale and technique for examination of nervous system in suspected infant victims of abuse. *Am J Forens Med Pathol* 2004;25:29-33.
10. Morad Y, Kim YM, Armstrong DC, et al: Correlation between retinal abnormalities and intracranial abnormalities in the shaken baby syndrome. *Am J Ophthalmol* 2002;134:354-359.

11. Kornberg AE: Skin and soft tissue injuries. *In:* Ludwig S, Kornberg AE (eds): *Child Abuse. A Medical Reference,* ed 2. Churchill Livingstone, New York, 1992, pp 91-104.

12. Hobbs CJ, Hanks HGI, Wynne JM: *Child Abuse and Neglect. A Clinician's Handbook.* Churchill Livingstone, London, 2000, pp 73-75.

13. Meadows R. *ABC of Child Abuse.* BMJ Publications, London, 1989, pp 199-248.

14. Case ME, Graham MA, Handy TC, et al: Position paper on fatal abusive head injuries in infants and young children. *Am J Forensic Med Pathol* 2001;22:112-122.

15. Geddes JF, Hackshaw AK, Vowles GH, et al: Neuropathology of inflicted head injury in children. I. Patterns of brain damage. *Brain* 2001;124:1290-1298.

16. DiRocco C, Velardi F: Epidemiology and etiology of cranio-cerebral trauma in the first two years of life. *In:* Raimondi AJ, Choux M, DiRocco C (eds): *Head Injuries in the Newborn and Infants.* Springer Verlag, New York, 1986, pp 125-139.

17. Coats B, Margulies SS: Material properties of human infant skull and suture at high rates. *J Neurotrauma* 2006;23:1222-1232.

18. Kleinman PK, Shelton YA: Hangman's fracture in an abused infant: imaging features. *Pediatr Radiol* 1997;27:776-777.

19. Hoffman GF, Naughten ER: Abuse or metabolic disorder? [letter]. *Arch Dis Child* 1998;78:399.

20. Allison JW, Davis PC, Sato Y, et al: Intracranial aneurysms in infants and children. *Pediatr Radiol* 1998;28:223-229.

21. Weissgold DJ, Budenz DL, Hood I, et al: Ruptured vascular malformation masquerading as shaken baby syndrome. *Surv Ophthalmol* 1995;39:509-512.

22. Rutty GN, Smith CM, Malia RG: Late-form hemorrhagic disease of the newborn: a fatal case report with illustration of investigations that may assist in avoiding the mistaken diagnosis of child abuse. *Am J Forensic Med Pathol* 1999;20:48-51.

23. O'Hare AE, Eden OB: Bleeding disorders and non-accidental injury. *Arch Dis Child* 1984;59:860.

24. vonKries R, Gobel U: Vitamin K prophylaxis and vitamin K deficiency, bleeding (VKDB) in early infancy. *Acta Pediatr* 1992;81:655-660.

25. Bilmire ME, Myers PA: Serious head injury in infants: accident or abuse? *Pediatrics* 1985;75:340-342.

26. Brown JA, Minns RA: Non-accidental head injury with particular reference to whiplash shaking injury and medico-legal aspects. *Dev Med Child Neurol* 1993;35:849-869.

27. Duhaime AC, Christian CW, Rorke LB, et al: Non-accidental head injury in infants – the "shaken-baby syndrome." *N Engl J Med* 1998;338:1822-1829.

28. Feldman KW, Bethel R, Shugerman RP, et al: The cause of infant and toddler subdural hemorrhage: a prospective study. *Pediatrics* 2001;108:636-646.

29. Blumbergs P, Reilly P, Vink R: Trauma. *In:* Love S, Louis DN, Ellison DW (eds): *Greenfield's neuropathology,* ed 8, Vol I. Hodder Arnold, London, 2008, pp 733-832.

30. Geddes JF, Tasker RC, Hackshaw AK, et al: Dural hemorrhage in non-traumatic infants: does it explain bleeding in "shaken baby syndrome"? *Neuropathol Appl Neurobiol* 2003;29:14-22.

31. Richards PG, Bertocci GE, Bonshek RE, et al: Shaken baby syndrome. *Arch Dis Child* 2006;91:205-206.

32. Haines DE: On the question of a subdural space. *Anat Rec* 1991;23:3-21.

33. Maxeiner H: Detection of ruptured bridging veins at autopsy. *Forensic Sci Int* 1997;89:103-110.

34. Maxeiner H: Lethal subdural bleedings of babies—accident or abuse? *Med Law* 2001;20:463-482.

35. Morrison CN, Minns RA: The biomechanics of shaking. *In:* Minns RA, Brown JK (eds): *Shaking and Other Non-accidental Head Injuries in Children.* Mac Keith Press, Cambridge, 2005, pp 106-146.

36. Lindenberg R, Freytag E: Morphology of brain lesions from blunt trauma in early infancy. *Arch Pathol* 1969;87:298-305.

37. Kelley BJ, Lifshitz J, Povlishock JT: Neuroinflammatory response after experimental diffuse traumatic brain injury. *J Neuropathol Exp Neurol* 2007;66:989-1001.

38. Strich SJ: Diffuse degeneration of the cerebral white matter in severe dementia following head injury. *J Neurol Neurosurg Psychiatry* 1956;19:163-185.

39. LeClercq PD, McKenzie JE, Graham DI, et al: Axonal injury is accentuated in the caudal corpus callosum of head-injured patients. *J Neurotrauma* 2001;18:1-9.

40. Graham DI, Saatman KE, Marklund N, et al: The neuropathology of trauma. *In:* Evans RW (ed): *Neurology and Trauma,* ed 2. Oxford University Press, New York, 2006, pp 45-94.

41. Povlishock JT, Becker DP, Cheng CLY, et al: Axonal change in minor head injury. *J Neuropath Exp Neurol* 1983;42:225-242.

42. Yam PS, Takesago T, Dewar D, et al: Amyloid precursor protein accumulates in white matter at the margin of a focal ischemic lesion. *Brain Res* 1997;760:150-157.

43. Dietrich WD, Kraydieh S, Prado R, et al: White matter alterations following thromboembolic stroke: a β-amyloid precursor protein immunocytochemical study in rats. *Acta Neuropathol* 1998;95:524-531.

44. Dolinak D, Smith C, Graham DI: Hypoglycemia is a cause of axonal injury. *Neuropath Appl Neurobiol* 2000;26:448-453.

45. Banker BQ, Larroche J-C: Periventricular leukomalacia of infancy. *Arch Neurol* 1962;7:386-410.

46. Bodian D: A new method for staining nerve fibers and nerve endings in mounted paraffin sections. *Anat Res* 1936;65:89-97.

47. Sherriff FE, Bridges LR, Gentleman SM: Markers of axonal injury in postmortem human brain. *Acta Neuropathol* 1994;88:433-439.

48. Dolinak D, Reichard R: An overview of inflicted head injury in infants and young children, with a review of β-amyloid precursor protein immunohistochemistry. *Arch Pathol Lab Med* 2006;130:712-717.

49. Starling SP, Patel S, Burke BL, et al: Analysis of perpetrator admissions to inflicted traumatic brain injury in children. *Arch Pediatr Adolesc Med* 2004;158:454-458.

50. Hadley MN, Sonntag VKH, Rekate HL, et al: The infant whiplash-shake injury syndrome: a clinical and pathological study. *Neurosurg* 1989;24:536-540.

51. Munger CE, Peiffer RL, Bouldin TW, et al: Ocular and associated neuropathologic observations in suspected whiplash shaken infant syndrome. A retrospective study of 12 cases. *Am J Forensic Med Pathol* 1993;14:193-200.

52. Swaiman KF: Neurologic examination after the newborn period until 2 years of age. *In:* Swaiman KF, Ashwal S (eds): *Pediatric Neurology Principles & Practice,* ed 3, Vol I. Mosby, St Louis, 1999, p 32.

53. Adams JH, Cameron HM: Obstetrical paralysis due to ischemia of the spinal cord. *Arch Dis Child* 1965;40:93-96.

54. Nacimiento W, Noth J: What, if anything, is spinal shock? *Arch Neurol* 1999;56:1033-1035.

55. Hubschmann OR, Krieger AJ: The pathophysiology of head trauma. *J Med Soc N J* 1983;3:181-183.

56. McIntosh TK, Smith DH, Meaney DF, et al: Neuropathological sequelae of traumatic brain injury: relationship to neurochemical and biomechanical mechanisms. *Lab Invest* 1996;74:315-342.

57. David TJ: Shaken baby (shaken impact) syndrome: non-accidental head injury in infancy. *J Soc Med* 1999;92:556-561.

58. Aldrich EF, Eisenberg HM, Saydjari C, et al: Diffuse brain swelling in severely head-injured children. A report from the NIH Traumatic Coma Data Bank. *J Neurosurg* 1992;76:450-454.

59. Minns RA, Brown JK: Neurological perspectives of non-accidental head injury and whiplash/shaken baby syndrome: an overview. *In:* Minns RA, Brown JK (eds): *Shaking and Other Non-Accidental Head Injuries in Children.* MacKeith Press, London, 2005, pp 1-105.

60. Toole JF: *Cerebrovascular Disorders,* ed 4. Raven Press, New York, 1990, pp 30-32.

61. Sane SM, Kleinman PK, Cohen RA, et al: Diagnostic imaging of child abuse. Section on Radiology. *Pediatrics* 2000;105:1345-1348.

62. Lonergan GJ, Baker AM, Morey MK, et al: From the archives of the AFIP. Child abuse: radiologic-pathologic correlation. *Radiographics* 2003;23:811-845.

63. Tung GA, Kumar M, Richardson RC, et al: Comparison of accidental and nonaccidental traumatic head injury in children on noncontrast computed tomography. *Pediatrics* 2006;118:626-633.

64. Steinbok P, Singhal A, Poskitt K, et al: Early hypodensity on computed tomographic scan of the head in an accidental pediatric head injury. *Neurosurgery* 2007;60:689-695.

65. Gilles FH: Hypotensive brainstem necrosis. Selective symmetrical necrosis of tegmental neuronal aggregates following cardiac arrest. *Arch Pathol* 1969;88:32-42.

66. Andrews A: Ocular manifestations of child abuse. *Pa Med* 1996;995:71-75.

67. Greenwald MJ, Weiss A, Oesterle CS, et al: Traumatic retinoschisis in battered babies. *Ophthalmology* 1986;93:618-625.

68. Giangiacomo J, Khan JA, Levine C, et al: Sequential cranial computed tomography in infants with retinal hemorrhages. *Ophthalmology* 1988;95:295-299.

69. Kivlin JD, Simmons KB, Lazoritz S, et al: Shaken baby syndrome. *Ophthalmology* 2000;107:1246-1254.

70. Schloff S, Mullaney PB, Armstrong DC, et al: Retinal findings in children with intracranial hemorrhage. *Ophthalmology* 2002;109:1472-1476.

71. Levin AV: Ophthalmic manifestations of inflicted childhood neurotrauma. *In:* Reece RM, Nicholson CE (eds): *Inflicted Childhood Neurotrauma.* American Academy of Pediatrics Press, Elk Grove Village, Ill, 2003, pp 128-159.

72. Block H: Abandonment, infanticide and filicide. *Am J Dis Child* 1988;142:1058-1060.

73. Caffey J: Multiple fractures in the long bones of infants suffering from subdural hematoma. *AJR Am J Roentgenol* 1946;56:163-173.

74. Caffey J: On the theory and practice of shaking infants. Its potential residual effects on permanent brain damage and mental retardation. *Am J Dis Child* 1972;124:161-169.

75. Annerbäck E-M, Lindell C, Svedin CG, et al: Severe child abuse: a study of cases reported to the police. *Acta Paediatr* 2007;96:1760-1764.

76. Leetsma JE: Case analysis of brain-injured admittedly shaken infants: 54 cases, 1969-2001. *Am J Forensic Med Pathol* 2005;26:199-212.

77. Squier W: Shaken baby syndrome: the quest for evidence. *Develop Med Child Neurol* 2008;50:10-14.

78. Talbert DG: Paroxysmal cough injury, vascular rupture and "shaken baby syndrome." *Med Hypoth* 2005;64:8-13.

79. Minns RA, Brown JK (eds): *Shaking and Other Non-Accidental Head Injuries in Children.* MacKeith Press, London, 2005.

80. Reece RM, Nicholson CE (eds): *Inflicted Childhood Neurotrauma.* American Academy of Pediatrics Press, Elk Grove Village, Ill, 2003.

46

BIOCHEMICAL MARKERS OF HEAD TRAUMA IN CHILDREN

Rachel P. Berger, MD, MPH

INTRODUCTION

Head trauma is a leading cause of death and disability in children and young adults in the United States.[1,2] Annually, approximately 3000 deaths, 50,000 hospitalizations, and 650,000 emergency department visits are due to head trauma.[3] The etiology of pediatric head trauma depends, in large part, on the patient's age. In infants, falls are the most common cause of head trauma, but child abuse is the most common cause of severe head trauma. In older children, head trauma of all severities is most often due to falls or recreational activities. In adolescents, motor vehicle crashes and assault are the most common etiologies of severe head trauma. In all age groups, head trauma rates for males are higher than for females.

Standard definitions for pediatric head trauma do not exist. It is difficult, therefore, to compare studies or perform meta-analyses since the definition of the condition being studied differs so significantly between studies. The most commonly used terms in the literature are head trauma, traumatic brain injury (TBI), head injury, closed head injury, and concussion. In some contexts, TBI refers only to children with head trauma who have a brain injury detected by computed tomography (CT). In other contexts, TBI denotes any child who has had trauma to the head with or without CT evidence of intracranial injury (ICI). In some studies, children with a skull fracture are considered to have a TBI, whereas in others, they are not. *Head trauma* is the most general term that encompasses all traumatic injuries to the head and is not dependent on CT evidence of ICI. In this chapter, the term *head trauma* is used to refer to patients with: (1) a history of traumatic injury to the head with or without radiologic evidence of injury, and/or (2) evidence of trauma to the head on either physical examination or by radiologic evaluation, but without any history of trauma. The lack of a requirement for a history of trauma is particularly important in children with head trauma resulting from abuse since caretakers of these children often do not report a history of trauma or are unaware of a traumatic event. The term *traumatic brain injury* will be used to refer to those patients with head injury in whom there is either a skull fracture or ICI on head CT. *Abusive head trauma* (AHT) will refer to children with TBI caused by child abuse.

The gold standard for clinical classification of the neurologic status of a patient with head trauma is the Glasgow Coma Scale (GCS) score (Table 46-1), a 15-point scale that evaluates brain injury severity based on motor, eye, and verbal responses. The range of scores is 3 to 15. A GCS score of 8 or less indicates severe head trauma, 9-12 indicates moderate head trauma, and 13-15 indicates mild head trauma. Although it is the gold standard for assessment of injury severity, the GCS score has several limitations. Most importantly, it is relatively insensitive to subtle brain injury. As a result, patients with a GCS score of 15 might still have underlying brain injury that is too subtle to result in a decrease in the GCS but can have long-term sequelae. The accuracy of the GCS score is particularly poor in young children in whom the verbal score is difficult to assign.[4,5] In these children the GCS score often underestimates injury severity. Although the infant face scale (IFS) was developed to address this limitation,[4] its use in infants and young children has not yet been validated.

Whereas the GCS score is the gold standard for classification of injury severity, the head CT is the gold standard for identification of ICI. Although CT is able to detect acute intracranial hemorrhage, it is much less sensitive to other abnormalities such as punctate hemorrhages, small contusions, or mild diffuse axonal injury. As a result, most children with head trauma have a normal head CT even though some of them might have ICI which cannot be visualized by CT. The significance of this problem, particularly as it relates to outcome prediction after mild head trauma, has become clearer as neuroimaging techniques have become more sensitive for detecting both anatomic and functional abnormalities. Magnetic resonance imaging (MRI), diffusion weighted imaging, magnetic resonance spectroscopy, diffusion tensor imaging, and proton emission technology are all more sensitive than head CT for identification of subtle ICI.[6-8] These neuroimaging techniques are not currently considered the gold standard for several reasons, including lack of accessibility, cost, the time to complete the tests, and for some tests, the need for sedation. In addition, MRI, the most easily accessible of the alternative imaging techniques, has the important limitation of being less sensitive than head CT for identifying skull fractures and acute hemorrhage.[9-12]

To address some of the limitations of the GCS and head CT in the areas of diagnosis and assessment of injury severity and outcome prediction, recent research has focused on the use of biomarkers of brain injury. The remainder of this chapter therefore focuses on the use of biomarkers to enhance the current gold standards for evaluating head trauma.

Table 46-1	Glasgow Coma Scale (GCS) Score

Assessed Response	Score
Eyes Open	
Spontaneously	4
To speech	3
To pain	2
No response	1
Best Verbal Response	
Oriented	5
Confused	4
Inappropriate words	3
Incomprehensible sounds	2
No response	1
Best Motor Response	
Obeys commands	6
Localizes pain	5
Withdraws	4
Abnormal flexion to pain	3
Abnormal extension to pain	2
No response	1

Table 46-2	The Use of Biochemical Markers of Injury in Various Organ Systems

Organ	Marker
Heart	Troponin, creatine phosphokinase (CPK)-MB fraction
Liver	Aspartate aminotransferase (AST), alanine aminotransferase (ALT) alkaline phosphatase, γ-glutamyl transpeptidase (GGPT)
Pancreas	Lipase, amylase
Muscle	CPK-MM fraction
Kidney	Blood urea nitrogen (BUN), creatinine (Cr)

THE USE OF BIOMARKERS OF INJURY IN THE FIELD OF PEDIATRICS

The Brain vs. Other Organs

Physicians routinely use biomarkers to diagnose disease, assess disease severity, assist in disease prognosis, and evaluate treatment efficacy in many organs other than the brain (Table 46-2). Injury and/or death to a cell often results in an increased concentration of a given biomarker, caused by either the release of that biomarker from the injured cell (e.g., creatine phosphokinase in patients with myocardial infarction) or the lack of excretion of a normally excreted chemical that results in its accumulation (e.g., blood urea nitrogen in patients with renal failure). Despite the robust biochemical response of the brain to injury (Figure 46-1) and a growing number of publications related to brain biomarkers (Figure 46-2), development of a useful brain biomarker has proved more difficult than the development of biomarkers for other organs. Perhaps the most important reason for the difficulty is the presence of the blood–brain barrier (BBB), which limits the amount of and size of the markers that can cross into the serum.

There are two possible sources for brain biomarkers. The first and most obvious source is the brain. After injury,

biomarkers are released from brain tissue and pass into the cerebrospinal fluid (CSF) and serum. The passage from brain to CSF and serum likely occurs through a transiently more permeable BBB, although there is evidence of other non-BBB–related mechanisms of biomarker transport.[13] Limited animal[14] and adult human[15] data suggest an increase in BBB permeability after head trauma, although the increase is likely variable and related to the location, severity, and type of injury.

One of the difficulties in evaluating a brain injury marker that is released from brain tissue is the issue of where to measure its concentration. Since it is not possible to directly measure biomarkers in the brain itself, the next best source would be the CSF, which bathes the brain. CSF is only available, however, in patients with severe head trauma in whom an extraventricular drain is placed for clinical care. Obtaining CSF in other head trauma patients is not routine and could be dangerous because of the possibility of herniation with lumbar puncture if increased intracranial pressure (ICP) is not recognized. In contrast, serum is easily available and routinely collected as part of clinical care after head trauma. One problem with measuring brain markers into the serum is that many of these markers (e.g., interleukins) are not specific to the brain and are also released by other organs. As a result, when these markers cross the BBB into serum, their concentration can be diluted by the background serum concentrations. This has been one of the barriers to identification of brain-derived serum markers.

The second source of brain biomarkers is the serum. In addition to the markers released from the brain after head trauma, there are also multiple signaling molecules and proteins that are released directly into the bloodstream from peripheral organs in response to head trauma.[16-18] There are two important advantages of markers that are released directly into the serum: they are often present in higher concentrations than markers that cross the BBB and they are often detected sooner after injury. Interest in these peripherally derived markers has been much more recent than the long-standing interest in brain-derived markers. Several recent studies evaluating these peripheral markers have been performed and will be discussed subsequently.[16-21]

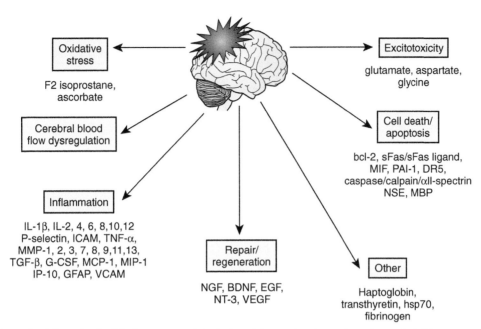

FIGURE 46–1 Schematic of the pathophysiologic response of the brain to injury and markers released as part of this response. *BDNF,* Brain-derived neurotrophic factor; *DR,* death receptor; *EGF,* epidermal growth factor; *G-CSF,* granulocyte colony stimulating factor; *GFAP,* glial fibrillary acidic protein; *ICAM,* intracellular adhesion molecule; *IL,* interleukin; *IP,* interferon inducing protein; *MBP,* myelin basic protein; *MCP,* monocyte chemoattractant protein; *MIF,* migration inhibitory factor; *MIP,* macrophage inflammatory protein; *MMP,* matrix metallopeptidase; *NGF,* nerve growth factor; *NSE,* neuron specific enolase; *NT,* neurotrophin; *PAI,* plasminogen activator inhibitor, alpha-II spectrin; *TGF,* transforming growth factor; *TNF,* tumor necrosis factor; *VCAM,* vascular cell adhesion molecule; *VEGF,* vascular endothelial growth factor. *(From Kochanek PM, Berger RP, Bayir H, et al: Biomarkers of primary and evolving damage in traumatic and ischemic brain injury: diagnosis, prognosis, probing mechanisms, and therapeutic decision making.* Curr Opin Crit Care *2008;14(2):135-141. Copyright 2008 Wolters Kluwer Health. All rights reserved.)*

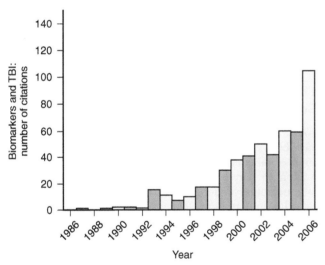

FIGURE 46–2 Number of citations in the published literature related to biomarkers of brain injury. *(Used with permission from Patrick Kochanek, MD.)*

Prior to discussing the potential roles of biomarkers in the care of children with head trauma, it is first helpful to review the biological properties of the brain-derived biomarkers that have been the focus of the published literature.

Candidate Biomarkers of Brain Injury: A 30-Year Odyssey Continues (Table 46-3)

Myelin-basic protein (MBP), one of the two most abundant proteins in myelin, was one of the earliest brain biomarkers

evaluated.[22,23] The few clinical studies of serum MBP[22-24] suggest that serum MBP is increased only after severe head trauma and/or intracranial hemorrhage. As a result of the small patient population in which it could be applied as well as development of more universally applicable biomarkers, MBP is no longer being actively pursued as a general biomarker of brain injury. In one specific clinical situation, however—the identification of AHT—MBP may be a useful biomarker. Unlike other biomarker concentrations that begin to rise immediately after injury and quickly decrease, serum MBP concentrations do not begin to increase until 24 to 48 hours after injury and remain increased for up to 2 weeks.[22] The late increase is likely related to the association of MBP with traumatic axonal injury; although axonal injury occurs at the time of head trauma, the Wallerian degeneration of the axon and release of MBP takes several days. Because of the late rise and prolonged presence in the serum, MBP might be useful in identifying nonacute intracranial hemorrhage in children in whom the concentrations of other biomarkers have already decreased.

As interest in MBP waned for the reasons discussed above, focus turned to the brain-specific fraction of creatinine phosphokinase (CPK-BB).[25-28] By the early 1990s, however, CPK was abandoned as a possible brain biomarker because of concern about its sensitivity and specificity. Almost all of the literature since that time has focused on two biomarkers: neuron-specific enolase (NSE) and S100B. NSE is a glycolytic enzyme localized primarily in neuronal cytoplasm, although it is also present in small quantities in platelets and red blood cells. It is a marker of neuronal death and is increased after head trauma of all severities.[24,26,29-33]

S100B is the major low-affinity calcium-binding protein in astrocytes.[34] It is released by astrocytes that die or are

Table 46-3	Characteristics of the Most Commonly Studied Biomarkers		
Biochemical Marker	**Abbreviation**	**Location**	**Serum Half-life**
Myelin-based protein	MBP	Myelin	12 hr
Creatinine phosphokinase—brain-specific fraction	CPK-BB	Brain, lungs	<1 hr
Neuron-specific enolase	NSE	Neurons, platelets, red blood cells, neuroendocrine cells	24 hr
S100B	Not applicable	Astrocytes, chondrocytes, adipocytes	<2 hr
Glial fibrillary acidic protein	GFAP	Glial cells	~1 week
Cleaved tau	c-tau	Axons of central nervous system neurons, proteolytically cleaved after release to form c-tau	Unknown
α-II spectrin/spectrin breakdown degradation products 120, 145, and 150	SBDP 120, 145, and 150	Cortical membrane cytoskeletal protein	Unknown
Hyperphosphorylated neurofilament heavy chain	pNFH	Axons	Unknown

irreversibly injured. Since the serum half-life of S100B is less than 100 minutes, increases in serum S100B after head trauma are transient. S100B concentrations can also be increased with significant noncranial injuries (e.g., pelvic fracture). This could limit its usefulness in the setting of multi-organ trauma.[35-38] An important limitation is the high normative concentrations of S100B in children less than 2 years of age.[29,39,40] Because of high baseline concentrations, a single value of S100B cannot be interpreted in young children with possible head trauma. However, serial concentrations in the same patient can provide important information about the progression and/or severity of injury as discussed later in this chapter.

Although the literature has focused on NSE and S100B, several papers have evaluated other brain-derived biomarkers including glial fibrillary acidic protein (GFAP)[41,42] and cleaved tau protein (c-tau).[43,44] There has also been a recent interest in structural markers of axonal injury, specifically, α-II spectrin and its degradation products, SBDP 120, 145 and 150[45-47] and hyperphosphorylated neurofilament heavy chain (pNFH).[48]

Although the number of different markers that have been evaluated is small, new techniques such as gel-based[49] and gel-free[20] proteomics, which can be performed both in the serum and CSF, allow for screening of the entire genome of patients with and without head trauma. These techniques, although technically difficult and markedly expensive, will likely identify additional brain-derived and peripherally derived biomarkers that are more sensitive and specific than those discussed previously. In a recently published feasibility study, Haqqani and colleagues[20] used gel-free proteomics to identify 95 uniquely expressed proteins in six children with severe head trauma compared with healthy adult controls. Although it is not possible to determine which of these proteins are brain-derived and which are peripherally derived,

the source of the markers and even the physiological explanation for their increase or decrease after head trauma is less important than their statistical association with head trauma. Although a significant amount of additional research is needed, these new techniques have the potential to revolutionize the field of biomarker development and validation.

The Potential Role of Serum Brain Biomarkers

For purposes of discussion, the potential roles of biomarkers have been divided into five categories: (1) diagnosis, (2) differentiation of head trauma and TBI, (3) assessment of head trauma severity/outcome prediction, (4) development of treatment interventions, and (5) evaluation of treatment efficacy. It is important to recognize, however, that this division is somewhat arbitrary and that the categories overlap considerably. Furthermore, studies that may focus on one specific role of biomarkers might have implications for future research and/or clinical care in a different category. The remainder of the chapter focuses on these roles in the context of pediatric head trauma with an emphasis on AHT. However, because of the dearth of pediatrics data, it will also be necessary to discuss some of the related adult literature.

Diagnosis of Head Trauma

In patients who can communicate and/or whose head trauma is witnessed, biomarkers are not needed to make a diagnosis. Infants and young children, however, cannot communicate, and since the etiology of their head trauma is often abuse, the history provided sometimes is not accurate. When used in the context of identification of head trauma, biomarkers would serve as a "point to the brain" test, much the same way that liver function tests can direct the treating physician to the liver as a possible source of the patient's symptoms. When used in this way, serum biomarkers might not provide information about the etiology of brain injury; an infant with hydrocephalus and one with AHT could both present with vomiting and both might have increased biomarkers.

The possible use of biomarkers to identify head trauma in infants and young children who present without a history of trauma and with nonspecific symptoms is the most well-studied application of biomarkers in this context. The clinical dilemma of how to differentiate the vomiting infant with a routine viral illness from the vomiting infant with head trauma presents itself hundreds of thousands of times every year in emergency departments (EDs) and pediatricians' offices throughout the United States. The problem in this situation is that in the correct context (e.g., when there is a history of or external evidence of trauma), the need for neuroimaging in these infants would be obvious. When there is a lack of history of trauma and/or a lack of findings on physical examination that suggest trauma, however, it is unlikely that a physician would even consider head trauma in the differential diagnosis of a vomiting or fussy infant. In the case of undisclosed head trauma, when the diagnosis of head trauma is not considered and is missed, an infant will be returned to a violent environment where he or she can be reinjured or killed. The magnitude of the problem of missed diagnosis of AHT has been estimated to be at least 30% to 40% based on several studies.[50-53] In a landmark study by Jenny and colleagues,[50] the authors determined based on a review of previous medical records that 31.2% (54/173) of children diagnosed with AHT in their hospital had been seen previously by a physician after AHT but had not been recognized as having AHT at that time. Remarkably, 27.8% of the AHT patients were reinjured in the time between misdiagnosis and eventual proper diagnosis, and at least four children died as a result of the delay in diagnosis. The high rate of reabuse after misdiagnosis demonstrates the critical importance of accurate and timely diagnosis.

A study by the author and colleagues[39] evaluated the possible use of serum biomarkers to screen for head trauma in high-risk infants. Children were eligible for the study if they were less than 1 year of age, had a temperature less than 38.3°C, and presented to the ED without a history of trauma and with symptoms that placed them at increased risk of having HT: vomiting without diarrhea, an apparent life-threatening event, irritability, fussiness, lethargy, or seizures or seizure-like activity.

Ninety-eight subjects were enrolled. Blood or CSF was collected at enrollment, frozen and batched for later measurement of NSE, S100B and MBP. A head CT was not performed as part of the study protocol, but was at the discretion of the treating physician. Because of the lack of a gold standard head CT in all subjects, all subjects were tracked by chart review and phone until 1 year of age or for 6 months after enrollment, whichever came later, to evaluate for subsequent evidence of possible child abuse. The authors hypothesized that if there was a missed case of AHT, it was likely that the child would be reinjured during the tracking period and re-present for medical care.

Based on the clinical diagnosis given at the time of discharge and follow-up data (i.e., the presence or absence of subsequent abuse), subjects were classified as: (1) AHT (i.e.,

the diagnosis of AHT was recognized at the time of enrollment), (2) no brain injury (NBI) (i.e., no brain injury was identified at enrollment or follow-up), (3) indeterminate (IND) (i.e., no brain injury was identified at enrollment, but the child was diagnosed with possible abuse during the follow-up period), or (4) "not classified" (i.e.. the child was identified with a brain injury that was not the result of AHT). The "not classified" group highlights the fact that if used as a "point to the brain" test, biomarkers would not provide information about the etiology of the brain injury: an infant with hydrocephalus and one with AHT could both present with vomiting and both might have increased biomarkers. An abnormal biomarker screen would simply suggest to the treating physician that neuroimaging should be considered.

Study subjects were then classified as true positives, false positives, true negatives, and false negatives based on whether biomarker concentrations were in agreement with clinical diagnosis. For example, a true negative would be a patient who was clinically identified as NBI and whose biomarker concentrations were normal. Sensitivity and specificity was calculated based on data from the NBI and AHT subjects only.

Of 98 subjects, 76% were classified as NBI, 14% as AHT, 5% as IND, and 5% as "not classified." As part of clinical care, 100% of the AHT and 28% of the NBI subjects had a head CT scan performed. Using previously derived cut-offs for abnormal biomarker concentrations,[29] NSE was 76% sensitive and 66% specific and MBP was 36% sensitive and 100% specific for AHT. S100B was increased in 90% of NBI subjects and therefore not specific for head trauma in this population. Of the five subjects who were identified at follow-up as possible victims of abuse (IND group), four had had an increased serum NSE concentration at enrollment, suggesting that these may have been missed cases of AHT. The results of this study suggest that NSE and MBP, but not S100B, might be able to identify children at high risk of AHT who would benefit from evaluation with head CT.

A more recent study measured the concentrations of peripherally derived brain markers after AHT.[17] Using multiplex bead technology to simultaneously screen 45 different serum biomarkers, the author and colleagues compared biomarker concentrations between infants with mild AHT and infants who presented with the same symptoms (e.g., vomiting) but who did not have brain injury. There were significant group differences in the concentrations of 9 of the 45 markers screened: vascular cellular adhesion molecule, interleukin-12, matrix metallopeptidase-9, intracellular adhesion molecule, eotaxin, hepatocyte growth factor, tumor necrosis factor receptor 2, interleukin-6, and fibrinogen. Several of these markers (i.e., matrix metallopeptidase-9, interleukin-6, and fibrinogen) have previously been identified as being increased in the serum after head trauma in adults.[54-56] It is not possible to determine whether the increase in serum concentrations of the biomarkers was due to increased leakage from brain into blood as a result of BBB dysfunction or as the result of a systemic response to brain injury. Knowing the source of the biomarkers (i.e., brain vs. peripheral), however, is not critical when they are being used in the context of a screening tool, since the goal is merely to identify that brain injury has occurred. It is important to recognize that several of these markers can be increased in the presence of fever[57,58] and in a wide variety of pediatric illnesses such as enteroviral meningitis (IL-6),[59] influenza (IL-6),[58] and rotavirus (IL-6, IL-10).[60] As a result, their specificity could be decreased if they are used in certain populations such as infants with febrile seizures or diarrhea.

These two studies suggest that there could be a wide variety of both brain and peripherally derived biomarkers that might be useful for AHT screening. Further research is essential in order to prospectively validate these markers. In addition, a study in which all subjects undergo the gold standard head CT is critical in order to truly assess the sensitivity and specificity of the biomarkers.

Differentiation of Head Trauma and TBI

In the clinical scenario in which biomarkers are used to differentiate head trauma and TBI, the treating physician already recognizes that head trauma might be the source of the patient's symptoms. The clinical dilemma is whether the possibility that the head CT will identify an ICI outweighs the radiation risk to the patient. The assumption is that a head CT is only necessary if it identifies TBI. Almost all of the literature related to using biomarkers to identify TBI has focused on S100B.

The use of biomarkers to differentiate head trauma from TBI initially focused on addressing a very specific clinical problem: how to differentiate adults with acute alcohol intoxication from those with alcohol intoxication and TBI without needing to perform a head CT on all of them. In one of the first studies to address this specific clinical problem, Mussack and colleagues[61] enrolled 139 subjects during the Munich Oktoberfest in 2000. All subjects underwent head CT and had serum NSE and S100B concentrations measured. S100B concentrations, but not NSE concentrations, were significantly higher in patients with TBI vs. those without TBI. It was possible to identify a cut-off value of S100B that provided 100% sensitivity and 50% specificity for identification of patients with TBI.

A recent multicenter study by the same group in Germany enrolled 1309 adults with mild head trauma. Mild head trauma in this study was defined as a history of head trauma, GCS score 13 to 15, and one or more clinical risk factors that included vomiting, intoxication, and severe headache. All subjects underwent head CT. The subset with ICI on head CT were identified by S100B with 99% sensitivity and 30% specificity using previously derived cut-offs for S100B.[62] The authors concluded that use of S100B could result in a 30% decrease in the use of head CT without missing any cases of ICI. Other adult studies have shown similar results.[63-65] In a study by Romner and colleagues,[63] the negative predictive value of an undetectable S100B serum level was 0.99, meaning that there was 99% probability that patients with a normal S100B did not have an ICI.

There is only a single pediatric study that has specifically addressed the ability of serum biomarkers to differentiate head trauma from TBI. A pilot study published in 2000 by Fridriksson and colleagues[66] reported on 50 children aged 0 to 18 years with head trauma. Forty-five percent of these children had ICI identified on head CT. In this population, an increased serum NSE concentration was 77% sensitive and 52% specific for ICI. Unfortunately, the authors did not report on the specificity at a sensitivity of 100%, and no follow-up study has been published.

Assessment of the Severity of Head Trauma/Outcome Prediction after Head Trauma

Outcome after head trauma is directly related to the severity of injury. After severe head trauma, outcome prediction is important for family counseling, for selection of patients who are most likely to benefit from rehabilitation services, and for decision-making, particularly as it relates to the extent of care to provide and whether to continue or withdraw care. After mild head trauma, outcome prediction is most important for identification of patients who are at highest risk of having sequelae from their injury and in whom early rehabilitation would be most helpful. Since only 10% to 15% of patients with mild head trauma have sequelae, it is neither possible nor appropriate to offer rehabilitation to all mild head trauma patients. The ability to predict outcome using biomarkers could have important implications for children with AHT. Access to rehabilitation services for children in foster care is notoriously poor, and the ability to identify those children who would benefit most from rehabilitation services would allow concerted effort to be directed toward those children. The ability to quantitatively predict outcome in cases of AHT could also have important legal implications in cases of AHT, since physicians are often asked in court to predict a given child's eventual outcome.

The adult literature related to biomarkers and outcome prediction is extensive and the interested reader is referred to a review article on the subject.[67] Very briefly, numerous markers have been assessed including NSE,[68,69] S100B,[41,70] MBP,[22] GFAP,[41,68] and cleaved tau protein.[71] Overall, the data demonstrate that higher serum biomarker concentrations are consistently correlated with worse outcome.

The pediatric literature is limited and is listed in its entirety in Table 46-4. As seen in that table, only a single study specifically focused on children with AHT.[72] This study evaluated the relationship between serum NSE, S100B, and MBP concentrations measured immediately after injury and neurocognitive outcome 6 months after injury in children less than 3 years of age with AHT compared with children less than 3 years of age with non-abusive head trauma. Eligible children with AHT (n = 15) were matched for gender, ethnicity, socioeconomic status, and injury severity with children with non-abusive head trauma. Outcome was assessed using the Glasgow Outcome Scale (GOS) score (1 = good outcome, 5 = death), the Vineland Adaptive Behavior Scale (VABS), and an age-appropriate IQ measure. Biomarker concentrations were measured every 12 hours for up to 5 days after injury. Initial, peak and "time to peak" (i.e., number of hours between the time of injury and the time of the peak biomarker concentration) were calculated for all three biomarkers. In cases of AHT, "time of injury" was defined as the time at which medical care was sought.

Overall, children with AHT had worse outcome on all three scales at 6 months compared with those with non-abusive head trauma, even though the subjects were matched for injury severity, socioeconomic status, gender, and ethnicity, and even though results were adjusted for age. "Time to peak" NSE, S100B, and MBP concentrations were all significantly longer after AHT vs. non-abusive head trauma. The difference in the serum "time to peak" concentrations between

Table 46-4	Serum Biomarkers and Outcome after Pediatric TBI			
Author (Year)	**Measured Outcome and When Outcome Was Measured**	**Conclusions**	**Significant Strengths**	**Significant Weaknesses**
Spinella et al[101]	Dichotomous PCPC score at hospital discharge and 6 mo	Significant difference in S100B concentration between poor and good outcome groups	First pediatric study	Sample size (n = 27), single marker, gross outcome measure
Bandyopadhyay et al[30]	GOS at hospital discharge	Significant difference in NSE between good and poor outcome groups	Larger study (n = 86)	Single marker, gross outcome measure
Beers et al[72]	GOS, VABS, IQ 6 mo after injury	Peak NSE and MBP and time to peak NSE inversely correlated with GOS, VABS, IQ; time to peak S100B inversely correlated with IQ, VABS	More refined outcome criteria, multiple markers/time points	Small sample size (n = 30)
Berger et al[102]	GOS, GOS-E Peds 0-3 mo, 4-6 mo, and 7-12 mo after injury	Peak NSE, S100B, and MBP inversely correlated with outcome, peak levels more strongly correlated than initial levels, earlier outcome assessment more strongly correlated than late outcome assessment	Large sample size (n = 152), multiple time-points/ biomarkers	Gross outcome measures
Piazza et al[103]	GOS-E 6 mo after injury	S100B concentrations do not correlate with outcome	None	Sample size (n = 15), outcome performed based on a phone call

From Berger R: The use of biomarkers to predict outcome after traumatic brain injury in adults and children. *J Head Trauma Rehabil* 2006;21(4):315-333. Copyright 2006 Wolters Kluwer Health. All rights reserved.
GOS, Glasgow Outcome Scale; *GOS-E*, GOS Extended; *GOS-E Peds*, GOS Extended-Pediatric; *MBP*, myelin-basic protein; *NSE*, neuron-specific enolase; *PCPC*, Pediatric Cerebral Performance Category; *VABS*, Vineland Adaptive Behavior Score.

AHT and non-abusive head trauma is indicative of prolonged neuronal, glial, and axonal injury and death in children with AHT, and is consistent with the moderate to strong inverse correlation between biomarker concentrations and outcome (e.g., high biomarker concentrations are associated with worse outcome). Higher peak and "time to peak" NSE concentrations were especially strongly correlated with poorer outcome on all three measures. Although the data in the literature are encouraging, significant work still needs to be done before biomarkers can be used to predict outcome after head trauma, particularly in children.

Development of Treatment Interventions

Despite numerous improvements in pediatric intensive care over the past 20 years, the mortality from head trauma has remained virtually unchanged.[73] As a result, one of the earliest recognized applications of biomarkers was to attempt to define the mechanisms that operated in the brains of children with severe head trauma and thereby develop effective interventions. These early studies used CSF from extraventricular drains placed for treatment of intracranial

hypertension. The results were instrumental in helping to define the evolution of secondary brain injury after severe head trauma and to highlight the importance of posttraumatic ischemia, excitotoxicity, energy failure, cerebral swelling, axonal injury, and inflammation.[74] These studies also provided some of the earliest evidence that the brain injury in AHT was different from the injury after non-abusive head trauma.[75-77] Several studies, for example, demonstrated increased CSF concentrations of neurotoxins[75,78] and decreased concentrations of neuroprotectants[76,79] after AHT *vs.* non-abusive head trauma. Although the reason for these differences is not yet understood, the results not only identify areas that might be therapeutic targets, but also suggest that treatment might need to be different for children with AHT *vs.* non-abusive head trauma.

A recent study by the author and colleagues[80] was the first to evaluate serum rather than CSF. In this study, serial serum samples were collected from 127 children with acute hypoxic-ischemic encephalopathy (HIE) (n = 27), AHT (n = 44), and non-abusive head trauma (n = 56). As in the previously described study, samples were collected upon arrival to the hospital and then every 12 hours for up to 5 days and NSE, S100B, and MBP concentrations were measured. Normal concentrations of each marker had been defined previously.[29]

The concentrations of all three markers in all three study groups were significantly increased compared with normal concentrations with the exception of MBP in subjects with HIE, consistent with the lack of traumatic axonal injury in this disease. The change in the concentration of markers over time differed significantly between groups and by marker (Figure 46-3). The change in NSE concentrations over time, for example, was significant after HIE and AHT, but not after non-abusive head trauma (see Figure 46-3, *A*). The "time to peak" NSE concentrations were longest after AHT, suggesting profound and ongoing neuronal injury after AHT. This could have important implications for the length of the therapeutic window for an intervention such as hypothermia, which might have an effect on the pathways that result in neuronal death.[81] There was no difference between initial and peak S100B concentrations for any group (see Figure 46-3, *B*), consistent with data that suggest S100B is released only at the time of the primary injury. Finally, the change in MBP concentrations over time was significant after both AHT and non-abusive head trauma, consistent with the importance of traumatic axonal injury in these types of injury (see Figure 46-3, *C*). Finally, the "time to peak" MBP concentrations were longer after AHT *vs.* non-abusive head trauma, suggesting more significant ongoing traumatic axonal injury after AHT.

The results of this study support the CSF data that suggest that there is a fundamental difference in the pathophysiology of AHT, HIE, and non-abusive head trauma. Specifically, the data demonstrate that the biochemical response of the brain to AHT is characterized by a combination of the neuronal injury seen with HIE and the traumatic axonal injury seen with non-abusive head trauma. Given the efficacy of hypothermia after HIE in both adults[3,82] and neonates,[83] these results suggest that on a theoretical basis, children with AHT might be particularly amenable to the therapeutic effects of hypothermia.

Evaluation of Treatment Efficacy

A final possible role for biomarkers is evaluation of treatment efficacy. In the few intervention trials that have been performed, treatment efficacy has been assessed by comparing outcomes of treated and nontreated patients.[84-86] Only gross measures of outcome (e.g., survival vs. mortality or GOS score) have routinely been assessed in these intervention studies, and the most accurate outcome assessments often cannot be performed for months to years after injury. Outcome measurement in infants and young children, the most common victims of AHT, is particularly problematic for multiple reasons: disabilities and functional deficits often are not known for years after injury; neuropsychological and neurocognitive studies are difficult to perform in young children; and well-established outcome measures, such as the GOS score, are adult oriented. A return to preinjury status, for example, is not relevant in children in whom expectations and developmental milestones are constantly changing. Biomarkers might be able to address at least some of these difficulties by serving as a surrogate for treatment efficacy and allowing for early assessment of clinical response to an

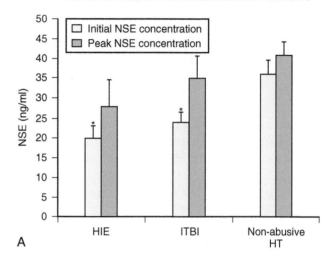

A

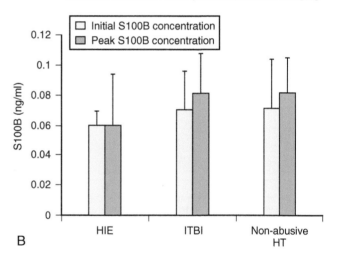

B

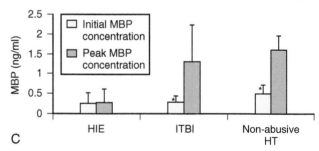

C

FIGURE 46-3 Mean initial and peak concentration of biomarkers after hypoxic-ischemic encephalopathy *(HIE)*, abusive head trauma *(AHT)*, and non-abusive head trauma *(HT)* **A,** NSE. **B,** S100B. **C,** MBP. Error bars represent standard error of the mean. *(From Berger RP, Adelson PD, Richichi R, Kochanek PM. Serum biomarkers after traumatic and hypoxemic brain injuries: insight into the biochemical response of the pediatric brain to inflicted brain injury. Dev Neurosci 2006;28(4-5):327-335. Copyright 2006 S. Karger AG. Basel. All rights reserved.)*

intervention. A study in adults after cardiac arrest, for example, demonstrated decreased serum NSE, but not S100B, concentrations immediately after injury in subjects treated with hypothermia compared with normothermia, suggesting decreased neuronal death in these patients.[87] Biomarkers have not been used previously to assess treatment efficacy in any clinical trials in head trauma patients, and therefore its use in this context is currently more theoretical than practical. As the treatment options for children with head trauma increase, biomarkers might play a progressively more important role as objective and rapid measures of efficacy.

SPECIFIC ISSUES RELATED TO BIOMARKERS AND AHT

In addition to the potential clinical uses of biomarkers described previously, there are several issues that are specific to the field of child abuse and deserve special mention. The first issue is whether biomarkers can be used to identify whether a given TBI is the result of abuse. It is clear based on significant CSF and serum literature over the past decade that significant differences exist in the biochemical response of the brain to AHT *vs.* non-abusive head trauma. It is critically important, however, to recognize that these are overall statistical differences and that these differences cannot be used on a case-by-case basis at this time. No single biomarker in any published study thus far has been able to accurately distinguish all patients with AHT from all those with non-abusive head trauma. This is likely related to the fact that AHT is not a homogenous disease or injury. Children with AHT have different types of injury (i.e., direct trauma vs. hypoxia vs. combinations of the two), different numbers of injuries (i.e., single vs. multiple events), and different times when medical care is sought relative to when the injury was sustained (i.e., immediate vs. delayed medical care). Each of these variables can affect biomarker concentrations and occur with varying severities and varying importance. Although it is possible that at some point in the future there will be a marker—or more likely, a pattern of biomarkers, which is highly suggestive of abuse. At this time, biomarkers cannot identify the etiology of TBI.

A second issue specific to AHT is the possible use of biomarkers to assist in timing of injury. The ability to time an injury could help identify possible perpetrators while excluding others based on when they were with the injured child. For example, since MBP concentrations do not rise until 48 to 72 hours after injury, it might be possible to assess that an injury is not acute in an infant who presents with increased MBP concentrations. Similarly, if peak NSE concentrations occur between 24 and 36 hours after injury and a child with AHT presents to the ED with a high NSE concentration that begins to decrease rather than increase after admission, it might be possible to assess that the injury was unlikely to have occurred in the previous 6 to 12 hours. Although the literature does suggest significant differences in the time course of both CSF and biomarkers in children with AHT *vs.* non-abusive heat trauma,[29,74,80] these differences are group differences and cannot currently be interpreted on a case-by-case basis. Thus, although this potential

use of biomarkers is exciting, significantly more research is needed.

Two final potential uses are related to the increasingly strong data that suggest that biomarkers are more sensitive to brain injury than head CT and might even be more sensitive than MRI.[63,88-90] This is not surprising, since the threshold for cellular brain injury is likely well below the threshold of imaging, as is true in other organs (e.g., liver). With additional research, it may be possible to use the presence of increased brain biomarkers as evidence of a concussion in the same way that increased liver function tests can often be used as evidence of abdominal trauma. This could be particularly important, for example, in an infant with isolated facial or ear bruises and a negative head CT. In cases of non-abusive head trauma, a patient with a witnessed (and therefore clearly not abusive) head trauma with symptoms such as vomiting and with a normal head CT would routinely be diagnosed with a concussion. The history of head trauma, however, is essential to make the diagnosis. Thus an infant without a history of head trauma, who presents with vomiting and facial bruising and a negative head CT, cannot currently be given a diagnosis of concussion. Because of the need for history of head trauma, the diagnosis of "concussion due to abuse" is very difficult, if not impossible, to make. Although infants with isolated bruising are often not well-protected by the child protection system, the additional diagnosis of a concussion might well prompt additional scrutiny of the child's safety.

Finally, if biomarkers are more sensitive than head CT, it might be possible to use biomarkers to identify those children with noncranial abuse and a negative head CT who should undergo brain MRI to further evaluate the possibility of head trauma that cannot be visualized by head CT. Although there is currently significant anecdotal evidence that some infants with noncranial abuse have normal head CTs and abnormal MRIs, identifying which infants with a negative head CT should undergo MRI is not evidence based. Research is needed to assess whether increased biomarker concentrations in children with negative head CT are sufficiently sensitive and specific to assist in selecting those children who should undergo MRI.

STRENGTH OF THE MEDICAL EVIDENCE

There are well-established methods for describing the strength of medical evidence in the context of evidence-based medicine. Data related to the quality, quantity, consistency, robustness, and magnitude of the effects observed are all important criteria. At this time, the strength of the evidence for the use of biomarkers in the care of patients with head trauma varies significantly depending on the patient population (i.e., adults vs. children) and the context in which the biomarkers are being used (e.g., differentiation of head trauma vs. TBI or assessment of treatment efficacy). Overall, the data suggest that biomarkers could have a significant clinical effect in the fields of both pediatric and adult head trauma and that there are potentially multiple contexts in which biomarkers might be useful and which require further study. Clearly use of biomarkers in the context of AHT is a very small part of a much larger field. In that regard, advances in the strength of the evidence will come much more quickly than if biomarkers were only useful in the context of AHT.

SUGGESTED DIRECTIONS FOR FUTURE RESEARCH

Given the morbidity and mortality of head trauma in children, the literature related to biomarkers after pediatric head trauma is surprisingly limited. The reasons for this are likely multifaceted, ranging from the generally less-extensive research infrastructure in pediatric vs. adult settings, the lack of pediatric clinical researchers, and the difficulty obtaining consent for research in infants and young children. The fact that AHT is an important cause of severe head trauma in infants and young children is an additional barrier since this group is traditionally difficult to consent and track as part of research studies, and institutional review boards are often hesitant to approve protocols involving victims of abuse. Although some of the adult biomarker data can be used to advance the pediatric field, a significant amount of research still needs to be performed in children. As clinicians who care for children are well aware, children, particularly children with brain injury, are not just little adults,[91] and what works in one age group might not work in another.

Although the volume of evidence related to biomarkers needs to increase, there also needs to be a focus on specific areas of biomarkers research. For example, almost all the previous studies have evaluated a single biomarker. Although a single biomarker or pair of biomarkers (e.g., troponin for myocardial infarction) has been sufficient in other organs, the brain is far more complex and less homogenous. Thus, injury to a small, critical area of the brain could result in a minimal increase in biomarker concentrations but has a significant effect on neurological status and/or long-term outcome. Likewise, injury to a larger, less-critical region of the brain might result in high biomarker concentrations, but have little effect on neurological status or outcome. As a result, it is unlikely that a single biochemical marker will be both sensitive and specific for all types of brain injury. Rather than pursuing a perfect marker, it therefore might be best to develop a panel of markers that would include markers of neuronal injury, glial cell injury, hypoxia, and inflammation—all important components of the brain's secondary response to injury.

Future research also needs to focus on a combination of biomarkers and other clinical tools. Prior to the focus on biomarkers, for example, there had been significant research in adults and children trying to determine whether demographic, clinical, and/or radiologic variables could be used to predict outcome.[92-99] Although most of these studies showed that certain variables correlate with outcome, the positive and/or negative predictive value of these variables were not high enough to dictate clinical decision-making. It is possible that although these clinical variables were not adequate by themselves, in combination with biomarkers, the sensitivity and specificity could be markedly enhanced.

If additional studies confirm the potential of biomarkers to provide important clinical information, research will need to focus on clinical availability. Although S100B can be measured quickly in a standard hospital laboratory in Europe,[100] there are currently no clinically available and/or FDA-approved point-of-care tests available for any of the serum biomarkers discussed previously. In order to be clinically useful in the acute care setting, tests of biomarker measurement will need to be easy to use and readily accessible. Once these tests are available, use of biomarkers will truly be able to move from the bench to the bedside.

References

1. Haller JA Jr: Pediatric trauma. The No. 1 killer of children. *JAMA* 1983;249:47.
2. Sosin DM, Sniezek JE, Waxweiler RJ: Trends in death associated with traumatic brain injury, 1979 through 1992. Success and failure. *JAMA* 1995;273:1778-1780.
3. Hypothermia after Cardiac Arrest Study Group: Mild therapeutic hypothermia to improve the neurologic outcome after cardiac arrest. *N Engl J Med* 2002;346:549-556.
4. Durham SR, Clancy RR, Leuthardt E, et al: CHOP Infant Coma Scale ("Infant Face Scale"): a novel coma scale for children less than two years of age. *J Neurotrauma* 2000;17:729-737.
5. Hahn YS, McLone DG: Risk factors in the outcome of children with minor head injury. *Pediatr Neurosurg* 1993;19:135-142.
6. van der Naalt J, Hew JM, van Zomeren AH, et al: Computed tomography and magnetic resonance imaging in mild to moderate head injury: early and late imaging related to outcome. *Ann Neurol* 1999;46:70-78.
7. Hofman PA, Stapert SZ, van Kroonenburgh MJ, et al: MR imaging, single-photon emission CT, and neurocognitive performance after mild traumatic brain injury. *AJNR Am J Neuroradiol* 2001;22:441-449.
8. Umile EM, Sandel ME, Alavi A, et al: Dynamic imaging in mild traumatic brain injury: support for the theory of medial temporal vulnerability. *Arch Phys Med Rehabil* 2002;83:1506-1513.
9. Kleinman P: *Diagnostic Imaging of Child Abuse*, ed 2. Mosby, St Louis, 1998.
10. Sato Y, Yuh WT, Smith WL, et al: Head injury in child abuse: evaluation with MR imaging. *Radiology* 1989;173:653-657.
11. Morad Y, Avni I, Benton SA, et al: Normal computerized tomography of brain in children with shaken baby syndrome. *J AAPOS* 2004;8:445-450.
12. Chabrol B, Decarie JC, Fortin G: The role of cranial MRI in identifying patients suffering from child abuse and presenting with unexplained neurological findings. *Child Abuse Negl* 1999;23:217-228.
13. Banks WA, Kastin AJ, Broadwell RD: Passage of cytokines across the blood-brain barrier. *Neuroimmunomodulation* 1995;2:241-248.
14. Adelson PD, Whalen MJ, Kochanek PM, et al: Blood brain barrier permeability and acute inflammation in two models of traumatic brain injury in the immature rat: a preliminary report. *Acta Neurochir Suppl (Wien)* 1998;71:104-106.
15. Kushi H, Katayama Y, Shibuya T, et al: Gadolinium DTPA-enhanced magnetic resonance imaging of cerebral contusions. *Acta Neurochir Suppl (Wien)* 1994;60:472-474.
16. Hergenroeder G, Redell JB, Moore AN, et al: Identification of serum biomarkers in brain-injured adults: potential for predicting elevated intracranial pressure. *J Neurotrauma* 2008;25:79-93.
17. Berger R, Ta'asan S, Rand A, et al: Multiplex assessment of serum biomarker concentrations in well-appearing children with inflicted traumatic brain injury. *Pediatr Res* 2009;65:97-102.
18. Kalsotra A, Zhao J, Anakk S, et al: Brain trauma leads to enhanced lung inflammation and injury: evidence for role of P4504Fs in resolution. *J Cereb Blood Flow Metab* 2007;27:963-974.
19. Rohlff C: Proteomics in molecular medicine: applications in central nervous systems disorders. *Electrophoresis* 2000;21:1227-1234.
20. Haqqani AS, Hutchison JS, Ward R, et al: Biomarkers and diagnosis; protein biomarkers in serum of pediatric patients with severe traumatic brain injury identified by ICAT-LC-MS/MS. *J Neurotrauma* 2007;24:54-74.
21. Sotgiu S, Zanda B, Marchetti B, et al: Inflammatory biomarkers in blood of patients with acute brain ischemia. *Eur J Neurol* 2006;13:505-513.
22. Thomas DG, Palfreyman JW, Ratcliffe JG: Serum-myelin-basic-protein assay in diagnosis and prognosis of patients with head injury. *Lancet* 1978;1:113-115.

23. Thomas DG, Hoyle NR, Seeldrayers P: Myelin basic protein immunoreactivity in serum of neurosurgical patients. *J Neurol Neurosurg Psychiatry* 1984;47:173-175.

24. Yamazaki Y, Yada K, Morii S, et al: Diagnostic significance of serum neuron-specific enolase and myelin basic protein assay in patients with acute head injury. *Surg Neurol* 1995;43:267-270.

25. Karpman RR, Weinstein PR, Finley PR, et al: Serum CPK isoenzyme BB as an indicator of brain tissue damage following head injury. *J Trauma* 1981;21:148-151.

26. Skogseid IM, Nordby HK, Urdal P, et al: Increased serum creatine kinase BB and neuron specific enolase following head injury indicates brain damage. *Acta Neurochir (Wien)* 1992;115:106-111.

27. Hans P, Born JD, Chapelle JP, et al: Creatine kinase isoenzymes in severe head injury. *J Neurosurg* 1983;58:689-692.

28. Rabow L, Hedman G: Creatine kinaseBB-activity after head trauma related to outcome. *Acta Neurochir (Wien)* 1985;76:137-139.

29. Berger RP, Adelson PD, Pierce MC, et al: Serum neuron-specific enolase, S100B, and myelin basic protein concentrations after inflicted and noninflicted traumatic brain injury in children. *J Neurosurg* 2005;103(1 Suppl):61-68.

30. Bandyopadhyay S, Hennes H, Gorelick MH, et al: Serum neuron-specific enolase as a predictor of short-term outcome in children with closed traumatic brain injury. *Acad Emerg Med* 2005;12:732-738.

31. Karkela J, Bock E, Kaukinen S: CSF and serum brain-specific creatine kinase isoenzyme (CK-BB), neuron-specific enolase (NSE) and neural cell adhesion molecule (NCAM) as prognostic markers for hypoxic brain injury after cardiac arrest in man. *J Neurol Sci* 1993;116:100-109.

32. Vazquez MD, Sanchez-Rodriguez F, Osuna E, et al: Creatine kinase BB and neuron-specific enolase in cerebrospinal fluid in the diagnosis of brain insult. *Am J Forensic Med Pathol* 1995;16:210-214.

33. Ross SA, Cunningham RT, Johnston CF, et al: Neuron-specific enolase as an aid to outcome prediction in head injury. *Br J Neurosurg* 1996;10:471-476.

34. Xiong Z, O'Hanlon D, Becker LE, et al: Enhanced calcium transients in glial cells in neonatal cerebellar cultures derived from S100B null mice. *Exp Cell Res* 2000;257:281-289.

35. Pelinka LE, Toegel E, Mauritz W, et al: Serum S 100 B: a marker of brain damage in traumatic brain injury with and without multiple trauma. *Shock* 2003;19:195-200.

36. Anderson RE, Hansson LO, Nilsson O, et al: High serum S100B levels for trauma patients without head injuries. *Neurosurgery* 2001;48:1255-1258.

37. Romner B, Ingebrigtsen T: High serum S100B levels for trauma patients without head injuries. *Neurosurgery* 2001;49:1490.

38. Rothoerl RD, Woertgen C: High serum S100B levels for trauma patients without head injuries. *Neurosurgery* 2001;49:1490-1491.

39. Berger RP, Dulani T, Adelson PD, et al: Identification of inflicted traumatic brain injury in well-appearing infants using serum and cerebrospinal markers: a possible screening tool. *Pediatrics* 2006;117:325-332.

40. Portela LV, Tort AB, Schaf DV, et al: The serum S100B concentration is age dependent. *Clin Chem* 2002;48:950-952.

41. Pelinka LE, Kroepfl A, Leixnering M, et al: GFAP versus S100B in serum after traumatic brain injury: relationship to brain damage and outcome. *J Neurotrauma* 2004;21:1553-1561.

42. Pelinka LE, Kroepfl A, Schmidhammer R, et al: Glial fibrillary acidic protein in serum after traumatic brain injury and multiple trauma. *J Trauma* 2004;57:1006-1012.

43. Bazarian JJ, Cimpello LB, Mookerjee S, et al: Predicting post concussion syndrome after mild traumatic brain injury using serum S100B and cleaved-tau. *Acad Emerg Med* 2004;11:516.

44. Begaz T, Kyriacou DN, Segal J, et al: Serum biochemical markers for post-concussion syndrome in patients with mild traumatic brain injury. *J Neurotrauma* 2006;23:1201-1210.

45. Cardali S, Maugeri R: Detection of αII-spectrin and breakdown products in humans after severe traumatic brain injury. *J Neurosurg Sci* 2006;50:25-31.

46. Ringger NC, O'Steen BE, Brabham JG, et al: A novel marker for traumatic brain injury: CSF alphaII-spectrin breakdown product levels. *J Neurotrauma* 2004;21:1443-1456.

47. Brophy G, Papa L, Liu M, et al: Alpha-II spectrin breakdown product kinetics in acute brain injury. *J Neurotrauma* 2008;25:902.

48. Blyth B, Bazarian J, Bazarian J, Shaw G: Differential patterns of release of UCHL-1 and PNFH into serum after severe traumatic brain injury. *J Neurotrauma* 2008;25:862.

49. Gao WM, Chadha MS, Berger RP, et al: Biomarkers and diagnosis; a gel-based proteomic comparison of human cerebrospinal fluid between inflicted and non-inflicted pediatric traumatic brain injury. *J Neurotrauma* 2007;24:43-53.

50. Jenny C, Hymel KP, Ritzen A, et al: Analysis of missed cases of abusive head trauma. *JAMA* 1999;281:621-622.

51. Laskey A: Shaken baby syndrome: a missed diagnosis. *In:* 1998 National Shaken Baby Conference, Salt Lake City, 1998.

52. Rubin DM, Christian CW, Bilaniuk LT, et al: Occult head injury in high-risk abused children. *Pediatrics* 2003;111:1382-1386.

53. Alexander R, Crabbe L, Sato Y, et al: Serial abuse in children who are shaken. *Am J Dis Child* 1990;144:58-60.

54. Suehiro E, Fujisawa H, Akimura T, et al: Increased matrix metalloproteinase-9 in blood in association with activation of interleukin-6 after traumatic brain injury: influence of hypothermic therapy. *J Neurotrauma* 2004;21:1706-1711.

55. Kossmann T, Hans VH, Imhof HG, et al: Intrathecal and serum interleukin-6 and the acute-phase response in patients with severe traumatic brain injuries. *Shock* 1995;4:311-317.

56. Conti A, Sanchez-Ruiz Y, Bachi A, et al: Proteome study of human cerebrospinal fluid following traumatic brain injury indicates fibrin(ogen) degradation products as trauma-associated markers. *J Neurotrauma* 2004;21:854-863.

57. Engel A, Kern WV, Murdter G, et al: Kinetics and correlation with body temperature of circulating interleukin-6, interleukin-8, tumor necrosis factor alpha and interleukin-1 beta in patients with fever and neutropenia. *Infection* 1994;22:160-164.

58. Kaiser L, Fritz RS, Straus SE, et al: Symptom pathogenesis during acute influenza: interleukin-6 and other cytokine responses. *J Med Virol* 2001;64:262-268.

59. Sato M, Hosoya M, Honzumi K, et al: Cytokine and cellular inflammatory sequence in enteroviral meningitis. *Pediatrics* 2003;112:1103-1107.

60. Jiang B, Snipes-Magaldi L, Dennehy P, et al: Cytokines as mediators for or effectors against rotavirus disease in children. *Clin Diagn Lab Immunol* 2003;10:995-1001.

61. Mussack T, Biberthaler P, Kanz KG, et al: Immediate S-100B and neuron-specific enolase plasma measurements for rapid evaluation of primary brain damage in alcohol-intoxicated, minor head-injured patients. *Shock* 2002;18:395-400.

62. Biberthaler P, Linsenmeier U, Pfeifer KJ, et al: Serum S-100B concentration provides additional information fot the indication of computed tomography in patients after minor head injury: a prospective multicenter study. *Shock* 2006;25:446-453.

63. Romner B, Ingebrigtsen T, Kongstad P, et al: Traumatic brain damage: serum S-100 protein measurements related to neuroradiological findings. *J Neurotrauma* 2000;17:641-647.

64. Savola O, Pyhtinen J, Leino TK, et al: Effects of head and extracranial injuries on serum protein S100B levels in trauma patients. *J Trauma* 2004;56:1229-1234.

65. Muller K, Townend W, Biasca N, et al: S100B serum level predicts computed tomography findings after minor head injury. *J Trauma* 2007;62:1452-1456.

66. Fridriksson T, Kini N, Walsh-Kelly C, et al: Serum neuron-specific enolase as a predictor of intracranial lesions in children with head trauma: a pilot study. *Acad Emerg Med* 2000;7:816-820.

67. Berger RP: The use of serum biomarkers to predict outcome after traumatic brain injury in adults and children. *J Head Trauma Rehabil* 2006;21:315-333.

68. Vos PE, Lamers KJ, Hendriks JC, et al: Glial and neuronal proteins in serum predict outcome after severe traumatic brain injury. *Neurology* 2004;62:1303-1310.

69. Lima JE, Takayanagui OM, Garcia LV, et al: Use of neuron-specific enolase for assessing the severity and outcome in patients with neurological disorders. *Braz J Med Biol Res* 2004;37:19-26.

70. Petzold A, Green AJ, Keir G, et al: Role of serum S100B as an early predictor of high intracranial pressure and mortality in brain injury: a pilot study. *Crit Care Med* 2002;30:2705-2710.

71. Shaw GJ, Jauch EC, Zemlan FP: Serum cleaved tau protein levels and clinical outcome in adult patients with closed head injury. *Ann Emerg Med* 2002;39:254-257.

72. Beers SR, Berger RP, Adelson PD: Neurocognitive outcome and serum biomarkers in inflicted versus non-inflicted traumatic brain injury in young children. *J Neurotrauma* 2007;24:97-105.

73. Pfenninger J, Santi A: Severe traumatic brain injury in children—are the results improving? *Swiss Med Wkly* 2002;132:116-120.

74. Kochanek PM, Clark RS, Ruppel RA, et al: Biochemical, cellular, and molecular mechanisms in the evolution of secondary damage after severe traumatic brain injury in infants and children: Lessons learned from the bedside. *Pediatr Crit Care Med* 2000;1:4-19.

75. Ruppel RA, Kochanek PM, Adelson PD, et al: Excitatory amino acid concentrations in ventricular cerebrospinal fluid after severe traumatic brain injury in infants and children: the role of child abuse. *J Pediatr* 2001;138:18-25.

76. Clark RS, Kochanek PM, Adelson PD, et al: Increases in bcl-2 protein in cerebrospinal fluid and evidence for programmed cell death in infants and children after severe traumatic brain injury. *J Pediatr* 2000;137:197-204.

77. Kochanek PM, Clark RS, Ruppel RA, et al: Cerebral resuscitation after traumatic brain injury and cardiopulmonary arrest in infants and children in the new millennium. *Pediatr Clin North Am* 2001;48:661-681.

78. Berger RP, Heyes MP, Wisniewski SR, et al: Assessment of the macrophage marker quinolinic acid in cerebrospinal fluid after pediatric traumatic brain injury: insight into the timing and severity of injury in child abuse. *J Neurotrauma* 2004;21:1123-1130.

79. Satchell MA, Lai Y, Kochanek PM, et al: Cytochrome c, a biomarker of apoptosis, is increased in cerebrospinal fluid from infants with inflicted brain injury from child abuse. *J Cereb Blood Flow Metab* 2005;25:919-927.

80. Berger RP, Adelson PD, Richichi R, et al: Serum biomarkers after traumatic and hypoxemic brain injuries: insight into the biochemical response of the pediatric brain to inflicted brain injury. *Dev Neurosci* 2006;28:327-335.

81. Kochanek PM, Berger RP, Bayir H, et al: Biomarkers of primary and evolving damage in traumatic and ischemic brain injury: diagnosis, prognosis, probing mechanisms, and therapeutic decision making. *Curr Opin Crit Care* 2008;14:135-141.

82. Bernard SA, Gray TW, Buist MD, et al: Treatment of comatose survivors of out-of-hospital cardiac arrest with induced hypothermia. *N Engl J Med* 2002;346:557-563.

83. Shah PS, Ohlsson A, Perlman M: Hypothermia to treat neonatal hypoxic ischemic encephalopathy: systematic review. *Arch Pediatr Adolesc Med* 2007;161:951-958.

84. McIntyre LA, Fergusson DA, Hebert PC, et al: Prolonged therapeutic hypothermia after traumatic brain injury in adults: a systematic review. *JAMA* 2003;289:2992-2999.

85. Kochanek PM, Safar PJ: Therapeutic hypothermia for severe traumatic brain injury. *JAMA* 2003;289:3007-3009.

86. Adelson PD, Ragheb J, Kanev P, et al: Phase II clinical trial of moderate hypothermia after severe traumatic brain injury in children. *Neurosurgery* 2005;56:740-754.

87. Tiainen M, Roine RO, Pettila V, et al: Serum neuron-specific enolase and S-100B protein in cardiac arrest patients treated with hypothermia. *Stroke* 2003;34:2881-2886.

88. Akhtar JI, Spear RM, Senac MO, et al: Detection of traumatic brain injury with magnetic resonance imaging and S-100B protein in children, despite normal computed tomography of the brain. *Pediatr Crit Care Med* 2003;4:322-326.

89. Berger R: Biomarkers or neuroimaging in central nervous system injury: will the real "gold standard" please stand up? *Pediatr Crit Care Med* 2003;4:391-392.

90. Ingebrigtsen T, Waterloo K, Jacobsen EA, et al: Traumatic brain damage in minor head injury: relation of serum S-100 protein measurements to magnetic resonance imaging and neurobehavioral outcome. *Neurosurgery* 1999;45:468-475.

91. Giza CC, Mink RB, Madikians A: Pediatric traumatic brain injury: not just little adults. *Curr Opin Crit Care* 2007;13:143-152.

92. Wagner AK, Hammond FM, Sasser HC, et al: Use of injury severity variables in determining disability and community integration after traumatic brain injury. *J Trauma* 2000;49:411-419.

93. Zafonte RD, Mann NR, Millis SR, et al: Posttraumatic amnesia: its relation to functional outcome. *Arch Phys Med Rehabil* 1997;78:1103-1106.

94. Cifu DX, Keyser-Marcus L, Lopez E, et al: Acute predictors of successful return to work 1 year after traumatic brain injury: a multicenter analysis. *Arch Phys Med Rehabil* 1997;78:125-131.

95. Keyser-Marcus LA, Bricout JC, Wehman P, et al: Acute predictors of return to employment after traumatic brain injury: a longitudinal follow-up. *Arch Phys Med Rehabil* 2002;83:635-641.

96. Feickert HJ, Drommer S, Heyer R: Severe head injury in children: impact of risk factors on outcome. *J Trauma* 1999;47:33-38.

97. Carter BG, Butt W: A prospective study of outcome predictors after severe brain injury in children. *Int Care Med* 2005;31:840-845.

98. Ong L, Selladurai BM, Dhillon MK, et al: The prognostic value of the Glasgow Coma Scale, hypoxia and computerised tomography in outcome prediction of pediatric head injury. *Pediatr Neurosurg* 1996;24:285-291.

99. McCullagh S, Oucherlony D, Protzner A, et al: Prediction of neuropsychiatric outcome following mild trauma brain injury: an examination of the Glasgow Coma Scale. *Brain Inj* 2001;15:489-497.

100. Mussack T, Kirchhoff C, Buhmann S, et al: Significance of Elecsys S100 immunoassay for real-time assessment of traumatic brain damage in multiple trauma patients. *Clin Chem Lab Med* 2006;44:1140-1145

101. Spinella PC, Dominguez T, Drott HR, et al: S-100 beta protein-serum levels in healthy children and its association with outcome in pediatric traumatic brain injury. *Crit Care Med* 2003;31:939-945.

102. Berger RP, Beers SR, Richichi R, et al: Serum biomarker concentrations and outcome after pediatric traumatic brain injury. *J Neurotrauma* 2007;24:1793-1801.

103. Piazza O, Storti MP, Cotena S, et al: S100B is not a reliable prognostic index in paediatric TBI. *Pediatr Neurosurg* 2007;43:258-264.

Conditions Confused with Head Trauma

Christopher S. Greeley, MD

INTRODUCTION

A cornerstone in the evaluation of suspected victims of abusive head trauma (AHT) is awareness of conditions with the potential to mimic findings seen in AHT. There are published guidelines for evaluation of children who are suspected to be victims of child abuse that can be used to guide medical professionals' evaluation of clinical and historical information.[1] The reported differential diagnosis of AHT is expansive.[2,3] It is important to recognize that the majority of the conditions cited are not true mimics of AHT, but instead are conditions in which intracranial bleeding and/or retinal bleeding have been described as a feature of their clinical spectrum (no matter how rare). This chapter does not focus on every possible condition in which intracranial or retinal hemorrhaging can occur, but instead discusses those conditions with findings that can truly be misconstrued as AHT.

Most conditions that mimic AHT fall into one of two categories. First are rare conditions that have clinical findings that can be mistaken for those seen in AHT. Second are relatively common conditions that rarely present with findings that also occur in AHT. In a convenience sample of 50 children mistakenly diagnosed with child abuse, the most common misstep was falsely attributing a normal finding, or normal variant, as being an inflicted injury. Dermal melanosis (Mongolian spots), impetigo, hemangiomata, and diaper dermatitis were the most common diagnoses.[4] A third possible category of mimics includes conditions that have been hypothesized as having features similar to AHT, but have limited clinical support for being true mimics. An example of this is scurvy. Scurvy (vitamin C deficiency) is cited as a mimic of AHT,[5] but a comprehensive medical evaluation, along with an understanding of the medical literature about and clinical features of scurvy will readily resolve any reasonable questions.

Contributing to confusion with AHT is the imprecise use of clinical terms. Terms such as "subdural hematoma," "retinal hemorrhage," and "rib fracture" can be used indiscriminately without more detailed descriptors. Improved precision of language will decrease the likelihood of incorrectly diagnosing AHT. For example, although retinal hemorrhages (RHs) in general have a very high level of specificity for AHT, the differential diagnosis for *any* RH is vast.[3,6] Precision of language and understanding of pathophysiology, in addition to a thorough understanding of the clinical literature, will facilitate accurately distinguishing AHT from potential mimics.

COAGULOPATHY AND HEMOSTASIS DEFECTS

Many coagulopathies can present with intracranial hemorrhage (ICH) as a clinical feature. The medical literature cites many case reports in which a true coagulopathy was diagnosed initially as a traumatic injury.[4,7-14] Of the major bleeding disorders, Vitamin K deficiency and Factor XIII deficiency are the most representative.

Vitamin K Deficiency

Vitamin K is a fat-soluble vitamin required for the carboxylation of certain clotting factors (II, VII, IX, X) in humans.[15] Vitamin K deficiency bleeding (VKDB) is one of the most commonly reported mimics of AHT.[7,9-12,14] It was initially described by Townsend[16] in 1894. At birth, the newborn pool of vitamin K is less than that required for robust production of vitamin K–dependent clotting factors. In the vast majority of infants, this relative lack of vitamin K stores remains clinically imperceptible,[15] although most symptomatic infants present within the first week of life. In 1939, administration of vitamin K was demonstrated to dramatically reduce the incidence of this potentially fatal condition.[17] The clinical manifestation of VKDB traditionally has been characterized by the timing of presentation: early (<24 hours of life), classic (1–7 days), and late (2–12 weeks). Typical symptoms of VKDB include rectal bleeding, bruising, hematemasis, and hemoptysis. The major source of vitamin K for the neonate is dietary. Maternal vitamin K deficiency can contribute to the development of VKDB in the fetus and newborn.[18,19] Medical conditions that impair the infant's absorption of vitamin K can increase the risk of VKDB in an infant. These include biliary atresia, liver dysfunction, cystic fibrosis, α-1-antitrypsin deficiency, malabsorption, and Alagille's syndrome.[20-23] Importantly, medications or exposure to toxins also need to be considered.[24,25]

In most developed nations, the vast majority of infants receive oral or intramuscular vitamin K supplementation. Vitamin K replacement has been shown to lower the incidence of ICH caused by VKDB.[26] The intramuscular route of administration is the preferred route because of reports of infants receiving only oral supplementation who have developed ICH from VKDB.[21,27-29] The administration of vitamin K does not completely prevent the development of VKDB,[23,30] or ICH from VKDB,[27] but the rates are dramatically lower.[21]

Breast milk provides inadequate vitamin K for the nursing infant. Infants fed cows' milk-based formula have a much lower risk of VKDB than those who are strictly breast fed. Breastfeeding increases the risk of VKDB in infants who have not received perinatal vitamin K supplementation.[14,23,28,31-34] Infants who have received parenteral vitamin K and are breast fed will have coagulation profiles similar to those infants who have received vitamin K and are bottle fed.[35] Although common in European countries, oral administration of vitamin K also has less of a protective effect than does parenteral administration.[27]

The most common presentation of the early form of VKDB is profound and potentially fatal intracranial bleeding.[12,15,36,37] Recent data support ICH (most commonly, subarachnoid hemorrhage) from VKDB as being limited to the first 12 weeks of life,[37] unless an underlying medical condition or hepatic disease is present.[11,14,20,21,28,30,31,33,34] In infants with VKDB-related ICH, RHs are rarely seen.[11,38] Whereas RHs have been noted in children with ICH from VKDB, no cases of retinoschisis or retinal folds have been reported. Infants with ICH from VKDB will have abnormal coagulation studies (PT, aPTT) including an elevated level of protein induced in vitamin K absence (PIVKA-II).[14,27,31] There have been no reported cases of ICH from VKDB in infants with normal PT, aPTT and PIVKA.

Factor XIII Deficiency

Factor XIII (FXIII) is found both in plasma and on platelets, and it is the last enzyme in the coagulation/thrombosis cascade. It has two major functions: to cross link fibrin monomers (essential in clot formation) and to cross-link α_2-antiplasmin to fibrin (essential in clot stability).[39] FXIII deficiency was first described in 1960[40] and is another recognized cause of bleeding in children to be mistaken for AHT.[8] The "classic" presentation of FXIII deficiency is delayed or prolonged bleeding from the umbilical stump (seen in >80% of infants with FXIII deficiency), along with delayed umbilical cord separation and bleeding during circumcision.[8,39,41,42] Although the majority of affected infants will have umbilical stump bleeding, the absence of this historical finding does not exclude the diagnosis.[43] As with most inherited disorders, consanguinity increases the risk of FXIII deficiency. Although most bleeding in FXIII deficiency involves the skin and soft tissues, the incidence of ICH is higher than that seen in other factor deficiencies.[39] ICH is the cause of death in 30% of those who die from hemorrhagic complications of their FXIII deficiency.[43] Since FXIII is integral to clot stability by protecting against dissolution, affected individuals are subject to prolonged and recurrent bleeding from a single event.[43] Although ICH has been described in children and adults with mildly suppressed levels (10-30% FXIII activity),[13,44] it is generally accepted that FXIII deficiency usually becomes clinically apparent with levels of less than 5% activity.[39] In the reported cases of infants and children with ICH in the presence of FXIII deficiency, RHs are either not mentioned,[8,13,41,44] or described as not present.[45] FXIII deficiency cannot be identified by routine coagulation testing (i.e., PT and aPTT); specific testing is required.

Hemophilia A (Factor VIII Deficiency)

The most common inherited coagulopathy that causes ICH is classic hemophilia A.[36] Birth-related ICH in hemophilia A occurs in 3% to 8% of those infants later found to have the condition, with mortality reported to be as high as 33%.[36,46,47] Early reports of the presence of ICH caused by birth in infants without an identified bleeding disorders stated that it occurred in approximately 0.11% of births,[46] although recent MRI studies of nonsymptomatic, normal newborns have shown much higher prevalences.[48,49] ICH in newborns can be the presenting symptom of infants with hemophilia A. More importantly, 1.9% of newborns with hemophilia A had *only* ICH without other clinical comorbidities. In older infants with hemophilia A, ICH presents without a history of trauma approximately 10% of the time, with those who have more severe hemophilia accounting for the majority. The diagnosis is usually not in question since these children all have profoundly abnormal coagulation studies (i.e., PT and aPTT).

Von Willebrand Disease

Von Willebrand disease (vWD) is the most common coagulopathy worldwide.[50] The majority with this condition have mild disease and are identified on asymptomatic routine screening (e.g., preoperative evaluation of coagulation). Broadly, vWD is classified into types 1, 2, and 3, with 80% of those affected having type 1. The diagnosis of vWD can be complex or nuanced, often involving relative levels of von Willebrand factor (vWF), von Willebrand factor ristocetin cofactor (vWF:RCo), and Factor VIII (FVIII). Given the importance of vWF in platelet function, testing for platelet defects can often reveal vWD.[51,52]

Compared with hemophilia A, vWD is not a commonly identified cause of ICH or RH in newborns and infants. One survey of the medical literature revealed only 23 reported cases of intracranial bleeding associated with vWD.[53] In a series of 42 boys with vWD,[54] one ICH was identified, a posttraumatic SDH in a 15-month-old who fell while running. Wetzstein and colleagues[55] reported a term newborn who presented with SDH and transverse sinus thrombosis who was subsequently diagnosed with vWD type 3. On presentation, the infant had a prolonged aPTT. Of note, the neonate did not receive vitamin K at birth. Only three reported cases of retinal bleeding associated with vWD exist.[56,57] These were in individuals 13, 19, and 33 years of age, none of whom had a history of trauma. There are no published reports of vWD being associated with RHs, retinoschisis, or retinal folds in infants or children.

Trauma-Related Coagulopathy

The presence of abnormal coagulation studies in children and adults with traumatic brain injury (TBI) is well described.[58-61] A meta-analysis of recently published reports identified an overall prevalence of coagulation abnormalities of 32.7% in patients with TBI, with reports of incidence as high as 60% in those with severe TBI.[60] In children specifically, the rate of coagulopathy associated with TBI has been reported to be as high as 77%.[61] Exposure of brain parenchyma to the circulation can initiate a cascade of both fibrinolysis and thrombosis. Systemic hypoperfusion likely plays an important role in augmenting the coagulopathy associated with TBI.[62] This cascade can be local and self limited, or it can lead to disseminated intravascular coagulation (DIC). The extent of resulting DIC is correlated to the severity of the brain injury.[59-61] The presence of other systemic injuries does not affect the likelihood of TBI resulting in a coagulopathy.[61] A prospective study of adults with TBI found a significant correlation between the serum level of fibrin degradation products (FDPs) and the severity of TBI.[59] As the FDP level increased, the prognosis worsened. Similar data were reported in a population of children diagnosed with AHT.[58] Hypoxia alone with normal perfusion (and without TBI) would not be expected to cause DIC (e.g., near-drowning). Prolonged hypoxia with systemic hypoperfusion, however, can itself trigger DIC. DIC can result in a nonspecific pattern of RHs.[63] However, retinal folds and retinoschisis do not occur in DIC alone without trauma as a component.

Coagulopathy associated with TBI has been described in children with AHT.[58] In the presence of concerning skeletal findings or historical data, brain injury with coagulopathy could be due to trauma. A normal FDP in a child with ICH would indicate the blood not being due to TBI-associated coagulopathy.[59]

Platelet Disorders

Defects of platelet function or number can be responsible for bruising or bleeding with routine activities. The most common clinical findings seen in children with abnormalities of platelets are mucocutaneous bleeding (e.g., epistaxis), ecchymoses, purpurae, and hemorrhagic surgical complications.[64,65] It is important to consider both the number and function of platelets in the evaluation of a platelet disorder. A normal platelet count is between 150,000 and 400,000 per mm^3. Size and shape of the platelets can be assessed by microscopic evaluation of the peripheral smear. In addition, there are functional tests available to investigate qualitative platelet defects (see below). An excellent guide outlining all platelet disorders and their clinical spectra is available.[64]

The most common pathological cause of bruising in childhood is idiopathic thrombocytopenic purpura (ITP). ITP is a self-limited autoimmune disease that results in destruction of platelets and is the most common coagulopathy mistaken for abuse.[4,7,10] Serious bleeding is very uncommon in children with ITP, although ICH can occur, specifically when platelet counts drop below 10,000 per mm^3.[66] RHs have been very rarely reported in children with ITP.[58,67] ITP should not be mistaken for abuse, since the definitive diagnostic test—a platelet count—is readily available and should be part of the very basic evaluation of a child with bleeding or bruising.

The two most common platelet dysfunction conditions in children are Glanzmann thrombasthenia (GT) and Hermansky-Pudlak syndrome (HPS). Although there are case reports of these conditions being mistaken for child abuse,[10,68] coagulation studies were abnormal in both instances. In GT, a surface platelet fibrinogen receptor defect results in poor platelet-platelet clumping (and clot formation). Most affected patients present with epistaxis, bruising, gingival bleeding,

and petechiae; ICH is rare.[64] Ocular findings are also quite rare in GT, and RHs have not been reported.[69]

HPS is often cited as a potential cause of retinal hemorrhaging in children. Only one report exists of an infant with HPS who had retinal and subdural hemorrhages.[68] In this report, a 7-week-old presented with seizure activity and was found to have an occipital SDH. The infant was found to have fewer than a dozen posterior pole hemorrhages on the right and a single macular hemorrhage on the left. The ocular findings (strabismus and nystagmus) in HPS are dependent upon the retinal pigment and macular function; the vascular integrity is not affected.[70] HPS is usually not a diagnostic dilemma, since affected individuals have albinism.

What Evaluation Should Be Performed to Rule Out Coagulopathy in Suspected Abuse Cases?

Inherited coagulopathies are a small but important cause of ICH in children. It is worth noting that the presence of a bleeding disorder does not preclude the diagnosis of AHT. One study of 50 children referred to a hematology service in Edinburgh, Scotland with suspected nonaccidental injury found eight (16%) with coagulation abnormalities.[9] The authors highlight that of the eight children, seven were confirmed to have been abused, with four of those having normalization of their screening tests upon repeat examination. Many general reviews of appropriate coagulopathy testing in suspected cases of abusive injuries have been published.[9,10,71-74] A detailed history and physical examination is the cornerstone for identification of a coagulopathy. An extensive history should include family history, medication history, prior hospitalization or surgeries, consanguinity, dietary history, and recurrent miscarriages in family members. For neonates and infants, a specific history of vitamin K administration and route is crucial. A history of umbilical stump bleeding and prolonged period to cord separation should be noted. A meticulous review of systems should include unexplained bruising, prolonged bleeding, epistaxis, gingival bleeding, and menorrhagia. The laboratory evaluation of a potential bleeding disorder should be carried out after all of this information is gathered.

An initial screening panel of labs should include the following:

- Complete blood count (CBC), with a platelet count
- Review of a peripheral smear (for assessment of platelet size and form)
- Activated partial thromboplastin time (aPTT)
- Prothrombin time (PT)
- Protein induced in vitamin K absence (PIVKA-II) (for infants under 3 months)

This initial battery of tests should exclude any significant predisposition to bleeding or severe factor deficiency.[74] However, some conditions might have a normal initial screening evaluation but may still be clinically relevant. These include mild hemophilia (A or B), FXIII deficiency, mild vWD, or functional platelet disorders.[64,74] If a bleeding predisposition is still a clinical concern, a secondary panel of labs should include:

- Specific Factor levels (specifically FXI and FVIII levels)
- Factor XIII activity level
- vWF antigen level
- vWF ristocetin cofactor assay (vWF:RCo)
- Platelet function testing (i.e., PFA-100)
- Thrombin time (TT)
- Fibrinogen assay

PIVKA-II

Historically, vitamin K deficiency was identified by correction of an elevated PT after administration of vitamin K. Currently, testing for vitamin K deficiency can be done in two ways: measuring serum vitamin K levels, and measuring levels of proteins induced in vitamin K absence (PIVKA-II).[15,75] Vitamin K levels do not correlate to the state of coagulopathy and can be misleading. PIVKA-II testing identifies an undercarboxylated prothrombin protein present in the serum of children who are vitamin K deficient.[75] PIVKA-II can be detectable in approximately 25% of all newborns, term or preterm.[75] PIVKA-II can be detected in up to 50% of cord blood samples while vitamin K levels in cord blood are negligible.[76] After parenteral vitamin K administration, PIVKA-II levels will be universally undetectable within 2 weeks, but vitamin K might not result in complete PIVKA-II suppression.[27] In vitamin K deficiency, PIVKA-II will be elevated prior to elevation of the PT or aPTT.[77] Medications (e.g., warfarin) or malabsorption (e.g., cystic fibrosis or liver disease) can result in elevated PIVKA-II despite a normal dietary vitamin K intake.

Since there are other causes of PT elevation, it is not a sensitive screen for vitamin K deficiency, but it can be used to screen for coagulopathy resulting from vitamin K deficiency. There have been no reported cases of VKDB in children with normal PIVKA-II.

Platelet Function Testing

Rarely, screening tests can miss a clinically relevant bleeding predisposition caused by platelet dysfunction. An excellent review of specific platelet conditions and their testing has recently been published.[64] Platelet functioning has historically been tested by an Ivy bleeding time (BT). The BT is performed by a technician using a standardized template creating a 10-mm long and 1-mm deep incision, typically on the forearm. As an operator-dependent test, BT results are difficult to standardize. The sensitivity and specificity of BT for identifying a bleeding disorder are unacceptably low.[52,78] For these reasons, in addition to the risk of scaring and infection, BT should no longer be part of routine coagulation testing in children. Platelet aggregometry testing is a series of challenge tests to patient whole-blood or serum. The patient sample is placed with aggregation agonists (i.e., ristocetin, thrombin), and time to platelet clumping is measured. Platelet response to *ex vivo* vascular shear injury is measured by the platelet function analyzer (PFA-100) (Dade Behring, Marburg, Germany).[51,74,79] This test uses collagen membranes over which the patient's citrated blood flows as an attempt to duplicate vascular injury. Time to cessation of flow is measured, with a prolonged time being abnormal.[65] Since this test measures occlusion of flow through a column, thrombocytopenia and anemia can confound the test results.

Because of significant overlap of reported normal ranges, true pathology (i.e., subtle qualitative platelet disorders) can be missed.[74] Any abnormal PFA-100 test needs to be clarified as to the precise abnormality. As noted earlier, platelet function testing can identify children with vWD.[51,52,79] In addition, testing with platelet flow cytometry and platelet nucleotide content is available but requires the guidance of an experienced pediatric hematologist.

Testing for Factor XIII Deficiency

Since FXIII is involved in clot formation and stability and is terminal in the coagulation cascade, PT and aPTT testing are normal in patients with FXIII deficiency, even with a profound predisposition to bleeding.[39,42,71] Patients with FXIII deficiency will have an unstable clot formed when placed in the $5M$ urea solution. The clot then stabilizes with the addition of normal serum.[41] Patients with normal PT, aPTT, and TT who have an abnormal clot solubility test are presumptively diagnosed with FXIII deficiency. The clot solubility test is a qualitative test and might only be positive in patients who have complete absence of FXIII. Although most people with inherited FXIII deficiency will be identified via this method, a quantitative FXIII assay might be beneficial.[39,80] In evaluating children with catastrophic ICH from an unknown etiology, testing for FXIII deficiency by clot solubility testing, FXIII assay, or both might identify rare cases of this deficiency. Of note, patients with FXIII do not form fibrin degradation products, since fibrin linkages are not formed. Hence, the presence of fibrin degredation products rules out significant FXIII deficiency.

TRAUMATIC EVENTS MISDIAGNOSED AS ABUSIVE HEAD TRAUMA

Accidents

One of the most common alternative explanations provided for AHT is that of a household accident, most typically a fall.[81] To fully appreciate the difference between the findings in AHT and those occurring in common household accidents, it is helpful to understand both the frequency of serious or fatal injuries from falls, as well as the specific injuries that usually occur with household accidents.

Serious and fatal injuries from household falls can and do occur, albeit rarely. Household accidents result in serious or fatal injuries at a rate that is markedly less than nonfatal or trivial injuries. This can be best appreciated by examining national data on fatalities in the United States. In 2004, the Centers for Disease Control and Prevention published the "Surveillance for Fatal and Nonfatal Injuries—United States, 2001 Report."[82] The data show that in 2001, there were 55 fatal falls in children 0 to 4 years of age in a population of 20 million children. In contrast, there were 1,039,275 emergency department (ED) visits for nonfatal falls. If it is estimated that the average toddler falls four times per week (with infants falling markedly less and school-aged children falling more than four times a week), then these 20 million children sustain over 1 billion falls per year. These falls resulted in 55 fatalities and more than 1 million ED visits. This rarity of fatal injuries from falls is consistent with another large study of over 11,000 infants.[83]

Studies of witnessed falls in children have indicated that short falls can occasionally result in skull and clavicle fractures, but serious or fatal injuries are unexpected.[84-87] It is important to recognize that the term "fall" is nonspecific and complex falls that can indeed injure children do occur. The two most common examples of complex falls are falls that involve stairs and falls that involve infant walkers. Falls involving stairways increase the risk for extremity injuries.[88,89] Falls involving walkers increase the likelihood of a severe brain injury.[90,91]

Denton and Mileusnic[92] reported a case of a 9-month-old who was noted to have a fatal short fall from a bed and who had a lucid interval of approximately 72 hours. Although this is an intriguing report, attributing the fatal intracranial injuries to the only witnessed fall is speculation. Given the long period between the witnessed event and death, there might have been other injuries (unwitnessed or inflicted) that could have exacerbated, or even been solely responsible for, the terminal injuries.

Plunkett[93] published a report on 18 deaths reported to the U.S. Consumer Product Safety Commission National Injury Information Clearinghouse. This database included information on reports of 75,000 injuries to children on playground equipment. Of the 18 fatalities reviewed, none were infants. Of the five deaths under 2 years of age, only one was witnessed. A 23-month-old who was videotaped falling off playground equipment was reported to be normal for approximately 5 minutes and then became obtunded. She was reported to have bilateral RHs (not further described but noted in the presence of papilledema) and an acute SDH. Most of the falls reported were from greater than 1.5 meters and were onto hard surfaces. Several involved children on swings or children with complicating preexisting conditions.

The entirety of the medical literature on injuries from falls in otherwise normal children indicates that fatal or devastating intracranial injuries from short falls are a profoundly rare event.[94] This is confirmed by Chadwick et al[95] in which the authors identified six such instances in a population of 2.5 million children.

Birth-Related Head Injuries

Injuries from the birthing process have been described since antiquity. Birth-related fatalities occur in 3.1 per every 1000 births.[96] Traumatic birth-related head injuries have been estimated to affect 3.1% of pregnancies.[97] Recognition of birth-related clavicular fractures and cervical nerve root palsies occasionally occur. Although the vast majority of neonates remain unscathed by the birthing process, significant injuries can rarely occur. Many more will have transient birth-related findings or injuries that resolve. The history in conjunction with the physical examination would readily exclude AHT from the differential. One series of 57,600 deliveries identified 17 cases of intracranial bleeding.[97] In only two of these cases was the delivery described as uneventful and free of instrumentation. Neonates with underlying medical (i.e., VKDB) or anatomical conditions (e.g., arachnoid cysts[98]) that could predispose to ICH would typically present in the newborn period with imaging or neurological findings supporting these conditions.

Whitby et al[99] published a report of 111 term babies who had brain MRI performed within 48 hours of birth. Nine of the 111 babies (8.1%) were found to have SDHs, all of which were clinically silent. Repeat MRI scans at 4 weeks of life demonstrated complete resolution of the intracranial blood without any residual collections or parenchymal injury. The authors conclude that SDHs that result from uneventful births are not clinically significant. These findings were confirmed by Vinchon et al.[97] Similarly, Looney et al[48] evaluated 88 infants with a 3.0T MRI at an average age of 3 weeks. Seventeen infants (26%) had ICH; 16 SDH, 2 SAH, and 6 parenchymal hemorrhage. The authors conclude that the birth-related ICHs are of a different pattern, such that mistaking them for AHT-associated intracranial bleeding is unlikely. Rooks et al[49] recently reported on 101 asymptomatic infants who received cranial MRIs within 72 hours of birth. Sixty-one percent had SDH, all in the posterior portion of the head. When followed up to 2 years of age, all had no physical signs or symptoms of head injury. All SDH resolved by 3 months of age.

RHs occur in up to one third of births[100,101] and have been described in multiple retinal layers.[101,102] RHs were most commonly seen in normal vaginal deliveries.[99] All of the hemorrhages noted by Hughes et al[100] were intraretinal, and in 51 of the 53 neonates, the hemorrhages resolved within 16 days. In the other two neonates the RHs were noted at 31 and 58 days; both had been delivered with vacuum assistance. Emerson et al[101] found that 86% of all RHs resolved within 2 weeks of birth, and all intraretinal hemorrhages by 1 month. The only hemorrhage noted at 4 weeks was a single subretinal hemorrhage that was not present at 6 weeks. RHs that are present after the first month of life are unlikely to be from birth.

OTHER CONDITIONS POSSIBLY MISTAKEN FOR AHT

Intracranial Fluid Collections

Physicians sometimes encounter a child with an enlarging head circumference who, upon head imaging, is noted to have large anterior hypodense, or mixed-density, collections. The differential diagnosis of large anterior hypodense collections includes chronic subdural hematomas, subdural hygroma, benign extraaxial fluid collection of infancy, or frontal cortical atrophy. Given the imprecision of the language used in the medical literature, limited information exists on accurately discriminating amongst these conditions in infants. What is clear from the literature is that in certain infants, the arachnoid space is larger than typical.[103-105]

Benign extraaxial fluid collection of infancy (BEAF) is asymptomatic and is often identified as an incidental finding on CT imaging. It likely represents a temporary imbalance between CSF production and absorption.[106] CT scanning alone is not able to reliably distinguish BEAF from a chronic subdural collection. Since BEAF is not traumatic in origin, a subdural neomembrane will not form. Subdural neomembranes are seen in infants and children with chronic SDH from either trauma or infection.[107,108] The neomembrane can be seen on autopsy, intraoperatively during surgery for ICH draining, or on contrast-augmented CT imaging. Because of the finer details on MRI scanning, neomembranes can also be identified on noncontrast MRI images.[109-111] The presence of a neomembrane would indicate that a hypodense collection is not uncomplicated BEAF. Much controversy exists about whether BEAF predisposes an infant to hemorrhage with routine care or after a trivial injury.[112,113] A recent finite element study demonstrated that increased extraaxial fluid in the subarachnoid space could actually *increase* the stability of bridging vessels and decrease the likelihood of subdural bleeding after injury.[114] This issue has not currently been resolved. Parenchymal, intraventricular, and retinal hemorrhages have not been reported with BEAF.

Infants can have mixed-density subdural collection identified on head imaging. Mixed-density collections have historically been described as being indicative of evidence of two distinct episodes of injury or bleeding ("acute on chronic"). Mixed-density collections, however, can appear either after a single significant traumatic event or with rebleeding of a chronic SDH. Single isolated traumatic events can result in an admixture of CSF and acute blood, giving the appearance of either rebleeding into a chronic collection, or multiple episodes of trauma.[115-117] The admixture of CSF and blood likely occurs via a tear in the arachnoid.[117,118] *Hyperacute* SDH can also appear to have multiple layers, perhaps representing the settling out of red blood cells, separating solid components of blood from serum.[119]

Chronic SDH in children can develop either as a maturation of an acute SDH[107,108] or as a result of extreme prematurity.[120] Chronic SDHs have also been described in neonates, likely the result of an intrauterine insult.[121,122] Acute intracranial bleeding in an infant presenting with a preexisiting chronic SDH raises the concern of reinjury as the cause of the fresh blood.

Trivial rebleeding into preexisting chronic SDH has been well described in animal models and adults.[123] This rebleeding occurs as a result of oozing from the outer subdural neomembrane and can be exacerbated by a new injury.[107,108,123,124] Because of open cranial sutures, bleeding from trivial oozing would not typically cause neurological symptoms. Since the bleeding from a chronic SDH is *intrahematoma*, intraparenchymal, intraventricular, or bleeding remote from the chronic SDH (i.e., RHs) could not be attributable to the preexisting collection.

Scurvy

Scurvy is the clinical manifestation of vitamin C deficiency. The typical findings of scurvy are generalized perifollicular petechial bleeding, commonly involving the lower extremities, associated with gingival hypertrophy and bleeding,[125-128] with 80% of the affected having anemia.[125] Pseudoparalysis caused by lower extremity pain and edema is a common feature. Because of poor collagen formation, affected individuals often have poor wound healing with hair that breaks easily and is described as "corkscrew."[126] The abnormal hair is similar to that found in Menke's disease, which is discussed below. Bone demineralization with preservation of the zones of provisional calcification (Frankel lines) along with Pelkan spurs (healing fractures through the zone of provisional calcification) are characteristic radiographic findings.[125,126,128] Additional radiographic findings include periosteal elevation from subperiosteal bleeding and linear epiphyseal lines (Wimberger ring).[125,126] ICHs in scurvy are quite rare. The review of the literature by Gilman and Tanzer[127] of ICH associated with scurvy identifies 13 definitive cases. Seven of

these were SDHs and five of the seven were in an infant or child. Of the reports described, all of the infants and children had additional unmistakable findings associated with scurvy.

Ophthalmological findings in scurvy are usually hemorrhagic in nature. Hemorrhage can occur in or around the orbit or in the globe. Conjunctival hemorrhage is the most common ophthalmological finding in scurvy.[129-132] Rare RHs have been described in adults with scurvy.[133,134] The adult patients reported in the literature had prolonged abnormal dietary history and exhibited extensive nonophthalmological manifestations of scurvy as well, such as cutaneous hemorrhage, cork-screw hairs, and gingival hypertrophy with bleeding. Only one report exists of RHs noted in a child with scurvy.[129] This 3-year-old child had induced dietary scurvy and presented with unilateral proptosis from a periosteal orbital hematoma. He had ipsilateral SRH and retinal detachment as well as other physical and radiographic stigmata of scurvy.

The diagnosis of scurvy in infants and children is largely clinical since testing for functional vitamin C deficiency is imprecise and clinically difficult. The most reasonable criterion for diagnosing symptomatic scurvy is rapid clinical response to appropriate vitamin C replacement.[128,129]

Severe and fatal cases of scurvy in infants and children have been described, including subdural and retinal hemorrhages, but clinical features characteristic of scurvy are always apparent.[129,135] Notably, there have been no reports in the medical literature of an infant whose only manifestation of scurvy was subdural and retinal hemorrhages, without cutaneous bruising, gingival changes, or bone and joint findings on examination or radiograph. Absent other findings, the diagnosis of scurvy would be purely speculative.

Glutaric Aciduria, Type 1

Glutaric acidemia type 1 (or "glutaric aciduria type 1," [GA1]) is an autosomal recessive metabolic disorder resulting from a mutation in the gene encoding the enzyme glutaryl-CoA dehydrogenase.[136] The enzymatic defect results in a significant movement disorder caused by basal ganglia neuronal loss. The neuronal loss can present with sudden encephalopathy after, or in conjunction with, a mild illness. This is often seen in the first 2 years of life. Prior to neurological decompensation, initial symptoms are minimal, with an increased head circumference in infancy (but not at birth) being a real but subtle finding.[136,137] Although the genetic mutation can be seen in many ethnicities, it has been noted to occur most prominently in those with northern European lineage.

The brain loss seen in GA1 can result in significant cerebral atrophy. The pattern of atrophy is quite typical and classically involves widening of the Sylvian fissures, regression of the temporal lobes, and characteristic lesions noted in the basal ganglia.[136] The cerebral atrophy results in expanded arachnoid and subdural spaces with the potential for hemorrhaging. Although SDHs are a described feature of GA1, they have not been described in the absence of frontal atrophy.[138] Retinal hemorrhaging (but not retinal folds or retinoschisis) has also been noted in up to 20% of children affected by GA1.[136,139,140]

GA1 has been reported as being mistaken for AHT.[136,138,141] Since affected children present with sudden, catastrophic, and seemingly unexplained collapse and can have acute and chronic subdural blood collections and RHs, inflicted injury would be an obvious concern. Since fractures are not a feature of GA1, the presence of any fractures would be of great importance in excluding this diagnosis. GA1 is diagnosed by testing urine for quantitative organic acids. High urinary levels of glutaric acid or 3-hydroxyglutaric acid are diagnostic in affected children. If urine testing is abnormal, specific enzyme assays can be required to identify the precise enzymatic defect.

Menkes Disease

Menkes disease (MD) has also been reported as a potential mimic of AHT.[142,143] Menkes disease, often called Menkes kinky hair syndrome, is an X-linked recessive disease resulting from a mutation that codes a copper transport enzyme.[144] The defect results in a systemic deficit of copper and subsequent global dysfunction of copper-dependent enzymes. This most notably results in poor collagen and elastin formation. Clinical hallmarks of MD are rapid and early neurological degeneration (within months of birth), poor growth, skeletal findings, and characteristic hair (pili torti). The hair in MD is short, friable, and twisted and has poor pigment, although fetal hair is unaffected. Blood vessels are tortuous and friable and are susceptible to rupture and bleeding with routine activities. This can result in intraabdominal or intracranial hemorrhage.[142,144] The skeletal manifestations include Wormian bones and metaphyseal defects (similar to the classic metaphyseal lesions associated with child physical abuse).[145] Long bone metaphyseal findings can also resemble those found in scurvy. The combination of ICH and metaphyseal fractures can pose as findings very similar to those of AHT.

The most common ophthalmologic findings described in MD include poor visual acuity and decreased retinal and iris pigmentation. RHs have not been a described feature of "classic" MD and thus may be crucial in distinguishing this condition from AHT.[146] Testing for MD can be done by simply microscopically examining scalp hairs for the characteristic pili torti. In addition, serum copper ceruloplasmin levels will be profoundly depressed. Infants with MD also have characteristic facies, including a high-arched palate, flat central face, and hypoplastic mandibles.

CONCLUSION

Abusive head injury is devastating to a child and family. Although medical providers can miss the findings of AHT,[81] there also exists instances when AHT is misdiagnosed. As noted earlier, many instances of misdiagnosed AHT have been reported, but the true degree to which it occurs is not definitely known. To minimize the misdiagnosis of AHT, medical providers need to be very familiar with, and able to comfortably exclude, a multitude of real and potential mimics.

References

1. Kellogg N and the Committee on Child Abuse and Neglect: Evaluation of suspected child physical abuse. *Pediatrics* 2007;119;1232-1241.
2. Fernando S, Obaldo RE, Walsh IR, et al: Neuroimaging of nonaccidental head trauma: pitfalls and controversies. *Pediatr Radiol* 2008;38:827-838.
3. David T: Non-accidental head injury—the evidence. *Pediatr Radiol* 2008;38:S370-S377.
4. Wheeler DM, Hobbs CJ: Mistakes in diagnosing non-accidental injury: 10 years' experience. *Br Med J* 1988;296:1233-1236.
5. Clemetson CAB: Is it "shaken baby" or Barlow's disease variant? *J Am Physicians Surg* 2004;9:78-80.
6. Levin AV: Retinal haemorrhages and child abuse. *In:* David TJ (ed): *Recent Advances in Paediatrics*, ed 18. Churchill Livingstone, Edinburgh, 2000, pp 151–219.
7. Harley JR: Disorders of coagulation misdiagnosed as nonaccidental bruising. *Pediatr Emerg Care* 1997;13:347-349.
8. Newman RS, Jalili M, Kolls BJ, et al: Factor XIII deficiency mistaken for battered child syndrome: case of "correct" test ordering negated by a commonly accepted qualitative test with limited negative predictive value. *Am J Hematol* 2002;71:328-330.
9. O'Hare AE, Eden OB: Bleeding disorders and non-accidental injury. *Arch Dis Child* 1984;59:860-864.
10. Taylor GP: Severe bleeding disorders in children with normal coagulation screening tests. *Br Med J* 1982;284:1851-1852.
11. Wetzel RC, Slater AJ, Dover GJ: Fatal intramuscular bleeding misdiagnosed as suspected nonaccidental injury. *Pediatrics* 1995;95:771-773.
12. Fenton LZ, Sirotnak AP, Handler MH: Parietal pseudofracture and spontaneous ICH suggesting nonaccidental trauma: report of 2 cases. *Pediatr Neurosurg* 2000;33:318-322.
13. Gordon M, Prakash N, Padmakumar B: Factor XIII deficiency: a differential diagnosis to be considered in suspected nonaccidental injury presenting with intracranial hemorrhage. *Clin Pediatr* 2008;47:385-387.
14. Brousseau TJ, Kissoon N, McIntosh B: Vitamin K deficiency mimicking child abuse. *J Emerg Med* 2005;29:283-288.
15. Lane PA, Hathaway WE: Vitamin K in infancy. *J Pediatr* 1985;106:351-359.
16. Townsend CW: The haemorrhagic disease of the newborn. *Arch Pediatr* 1894;11:559-565.
17. Waddell WW, Guerry D: The role of vitamin K in the etiology, prevention, and treatment of hemorrhage in the newborn infant. *J Pediatr* 1939;15:802-811.
18. Hirose M, Akiyama M, Takakura K, et al: Active Crohn disease with maternal vitamin K deficiency and fetal subdural hematoma. *Obstet Gynecol* 2001;98:919-921.
19. Sakai M, Yoneda S, Sasaki Y, et al: Maternal total parenteral nutrition and fetal subdural hematoma. *Obstet Gynecol* 2003;101:1142-1144.
20. Akiyama H, Okamura Y, Nagashima T, et al: Intracranial hemorrhage and vitamin K deficiency associated with biliary atresia: summary of 15 cases and review of the literature. *Pediatr Neurosurg* 2006;42:362-367.
21. Ijland MM, Pereira RR, Cornelissen EAM: Incidence of late vitamin K deficiency bleeding in newborns in the Netherlands in 2005: evaluation of the current guideline. *Eur J Pediatr* 2008;167:165-169.
22. Vorstman EBA, Anslow P, Keeling DM, et al: Brain haemorrhage in five infants with coagulopathy. *Arch Dis Child* 2003;88;1119-1121.
23. Miyasaka M, Nosaka S, Sakai H, et al: Vitamin K deficiency bleeding with intracranial hemorrhage: focus on secondary form. *Emerg Radiol* 2007;14:323-329.
24. Babcock J, Hartman K, Pedersen A, et al: Rodenticide-induced coagulopathy in a young child. *Am J Pediatr Hematol Oncol* 1993;15:126-130.
25. Oswal K, Agarwal A: Warfarin-induced fetal intracranial subdural hematoma. *J Clin Ultrasound* 2008;36:451-453.
26. Matsuzaka T, Yoshinaga M, Tsuji Y, et al: Incidence and causes of intracranial hemorrhages in infancy: a prospective surveillance study after vitamin K prophylaxis. *Brain Devel* 1989;11:384-388.
27. Suzuki K, Fukushima T, Meguro K, et al: Intracranial hemorrhage in an infant owing to vitamin K deficiency despite prophylaxis. *Childs Nerv Syst* 1999;15:292-294.
28. Flood VH, Galderisi FC, Lowas SR, et al: Hemorrhagic disease of the newborn despite vitamin K prophylaxis at birth. *Pediatr Blood Cancer* 2008;50:1075-1077.
29. Ekelund H: Late hemorrhagic disease in Sweden 1987-1989. *Acta Paediatr Scand* 1991;80:966-968.

30. Cekinmez M, Cemil T, Cekinmez EK, et al: Intracranial hemorrhages due to late-type vitamin K deficiency bleeding. *Childs Nerv Syst* 2008;24:821-825.
31. Behrmann BA, Chan WK, Finer NN: Resurgance of hemorrhagic disease of the newborn: a report of three cases. *CMAJ* 1985;133: 884-885.
32. Demirören K, Yavuz H, Çam L: Intracranial hemorrhage due to vitamin K deficiency after the newborn period. *Pediatr Hematol Oncol* 2004;21:585-592.
33. Per H, Kumandas S, Özdemir MA, et al: Intracranial hemorrhage due to late hemorrhagic disease in two siblings. *J Emerg Med* 2006;31:49-52.
34. Hubbard D, Tobias J: Intracerebral hemorrhage due to hemorrhageic disease of the newborn and failure to administer vitamin K at birth. *South Med J* 2006;99:1216-1220.
35. Jimenez R, Navarrete M, Jimenez E, et al: Vitamin K-dependant clotting factors in normal breast fed infants. *J Pediatr* 1982;100: 424-426.
36. Mishra P, Naithani R, Dolai T, et al: Intracranial hemorrhage in patients with congenital haemostatic defects. *Haemophilia* 2008: 14;1-4.
37. Chaou WT, Chou ML, Eitzman DV: Intracranial hemorrhage and vitamin K deficiency in early infancy. *J Pediatr* 1984;105:880-884.
38. Rutty GN, Smith CM, Malia RG: Late-form hemorrhagic disease of the newborn: a fatal case report with illustrations of investigations that may assist in avoiding the mistaken diagnosis of child abuse. *Am J Forensic Med Pathol* 1999;20:48-51.
39. Anwar R, Miloszewski KJA: Factor XIII deficiency. *Br J Haematol* 1999;107:468-484.
40. Duckert F, Jung E, Shmerling DH: A hitherto undescribed congenital hemorrhagic diathesis probably due to fibrin stabilising factor deficiency. *Thromb Diath Haemorrh* 1960;5:179-186.
41. Almeida A, Khair K, Hann I: Unusual presentation of factor XIII deficiency. *Haemophilia* 2002;8:703-705.
42. Bhattacharya M, Biswas A, Ahmed RPH, et al: Clinico-hematologic profile of factor XIII–deficient patients. *Clin Appl Thromb Hemost* 2005;11:475-480.
43. Vural M, Yarar C, Durmaz R: Spontaneous acute subdural hematoma and chronic epidural hematoma in a child with F XIII deficiency. *J Emerg Med* 2010;38:25-29.
44. Albanese A, Tuttolomondo A, Anile C, et al: Spontaneous chronic subdural hematomas in young adults with a deficiency in coagulation factor XIII: report of three cases. *J Neurosurg* 2005;102:1130-1132.
45. Larson PD, Wallace JW, Frankel LS, et al: Factor XIII deficiency and intracranial hemorrhages in infancy. *Pediatr Neurol* 1990;6:277-278.
46. Tarantino MD, Gupta SL, Brusky RM: The incidence and outcome of intracranial haemorrhage in newborns with haemophilia: analysis of the Nationwide Inpatient Sample database. *Haemophilia* 2007;13: 380-382.
47. Stieltjes N, Calvez T, Demiguel V, et al: French ICH Study Group. Intracranial hemorrhages in French haemophilia patients (1991–2001): clinical presentation, management and prognosis factors for death. *Haemophilia* 2005;11:452-458.
48. Looney CB, Smith JK, Merck LH, et al: Intracranial hemorrhage in asymptomatic neonates: prevalence on MR images and relationship to obstetric and neonatal risk factors. *Radiology* 2007;242:535-545.
49. Rooks VJ, Eaton JP, Ruess L, et al: Prevalence and evolution of intracranial hemorrhage in asymptomatic term infants. *AJNR Am J Neuroradiol* 2008;29:1082-1089.
50. Robertson J, Lillicrap D, James PD: von Willebrand disease. *Pediatr Clin North Am* 2008;55:377-392.
51. Harrison P, Robinson M, Liesner R, et al: The PFA-100: a potential rapid screening tool for the assessment of platelet dysfunction. *Clin Lab Haematol* 2002;24:225-232.
52. Triplett DA: Coagulation and bleeding disorders: review and update. *Clin Chem* 2000;46:1260-1269.
53. Mizoi K, Onuma T, Mori K: Intracranial hemorrhage secondary to von Willebrand's disease and trauma. *Surg Neurol* 1984;22:495-498.
54. Ziv O, Ragni MV: Bleeding manifestations in males with von Willebrand disease. *Haemophilia* 2004;10:162-168.
55. Wetzstein V, Budde U, Oyen F, et al: Intracranial hemorrhage in a term newborn with severe von Willebrand disease type 3 associated with sinus venous thrombosis. *Haematologica* 2006;91:e163-e165.
56. Herrmann WA, Lohmann CP, Demmler-Hackenberg W, et al: Von Willebrand's disease type 1 as cause for subvitreal, retinal and sub-

retinal hemorrhages. *Graefes Arch Clin Exp Ophthalmol* 2005;243:383-385.
57. Shiono T, Abe S, Watabe T, et al: Viterous, retinal and subretinal hemorrhages associated with von Willebrand's syndrome. *Graefes Arch Clin Exp Ophthalmol* 1992;230:496-497.
58. Hymel KP, Abshire TC, Luckey DW, et al: Coagulopathy in pediatric abusive head trauma. *Pediatrics* 1997;99:371-375.
59. Olson JD, Kaufman HH, Moake J, et al: The incidence and significance of hemostatic abnormalities in patients with head injuries. *Neurosurgery* 1989;6:825-832.
60. Harhangi BS, Kompanje EJO, LeeBeek FWG, et al: Coagulation disorders after traumatic brain injury. *Acta Neurochir (Wien)* 2008:150:165-175.
61. Affonseca CA, Carvalho LFA, Guerra SD, et al: Coagulation disorder in children and adolescents with moderate to severe traumatic brain injury. *J Pediatr (Rio J)* 2007;83:274-282.
62. Cohen MJ, Brohi K, Ganter MT, et al: Early coagulopathy after traumatic brain injury: the role of hypoperfusion and the protein C pathway. *J Trauma* 2007;63:1254-1262.
63. Dinakaran S, Chan TKJ Rogers NK, et al: Retinal hemorrhages in meningococcal septicemia. *J AAPOS* 2002;6:221-223.
64. Bolton-Maggs PHB, Chalmers EA, Collins PW, et al: A review of inherited platelet disorders with guidelines for their management on behalf of the UKHCDO. *Br J Haematol* 2006;135:603-633.
65. Biousse V: Coagulation abnormalities and their neuro-ophthalmologic manifestations. *Curr Opin Ophthalmol* 1999;10:382-393.
66. Neunert C, Buchanan G, Imbach P: Severe hemorrhage in children with newly diagnosed immune thrombocytopenic purpura. *Blood* 2008;112:4003-4008.
67. Frankel CA, Pastore DJ: ITP with intracranial hemorrhage and vitreous hemorrhage. *Clin Pediatr (Phila)* 1990;29:725-728.
68. Russell-Eggitt IM, Thompson DA, Khair K, et al: Hermansky-Pudlak syndrome presenting with subdural haematoma and retinal haemorrhages in infancy. *J Royal Soc Med* 2000;93:591-592.
69. Kamburoğlu G, Kiratli H: Recurrent traumatic hyphema in a patient with Glanzmann thrombasthenia. *J AAPOS* 2006;10:186-187.
70. Izquierdo NJ, Townsend W, Hussels IE: Ocular findings in the Hermansky–Pudlak syndrome. *Trans Am Ophthalmol Soc* 1995;93: 191-200.
71. Lee ACW: Bruises, blood coagulation tests and the battered child syndrome. *Singapore Med J* 2008;49:445-449.
72. Thomas AE: The bleeding child; is it NAI? *Arch Dis Child* 2004;89:1163-1167.
73. Acosta M, Edwards R, Jaffe EI Yee, et al: A practical approach to pediatric patients referred with an abnormal coagulation profile. *Arch Pathol Lab Med* 2005;129:1011-1016.
74. Liesner R, Hann I, Khair K: Non-accidental injury and the haematologist: the causes and investigation of easy bruising. *Blood Coag Fibrinol* 2004;15:S41-S48.
75. Kumar D, Greer FR, Super DM, et al: Vitamin K status of premature infants: implications for current recommendations. *Pediatrics* 2001;108:1117-1122.
76. Greer FR, Costakos DT, Suttie JW: Determination of des-gamma-carboxy-prothrombin (PIVKA II) in cord blood of various gestational ages with the STAGO antibody: a marker of vitamin K deficiency? *Pediatr Res* 1999;45:283A.
77. Widdershoven J, van Munster P, De Abreu R, et al: Four methods compared for measuring des-carboxy-prothrombin. *Clin Chem* 1987;33:2074-2078.
78. Khair K, Liesner R: Bruising and bleeding in infants and children—a practical approach. *Br J Haemat* 2006;133:221-231.
79. Harrison P: The role of PFA-100 testing in the investigation and management of haemostatic defects in children and adults. *Br J Haematol* 2005;130:3-10.
80. Schroeder V, Durrer D, Meili E, et al: Congenital factor XIII deficiency in Switzerland: from the worldwide first case in 1960 to its molecular characterisation in 2005. *Swiss Med Week* 2007;137:272–278.
81. Jenny C, Hymel KP, Ritzen A, et al: Analysis of missed cases of abusive head trauma. *JAMA* 1999;281:621-626.
82. Vyrostek SB, Annest JL, Ryan GW: Surveillance for fatal and nonfatal injuries—United States, 2001. *MMWR Surveill Summ* 2004;53:1-57.

83. Warrington SA, Wright CM, Team AS: Accidents and resulting injuries in premobile infants: data from the ALSPAC study. *Arch Dis Child* 2001;85:104-107.

84. Helfer RE, Slovis TL, Black M: Injuries resulting when small children fall out of bed. *Pediatrics* 1977;60:533-535.

85. Lyons TJ, Oates RK: Falling out of bed: a relatively benign occurrence. *Pediatrics* 1993;92:125-127.

86. Nimityongskul P, Anderson LD: The likelihood of injuries when children fall out of bed. *J Ped Orthop* 1987;7:184-186.

87. Williams RA: Injuries in infants and small children resulting from witnessed and corroborated free falls. *J Trauma* 1991;31:1350-1352.

88. Joffe M, Ludwig S: Stairway injuries in children. *Pediatrics* 1998;82:457-461.

89. Chiaviello CT, Christoph RA, Bond GR: Stairway-related injuries in children. *Pediatrics* 1994;94:679-681.

90. Chiaviello CT, Christoph RA, Bond GR: Infant walker-related injuries: a prospective study of severity and incidence. *Pediatrics* 1994;93:974-976.

91. Smith GA, Bowman MJ, Luria JW, et al: Babywalker-related injuries continue despite warning labels and public education. *Pediatrics* 1997;100:E1.

92. Denton S, Mileusnic D: Delayed sudden death in an infant following an accidental fall: a case report with review of the literature. *Am J Forens Med Pathol* 2003;24:371-376.

93. Plunkett J: Fatal pediatric head injuries caused by short-distance falls. *Am J Forens Med Pathol* 2001;22:1-12.

94. Case ME, Graham MA, Handy TC, et al: Position paper on fatal abusive head injuries in infants and young children. *Am J Forens Med Pathol* 2001;22:112-122.

95. Chadwick DL, Bertocci G, Castillo E, et al: Annual risk of death resulting from short falls among young children: less than 1 in 1 million. *Pediatrics* 2008;121:1213-1224.

96. Leestma JE: Forensic neuropathology. *In:* Duckett S (ed): *Pediatric Neuropathology.* Williams & Wilkins, Baltimore, 2002, pp 243-283.

97. Vinchon M, Pierrat V, Tchofo PJ, et al: Traumatic intracranial hemorrhage in newborns. *Childs Nerv Syst* 2005;21:1042-1048.

98. Gosalakkal JA: Intracranial arachnoid cysts in children: a review of pathogenesis, clinical features, and management. *Pediatr Neurol* 2002;26:93-98.

99. Whitby EH, Griffiths PD, Rutter S, et al: Frequency and natural history of subdural hemorrhages in babies and relation to obstetric factors. *Lancet* 2004;363:846-851.

100. Hughes LA, May K, Talbot JF, et al: Incidence, distribution, and duration of birth-related retinal hemorrhages: a prospective study. *J AAPOS* 2006;10:102-106.

101. Emerson MV, Pieramici DJ, Stoessel KM, et al: Incidence and rate of disappearance of retinal hemorrhage in newborns. *Ophthalmology* 2001;108:36-39.

102. Kaur B, Taylor D: Fundus hemorrhages in infancy. *Surv Ophthalmol* 1992;37:1-17.

103. Narli N, Soyupak S, Yildizdaş HY, et al: Ultrasonographic measurement of subarachnoid space in normal term newborns. *Eur J Radiol* 2006:58:110-112.

104. Raul J-S, Roth S, Ludes B, et al: Influence of the benign enlargement of the subarachnoid space on the bridging vein strain during a shaking event: a finite element study. *Int J Legal Med* 2008;122:337-340.

105. Alper G, Ekinci G, Yilmaz Y, et al: Magnetic resonance imaging characteristics of benign macrocephaly in children. *J Child Neurol* 1999;14:678-682.

106. Fessell DP, Frankel D, Wolfson WP: Sonography of extraaxial fluid in neurologically normal infants with head circumference greater than or equal to the 95th percentile for age. *J Ultrasound Med* 2000;19:443-447.

107. Wolpert, SM, Barnes PD: *MRI in Pediatric Neuroradiology.* Mosby-Year Book, Philadelphia, 1992.

108. Schachenmayr W, Friede RL: The origin of the subdural neomembrane: fine structure of the dura-arachnoid interface in man. *Am J Pathol* 1978;92:53-68.

109. Freide RL, Schachenmayr W: The origin of the subdural neomembrane: fine structure of neomembranes. *Am J Pathol* 1978;92:69-84.

110. Wilms G, Vanderschueren G, Demaerel PH, et al: CT and MRI in infants with pericerebral collections and macrocephaly: benign enlargement of the subarachnoid spaces versus subdural collections. *Am J Neuroradiol* 1993;14:855-860.

111. Kleinamn PK, Ragland RL: Gadolinium dimeglumine-enhanced MR imaging of subdural hematoma in an abused infant. *AJR Am J Radiol* 1996;166:1456-1458.

112. Blitshteyn S, Mechtler LL, Bakshi R: Diffuse dural gadolinium MRI enhancement associated with bilateral chronic subdural hematomas. *Clin Imag* 2004;28:90-92.

113. Pittman T: Significance of a subdural hematoma in a child with external hydrocephalus. *Pediatr Neurosurg* 2003;39:57-59.

114. Hymel K, Jenny C, Block R: Intracranial hemorrhage and rebleeding in suspected victims of abusive head trauma: addressing the forensic controversies. *Child Maltreat* 2002;7:329-348.

115. Vinchon M, Noulé N, Tchofo PJ, et al: Imaging of head injuries in infants: temporal correlates and forensic implications for the diagnosis of child abuse. *J Neurosurg* 2004;101:S44-S52.

116. Dias MS, Backstrom J, Falk M, et al: Serial radiography in the infant shaken impact syndrome. *Pediatr Neurosurg* 1998;29:77-85.

117. Joy HM, Anscombe AM, Gawne-Cain ML: Blood-stained, acute subdural hygroma mimicking a subacute subdural haematoma in non-accidental head injury. *Clin Radiol* 2007;62:703-706.

118. Zouros A, Bhargava R, Hoskinson M, et al: Further characterization of traumatic subdural collections of infancy. Report of five cases. *J Neurosurg* 2004;100:512-518.

119. Barnes PD, Robson CD: CT findings in hyperacute nonaccidental brain injury. *Pediatr Radiol* 2000;30:74-81.

120. Lorch SA, D'Agostino JA, Zimmerman R, et al: "Benign" extra-axial fluid in survivors of neonatal intensive care. *Arch Pediatr Adolesc Med* 2004;158:178-182.

121. Powers CJ, Fuchs HE, George TM: Chronic subdural hematoma of the neonate: report of two cases and literature review. *Pediatr Neurosurg* 2007;43:25-28.

122. Hadzikaric N, Al-Habib H, Al-Ahmad I: Idiopathic chronic subdural hematoma in the newborn. *Childs Nerv Syst* 2006;22:740-742.

123. Lee KS: Natural history of chronic subdural haematoma. *Brain Inj* 2004;18:351-358.

124. Wilberger JE: Pathophysiology of evolution and recurrence of chronic subdural hematomas. *Neurosurg Clin North Am* 2000;11:435-438.

125. Tamura Y, Welch DC, Zic JA, et al: Scurvy presenting as painful gait with bruising in a young boy. *Arch Pediatr Adolesc Med* 2000;154:732-735.

126. Larralde M, Santos Muñoz A, Boggio P, et al: Scurvy in a 10-month-old boy. *Int J Dermatol* 2007;46:194-198.

127. Gilman BB, Tanzer RC: Subdural hematoma in infantile curvy: report of a case with review of literature. *JAMA* 1932;99:989-991.

128. Olmedo JM, Yiannias JA, Windgassen EB, et al; Scurvy: a disease almost forgotten. *Int J Dermatol* 2006;45;909-913.

129. Verma S, Sivanandan S, Aneesh MK, et al: Unilateral proptosis and extradural hematoma in a child with scurvy. *Pediatr Radiol* 2007;37:937-939.

130. Sullivan TJ, Wright JE: Non-traumatic orbital haemorrhage. *Clin Exp Ophthalmol* 2000;28:26-31.

131. Hood J, Hodges RE: Ocular lesions in scurvy. *Am J Clin Nutr* 1969;22:559-567.

132. Snow I: Eye symptoms of infantile scurvy. A case of infantile scurvy with extreme protrusion of the right eyeball, shown by autopsy to be due to a large retrobulbar hematoma. Transactions Am Pediatr Soc, 17th Session 1905:78-82.

133. Bloxham CA, Clough C, Beevers DG: Retinal infarcts and haemorrhages due to scurvy. *Postgrad Med J* 1990;66:687.

134. Adetona N, Kramarenko W, McGavin CR: Retinal changes in scurvy. *Eye* 1994;8:709-710.

135. Mimasaka S, Funayama M, Adachi N, et al: A fatal case of infantile scurvy. *Int J Legal Med* 2000;114:122-124.

136. Strauss KA, Puffenberger EG, Robinson DL, et al: Type I glutaric aciduria, part 1: natural history of 77 patients. *Am J Med Genet C Semin Med Genet* 2003;121C:38-52.

137. Hartley LM, Khwaja OS, Verity CM: Glutaric aciduria type 1 and nonaccidental head injury. *Pediatrics* 2001;107:174-175.

138. Morris AAM, Hoffmann GF, Naughten ER, et al: Glutaric aciduria and suspected child abuse. *Arch Dis Child* 1999;80:404-405.

139. Gago L, Wegner R, Capone A, et al: Intraretinal hemorrhages and chronic subdural effusions: glutaric aciduria type 1 can be mistaken for shaken baby syndrome. *Retina* 2003;23:724-726.

140. Kafil-Hussain NA, Monavari A, Bowell R, et al: Ocular findings in glutaric aciduria type 1. *J Pediatr Ophthalmol Strabismus* 2000;37:289-293.

141. Juul K, Andersen J, Basile Cvitanich V, et al: Case 2: Suspected non-accidental injury. *Acta Paediatr* 2006;95:1323-1325.

142. Nassogne MC, Sharrard M, Hertz-Pannier L, et al: Massive subdural haematomas in Menkes disease mimicking shaken baby syndrome. *Childs Nerv Syst* 2002;18:729-731.

143. Bacopoulou F, Henderson L, Philip SG: Menkes disease mimicking non-accidental trauma. *Arch Dis Child* 2006;91:919.

144. Jankov RP, Boerkoel CF, Hellmann J, et al: Lethal neonatal Menkes' disease with severe vasculopathy and fractures. *Acta Paediatr* 1998;87:1297-1300.

145. Pinto F, Calderazzi A, Canapicchi R, et al: Radiological findings in a case of Menke's disease. *Childs Nerv Syst* 1995;11:112-114.

146. Gasch AT, Caruso RC, Kaler SG, et al: Menkes' syndrome: ophthalmologic findings. *Ophthalmology* 2002;109:1477-1483.

48

OUTCOME OF ABUSIVE HEAD TRAUMA

Linda Ewing-Cobbs, PhD, and Mary R. Prasad, PhD

INTRODUCTION

Since Caffey[1] and Kempe et al's[2] groundbreaking reports linking battering and shaking of infants to cerebrovascular lesions and mental retardation, numerous studies have examined mechanisms of injury and predictors of outcome in this most vulnerable population of children. Assessment of specific outcomes across different clinical populations varies depending on the level of analysis and time frame. The six major areas of outcome research include death, disease, disability, discomfort, dissatisfaction, and destitution.[3,4] In acute care studies, death and disease are used as outcome markers, although post-acute studies typically examine disability, impairment, and health-related quality of life. This chapter examines the literature regarding post-acute outcomes in children with abusive head trauma (AHT). To facilitate evaluation of the strength of the empirical foundation for determining outcomes, findings are examined in relation to study methodology. Outcomes from studies examining prospectively recruited samples of children with AHT evaluated using rating scales and/or standardized measures of cognition and behavior are compared with outcomes of children with noninflicted head trauma (NHT) or to sociodemographically similar community comparison children. Findings from descriptive studies examining rates of disability and impairment are also examined. Predictors of post-acute outcomes, including coma rating scales, biomarkers, neuroimaging findings, and family factors, are reviewed. Finally, directions for future research on outcomes following early brain injury are discussed.

NEUROBEHAVIORAL AND NEUROPSYCHOLOGICAL OUTCOMES

Studies examining outcomes after inflicted childhood neurotrauma vary along several key dimensions, including determination of the external cause of injury, recruitment and follow-up methodology, and the specific outcome domains evaluated. Determination of the presence of AHT is difficult since the history is often not provided or is incompatible with the clinical presentation. Different approaches to identifying AHT have attendant strengths and weaknesses

and can introduce different biases. Several investigators applied an algorithm similar to Duhaime et al[5] to categorize injuries as presumptive or suspicious for AHT based on the presenting injury in relation to the history and associated findings.[6-8] This approach is affected by the circular reasoning inherent in using specific clinical findings often associated with abusive injury to support diagnosis of abusive injury. Hymel et al[9] used a priori criteria, including admitted abusive acts, infants with acute cardiorespiratory compromise linked to traumatic injuries, developmentally inconsistent histories, changing explanations of the trauma, and presence of at least two noncranial injuries considered moderately or highly associated with abuse. Application of these criteria in a multicenter study resulted in classification of the external cause of injury as "undetermined" in 24%. Developmental outcomes of the undetermined group were significantly more favorable than in children classified as either AHT or NHT.[9] Because of the difficulty diagnosing putative inflicted injury in milder cases, a bias exists toward inclusion of children with more severe traumatic brain injury (TBI) in the inflicted injury group. This bias is most likely to affect retrospective studies.

Post-acute outcome studies are unavoidably biased by the willingness of parents and guardians to volunteer to participate. High rates of attrition approaching 50% within 6 months to 1 year after injury are common. Long-term outcome studies are likely to retain children from intact families who have resources to facilitate participation, in situations in which the perpetrator is not a close relative, and in children with very poor outcomes who continue to require medical care.

Outcomes in children with AHT who have been assessed from subacute to chronic stages of recovery include neurological findings, global outcome ratings, or specific neurodevelopmental outcomes assessed using standardized instruments. Table 48-1 provides findings from studies examining outcome using rating scales and standardized mental, motor, and/or adaptive behavior outcomes in children with AHT. The Glasgow Outcome Scale (GOS)[10] and pediatric variants (Pediatric Outcome Performance Category)[4] are rating scales that assess outcome on a five- or six-point scale ranging from good outcome to death. Standard scores have a mean of 100 and a standard deviation of 15 or 16.

The table of outcome studies and the following review are organized according to study methodology.

Acknowledgements: Preparation of this chapter was supported in part by National Institute of Neurological Disorders and Stroke grants R01 NS 46308, R01 NS 29462, and Department of Education grant H133G040279.

Table 48-1 Outcomes in Children with Abusive Head Trauma by Study Design

Author	Sample Size	Months of Age at Injury (Range) Mean	Study Design	Follow-Up Interval	Glasgow Outcome Scale or Pediatric Outcome Performance Category (%)					Standardized Assessment (M)		
						Good/ mild	Moderate	Severe	PVS	Mental	Motor	Adaptive
Comparison of Abusive Head Trauma to Noninflicted TBI and/or Control Groups												
Beers (2007)	a = 15 n = 15	a = 5.8* n = 17.2	Prospective cross-sectional cohort	6 mo						a = 69.0* n = 97.3	— —	95.9* 115.8
Ewing-Cobbs (1998)	a = 20 n = 20	(0-59) a = 10.6* n = 35.6	Prospective longitudinal cohort	1.3 mo	a: n:	20 55	65 25	15 20	0* 0	a = 78.2* n = 87.7	80.3* 84.3	— —
Ewing-Cobbs (1999)	a = 28 c = 28	(0-42) a = 9.3 c = 9.4	Prospective longitudinal cohort	4.6 mo	a:	25	61	14	0	a = 82.1* c = 97.7	81.9* 100.5	— —
Hymel (2007)	a = 11 n = 30 ? = 13	(0-35) a = 10.5 n = 9.0 ? = 11.5	Prospective longitudinal cohort and convenience sample	6 mo follow-up in: 4 iTBI, 16 nTBI, 6 ?TBI						a = 60.0* n = 94.4 ? = 107.3	59.8* 101.8 102.2*	— — —
Keenan (2004)	a = 62 n = 50	(0-23) a = 4.0* n = 7.5	Prospective population-based longitudinal cohort	Discharge	a: n:	55 82	45* 18					
					(Dichotomized into good/mild *vs* moderate/severe)							
Keenan (2006a)	a = 41 n = 31		Follow-up of prospective population-based longitudinal cohort	1 y	a: n:	53 77	20 16	27 7	0* 0	— —	— —	96.4* mdn 100.0 mdn
Keenan (2007)	a = 25 n = 23 c = 31		Follow-up of prospective population-based longitudinal cohort	1-3 y						a = 68* n = 84	55* 92	94 100
Descriptive Studies of Inflicted TBI												
Barlow (2005)	a = 25	(0-34) 2.3 mdn	Cross-sectional and prospective longitudinal	59 m		48	16	36	—			
Bonnier (2003)	a = 25	(0-13) 4.2	Retrospective cohort	6 y (2.5-13 y)		4	35	48	12	a = 63.3		
Duhaime (1996)	a = 14	(1-24) 6.4	Follow-up of prospective cohort	9 y		14	36	43	7			
Ghahreman (2005)	a = 56	(0.5-46) 8.2	Retrospective record review	Mdn 20 mos		39	19	26	10			
Johnson (1995)	a = 28	5	Retrospective record review	—		32	25	42	4			

Note: * = Statistically significant group comparison; ? = uncertain mechanism of injury; *a* = abusive head trauma; *c* = community comparison group; *m* = mean; *mdn* = median; *mo* = months; *n* = noninflicted *TBI*; PVS = persistent vegetative state; *y* = year.

Outcome of Abusive Head Trauma in Relation to Noninflicted Head Trauma or Community Comparison Groups

In one of the first prospective follow-up studies, Ewing-Cobbs and colleagues[7] examined outcomes of 20 children with AHT and 20 with NHT in relation to injury severity measures and neuroimaging findings. The Glasgow Coma Scale (GCS),[11] which is commonly used to assess the severity of acute TBI, is composed of three scales assessing eye, motor, and verbal responses. Children with AHT and NHT had comparable injury severity in terms of initial GCS scores and duration of impaired consciousness. However, the NHT group was significantly older than the AHT group. At 1 month after TBI, GOS scores indicated significant differences in functional outcome related to the external cause of TBI. Severe disability occurred with similar frequency across groups; children with AHT, however, had a significantly higher rate of moderate disability (65% vs. 20%) and a lower rate of good recovery (20% vs. 55%) than those with NHT. General cognitive outcomes were related to the external cause of TBI. At 1 month after injury, 45% of children with AHT and only 5% of those with NHT scored below the second percentile. Motor scores were similar in both TBI groups, with mean percentiles of 9 and 14 for the AHT and NHT groups, respectively.

Twenty-eight children in the AHT group were examined at 1 and 3 months after TBI using the Bayley Scales of Infant Development.[12] Comparison of their developmental outcomes in relation to those of a sociodemographically similar community comparison group indicated that mean mental developmental scores of children in the AHT group did not change across the follow-up interval and remained significantly below those from the comparison group.[13] This lack of improvement in test scores suggests no short-term recovery of function. Relative to the comparison group, the children with AHT had significantly lower mental and physical developmental scores that persisted from 1 to 3 months after the injury. At the 3-month interval, the mean mental and physical developmental indexes indicated substantial persistent morbidity. Behavior ratings identified a significantly higher rate of impairment in the AHT than in the comparison group on motor quality, orientation/engagement, and emotional regulation. Persistent difficulties in motor tone, fine and gross motor control, and movement quality were identified. In addition, the level and consistency of arousal and alertness, as well as the child's interest, initiative, and exploration of materials during assessment activities, were significantly reduced. GOS scores were stable across the assessment interval. The majority of the children had a moderate disability (61%). By 3 months after AHT, the rates of behavioral difficulties remained strikingly high. Approximately 40% of infants and children had impairments in energy, interest, and toy exploration, 54% had deficits in motor tone or coordination, 85% had deficits in attention or arousal, and 48% had deficits in regulation of affect, frustration tolerance, and adaptation to change.[13]

Examination of the social competence of children with AHT revealed significant deficits in multiple social and cognitive areas that are cornerstones of early learning and social interaction. Children with AHT showed reduced competence in several key areas, including initiation of and response to social overtures, display of positive affect, coordinating their attention in social learning interactions with an examiner, establishing mutual gaze, and complying with requests.[14] Impairment in these early social and cognitive skills following AHT are of concern since they are precursors to more elaborate executive processing skills essential for regulating behavior and emotions.[15] Further longitudinal follow-up studies completed 5 to 8 years after both AHT and NHT in the same cohorts of children revealed persistent reduction in IQ scores (M = 83.0, SD = 14.0) relative to a community comparison group (M = 95.7, SD = 10.5). In addition, children with early TBI had significantly lower scores than the comparison group on standardized measures of reading, math, and language.[16]

Hymel and colleagues[9] enrolled a prospective sample of 27 children with AHT and NHT who were hospitalized at two sites and an additional convenience sample of 27 eligible patients from seven additional sites. Twenty-seven of the 52 surviving children less than 3 years of age completed follow-up procedures 6 months after the injury. The Bayley Scales of Infant Development[12] mental development score was significantly lower in the four children with AHT than in the 16 with NHT. Similarly, mean gross motor performance was below the first percentile in six children with AHT and at approximately the 50th percentile in 11 with NHT.

In a series of well-designed population-based studies, Keenan and colleagues[8] examined early and late outcomes after serious AHT or NHT sustained prior to 3 years of age. This is a unique cohort because the children were drawn from a population-based sample of children injured in North Carolina from 2000 to 2001. Serious TBI was defined as an intracranial injury verified by neuroimaging or pathologic studies. Fifty-three percent of the sample was categorized in the AHT group. Pediatric Outcome Performance Category scores[4] were based on medical record review of the child's status at discharge. Even though the children with NHT had more severe injuries, outcome scores were less favorable in children with AHT.[8]

Keenan and colleagues followed the above cohort and reported outcomes at 1 year[17] and 2 years[18] after TBI. At the 1-year follow-up, children in the AHT group continued to have worse outcome than those with NHT (see Tables 48-1 and 48-2). Twenty-seven percent were severely disabled whereas only 6.5% of the children with NHT were rated with severe disability. Children with AHT were more likely to have chronic health problems than those in the NHT group. Children with poor outcomes used more rehabilitation services than those with good or mild disabilities; those with inflicted injuries were somewhat more likely to be high users or resources than children with NHT.

At the 2-year follow-up interval, 66.7% of children retained their classification based on outcome ratings. For children whose scores changed, improvement was as likely as deterioration. When scores were examined at discharge, 1 year, and 2 years after TBI, children with NHT were more likely than those with AHT to show improvement over time. Ratings of chronic health problems were stable from 1 to 2 years after TBI irrespective of the mechanism of injury. One fourth of the sample continued to receive rehabilitation therapies, with an increase in the number of children receiving speech therapy during the second year after injury.[18]

Keenan and colleagues[19] examined the same cohort of children at 3 years of age. Based on the Mullen Scales of Early Learning,[20] the AHT group scored significantly lower than the NHT group on the composite score, as well as on component subtests evaluating visual reception, fine motor, receptive language, and expressive language outcomes. The median composite standard score was 68 (first percentile) for the AHT and 84 (14th percentile) for the NHT groups. Clearly, the children with AHT had very significant and persistent cognitive and motor sequelae. Median adaptive behavior scores were similar in both TBI groups and fell in the average range, but were lower than scores from a healthy comparison group.

Descriptive Studies of Abusive Head Trauma

As apparent in Table 48-1, descriptive studies are more likely than psychometric studies to include children with severe disabilities and/or those in a persistent vegetative state. Barlow and colleagues[6] examined long-term outcomes an average of 59 months after AHT in 25 children recruited from both cross-sectional and prospective Scottish cohorts. Outcome ratings suggested a good recovery in 48%, moderate disability in 16%, and a severe disability in 36%. Visual impairment, including cortical blindness, visual field defects, and/or reduced acuity, was reported in 48%. Relative to normative standards, general cognitive scores were substantially reduced in most children; one third of the children either scored below the 0.1 percentile or were untestable. Adaptive behavior scores also indicated significant difficulty in communication, daily living, and socialization domains. Behavior problems were present in 52% of the children, with problematic behaviors often developing between ages 2 and 3.

Bonnier and colleagues[21] completed extended follow-up in 23 cases of confirmed AHT identified through retrospective chart review. The children were ages 3 weeks to 13 months at the time of injury and were at least 3 years of age at follow-up. Neuroimaging studies obtained during the first 3 months after injury revealed subdural or subarachnoid hemorrhage, parenchymal edema, lobar atrophy involving both gray and white matter, arterial infarcts, and subcortical gliotic scars. Outcomes were unfavorable in 60% of the sample, who had GOS ratings of severe disability or persistent vegetative state. An additional 35% had moderate disabilities, with good recovery occurring in only one case (4%). Similarly, a high rate of unfavorable long-term outcomes was reported in 14 children an average of 9 years after AHT.[22] Although outcomes were variable, the majority of patients had outcome ratings of moderate (36%) or severe (43%) disability. Other studies converge in identifying major neurological sequelae following severe AHT. Microcephaly, visual impairment, characterized by homonymous hemianopia or cortical blindness, and motor impairment, characterized by either hemiparesis or quadriparesis, occur in a high proportion of survivors of severe AHT.[23-26]

These studies suggest that the consequences of early TBI in general, and AHT in particular, are significant and persistent and affect multiple domains of cognitive, motor, and behavioral functioning. No studies have identified significant, sustained improvement in performance over time.

Rather, children who incur severe AHT early in life have a high likelihood of developing deficits that persist throughout the lifespan.

MECHANISM OF INJURY, NEUROIMAGING FINDINGS, AND BIOMARKERS IN RELATION TO OUTCOME

The mechanisms involved in AHT are not well understood. The often devastating injury to the central nervous system in children with severe AHT typically reflects a combination of focal and diffuse injury. Although there is agreement that children with AHT sustain diffuse cerebral injury, there is debate regarding the degree to which the injury is primarily traumatic or hypoxic-ischemic in nature.[27-30] The immature brain appears to recover relatively well following focal injury; however, it appears to be less resilient following diffuse injury from a variety of mechanisms, including infections, radiation, and traumatic injury.[31-33]

Several studies examined the role of neuroimaging findings in relation to outcomes. Hymel and colleagues[9] examined the mechanism of injury as a predictor of outcome 6 months after injury in a prospective sample of four children with AHT and 16 children with NHT. Mechanisms included: contact (limited craniofacial bruising and/or laceration, subgaleal hematoma, skull fracture, or epidural hematoma); noncontact (acute concussion, diffuse axonal injury, interhemispheric hematoma); combined; and undetermined categories (subarachnoid hemorrhage, brain contusions, subdural collection that does not extend to the interhemispheric space). Standardized cognitive and motor outcomes were differentially related to the predictor variables. Both cognitive and motor outcomes were strongly related to external cause of injury (abusive vs. noninflicted), depth of injury (depth of visible injury on CT/MRI of the brain), acute cardiorespiratory compromise, and initial GCS score. Motor scores were also predicted by the mechanism of injury and duration of impaired consciousness. Other studies have not identified mechanism of injury, defined as whiplash shaking with or without evidence of impact, to be related to a global outcome measure.[6]

In a retrospective record review of 23 children with AHT, Bonnier and colleagues[21] also found that intraparenchymal lesions were associated with poor outcome. Intraparenchymal lesions included atrophy, arterial infarcts, subcortical gliotic scars in the white matter, lesions of the corpus callosum, and lesions of the cerebellum. Children with diffuse lesions had more significant intellectual impairments. GOS scores were also significantly associated with the initial GCS score, presence of retinal hemorrhages, and presence of skull fracture. Similar findings were found in a retrospective study conducted by Gilles and Nelson.[24] They identified two subgroups based on acute CT scan findings: those with diffuse cerebral hypoattenuation (n = 7) and those with focal hypodensity (n = 7) who were followed for at least 3 months after hospital discharge. Cerebral infarctions developed in all children. Diffuse brain swelling was associated with worse standardized developmental outcomes. Several studies noted a high rate of deceleration of head growth or microcephaly in a large proportion of children with AHT, associated with cortical atrophy and a greater likelihood of a poor outcome.[24,34]

Prasad and colleagues[35] examined the relationship between clinical and neuroimaging variables and multiple outcome measures in a longitudinal, prospective group of 60 children less than 6 years of age who sustained either AHT or NHT. Modified GCS score, duration of impaired consciousness, and the number of intracranial lesions visualized on CT/MRI accounted for a significant amount of the variance in the GOS, cognitive, and motor scores at baseline, 3-, and 12-month postinjury evaluations. The presence or absence of cerebral infarcts accounted for significant variability in outcomes. In the follow-up of this cohort, children with cerebral infarcts had decreasing physical developmental scores from baseline to 3 months after injury and were more likely to be rated as having suboptimal behavioral regulation than children without infarcts.[13]

The impact that abusive neurotrauma exerted on motor and cognitive outcomes, above and beyond the effect of TBI, was examined in the same sample. Across the follow-up period, motor scores were consistently related to injury severity (depth of unconsciousness and duration of unconsciousness) as well as to pupillary responsiveness. The presence of AHT did not significantly contribute to prediction of motor outcome after inclusion of injury severity in the regression model. In contrast, the presence of AHT did significantly predict cognitive outcomes beyond the influence of injury severity. This difference in the impact of abuse on cognitive and motor outcome suggests that cognitive outcome might be more influenced by psychosocial factors whereas motor outcome may be more directly related to neurological variables such as prolonged unconsciousness and the depth of the unconsciousness.

As noted in Chapter 46, "Biochemical Markers of Head Trauma in Children," cerebrospinal fluid (CSF) and serum biomarkers show promise in accounting for variability in outcomes. In a prospective cross-sectional sample of 15 infants and young children with AHT and 15 with NHT, Beers et al[36] identified significantly less favorable GOS scores, lower IQ scores, and reduced adaptive behavior in the AHT group when assessed 6 months after TBI. All outcome scores were significantly correlated with time to peak for serum biomarkers, including neuron-specific enolase, S100B, and myelin-basic protein. Shore and colleagues[37] noted that neuron-specific enolase and S100B derived from CSF were significantly correlated with GOS scores only in children older than 4 years of age and did not distinguish between children with AHT and NHT.

FAMILY ENVIRONMENT

Surprisingly little is known about the effect of the family environment on outcome from AHT. Work with maltreated children conducted by Cicchetti and others[38] has highlighted the deleterious impact of an abusive home environment on the psychological and social development of children. Prasad and colleagues[39] examined a prospective sample of 19 children who had been hospitalized for physical abuse and who had no known history of brain injury. Relative to a socio-economically similar comparison group, the physically abused children scored significantly lower on standardized tests of cognitive functioning, motor skills, and language

skills.[39] The average general cognitive functioning scores for the physically abused and comparison groups were at the 16th and 37th percentiles, respectively. Although no child in the physical abuse group had any indication of head injury at the time of hospitalization, MRI of the brain revealed cerebral abnormalities in 2 of 15 children. Both children were found to have significant cerebral atrophy of unknown etiology. It is possible that the atrophy was a result of occult or prior head injury caused by abusive head trauma that was not reported to medical personnel. It is important to note that both children scored within the average range on measures of cognitive functioning. The majority of children in the physical abuse group had normal MRI scans yet performed significantly lower on measures of cognitive and motor outcome than the comparison group. These findings highlight the deleterious effects of physical abuse and the family environment on the development of children even in the absence of brain injury.

In the population followed by Keenan and colleagues, families of children with AHT and NHT did not differ in percentage of unmarried mothers, minority group membership, or employment. Social capital (the maternal caregiver's social relationship in her family and community) was also similar in both groups. Children with AHT were more likely to be receiving chronic medication treatment, usually anticonvulsants. Children with AHT had greater use of services such as home health, physical therapy, and occupational therapies at 1 year after injury. At 2 and 3 years after injury,[17,19] a significant number of families of children with both AHT and NHT lived below the poverty level and had low social capital. At 3 years after injury, Keenan and colleagues[19] found that posttraumatic seizures, GCS less than 13, low social capital, and poverty were associated with worse outcomes.

ILLUSTRATIVE CASE REPORT

A 3-month-old female is brought into the emergency department (ED) of a Level 1 trauma center by her biological mother because of depressed consciousness. Her mother reported that the infant had been dropped by her boyfriend. Upon admission to the ED, the child was responsive, moved all extremities, and received an admission GCS score of 15. By the next day, she began having focal seizures. MRI of the brain revealed a large right-sided subdural hematoma with midline shift (Figure 48-1, A). MRI of the brain 1 year after injury revealed right hemiatrophy and encephalomalacia in the right parietal occipital region; atrophy of the corpus callosum was notable (Figure 48-1, B). Follow-up MRI 5 years after injury revealed ex-vacuo ventriculomegaly, marked right hemisphere cortical and subcortical atrophy, and encephalomalacia in the posterior right hemisphere, as well as mild atrophy of the left cerebral hemisphere (Figure 48-1, C).

The case was evaluated by Child Protective Services and she was released to the care of her mother. As demonstrated in Figure 48-2, her baseline cognitive scores were in the average range and age appropriate, whereas her motor skills were quite impaired. By 1 year after injury, cognitive and motor functioning were in the average range. Her significant improvement in gross motor skills was likely due to physical therapy services she received until the age of 1 year, when

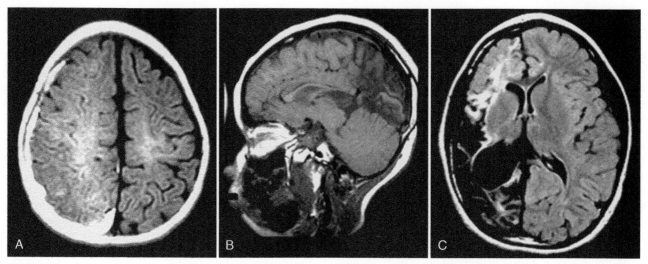

FIGURE 48-1 Changes in imaging studies in a victim of abusive head trauma. **A,** Initial MRI of the brain shows a large right-sided subdural hematoma with midline shift. **B,** Follow up MRI 1 year post-injury revealed encephalomalacia secondary to an infarction in the right parietal region. **C,** Follow-up MRI 5 years after injury revealed ex-vacuo ventriculomegaly, marked right hemisphere cortical and subcortical atrophy, and encephalomalacia in the posterior right hemisphere.

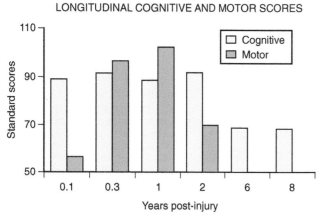

FIGURE 48-2 Changes in cognitive and motor functioning during the 8 years after an episode of abusive head trauma in the case shown in Figure 48-1.

she no longer qualified for services. By 2 years after injury, her scores began to decline and by the age of 6 years, she was functioning in the deficient range for cognitive and motor skills. The child repeated kindergarten three times. Her mother was unable to provide a stable home environment, resulting in frequent moves during the school year. At the age of 9 years, she was in the first grade and receiving special education services.

This case illustrates the challenges facing children with severe AHT. The infant discussed here sustained a devastating brain injury despite presenting with a GCS score of 15 at the time of admission. The decline in her performance with maturation reflects the cumulative impact of severe early brain injury; damage to neural systems reduces the rate of new learning and impairs the acquisition of later developing skills such as reading.[40] Her academic struggles were exacerbated by an unstable home environment and she did not receive appropriate educational or therapeutic interventions.

STRENGTH OF THE EVIDENCE

The evidence base for research on the outcome of AHT is nascent. Recent studies have directly examined performance in children classified as AHT relative to those classified as NHT or to typically developing children, examined physiological and neuroimaging differences in these groups, and have tracked development longitudinally. Despite different approaches to categorization of the external cause of injury and different measures of cognitive, motor, and behavioral outcomes, the studies converge in reporting significant, persistent, and pervasive sequelae in children who survive AHT.

SUGGESTIONS FOR FUTURE RESEARCH

To develop the sparse literature on outcome after AHT, future studies should address several areas. First, developmentally appropriate scales for assessing injury severity and disturbance of consciousness need to be developed and validated. Existing coma scales may underestimate the severity of initial brain injury in infants. Second, serial neuroimaging studies that permit evaluation of the acute brain injury, as well as assessment of the impact of primary and secondary injuries on subsequent brain development are needed. Third, it is essential to use norm-based outcome measures that appropriately assess key developmental outcomes and permit longitudinal investigation of developmental trajectories in different ability areas.

Future studies need to carefully address determination of the external cause of TBI and examination of the specific roles that interactions between traumatic axonal, hypoxic-ischemic, and vascular injuries play in determining outcomes. Multivariate models are needed to examine the contribution of different, yet often correlated, predictor variables in relation to well-defined outcome domains. Large, prospective multicenter studies that emphasize longitudinal imaging and quantitative developmental follow-up are needed to assess the pathways through which imaging, physiological, and socioenvironmental variables shape outcomes.

References

1. Caffey J: Multiple fractures in the long bones of infants suffering from subdural hematoma. *Am J Roentgenol* 1946;56:163-173.
2. Kempe CH, Silverman FN, Steele BF: The battered child syndrome. *JAMA* 1962;181:17-24.
3. Lohr KN: Advances in health status assessment. Overview of the conference. *Med Care* 1989;27:S1-11.
4. Fiser DH, Long N, Roberson PK, et al: Relationship of pediatric overall performance category and pediatric cerebral performance category scores at pediatric intensive care unit discharge with outcome measures collected at hospital discharge and 1- and 6-month follow-up assessment. *Crit Care Med* 2000;28:2616-2620.
5. Duhaime AC, Alario AJ, Lewander WJ: Head injury in very young children: mechanisms, injury types, and ophthalmologic findings in 100 hospitalized patients younger than two years of age. *Pediatrics* 1992;90:179-185.
6. Barlow KM, Thomson E, Johnson D, et al: Late neurologic and cognitive sequelae of inflicted traumatic brain injury in infancy. *Pediatrics* 2005;116:e174-e185.
7. Ewing-Cobbs L, Kramer L, Prasad M, et al: Neuroimaging, physical, and developmental findings after inflicted and noninflicted traumatic brain injury in young children. *Pediatrics* 1998;102:300-307.
8. Keenan HT, Runyan DK, Marshall SW, et al: A population-based comparison of clinical and outcome characteristics of young children with serious inflicted and noninflicted traumatic brain injury. *Pediatrics* 2004;114:633-639.
9. Hymel KP, Makoroff KL, Laskey AL, et al: Mechanisms, clinical presentations, injuries, and outcomes from inflicted versus noninflicted head trauma during infancy: results of a prospective, multicentered, comparative study. *Pediatrics* 2007;119:922-929.
10. Jennett B, Bond M: Assessment of outcome after severe brain damage. *Lancet* 1975;1:480-487.
11. Teasdale G, Jennett B: Assessment of coma and impaired consciousness: a practical scale. *Lancet* 1974;2:81-84.
12. Bayley N: *Bayley Scales of Infant Development*, ed 2. The Psychological Corporation, San Antonio, 1993.
13. Ewing-Cobbs L, Prasad M, Kramer L, et al: Inflicted traumatic brain injury: relationship of developmental outcome to severity of injury. *Pediatr Neurosurg* 1999;31:251-258.
14. Landry SH, Swank PR, Steubing K, et al: Social competence in young children with inflicted traumatic brain injury. *Dev Neuropsychol* 2004;26:707-733.
15. Ewing-Cobbs L, Prasad M, Landry SH, et al: Executive functions following traumatic brain injury in young children: a preliminary analysis. *Dev Neuropsychol* 2004;26:487-512.
16. Ewing-Cobbs L, Prasad M, Kramer L, et al: Late intellectual and academic outcomes following traumatic brain injury sustained during early childhood. *J Neurosurg* 2006;105:S287-S296.
17. Keenan HT, Runyan DK, Nocera MA: Child outcomes and family characteristics 1 year after severe inflicted or noninflicted traumatic brain injury. *Pediatrics* 2006;117:317-324.
18. Keenan HT, Runyan DK, Nocera MA: Longitudinal follow-up of families and young children with traumatic brain injury. *Pediatrics* 2006;117:1291-1297.
19. Keenan HT, Hooper SR, Wetherington CE, et al: Neurodevelopmental consequences of early traumatic brain injury in 3-year-old children. *Pediatrics* 2007;119:e616-e623.
20. Mullen EM: *Mullen Scales of Early Learning*. American Guidance Service, Circle Pines, Minn, 1995.
21. Bonnier C, Nassogne M, Saint-Martin C, et al: Neuroimaging of intraparenchymal lesions predicts outcome in shaken baby syndrome. *Pediatrics* 2003;112:808-814.
22. Duhaime AC, Christian CW, Moss E, et al: Long-term outcome in infants with the shaking-impact syndrome. *Pediatr Neurosurg* 1996;24:292-298.
23. Ghahreman A, Bhasin V, Chaseling R, et al: Nonaccidental head injuries in children: a Sydney experience. *J Neurosurg* 2005;103:213-218.
24. Gilles EE, Nelson MD Jr: Cerebral complications of nonaccidental head injury in childhood. *Pediatr Neurol* 1998;19:119-128.
25. Johnson DL, Boal D, Baule R: Role of apnea in nonaccidental head injury. *Pediatr Neurosurg* 1995;23:305-310.
26. Kivlin JD: A 12-year ophthalmologic experience with the shaken baby syndrome at a regional children's hospital. *Trans Am Ophthamol Soc* 1999;97:545-581.
27. Taylor S, Eisenberger NI, Saxbe D, et al: Neural responses to emotional stimuli are associated with childhood family stress. *Biol Psychiatry* 2006;60:296-301.
28. Geddes JF, Hackshaw AK, Vowles GH, et al: Neuropathology of inflicted head injury in children I: Patterns of brain damage. *Brain* 2001;124:1290-1298.
29. Berger RP, Adelson PD, Richichi R, et al: Serum biomarkers after traumatic and hypoxemic brain injuries: insight into the biochemical response of the pediatric brain to inflicted brain injury. *Dev Neurosci* 2006;28:327-335.
30. Duhaime AC, Gennarelli TA, Thibault LE, et al: The shaken baby syndrome. A clinical, pathological, and biomechanical study. *J Neurosurg* 1987;66:409-415.
31. Anderson V, Smibert E, Ekert H, et al: Intellectual, educational, and behavioral sequelae after cranial irradiation and chemotherapy. *Arch Dis Child* 1994;70:476-483.
32. Ewing-Cobbs L, Fletcher JM, Levin HS, et al: Longitudinal neuropsychological outcome in infants and preschoolers with traumatic brain injury. *J Int Neuropsychol Soc* 1997;3:581-591.
33. Taylor HG, Barry C, Schatschneider C: School-aged consequences of Haemophilus influenzae Type b meningitis. *J Clin Child Psychol* 1993;22:196-206.
34. Bonnier C, Marique P, Van Hout A, et al: Neurodevelopmental outcome after severe traumatic brain injury in very young children: role for subcortical lesions. *J Child Neurol* 2007;22:519-529.
35. Prasad M, Ewing-Cobbs L, Swank PR, et al: Predictors of outcome following traumatic brain injury in young children. *Pediatr Neurosurg* 2002;36:64-74.
36. Beers SR, Berger RP, Adelson PD: Neurocognitive outcome and serum biomarkers in inflicted versus non-inflicted traumatic brain injury in young children. *J Neurotrauma* 2007;24:97-105.
37. Shore PM, Berger RP, Varma S, et al: Cerebrospinal fluid biomarkers versus Glasgow Coma Scale and Glasgow Outcome Scale in pediatric traumatic brain injury: the role of young age and inflicted injury. *J Neurotrauma* 2007;24:75-76.
38. Cicchetti D, Blender JA: A multiple-levels-of-analysis approach to the study of developmental processes in maltreated children. *Proc Natl Acad Sci U S A* 2004;101:17325-17326.
39. Prasad M, Kramer A, Ewing-Cobbs L: Cognitive and neuroimaging findings in physically abused preschoolers. *Arch Dis Child* 2005;90:82-85.
40. Ewing-Cobbs L, Barnes MA, Fletcher JM: Early brain injury in children: development and reorganization of cognitive function. *Dev Neuropsychol* 2003;24:669-704.

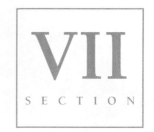

PSYCHOLOGICAL ASPECTS
OF CHILD MALTREATMENT

Lisa Amaya-Jackson, MD, MPH, and Judith A. Cohen, MD

PSYCHOLOGICAL IMPACT AND TREATMENT OF SEXUAL ABUSE OF CHILDREN

Brooks R. Keeshin, MD, and David L. Corwin, MD

INTRODUCTION

Sexually abused children experience a wide range of psychological and behavioral sequelae ranging from little discernable impact to a variety of psychiatric disorders and serious behavioral problems. Among the most common reactions in children are increased anxiety, depression, posttraumatic stress disorder (PTSD), inappropriate sexual behaviors, nightmares, behavioral regression, learning problems, increased distrust, and fearfulness. Recent research has also found strong associations between adverse childhood experiences (including child sexual abuse) and many of the most serious long-term chronic illnesses, including the top 10 causes of death in the United States.[1] The heterogeneous nature of sexual abuse, differing reactions of caregivers, individual strengths and vulnerabilities—both biological and social—and differing access to mental health care among children are the most likely sources of this variability of reactions to child sexual abuse. As Putnam[2] noted in his 2003 review of child sexual abuse, "Childhood sexual abuse is a complex life experience, not a diagnosis or a disorder."

Despite and perhaps because of the heterogeneity of psychological and behavioral reactions to child sexual abuse, a number of treatments have demonstrated some effectiveness in diminishing the impacts of this abuse. A recent meta-analysis[3] reviewed 28 studies describing the effectiveness of cognitive-behavioral, play, supportive, group, abuse-specific, individual, and family therapy for children who have experienced sexual abuse. As detailed later in this chapter, the authors found that these different treatments appear more effective for some sequelae than others and that careful assessment of the effects of sexual abuse on individual children is the best way to decide which specific treatments are most likely to help that child. They also found that longer duration of treatment was associated with greater treatment effectiveness.

HISTORY OF AWARENESS

The recent history of our knowledge and understanding of childhood sexual abuse (CSA) includes several cycles of discovery and resuppression. Its complexity, disturbing nature, and serious ramifications of confronting CSA underlie these cycles.[4]

Early in his career, Sigmund Freud was influenced by the work of French physicians like Ambroise Auguste Tardieu, whose forensic records beginning in the 1850s demonstrated that contrary to previous beliefs, sexual abuse was common and occurred in all socioeconomic levels. Toward the end of the nineteenth century, Freud[5] presented *The Aetiology of Hysteria*, a paper in which he described adult onset hysteria, obsessions, chronic paranoia, and other psychoses to women's experiences of CSA. At the same time, Pierre Janet was observing dissociative symptoms among individuals who had experienced significant trauma. The widespread nature of hysteria in Europe, especially among the upper classes, implied that abuse and incestual relationships were abundantly more common than the intellectual or religious communities believed or could tolerate.

Freud was met with great hostility for his "seduction hypothesis" and within a few years he completely repudiated his hypothesis, stating instead that these sexual abuse disclosures were memories of sexual fantasies rather than actual experiences.[4] Furthermore, psychological trauma was not seen as central to psychiatry at that time, resulting in Janet's findings being ignored for decades.[6] In 1932, one of Freud's closest psychoanalytic disciples, Sandor Ferenczi, reasserted the "seduction hypothesis" based on confessions from adults he treated regarding their sexual abuse as children. His paper, "Confusion of tongues between adults and the child," is one of the most insightful and prophetic descriptions of the occurrence and harms associated with child sexual abuse preceding our present era. Ironically, Freud was one of the primary critics expressing skepticism about Ferenczi's observations. Sexual abuse and childhood trauma were again disregarded by the medical community.

It was not until the feminist movement in the United States during the 1960s, primarily out of their work with rape survivors and the medical "rediscovering" of child abuse, that the subject of CSA again received attention. Dr. C. Henry Kempe, a leader in the recognition of child physical abuse, gave a speech in 1977 to the American Academy of Pediatrics on child sexual abuse,[7] marking a turning point within the modern medical community on the awareness and responsibility of physicians to care for victims of sexual abuse. In the last several decades, the combination of increased research, high-profile cases, and mandatory reporting has established the widespread nature and psychological effects of CSA about which Freud briefly theorized. This has lead to research addressing psychological effects, prevention, and treatment of CSA. Although the descriptions of psychological effects are more specific, the research is much more developed, and the treatment evidence based, the profound effects of CSA found by current research are very similar to the observations of Freud, Janet, and Ferenczi decades earlier.

EFFORTS TO CHARACTERIZE CHILD SEXUAL ABUSE AND ASSOCIATED IMPACTS

Child Sexual Abuse Accommodation Syndrome

One of the most influential articles on the phenomenology of CSA is Roland Summit's child sexual abuse accommodation syndrome (CSAAS) published in 1983.[8] Through describing the CSAAS, Summit sought to "... disabuse judges and jurors from commonly held misconceptions about child sexual abuse." CSAAS includes the *secrecy;* the *helplessness* of children; *entrapment* of the child; *accommodation* to the sexual abuse; a *delayed, inconsistent, and unconvincing disclosure* of the abuse; and for those who do disclose abuse, frequent *retraction* of their prior disclosures.

The first aspect of CSAAS is *secrecy.* Summit[8] observed that sexual abuse, unlike other forms of maltreatment, is more secretive in nature. There are typically no witnesses, the perpetrator uses threats or guilt to quiet the child, and the child relies on the perpetrator to explain the experience since the child is typically sexually naïve. Psychologically, this places the responsibility on the child to maintain the status quo. By the secretive nature of the experience, the child discerns the action is bad or wrong, but is also quite aware, either through direct or implied threat, that disclosing the abuse would cause serious negative consequences. Furthermore, the perpetrator often reinforces the silence of the child by telling him or her that no one would believe a disclosure, or that others would perceive the abuse as the child's fault.

Helplessness is the second aspect of the syndrome. Summit observes that most adults assume that a child who suffers abuse would simply tell of the abuse at the first possible chance. This thought process, however, does not respect the naturally dependent nature of the child, especially since the majority of CSA is perpetrated by people known to the child and not by strangers. Typically, children lack the authority within the framework of the family to effectively oppose an adult caregiver or another authority. Therefore, most children do not kick or scream out when sexually assaulted, but instead implore tactics such as pretending to be asleep, hiding, or simply dissociating from the experience.

Entrapment and accommodation is the next part of CSAAS. Since the sexual abuse is rarely a one-time occurrence, and the child is already overcome by feelings of secrecy and helplessness, the child becomes entrapped in a cycle of abuse and must learn to accommodate psychologically. This is partly why CSA often continues until the child matures or a third party discovers the abuse. In some ways, this is an attempt by the child to gain some feeling of control of the situation, usually by placing the blame on himself or herself, which can lead to self-hate and self-debasement. Children can further accommodate psychologically through fragmentation, dissociation, and in some extreme cases, the development of dissociative identity disorder.

Delayed, conflicted, or unconvincing disclosure is the fourth principle in CSAAS. Even though studies show that it is quite normal for children to delay their report of sexual abuse, this delay—in combination with the fact that describing chronic abuse long after it began can appear conflicted or unconvincing—leads to questioning the truthfulness of the child. Furthermore, the child's coping strategies, either positive or negative, can be used as further evidence of the factitious nature of the disclosure. Children are often not considered to be reliable when they have begun to use drugs, engage in self-mutilation behavior, have explosive outbursts, be delinquent, or dissociate as part of their accommodation. Conversely, a child who has maintained good grades, appropriate social skills, and other successes does not *appear* to be a victim of abuse, leading to dismissive reactions from adult figures. In either context, this lack of congruency with the expected appearance of a "true victim" and a delayed or conflicting disclosure fosters a skeptical response from many adults. This may be the case especially if acknowledging the true nature of the disclosure significantly diminishes that adult's prior self concept as protector of the child.

Retraction is the final element of CSAAS. Often children who do disclose will recant their previous statement when they discover that many of their previous fears about disclosing were warranted. Nonoffending family members often do not believe disclosures, the perpetrator abandons and blames the child, and the family can fragment when a report of sexual abuse is made. Again the child is faced with the decision to preserve one's self or the family, and often the child chooses the family. To many adults, the retraction appears much more convincing than the original disclosure because at the moment of retraction, all of the doubts and questions of the adults are answered and the integrity of the family is restored.

Overall, CSAAS describes the phenomenon of CSA for many sexually abused children, especially prolonged, interfamilial forms of CSA. CSAAS is neither a diagnostic checklist nor appropriate evidence to prove CSA. Its value in the legal, investigative, and clinical arenas is to counter attempts to use delayed disclosure and recantation to disprove other evidence of sexual abuse, such as detailed disclosures and testimony by child victims. The syndrome further elucidates the countertransference and projection experienced by nonoffending family members and professionals alike when confronted by reports of CSA. It explains developmentally understandable beliefs and coping strategies of children when they become victims of CSA. The clinician must remember that a child's experience and reaction to trauma, especially the trauma associated with CSA, is often different than an adult's expectation of what a reaction should look like. Understanding this juxtaposition is essential to appropriately working with many victims of CSA.

Traumagenic Dynamics

A frequently cited conceptual model for organizing the various effects observed in studies of sexually abused children was proposed by Finkelhor and Browne.[9] It describes four *"traumagenic dynamics"*—traumatic sexualization, betrayal, stigmatization and powerlessness—as the core psychological injuries associated with child sexual victimization. Finkelhor and Browne believed that by understanding these core dynamics, one could anticipate and understand the origin of psychological reactions to child sexual abuse, with a child's manifestation of symptoms categorized by one or more of the dynamics described. The child's own psychological predispositions, environment, and type of trauma affect how the child reacts to the different dynamics. This theory helped focus research presented later describing the childhood and long-term psychological sequelae of CSA. When reviewing the effects of CSA, it is useful to consider which traumagenic dynamics are most salient to the individual child's reaction.

Traumatic sexualization refers to the changes that occur in the child's feelings and attitudes toward sex and sexuality. Often when children are victims of CSA, they are rewarded, taught misconceptions about sexual behavior, or are conditioned to perceive sexual activity with negative emotions or memories. This results in increased knowledge of sexual issues and premature and distorted sexualization. Sexually abused children sometimes demonstrate increased sexual behaviors and interest or avoidance and sexual inhibition.

Betrayal is experienced by many CSA victims in two principle scenarios. First, if the CSA is intrafamilial, the perpetrator, a caregiver on whom the child depended, causes direct harm to the child. Second, in either intrafamilial or extrafamilial CSA, when the child discloses the abuse, nonoffending caregivers either cannot believe the child or change their attitude toward the child. Again, the child feels betrayed by someone that they previously viewed as a protector with whom the child felt safe and secure. A lack of trust in the caregiver can be an impetus for depression, extreme dependency or mistrust, anger, and an inability to judge trustworthiness in others.

CSA victims experience *stigmatization* when they are blamed for the abuse and told to keep the abuse secret by either the abuser or nonoffending caregivers. Furthermore, victims are given the impression, either directly or indirectly, that they are "damaged goods." The child learns to feel shame and guilt as a result of the abuse and often views himself or herself as different from others, leading to either isolation or maladaptive behaviors that originate from an increased need for acceptance. A significantly stigmatized child might even engage in self-mutilation or suicidal behavior.

The dynamic of *powerlessness*, or lack of control, results from the child's inability to prevent the invasion of his or her body, lack of efficacy in stopping the abuse, and the continual fear that many children experience in CSA. This dynamic can be exacerbated if attempts to disclose are not believed. Powerlessness can result in anxiety, fear, and lower self-esteem or an increased need for control and identification with the aggressor.

RISK FACTORS

Given the ubiquitous nature of CSA in the United States, where in any given year 1 out of every 12 children is sexually abused,[10] all children are at some risk for becoming a victim. However, some retrospective data are available to help guide the practitioner in identifying qualities that make a patient more at risk for sexual abuse.

The first and most well-documented risk factor is gender, with girls being victimized disproportionately more often than boys in both intrafamilial and extrafamilial CSA. Furthermore, it appears that children are at greatest risk to being a victim of sexual abuse when they are between the ages of 8 and 12.[10]

Parental issues, such as conflicted parent-child relationships, living apart from one's parents, parental mental illness or substance abuse problems, and marital conflict have all been associated with a higher risk of CSA.[11] Experiencing other forms of abuse, either physical or emotional, also increases one's risk for sexual abuse.[12] Other studies that have only looked at risk factors for women have found that parental drinking and a perception that one's parents were rejecting rather than loving were risk factors for CSA.[13] Maternal history of CSA is also a risk factor for daughters to be sexually abused, which has led some to speculate that there is an intergenerational transmission of risk through either psychological or environmental factors.[14] Furthermore, when a mother has both a history of sexual abuse and drug use, the co-occurrence of these two risk factors significantly increases the risk that her child will be a victim of sexual abuse.[15]

Children with developmental disability are more at risk for CSA.[14] Specifically, studies have shown that children with mental retardation, behavior problems, and developmental disability have a higher rate of abuse, which may be an underrepresentation of the true rates of abuse, given the difficulty or inability to disclose among disabled children. Disabled children tend to be abused earlier than nondisabled children. Overall, disabled children have been found up to three times more likely to be sexually abused than their nonabused peers.

Of note, socioeconomic status and ethnicity have not been consistently or strongly associated with risk of CSA, indicating that CSA transcends ethnic and economic lines.[10]

SEXUAL BEHAVIOR

Children's sexual development begins in early childhood and continues through adolescence. Abnormal sexual behavior in a child can be a symptom of increased stress on the child. This stress can arise from a number of origins, including but not limited to major life changes, family dysfunction, and being a victim of abuse. Child sexual development can be quite distressing to parents, making sexual behaviors a common concern in pediatric visits. Furthermore, many parents are concerned that a child who is asking questions of a sexual nature or engaging in sexual activities such as masturbation might be a victim of CSA. It is up to the clinician to be aware of what constitutes normal vs. abnormal and developmentally inappropriate sexual behavior, and to understand that although approximately one third of victims of CSA demonstrate increased sexual behavior, precocious sexual behavior may have other origins.

William Friedrich[16] contributed much to our understanding of sexual behavior development in children by studying sexual behavior in victims of sexual abuse in comparison to other groups of children. Friedrich developed the Child Sexual Behavior Inventory (CSBI), a scale that compares the sexual behavior of normal, psychiatric, and sexually victimized children between 2 and 12 years of age.[16] Friedrich's work demonstrates that normal young children exhibit sexual behavior and that their sexual behavior increases until about the age of 5 or 6, at which point observed sexual behavior significantly declines until right before adolescence. Specifically, Friedrich observed that it is developmentally appropriate for 2- to 5-year-olds to be sexually intrusive, standing too close to others, touching the breasts/genitalia of themselves or others, or attempting to look at other's genitalia. Furthermore, even though the overall rate dropped, Friedrich noted that greater than 20% of both boys and girls continued to touch themselves in private and look at others while undressing from the ages of 6 to 9 even though they are considered to be in their "latency" stage of sexual development. Finally, by the time children reached 10 to 12 years old, sexually intrusive behavior had greatly decreased and the only normative sexual behavior was being very interested in the opposite sex.

Age-inappropriate sexual behavior is strongly associated with CSA. However, physical abuse, neglect, exposure to domestic violence, excessive life stress and exposure to family sexuality can also result in inappropriate sexual behavior.[17] Among preschool-age children, changes in sexual behavior are more common because of a lack of understanding concerning social sexual norms. However, only one third of preschool-age CSA victims demonstrate abnormal sexual behavior.[18]

There is some evidence to suggest that age-inappropriate sexual knowledge and emotional reactions might be more specific markers for CSA among young children.[18] When children learn about sex and sexuality in the context of a strong emotion-evoking experience such as CSA, sexuality becomes part of their knowledge base. This is in contrast to nonabused preschoolers who lack sexual knowledge and accompanying emotional reactions. Therefore, when asked about potentially sexual topics such as genitals or nudity, or when shown pictures of people interacting in potentially sexual ways, nonabused children respond naïvely. The CSA victim, however, is more likely to demonstrate knowledge of sexual behavior and function that is beyond their developmental stage. In the CSBI, inappropriate sexual knowledge is one of the most distinguishing factors between sexually abused and nonabused children.[17]

SHORT-TERM EFFECTS

Victims of CSA show a variety of short-term psychological outcomes. These outcomes are quite varied in nature and are most likely dependent on a number of factors including the age of the child, the type and duration of the sexual abuse, the other types of abuse that the child has endured, and the relationship of the child to the perpetrator. Protective factors, such as having a supportive and stable family, feeling safe, and having access to resources, can also play a role in the manifestations of psychological outcomes of sexual abuse. Finally, a large percentage of children, as high as 40%, will have no discernable changes in their affect or behavior following confirmed sexual abuse.[19] This lack of symptomatology, which has been called the "sleeper effect,"[20] does not mean that the victim will never have any short-term psychological effects of the abuse, with as many as 20% of these children being positive for psychological morbidity at 12 to 18 months' follow-up.[19] This process of a "sleeper effect" seems to occur more often with children who are victims of less severe forms of CSA.[20]

In New Zealand, a longitudinal study looked at factors that correlated with victims of CSA either having symptoms later in childhood or being symptom free from their traumatic experience.[21] The study demonstrated that with increased severity of sexual abuse (i.e., physical restraint or penetration), there was a linear association with increase in emotional and behavioral symptoms. They further observed that there was a statistically greater chance for adjustment problems if the victim was younger than 10 at the time of the abuse, if there was less paternal care and if the victim's peers engaged in substance abuse. Interestingly, the study found that there was no significant association between adjustment outcomes and intrafamilial vs. extrafamilial abuse, gender of the victim, maternal or paternal protection, or peer attachment. In their cohort, by the age of 18, nearly 25% of all victims of CSA had no discernable adjustment symptoms.[21]

Maternal relationships tend to impact the manifestations of CSA. In one study, there was a direct correlation between the quality of the mother-daughter relationship and the development of internalizing and externalizing symptoms in a group of sexually abused girls.[22] Furthermore, family adaptability and paternal response to abuse have been related to the severity of behavior problems after the discovery of CSA.[23] As will be covered in greater detail in the treatment section of this chapter, parents not only affect the manifestations of CSA, but are important to the effectiveness of treatment as well.

Dissociation, which Summit and others have observed in victims of CSA,[8] recently has been seen not just a symptom of sexual abuse, but also a mediator of psychopathology related to sexual abuse. It has been well established that victims of CSA on average score higher than norms on child dissociative scales.[24] This means that in general, victims of CSA experience disruptions in the normally integrated functions of consciousness, memory, identity, and perception of the environment, even though they may not meet full criteria for dissociative disorder. It has been shown that unlike physical abuse, dissociation is significantly associated with sexual abuse.[25] Further analysis demonstrates that in areas such as increased internalizing and externalizing problems, increased psychiatric illness scales and increased suicidality, dissociation was a significant covariate; when dissociation was controlled, the significant effect of sexual abuse disappeared, indicating that dissociation can be a common adaptation in symptomatic victims of sexual abuse.

Early Childhood (2-6)

In early childhood, children known to have been sexually abused have been observed to have a variety of changes in their behaviors, and these changes are generally the same whether or not the perpetrator is intrafamilial or extrafamilial.[21] Sexually abused children in this age range show higher rates of inappropriate sexual behaviors, demonstrate lower intellectual abilities, and often show evidence of PTSD compared with nonabused children.[26] Three- to 6-year-old CSA victims tend to express more depression and anxiety and to exhibit more symptoms of social withdrawal compared with nonabused children.[26] These children tend to overrate their social competence compared with their peers.[27] Younger children tend not to exhibit increases in nonsexual-related behaviors compared with norms unless there are other stressors in the home such as father's use of alcohol or a maternal history of sexual abuse.[26]

Middle Childhood (7-12)

Latency-aged children continue to exhibit increased symptoms of depression, anxiety, and PTSD.[28] This age group has increased rates of suicidal ideation. Increased sexual anxiety and inappropriate sexual behavior are also noted in this age range,[28] including sexual aggression.[25] In this age range, the child's coping strategies and family/peer support appear to play a significant role in the psychological manifestations of their abuse.[21] Also, unlike younger children, children in this age group tend to underrate their social competence.[27] Although no clear evidence of eating disorders has been reported, some studies suggest that body and weight dissatisfaction as well as purging and dietary restriction can begin in this age range among victims of CSA.[29]

Adolescence/Young Adult (13-18)

The psychological effects of child sexual abuse on adolescents are the most studied of the different developmental periods. Just as in the previous developmental periods, depression, anxiety, and PTSD are well documented within this age group.[21,30,31] Adolescents experience higher rates of depressive symptoms and lower global self-worth compared with younger children, and the risk of having an affective disorder appears to be strongly related to the severity of their abuse. Suicidal ideation and completed suicide are increased among victims of CSA, with males having more suicidal tendencies than females.[28] Self-harm was also noted to be four times higher among adolescent females compared with controls.[32]

Negative beliefs and emotions about one's self have been shown to be highly correlated with the symptoms and severity of PTSD in victims of CSA. Specifically, anger, shame, and humiliation have been directly linked to CSA.[33] This negative system of emotions is believed to be based on the feeling of being attacked and defeated, leading to lack of self-worth and self-efficacy. Victims of CSA then tend to engage in activities that reinforce low self-worth, perpetuating negative internalized emotions.[9] The associated sexual behavior reported in this age group is no longer defined by the CSBI observed ratings scales that deal with inappropriate sexualized behavior, but rather come under the definition of risky sexual behavior. For example, adolescents who have been sexually abused are more likely to have had intercourse, have more frequent intercourse, and report an earlier age of onset of intercourse than their peers who have not been sexually abused.[32,34] Furthermore, there is a higher rate of sexually transmitted diseases, including HIV, and teen pregnancy.[32] Although many of the sexually related co-morbidities can be linked to increased sexual activity and risky sexual activity, some speculate that the increase in pregnancy is multifactorial and includes a desire by some female victims of CSA to conceive.[34] CSA victims who become pregnant as adolescents have an increased risk for pregnancy complications including preterm birth.[32] CSA victims also

report having more difficulty establishing and maintaining relationships within their peer groups.[34,35]

Sleep disturbances are more common in victims of CSA compared with controls. Although sleep disturbances (insomnia, hypersomnia) are a common symptom for other psychiatric illnesses such as PTSD and depression, it has been shown that in adolescence, problems with sleep are independently associated with victimization.[36]

Sexually abused teens also have a higher rate of antisocial traits and other nonsexual behavior problems.[37] These documented findings include being greater likelihood to run away from home[38] and gang affiliation.[39] There is also clear evidence to suggest an association between disordered eating and CSA among adolescents. These behaviors include frequent dieting, binge eating, and preoccupation with weight.[40]

Substance abuse is higher among adolescents with a history of sexual abuse.[37] Alcohol abuse, including binge drinking, is also higher among CSA victims. Victims tend to start using substances earlier, use more frequently, use a greater variety of substances, and report more reasons for using substances than their peers. The risk of substance abuse among adolescents increases even more if one is a victim of both physical and sexual abuse. Reasons for using include coping with previous traumatic memories and emotional problems. In general substance abusers with a history of abuse are more likely than nonvictims to express a specific reason why they abuse substances.

Although some of the relationships between psychological and behavioral co-morbidities with CSA appear clear, the manner in which they are related is far more complex. This is demonstrated by the difficulty in replicating identified relationships in subsequent studies. Adverse childhood experiences such as physical abuse or family dysfunction can increase the risk of adverse psychological outcomes. Sometimes children demonstrate minimal to no effects of CSA when strong family support or internal resiliency is demonstrated. Therefore, many in the field wonder about the mechanism by which CSA leads to its outcomes. To that point, many have begun to look at commonalities that could be used to better predict psychological outcomes associated with CSA. Some have taken a biological approach, looking at serum markers of different hormones associated with psychological distress such as cortisol levels and ACTH. Others have used imaging techniques to compare the brain volume, blood flow, and function in abused and nonabused children. Finally, others have developed theoretical psychological models that attempt to break down the factors that increase or decrease the rate of psychological distress associated with CSA.

CHILD SEXUAL ABUSE AND PSYCHIATRIC DIAGNOSIS

A 1985 effort to describe the characteristics of sexually abused children that might be useful for distinguishing them from nonsexually abused children[41] highlighted the limitations of DSM-III psychiatric diagnoses to adequately describe the diverse psychological and behavioral changes observed among sexually victimized children. Subsequent work focused upon the common reactions among victims of interpersonal violence and exploitation including child sexual abuse, rape, and intimate partner violence. Van der Kolk and others[42] developed the concept of complex PTSD to better describe this population. This more pervasive impact of interpersonal victimization is described in the "Associated Features and Disorders" section on PTSD in DSM-IV as follows:

"The following associated constellation of symptoms may occur and are more commonly seen in association with an interpersonal stressor (e.g. childhood sexual or physical abuse, domestic battering): impaired affect modulation; self-destructive and impulsive behavior; dissociative symptoms; somatic complaints; feelings of ineffectiveness, shame, despair, or hopelessness; feeling permanently damaged; a loss of previously sustained beliefs; hostility; social withdrawal; feeling constantly threatened; impaired relationships with others; or a change from the individual's previous personality characteristics."[43]

LONG-TERM OUTCOMES OF CHILDHOOD SEXUAL ABUSE

Like the psychological impact and behaviors associated with children who have been sexually abused, a variety of psychological outcomes have been observed at higher prevalence rates in adults with a history of CSA. Again, many factors affect the manifestation of symptoms, including severity of the trauma, biological predispositions in the victim, overall family dysfunction, co-morbid illnesses, and additional traumas. Researchers have also identified factors such as shame, interpersonal difficulties, and avoidant coping strategies that can mediate the expression of adult outcomes.[44] Furthermore, although over time the percentage of victims who have symptoms increases, there will continue to be a cohort of individuals who have no discernable sequelae related to the trauma.

Research on treatment for CSA victims is showing promise but still early in its development. Cognitive-behavioral therapy (CBT) and other treatments have been shown to decrease psychological symptoms in childhood. However, there is still no evidence to demonstrate that childhood treatment will affect or modify psychological manifestations in adulthood.

There are few longitudinal studies that look at the effects of CSA in adulthood; therefore, much of the information that we have regarding long-term outcomes is based on cross-sectional retrospective analyses. The usefulness of this information to health care professionals (HCPs) is not to report to parents what will happen to their children when they are adults, but rather to provide a general framework for the types of issues that some individuals struggle with for years after the abuse has ended.

Posttraumatic Stress Disorder

PTSD is one of the more common long-term effects of CSA. Specific symptoms associated with late-evolving PTSD typically include flashbacks, intrusive thoughts, hyperarousal states, cognitive distortions, misperception of normal social transactions as threatening, and avoidance of situations or stimuli that might be, in some way, reminiscent of the abuse.

PTSD is more common among victims who had a delay in their disclosure than those who disclosed within 1 month of the abuse.[45]

PTSD is a type of anxiety disorder, and therefore it makes sense that survivors of CSA would be more prone to develop not only PTSD, but also a wide range of anxiety disorders. Patients with an anxiety disorder and a history of CSA are likely to have more severe anxiety as well as co-morbid depression.[46] Women with histories of severe CSA have been shown to have increased risk of generalized anxiety disorder and social phobia.[47]

Depression

Depression is another psychiatric disorder commonly encountered among adults with histories of CSA.[45] Twin studies demonstrate that when controlled for genetics and environment, CSA is an independent risk factor for adult depression, along with suicide attempts.[48] Although depressive symptoms were first noted in samples of female victims,[49] subsequent research has demonstrated that both male and female victims of CSA suffer equally from depressive symptoms.[50] Depressed individuals with histories of CSA tend to score higher on self-report depression scores and to demonstrate more personality dysfunction and more borderline personality traits than depressed individuals without a history of CSA.[51]

Domestic Violence/Revictimization

Domestic violence,[52,53] other violent relationships, more severe violence, and relationship violence initiated by women occur more frequently in victims of CSA.[35] Domestic violence was four times more likely if CSA involved intercourse.[53] In males who were victims of contact CSA, there is a threefold increase in the risk of becoming a perpetrator of domestic violence and an increased risk of aggressive behavior in general in their relationships.[53] Many studies have found an increase in the incidence of rape among survivors of CSA, with one study showing a threefold increase in the report of being raped.[54] Non-violent marital problems[55] and divorce are also significantly more common among victims of CSA.

Eating Disorders

CSA has been associated with various eating problems but not eating disorders as defined by DSM-IV. However, CSA has been associated with excessive eating,[54] and women with a history of severe CSA are more likely than nonabused women to suffer from bulimia nervosa.[56]

General Mental Health

Women with a history of CSA, especially severe CSA, have lower overall levels of perceived mental health and self esteem.[54,57] There is also a higher rate of psychiatric hospitalizations among women with a history of CSA.[57] Both genders have demonstrated overall increases in measures that quantify mental health problems, with symptoms such as paranoia, psychoticism, and hostility significantly more common in this population.[50]

Substance Abuse/Dependence

Women with a history of CSA have a higher rate of alcohol dependence.[58] Furthermore, it appears that there is an overall increase in addiction to tobacco and illicit substances among CSA survivors.[58] Substance abusers with a history of CSA tend to have more severe addictions and greater difficulty maintaining sobriety in treatment programs.[59] The rate of drug and alcohol dependence tends to be more common if the CSA involved intercourse.

Parenting

Much concern is given to the risk that a childhood victim of CSA will become a perpetrator of abuse as a parent. Female survivors tend to have a more negative perception of themselves as parents and are more likely to use physical methods of punishment.[60] Furthermore, CSA victims tend to be less comfortable with the more intimate aspects of parenting, including diaper changing.[61] Mothers who were victims themselves also tend to have more involvement with child protective services in regards to their own children.[62] However, it does not appear that a history of sexual abuse leads to poor or abusive parenting. Rather, potential long-term outcomes of CSA such as depression and a decreased locus of control explain much of the parenting difficulties,[63] meaning that in the absence of such sequelae, CSA victims function no differently than other parents.

Medical Problems

Long-term medical problems with psychological components have been observed in adults who have a history of CSA. There is an overall increased use of medical services among distressed adults with histories of CSA,[64,65] increased reports of nonspecific pelvic pain, pain during intercourse,[66] general sexual problems,[55,58] urinary retention, irritable bowel syndrome, fibromyalgia,[65] premenstrual distress, menstrual problems including excessive bleeding and painful menstruation,[66] poor or excessive prenatal weight gain, increased depression and anxiety while pregnant,[67] increased incidence of abortions,[55] increased occurrence of sexually transmitted infections, and increased HIV risk behaviors.[68] Although there is an overall increase in use of medical services and medical costs, there is a decreased use of pap smears to screen for cervical cancer among abuse survivors.[69]

The Adverse Childhood Experiences (ACE) Study demonstrated strong dose-related associations between several adverse childhood experiences, including CSA and many serious long-term health problems.[1] ACE investigators Felitti and Anda looked at the childhood experiences of a cohort of 17,000 members of a California-based HMO. They screened for nine potential adverse experiences, including histories of sexual, physical, and psychological abuse; neglect; witnessing domestic violence; substance abuse and mental illness in the home; and missing or incarcerated parents. They found that of the respondents who claimed at least one ACE, 87% reported at least one other.[12] This fact demonstrates the interrelatedness of different adverse childhood events, explaining the difficulty that researchers have in identifying experiences such as sexual abuse as the only

cause of an adverse outcome. ACE research has generated articles that link common medical ailments such as obesity, chronic obstructive pulmonary disease, heart disease, and liver disease to adverse childhood events including CSA. This research demonstrates that childhood trauma such as sexual abuse can significantly impact adult health.

GENDER DIFFERENCES IN THE EFFECTS OF SEXUAL ABUSE

Boys are sexually abused at a significantly lower rate than girls, with most experts estimating the lifetime prevalence of sexual abuse for boys to be somewhere around 10% to 15%, which is one reason why more attention has been paid to the effects of CSA in females. Boys and girls both demonstrate similar adverse sequelae when they are victims of sexual abuse. Both consistently exhibit internalizing (i.e., depression and anxiety) and externalizing (i.e., behavior problems and sexually acting out) symptoms; however, boys demonstrate more externalizing problems than girls, including more suicide attempts and binge drinking.[31] Boys are also more likely to have concerns about homosexuality than female victims of CSA.[70] Reasons for these differences might be attributable to the differences in sexual abuse experiences between boys and girls. Males constitute the large majority of perpetrators against both females and males, hence boys' sexual abuse is most often homosexual and girls' heterosexual. CSA among boys is typically more physical in nature, involves more acts of penetration, and is co-morbid with physical abuse more often than with girls. Boys are more likely to be sexually abused by someone outside the family, and the duration of the abuse is typically shorter for boys than girls. The nature of the disclosure is also quite different between genders, with boys being less willing to disclose abuse, experiencing more conflict with issues concerning gender identity, demonstrating more ambivalence as to whether they disapproved of the sexual abuse, and are more likely to feel that their being victimized was due to their own weakness.[70]

Since the large majority of CSA perpetrators are male, it is important to recognize the minimal and incomplete data concerning the relationship between being a male victim of CSA and the likelihood of later becoming a perpetrator. It is well established that perpetrators of CSA and other crimes of sexual violence are more likely to be victims of CSA themselves.[71] However, many sexual predators suffered from other forms of adverse childhood experiences as well, including physical abuse and neglect, and they generally come from homes with significant pathology and family dysfunction. Most sexually abused boys do not become child sexual abusers.[72]

DISCLOSURE

CSA victims rarely have physical symptoms pathognomonic for CSA. Instead, a large percentage of discovered cases of sexual abuse are due to patient disclosures. Approximately 10% of all confirmed cases of CSA reports were made by medical professionals in 2005.[73]

HCPs realize that although their primary responsibility is to the patient, they must work to maintain a relationship with the entire family as well. This relationship can be difficult during times of severe stress, such as when disclosures of sexual abuse are made, since over 50% of confirmed cases of sexual abuse are perpetrated by either parents or other family members. Although the HCP is not an investigator, since the late 1970s, it has been the law in all 50 states for adults who are responsible for the care of children (i.e., teachers, doctors, day care professionals) to report all suspected abuse to the proper governmental agency, typically a child abuse hotline. Being upfront and explaining to the family one's legal obligation to report any suspicion of abuse is typically the best way to keep the lines of communication open and to maintain a relationship with the family. Furthermore, if the practitioner takes the time to explain the process that the parents will typically go through during a child protective services investigation, less damage is done to the relationship between the practitioner and the family.

Many factors go into timing and circumstance of disclosure. Reports indicate a generally longer lapse between incident and disclosure if the patient is young, if the sexual abuse occurs multiple times, or if the perpetrator is a family member. Disclosure typically occurs more quickly if the perpetrator is a stranger. The severity of the abuse has been shown in multiple studies to have little to no effect on the timing of the disclosure. Overall, one must remember that delay is more often the rule than the exception. Parents will question why their child waited, especially in cases of chronic sexual abuse, to disclose to a parent or to another responsible adult. It is the job of the pediatrician or the child abuse team to reassure the parents that this delay is normal (see previous discussion on CSAAS) and is not a reflection of the validity of the allegations. In a national survey via telephone, 75% of women who reported at least one episode of sexual abuse before the age of 18 waited at least 5 years to tell another person, with nearly 25% of all victims reporting their abuse for the very first time during the telephone interview.[74]

HCPs must also realize that the disclosure of sexual abuse affects the whole family, not just the victim. It is quite common for parents to become emotional when a child makes a disclosure of sexual abuse. The emotion varies depending on the nature of the parent and the parent–child relationship as well as the parents' own experiences and problems. Since the outcome for the child in cases of CSA is related to the reaction and support of his or her parents, it is vital that the practitioner take time with the parent and make sure that their immediate concerns are heard and that they have options for support when they leave the office.

Reporting to Child Protective Services

In CSA, the primary objective after ensuring the appropriate medical work-up of the patient is to plan with nonoffending parents a safe and appropriate environment for the patient. While the patient is still in the office or emergency department, it is important to screen nonoffending parents for other home safety issues such as parental drug use, history or threat of physical abuse, and history or threat of domestic violence. Depending on the age of the child, severity of CSA, the possible perpetrator, and other factors that increase the physical risk to the patient, possible immediate outcomes of

a referral to child protective services (CPS) include going home with a follow-up visit from CPS, the child being placed in the care of a safe family member, or the child being taken into state custody. Usually the CPS case worker, after hearing the referral, can advise the HCP what the probable short-term outcome will be, allowing the provider to inform the parents. However, the role of CPS is to provide for the safety of children, and so as new information becomes available, the level of intervention may change. It is important not to make promises to the family that are beyond the control of the HCP.

Concerning responsibility to report, there are several factors to consider. First and foremost, all should be familiar with their own state laws that delineate the requirements on referral and documentation. When documenting suspected abuse, HCPs should list both the specific questions as well as the patient's response in the note, any significant behaviors or interactions observed during the visit, and a detailed note describing the physical examination. Second, in making the decision whether to report, the American Academy of Pediatrics[75] has published guidelines that incorporate history, physical, and laboratory findings to aid pediatricians in accurately assessing their level of suspicion and their duty to report.

Medical Examination and Interaction with Child Abuse Team

Most authorities agree that a physical examination, specifically the anogenital examination, should be performed in a child-friendly setting. The examination should never be forced or involve restraints. Gullay and colleagues[76] found that of nonabused preschool children, only 7.7% rated the anogenital examination as somewhat negative even though it was significantly more distressing than the examination of the ears or mouth. One study showed that allowing children to watch the videocolposcopy in real time during the examination was tolerable, especially in children who had disclosed sexual abuse. Furthermore, studies have shown that appropriate professional preparation leads to decreased distress during the anogenital examination. Dubowitz[77] in his review in 1998 concluded that no data exist to support that an examination performed by an experienced practitioners would lead to long-term emotional trauma.

Gully[76] developed the Genital Examination Distress Scale (GEDS) to measure the emotional distress during genital examinatiion. GEDS is a simple-to-use scale for children age 1 to 17 that uses verbally expressed and physiological responses to gauge the distress of the child during the examination. Although there are no long-term outcomes associated with the GEDS measure, the tool can be used both for research as well as clinical purposes as child abuse centers continue to look at how to improve the comfort of children undergoing evaluation for abuse.[78] Recent research shows promising results for increasing the value of the forensic medical examination for possible CSA by educating caregivers about evidence-based psychological treatments at the time of the medical evaluation. Educating caregivers about psychological treatments was associated with greater awareness of options available and overall increased satisfaction with the medical examination.[79]

Disclosure *vs.* Forensic Interview

It is vital that HCPs understand the difference between their interview with the child and a forensic interview. The job of the HCP is to obtain enough information from the child and the family to make informed clinical decisions on the child's behalf. Once the standard of suspicion of sexual abuse has been met, the HCP is obligated to report to CPS. Any additional information providers collect is for the medical treatment, current safety, and appropriate referral of the patient. Many large cities have specialized interviewers, either social workers or police officers, who have been specially trained to interview suspected victims of sexual abuse. It is their responsibility to collect information in an open-ended and non-suggestive manner so that information received may be used in potential legal proceedings. The duty of the HCP is to provide medical evaluation and care to the patient and to thoroughly document all findings obtained in the history and physical examination that might be needed to ensure the patient's safety.

TREATMENT

The identification of effective modes of treatment for victims of CSA is still in its early stages of development. The varied treatment modalities available and the variation in the presentation of abuse victims have impeded rapid progress in the evaluation of treatment effectiveness. Furthermore, the severity, background, and co-morbidities of the abused have been difficult confounders to deal with in the context of small cohort studies. The first studies that attempted to use pretreatment and posttreatment scores to identify effectiveness date to the mid-1980s. Not all published studies have used control groups, and those that have used controls have suffered from the fact that even without treatment, children tend to improve over time, making it difficult to demonstrate significant effects of treatment. As the number of studies have increased, however, metaanalyses have increased the power of study findings. It now appears that children who participate in treatment tend to do better in targeted areas of difficulty or "secondary problems" associated with their victimization.[3] The major secondary problems targeted in most studies include behavior problems, social functioning, low self-concept, and psychological distress. In general, the longer the treatment lasts, the more the child improves on the secondary problems observed. The following is a brief description of studied therapies that either alone or in combination with other modalities have demonstrated some effectiveness in treating the secondary problems associated with CSA.

Play Therapy

Play therapy is a modality that encourages natural expression of feelings associated with abuse through normal child activities such as play. It provides a comfortable environment for the child to express oneself and work through inner conflicts, even if the child is developmentally unable to verbally express the conflicts themselves. In a group setting, play therapy can encourage the formation of safe relationships with other peers that have had similar experiences. Only a few studies have looked at the efficacy of play therapy on victims of sexual abuse. Most of these studies focus on or include younger children, and most are small studies. In metaanalysis, play therapy seemed to have the greatest effect in dealing with difficulties of social functioning. This might be explained by the inherent socialization found in the act of play itself, either with an individual therapist or in a group setting.[3]

Trauma-focused play therapy is one such technique that is used with children who have experienced trauma. Developed by Eliana Gil,[80] sessions generally last for several months. The therapy involves the use of toys that are selected based on the child's traumatic experience. The child is permitted to move at the child's own pace, and when appropriate, the play is used to expand the child's own trauma narrative, allowing for a gradual desensitization to the trauma. The goal of therapy is reduction of anxiety and fear related to the trauma.

Abuse Specific Therapy

Goals for abuse specific therapy are to provide safety, support, and education for the child as it pertains to their victimization, with the objectives of increasing safety, preventing re-abuse, and decreasing the psychological sequelae of sexual abuse. There are several small studies in which abuse-specific therapy has been compared to controls or has been studied in both individual and group settings. Metaanalysis has demonstrated that abuse-specific therapy was effective in the treatment of psychological distress, behavior, and self-concept problems.[3] Since the majority of the studies looked at abuse-specific therapy in the context of a group setting, it is hard to know whether the benefits of the therapy were related to the modality or the group process and peer interaction. Regardless, there appears to be benefit gained by victims dealing directly with their experiences of abuse.

Trauma-focused integrative-eclectic therapy (IET), developed by William Friedrich,[80] has been implemented with disadvantaged families that are both therapy naïve and avoidant. The therapy identifies the trauma that affects not only the child, but also their relationships within the family structure. IET addresses attachment of the child to nonoffending parents by fostering sensitivity, improving the quality of parent–child play and positive attention, and decreasing intrusive parental behavior. Dysregulation and misperceptions of self caused by the trauma are the other main focuses of therapy, using primarily CBT methods to integrate thoughts, feelings, and emotions by enhancing coping strategies of the patient and appropriate behavior management strategies used by the parents.

Symptom-Focused Therapy

Some therapies are specifically geared toward symptoms and behaviors that are common among victims of CSA, but are not necessarily abuse specific therapies. "Cognitive-Behavioral and Dynamic Play Therapy for Children with Sexual Behavior Problems and their Caregivers" is a 12-session program that incorporates both CBT and play therapy techniques.[80] The therapy includes development of sexual behavior rules, understanding of impulse control, and age-appropriate sexual education. The play therapy component allows the child to reflect, interpret, and express feelings in a safe environment and facilitates the improvement of peer relationships, which often are strained when children have inappropriate sexual behavior.

CSA victims with significant dissociative symptoms might benefit from the "integrative developmental model for treatment of dissociative symptomatology."[80] This model emphasizes self-awareness and affects regulation in order to more effectively interrupt automatic dissociative withdrawal.[80] This treatment approach includes the family by improving communication skills, tolerance, and acceptance of feelings and by empowering the parental figures to use appropriate behavior management techniques, even when the child is in a dissociative state.

Supportive Therapy

Supportive therapy is used by therapists to maintain or improve a patient's self-esteem, to minimize the recurrence of symptoms or distress, and to empower the patient's capacity to deal with adversity. Theoretically, there is much value to these objectives in treating victims of sexual abuse, and in reality most therapeutic modalities provide some degree of support from the therapist toward the patient. When combined with other modalities or compared with no treatment at all, supportive therapy has been shown to be effective in treating behavior problems.[3] However, as an independent modality, supportive therapy has, by itself, not achieved the results of other modalities such as CBT.

Cognitive-Behavioral Therapy

CBT is the modality of treatment that has been most extensively studied in populations of sexual abuse victims, both in group and individual settings. At its core, CBT is based on the theory that a significant amount of emotional deregulation stems from learned behaviors and thinking patterns. The goal of therapy is to learn how to identify, correct, and prevent these maladaptive thoughts and behaviors. CBT has been studied and validated in the treatment of many different psychiatric illnesses, either alone or in conjunction with pharmacotherapy. Although manualized versions of CBT exist, many practitioners use pieces or aspects of CBT in their therapeutic repertoire, making the application of CBT quite diverse. Overall, metaanalysis demonstrates that CBT has been shown to be effective in the treatment of behavior problems, psychological distress, and low self-concept among victims of CSA.[3]

Cognitive processing therapy (CPT), a brief 12- to 16-week therapy, has been demonstrated to effectively treat the depressive symptoms associated with victims of traumatic experiences, including sexual assault.[80] This CBT approach addresses the premise that after traumatic experiences, inappropriate coping strategies of assimilation and over-accommodation disrupt the individual's ability to learn and process new information and lead to depressive feelings of self-blame, guilt, and shame. CPT works to correct these cognitive errors through appropriate accommodation and processing of the traumatic experience.

Trauma-focused CBT (TF-CBT) has been the most studied of the CBTs and is the most widely accessible manualized method. TF-CBT is a stepwise approach for the treatment of individuals who have been traumatized, either acutely or chronically, and who suffer psychiatric and/or behavioral complications from their trauma.[81] Patients who would benefit from TF-CBT include those with PTSD, anxiety, depressive behavior, and self-image changes that have occurred as a result of a traumatic event or series of traumas. In the treatment of sexually abused individuals, TF-CBT uses a combination of abuse-specific and age-appropriate sex education, relaxation, and narrative techniques that empower the child to better cope with remembering the trauma, process the trauma(s), and become desensitized to these memories. The therapist works with both the patient and the nonoffending parents, helping to address misconceptions about sexual abuse and enabling each other to communicate about the trauma by providing structure and a safe environment to share the narrative. This method has been demonstrated in several studies to be effective for children ages 3 to 17, as the therapist adjusts the material and tasks to the developmental level of the child.

TF-CBT is comprised of eight main components including psycho-education, relaxation techniques, affect expression, cognitive coping, trauma narrative, cognitive processing, parenting skills, and parent–child sessions.[81] Although the method is manualized, it is not intended to be rigid. Therapists are encouraged to allow the child to take the lead, and to spend a greater percentage of time in areas or skills where the child or parents are having significant difficulty. The core values of demonstrating respect for the victim and family, adapting to the needs of the individual, encouraging family involvement when appropriate, developing strong therapeutic relationships, and fostering self-efficacy in both the child and the parent are interwoven in all aspects of the therapy. The following is a brief summary of the principal components of TF-CBT.

Psycho-Education

Education is initially given to victims to help them better understand trauma and the symptoms associated with the trauma. Quite often victims experience changes in their emotions and behaviors as being peculiar or unnatural, and it is up to the therapist to inform the patient about the normalcy of their reaction to the traumatic experience. Furthermore, both parents and patients will need to be educated about the process of therapy itself, since many victims of sexual abuse will be "therapy naïve" and might be intimidated by the process.

Relaxation Techniques

Before the therapist can engage the child in his or her traumatic experience, it is important to provide the child with the skills necessary to deal with troubling thoughts or emotions. The therapist works with the child to teach him or her self-relaxation techniques (e.g., controlled breathing) and mind techniques (e.g., thought stopping). This gives children feelings of control over their ability to experience and modulate emotions.

Affect Expression

In order to better manage emotions and anxiety, especially as it relates to their trauma, children often need to be taught how to label emotions and identify levels of intensity. This can be done at the appropriate developmental level of the child.

Cognitive Coping

Many children who have been traumatized have unhelpful and inaccurate thoughts and beliefs concerning the trauma or the effects of the trauma. Both children and parents can have these "thinking errors." It is important for the therapist to educate the child and parent about the relationship between thoughts, feelings, and behaviors demonstrated in the cognitive triangle. At first, the therapist will use non-trauma-related examples to demonstrate the relationship so that when it is time to tackle the issue of the trauma, the child and parent are better prepared to see the "think-feel-do relationship."

Trauma Narrative

The formation of a detailed trauma narrative is a critical step in enabling the child to work through his or her experience. This aim of the trauma narrative is to better enable the patient to control thought intrusions, reduce avoidance of things related to the trauma, and prepare for potential triggers or reminders of the trauma. This is accomplished by breaking apart the association of thoughts, reminders, and discussions of the trauma from the intense negative emotions experienced by the patient. Eventually, with the help of the therapist, the child will share the personal narrative with the parent.

Cognitive Processing

Cognitive processing is a technique that teaches patients how to challenge and modify their thoughts. This is accomplished by exploring the thoughts of the patient with the goal of eventually changing his or her understanding of the experience so that it might be placed in perspective, that the trauma is only one aspect of the patient's life, not a defining one.

Parenting Skills

After a traumatic event, oftentimes parents find it difficult to control the child's behavior because of the guilt that the parents feel related to the traumatic event. These skill-building sessions are done with the parent to not only positively manage the behavior of the child, but also to address the parent's own distress about the child's abuse and improve the parent–child relationship.

Parent–Child Sessions

These sessions allow the child and parent to communicate successfully about the traumatic event and for the parent to model appropriate coping strategies and demonstrate support for their child. This is an important step for enabling the child to effectively communicate emotions to parents or other supportive adult figures after the therapy has terminated.

Group Therapy

Group therapy is a modality that has many benefits when treating a population of victims of CSA. First, many therapists are trained in group therapy who can provide these services, making group therapy common and typically easy to find. Second, in areas with scarce resources, especially scarce mental health resources, group therapy is a practical way to provide services to many victims in an efficient manner. Some of the concerns about group therapy deal with the possible revictimization that could occur by hearing the stories of other victims; the literature, however, does not bear this out. Group therapists believe that the nature of the group itself is therapeutic, specifically addressing the common feelings of isolation and stigma of being a victim of CSA by working with other victims. To meet this objective, groups are typically small and usually consist of children approximately the same age range. Reeker et al[82] reviewed the literature and performed a metaanalysis reviewing efficacy on 15 studies that had some type of pretreatment and posttreatment measures. Most of the group approaches studied used a multimodality approach, although some groups used either CBT or play therapy as the core aspect of the therapy. Overall, they found that groups demonstrated a mean effect size of 0.79, indicating their usefulness in the treatment of CSA.[82]

Involvement and Treatment of Nonoffending Parents

The parental response to children's disclosure of sexual abuse has received a significant amount of attention over the last 25 years. Adams-Tucker[83] observed in 1982 that sexually abused children appeared to be less symptomatic if they received emotional support from a nonoffending parent. Since the type and severity of abuse is not amenable to change except through disclosure and protection, this was the first clue that mediating factors existed on the effects of sexual abuse that could be impacted.

Just as a positive, supportive emotional response leads to decreased behavior problems and symptoms among sexually abused children, it was also found that negative maternal reactions correlated with more severe behavior problems, especially sexual behavior problems if the victims have decreased family support. Furthermore, if the family was not supportive of itself and cohesive, there is a greater chance of the victim having behavior problems.[84] Although the incorporation of parents into therapy for children varies greatly over the different modalities, retrospective analyses suggest that including the parents in the child's treatment leads to more successful outcomes.[85]

Women who were abused themselves as children might respond less supportively to their sexually abused children and can exhibit more anxiety and depressive symptoms related to their child's disclosure.[86] Therefore, when the practitioner is attempting to estimate the risk that the child has for poor psychological outcomes related to her sexual abuse, it might be helpful to obtain a complete family sexual abuse history. Such a history will give the practitioner clues as to the presence of family dysfunction and the ability of nonoffending parents to be emotionally supportive of the victim. This information is vital in guiding therapy modalities that can address not only the trauma, but the family system as well.

The abuse history of nonoffending parents can be a factor in their response to the disclosure of sexual abuse. Although percentages vary greatly, most experts agree that women who were victims of abuse themselves are more likely to have children who will be abused, especially mothers who suffered more severe forms of abuse. This is seen as intergenerational transmission of abuse. The discovery by a parent that his or her child is a victim of sexual abuse is in itself a crisis that can have long-lasting psychological impact on the nonoffending parent.[87] Since CPS has the safety of the child as its utmost priority, nonoffending parents in newly reported cases of sexual abuse are often confronted by accusations of failure to protect and implications of collusion. Mothers have been called untruthful, have been accused of prompting their children to make false allegations, and at times are saddled with the culpability of having allowed the abuse to take place. Among mothers, there is often a strong dissatisfaction with the overall system designed to handle such cases.[88] The uncertainty of dealing with the criminal justice and family protection systems can further exacerbate the underlying frustration.

Protective parents often feel overwhelmed by the system, and many who have gone through the process recommend the importance of having good legal counsel and appropriate emotional support of their own, in the form of family, friends, or professional support. Parental reaction and emotional stability, however, have a significant effect on the psychological outcome of CSA. Therefore, providers who offer a safe, supportive environment and acknowledge the difficulties faced by mothers required to interact with child welfare agencies will more often form alliances that could positively affect the victim's outcome.

Since the psychological outcomes of the victims are significantly affected by the parental response, it makes sense that providing support and treatment for nonoffending parents would be in the patient's best interest. The TF-CBT model of treatment provides for education and support of the nonoffending parent(s) as part of the manualized treatment of sexual abuse. In England, several researchers have looked at group therapy and support groups to meet the needs of parents as well. The observation is that a group that consists of victims' mothers can be beneficial and allow the women to process their common feelings of guilt, anger, and lack of trust.[87] A group that focused on mothers whose children were victims of incest noted a common progression of emotions.[89] First, mothers expressed anger toward the perpetrator. Next, mothers were able to talk about their own past experiences in dysfunctional families and how that affected their reaction to the abuse. By realizing how their own history interacted with the abuse of their children, mothers were then able to gain confidence in their ability to prevent abuse in the future.

Family Therapy

Family resolution therapy (FRT) is designed to work with families of victims of physical or sexual abuse who have already demonstrated progress in victim and offender treatment programs.[80] The goal of FRT is to construct safe, functional, and stable family dynamics. This is accomplished over 6 to 18 months through psycho-education regarding abuse experiences and reactions, revamping of family structure, boundaries that enabled the abuse, and cognitive and behavioral techniques to alter family processes, relationships, and hierarchy. FRT uses close monitoring and collateral information to assess therapeutic response. The eventual outcome is based on the family's progression through the therapy, which can range from family reunification and maintenance to a complete ending of parent–child relationship.

Focused treatment interventions (FTI) are based on the premise that the parents are ultimately responsible for the safety of their children.[80] Through a comprehensive assessment including forensic medical examination and interview as well as extensive social history, the child maltreatment is identified along with any social factors that increase the risk of subsequent maltreatment (i.e., parental alcohol abuse, mental illness). Interventions, including family therapy, are then focused on working with the parents to reduce risk factors and increase safety for the child.

Intensive family preservation services (IFPS) are home-based, primarily cognitive-behavioral approaches designed to decrease the rate of family separation in cases of maltreatment or high risk of maltreatment.[80] The program focuses on parental skill deficits, child behavior problems, and dysfunctional or violent family relationships. Although the treatment does not appear to reduce the risk of out-of-home placement, it tends to decrease subsequent maltreatment and accelerates reunification.

Pharmacological Treatments

No medicine is currently recommended for the treatment of children who are victims of sexual abuse. Only one study has looked at the treatment of children using an antidepressant, sertraline, which is a first-line drug in the treatment of adult PTSD.[90] That study looked at two groups receiving TF-CBT, with only one of the groups receiving sertraline. Since both groups showed improvement in symptoms and the normal onset of efficacy for a selective serotonin reuptake inhibitor is 4 to 12 weeks, it is difficult to say from where the benefits arose. The authors concluded that TF-CBT continues to be the first-line treatment for victims of sexual abuse.

A number of sexually abused children have significant co-morbidities, some of which may not be adequately addressed by psychological therapies alone. In those cases it is important that a referral to a child psychiatrist be made. The decision to use pharmacotherapy in children with mental illness is always a difficult choice, where one weighs the current effect, severity, and duration of the illness on the child. A child who has been traumatized by sexual abuse makes the decision to treat with medicine even more complicated. On one hand, practitioners want to be conservative in their treatment, limiting the child's exposure to medicine if there are little data demonstrating long-term effects as well as knowledge of rare but well-known risks such as increased suicidal ideation with many psychotropic medications such as SSRIs. However, an abuse survivor who suffers from significant co-morbid attention deficit hyperactivity disorder (ADHD), depression, anxiety, or PTSD is at risk of experiencing delays in development that could carry with it long-term sequelae in areas of relationships, education, and quality of life, not to mention an increased risk of suicidal ideation and completed suicide. Child psychiatrists are best trained to deal with the complex treatment of these patients.

STRENGTH OF THE MEDICAL EVIDENCE

In 2004, Saunders, Berliner and Hanson[80] revised the *Child Physical and Sexual Abuse: Guidelines for Treatment* of the National Crime Victims Research and Treatment Center. This study looked at all of the published methods used in the treatment of victims of physical and sexual abuse. They then reviewed all published outcomes data on each method to provide an evidence-based score. Although not specific to CSA, this is the most comprehensive review of the evidence behind different treatment modalities. Only trauma-focused CBT received a score of 1, indicating "well-supported, efficacious treatment," signifying that the benefits had been well proven in the literature.[80] Most of the named treatment modalities dealing with abuse victims—including CBT/Psychodynamic Children with Sexual Behavior Problems, Cognitive Processing Therapy, Eye Movement Desensitization and Reprocessing Therapy, Resilient Peer Training Intervention, Therapeutic Child Development Program and Trauma-Focused Integrative-Eclectic Therapy—all received a score of 3, indicating that they were "supported and acceptable treatment."[80] This score does not indicate that there is any well-documented efficacy associated with the treatment in the literature.

FUTURE RESEARCH AND DEVELOPMENT

It is clear that victims of CSA are members of a heterogeneous group that react to their trauma in varied ways. Furthermore, we are increasing our knowledge of co-factors that appear to mediate the expression of symptoms in CSA victims. Unfortunately, there are very few studies that are longitudinal in nature and adequately powered to look at how factors other than the CSA affect immediate and long-term outcomes. Ideally, large longitudinal studies will provide additional community-based data on mediators and effects of CSA.

With the development of manualized protocols, there has been a significant increase in the amount of evidence regarding the treatment of CSA. Previous research was hampered by small numbers, lack of control groups, and ill-defined outcome measures. There are now a large number of techniques that have promising theories but lack a significant body of literature to support their outcomes. Because of the varied nature of the effects of CSA, outcome measures need to be comprehensive and specific so that techniques of individual practitioners and the manuals in general can be modified over time to improve outcomes. Furthermore, educating medical personnel, law enforcement and social services as well as the public in general about the potentially serious outcomes and effective treatments available to victims of CSA will increase the access to a broader population of CSA victims, enhancing the validity of future studies.

The National Child Traumatic Stress Network is a U.S. Substance Abuse and Mental Health Service Administration (SAMHSA)–funded national program whose mission is to increase the availability of evidence-based treatments to traumatized children and families. Their website, www.NCTSN.org, has a wealth of useful information for both providers and families.

References

1. Felitti VJ, Anda RF, Nordenberg D, et al: Relationship of childhood abuse and household dysfunction to many of the leading causes of death in adults. The Adverse Childhood Experiences (ACE) Study. *Am J Prev Med* 1998;14:245-258.
2. Putnam F: Ten-year research update review: child sexual abuse. *J Am Acad Child Adolesc Psychiatry* 2003;42:269-278.
3. Hetzel-Riggin M, Brausch A, Montgomery B: A meta-analytic investigation of therapy modality outcomes for sexually abused children and adolescents: An exploratory study. *Child Abuse Negl* 2007;31:125-141.
4. Olafson E, Corwin DL, Summit RC: Modern history of child sexual abuse awareness: cycles of discovery and suppression. *Child Abuse Negl* 1993;17:7-24.
5. Masson J: *The Assault on Truth*. Random House, New York, 1984.
6. van der Kolk BA, van der Hart O: Pierre Janet and the breakdown of adaptation in psychological trauma. *Am J Psychiatry* 1989;146:1530-1540.
7. Kempe CH: Sexual abuse, another hidden pediatric problem: the 1977 C. Anderson Aldrich lecture. *Pediatrics* 1978;62:382-389.
8. Summit R: The child sexual abuse accommodation syndrome. *Child Abuse Negl* 1983;7:177-193.
9. Finkelhor D, Browne A: The traumatic impact of child sexual abuse: A conceptualization. *Am J Orthopsychiat* 1985;55:530-541.
10. Finkelhor D, Ormrod R, Turner H, et al: The victimization of children and youth: A comprehensive, national survey. *Child Maltreat* 2005;10:5-25.
11. Finkelhor D, Hotaling G: Sexual abuse in the National Incidence Study of Child Abuse and Neglect: an appraisal. *Child Abuse Negl* 1984;8:23-32.
12. Edwards VJ, Holden GW, Felitti VJ, et al: Relationship between multiple forms of childhood maltreatment and adult mental health in community respondents: results from the adverse childhood experiences study. *Am J Psychiatry* 2003;160:1453-1460.
13. Vogeltanz N, Wilsnack S, Harris T, et al: Prevalence and risk factors for childhood sexual abuse in women: national survey findings. *Child Abuse Negl* 1999;23:579-592.
14. Sullivan P, Knutson J: Maltreatment and disabilities: A population-based epidemiological study. *Child Abuse Negl* 2000;24:1257-1273.
15. McCloskey L, Bailey J: The intergenerational transmission of risk for child sexual abuse. *J Interpers Violence* 2000;15:1019-1035.
16. Friedrich W, Fisher J, Broughton D, et al: Normative sexual behavior in children: a contemporary sample. *Pediatrics* 1998;101:e9.
17. Friedrich W, Fisher J, Dittner C, et al: Child Sexual Behavior Inventory: Normative, psychiatric and sexual abuse comparisons. *Child Maltreat* 2001;6:37-49.
18. Brilleslijper-Kater S, Friedrich W, Corwin D: Sexual knowledge and emotional reaction as indicators of sexual abuse in young children: theory and research challenges. *Child Abuse Negl* 2004;28:1007-1017.
19. Finkelhor D, Berliner L: Research on the treatment of sexually abused children: a review and recommendations. *J Am Acad Child Adolesc Psychiatry* 1995;34:1408-1423.
20. Trickett P, Noll J, Reiffman A, et al: Variants of intrafamilial sexual abuse experiences: implications for short- and long-term development. *Dev Psychopathol* 2001;13:1001-1019.
21. Lynskey M, Fergusson D: Factors protecting against the development of adjustment difficulties in young adults exposed to childhood sexual abuse. *Child Abuse Negl* 1997;21:1177-1190.
22. Hazzard A, Celano M, Gould J, et al: Predicting symptomatology and self-blame among child sex abuse victims. *Child Abuse Negl* 1995;19:707-714.

23. Mannarino A, Cohen J: Family-related variables and psychological system formation in sexually abused girls. *J Child Sex Abuse* 1996;5:105-119.

24. Putnam F: *Dissociation in Children and Adolescents—A Developmental Perspective.* Guilford Press, New York, 1997.

25. Kisiel C, Lyons J: Dissociation as a Mediator of Psychopathology among sexually abused children and adolescents. *Am J Psychiatry* 2001;158:1034-1039.

26. Mian M, Marton P, LeBaron D: The effects of sexual abuse on 3- to 5-year-old girls. *Child Abuse Negl* 1996;20:731-745.

27. Black M, Dubovitz H, Harrington D: Sexual abuse: developmental differences in children's behavior and self-perception. *Child Abuse Negl* 1994;18:85-95.

28. Tyler K: Social and emotional outcomes of childhood sexual abuse—A review of recent research. *Aggress Violent Behav* 2002;7:567-589.

29. Wonderlich S, Crosby R, Mitchell J, et al: Relationship of childhood sexual abuse and eating disturbance in children. *J Am Acad Child Adolesc Psychiatry* 2000;39:1277-1283.

30. Silverman A, Reinherz H, Giaconia R: The long-term sequelae of child and adolescent abuse: A longitudinal community study. *Child Abuse Negl* 1996;20:709-723.

31. Garnefski N, Arends E: Sexual abuse and adolescent maladjustment: differences between male and female victims. *J Adolesc* 1998;21:99-107.

32. Noll J, Horowitz L, Bonanno G, et al: Revictimization and self-harm in females who experienced childhood sexual abuse: results from a prospective study. *J Interpers Violence* 2003;18:1452-1471.

33. Negrao C, Bonanno G, Noll J, et al: Shame, humiliation, and childhood sexual abuse: distinct contributions and emotional coherence. *Child Maltreat* 2005;10:350-363.

34. Fergusson D, Horwood L, Lynskey M: Childhood sexual abuse, adolescent sexual behaviors and sexual revictimization. *Child Abuse Negl* 1997;21:789-803.

35. Dilillo D, Giuffre D, Tremblay G, et al: A closer look at the nature of intimate partner violence reported by women with a history of child sexual abuse. *J Interpers Violence* 2001;16:116-132.

36. Noll J, Trickett P, Susman E, et al: Sleep disturbances and childhood sexual abuse. *J Pediatr Psychol* 2006;31:469-480.

37. McClellan J, Adams J: Clinical characteristics related to severity of sexual abuse: a study of seriously mentally ill youth. *Child Abuse Negl* 1995;19:1245-1254.

38. Kaufman J, Widom C: Childhood victimization, running away, and delinquency. *J Res Crime Delinq* 1999;36:347-370.

39. Thompson K, Braaten-Antrim R: Youth maltreatment and gang involvement. *J Interpers Violence* 1998;13:328-345.

40. Ackard D, Neumark-Sztainer D, Hannan P, et al: Binge and purge behavior among adolescents: associations with sexual and physical abuse in a nationally representative sample: the Commonwealth Fund survey. *Child Abuse Negl* 2001;6:771-785.

41. Corwin DL: Early diagnosis of child sexual abuse: diminishing the lasting effects. *In:* Wyatt G, Powell G (eds): *The Lasting Effects of Child Sexual Abuse.* Sage Publications, Newbury Park, Calif, 1988, pp 251-270.

42. Van der Kolk B, Roth S, Pelcovitz D et al: Disorders of extreme stress: the empirical foundation of a complex adaptation to trauma. *J Trauma Stress* 2005;18:389-399.

43. American Psychiatric Association: *Diagnostic and Statistical Manual of Mental Disorders* (ed 4 rev). American Psychiatric Association, Washington, DC, 2000, p 465.

44. Whiffen V, MacIntosh H: Mediators of the link between childhood sexual abuse and emotional distress: a critical review. *Trauma Violence Abuse* 2005;6:24-39.

45. Ruggiero K, Smith D, Hanson R, et al: Is disclosure of childhood rape associated with mental health outcome? Results from the National Women's Study. *Child Maltreat* 2004;9:62-77.

46. Mancini C, Van Ameringen M, MacMillan H: Relationship of childhood sexual and physical abuse to anxiety disorders. *J Nerv Ment Dis* 1995;183:309-314.

47. Kendler K, Bulik C, Silberg J, et al: Childhood sexual abuse and adult psychiatric and substance use disorders in women. *Arch Gen Psychiatry* 2000;57:953-959.

48. Nelson E, Heath A, Madden P, et al: Association between self-reported childhood sexual abuse and adverse psychosocial outcomes. *Arch Gen Psychiatry* 2002;59:139-145.

49. Browne A, Finkelhor D: Impact of child sexual abuse: a review of the research. *Psychol Bull* 1986;99:66-77.

50. Young M, Harford K, Kinder B, et al: The relationship between childhood sexual abuse and adult mental health among undergraduates: victim gender doesn't matter. *J Interpers Violence* 2007;22:1315-1331.

51. Gladstone G, Parker G, Wilhelm K, et al: Characteristics of depressed patients who report childhood sexual abuse. *Am J Psychiatry* 1999;156:431-437.

52. Coid J, Petruckevitch A, Feder G, et al: Relation between childhood sexual and physical abuse and risk of revictimisation in women: a cross-sectional survey. *Lancet* 2001;358:450-454.

53. Whitfield C, Anda R, Dube S, et al: Violent childhood experiences and the risk of intimate partner violence in adults. *J Interpers Violence* 2003;18:166-185.

54. Fleming J, Mullen P, Sibthorpe B, et al: The long-term impact of childhood sexual abuse in Australian women. *Child Abuse Negl* 1999;23:145-159.

55. Dube S, Anda R, Whitfield C, et al: Long-term consequences of childhood sexual abuse by gender of victim. *Am J Prev Med* 2005;28:430-438.

56. Rayworth B, Wise L, Harlow B: Childhood abuse and risk of eating disorders in women. *Epidemiology* 2004;15:271-278.

57. Mullen P, Martin J, Anderson J, et al: The long-term impact of the physical, emotional, and sexual abuse of children: a community study. *Child Abuse Negl* 1996;20:7-21.

58. Nelson E, Heath A, Lynskey M, et al: Childhood sexual abuse and risks for licit and illicit drug-related outcomes: a twin study. *Psychol med* 2006;36:1473-1483.

59. Pirard S, Sharon E, Kang S, et al: Prevalence of physical and sexual abuse among substance abuse patients and impact on treatment outcomes. *Drug Alcohol Depend* 2005;78:57-64.

60. Banyard V, Williams L, Siegel J: The impact of complex trauma and depression on parenting: an exploration of mediating risk and protective factors. *Child Maltreat* 2003;8:334-349.

61. Douglas A: Reported anxieties concerning intimate parenting in women sexually abused as children. *Child Abuse Negl* 2000;24:425-434.

62. Dilillo D, Damashek A: Parenting characteristics of women reporting a history of childhood sexual abuse. *Child Maltreat* 2003;8:319-333.

63. Mapp S: The effects of sexual abuse as a child on the risk of mothers physically abusing their children: a path analysis using systems theory. *Child Abuse Negl* 2006;30:1293-1310.

64. Arnow B, Hart S, Scott C, et al: Childhood sexual abuse, psychological distress, and medical use among women. *Psychosom Med* 1999;61:762-770.

65. Finestone H, Stenn P, Davies F, et al: Chronic pain and health care utilization in women with a history of childhood sexual abuse. *Child Abuse Negl* 2000;24:547-556.

66. Sack M, Lahmann C, Jaeger B, et al: Trauma prevalence and somatoform symptoms. *J Nerv Ment Dis* 2007;195:928-933.

67. Lang A, Rodgers C, Lebeck M: Associations between maternal childhood maltreatment and psychopathology and aggression during pregnancy and postpartum. *Child Abuse Negl* 2006;30:17-25.

68. Bensley L, Van Eenwyk J, Simmons K: Self-reported childhood sexual and physical abuse and adult HIV-risk behaviors and heavy drinking. *Am J Prev Med* 2000;18:151-158.

69. Farley M, Golding J, Minkoff J: Is a history of trauma associated with a reduced likelihood of cervical cancer screening? *J Fam Pract* 2002;51:827-831.

70. Romano E, DeLuca R: Male sexual abuse: a review of effects, abuse characteristics, and links with later psychological functioning. *Aggress Violent Behav* 2001;6:55-78.

71. Holmes W, Slap G: Sexual abuse of boys—definition, prevalence, correlates, sequelae, and management. *JAMA* 1998;280:1855-1862.

72. Whitaker D, Le B, Hanson R, et al: Risk factors for the perpetration of child sexual abuse: a review and meta-analysis. *Child Abuse Negl* 2008;32:529-548.

73. Gaudiosi JA: *Child Maltreatment 2006.* U.S. Department of Health and Human Services, Washington, DC, 2006.

74. Smith D: Delay in disclosure of childhood rape: results from a national survey. *Child Abuse Negl* 2000;24(2):273-287.

75. Kellogg N and the American Academy of Pediatrics Committee on Child Abuse and Neglect: The evaluation of sexual abuse in children. *Pediatrics* 2005;116:506-512.

76. Gully K, Fenheim G, Myhre A: Non-abused preschool children's perception of an anogenital examination. *Child Abuse Negl* 2007;31: 885-894.

77. Dubowitz H: Children's responses to the medical evaluation for child sexual abuse. *Child Abuse Negl* 1998;22:581-584.

78. Gully K, Britton H, Hansen K, et al: A new measure for distress during child sexual abuse examinations: The Genital Examination Distress Scale. *Child Abuse Negl* 1999;23:61-70.

79. Gully K, Price B, Johnson M: Increasing abused children's access to evidence-based treatment: diffusion via parents as consumers. *Child Maltreat* 2008;280-288.

80. Saunders BE, Berliner L, Hanson RF (eds): *Child Physical and Sexual Abuse: Guidelines for Treatment* (Revised Report: April 26, 2004). National Crime Victims Research and Treatment Center, Charleston, SC, 2004.

81. Cohen JA, Mannarino AP, Deblinger E: *Treating Trauma and Traumatic Grief in Children and Adolescents*. Guilford Press, New York, 2006.

82. Reeker J, Ensing D, Elliott R: A meta-analytic investigation of group treatment outcomes for sexually abused children. *Child Abuse Negl* 1997;21:669-680.

83. Adams-Tucker C: Proximate effects of sexual abuse in childhood: a report on 28 children. *Am J Psychiatry* 1982;139:1252-1256.

84. Leifer M, Kilbane T, Grossman G: A three-generational study comparing the families of supportive and unsupportive mothers of sexually abused children. *Child Maltreat* 2001;6:353-364.

85. Hill A: Patterns of non-offending parental involvement in therapy with sexually abused children: a review of the literature. *J Soc Work* 2005;5:339-358.

86. Paredes M, Leifer M, Kilbane T: Maternal variables related to sexually abused children's functioning. *Child Abuse Negl* 2001;25:1159-1176.

87. Hill A: "No-one else could understand": women's experiences of a support group run by and for mothers of sexually abused children. *Br J Soc Work* 2001;31:385-397.

88. Plummer C, Eastin J: System intervention problems in child sexual abuse investigations: the mothers' perspectives. *J Interpers Violence* 2007;22:775-787.

89. Hildebrand J, Forbes C: Group work with mothers whose children have been sexually abused. *Br J Soc Work* 1987;17:285-304.

90. Cohen J, Mannarino A, Perel J, et al: A pilot randomized controlled trial of combined trauma-focused CBT and sertraline for childhood PTSD symptoms. *J Am Acad Child Adolesc Psychiatry* 2007;46:811-819.

50

PSYCHOLOGICAL IMPACT AND TREATMENT OF PHYSICAL ABUSE OF CHILDREN

David J. Kolko, PhD, ABPP, and Rachel P. Kolko, BA

INTRODUCTION

This chapter presents a basic overview of the empirical status of methods designed to assess and treat child physical abuse (CPA) and its consequences in children and adolescents. Relevant evidence-based treatments (EBT) will be described, which offer empirical evaluations of specific practices. We focus on information that could help the health care professional (HCP) to better understand and support intervention efforts with these cases.[1-3] Because many children with a history of CPA or their caregivers do not spontaneously report abusive experiences or any resulting consequences, including trauma symptoms, HCPs may be in the best position to identify these children and to offer suggestions about possible interventions. Thus, it is important for HCPs to be aware of the various forms and characteristics of CPA, to be prepared to evaluate abused children and suspected caregivers in the health care setting, and to serve as knowledgeable referral sources to EBTs that deal with this problem.[1] To facilitate this understanding, we cover the following topics: definitions and prevalence, characteristics and consequences, screening and assessment, service referral and access, intervention and treatment, and prevention. A summary is provided of the implications of this research for practice and research as well as topics for further exploration.

CHILD PHYSICAL ABUSE AND THE CONTINUUM OF FORCE

Definitions

The nature and extent of CPA has been described using various definitions. The National Incidence Study (NIS-3)[4] defined CPA as present when a child younger than 18 years of age has experienced an injury (harm standard) or risk of an injury (endangerment standard) as a result of having been hit with a hand or other object or having been kicked, shaken, thrown, burned, stabbed, or choked by a parent or parent-surrogate. In contrast, the definitions used in the National Child Abuse and Neglect Data Study (NCANDS) were based on separate state definitions, but the item used to capture physical abuse information reflected the "number of victims of physical acts that caused or could have caused

physical injury."[5] For purposes of clarification, this review includes literature on a related topic, namely, corporal punishment (CP), which includes "the use of physical force with the intention of causing a child pain, but not injury, for the purposes of correction or control of the child's behavior."[6]

As highlighted by these few definitions, what constitutes CPA varies by local standards and official definitions, the context in which abusive behavior is being examined, and the level of empirical rigor used in crafting a definition. Thus, CPA may reflect a range of behaviors that differ in behavioral topography, frequency, severity, and temporal stability, not to mention informant source. In light of the breadth of this topic and the many forms and definitions of abuse, it is important to keep in mind that there is a continuum of physical force that includes the more serious, substantiated cases of physical abuse (CPA), as well as other acts that might be viewed as general forms of child physical maltreatment (CPM), and the use of CP or physical discipline.[7]

Prevalence/Scope

CPA continues to reflect a significant physical and mental health concern in this country. Based on reports from the states to the Department of Health and Human Services in 2005, physical abuse accounted for 16.6% of all reports, which is second only to reports of neglect (62.8%).[8] The National Survey of Child and Adolescent Well-Being (NSCAW) is a study of children and adolescents who came to the attention of the child welfare system for suspected abuse or neglect.[9] Based on the recently released NIS-4 survey using data from 2005–2006, an estimated 323,000 children met the harm standard and an estimated 476,000 children met the endangerment standard for child physical abuse.[4] These numbers represent 23% and 29% reductions in the rates reported for physical abuse cases relative to the rates reported in the prior NIS survey for cases meeting the harm and endangerment standards, respectively. Among all abuse reports, physical abuse accounted for the majority of reports (58%). As these figures suggest, the physical abuse of children still remains all too common.

Understandably, estimated rates of prevalence and incidence are influenced by the specificity of the definition used to identify cases of CPA, given the absence of a clear consensus definition. Unlike the use of medical or mental health diagnoses, the determination of child abuse reflects a social judgment process that seeks to integrate several social-demographic details (e.g., risk factors, safety issues) with the child's physical/medical status and severity of injury.[10] In many cases, it is difficult to determine when an incident involving physical force by a caregiver represents actual CPA or extreme parent-to-child discipline (e.g., beating vs. spanking/slapping), which often blurs the distinctions among abusive, subabusive, or nonabusive behavior. Reporting rates are also subject to variation in the interpretation of county or state definitions, as well as other case (e.g., prior history of agency involvement), caseworker (e.g., caseload, history of experience, training), and/or social service system factors (e.g., degree of supervision/monitoring, population size), among other variables.[11]

Health and other officials recognize that cultural and personal attitudes about the use of CP play a substantial role in shaping one's views about identifying and reporting CPA, among other influences. Although few positive developmental outcomes, if any, have been found associated with the use of CP,[12,13] most individuals view various forms of CP, such as spanking, as appropriate and effective methods of correction. In fact, 62% of Americans in general, and 61% of American parents in particular, view spanking as a favorable form of discipline.[14] In addition, more than 90% of parents in various countries frequently hit toddlers.[15]

Although CP is not tantamount to child abuse, the line between abusive and proper discipline often remains obscure. As noted by Straus,[15] about two thirds of all cases of CPA begin as CP, which escalates into abusive behavior. Thus, the task of determining when a specific parental behavior or set of behaviors qualifies as CPA and deserves to be reported is complex and multidetermined and requires a concerted effort to understand the broader continuum of physical force. These and other judgments about the various forms of physical discipline in which caregivers engage are among the reasons for different rates of substantiation across states in the United States.[16]

HCPs clearly recognize that children's exposure to excessive or harmful punishment or ineffective physical discipline takes numerous forms and often defies easy identification or a simple or precise definition. After all, these experiences are frequently not reported by the family, even when physical signs or symptoms are evident. Also, many children or parents offer alternative descriptions when asked about the nature and contributors to a child's physical symptoms or pain. Thus, the classification of punishment as abuse can be difficult, especially given the serious consequences for parents and children when CPA is confirmed.

Chapter 2, "Epidemiology of Physical Abuse," outlines factors in children, parents, family, and environment that increase the likelihood of abuse. By identifying the individual features that increase the risk for CPA, past and current abuse can be more easily addressed, and future abuse is more likely to be prevented.

CHARACTERISTICS AND CONSEQUENCES

In addition to its health and medical effects, another important area for HCPs to consider is the range of clinical consequences that may be experienced by physically victimized children. Although CP appears to have few beneficiary effects, the literature reveals a variety of associations between CP and impaired or disrupted development.[1] Children and adolescents who have experienced CP or CPA often develop externalizing or internalizing problems that can promote other behavior problems.[17] Many of these behavioral and emotional problems surface by late childhood and adolescence, although some may be apparent earlier.[17]

Cognitive/Learning and Attributions

CPA affects how children understand relationships, often creating maladaptive attribution patterns. Girls who have been abused attribute less power to themselves than to parents, and women who were abused as children attribute less power to themselves than to children.[18] Often, victims of CPA develop distorted social cognition schemas, which lead them to accept violence in future relationships.[19]

As shown by recent neurophysiological research, abused children process information relating to emotion differently than normal children.[20] They are more attentive to visual and auditory anger cues and potential threats, which places them at a greater risk for anxiety than nonabused children.[20] They are also more likely to display depressive symptoms.[17]

CPA has been found to produce detrimental effects upon adaptive functioning. Even in children who face multiple adversities (e.g., low socioeconomic status, minority status), those who experienced CPA show a greater degree of maladaptive functioning than their nonabused counterparts.[21] Given that some of the parents who abuse their children were victims of physical abuse during their childhood, one of the most damaging consequences of CPA is the increased likelihood that such victims will later abuse their own children.[6,22]

Behavior and Mental Health Problems

Quite possibly, the most common consequences of CPA that arise during childhood and adolescence involve externalizing (aggression or antisocial behavior) and, to a lesser extent, internalizing problems (depression or anxiety).[2,17] Such dysfunctional behavior patterns can, at times, reflect serious antisocial or dangerous behaviors, such as firesetting behavior.[23] In terms of the externalizing patterns, the victims of CPA are more likely to display aggressive or antisocial behavior,[24] develop oppositional defiant disorder,[25] or abuse drugs and/or alcohol.[26] Physical abuse can also worsen behavior problems, possibly by elevating the emotional and behavioral difficulties that often lay at the root of maladaptive behavior. For example, juvenile firesetters who have experienced CPA tend to display more severe behavior problems than their nonabused counterparts,[23] and children with a history of CPA may be more likely to start drinking earlier and to use alcohol to cope rather than for pleasure or social reasons.[27] Externalizing behavior problems related to CPA can occur as early as the late toddlerhood years.[17]

As for internalizing disorders, the most frequently documented consequence of CPA exposure is depression.[26,28] Other research suggests that experiencing CPA leads to increased risks of suicidality,[29] suicide attempts, and general mental health problems.[30]

Social/Interpersonal Competence and Relationship Skills

Individuals with a history of CPA tend to have more difficulties with interpersonal relationships than nonabused individuals. CPA increases the greater risk for violent or aggressive behavior in relationships[31] and impaired interpersonal functioning.[32] Maltreated children may be less communicative, less warm, and more conflicted in their interpersonal relationships than nonabused children,[21] and they experience more conflict with peers and partners.[33] Victims of CPA do not always become the aggressor; sometimes people who experienced CPA are more willing to accept violence in their future relationships than nonabused people.[19] Essentially, the people who experienced CPA are at a greater risk for continuing the vicious cycle of abuse, either as a perpetrator or a victim, which also affects the lives of their families.

Posttraumatic Stress Disorder

Some physically abused children may experience posttraumatic stress disorder (PTSD) as a result of exposure to a specific traumatic event or series of events.[34] PTSD consists of five core components.[35] The child must *experience a traumatic event* that qualifies as a serious traumatic stressor, possibly one that was either objectively or subjectively related to threats to life or physical integrity.[36,37] The three core symptom clusters of PTSD are *reexperiencing* (e.g., symptoms include upsetting feelings when memories or reminders of the traumatic event recur), *avoidance/numbing*, and *hyperarousal*. In order to meet full PTSD criteria, children must have at least one reexperiencing symptom (e.g., recurrent and distressing memories or thoughts of the event, physiological reactivity to trauma reminders), three avoidance symptoms (e.g., efforts to avoid thoughts, feelings, or talking about the traumatic event; avoiding activities, places, people, or situations that serve as trauma reminders), and two hyperarousal symptoms (e.g., difficulty falling or staying asleep, irritability, or temper outbursts).[35] Finally, these symptoms must be present for at least a month and must cause functional impairment in social, school, family, health, or another important area of daily living.[35] Even if a child has only a few PTSD symptoms, the case may warrant a referral for further evaluation if the symptoms are of sufficient severity to cause functional impairment.[38]

Health/Medical

In a large telephone interview study of adult women, the poorest health was found among women with a history of both sexual and physical abuse in childhood (e.g., severe depression, physical symptoms, joint pain, nausea/vomiting, fair/poor health, lower functionality). Those with either form of abuse also had modest levels of these problems.[39]

Summary

CPA produces an environment that is stressful to the child, which increases the likelihood of internalizing and externalizing behavior problems.[40] Thus, when HCPs recognize internalizing or externalizing behavior problems, specifically aggressive or antisocial behavior or depression, they should consider inquiring about the child's exposure to CP — and possibly CPA. Furthermore, it is important to recognize that CPA often occurs with exposure to another type of adverse situation, such as psychological, sexual, or substance abuse.[41] HCPs should then consider the breadth of factors and consequences related to CPA and harsh physical discipline, since such experiences can have severe physical, psychological, and cognitive effects on these children and their families. Reporting and intervening in cases of physical abuse can help the child and the surrounding family members. By understanding some of the risk factors, consequences, and related problems and disorders associated with CPA, HCPs will be in a better position to recognize and aid the victims of physical abuse and to help to prevent future abuse.

SCREENING AND ASSESSMENT/EVALUATION

Interview Probes for Exploring Exposure to Physical Discipline and Child Physical Abuse

There is clearly no standard protocol, procedure, or set of questions for learning about a child's potential history of child abuse. Instead, one can only attempt to establish interview conditions that are conducive to the conduct of an accurate and comfortable interview and to ask simple, clear, and nonleading questions that seek helpful information.[42] Setting the stage for a productive conversation like this requires an understanding of the child's developmental history and family circumstances, sensitivity to the topic, and patience in responding to the child's or parent's answers. Another important condition involves establishing the purpose and limits of confidentiality for an interview so that the informant is aware of how the information will be used.

Due to the context in which physical discipline often occurs, it is helpful to ask open-ended questions and to normalize the use of punishment and various forms of discipline. Key initial questions could solicit information about the child's exposure to punishment (e.g., how often punished, what happens), including physical punishment (e.g., spanking, slapping, grabbing, pushing) and most extreme or serious kinds of punishment or discipline used with the child. In some cases, it may then be important to ask if a child is worried about parental loss of control and the possibility of being physically hurt.

Details need to be obtained for all reported incidents of child maltreatment or abuse. Common parameters of such incidents reflect the perpetrator and relationship to child, possible contributors to the incident, the specific acts or behaviors involved, the setting, and any consequences or reactions in the child (e.g., pain, injuries, medical services) and perpetrator (e.g., threats to maintain secrecy). The child's overall impressions regarding the reasons for the incident may also be relevant to examine. Generally, it is helpful to ask open-ended questions, which solicit more complete details, although there are times when a reluctant or low-functioning informant may benefit from more close-ended questions. Clearly, one implication of such careful questioning is the need to carefully document the child's or parent's statements, and the possibility of needing to report the incident to child protective services. Further, it might be necessary to consider what, if any, safety plans are needed immediately based on an approximation of the child's level of risk.

Some HCPs feel comfortable asking children about exposure to physical abuse or other types of events. Generally, children and parents should be asked these questions separately and privately, mindful of any reporting requirements. A few general questions designed to elicit information about a child's general exposure to traumatic events might be helpful, such as (1) Has there been any significant change in the child's life or functioning since the last visit? (2) Did anything unusual happen to the child? (3) Has there been any significant change in the child's behavioral or emotional functioning? and (4) Has anyone reported or observed any sudden changes in the child's behavior or mood? These questions could also be directed toward identifying the child's exposure to specific types of noninterpersonal traumas (e.g., bad accidents, medical illness/procedures, natural disasters), and interpersonal traumas (e.g., physical violence, physical abuse, sexual abuse, domestic violence, traumatic death), and other frightening events (e.g., kidnapping, terrorism, etc.).[38]

When assessing children for the presence of PTSD symptoms, it is important to anchor the symptoms to a specific stressor. If the HCP is interviewing the child, he or she should ask the child whether any of the above experienced events was very upsetting or scary to the child. If the child reports that any of these events were distressing, it is then important to determine which one was most traumatic *from the child's perspective*, and then assess the child for the presence of the PTSD symptoms described above. However, interviewing children for PTSD symptoms is a challenging task, particularly asking about avoidance. Children and parents should ideally be asked about the child's symptoms separately to obtain optimal information, since inclusion of parental report has been shown to improve the rate of accurate diagnosis.[37]

In most practices, time demands will preclude clinicians from conducting personal interviews to assess PTSD symptoms. As described in the next section, self-report instruments are available for inquiring about trauma exposure.

Formal Instruments/Tools

Numerous instruments have been reported to facilitate screening and assessment of CPA. We have identified certain ones that seem applicable to the HCP and the setting in which this activity would be conducted. Some measures examine broad clinical concerns that can co-occur following abuse, such as PTSD, depression, anxiety, and behavioral problems.[43] Consequently, it may be necessary to include other instruments to evaluate a child's clinical needs or psychosocial status. In some cases, parents identify other clinical concerns that relate to the child's recent exposure to traumatic events, beyond CPA. What follows are some brief descriptions of potentially relevant instruments that have adequate psychometric properties.

Injury/Re-Abuse (Recidivism) and High-Risk Behaviors

The Traumatic Events Screening Inventory (TESI) can serve as a general screen to identify a child's recent exposure to various traumatic experiences.[44] The measure includes several primary domains that reflect both interpersonal and noninterpersonal events (e.g., direct exposure to or witnessing of severe accidents, illness, disaster, family or community conflict or violence, sexual molestation). The measure has good psychometrics and is recommended as an interview, especially since it has follow-up probes designed to solicit more details when a given trauma is identified.

Focusing more on possible physical abuse, a treatment provider might prefer to administer a few, brief questions to caregivers or children to determine if the child is exposed to high-risk parental behaviors. The Weekly Report of Abuse Indicators (WRAI) captures a few high-risk parental behaviors to assess risk status and monitor treatment course.[45,46] The three items reflect the severity of parental anger (1-5 point scale), any parental use of threats or physical force/discipline, and the severity of any recent family problems (1-3 point scale). Parents are also asked to report whether they thought about using physical force.

The Brief Child Abuse Potential Inventory (B-CAPI) was recently developed to provide an efficient tool for screening parents at risk for CPA or mistreatment of their children.[47] The B-CAPI consists of a 24-item abuse risk scale with a recommended risk cutoff (12) and a 9-item validity scale. Scores on the risk scale relate to future child protective services reports. Thus, this tool may help to inform an HCP's concerns about parental risk for physical abuse.

HCPs could also request information from official child welfare system records in order to learn more about histories of both caregivers and their children in terms of child welfare involvement and outcome. This could include incidents involving child maltreatment, physical injury, court involvement, and placement stability or disruption. Relevant parameters of these experiences have been coded using the Maltreatment Classification System (MCS) to help identify key incident details (e.g., type, perpetrator, frequency, severity).[48,49] Given the often modest to high recidivism rates, such information may be useful in highlighting children at risk for continued involvement in abuse or neglect.[50,51] It should be noted that some agencies will be reluctant to share this type of information outside of the environment of a community/hospital multidisciplinary team.

Clinical Problems/Symptoms

The Trauma Symptom Checklist for Children (TSC-C) is one of the few clinical instruments developed to assess children's and adolescents' responses to unspecified traumatic events in an array of symptom domains.[52] The scales include posttraumatic stress, anger, anxiety, depression, sexual concerns and preoccupation, and dissociation. The child is asked to indicate how often each item happens to him or her using a four-point scale (0 = never; 1 = sometimes; 2 = lots of times; 3 = almost all the time). One advantage of the TSCC is that it can efficiently assess posttraumatic stress symptoms and other symptoms related to exposure to physical abuse. In particular, the posttraumatic stress scale consists of 10 posttraumatic stress symptoms (e.g., intrusive recollections of traumatic events, sensory reexperiencing and nightmares, dissociative avoidance, fears), and has high good psychometric properties. The TSCC was standardized on a large sample of racially and economically diverse children from urban and suburban settings, and provides norms according to age and gender (T-score mean = 50) as well as clinical cutoff scores.

The nine-item Abbreviated UCLA PTSD Index[53] provides a brief evaluation of the severity of PTSD symptoms. A score of 20 correlates highly with a diagnosis of PTSD,[53] although children with scores of 8 to 10 likely have clinically meaningful symptoms of PTSD that, if accompanied by functional impairment, may also merit clinical referral for further evaluation.[37] The validity of this measure has been demonstrated in school settings following disasters such as the September 11, 2001 terrorist attacks.[36]

Functional Impairment

HCPs may find it helpful to use the 13-item Columbia Impairment Scale (CIS)[54] with parents or children to capture the child's overall impairment in four areas of functioning (i.e., family, peers, work, school). Items are rated on five-point Likert-scales ("no problem" = 0; "big problem" = 4), with a range of 0 to 52. The measure has good internal consistency, reliability, and validity in clinic samples.

Environmental Context

Concerns about the presence of negative and absence of positive parenting activities might warrant administration of the Alabama Parenting Questionnaire (APQ).[55] The APQ evaluates six dimensions of parenting practices and activities (i.e., involvement, positive parenting, poor monitoring/supervision, inconsistent discipline, corporal punishment, other discipline practices) that may help to identify common responses to various child behaviors. This scale has good psychometric properties.

The Parent-Child Conflict Tactics Scales (CTSPC)[56] provides a more focused and comprehensive assessment of mild to serious forms of parental verbal, psychological, and physical discipline (non-violent discipline, physical assault) during child conflicts. Some of the items in this tool represent parental actions that may cause severe forms of physical abuse (e.g., using a knife or gun). The scales possess excellent reliability and good validity with children and parents.[57,58]

The Family Environment Scale (FES-A)[59] includes three subscales (e.g., cohesion, expressiveness, conflict) that reflect a general family relationships index. The scale has been used with several clinic samples of varying ethnic backgrounds with good results in terms of reliability, stability over time, and predictive validity. The conflict and cohesion subscales are particularly useful in evaluating the environment in which harsh or coercive parent–child interactions emerge.

For families with adolescents, the 20-item Conflict Behavior Questionnaire (CBQ) can be used to evaluate parent–child hostility and discord,[60] given that negative communication is a common correlate of CPA. Scores can be interpreted using a normative cutoff. The CBQ has high reliability, internal consistency, and treatment sensitivity.[60]

Services or Intervention Experience

To learn about a family's recent involvement in treatment or other services, the Service Assessment for Children and Adolescents (SACA) can be administered to parents to evaluate the extent of a child's recent service use in several major domains (e.g., overnight, outpatient, school), as well as some service-related parameters (e.g., usefulness) and obstacles (e.g., agency policies) that might affect the child's current status.[61] It might be important to learn what concurrent services are being received (e.g., medication, care management) or whether families might benefit from more intensive services (crisis intervention, placement) after an evaluation.

Summary

Since HCPs often see cases involving suspected CPA, this section offers brief recommendations to facilitate recognition and evaluation of these children.[38] It is important, however, to realize that they may not always report such cases to the authorities or be fully aware of reporting requirements.[62] Consequently, there may be potential benefit to providing both education and support to HCPs as a way of reducing any barriers to recognizing and reporting physical abuse.

SERVICE REFERRAL, ACCESS, AND USE

In advance of describing the nature and impact of various interventions or treatment approaches, it is important to highlight the issue of service referral, access, and use or involvement given persistent problems with engagement, compliance, and dropout among abusive families.[63,64] A fundamental concern is the fact that many families fail to receive needed mental health services, since many victims of CPA are not referred for treatment.[65] One reason for limited service referral is the variability in the timeliness with which caseworkers' risk assessments are completed by accepted deadlines.[49] In addition, this study found that caseworkers' risk assessment reports for a subset of cases did not appear related to the results of a battery of clinical assessment measures collected by independent research assistants, which suggests that the client's mental health needs might not have been clearly identified as a basis for referral.

The relatively low rates of service use among CPA victims and their families are well documented. An administrative record review study found that between 40% and 60% of all cases in which maltreatment was substantiated appeared to receive no subsequent services.[66] A survey of practitioners found that CPA victims received only 7 of a total of 23 sessions of services that were conducted to reduce the negative consequences of this experience.[67] In terms of other services, fewer than half of a small sample of physically abused children had received a medical evaluation related to CPA, although the majority had received wellness care.[68] Half of these cases were heard in family court and fewer than half were receiving mental health services. Children were more likely to receive services if the maltreating caregiver was not in the home. Caregivers were more likely to receive services if they acknowledged the abuse. Similar results were reported based on a chart review for a sample of CPA victims in Sweden,[69] in which about half of these children had received services prior to the abuse, but one fourth of the charts had no mention of the CPA and only 6 of 126 had received individual therapy. Interestingly, formal intervention by the department of social services prior to the abuse was related to receiving interventions by the department up to 4 years later.[69]

One study of families referred to CPS following an incident of child physical or sexual abuse examined the treatment experiences of the sample upon intake and at a second assessment following an initial service about 6 months later.[49] Based on standardized clinical assessments conducted with child victims and their caregivers, several findings were reported, including: (1) 30% of the caregivers and children had a past history of psychiatric hospitalization, and (2) at the follow-up assessment, children and their caregivers reported high rates of family (47%, 39%) and parent counseling (33%, 48%), but lower rates for child treatment (17%, 19%), respectively. Four variables predicted higher overall family service use at intake: white race, low child anxiety, parental distress, and parental abuse history as a child. Such findings highlight the low rate of service involvement of this sample and a few of the background characteristics that may increase service referral.

One of the few national studies of children referred to child welfare services for allegations or abuse or neglect reported a population estimate of service use.[9] Nearly one half of youths ages 2 to 14 years with a completed child welfare investigation had clinically significant behavioral or emotional problems. These youths were much more likely to receive mental health services in the prior 12 months, but only one fourth of such youths received any specialty mental health care. One implication of these findings is the need for more routine screening and treatment referral of youth with recent child welfare referral, especially those with clinical need. Active HCP referral may be particularly necessary given that many parents who think about getting professional counseling for their children do not follow through on their considerations.[70] In fact, only 20% of juvenile crime victims actually received services. In addition, parental help-seeking was influenced by outside advice, suggesting the potential benefit of HCP input or recommendations for mental health consultation.

Even when families are referred and get involved, participation rates are variable. For example, one program evaluation report documented a 38% no-show rate at home, a 66% no-show rate in the clinic, and a 36% dropout rate among 45 families.[71] A similar dropout rate (44%) has been reported in a study of specialty family treatment.[72] Further, participation in child treatment is not always associated with clinical benefit.[73] In this study of 68 children referred to community agency providers after a report of child physical or sexual abuse, child treatment was received by 19% and 50% of the children by 1- and 2-year follow-up, respectively. Initial child treatment was not associated with significant gains in child outcomes; child improvement in abuse-related outcomes was associated with having PTSD and lower adjustment at intake. Initial child treatment was also unrelated to re-abuse or out-of-home placement documented by 2-year follow-up. Other reports indicate mixed benefits following child treatment.[68]

Among the many potential alternatives to increasing service access and use, one novel alternative involves discussing key obstacles to EBT access by a trained professional.[74] This protocol involved the administration of a 29-item checklist of potential barriers, which was then discussed with parents to provide useful information and suggestions to enhance parental expectations of benefit following exposure to an EBT. Results indicated that parents demonstrated an increase in knowledge about and rapport during a medical evaluation, and showed an increase in satisfaction with the routine after the protocol. This application based on a brief interaction between professional and parent highlights one viable approach to enhancing diffusion and use of EBTs in community settings.

INTERVENTION AND TREATMENT

There are a number of alternative interventions and treatment approaches to serving the needs of physically abused children and their families, in part because of demographic and clinical heterogeneity of this client population.[75] These approaches emphasize different clients (e.g., parent/family *vs.* child centered), targets (e.g., child management, anger management), content or methods (parenting skills *vs.* peer social support), or modalities (cognitive-behavioral therapy [CBT] *vs.* family therapy). The following section provides a brief overview of selected intervention approaches and studies whose outcomes bear treatment implications. Where available, outcome evidence will be reported. For further information, several online sources can be consulted.[76-78]

One exceptional source of relevant information about treatment and services is the National Child Traumatic Stress Network (NCTSN),[76] a national network of over 60 sites that provide community treatment and services across the United States, which was established by the Substance Abuse and Mental Health Services Administration (SAMHSA) in 2001 to improve the standard of care for traumatized children, adolescents, and their families. The NCTSN maintains a website with downloadable and printable information about abuse and neglect, as well as PTSD, which can be given to parents and children in the practitioner's office. The website includes some new materials related to CPA, including a "Q&A" interview designed to address common concerns about physical abuse, some handouts relevant for professionals or caregivers interested in services, and other related information on trauma in children. A full set of resources for specialized mental health referrals across the United States is available from this resource. To access the NCTSN website, go to www.NCTSNet.org.

Child-Focused Intervention

Children involved in physical abuse might benefit from participation in services, even though the amount of attention paid to descriptions or evaluations of child treatments is limited.[2,79] Generally, child intervention is one element of a more broad-based family or parent-directed intervention.[50]

Intensive day and residential treatment programs, primarily for maltreated preschoolers, have offered access to different developmentally appropriate and therapeutic activities (e.g., recreation, learning, play) and modalities (e.g., child play groups, family counseling) with trained staff who work closely with each group.[80,81] Clinical reports based on this work document improvements in several developmental skill areas. For example, a program in Australia consisting of a therapeutic preschool and home visitation found improved intellectual functioning and receptive language at discharge 1 year later.[82]

A more intensive, group-based treatment program was aimed at encouraging supportive peer relationships and identification of personal feelings, along with play, speech, and physical therapy.[83] The program incorporated other family services (e.g., family and individual therapy, support group counseling, parent education, crisis line). Relative to a control group, treated children saw themselves as having higher cognitive competence, peer acceptance, and maternal acceptance, and they received higher developmental quotients on standardized measures. Teacher ratings supported these improvements. Still, most children scored below the "normal" range in most areas. Day or residential treatment programs that combine skills training and experiential methods might be most useful in targeting the diverse social-psychological problems of the more seriously dysfunctional child victim and family.

A second approach reflects the application of specific behavioral and social learning procedures directed toward improving peer relations and social adjustment of young child victims by arranging play-buddy sessions in which withdrawn maltreated children were exposed to social initiation techniques demonstrated by trained peer confederates, called resilient peer treatment (RPT).[84] Studies have shown that RPT is more effective than adult initiations in improving children's social adjustment and peer initiations,[85,86] and is more beneficial for withdrawn, than aggressive, children.[84-86] Maintenance effects 2 months fter RPT have also been documented.[87] This intervention may be especially relevant for children who demonstrate clear social or interpersonal deficits.

A preliminary report was made of a cognitive-behavioral group conducted over a 16-week period with six physically abused children, four of whom completed the group.[88] The program emphasized content in three primary domains (i.e., trauma-specific work, anger management, social skills training). Outcome assessment based on child reports revealed improvements for some but not all group participants (anger reactions, posttraumatic symptoms), with parent reports indicating some increase in emotional and behavioral problems after treatment. Advantages to group work include the ability to draw upon shared group experiences and problems, although it is not always easy to find suitable group members at a given time.

Parent-Focused Intervention

Perhaps the most common intervention strategies for CPA involve training parents in positive and nonviolent child management practices.[63,79] Training is often directed toward helping parents learn to monitor their child's behavior, to issue clear and effective instructions, to use attention and ignoring at the right time, to say positive things or deliver positive consequences (reinforcement), to apply time-out and response cost as alternatives to physical discipline, and to establish and maintain home-based behavioral programs.

Interventions that include training in these parenting principles have reported improved parental repertoires and parent–child outcomes (e.g., more prosocial interaction, conflict resolution) that have often been maintained at follow-up. For example, one approach that integrated individualized parent training in various child management procedures with parent–child stimulation training reported improvements in both parent (e.g., child abuse potential, parental depression) and child (e.g., behavior problems) targets,[50] although there was less improvement in family interaction.

Interventions for parents have broadened beyond the focus on child management by targeting parents' cognitive-behavioral repertoires to deal with a variety of clinical problems. Several CBT procedures have been directed toward changing parental dysfunction related to the use of distorted beliefs or attributions, limited problem-solving skills, and heightened anger reactivity, each of which can contribute to parental aggression.[89] These procedures help parents become aware of their negative self-statements and to generate prosocial alternatives to these statements, promote realistic developmental expectations,[90] encourage the use of coping self-statements and relaxation skills,[91] or interact using appropriate communication and problem-solving skills.[92,93] The addition of cognitive restructuring and problem-solving to other stress management methods has been associated with reduced child assault and anger arousal and higher empathy in parents, as well as fewer complaints concerning child behavior problems.[92,94] Their clinical merit notwithstanding, some of these studies were uncontrolled reports and none of these studies reported follow-up or abuse recidivism data.

Providing parental education and support is another general approach that has been used with at-risk parents and their young children.[95] For example, one program incorporated several procedures in a community-based center (e.g., respite, support groups, training in discipline and developmental expectations, parent and child sessions), which was associated with clinical improvements on some measures (parental depression and stress) but not others (social support, child misbehavior). Controlled studies need to document the efficacy of this intervention approach with abusive families. A related program that provides exposure to a parenting curriculum (Systematic Training for Effective Parenting [STEP]) has also demonstrated a significant increase in positive perceptions of their children and a reduction in child abuse potential, relative to a control group.[96]

Parent–Child and Family-Focused Treatment

Many intervention approaches integrate parent and child components, including interventions that focus upon the family, in recognition of the interaction between various parent and child factors. Therefore, early studies have reported some benefits to family casework (e.g., discussion of individualized family treatment plans, training in behavioral parenting techniques) in reducing coercion in physically abusive families.[72]

Parent-Child Interaction Training (PCIT)[97] has been adapted for use with physical abuse based on its long history of application to the treatment of behavior problems in young children.[98] PCIT addresses issues related to harsh or ineffective parental discipline and heightened behavioral dysfunction in children by providing parents opportunities to develop more positive relationships with their children and to learn appropriate parenting techniques through ongoing coaching efforts during observed interactions. Outcome evidence in a recent study in abused children and their caregivers showed that PCIT was associated with lower official recidivism rates than a condition consisting of both PCIT and supplemental family services or a condition involving routine parenting classes conducted in the community.[51] PCIT is noteworthy for its attention to various stages in the treatment process, ranging from assessment and the training of behavioral play skills to the training of discipline skills and use of booster sessions.

Some approaches promote greater integration of interventions for caregivers and children/adolescents. For example, Alternatives for Families: A Cognitive-Behavioral Therapy (AF-CBT) seeks to reduce caregiver/family risk factors for physically abusive or coercive behavior and ameliorate the consequences of these experiences for children, at both the individual and family-context levels. AF-CBT incorporates individual CBT methods for parents and children with family-system procedures.[3] Each of these elements has been associated with improvements in child behavior problems, caregiver abuse risk/behavior, and family conflict/cohesion, and with low recidivism rates at follow-up.[45,46] It is important to note that 20% to 23% of all children and their parents independently reported high levels of physical discipline/force during the early and late phases of treatment, as well as heightened parental anger and family problems,[45] suggesting the importance of targeting parent–child coercion and use of force.

A related CBT-based intervention called Combined Parent-Child Cognitive Behavioral Therapy has integrated individual and group components for parents and their children.[99] The intervention includes elements from several treatments, including trauma-focused CBT, AF-CBT, and other methods, and could be especially useful in cases in which children report at least some symptoms of PTSD. Anecdotal evidence suggests some initial improvements among families who have participated in this program.

Most of the aforementioned treatments are administered in clinic settings, but other interventions have been applied in the home, on an intensive basis, and directed toward multiple family participants.[100] Such ecologically based and family-centered services generally have targeted contextual risk factors associated with abuse, specific skills deficits, and/or personal competencies. For example, intensive family-based reunification services (vs. routine reunification services) have been found to improve reunification rates,[101,102] possibly because of the provision of in vivo services and training in CBT skills (e.g., problem-solving, communication). Evidence on family preservation and support programs, however, did not support their effectiveness in preventing future child maltreatment cases.[103]

Additional multicomponent clinical interventions have targeted diverse individual, family, and systemic problems in the home and community. For example, multisystemic therapy (MST) targets problems in the child, parent, family, and social systems (e.g., peer training, child management,

family communication) following an individualized family assessment and in accord with a set of treatment principles (e.g., ecologically based, individualized, intensive). An early study found that MST was associated with improved parent–child relationships (parental efforts to control child, child compliance), whereas parent training was more effective in reducing identified social problems.[104]

Other programs conducted in the child's ecology emphasize the application of individualized skills training methods to problems specific to the family (e.g., child management training, social support, assertion training, job training, home safety/finances training). For example, Project Safe-Care incorporates three primary interventions from several originally examined in Project 12-Ways designed to address the common behavioral deficiencies of abusive parents (infant and child health care, home safety, stimulation/bonding, or parent–child interaction). Results from Project SafeCare[105] indicated improvements in parent-identified goals, but mixed evidence in terms of reduced re-abuse rates.[106] The strong emphasis upon careful assessment and then individualized home-based training is a significant strength of this program. Such comprehensive interventions underscore the need to provide multiple services to stabilize the home environment and promote improvements in parent–child relations with abusive families, many of which exhibit considerable family dysfunction.

A more recent intervention, child–parent psychotherapy (CPP), is noteworthy for its unique effort to integrate the treatment of young children exposed to domestic violence and their caregivers.[107] CPP combines several therapeutic elements, including play, developmental guidance, trauma-focused interventions, and concrete assistance to promote children's well-being and parent's capacity to both nurture and protect. For example, parents learn how to respond to children's emotional and developmental needs, and create a safe family environment. Relative to the provision of case management and community referral for individual treatment, CPP was found associated with significantly greater reductions in child's behavior problems and mother's general distress.[108] This is one of the few EBTs for traumatized preschoolers and their mothers.

It is worth mentioning that other treatments have been developed to address PTSD or related symptoms in children or adolescents exposed to traumatic events, including sexual or physical abuse, family or community violence, loss and grief, and natural disasters, among others. Perhaps the best known treatment for trauma is trauma-focused cognitive-behavior therapy (TF-CBT).[109] TF-CBT has been most extensively examined in the treatment of CSA, where it has yielded reductions in symptoms of PTSD, depression, and anxiety in several studies, but it bears relevance to an array of other traumatic experiences. The treatment includes several key components designed to address the experience of traumatic reactions (e.g., trauma narrative, psycho-education, relaxation, promotion of child safety and support). A related intervention, cognitive behavioral intervention for trauma in schools (CBITS), has been applied on a group basis in schools and has been found to reduce PTSD symptoms in adolescents exposed to violence.[110] Although the intervention has been developed for exposure to community violence, it might be appropriate for dealing with PTSD following physical abuse.[111]

Summary

What are some of the implications of this review of treatment approaches and outcomes? First, these findings provide additional, albeit qualified, support for the continued development of individual, group, and family treatments involving child victims of physical abuse. Second, it seems necessary to address caregivers' parenting practices in order to develop a more effective disciplinary repertoire. Third, integrated interventions that can adequately target the broad clinical features of abused children and their parents/families might help to improve positive outcomes. In terms of clinical approaches, most interventions have applied CBT and parenting skills training procedures to specific competencies and clinical problems.[1] This general focus is consistent with the four suggested CBT strategies recommended for the treatment of traumatized children and their parents: exposure to the traumatic event, stress management and coping skills training, exploration and correction of cognitive distortions related to the traumatic event, and interventions with parents.[112] Several potential targets exist for parents (e.g., negative child perceptions, developmentally appropriate expectations, self-control, affect or stress management, positive discipline, social support) and children (e.g., anger identification and control, relaxation, social skills, peer play activities, misattributions, academic competencies, problem-solving).[2]

Fourth, providing treatment in the natural environment can be beneficial, but successful treatment has also been conducted in clinic settings where safety and comfort can be provided. Setting type must be determined based on both program and parental input, but can be influenced by the varying needs of the population found in different geographic regions such as rural areas.[113] Fifth, there may be times when a family needs different services, such as crisis intervention or concrete or support services (e.g., Homebuilders).[114] Since intervention studies have shown mixed evidence for the maintenance of treatment gains,[50,106] an examination of therapeutic methods that promote greater scope and stability of improvements seems warranted (e.g., "check-ups," service calls). Much work still needs to be done to promote the development, application, and evaluation of psychosocial interventions designed to modify both the sequelae of an abusive experience and the risk of re-abuse.[63]

PREVENTION

The available literature on primary prevention highlights a number of alternative programs and activities.[115,116] Numerous prevention programs have been directed toward reducing a variety of risk factors for abuse (see Chapter 64, "The Prevention of Child Abuse and Neglect"). Klevens and Whitaker[115] conducted a literature review that identified the types of risk factors that were targeted (e.g., individual, family, community) and whether or not the program was evaluated. One-half of the programs were delivered in the home or community, with some programs conducted in hospitals and schools. One third of the programs targeted three or more risk factors, which were highly diverse (poor early bonding, knowledge of child abuse, lack of child care, harsh discipline, poverty, unemployment). Only one fourth of the programs, however, included a rigorous evaluation.

On the positive side, programs targeting certain risk factors did report some reduction in abusive behavior (e.g., low education, unwanted pregnancy, poor bonding, expectations, substance abuse, dysphoria, parenting, stress, isolation). Many worthy risk factors, however, were generally ignored and deserve further attention in prevention programs, such as social norms regarding physical discipline, poverty, partner violence, and the young age of parents. Each of these factors could be addressed, at least to some extent, by anticipatory guidance or other brief encounters within the primary care setting.

One of the more commonly evaluated approaches involves home visitation to new parents. An early version of this approach involved establishing nurse–family partnerships in which visiting nurses provided educational information, support, some counseling, and referral information over a lengthy period. Controlled studies showed beneficial maternal and child outcomes, which have been extended to follow-ups of between 4 and 15 years. Positive outcomes included reduced rates of child maltreatment.[117] Interestingly, use of paraprofessionals was associated with about one half of the benefits obtained using nurses as home visitors. Indeed, several home visiting programs that rely upon paraprofessionals have been conducted. The effects of these programs have been limited to short-term benefits in self-reported clinical problems or abusive behavior, but no significant improvements in reducing official child abuse reports.[116] It also bears mentioning that mixed evidence has sometimes been found using public health nurses.[118]

Parent training programs have also been used to address parental comfort with and competence in parenting skills.[119] Such programs often address parenting skills training and parental coping and may include alternative teaching methods (e.g., seminars) and targets (e.g., stress management). Evidence suggests improvements in attitudes and emotional well-being, but only minimal evidence exists regarding the prevention of child maltreatment. The importance of targeting these types of skills is supported by a recent study in which mothers of 3-year-olds were interviewed about disciplinary situations that elicited their strongest reactions, including a situation in which physical punishment occurred.[120] The predictors of physical punishment were found to be maternal attitudes toward physical punishment, maternal perception of the seriousness and intent of the child's misbehavior, and maternal anger in response to the child's misbehavior. Such findings highlight the potential benefit of targeting mother's cognitive and affective repertoires in reducing the decision to use physical punishment.

WHAT CAN HEALTH CARE PROVIDERS DO?

In terms of specific efforts that can be made in office and hospital practice, the HCP is in a unique position to identify, report, and intervene following incidents involving physically coercive, inappropriate, or abusive parental behavior. A first step toward addressing the problem of physical abuse is to become more familiar with its origins, risks, characteristics, consequences, and treatment in order to better recognize situations in which abuse might be likely.[3] There is a need for better training in background information that emphasizes the signs and symptoms of physical abuse, as well as greater HCP participation in reporting appropriate cases to child protection agencies.[121]

In terms of possible case identification, the HCP is often among the first professionals to learn about such incidents and to have an opportunity to provide medical attention and offer feedback designed to discourage further involvement in such behavior. Participant event monitoring (PEM)[122] is a structured process for asking questions about recent injury events and understanding parental interventions used to address these events that may help HCPs incorporate such a routine in their clinical practice. PEM offers a set of interview probes that can help to prevent further injuries to children through systematic tracking of the events themselves and the responses made to them (e.g., what was the child doing at the time of the injury, rate severity of the injury, what was done to help your child afterwards, rate how much the event was due to the caregiver). HCPs may find this structured approach useful in providing clues about prevention efforts at various levels of injury severity.

One other implication of the results from prevention studies for HCPs in the ability to discourage the use of CP, which has been promoted at the policy level in several countries.[21,123] Although the available evidence for a legal ban on CP is mixed,[116] it is certainly feasible for HCPs to ask questions about parenting repertoires and child outcomes when parents begin to discuss either child management frustrations or actual use of physical discipline. Such interactions may provide the context for a discussion of more effective child management techniques and actual training or instructions in the use of a different approach.

Avenues for encouraging service participation are also available to the HCP. Schools are a major gateway for mental health referral of crime victims,[70] so HCPs may be able to partner with school officials or teachers to facilitate access to care. In addition, child advocacy centers (CAC) can provide support to primary care providers,[124] especially given some modest evidence showing increased use of medical examinations, law enforcement involvement, and case substantiation among CAC compared with standard services.[125] CACs offer a multidisciplinary approach to investigation, management, treatment, and prosecution of child abuse cases, and are a helpful resource to the HCP for information and medical collaboration. Other approaches include direct efforts to enhance the capacity of primary care provider practices to adopt and implement novel child abuse prevention programs, such as Practicing Safety.[126] In this report, a combination of organizational change approaches and specialized assessment procedures was used to facilitate practice innovation and implementation of the program. Specific safety tools were found to be integrated into the daily repertoires of the pediatricians, including new patterns of communication with patients. This practice-level intervention might provide pediatric settings with new tools to address the problem of CPA and, more generally, child maltreatment.

Finally, in those cases in which significant physical injury or trauma has occurred, the HCP would be able to promote an initial sympathetic response to the child who has been exposed to traumatic events and who exhibits the symptoms of PTSD.[38] Observations of the child during routine physical examinations and related physical evidence can help to identify traumatic exposure and symptoms, which could be corroborated by parental interview using questions that examine the child's experiences and the timing of any these events. The HCP can also help to prevent further physical injuries and possible PTSD by suggesting to parents when children appear to be at risk for traumatic exposure or experiences, such as when they are exposed to high-risk situations (e.g., new parents who are overwhelmed, escalating use of coercive caregiver practices, reports of increased frustration or physical force during child management or disciplinary interactions, caregiver use of drugs and alcohol). Certainly, the HCP can offer advice regarding steps that may minimize a child's exposure to high-risk situations and encourage parents to monitor and promote child safety, both in and out of the home.

STRENGTH OF THE EVIDENCE

This literature review highlights recent developments in understanding and treating CPA and the somewhat variable level of evidentiary support found in different topic areas. For example, far more rigorous research exists regarding certain risk factors for and consequences of CPA than its treatment or prevention. Numerous prior studies have examined an array of consequences associated with CPA relative to nonabused samples or samples of nonphysically abused children. More recent studies have begun to shed light on neuropsychological, neurophysiological, and neuroanatomical consequences using rigorous methodologies, which elucidate key functional and structural problems related to a history of CPA.[127]

Less research has been conducted examining interviewing and screening methods in primary care and the role of HCPs in the identification and management of such cases. Some work has been devoted to understanding HCPs as expert witnesses or the sources of their judgments regarding decisions to report a case to child protective services. Further, there has been a modest increase in the number of intervention approaches that have been subject to empirical evaluation. The findings of those studies suggest greater optimism regarding the impact of treatment on parental repertoires and parent–child or family interaction. Still, few alternative treatment models or approaches have been compared. We also need to study methods to enhance motivation, disclosure, and processing of the abusive incident, given high rates of parental denial or reluctance to discuss what happened and why. Also, it is not clear whether explicit, direct attention to understanding and processing the child's abusive experiences (incident) or its consequences is important for either child or parent improvement. Most studies do not include evaluations of both clinical problems and recidivism, with some exceptions.[45,50]

Finally, the evidence base regarding efforts to prevent CPA are to some extent equivocal. Whereas some studies show benefits (e.g., home visits by professional nurses), other evidence suggests either more modest benefits or no benefits in terms of reductions in child maltreatment rates. The limitations of these studies include limited retention or participation rates, complicated or lengthy intervention programs, and restricted assessment measures or outcomes. In particular, many studies to do not include direct measures of child abuse or neglect recidivism. Thus, it is somewhat unclear as to whether prevention requires a comprehensive and intensive approach (e.g., nurse visitation) or a more focused intervention directed toward specific topics (e.g., skills training).

DIRECTIONS FOR FUTURE RESEARCH

Listed below are a few of the more important topics that merit further empirical examination or evaluation in relation to the HCP's role in addressing the problem of CPA. Since HCPs may be among the first professionals to identify and assess new cases, studies should carefully evaluate the most efficient and useful methods for interviewing and screening for a history of CPA, and to understand how both parents and victims describe/explain their experiences. Such information could help the HCP serve as an effective sentinel for new incidents and as an effective referral source for services. Models of the origins and maintenance of abusive behavior may also benefit from this work.

Studies of the developmental, health-related, and physical effects of CPA would shed further light on the general medical consequences and long-term effects of CPA. Such information would highlight the greater role that HCPs and medical experts play in the management of this problem, and the possibility that such input might affect the selection of both psychological and educational interventions for certain victims and their families. The presence of long-term continuity in several forms of dysfunction following early CPA provides further support for the potential relevance of medical research.

Many children and their parents are not referred for services or, if they are referred, fail to engage in treatment for an adequate length of time. Studies must begin to more carefully articulate the clinical and nonclinical needs of children exposed to CPA and their families, rather than reporting generally vague or broad statements of mental health dysfunction.

As suggested by Staudt,[128] it would be important to identify specific types of mental health need and to suggest appropriate types of services and treatment experiences likely to address these needs, including informal and nontraditional methods. Clearly, studies are needed that examine different parameters of services, including treatment duration, participants, foci or targets, outcomes, and barriers.

In terms of intervention, it seems necessary to extend existing evidence by comparing alternative EBTs and evaluating their impact on several types of key outcomes, including clinical symptoms/functioning, family stability and support, and abuse recidivism.[1] Little information has been reported regarding predictors of successful service involvement and treatment outcome, including treatment moderators and mediators.[129]

Research needs to determine which background or treatment variables contribute to a significant reduction in a child's risk for repeated CPA or exposure to coercive physical discipline. Other worthy research targets include comparisons of single vs. multicomponent interventions, since many recent treatments include diverse treatment components. Perhaps more streamlined and focused interventions, such as having HCPs provide brief parenting guidelines and psycho-education about the consequences of abuse could enhance both participation and ultimate outcome. In general, few intervention studies relevant to HCPs and the primary care setting have been conducted in the past decade.

Research should be directed toward evaluating prevention approaches in the context of pediatric primary care. Such approaches might be focused on the use of CP, harsh or coercive treatment of children, and parental misunderstandings of common children's behavioral and emotional reactions. Primary care providers could also be important links to a more comprehensive public health approach to prevention that integrates other methods, such as home visitation, collaborative care management, Internet-based educational programs, and involvement with local children's advocacy centers.[125]

SUMMARY

This chapter provides a brief summary of recent empirical research regarding the prevalence and consequences, assessment, treatment, and prevention of CPA and the use of physical discipline relevant to HCPs. HCPs are in a special position to recognize, respond to, and refer children who are exposed to CPA, especially given their involvement with children at their earliest ages. The HCP is often the first adult or professional to learn about children who receive physical punishment, suffer from injuries or pain varying in severity, and/or experience significant traumatic reactions in light of these events, which could be facilitated by their ability to obtain evidence that can support this clinical impression. Being more familiar with the content of this chapter will enable the HCP to more effectively ascertain relevant information about an incident of abuse, offer service recommendations, and provide directive feedback designed to discourage the use of harsh or abusive physical discipline. In promoting more focused assessment and treatment efforts, the basic tools described here might help to initiate a more timely and responsive process of professional support of the physically abused child and his family.

References

1. Kolko DJ: Child physical abuse. *In:* Meyers JEB, Berliner L, Buckley JA, et al (eds): *APSAC Handbook of Child Maltreatment,* ed 2. Sage Publications, Thousand Oaks, Calif, 2002, pp 21-54.
2. Kolko DJ, Swenson CC: *Assessing and Treating Physically Abused Children and their Families: A Cognitive Behavioral Approach.* Sage Publications, Thousand Oaks, Calif, 2002.
3. Stirling J, Amaya-Jackson L, and the American Academy of Pediatrics Committee on Child Abuse and Neglect: Understanding the behavioral and emotional consequences of child abuse. *Pediatrics* 2008; 122:667-673.
4. Sedlak AJ, Mettenburg J, Basena M, et al: *Fourth National Incidence Study of Child Abuse and Neglect (NIS-4): Report to Congress.* U.S. Department of Health and Human Services, Washington, DC, 2010.
5. Child Maltreatment 1998: *Reports from the states to the National Child Abuse and Neglect Data System.* U.S. Department of Health and Human Services, Washington, DC, 2000, Appendix B, p 8.
6. Straus MA: *Beating the Devil Out of Them: Corporal Punishment in American Families.* Lexington Books, Lexington, Mass, 1994, p 4.
7. Cousins J: Macrotheories: child physical punishment, injury and abuse. *Community Pract* 2005;78:276-279.
8. Gaudiosi JA: *Child maltreatment 2005.* U.S. Department of Health and Human Services, Administration on Children Youth and Families, Washington, DC, 2007.
9. Burns BJ, Phillips SD, Wagner HR, et al: Mental health need and access to mental health services by youth involved with child welfare: a national survey. *J Am Acad Child Adolesc Psychiatry* 2004;43:960-970.

10. Emery RE, Laumann-Billings L: An overview of the nature, causes and consequences of abusive family relationships: toward differentiating maltreatment and violence. *Am Psychol* 1998;53:121-135.

11. Levine M, Doueck HJ: *The Impact of Mandated Reporting on the Therapeutic Process.* Sage Publications, Thousand Oaks, Calif, 1995.

12. Gershoff ET: Corporal punishment by parents and associated child behaviors and experiences: a meta-analytic and theoretical review. *Psychol Bull* 2002;128:539-579.

13. Smith JR, Brooks-Gunn J: Correlates and consequences of harsh discipline for young children. *Arch Pediatr Adolesc Med* 1997;151:777-786.

14. What grown-ups understand about child development: A national benchmark survey. DYG, Danbury, Conn, 2000. Available at http://www.eric.ed.gov/ERICDocs/data/ericdocs2sql/content_storage_01/0000019b/80/16/c6/5c.pdf. Accessed March 30, 2009.

15. Straus MA: Commentary: The special issue on prevention of violence ignores the primordial violence. *J Interpers Violence* 2008;23:1314-1320.

16. American Humane Fact Sheet. Child Physical Abuse. American Humane, Denver, 2007. Available at http://www.americanhumane.org/assets/docs/about-us/AU-FS-child-physical-abuse.pdf. Accessed March 30, 2009.

17. Mulvaney MK, Mebert CJ: Parental corporal punishment predicts behavior problems in early childhood. *J Fam Psychol* 2007;21:389-397.

18. Bugental DB Shennum W: Gender, power, and violence in the family. *Child Maltreat* 2002;7:56-64.

19. Ponce AN, Williams MK, Allen GJ: Experience of maltreatment as a child and acceptance of violence in adult intimate relationships: mediating effects of distortions in cognitive schemas. *Violence Vict* 2004;19:97-108.

20. Shackman JE, Shackman AJ, Pollak SD: Physical abuse amplifies attention to threat and increases anxiety in children. *Emotion* 2007;7:838-852.

21. Flores E, Cicchetti D, Rogosch FA: Predictors of resilience in maltreated and nonmaltreated Latino children. *Dev Psychol* 2005;41:338-351.

22. Medley AN, Sachs-Ericsson N: Predictors of parental physical abuse: The contribution of internalizing and externalizing disorders and childhood experiences of abuse. *J Affect Disord* 2009;113:244-254.

23. Root C, Mackay S, Henderson J, et al: The link between maltreatment and juvenile firesetting: correlates and underlying mechanisms. *Child Abuse Negl* 2008;32:161-167.

24. Grogan-Kaylar A: Relationship of corporal punishment and antisocial behavior by neighborhood. *Arch Pediatr Adolesc Med* 2005;159:938-942.

25. Steiner H, Remsing L, and Work Group on Quality Issues: Practice parameter for the assessment and treatment of children and adolescents with oppositional defiant disorder. *J Am Acad Child Adolesc Psychiatry* 2007;46:124-141.

26. Schilling EA, Aseltine RHJ, Gore S: Adverse childhood experiences and mental health in young adults: A longitudinal survey. *BMC Public Health* 2007;7:30.

27. Rothman EF, Edwards EM, Heeren T, et al: Adverse childhood experiences predict earlier age of drinking onset: Results from a representative sample of current or former drinkers. *Pediatrics* 2008;122:298-304.

28. Fogarty CT, Fredman L, Heeren TC, et al: Synergistic effects of child abuse and intimate partner violence on depressive symptoms in women. *Prev Med* 2008;46:463-469.

29. Salzinger S, Rosario M, Feldman RS, et al: Adolescent suicidal behavior: Associations with preadolescent physical abuse and selected risk and protective factors. *J Am Acad Child Adolesc Psychiatry* 2007;46:859-866.

30. Fergusson DM, Boden JM, Horwood J: Exposure to childhood sexual and physical abuse and adjustment in early adulthood. *Child Abuse Negl* 2008;32:607-619.

31. Finzi R, Ram A, Har-Even D, et al: Attachment styles and aggression in physically abused and neglected children. *J Youth Adolesc* 2001;30:769-786.

32. Harkness LH, Lumley MN, Truss AE: Stress generation in adolescent depression: The moderating role of child abuse and neglect. *J Abnorm Child Psychol* 2008;36:421-432.

33. Egeland B, Yates T, Appleyard K, et al: The long-term consequences of maltreatment in the early years: A developmental pathway model to antisocial behavior. *Child Serv Soc Policy Res Pr* 2002;5:249-260.

34. Kolko DJ, Brown EJ, Berliner L: Children's perceptions of their abusive experience: measurement and preliminary findings. *Child Maltreat* 2002;7:42-55.

35. American Psychiatric Association: *Diagnostic and Statistical Manual of Mental Disorder, ed 4-TR.* American Psychiatric Association, Washington, DC, 2000.

36. Applied Research and Consulting, LLC: *Effects of the World Trade Center Attack on NYC Public School Students: Initial Report to the New York City Board of Education.* Columbia University Mailman School of Public Health, New York State Psychiatric Institute, New York, 2002.

37. Scheeringa MS, Wright MJ, Hunt JP, et al: Factors affecting the diagnosis and prediction of PTSD symptomatology in children and adolescents. *Am J Psychiatry* 2006;163:644-651.

38. Cohen JA, Kolko DJ: Transforming trauma: recognizing and responding to posttraumatic stress disorder symptoms in children and adolescents, *In:* McInerny TK, Adam HM, Campbell DE, et al (eds): *American Academy of Pediatrics Textbook of Pediatric Care.* American Academy of Pediatrics, Elk Grove Village, Ill, 2009.

39. Bonomi AE, Cannon EA, Anderson ML, et al: Association between self-reported health and physical and/or sexual abuse experienced before age 18. *Child Abuse Negl* 2008;32:693-701.

40. Turner HA, Finkelhor D: Corporal punishment as a stressor among youth. *J Marriage Fam* 1996;58:155-166.

41. Felitti VJ, Anda RF, Nordenberg D, et al: Relationship of childhood abuse and household dysfunction to many of the leading causes of death in adults. The Adverse Childhood Experiences (ACE) study. *Am J Prev Med* 1998;14:245-258.

42. Kolko DJ: Treatment research in child maltreatment: clinical and research directions. *In:* Ward SK, Findelhor D (eds): *Program Evaluation and Family Violence Research.* The Hawthorne Press, Binghamton, NY, 2000, pp 139-164.

43. Kilpatrick DG, Ruggiero KJ, Acierno R, et al: Violence and risk of PTSD, major depression, substance abuse/dependence, and comorbidity: results from the National Survey of Adolescents. *J Consult Clin Psychol* 2003;71:692-700.

44. Ford JD, Racusin R, Daviss WB, et al: Trauma exposure among children with oppositional defiant disorder and attention deficit-hyperactivity disorder. *J Consult Clin Psychol* 1999;67:786-789.

45. Kolko DJ: Clinical monitoring of treatment course in child physical abuse: psychometric characteristics and treatment comparisons. *Child Abuse Negl* 1996;20:23-43.

46. Kolko DJ: Individual cognitive-behavioral treatment and family therapy for physically abused children and their offending parents: a comparison of clinical outcomes. *Child Maltreat* 1996;1:322-342.

47. Ondersma SJ, Chaffin MJ, Mullins SM, et al: A brief form of the child abuse potential inventory: development and validation. *J Clin Child Adolesc Psychol* 2005;34:301-311.

48. Manly JT, Cicchetti D, Barnett D: The impact of subtype, frequency, chronicity, and severity of child maltreatment on social competence and behavior problems. *Dev Psychopathol* 1994;6:121-143.

49. Kolko DJ: CPS operations and risk assessment in child abuse cases receiving services: initial findings from the Pittsburgh Service Delivery Study. *Child Maltreat* 1998;3:262-275.

50. Wolfe DA, Edwards B, Manion I, et al: Early intervention for parents at risk of child abuse and neglect: a preliminary investigation. *J Consult Clin Psychol* 1988;56:40-47.

51. Chaffin M, Silovsky JF, Funderburk B, et al: Parent-child interaction therapy with physically abusive parents: efficacy for reducing future abuse reports. *J Consult Clin Psychol* 2004;72:500-510.

52. Briere J: *Trauma Symptom Checklist for Children: Professional Manual.* Psychological Assessment Resources, Odessa, Fla, 1996.

53. Steinberg AM, Brymer MJ, Decker KB, et al: The University of California at Los Angeles Post-traumatic Stress Disorder Reaction Index. *Curr Psychiatry Rep* 2004;6:96-100.

54. Bird HR, Shaffer D, Fisher P, et al: The Columbia Impairment Scale (CIS): pilot findings on a measure of global impairment for children and adolescents. *Int J Methods Psychiatr Res* 1993;3:167-176.

55. Shelton KK, Frick PJ, Wootten J: Assessment of parenting practices in families of elementary school-age children. *J Clin Child Psychol* 1996;25:317-329.

56. Straus MA, Hamby SL, Boney-McCoy S, et al: The Revised Conflict Tactics Scales (CTS2): development and preliminary psychometric data. *J Fam Issues* 1996;17:283-316.

57. Straus MA: Measuring intrafamily conflict and violence: the Conflicts Tactics (CT) Scales. *In:* Straus MA, Gelles (eds): *Physical Violence in American Families. Risk Factors and Adaptations to Violence in 8145 Families.* Transaction Publishers, New Brunswick, NJ, 1990, pp 29-47.

58. Kolko DJ, Kazdin A, Day BT: Children's perspectives in the assessment of family violence: Psychometric characteristics and comparison to parent reports. *Child Maltreat* 1996;1:156-167.

59. Moos RH, Insel PM, Humphrey B: *Family Work and Group Environment Scales.* Consulting Psychologists Press, Palo Alto, Calif, 1974.

60. Robin AL, Foster SL: *Negotiating Parent-Adolescent Conflict: A Behavioral-Family Systems Approach.* The Guilford Press, New York, 1989.

61. Horowitz LA, Putnam FW, Noll JG, et al: Factors affecting utilization of treatment services by sexually abused girls. *Child Abuse Negl* 1997;20:35-48.

62. Lazenbatt A, Freeman R: Recognizing and reporting child physical abuse: a survey of primary healthcare professionals. *J Adv Nurs* 2006;56:227-236.

63. Chaffin M, Schmidt S: An evidence-based perspective on interventions to stop or prevent child abuse. *In:* Lutzker JR (ed): *Preventing Violence: Research and Evidence-Based Intervention Strategies.* American Psychological Association, Washington, DC, 2006, pp 49-68.

64. Cohn AH, Daro D: Is treatment too late: What ten years of evaluative research tell us. *Child Abuse Negl* 1987;11:433-442.

65. Kaplan SJ, Pelcovitz D, Labruna V: Child and adolescent abuse and neglect research: a review of the past 10 years. Part I: Physical and emotional abuse and neglect. *J Am Acad Child Adolesc Psychiatry* 1999;38:1214-1222.

66. English DJ: The extent and consequences of child maltreatment. *Future Child* 1998;8:39-53.

67. Greenwalt BC, Sklare G, Portes P: The therapeutic treatment provided in cases involving physical child abuse: a description of current practices. *Child Abuse Negl* 1998;20:71-78.

68. Swenson CC, Brown EJ, Sheidow AJ: Medical, legal, and mental health service utilization by physically abused children and their caregivers. *Child Maltreat* 2003;8:138-144.

69. Lindell C, Svedin CG: Mental health services provided for physically abused children in Sweden. A 4-year follow-up of child and adolescent psychiatric charts. *Nord J Psychiatry* 2005;59:179-185.

70. Kopiec K, Finkelhor D, Wolak J: Which juvenile crime victims get mental health treatment? *Child Abuse Negl* 2004;28:45-59.

71. Warner JD: *An examination of demographic and treatment variables associated with session attendance of maltreating families.* Annual Conference of the Association for the Advancement of Behavior Therapy, San Francisco, November, 1990.

72. Nicol AR, Smith J, Kay B: A focused casework approach to the treatment of child abuse: a controlled comparison. *J Child Psychol Psychiatry* 1988;29:703-711.

73. Kolko DJ, Baumann BL, Caldwell N: Child abuse victims' involvement in community agency treatment: service correlates, short-term outcomes, and relationship to reabuse. *Child Maltreat* 2003;8:273-287.

74. Gully KJ, Price BL, Johnson MK: Increasing abused children's access to evidence-based treatment: diffusion via parents as consumers. *Child Maltreat* 2008;13:280-288.

75. Barlow J, Johnston I, Kendrick D, et al: Individual and group-based parenting programmes for the treatment of physical child abuse and neglect. *Cochrane Database Syst Rev* 2006;3:CD005463.

76. The National Child Traumatic Stress Network. Available at http://www.nctsnet.org/nccts/nav.do?pid=hom_main. Accessed March 31, 2009.

77. National Association of Cognitive-Behavioral Therapists: NACBT Online Headquarters. Available at http://www.nacbt.org/whatiscbt.htm. Accessed March 31, 2009.

78. Child Welfare Information Gateway. Administration for Children and Families, U.S. Department of Health and Human Services, Washington, DC. Available at http://www.childwelfare.gov/. Accessed March 31, 2009.

79. Azar ST, Wolfe DA: Child physical abuse and neglect. *In:* Mash EJ, Barkley RA (eds): *Treatment of Childhood Disorders.* Guilford Press, New York, 2006, pp 595-646.

80. Culp RE, Heide JS, Richardson MT: Maltreated children's developmental scores: treatment versus nontreatment. *Child Abuse Negl* 1987;11:29-34.

81. Sankey CC, Elmer E, Halechko AD, et al: The development of abused and high-risk infants in different treatment modalities: residential versus in-home care. *Child Abuse Negl* 1985;9:237-243.

82. Oates RK, Bross DC: What have we learned about treating child physical abuse? A literature review of the last decade. *Child Abuse Negl* 1995;19:463-473.

83. Culp RE, Little V, Letts D, et al: Maltreated children's self-concept: effects of a comprehensive treatment program. *Am J Orthopsychiatry* 1991;61:114-121.

84. Fantuzzo JW, Stovall A, Schnachtel D, et al: The effects of peer social initiations on the social behavior of withdrawn maltreated preschool children. *J Behav Ther Exp Psychiatry* 1987;18:357-363.

85. Davis S, Fantuzzo JW: The effects of adult and peer social initiations on social behavior of withdrawn and aggressive maltreated preschool children. *J Fam Violence* 1989;4:227-248.

86. Fantuzzo JW, Jurecic L, Stovall A, et al: Effects of adult and peer social initiations on the social behavior of withdrawn, maltreated preschool children. *J Consult Clin Psychol* 1988;56:34-39.

87. Fantuzzo JW, Sutton-Smith B, Atkins M, et al: Community-based resilient peer treatment of withdrawn maltreated preschool children. *J Consult Clin Psychol* 1996;64:1377-1386.

88. Swenson CC, Brown EJ: Cognitive behavioral group treatment for physically abused children. *Cogn Behav Pract* 1999;6:212-220.

89. Mammen OK, Pilkonis PA, Kolko DJ, et al: Anger and anger attacks as precipitants of aggression: What we can learn from child physical abuse. *In:* Cavell TA, Malcolm KT (eds): *Anger, Aggression and Interventions for Interpersonal Violence.* Lawrence Erlbaum Associates, Mahwah, NJ, 2007, pp 283-311.

90. Barth RP, Blyth BJ, Schinke SP, et al: Self-control training with maltreating parents. *Child Welfare* 1983;62:313-324.

91. Egan KJ: Stress management and child management with abusive parents. *J Clin Child Psychol* 1983;12:292-299.

92. Acton RG, During SM: Preliminary results of aggression management training for aggressive parents. *J Interpers Violence* 1992;7:410-417.

93. Nuris PS, Lovell M, Edgar M: Self-appraisals of abusive parents: a contextual approach to study and treatment. *J Interpers Violence* 1988;3:458-467.

94. Whiteman M, Fanshel D, Grundy JG: Cognitive-behavioral interventions aimed at anger of parents at risk of child abuse. *Soc Work* 1987;32:469-474.

95. Whipple EE, Wilson SR: Evaluation of a parent education and support program for families at risk of physical child abuse. *Fam Soc* 1996;77:227-239.

96. Fennell DC, Fishel AH: Parent education: an evaluation of STEP on abusive parents' perceptions and abuse potential. *J Child Adolesc Psychiatr Nurs* 1998;11:107-120.

97. Eisenstadt TH, Eyberg S, McNeil CB, et al: Parent-child interaction therapy with behavior problem children: relative effectiveness of two stages and overall treatment outcome. *J Clin Child Psychol* 1993;22:42-51.

98. Herschell AD, McNeil CB: Theoretical and empirical underpinnings of parent-child interaction therapy with child physical abuse populations. *Educ Treat Child* 2005;28:142-162.

99. Runyon MK, Deblinger E, Schroeder CM: Pilot evaluation of outcomes of combined parent-child cognitive-behavioral group therapy for families at risk for child physical abuse. *Cogn Behav Pract* 2009;16:101-118.

100. Corcoran J: Family interventions with child physical abuse and neglect: a critical review. *Child Youth Serv Rev* 2000;22:563-591.

101. Fraser MW, Walton E, Lewis RE, et al: An experiment in family reunification: correlates of outcomes at one-year follow-up. *Child Youth Serv Rev* 1996;18:335-361.

102. Walton E, Fraser MW, Lewis RE, et al: In-home family-focused reunification: an experimental study. *Child Welfare* 1993;72:473-487.

103. Chaffin M, Bonner BL, Hill RF: Family preservation and family support programs: child maltreatment outcomes across client risk levels and program types. *Child Abuse Negl* 2001;25:1269-1289.

104. Brunk M, Henggeler SW, Whelan JP: Comparison of multisystemic therapy and parent training in the brief treatment of child abuse and neglect. *J Consult Clin Psychol* 1987;55:171-178.

105. Lutzker JR, Bigelow KM, Doctor RM, et al: An ecobehavioral model for the prevention and treatment of child abuse and neglect. History and applications. *In:* Lutzker JR (ed): *Handbook of Child Abuse Research and Treatment.* Plenum Press, New York, 1998, pp 239-266.

106. Wesch D, Lutzker JR: A comprehensive 5-year evaluation of Project 12-Ways: an ecobehavioral program for treating and preventing child abuse and neglect. *J Fam Violence* 1991;6:17-35.

107. Lieberman AF Van Horn P: *Psychotherapy with Infants and Young Children: Repairing the Effects of Stress and Trauma on Early Attachment.* Guilford Press, New York, 2008.

108. Lieberman AF, Ippen CG, Van Horn P: Child-parent psychotherapy: 6-month follow-up of a randomized controlled trial. *J Am Acad Child Adoles Psychiatry* 2006;45:913-918.

109. Cohen JA, Deblinger E, Mannarino AP (eds): *Treating Trauma and Traumatic Grief in Children and Adolescents.* Guilford Press, New York, 2006.

110. Stein BD, Jaycox LH, Kataoka SH, et al: A mental health intervention for schoolchildren exposed to violence: a randomized controlled trial. *JAMA* 2003;290:603-611.

111. National Child Traumatic Stress Network: Empirically supported treatments and promising practices. 2008. Available at http://www.nctsnet.org/nccts/nav.do?pid=ctr_top_trmnt_prom. Accessed March 31, 2009.

112. Cohen JA, Mannarino AP, Murray LK, et al: Psychosocial interventions for maltreated and violence-exposed children. *J Soc Issues* 2006;62:737-766.

113. Paul LA, Gray MJ, Elhai JD, et al: Promotion of evidence-based practices for child traumatic stress in rural populations: identification of barriers and promising solutions. *Trauma Violence Abuse* 2006;7:260-273.

114. Whittaker J, Kinney JK: *Reaching High-Risk Families: Intensive Family Preservation in Human Services.* Aldine de Guyter, New York, 1990.

115. Klevens J, Whitaker DJ: Primary prevention of child physical abuse and neglect: gaps and promising directions. *Child Maltreat* 2007;12:364-377.

116. Krugman SD, Lane WG, Walsh CM: Update on child abuse prevention. *Curr Opin Pediatr* 2007;19:711-718.

117. Olds DL, Robinson J, O'Brien R, et al: Home visiting by paraprofessionals and by nurses: a randomized controlled trial. *Pediatrics* 2002;110:486-496.

118. MacMillan HL, Thomas BH, Jamieson E, et al: Effectiveness of home visitation by public-health nurses in prevention of the recurrence of child physical abuse and neglect: a randomised controlled trial. *Lancet* 2005;365:1786-1793.

119. Sanders MR, Cann W, Markie-Dadds C: The Triple-P Positive Parenting Programme: a universal population-level approach to the prevention of child abuse. *Child Abuse Rev* 2003;12:155-171.

120. Ateah CA, Durrant JE: Maternal use of physical punishment in response to child misbehavior: implications for child abuse prevention. *Child Abuse Negl* 2005;29:169-185.

121. Vandeven AM, Newton AW: Update on child physical abuse, sexual abuse, and prevention. *Curr Opin Pediatr* 2006;18:201-205.

122. Straus MA: Corporal punishment and primary prevention of physical abuse. *Child Abuse Negl* 2000;24:1109-1114.

123. Peterson L, Brown D, Bartelstone J, et al: Methodological considerations in participant event monitoring of low-base-rate events in health psychology: children's injuries as a model in health psychology. *Health Psychol* 1996;15:124-130.

124. Hornor G: Child advocacy centers: providing support to primary care providers. *J Pediatr Health Care* 2008;22:35-39.

125. Smith DW, Witte TH, Fricker-Elhai AE: Service outcomes in physical and sexual abuse cases: a comparison of child advocacy center-based and standard services. *Child Maltreat* 2006;11:354-360.

126. Abatemarco DJ, Kairys SW, Gubernick RS, et al: Expanding the pediatrician's black bag: a psychosocial care improvement model to address the "new morbidities." *Jt Comm J Qual Patient Saf* 2008;34:106-115.

127. Staudt MM: Mental health services utilization by maltreated children: research findings and recommendations. *Child Maltreat* 2003;8:195-203.

128. Watts-English T, Fortson BL, Gibler N, et al: The psychobiology of maltreatment in childhood. *J Soc Issues* 2006;62:717-736.

129. Silverman WK, Pina AA, Viswesvaran C: Evidence-based psychosocial treatments for children and adolescents exposed to traumatic events. *J Clin Child Adolesc Psychol* 2008;37:156-183.

51

PSYCHOLOGICAL IMPACT AND TREATMENT OF NEGLECT OF CHILDREN

Maureen M. Black, PhD, and Sarah E. Oberlander, PhD

INTRODUCTION

Child neglect is the most common type of maltreatment. The National Child Abuse and Neglect Data System (NCANDS),[1] the primary source of information on children who have been reported to child protective service (CPS) agencies, has reported that 62.8% (564,765) of the approximately 899,000 children reported to CPS agencies in 2005 experienced neglect alone. (See Chapter 5, "Epidemiology of Child Neglect.") The Federal Child Abuse, Prevention, and Treatment Act (CAPTA)[2] defines neglect as the failure to ensure that children's basic needs are met. Professionals frequently refer to four types of neglect: physical, educational, emotional/psychological, and medical. (See Chapter 55, "Definitions and Categorization of Child Neglect.")

Physical neglect, the most prevalent form of neglect, refers to the failure to provide basic necessities, such as food, clothing, and shelter. Physical neglect also includes abandonment, inadequate supervision, and lack of protection. *Educational neglect* implies that the child's educational needs have not been met, often by not enrolling the child in an appropriate school, not allowing the child to participate in educational activities, or chronic truancy. *Emotional/psychological neglect* refers to exposing the child to conditions that could result in psychological harm or extremely poor self-image, such as frequently berating the child, ignoring the child's need for stimulation, verbally assaulting the child, isolating the child from others, threatening the child, or involving the child in illegal activities. *Medical neglect* refers to the lack of appropriate medical or mental health care or treatment. In this chapter, we examine: (1) the predictors of neglect, (2) the psychological consequences of neglect, (3) the mechanisms linking neglect with children's psychological functioning, (4) programs and policies that have alleviated the negative effects of neglect on children's psychological functioning, (5) long-term consequences of neglect, and (6) recommendations for future research, programs, and policies to reduce the negative consequences of neglect on children's psychological functioning.

PREDICTORS OF NEGLECT

The predictors of child neglect are organized based on developmental-ecological theory, which conceptualizes child development from distal to proximal, beginning with community level variables and ending with child level variables.[3]

Most of the research conducted to identify "predictors" of neglect has been collected from cross-sectional studies, making it difficult to separate predictors from consequences. For example, although withdrawal has been identified as a predictor of neglect,[4] children with chronically inappropriate or dirty clothing might be ignored by their peers and become withdrawn as a result.[5]

Poverty

Neglect is more directly associated with poverty than other types of child maltreatment.[6,7] Children living in high poverty areas are six times as likely to experience neglect, compared with children living in low poverty areas.[8] Impoverished neighborhoods are often characterized by high levels of unemployment and vacant housing, which are associated with high maltreatment rates.[9] Population loss in some impoverished neighborhoods leads to low levels of social contact and support, which are associated with neglect.[9] Families living in impoverished neighborhoods often have fewer opportunities to meet children's needs than families living in middle-income communities, particularly if population loss is accompanied by reductions in services such as hospitals, schools, playgrounds, and transportation. Families in low-income communities also have few resources to adequately meet their children's physical needs of nutrition, clothing, and personal hygiene.[10] Poverty exacerbates other risk factors for neglect, such as food insecurity, poor maternal nutrition, maternal depression, and stressful life events.[11]

Food Insecurity

Food security is defined as access to enough food for an active, healthy life for all household members, and *food insecurity* is defined as limited or uncertain access to enough food to meet basic needs for household members at all times.[12,13] These definitions capture both the availability of food and the anxiety or concern regarding limited food availability. Food insecurity has been associated with negative consequences for children in the first 3 years of life, including worse caregiver-reported health, more hospitalizations,[14] a higher likelihood of developmental risk,[15] and behavioral problems.[16] The mechanisms linking food insecurity with negative consequences for children include both nutritional pathways (compromised with both the quantity and quality of food available) and nonnutritional pathways (increased anxiety and stress related to the inconsistent availability of food).[17] Thus, food insecurity threatens children's physical and psychological health, serving as a form of both physical and emotional neglect.

Poor Maternal Nutrition

Recent research has suggested that maternal nutritional status may be related to parenting behavior, and specifically to child neglect. For example, iron deficiency, the most prevalent single nutrient deficiency in the world,[18] is associated with reduced work capacity, poor immune function, and changes in cognition, emotions, and behavior. Although most of the research has focused on young children, there are reports of altered cognition and behavior in iron-deficient women of reproductive age.[19] Behavioral symptoms associated with iron deficiency in adults include irritability, apathy, fatigue, depressive symptoms, and hypoactivity. Two reports from South Africa included anemic and nonanemic mothers evaluated at 10 weeks and 9 months postpartum.[20,21] Not only was iron status associated with measures of cognition, anxiety, stress, and depression, but anemic mothers who received iron treatment experienced a 25% improvement ($P < .05$) in measures of cognition, depression, and stress, compared with anemic mothers who received placebo.[21] In addition, infants of anemic mothers demonstrated developmental delays at 10 weeks that were sustained through 9 months in spite of iron treatment. At 9 months, anemic mothers were significantly more negative toward their babies, with less goal setting and responsivity than nonanemic mothers. In contrast, anemic mothers who received iron treatment had similar behavioral observation scores to nonanemic mothers, suggesting the protective effects of iron on maternal parenting behavior.[21] Thus, iron-deficient mothers appear to be at risk for neglecting their children.

Maternal Depression

Maternal depression has been identified as a predictor of neglect.[22,23] Between 10% and 15% of postpartum women experience depressive symptoms, and postpartum depression has been identified as a predictor of neglect.[24] Depression can interfere with mothers' ability to provide consistent affectionate and stimulating contact to their infants; in extreme cases, mothers are unable to respond to their children's needs at all.[25] In a metaanalysis, Lovejoy and colleagues[26] found that the relation between maternal depression and negative maternal parenting behavior was moderated by timing of the depression, with the strongest effects for current, as opposed to past, depression. In addition, effects were strongest for low-income women and mothers of infants, highlighting the vulnerability early in life when women are transitioning to a new role and can have limited support and confidence, particularly in low-income communities.

Stressful Life Events

Stressful life events are predictors of neglect.[27] Kotch et al[23] found an interaction between stress and social support, such that children in families with high stress and low social support were the most at risk for child maltreatment. Financial difficulties, substance abuse, illness, and daily stressors strain a family's resources, exacerbate family conflict, and potentially lead to neglect.[28-30]

Interpersonal Violence

Interpersonal violence has consistently been identified as a life event that is a predictor of neglect.[31] More than one third (35%) of neglect cases also include reports of interpersonal violence.[32] Perpetrators of interpersonal violence might not be focused on the physical or emotional needs of their children, and victims of interpersonal violence might be fearful and unable to adequately meet their children's needs.[33]

Child Temperament

Child characteristics have been identified as factors associated with neglect, although the direction of the association is not clear. Neglect is associated with maternal report of difficult temperament.[34,35] Mothers who described their infants as temperamentally difficult were more likely than other mothers to have a reported incident of neglect 2 years later.[34] Harrington et al[35] found that maternal reports of temperamental difficulty were associated with emotional neglect, but not physical neglect. It is not clear whether mothers who neglect are more likely to perceive their child as difficult, or whether children with a difficult temperament make it more difficult for mothers to meet their emotional and physical needs.

Child Development and Behavior

Multiple investigators have found that children with disabilities are at increased risk for maltreatment,[36] possibly through the challenges and stress facing their families.[37,38] A recent investigation of the administrative records of over 100,000 children under age 6 years in Illinois receiving Medicaid between 2000 and 2006 found that children with chronic health conditions or behavioral/emotional problems were at increased risk for abuse and neglect, particularly if they had been maltreated in the past.[39] A diagnosis of developmental delay/mental retardation, however, did not increase the risk of maltreatment. In contrast, other investigators have found that infants with low mental and motor development scores at 9 months of age were more likely to have experienced neglect by age 2 than other infants.[34] The discrepancy may be partially explained by the data source. Administrative records include diagnosed problems, rather than caregiver-identified problems, that might be as yet undiagnosed among children under age 6.

PSYCHOLOGICAL CONSEQUENCES OF NEGLECT

The impact of neglect on children's psychological development is best understood when evaluated with respect to general theories of child development. Children proceed through a series of developmental tasks from infancy through adolescence.[40] These stages begin with attachment during the first year of life, the enduring and predictable relationships infants form with their caregivers. Autonomy and self-regulation are the primary tasks of the second and third years as toddlers acquire skills that contribute to their independence in both functional areas (eating, toileting) and interpersonal relationships (language). Peer relationships, the tasks of early childhood, become increasingly important as children attend preschool and elementary school. Finally, during middle childhood, the child has to integrate the earlier tasks to develop the interpersonal skills necessary for satisfying relationships during adolescence.[41] Although each task is associated with a specific age range, the tasks are not limited to that period and extend throughout childhood from infancy through adolescence.

Infancy

Most of the maltreatment that occurs during infancy is neglect, given the dependency needs of infants. The interdependence between infants and their primary caregivers is well documented.[42] Early infancy begins as a period of dependence as infants learn about their social-emotional environment through interactions with their primary caregivers. As infants and caregivers develop mutuality through a reciprocal process of looking to one another for affective cues and responses, they develop a synchrony in which responses stimulate expectations for subsequent interactions.[42] Under ideal conditions, infants and caregivers develop a mutually satisfying pattern of interactions that facilitates healthy physical and psychological development in the infant. Infants learn that their needs will be met according to predictable cues, and they learn to trust their caregivers. When caregivers are not consistent in their responses, infants can be denied models to imitate and contingent feedback. Without satisfying interactions, infants might have difficulty developing trust and a secure attachment with their primary caregivers and are at risk for subsequent emotional and relational problems.[43]

Research from the 1940s demonstrated that institutionalized infants experienced severe and often permanent declines in their health and development, even when they had adequate food.[44] The lack of nurturance and stimulation disrupted the children's cognitive and psychological development. Data from Romanian orphanages characterized by few staff and limited opportunities for nurturance and stimulation have shown that by age 3 years, infants experience poor growth, cognitive delays, and multiple psychological problems including attachment disorders, autistic-like behaviors, and poor social skills.[45] These findings highlight the negative consequences of severe emotional neglect on children's psychological functioning very early in life.

In a recent application of developmental-ecological theory among very low income, inner-city families of infants and toddlers, the relationships between neglect and child and family functioning differed by the type of neglect.[35] Emotional neglect was associated with a path from family functioning through perceptions of child temperament. There were no direct links from family functioning, support, or life events to emotional neglect, but mothers who were involved in well-functioning families were more likely to regard their child as having an easy temperament, and children who were perceived as being relatively easy were less likely to experience emotional neglect. These findings

illustrate the importance of conceptualizing neglect from a developmental–ecological perspective that incorporates the family and the child's contributions through their temperament. The link between mothers' perceptions of their children's temperament and child neglect suggests that maternal perceptions of children's temperament are an important component of neglect that should be incorporated into intervention strategies. In contrast, when physical neglect was considered, there were no associations with child temperament and family context. Thus, different factors are associated with physical and emotional neglect.

School-Aged Children

Several investigators have shown that neglected children are more likely to exhibit developmental, emotional, and behavioral problems than are nonneglected children.[46] There is variation, however, in the specific behavior problems shown by neglected children. Investigators have noted that at times neglected children are passive and withdrawn, and at other times, they are aggressive.[47] Thus, children who have been neglected might have dysfunctional working models of social interactions, and in response to routine peer play, display both withdrawn and aggressive behavior.

Egeland et al[46,48] followed four groups of mother–child pairs (abusive, neglectful, psychologically unavailable, and non-maltreating controls) and reported that children of neglectful and psychologically unavailable mothers were more likely to be anxiously attached when compared with non-maltreated children. Without a secure attachment relationship with the primary caregiver, the tasks of autonomy and self-development and the ability to form trusting relationships with peers are threatened.[49] Neglected children have fewer positive social interactions with peers than do non-neglected peers and are often less self-assured.[50]

The vulnerability of neglected children has been well described in a longitudinal follow-up study.[47] By early school age, neglected children had deficits in cognitive performance, academic achievement, classroom behavior, and personal social interactions with peers and adults. The neglected children rarely expressed positive affect and demonstrated more developmental problems than any other subgroup of maltreated children. Several authors have found that children with a history of neglect have more school absences,[51] more retentions, and lower grades than do non-neglected children.[52]

Risk and compensatory factors also influence children's adjustment to neglect. For example, a child who is intelligent, attractive, or talented may be more able to withstand neglectful situations than one who is not intelligent, not attractive, and has low self-esteem.[53] Although protective factors can mitigate against some of the negative sequelae associated with neglect, Farber and Egeland[53] argued that the environmental challenges associated with maltreatment, and particularly with neglect or psychological unavailability, tend to overpower these protective factors, thereby increasing children's vulnerability.

Adolescents

The adolescent period is marked by transition as the dependency of childhood evolves into the independence (or interdependence) of adulthood. The primary tasks of adolescence are to form multiple attachment relationships, to internalize standards of morality, and to assume responsibility for personal actions.[54] Adolescents who have experienced prior neglect are at risk for emotional and behavioral problems if they have not mastered earlier developmental tasks successfully.

Neglect during adolescence can be particularly difficult to define, because the boundaries between adolescent independence and parental responsibility are unclear. As children age, the influence of parents is supplemented and sometimes replaced by the influence of peers and other forces in the community. Although adolescents do not require the close supervision required by younger children, they continue to require parental guidance and monitoring.[38] Adolescents benefit from clear parental demands that are established using a warm, democratic, and respectful approach.[40] Without access to parents who provide both supervision and nurturance, adolescents can be at increased risk for behavioral and emotional problems, such as engaging in high-risk behaviors (e.g., early initiation of sexual activity, substance abuse).

MECHANISMS LINKING NEGLECT WITH CHILDREN'S PSYCHOLOGICAL FUNCTIONING

Several possible mechanisms link neglect with children's psychological functioning, including biological theories of stress and psychosocial theories of development.

Biological Stress Response

Animal studies have suggested that neglect in the form of maternal deprivation is associated with disruptions to the development of the biological stress response.[55] DeBellis[56] explains that children process neglect as intense anxiety and stress, which activates their neurotransmitter systems, neuroendocrine system, and immune system. The major brain catecholamine neurotransmitters are serotonin and dopamine. Serotonin plays an important role in mood and behavior regulation. Low and dysregulated levels of serotonin have been associated with depression, aggressiveness, impulsivity, and suicide. Primate studies have shown that in response to chronic stress, serotonin levels in the prefrontal cortex drop, although they might increase in other areas of the brain. In response to stress, dopamine prefrontal cortical function is enhanced to prepare for a response to the stress. In response to *chronic* stress, however, there can be an overproduction of dopamine-impairing prefrontal cortical functioning rather than enhancing it, leading to inattention, hypervigilance, cognitive problems, and paranoia.

Recent advances in behavioral neuroscience have shown the important role that experiences, such as neglect, can have on brain development. Brain development begins prenatally with an overproduction of neurons and continues through school years.[57] Brain development begins with the formation of brain cells, followed by cell migration and differentiation, the development of synapses to enable cells to communicate with one another, and the formation of myelin, supportive tissue that protects the nerve cells and facilitates

communication.[58] During the first 4 years of life, there is selective pruning of synapses, along with myelination.[59]

The process of forming and eliminating synapses is influenced by individual experiences.[58] Greenough and colleagues[59] argue for the distinction between two types of experiences: experience-expectant and experience-dependent. Experience-expectant refers to species-specific development, such as sensory and motor systems. The maturational influences that guide development are operationalized by experiences that are expected, such as adequate care. Expected experiences "influence the brain by causing chemical changes within cells that influence cell function and structure."[58]

In contrast, experience-dependent development occurs in the context of unique experiences. They enable children to adapt to specific cultures and the demands of their environment. When children are denied such experiences (e.g., through neglect), they might not develop the synapses necessary for optimal functioning. Structural changes in synaptic formation appear to be dependent on neurochemical-receptor systems that, in turn, are influenced by basic caregiving experiences.[58]

The timing of early developmental experiences has been a central issue in studying behavioral neuroscience. The critical or sensitive period hypothesis suggests that if an event, such as neglect, occurs during a specified period, often during periods of rapid development, it will have specific effects on the organism.[60] In addition, since components of the central nervous system develop along differing schedules, the sensitive periods of the components likely vary with respect to onset and duration.

The field of behavioral neuroscience is emerging with the development of safe procedures to conduct neuroimaging studies in children (see Chapter 54, "Effects of Abuse and Neglect on Brain Development"). In a recent review, DeBellis[56] identified several studies using magnetic resonance imaging (MRI) to examine brain structure in children who experienced child neglect. The adverse effects of neglect on brain structure appeared to be particularly prominent among children (especially males) with maltreatment-related PTSD. Future research, using techniques such as functional MRI, will be helpful in understanding differential patterns of brain activation related to neglect.

Developmental Systems Theory

Developmental systems theories (DSTs)[3,61] can also be helpful in understanding the multiple mechanisms linking neglect with children's psychological functioning. DST is based on ecological theory and conceptualizes interactions across multiple levels, extending from basic biological processes to interactions at individual, family, school, community, and cultural levels. As with any systems model, interactions are bidirectional, such that changes in one aspect of the system may affect relations and processes throughout the system.

Direct Effects of Neglect

In a direct effects model, neglect influences children's psychological functioning by increasing risk factors and limiting protective factors and opportunities for stimulation and enrichment. Evidence suggests that many of the negative effects of neglect on children are influenced by co-occurring risk factors, such as family income. Low-income families often have limited education, thereby detracting from the human capital and opportunities available to their children.[62] For example, low-income families limit their children's linguistic environment by using language that is dominated by commands and simple structure, rather than by explanations and elaboration.[63] In addition, low-income families tend to use harsh parenting styles that are based on parental control, rather than reciprocal, interactive styles that promote emotional development and social competence.[64]

Moderated Effects of Neglect

A moderated effect means that the effects of neglect vary across characteristics of families or children. For example, families who are poorly educated with poor decision-making skills may have more difficulty protecting their children from the effects of neglect than families who are better educated with rational decision-making skills.[65] Moderated effects might also operate by conferring protection on children. For example, the Family Investment Model[66] proposes that parents who are better educated or have access to financial resources invest in their children through educationally enhancing materials (e.g., books) and activities (e.g., reading), thus potentially protecting their children from some of the negative consequences of neglect.

Family characteristics may also influence the association between neglect and children's psychological functioning through a process known as "social selection."[67] The social selection perspective hypothesizes that individual differences in parental traits lead to differences in parenting and in turn impact children's psychological functioning. For example, parents who have prosocial attributes, such as honesty, integrity, and dependability, transmit these values to their children, thus conferring protection even in the face of neglect.[68]

Mediated Effects of Neglect

In mediated models, the effects of neglect are felt through disruptions in family functioning, which in turn have negative repercussions on the children. This model is extended from studies of the effects of the Depression of the 1930s on families and on children.[69] It is consistent with the Family Stress Model,[70] in which poverty associated with economic hardship leads to family stress and has a negative impact on parental emotional well-being and mental health, undermining parenting behavior and increasing the likelihood of parents using either harsh and controlling parenting or neglectful parenting. The result is behavioral and developmental problems for the children. In other words, parents who are stressed and overwhelmed with the pressures of poverty might be unable to meet the emotional, cognitive, and caregiving needs of their children.

Transactional Effects of Neglect

In transactional models, the effects of neglect reverberate through the relations between families and children,

incorporating both moderated and mediated processes. Just as parental characteristics can moderate the impact of neglect on children's psychological functioning, children's characteristics can play a similar role. For example, caregivers of temperamentally difficult children are less likely to exhibit sensitive-responsive caregiving and more likely to report depressive symptoms than caregivers of temperamentally easy children.[71,72] The negative consequences of maternal depressive symptoms on children's psychological functioning are exacerbated in the face of raising a temperamentally difficult child,[73] suggesting a similar relationship in the context of neglect. In contrast, the Family Investment Model[66] would predict that caregivers are likely to invest in educational resources, even in times of poverty and neglect, if they perceive their children to be bright or academically talented.

Thus, although caregivers may experience stress related to neglect, resulting in mental health problems and interfering with the quality of their interactions with their children, they are also influenced by their perceptions of their children's skills and their children's behavior. Likewise, children are influenced by multiple processes. In addition to the direct effects of a lack of resources or other risk factors associated with neglect, there are also negative effects of caregiver behavior, including inconsistent caregiving or harsh parenting. The cycle continues as caregivers react to their children's behavior.

Community Influences on Neglect

DST also highlights the effects of neighborhood, community, and cultural influences on neglect. Low-income families, at risk for neglect, tend to live in low-income neighborhoods, often characterized by high density, crime, and few opportunities for academic socialization.[74] Schools are often underfunded, beset by disciplinary problems, staffed by poorly equipped teachers, and confronted with difficulties meeting their educational mandates.[75] Although community level variables related to neglect contribute to children's academic performance (and sometimes educational neglect), they typically account for less variance than family-level variables,[76] suggesting that as with the Family Stress Model, the effects of community level variables may be mediated through family relations.

PROGRAMS AND POLICIES RELATED TO CHILD NEGLECT

Many intervention programs to address child abuse and neglect have been described in the literature. Few, however, have been evaluated, and even fewer have specifically reported outcomes for child neglect. Several interventions with experimental designs are discussed, including play therapies, family interventions, and home visitation programs.

Play Therapy

Allin et al[77] conducted a systematic review of the literature on the treatment of child neglect between 1980 and 2003. They identified 54 studies that met the content-specific selection criteria of (1) including children and families who had experienced neglect, (2) describing an intervention, and (3) measuring an outcome. Only 14 studies had an observational or experimental design that included a comparison group; two were rated as good, three as fair, and nine as poor. Both of the studies rated as good evaluated play therapy for children who had been neglected.

First, Fantuzzo et al[78] conducted a randomized controlled trial of resilient peer treatment. Their sample included 46 African American children from Head Start centers who had been identified as socially isolated by teachers and independent classroom observers. Twenty-two children in the sample had a documented history of physical abuse, neglect, or both. Children in the experimental group were each matched with a resilient peer. Resilient peers were identified by observers as engaging in high levels of positive play with other children in the classroom. Head Start parent volunteers served as play supporters, and they encouraged peer dyads to play in a designated corner of the classroom for 15 sessions over 2 months. Play supporters observed the play and offered supportive comments to the dyad. Children in the control condition were matched with a peer with average play ability for 15 sessions and the play supporter observed the play sessions, but did not encourage peer play. At 2 weeks after intervention, classroom observers blind to the treatment condition rated children in the experimental group (both those with and without a history of maltreatment) as engaging in more positive play and less solitary play than children in the control condition. At 2 months after intervention, teachers rated children in the experimental group as exhibiting fewer internalizing and externalizing behaviors than children in the control condition.

Second, Udwin[79] completed a randomized controlled trial of imaginative play with a sample of 34 preschool children who had experienced neglect, abuse, or both, and had been removed from their homes. Half of the sample was assigned to the experimental condition, which consisted of 10 30-minute imaginative play sessions led by a facilitator. The other half of the sample was assigned to a control condition that consisted of 10 30-minute play sessions with no active training in imaginative play. At 4 weeks after intervention, independent student observers rated children in the experimental group as exhibiting better peer interactions and cooperation, imagination, positive affect, divergent thinking, and less aggressive play, compared with children in the control group.

Family Interventions

Brunk et al[80] compared multisystemic therapy (MST) and parent training (PT) in the treatment of child abuse and neglect. Families who were court-ordered to receive counseling following an incident of child abuse or neglect were offered the opportunity to participate in the research study, and half of the families agreed to participate. The 43 participating families were randomly assigned to either MST or PT. Both groups received 1.5-hour therapy sessions once a week, lasting for 8 weeks.

Families in the MST group received individual therapy at their home or in a health clinic. MST was tailored to the family's needs; for example, neglectful parents received instruction on performing executive functions. Most families received education about child management strategies and behavioral expectations. Therapists served as advocates with outside agencies with about half of the families. PT was conducted with groups of parents in a health care clinic. Multiple therapists were present during PT, and sessions focused on instructing parents about human development and child management techniques. Families identified specific problem behaviors and therapists discussed behavior management programs.

Families were assessed before entering treatment and within 1 week following their final therapy session. Parents completed self-report questionnaires and were videotaped interacting with their child completing block design tasks. Results indicated that parents in both treatment groups reported reduced overall stress and a reduction in the severity of family problems. Independent coding of the parent–child observational task suggested that following the intervention, parents in the MST group showed increased effectiveness in their attempts to control their children's behavior, children in the MST group were less passive, and neglectful parents became more responsive to their children's behavior.

Meezan and O'Keefe[81,82] compared the effectiveness of a multifamily group therapy with the normal course of family therapy available to families with a history of child maltreatment. The sample included 81 families with an open case of child abuse or neglect with the Los Angeles County Department of Children and Family Services. The multifamily group therapy, Family-to-Family, was designed to alter intrafamilial interaction patterns and increase parental responsiveness to prevent and treat child maltreatment. The program was tailored to meet the needs of the individual family. Families in the Family-to-Family group met with a team of four clinicians for 2.5 hours per week over 8 months. Family-to-Family included six themes: (1) physical, emotional/social, and cognitive development, (2) discipline, responsibility, and self-regulation, (3) value, character building, and self-respect, (4) focus on feelings, (5) person, partner, and parents … plus, and (6) productive communication and relationship building. The program also included a case management approach that linked families to community resources, such as food banks.

Families in the comparison group received the course of family therapy that was typically available to families with an open child maltreatment case. The comparison treatment included structural family therapy, behavior modification, cognitive-behavioral therapy, and case management. Families attended about 10 1-hour individual family therapy sessions. The main outcome of this study was child abuse potential and appropriate discipline, measured by the Child Abuse Potential Inventory (CAP).[83] These data were collected through self-report questionnaires completed at pre- and post-intervention. Both therapy groups had high child abuse potential scores above the clinical cutoff at pretest. After the intervention, CAP scores in the experimental group decreased significantly, ending below the clinical cutoff. Scores in the comparison group decreased slightly but remained above the clinical cutoff.

Home Visitation

The Nurse Home Visitation Program designed by Olds and colleagues[84,85] is one of the most well-known long-term follow-ups of a randomized trial to prevent problems among new mothers, including child abuse and neglect. The original sample included 400 first-time mothers recruited before the 30th week of pregnancy, 85% of whom were unmarried, adolescent, or poor. Families were randomly assigned to one of four treatment conditions: (1) no services during pregnancy, and infant screening between 1 and 2 years of age, (2) free transportation to prenatal care and well-child visits, and infant screening, (3) biweekly nurse home visitation during pregnancy, transportation, and infant screening, and (4) nurse home visitation during pregnancy and through 2 years postpartum, transportation, and infant screening. Nurse home visitors provided family support and education regarding fetal and infant development and linked families with services.

During the first 2 years postpartum, Department of Social Service records indicated that 19% of highest-risk mothers (poor and unmarried adolescents) in the comparison group had an officially reported incident of child abuse or neglect, compared with 4% of highest-risk mothers in the nurse visitation group. Among participants in the comparison group, incidence of maltreatment was associated with low maternal sense of control. This association was not statistically significant among mothers in the nurse visitation treatment groups.

Project SafeCare is a home visiting program that was designed to address three factors closely linked with child neglect: (1) home safety, (2) infant and child health care, and (3) stimulation/bonding or parent–child interaction.[86,87] Families in the intervention were either referred by a child protective service agency following a report for child abuse or neglect or referred by a local hospital's maternal health education office. Children of families in the latter group were identified as at risk for maltreatment, because parents were young, single, and/or poor. More than 40% of the participants in Project SafeCare spoke Spanish exclusively. Project SafeCare families were matched with comparison families from the same child protective service offices that were referred to other services.

The Project SafeCare model includes 15 weeks of intervention with 5 weeks concentrating on each area, conducted on a one-on-one basis with nurses or research assistants. Interventionists provide education about developmentally appropriate skills and activities, safety hazards, cleanliness, locks, and how to respond when a child is ill. Substantiated incidents of abuse and neglect were used as the outcome measure in this study, and program evaluations indicate that families in Project SafeCare were less likely to experience neglect during the intervention period and during the 2 years following the intervention.

Family Connections

Few interventions have specifically targeted child neglect, so it is unclear how successfully the programs presented above prevented different forms of child maltreatment. To our knowledge, Family Connections is the first prevention program expressly targeting child neglect.[88] One-hundred fifty-four families were randomly assigned to receive a 3-month (FC3) or 9-month (FC9) intervention. Targeted families lived in Baltimore, Maryland's Westside Empowerment Zone, an area experiencing extreme poverty, unemployment, and economic distress. Eligible families had the

following characteristics: (1) a referrer was concerned that neglect was occurring at a low level not yet reportable to CPS, (2) at least two risk factors for neglect related to the child (e.g., behavior problems, disabilities) or caregiver/ family (e.g., substance abuse, homelessness), (3) no current CPS involvement, and (4) a willingness to participate. Prior CPS involvement was not an exclusion criterion for inclusion in the study. Families were referred by schools, community-based organizations, clinics, public social services, or self referred. After a baseline assessment, families were randomized into a treatment group and then connected with their interventionist, a social work intern. Families in both treatment groups received approximately 1 hour of services per week. Self-report data were collected via an audio computer-assisted self-interview.

Family Connections was developed using Bronfenbrenner's[3] theory of social ecology. The nine principles of the program are community outreach, individualized family assessment, tailored interventions, helping alliance, empowerment approaches, strengths perspective, cultural competence, developmental appropriateness, and outcome-driven service plans. The program has four core components. First, emergency assistance allowed interventionists to quickly assess a family's critical needs and provide resources during a time of crisis (e.g., eviction notice). Goods and services were provided by resource directories, in-kind resources, and an emergency fund. Second, the home-based family intervention was tailored to the needs of each family after determining their specific risk factors. Third, service coordination was provided by interventionists who helped families access services. Fourth, multifamily supportive recreational activities were held at least four times a year to promote local, cultural, and recreational activities. Families also received newsletters with parenting tips and advertisements for free or low-cost family events. Family Connections is a unique program that combines graduate student education with service to the community. Graduate student social work interns serve as interventionists, with supervision provided by faculty members.

Three risk factor domains were assessed at pre- and post-intervention: caregiver depressive symptoms, parenting stress, and everyday stress. The four protective factor domains assessed included parenting attitudes, parenting sense of competence, family functioning, and social support. Child safety and child behavior were assessed through caregiver report. Child abuse or neglect reports were assessed by searching official child abuse and neglect records.

Prior to the Family Connections intervention, CPS had received 274 reports related to 87 of the 154 families in the sample. There were no significant differences in pre-intervention CPS reports between the FC3 and FC9 families. Twenty-four CPS reports were made related to 17 families during the intervention period and 11 reports were made regarding 11 families during the 6 months after intervention. There were no differences in the number of reports made regarding FC3 or FC9 families.

Caregiver depressive symptoms and parenting stress scores decreased over time in both treatment groups. Some improvements were noted in social support, parenting attitudes, and parenting sense of competence. Family functioning did not change over time in either group. Independent observers noted improvements in crowding and household sanitation over time in both groups. Children's behavior problems decreased across both groups, although caregivers in the FC9 group reported greater improvements in child internalizing behavior than caregivers in the FC3 group.

DePanfilis and Dubowitz[88] noted few differences in risk or protective factor changes between the FC3 and FC9 groups. Families in the FC9 condition reported being less satisfied with the program than FC3 families, and fewer FC9 families completed the program. The authors note that the burden of participating in a 9-month intervention might have been excessive for some families. Alternatively, interventionists might have worked with greater intensity among FC3 families, given the shorter intervention period.

Between 30% and 80% of families most at risk for child maltreatment complete prevention programs.[89] Eighty-nine percent of families in the FC3 condition and 46% of families in the FC9 condition completed the Family Connections intervention.[90] Girvin et al[90] explored predictors of program completion. Results of multivariate quantitative analyses revealed that FC3 families were more likely to complete the program than FC9 families, but few depressive symptoms and high satisfaction with the service provider also increased the odds that a family would adhere to the program. Family Connections staff attributes their success to focusing on concrete needs first and then continuing to develop higher level skills that reduce the risk of child maltreatment. Future research is needed to measure less tangible factors that may be associated with adherence, such as motivation and engagement.[90]

DePanfilis and colleagues[91] have also investigated the cost-effectiveness of Family Connections. During one typical month of the intervention, staff spent 20.9 hours serving a typical FC3 family and 15.9 hours serving a typical FC9 family. During that month, 54 families were served at a total cost of $28,955. The total cost includes three staff salaries ($13,923), salaries for 12 social work interns ($13,206), rent and utilities ($722), supplies and copying ($298), transportation ($163), and client family expenditures ($643). The monthly cost per family was $607 for FC3 families (or $1,821 for 3 months) and $477 per FC9 family (or $4,194 for 9 months). Many of the pre- to post-intervention gains were similar between the FC3 and FC9 groups, which may suggest that the FC3 intervention was more cost-effective. Differences in child behavior scores were greater in the FC9 group, and the cost of a one-unit change in the child behavior score among FC9 families ($276) was slightly lower than the cost of the same change among FC3 families ($337).

Family Connections is an exemplary program for combining education with service, using a theoretical foundation, and conducting rigorous empirical testing. Without a comparison group that did not receive a Family Connections intervention, however, it is difficult to attribute changes over time to the program. Family Connections is currently undergoing a 5-year multisite replication. The cross-site evaluation will provide further empirical testing of the intervention.

LONG-TERM FOLLOW-UP

Several investigations have focused on the long-term follow-up of childhood abuse and neglect, although most do not separate the two conditions. Although children with a history of abuse or neglect are at risk for violent criminal behavior,[92] children who experience an onset of abuse or neglect early in life are at risk for anxiety and depression as adults, and children who experience an onset of abuse or neglect during the school-age years are at risk for behavior problems as adults.[93] These findings are consistent with developmental-ecological theory and illustrate the importance of considering children's development.

Resilience has also been investigated in the face of abuse and neglect. One investigator found that approximately 22% of neglected children were resilient as adults.[94] Resilience was defined as success in six of eight domains, including psychiatric disorders, employment, education, homelessness, social activity, substance abuse, official reports of criminal behavior, and self-reports of criminal behavior. Children with a history of abuse or neglect had more negative scores than comparison children in six of the eight domains. When overall resilience was considered, 27% of abused/neglected females and 33% of abused/neglected males met the criterion for resilience.

As Widom[95] has shown, children who have experienced child neglect are at increased risk for exposure to subsequent traumatic events, such as physical assault or rape. Although a history of neglect is associated with symptoms of PTSD, it is not significantly associated with lifetime PTSD when covariates, such as history of behavior problems, divorce or separation, and alcohol or drug dependence are introduced into the model. Thus, the connection between neglect and PTSD is not direct, but partially explained through child, family, and lifestyle variables.

RECOMMENDATIONS FOR PRACTICE AND FUTURE RESEARCH

The literature on neglect repeatedly claims that there has been "neglect of neglect." The field is beset with confusion, beginning with a lack of definitional clarity, including whether to rely on CPS definitions that vary across jurisdictions, whether to focus on children's needs, or whether to focus on caregiver behavior. Because neglect frequently occurs with abuse, the two are often entangled, both in practice and in research. The prevalence of neglect is highest among the youngest children, those least able to report or explain what has or has not happened. Finally, there is a paucity of research focused on neglect. For at least 15 years, there has been a call for rigorous research that addresses neglect, focusing on the precursors, consequences, prevention, and treatment.[96] The following recommendations focus on the psychosocial impact and treatment of neglect of children.

1. Comprehensive evaluation: When neglect is suspected, children are at risk for psychological problems. Thus, evaluations of neglected children should address their psychological and developmental functioning.
2. Ensure safety: Ensuring children's safety is paramount. Every state has a child protective services agency to assist with evaluations and interventions, as necessary. Working with the local CPS agency can be very helpful in understanding the services available.
3. Interdisciplinary intervention with follow-up and ongoing monitoring: Neglect often crosses multiple systems,

including medical, psychological, and social, thus requiring intervention through multiple disciplines.

4. Clarity of definition: Definitional clarity is fundamental to understanding the psychological consequences of neglect. Investigators should clarify the definitions they are using. If they are relying on CPS definitions, they should clarify the details of the definition, including the prevalence of neglect in the population under investigation.

5. Theory-driven research: As opposed to abuse, which can be a single event or multiple events, neglect is often a chronic situation in which children's basic needs are not met. Interpreting the psychological consequences of neglect from the perspective of theories of child development enables investigators to understand how the absence of support affects children's development, thereby providing both additional information on children's development and guidance on intervention strategies. DST forms a theoretical basis that is very relevant to child neglect because it incorporates children, families, communities, and culture.

6. Indirect effects: DST emphasizes that models should incorporate both direct and indirect effects. For example, the effects of neglect are often heightened when they co-occur with other threats. Children who are exposed to multiple conditions (both neglect and failure-to-thrive) often have worse outcomes than children exposed to neither or only one condition.[97,98]

7. Prevention research: There is a paucity of research devoted to preventing neglect. Admittedly it is difficult to investigate events before they occur, but there is enough known about the risk factors for neglect to identify families at risk. Prevention research should follow the guidelines of prevention science, as outlined by the Society of Prevention Research,[99] including rigorous designs that include a control or comparison group. Strategies such as waitlist control or comparison of two interventions may provide a comparison while ensuring an intervention for all participants.

8. Treatment research: Little is known about effective treatment for children who have experienced neglect. Again, rigorous scientific methods are needed to evaluate the effectiveness of treatment programs.

For front-line health care providers caring for high-risk families of young children, the following are principles that should apply to their practices.

1. Prevent child neglect and promote children's health and well-being by promoting developmentally appropriate parenting practices through anticipatory guidance.[100]

2. Provide written recommendations and guidelines when counseling patients and parents.[100]

3. For questions related to safety seats for children, access sources such as the American Academy of Pediatrics for up-to-date information on car seat safety.[101]

4. Give families information on emergency services available in their communities, such as food pantries, Parents Anonymous, and poison control.

5. Screen for predictors of neglect, including poverty, food insecurity, maternal mental health and nutrition, stressful life events, and child temperament, development, and behavior.

6. Screen for food insecurity. The U.S. Department of Agriculture developed a six-item food insecurity screening questionnaire.[102]

7. Encourage parents to use principles of modeling to help their children establish daily routines (brushing their teeth, regular bed times).

8. Screen for maternal depression. Kemper and Babonis[103] identified a three-item screening questionnaire that identifies depression. Other longer measures also exist.

9. Screen for children's developmental risks. The 10-item Parents' Evaluation of Developmental Status[104] helps identify children at risk for school problems and developmental and behavioral disabilities.

10. Gather information directly from children and adolescents. Observe children for signs of poor hygiene or care. Plot children's growth to compare with normal growth curves.

11. Consider and employ family strengths and supports. Inquire about family resources, such as extended family members.

12. Understand eligibility criteria and provide referrals to services (e.g., medical assistance, housing assistance, WIC, Food Stamps). Follow up on referrals to services.

13. Physicians in all states are mandated to report suspected child abuse and neglect. Work with Child Protective Services to understand how to make reports and what family functioning services are available.

References

1. Child Maltreatment 2006. U.S. Department of Health and Human Services, Administration for Children and Families, Washington, DC, 2008. Available at http://www.acf.hhs.gov/programs/cb/pubs/cm06/cm06.pdf. Accessed April 9, 2009.

2. Child Abuse Prevention and Treatment Act, 42 U.S.C. 5106g, §Sec. 111-2.

3. Bronfenbrenner U (ed): *The Ecology of Human Development*. Harvard University Press, Cambridge, Mass, 1979.

4. Brown J, Cohen P, Johnson JG, et al: A longitudinal analysis of risk factors for child maltreatment: findings of a 17-year prospective study of officially recorded and self-reported child abuse and neglect. *Child Abuse Negl* 1998;22:1065-1078.

5. DePanfilis D: How do I determine if a child is neglected? *In:* Dubowitz H, DePanfilis D, (eds): *Handbook for Child Protection Practice*. Sage Publications, Thousand Oaks, Calif, 2000.

6. Garbarino J, Sherman D: High-risk neighborhoods and high-risk families: the human ecology of child maltreatment. *Child Dev* 1980;51:188-198.

7. Pelton CL: Family violence—child abuse and neglect. *S D J Med* 1981;34:23-28.

8. Lee BJ, Goerge M: Poverty, early childbearing, and child maltreatment: a multinomial analysis. *Child Youth Serv Rev* 1999;21:755-768.

9. Coulton CJ, Korbin JE, Su M, et al: Community level factors and child maltreatment rates. *Child Dev* 1995;66:1262-1276.

10. Ernst JS, Meyer M, DePanfilis D: Housing characteristics and adequacy of the physical care of children: an exploratory analysis. *Child Welfare* 2004;83:437-452.

11. Slack KS, Holl JL, McDaniel M, et al: Understanding the risks of child neglect: an exploration of poverty and parenting characteristics. *Child Maltreat* 2004;9:395-408.

12. Nord M, Andrews M, Carlson S: Household Food Security in the United States, 2004. U.S. Department of Agriculture, Washington, DC, 2005. Available at http://www.ers.usda.gov/publications/err11/err11.pdf. Accessed April 4, 2009.

13. Nord M, Andrews M, Winicki J: Frequency and duration of food insecurity and hunger in U.S. households. *J Nutr Educ Behav* 2002;34:194-200.

14. Cook JT, Frank DA, Berkowitz C, et al: Food insecurity is associated with adverse health outcomes among human infants and toddlers. *J Nutr* 2004;134:1432-1438.

15. Rose-Jacobs R, Black MM, Casey PH, et al: Household food insecurity: associations with at-risk infant and toddler development. *Pediatrics* 2008;121:65-72.

16. Whitaker RC, Phillips SM, Orzol SM, et al: The association between maltreatment and obesity among preschool children. *Child Abuse Negl* 2007;31:1187-1199.

17. Zaslow M, Bronte-Tinkew J, Capps R, et al: Food security during infancy: implications for attachment and mental proficiency in toddlerhood. *Matern Child Health J* 2009;13:66-80.

18. United Nations Administrative Committee on Coordination: 4th Report on The World Nutrition Situation. World Health Organization, Geneva, 2000. Available at http://www.unscn.org/layout/modules/resources/files/rwns4.pdf. Accessed April 11, 2010.

19. Murray-Kolb LE, Beard JL: Iron treatment normalizes cognitive functioning in young women. *Am J Clin Nutr* 2007;85:778-787.

20. Beard JL, Hendricks MK, Perez EM, et al: Maternal iron deficiency anemia affects postpartum emotions and cognition. *J Nutr* 2005;135:267-272.

21. Perez EM, Hendricks MK, Beard JL, et al: Mother-infant interactions and infant development are altered by maternal iron deficiency anemia. *J Nutr* 2005;135:850-855.

22. Chaffin M, Kelleher K, Hollenberg J: Onset of physical abuse and neglect: psychiatric, substance abuse, and social risk factors from prospective community data. *Child Abuse Negl* 1996;20:191-203.

23. Kotch JB, Browne DC, Ringwalt CL, et al: Risk of child abuse or neglect in a cohort of low-income children. *Child Abuse Negl* 1995;19:1115-1130.

24. Reck C, Hunt A, Fuchs T, et al: Interactive regulation of affect in postpartum depressed mothers and their infants: an overview. *Psychopathology* 2004;37:272-280.

25. Crittendon PM: Child neglect: causes and contributions. *In:* Dubowitz H (ed): *Neglected Children: Research, Practice, and Policy.* Sage Publications, Thousand Oaks, Calif, 1999.

26. Lovejoy MC, Graczyk PA, O'Hare E, et al: Maternal depression and parenting behavior: a meta-analytic review. *Clin Psychol Rev* 2000;20:561-592.

27. Goldman J, Salus MK, Wolcott D, et al: *A Coordinated Response to Child Abuse and Neglect: The Foundation for Practice.* Department of Health and Human Services, National Center on Child Abuse and Neglect, Washington, DC, 2003.

28. Gaines R, Sandgrund A, Green AH, et al: Etiological factors in child maltreatment: a multivariate study of abusing, neglectful, and normal mothers. *J Abnorm Psychol* 1978;87:531-540.

29. Rycus JS, Hughes RC: *Field Guide to Child Welfare: Volume I. Foundations of Child Protective Services.* CWLA Press, Washington, DC, 1998.

30. Williamson JM, Bordin CM, Howe BA: The ecology of adolescent maltreatment: a multilevel examination of adolescent physical abuse, sexual abuse, and neglect. *J Consult Clin Psychol* 1991;59:449-457.

31. Crosson-Tower C: *Understanding Child Abuse and Neglect.* Pearson, Boston, 2008.

32. Shepard M, Raschick M: How child welfare workers assess and intervene around issues of domestic violence. *Child Maltreat* 1999;4:148-156.

33. Bancroft L, Silverman JG (eds): *The Batterer as Parent: Addressing the Impact of Domestic Violence on Family Dynamics.* Sage Publications, Thousand Oaks, Calif, 2002.

34. Brayden RM, Altemeier WA, Tucker DD, et al: Antecedents of child neglect in the first two years of life. *J Pediatr* 1992;120:426-429.

35. Harrington D, Black MM, Starr RH Jr, et al: Child neglect: relation to child temperament and family context. *Am J Orthopsychiatry* 1998;68:108-116.

36. Little L (ed): *Victimization of Children with Disabilities.* American Psychological Association, Washington, DC, 2004.

37. Hibbard RA, Desch LW, American Academy of Pediatrics Committee on Child Abuse and Neglect, et al: Maltreatment of children with disabilities. *Pediatrics* 2007;119:1018-1025.

38. Sullivan PM, Knutson JF: Maltreatment and disabilities: a population-based epidemiological study. *Child Abuse Negl* 2000;24:1257-1273.

39. Jaudes PK, Mackey-Bilaver L: Do chronic conditions increase young children's risk of being maltreated? *Child Abuse Negl* 2008;32:671-681.

40. Steinberg L: Cognitive and affective development in adolescence. *Trends Cogn Sci* 2005;9:69-74.

41. Cicchetti D: *How Research or Child Maltreatment Has Informed the Study of Child Development: Perspectives from Developmental Psychopathology.* Cambridge University Press, New York, 2004.

42. Belsky J, Rovine M, Taylor DG: The Pennsylvania Infant and Family Development Project, III: the origins of individual differences in infant-mother attachment: maternal and infant contributions. *Child Dev* 1984;55:718-728.

43. Ainsworth MD: Infant–mother attachment. *Am Psychol* 1979;34:932-937.

44. Spitz RA: Hospitalism: An inquiry into the genesis of psychiatric conditions in early childhood. *Psychoanal Study Child* 1945;1:53-74.

45. O'Connor TG, Rutter M: Attachment disorder behavior following early severe deprivation: extension and longitudinal follow-up. English and Romanian Adoptees Study Team. *J Am Acad Child Adolesc Psychiatry* 2000;39:703-712.

46. Egeland B, Sroufe A: Developmental sequelae of maltreatment in infancy. *New Dir Child Adolesc Dev* 1981;1981:77-92.

47. Erikson MF, Egeland B, Pianta R (eds): *The Effects of Maltreatment on the Development of Young Children.* Cambridge University Press, New York, 1989.

48. Egeland B, Sroufe LA, Erickson M: The developmental consequence of different patterns of maltreatment. *Child Abuse Negl* 1983;7:459-469.

49. Sroufe LA, Waters E: Attachment as an organizational construct. *Child Dev* 1977;48:1184-1189.

50. Hoffman-Plotkin D, Twentyman CT: A multimodal assessment of behavioral and cognitive deficits in abused and neglected preschoolers. *Child Dev* 1984;55:794-802.

51. Wodarski JS, Kurtz PD, Gaudin JM Jr., et al: Maltreatment and the school-age child: major academic, socioemotional, and adaptive outcomes. *Soc Work* 1990;35:506-513.

52. Eckenrode JJ, Laird M, Doris J: School performance and disciplinary problems among abused and neglected children. *Dev Psychol* 1993;29:53-62.

53. Farber FA, Egeland B. *Invulnerability among Abused and Neglected Children.* Guilford, New York, 1987.

54. Lamborn SD, Mounts NS, Steinberg L, et al: Patterns of competence and adjustment among adolescents from authoritative, authoritarian, indulgent, and neglectful families. *Child Dev* 1991;62:1049-1065.

55. Sanchez MM, Ladd CO, Plotsky PM: Early adverse experience as a developmental risk factor for later psychopathology: evidence from rodent and primate models. *Dev Psychopathol* 2001;13:419-449.

56. DeBellis MD: The psychobiology of neglect. *Child Maltreat* 2005;10:150-172.

57. Thompson RA, Nelson CA: Developmental science and the media. Early brain development. *Am Psychol* 2001;56:5-15.

58. Shonkoff JP, Phillips DA (eds): *From Neurons to Neighborhoods: The Science of Early Childhood Development.* National Academy Press, Washington, DC, 2000.

59. Greenough W: The nature and nurture of behavior: developmental psychobiology. *In:* Freeman WH (ed): *Readings from Scientific American,* W.H. Freeman, San Francisco, 1973.

60. Bornstein MH: Sensitive periods in development structural characteristics and causal interpretations. *Psychol Bull* 1989;105:179-197.

61. Sameroff AJ: Developmental systems and psychopathology. *Dev Psychopathol* 2000;12:297-312.

62. Coleman J: *Equality and Achievement in Education.* Westview Press, Boulder, Colo, 1990.

63. Hart B, Risley TR: *Meaningful Differences in the Everyday Experience of Young American Children.* Paul H. Brookes Publishing, Baltimore, MD, 1995.

64. Steinberg L, Dornbusch SM, Brown BB: Ethnic differences in adolescent achievement. An ecological perspective. *Am Psychol* 1992;47:723-729.

65. Shipler DK: *The Working Poor: Invisible in America.* Knopf Publishing Group, New York, 2004.

66. Yeung WJ, Linver MR, Brooks-Gunn J: How money matters for young children's development: parental investment and family process. *Child Dev* 2008;73:1861-1879.

67. Conger RD, Donnellan MB: An interactionist perspective on the socioeconomic context of human development. *Annu Rev Psychol* 2007;58:175-199.

68. Mayer M, Dufour S, Lavergne C, et al: *Comparing Parental Characteristics Regarding Child Neglect: An Analysis of Cases Retained by Child Protection Services in Quebec.* Centres of Excellence in Child Well-Being, Montreal, 2003.

69. Elder GH, Caspi A: Economic stress in lives: developmental perspectives. *J Soc Issues* 1988;44:25-45.

70. Conger RD, Wallace LE, Sun Y, et al: Economic pressure in African American families: a replication and extension of the family stress model. *Dev Psychol* 2002;38:179-193.

71. Hyde JS, Else-Quest NM, Goldsmith HH, et al: Children's temperament and behavior problems predict their employed mothers' work functioning. *Child Dev* 2004;75:580-594.

72. Wachs TD: The what, why and how of temperament: a piece of the action. *In:* Balter L, Tamis-Lemonda C (eds): *A Handbook of Contemporary Issues.* Psychology Press, Philadelphia, 1999, pp 23-44.

73. Black MM, Baqui AH, Zaman K, et al: Depressive symptoms among rural Bangladeshi mothers: implications for infant development. *J Child Psychol Psychiatry* 2007;48:764-772.

74. Black MM, Krishnakumar A: Children in low-income, urban settings. Interventions to promote mental health and well-being. *Am Psychol* 1998;53:635-646.

75. Murnane RJ, Steele JL: What is the problem? The challenge of providing effective teachers for all children. *Future Child* 2007;17:15-43.

76. Leventhal T, Brooks-Gunn J, McCormick MC, et al: Patterns of service use in preschool children: correlates, consequences, and the role of early intervention. *Child Dev* 2000;71:802-819.

77. Allin H, Wathen CN, MacMillan H: Treatment of child neglect: a systematic review. *Can J Psychiatry* 2005;50:497-504.

78. Fantuzzo J, Sutton-Smith B, Atkins M, et al: Community-based resilient peer treatment of withdrawn maltreated preschool children. *J Consult Clin Psychol* 1996;64:1377-1386.

79. Udwin O: Imaginative play training as an intervention method with institutionalised preschool children. *Br J Educ Psychol* 1983;53 Pt 1:32-39.

80. Brunk M, Henggeler SW, Whelan JP: Comparison of multisystemic therapy and parent training in the brief treatment of child abuse and neglect. *J Consult Clin Psychol* 1987;55:171-178.

81. Meezan W, O'Keefe M: Evaluating the effectiveness of multifamily group therapy in child abuse and neglect. *Res Soc Work Pract* 1998;8:330-353.

82. Meezan W, O'Keefe M: Multifamily group therapy: impact on family functioning and child behavior. *Fam Soc* 1998;79:32-44.

83. Milner JS: Applications and limitations of the CAP inventory. *Early Child Dev Care* 1989;42:85-87.

84. Olds DL, Henderson CR Jr, Chamberlin R, et al: Preventing child abuse and neglect: a randomized trial of nurse home visitation. *Pediatrics* 1986;78:65-78.

85. Olds DL, Henderson CR Jr, Kitzman HJ, et al: Prenatal and infancy home visitation by nurses: recent findings. *Future Child* 1999;9:44-65, 190-191.

86. Lutzker JR: *Handbook of Child Abuse Research and Treatment.* Plenum Press, New York, 1998.

87. Lutzker JR, Bigelow KM: *Reducing Child Maltreatment: A Guidebook for Parent Services.* Guilford Press, New York, 2002.

88. DePanfilis D, Dubowitz H: Family connections: a program for preventing child neglect. *Child Maltreat* 2005;10:108-123.

89. Lundquist LM, Hansen DJ (eds): *Enhancing Treatment Adherence, Generalization, and Social Validity of Parent-Training with Physically Abusive and Neglectful Families.* Plenum Press, New York, 1998.

90. Girvin H, DiPanfilis D, Daining C: Predicting program completion among families enrolled in a child neglect preventitive intervention. *Res Soc Work Pract* 2007;17:674-685.

91. DePanfilis D, Dubowitz H, Kunz J: Assessing the cost-effectiveness of Family Connections. *Child Abuse Negl* 2008;32:335-351.

92. Widom CS: The cycle of violence. *Science* 1989;244:160-166.

93. Kaplow JB, Widom CS: Age of onset of child maltreatment predicts long-term mental health outcomes. *J Abnorm Psychol* 2007;116:176-187.

94. McGloin JM, Widom CS: Resilience among abused and neglected children grown up. *Dev Psychopathol* 2001;13:1021-1038.

95. Widom CS: Posttraumatic stress disorder in abused and neglected children grown up. *Am J Psychiatry* 1999;156:1223-1229.

96. National Research Council: *Understanding Child Abuse and Neglect.* National Academy Press, Washington, DC, 1993.

97. Kerr MA, Black MM, Krishnakumar A: Failure-to-thrive, maltreatment and the behavior and development of 6-year-old children from low-income, urban families: a cumulative risk model. *Child Abuse Negl* 2000;24:587-598.

98. Mackner LM, Starr RH Jr., Black MM: The cumulative effect of neglect and failure to thrive on cognitive functioning. *Child Abuse Negl* 1997;21:691-700.

99. Flay BR, Biglan A, Boruch RF, et al: Standards of evidence: criteria for efficacy, effectiveness and dissemination. *Prev Sci* 2005;6:151-175.

100. Hagan JF Jr, Shaw JS, Duncan P: *Bright Futures Guidelines for Health Supervision of Infants, Children, and Adolescents,* ed 3. American Academy of Pediatrics, Elk Grove Village, Ill, 2008.

101. American Academy of Pediatrics: Car Seat Safety: A Guide for Families. American Academy of Pediatrics, Elk Grove Village, Ill, 2009. Available at http://aap.org/family/carseatguide.htm. Accessed April 4, 2009.

102. Bickel G, Nord M, Price C, et al: Guide to Measuring Household Food Security. United States Department of Agriculture, Washington, DC. Available at http://www.fns.usda.gov/fsec/files/fsguide.pdf. Accessed April 4, 2009.

103. Kemper KJ, Babonis TR: Screening for maternal depression in pediatric clinics. *Am J Dis Child* 1992;146:876-878.

104. Glascoe FP: Collaborating with Parents: Using Parents' Evaluation of Developmental Status to Detect and Address Developmental and Behavioral Problems. Ellsworth & Vandermeer Press, Nashville, 1998.

52

Psychological Impact on and Treatment of Children Who Witness Domestic Violence

Patricia Van Horn, JD, PhD, and Alicia F. Lieberman, PhD

INTRODUCTION

It is well established that exposure to domestic violence has a significant negative impact on children's development, affecting their emotional, social, and cognitive functioning and interfering with their ability to learn. Children are affected by violence as early as infancy. For more than 30 years, researchers have published accounts about children exposed to domestic violence, with the rate of publication increasing dramatically in the past 10 years. Numerous books and countless papers and articles have described the cognitive, emotional, and behavioral impact of witnessing violence on children as well as the mediators and moderators of these effects.[1-6] The sheer volume of this material has given rise to conceptual and methodological disagreements about the optimal course of research in this area. It has been challenging at times to draw definitive conclusions from the numerous studies because there is a lack of agreement about what descriptive terms are best and the meanings of these terms.[7,8] Methodological differences have also delayed consensus because researchers have drawn on different samples and have not consistently examined conditions such as poverty, parental mental illness, parental substance abuse, and child maltreatment that often co-exist with domestic violence and have independent impact or act as moderators of children's functioning.[9-11] Even with these limitations, it is well established that exposure to domestic violence has independent effects relative to other negative factors in the child's environment.

In this chapter we briefly review the incidence and prevalence of exposure to domestic violence and describe some of the challenges that inconsistent terminology brings to the research. We also examine the ecological contexts that mediate and moderate the impact of exposure to domestic violence and review, by developmental stage, the known impacts of exposure. We describe models of intervention shown to be effective with exposed children and discuss the features that these intervention models have in common. Finally, we will evaluate the strength of the evidence about children's exposure and suggest directions for future research.

TERMINOLOGY AND TAXONOMY

In spite of two excellent critiques published 14 years apart,[7,8] the field still struggles with inconsistency in how to think about what it means to witness or be exposed to domestic violence and what we mean by domestic violence. These inconsistencies present interpretive challenges. Holden[8] notes that the move to the use of the word "exposed" rather than "witnessed" or "observed" is an improvement in describing children's experience of domestic violence because the term is inclusive of different types of experience and does not assume that the child must actually see the violence to be affected. Many studies, however, do not describe the nature of the participating children's exposure. One review of 22 studies published between 1987 and 1997 found that only 43% included a description of the nature of the exposure.[12]

To improve reporting of the nature of exposure, Holden[8] proposes a 10-category descriptive taxonomy of children's exposure to domestic violence. The categories are: (1) prenatal exposure, (2) intervening verbally or physically to stop the assault, (3) being physically or verbally assaulted during a domestic violence incident, (4) joining the assault, either through force or voluntarily, (5) being an eyewitness to the assault, (6) hearing, but not seeing, the assault, (7) seeing the immediate consequences of the assault, (8) experiencing life changes as a result of the assault, (9) being told or overhearing conversation about the assault, and, (10) being ostensibly unaware of the assault.

The second definitional challenge is the lack of unanimity in the literature about what constitutes domestic violence. Based on a review of the research, Holden[8] suggests nine dimensions around which domestic violence can be organized, and suggests that researchers use these descriptive dimensions when reporting study findings. The first dimension describes the type of violence that occurred, including whether the violence is physical or psychological,[13] minor or severe,[14] or mutual vs. male-initiated violence.[15] The second dimension is the nature of the particular act of violence that occurred and whether the perpetrator of the violence intended injury. The third dimension considers the nature and severity of injuries. The fourth dimension consists of timing variables such as the frequency of violence, the duration of single incidents of violence, the child's age at the time the exposure began (important because duration of exposure has a significant effect on the accumulation of posttraumatic stress disorder [PTSD] symptoms),[16] and the amount of time that elapses between assaults. The fifth dimension captures the extent to which incidents escalate in frequency or intensity over time. The sixth dimension examines the type of perpetrator, using the typology proposed by Holtzworth-

Munroe and Stuart[17] of family assaults only, antisocial, and dysphoric/borderline. The seventh, eighth, and ninth dimensions describe, respectively, the perpetrator's relationship to the child, the victim's role in the assault, and the way in which the assault is resolved.

These two taxonomies, describing the nature of the child's exposure and the nature of the violence itself, are based on research studies but require empirical validation. If researchers consistently gathered and reported study data along these descriptive dimensions, more definitive conclusions could be drawn from the literature describing the cognitive, behavioral, and emotional impact of children's exposure to domestic violence. The taxonomies can also be used by clinicians to collect information about an individual child's experience that will enable them to choose the interventions most likely to be effective.

In this chapter, we include in our literature review only work that describes the psychological impact of children's exposure to violence between the child's mother and a current or former adult partner. Other forms of violence to which children may be exposed in their homes, such as violence between siblings or physical violence directed at the child, are outside the scope of this chapter.

PREVALENCE OF CHILDREN LIVING IN VIOLENT HOUSEHOLDS

An accurate estimate of the prevalence of children's exposure to domestic violence is challenging because researchers have used different definitions of domestic violence, different measures for collecting data, and different methodologies. Field and Caetano[18] reviewed nationally representative estimates of assaultive behavior between partners in the United States and found generally low prevalence rates (e.g., < 1%) when respondents must self-identify as crime victims before questions about domestic violence are asked. In contrast, survey instruments that measure behaviors in the context of family rather than crime generally result in higher prevalence rates (e.g., 12-20%). This is not necessarily a consistent pattern, however; for example, the National Violence Against Women Survey[19] used behavioral queries and found a prevalence rate of 1.4%, only slightly greater than the crime surveys.

One early attempt to estimate the number of children living in violent households was Carlson's 1984 study,[20] still frequently cited by researchers and policy makers. Extrapolating from the 1975 National Family Violence Survey[21] and U.S. Census data, Carlson estimated that approximately 3.3 million children in the United States are exposed to domestic violence each year. Because this estimate was created in the context of an early literature review and with limited data available, it is beset with a number of methodological challenges that are acknowledged by the author. First, Carlson's estimate was based on reports from one family member. Disagreement between partners on the occurrence of acts of domestic violence is common,[22] casting doubt on the reliability of data from a single reporter. Second, the estimate was limited to households with a child between 3 and 17 years of age, which could be problematic because children 5 years old or younger appear to be disproportionately represented in homes with domestic violence.[23,24] Finally, Carlson considered only acts of severe violence (e.g., punching, kicking,

threat or actual use of weapons), acts that are less common than milder forms of violence (e.g., pushing, slapping, grabbing). These milder forms of violence, however, are associated with behavioral problems in children exposed to them.[25] All the methodological flaws of this early review tend to underestimate prevalence of domestic violence.

More recent population-based surveys attempt to find a more accurate estimate of the extent of children's exposure. McDonald et al[26] estimated that 15.5 million children (29.4%) are exposed to domestic violence annually, including 7 million children (13.3%) exposed to severe violence in their homes. The researchers conducted in-home interviews with 1615 married or cohabiting couples. Both members of the couple were interviewed about specific violent behaviors, both mild and severe, that they had committed or sustained in the year preceding the interview. This study revealed that there is more likely to be domestic violence in households with children; it does not, however, report the ages of children living in the home, so it cannot be used to confirm earlier findings that children under 6 are disproportionately exposed to domestic violence.[23,24] Nor does it report on number and frequency of violent events or other contextual risk factors such as community violence, poverty, or child maltreatment.

Finkelhor and colleagues[27] examined exposure to domestic violence as one of a variety of types of victimization in 2030 children age 2 to 17 years living in the United States. This survey found that 71 children per 1000 witness domestic violence each year, or 2,190,000 children. Girls were more likely to witness domestic violence than boys, and children under 13 were more likely to be exposed.

Several methodological differences between McDonald[26] and Finklehor[27] may explain the lower prevalence rate in the latter study. First, Finklehor eliminated children aged birth to 2 years from the sample. Second, domestic violence was defined far more narrowly in Finklehor's study, with a single question asking whether the child had seen a parent get hit (e.g., slapped, hit, punched, or beat up) by another parent or by the parent's boyfriend or girlfriend in the past year. All types of exposure except direct observation were eliminated, as were all types of violence except hitting. Other questions covered the child's direct observation of assaults with weapons and the murder of someone close to the child. These types of victimization might have involved domestic assaults or murders, but they were not included in the domestic violence totals.

Fantuzzo and his colleagues[24] took a public health approach to estimating the prevalence of children exposed to domestic violence crimes investigated by police officers. Prevalence findings showed that children were present for 44% of the investigated domestic violence incidents, with slightly over 1000 children exposed across the period of the study. Children under 6 were overrepresented. Of the children present during the domestic violence event, 81% were assessed by the investigating police officer to have experienced direct sensory exposure to the event; 4% of the exposed children were physically injured in the domestic violence event.

These three recent studies use divergent methodologies and, not surprisingly, find different prevalence rates. They leave no doubt, however, that large numbers of children are exposed to domestic violence each year.

DOMESTIC VIOLENCE EXPOSURE IN AN ECOLOGICAL CONTEXT

Children's development is shaped by a vast array of factors, and domestic violence is not generally an isolated stressor. These two statements point to the undeniable truth that when children present with cognitive, emotional, or behavioral problems, the quest to understand the etiology of the problems does not end with asking about whether the child has been exposed to violence at home. This is an important factor, but only one of many that must be assessed. Bronfenbrenner[28,29] and others[30] proposed an ecological-transactional approach to understanding children's development that conceptualizes the child's developmental environment as an interaction among the immediate settings in which the child develops (*microsystems*), the relationships between these microsystems (*mesosystems*), and settings in which children are not necessarily found (e.g., government agencies, parent's workplaces) but that affect their development in important ways (*exosystems*). The decisions at the level of exosystems can have profound impacts on microsystems, as when a legislative body passes funding to subsidize child care for young children, which in turn alleviates economic stress in children's immediate families.

In an ecological-transactional analysis of development, children are at the heart of the interlocking relationships between systems at these multiple levels. Metaphorically, it can also be said that children are themselves microsystems. Children's temperaments, personalities, patterns of attachment, capacities for self-regulation, and cognitive potential are all the result of an interplay between children's genetic makeup and the environment in which that genetic makeup is expressed. Development, even at the cellular level, is experience dependent,[31] and all of the environmental contexts that, directly or indirectly, affect children have a role in determining who the child will become.

Factors Intrinsic to the Child

Pynoos and colleagues[32] suggest a number of factors intrinsic to the child that may affect children's responses to potentially traumatic stressors such as exposure to domestic violence. These include the child's genetic makeup, temperament, quality of attachment, repertoire of coping strategies, acquired developmental competencies, and a range of attributes having to do with the organization of the child's stress response system. (See Chapter 54, "Effects of Abuse and Neglect on Brain Development.") Even these so-called intrinsic factors, however, develop in relationships with caregivers,[33] and parents hold a central place within the ecological world of the developing child. Especially for young children, parents place their imprint on every aspect of the child's development, both directly through their behavior toward the child and indirectly as they bring the influences that the larger world has upon them into their relationships with their children.

The Power of Parents

Parents have the most powerful direct effect on children's development and are themselves acted upon by interlocking systems that determine their individual and parental functioning. Belsky[34] proposed three factors that interact with one another, predicting compromised parenting in families where there is violence. First, parenting quality is tied to the parent's personal psychological resources, and both victims[35,36] and perpetrators[33,34,37] of violence often have diminished psychological well-being. Second, children's behavior has a powerful role in shaping parenting, and the behavioral difficulties of children exposed to violence may lead parents to adopt authoritarian parenting strategies.[38] Third, a satisfying relationship between the parents, lacking in violent families, provides a major contextual support for good parenting. Other models of the determinants of parenting behavior include additional factors (e.g., the parents' social network, parents' view of the child), but all of the models give parents' functioning and behavior a central place in children's development.[39-41] These theoretical models are supported by ample empirical evidence of the importance of the quality of the parent–child relationship in mediating and moderating children's outcomes after exposure to violence.

Factors Outside the Family: Society and Culture

James Garbarino[42] labels as "socially toxic" the combination of social-cultural conditions that combine to deprive children of opportunities to learn and thrive. These conditions include economic inequality, racism, community violence, and the legitimization of aggression and violence in the mass media. These societal risk factors act together, with children from racial minorities more likely to be poor, more likely to be exposed to violence and aggression in the home and the community, and less likely to have access to services.[43] The impact of social toxicity on children is nowhere clearer than in the stark differences in the incidence of domestic violence among socioeconomic groups. The likelihood of domestic violence increases as family income decreases. The incidence of domestic violence is 3% for families with a yearly income of more than $75,000 a year, and rises to 20% in families with a yearly income of less than $7500.[44]

These social forces act on children's development both through direct exposure and as the communities in which parents live and work affect parents' moods and sense of support and security, feelings that are brought to their parenting. To buffer children from stress,[32] parents need to rely on society as a whole to help them protect their children from the toxic effects of violence and inequality. When society fails families, the reverberations are felt at every level.[45]

Children's roles in their families, the meaning of their experiences, and the meanings that their caregivers attach to the supports and stressors in the larger community are determined by cultural factors. To give the force of culture its due in an ecological model, we must go beyond an assessment of the family's current environment and ask additional questions: From where did the family come; why, how, and when did it get here; and how does its culture view and cope with stressful and potentially traumatic experiences?[46]

Co-Occurrence of Stressors

Domestic violence generally occurs as one of several stressors with which families and children must cope. As stated earlier, children exposed to domestic violence are more likely to suffer poverty and racial inequities.[43,44] In addition, children exposed to domestic violence are more likely than nonexposed children to suffer child maltreatment.[9,47,48] In a meta-analysis of the literature related to children's exposure to domestic violence, Kitzmann and colleagues[9] found a 50% overlap between child maltreatment and child exposure to domestic violence. Researchers[48] have offered two theoretical models for these high rates of co-occurrence. The first is that particular person-based variables are responsible for both types of aggression. These variables may include some that are intrinsic to the parent (personality characteristics such as impulsivity or hostility, biological characteristics such as genetic loading for aggression or physiological reactivity to stress, psychological functioning, and historical risk factors), and some that are environmental or contextual risk factors (stressful events, financial stress, and lack of social support). The second model is the spillover hypothesis, positing that one type of aggression contributes to the other (e.g., that the impact of victimization increases the victimized parent's potential for maltreating the child).

Domestic violence and child maltreatment are not the only co-occurring stressors that children suffer. Finklehor and colleagues[27] measured a variety of assaults and violence to which children are exposed, including exposure to domestic violence, and found that any child who reported being victimized had an average of three types of victimization within the year. They also found, consistent with other research, that poor and minority children were more likely to report victimization in the forms of sustaining or witnessing violence. This finding is of critical importance because a substantial body of research indicates that victimized children's risk for poor outcomes both during childhood[49,50] and adulthood.[51]

Given the complexity of the variables that contribute to creating challenges and vulnerabilities in children's developmental outcomes, it stands to reason that isolating exposure to domestic violence as the responsible variable would be a difficult task. Nevertheless, three metaanalytic studies using different methodologies and selecting studies from different periods established that exposure to domestic violence makes a contribution to the variance in children's outcomes over and above the variance contributed by other factors.[9-11]

MECHANISMS OF ACTION: THE DUAL LENSES OF ATTACHMENT AND TRAUMA

Whether exposure to domestic violence is traumatic for a particular child depends upon an array of constitutional and experiential factors.[32] Exposure often raises to the level of traumatic stress, as evidenced by the high number of exposed preschool children[52] as well as school-age children and adolescents[53-55] who meet criteria for PTSD. For children younger than 4 years old, witnessing assaults against their mothers is associated with more symptoms than are other types of traumas, including assaults sustained by the children themselves.[56] These high rates of PTSD suggest that for children of all ages, exposure to acts of violence between their parents can give rise to the kind of overwhelming fear and terror that, by definition, accompanies a traumatic

event.[57] Such events, with their overwhelming sights, sounds, and even smells, shatter the child's developmentally based expectation that their caregivers will protect them from pain and injury. This is especially the case for young children, who are unprepared to appraise risk and take protective action on their own.[32,58]

Young children's experience of domestic violence must be viewed through the dual lenses of attachment and trauma because young children organize their responses to fear and danger around their relationships with their attachment figures, seeking protection from their caregivers in times of threat.[59-62] Attachment figures can be the child's strongest buffer against stress, but can also present children with developmentally salient challenges. An attachment figure who is available to the child under conditions of risk and stress can buffer the child's response, both physiologically[63] and emotionally,[64,65] contributing to the child's recovery after the traumatic event. In contrast, an attachment figure who is not attuned and reassuring or who is the source of the child's fears can exacerbate the child's response.[63,66] Although intertwined, attachment and trauma also exert separate influences on children's development, but research and clinical thought in each of these two areas have, until recently, proceeded without regard to the impact of the other.[61,62]

The Attachment Lens

Attachment theory posits that a primary mother figure is central to normal early development, asserting that systematic links exist between quality of caregiving, resulting patterns of attachment, and the developing child's emotional health.[67] The original research establishing the connection between quality of attachment and infant mental health was based on careful observation of infant behavior in a variety of ecologically valid settings.[59,67] Main and colleagues[68,69] greatly increased the clinical relevance of attachment theory when they moved away from purely behavioral observations and toward the conceptualization of states of mind related to attachment in both adults and children. They asserted that frightening or frightened behavior in the parent—the hallmark of caregiving behaviors linked to disorganized behavior and increased risk for mental health disturbances in the child—stemmed from the parent's unresolved state of mind about her own traumatic childhood experiences. Thus, an attachment-based understanding of young children's symptoms holds that frightening or frightened parental behavior is the mechanism responsible for transmitting from parent to child incoherent and contradictory states of mind regarding attachment. These contradictory states of mind, in turn, are manifested in the child by disorganized behavior as the child attempts to resolve the paradox of fearing the person from whom protection is sought.

Lyons-Ruth and colleagues[70] elaborated these ideas in a way that is particularly relevant to the child's direct exposure to traumatic events such as domestic violence. They propose a relationship diathesis model that focuses on the modulation of fear and places it in a relational context. In the relationship diathesis model, vulnerability to stress-related dysfunction is determined by at least three factors: the characteristics of the stressor, the individual's genetic vulnerability to stress, and the capacity of the attachment system to modulate the high levels of arousal that accompany stress. Children's emotional and behavioral symptoms emerge when the stressor is too overwhelming or when the attachment relationship is unable to modulate the child's overwhelming affective response to the stressor. The authors proposed that parents with unresolved fear dating back to childhood traumatic experiences have difficulty helping their children modulate strong emotions such as fear because the parents curtail their conscious attention to the child's fear signals in order to not reevoke their own early traumatic responses. Fear signals left unattended are not modulated in the relationship, leaving children alone with their own unresolved traumatic experiences.

Attachment theory thus predicts two explanations for young children's symptoms. The first is rooted in children's responses to their parents' frightened/frightening behavior, stemming in turn from the parents' unresolved childhood traumatic experiences of trauma. The second, explicated in the relationship diathesis model, predicts that the parent's own experiences of childhood trauma interfere with the parent's capacity to soothe the child in the face of present stress, leading to emotional and behavioral dysfunction in the child. The relationship diathesis model provides a bridge to trauma theory, which offers its own explanation for children's symptoms after a stressful event.

The Trauma Lens

Trauma theory addresses the individual's response to direct exposure to an overwhelming stressor. The specific symptoms and developmental challenges that a child may face after a trauma depend, among other factors, on the child's developmental stage at the time of the experience.[32] Infants, toddlers, and preschoolers may be particularly negatively affected because of the impact that trauma has on every aspect of the infant and young child's development. There are three fundamental developmental tasks in infancy and early childhood: forming a hierarchy of attachment relationships and other close interpersonal relationships; developing the capacity to experience, regulate, and express a variety of emotions; and exploring the environment and learning. Trauma, which involves multiple and intense negative emotions, can damage the developing mechanisms of emotional regulation. It threatens the developing child's ability to maintain a sense of security in attachment relationships as the child experiences failure of protection at the moment of trauma and grows to expect that the pain and fear of the original trauma will be repeated in other relationships.[71] Finally, children's ability to explore the environment and learn can be diminished by the fearfulness, constricted and repetitive play, and hypervigilance that can follow trauma. As the child grows, reminders of the original trauma reawaken the negative emotions that were part of the original event, further distorting the child's development.[32]

The Dual Lens

Trauma theory posits that symptoms flow from the dysregulation, relational disturbances, and inhibitions of exploration that are part of the trauma response not only in early childhood but at all developmental stages. Attachment theory sees the source of children's symptoms as misattuned caregiving patterns in which frightened or frightening parents do not meet the children's needs for comfort but are, instead, the source of their fear. We argue that in order to understand the source of any individual child's difficulties and intervene effectively, clinicians should perform their assessments using both attachment and trauma lenses because children's attachment relationships and their responses to traumatic events are inextricably intertwined. Whether the traumatic experience is exposure to domestic violence or some other event, it is essential to examine the quality of the child's caregiving relationships before the trauma in order to understand the degree of interpersonal security that the child brings to the experience and how the child's relationships might assist or derail recovery. It is also essential to understand the nature of the traumatic stressor, the child's experience of the event itself, the developmental and constitutional coping resources that the child possesses, and the social and cultural context in which the trauma took place.

CHILDREN'S RESPONSES TO DOMESTIC VIOLENCE

Understanding the effect of domestic violence on children is a complex enterprise that demands understanding of the nature and extent of the violence, the nature of children's sensory experience of the violence, the quality of caregiving relationships, the extent to which the violence co-occurs with other stressors, and the environmental and cultural context within which the violence occurs. As we examine the effects of domestic violence on children, we will, therefore, focus on three questions: (1) Is exposure to domestic violence associated with negative outcomes for children even when controlling for the impact of other stressors? (2) Are there variables that mediate or moderate the impact of exposure to violence for children generally or for particular groups of children? and (3) Are there differences in the effect of exposure to violence across developmental stages?

It is clear from the literature that children exposed to violence generally have worse outcomes than nonexposed children. An excellent way to understand the effect of violence generally is to examine metaanalyses—namely, studies that examine a number of individual studies in an area of interest in order to determine effect sizes in the population. Three recent metaanalyses examine children's exposure to domestic violence as the variable of interest.[9-11] Kitzmann et al[9] included in their metaanalysis shelter samples, community samples, and clinical samples. They reported no significant differences in effect sizes among the samples and found that across the samples, about 63% of children exposed to domestic violence were faring more poorly than nonexposed children. This finding is consistent with earlier studies of shelter samples indicating that about one third of children in shelter were functioning as well as nonexposed children.[72,73] This metaanalysis and two others[10,11] examined age and gender as moderators of children's internalizing problems (anxious, depressed, and withdrawn behaviors) and externalizing problems (aggressive and destructive behaviors) and found no significant differences by either age or gender. There was an indication, however, that preschool girls exposed to domestic violence had lower scores on measures of social competence and showed greater distress in response to adult conflict than did nonexposed preschool girls. This finding did not exist for preschool boys or for girls in middle childhood.

One striking result from the two metaanalyses that obtained effect sizes for symptoms of PTSD in addition to internalizing and externalizing behaviors was that the effect sizes for PTSD were larger.[9,11] This leads to the question of whether internalizing and externalizing behaviors, the most commonly used measures of child functioning in the literature on children exposed to violence, are the most valid measures of outcome.

Kitzmann et al[9] also examined the impact of other adversities in addition to child exposure to physical violence. They found that children exposed to physical violence had more negative outcomes than children who were exposed only to verbal discord in their homes, but the outcomes of children exposed to physical violence between their parents did not differ significantly from the outcomes of physically abused children or of children who were both exposed to interparental violence and physically abused. The same metaanalysis found, however, that when individual studies controlled for the presence of multiple stressors, they found smaller effect sizes for exposure to domestic violence than did studies that did not control for these variables. This finding leads to the conclusion that multiple stressors have a cumulative effect on children's development.

These three metaanalyses offer strong support for the proposition that children exposed to domestic violence fare generally worse than do nonexposed children; that across samples, children of all ages and boys and girls are equally affected; and that PTSD symptoms may be a stronger predictor of outcome than internalizing and externalizing behaviors. One of them[9] begins to answer the first question posed above with the finding that significant effects of exposure to domestic violence remain even when controlling for co-occurring stressors, although the effects are attenuated. The other questions, however, remain unanswered. The metaanalyses do not examine moderators other than age and gender, nor do they take into account that violence might affect children differently at different developmental stages.

Developmental psychopathology[74] and trauma theory[32] both suggest that childhood exposure to violence should be viewed in the context of normal development. At each stage of development, children are faced with different challenges, and exposure to violence may disrupt a child's capacity to meet those stage-specific challenges.[75,76] In the sections that follow, we examine the literature on children's exposure to domestic violence across three different developmental stages: (1) infancy and early childhood, (2) middle childhood, and (3) adolescence.

Exposure to Violence in Infancy and Early Childhood

Children are affected by exposure to violence as early as infancy. Because of their physical vulnerability, infants and very young children are at increased risk for physical injury during episodes of violence; in addition, they are faced during these episodes with the unsolvable problem of needing to seek protection from the very caregivers who are the source of their fear. One of the elementary developmental

tasks of infancy and early childhood is forming trusting, secure relationships with attachment figures. Infants and young children rely on their attachment figures to protect them from danger and to make the world predictable for them. Domestic violence can shatter the developing trust that young children have in their caregivers, leading to insecurities not only in their attachments, but in other relationships in their lives.[77] In addition to forming attachment relationships, infants and young children must navigate a series of anxieties that emerge sequentially as they develop. These are anxiety about loss of the caregiver, anxiety about loss of the caregiver's love, anxiety about physical damage to the self, and anxiety about not meeting social standards that takes the form of guilt and shame.[75] Witnessing domestic violence during infancy and early childhood can interact with these developmentally normative anxieties and amplify them because witnessing actual assaults on caregivers makes the child's internal fears all too real. The exacerbation of developmentally expectable fears may be at the root of the symptoms that have been observed clinically, including irritability and difficulty being soothed, sleep disturbances, emotional distress, somatic complaints, fears of being alone, and regression in language and toileting.[78-80] Finally, one of the most salient developmental tasks of toddlerhood is managing the conflict between emerging urges toward independence and autonomy and the wish to stay close to and protected by the attachment figure. Assaults on an attachment figure at this stage of development can make a child so anxious about the attachment figure's safety that the child's developmental push for autonomy is derailed.

Empirical evidence exists that the risk to infants from domestic violence begins before birth. Pregnant women who are victims of domestic violence have more difficult time bonding with their babies,[81] increased potential for perpetrating acts of child abuse,[82] and higher rates of child abuse and punitive parenting, with young minority mothers having increased risks.[83,84]

This risk continues after the birth of the baby. Consistent with attachment theory, most studies of the impact of domestic violence on the youngest children indicate that negative outcomes are tied to parenting behaviors and/or the quality of the parent–child relationship. In one community sample of 203 12-month-old infants and their mothers, the infants' direct and indirect risk and protective factors for externalizing behaviors included exposure to domestic violence, maternal parenting behavior, maternal mental health, and maternal social support.[85] The occurrence of domestic violence was measured twice. During the third trimester of pregnancy, domestic violence prior to and during pregnancy was assessed (past domestic violence); when the baby was 12 months old, domestic violence during the first postpartum year was assessed (current domestic violence). Although both past and current domestic violence were associated with mental health problems in the mothers, only current domestic violence was related to observed parenting. Women who suffered domestic violence during the postpartum period were less able to respond warmly and sensitively to their babies, showed more hostility toward the child, and demonstrated more emotional disengagement in the mother–child relationship. On the other hand, infant externalizing behavior was predicted independently by both current and past domestic violence, raising the possibility that past domestic violence occurring during pregnancy affected the fetus through stress-induced cortisol changes that are still manifested in externalizing behavior at age 1.[86]

Researchers have also considered the impact of violence exposure on infants' internalizing behaviors. Crockenberg and colleagues[87] suggest a possible mechanism for development in infancy of internalizing behavior in response to marital aggression. She found that infants exposed to paternal aggression displayed distress at novel stimuli and withdrew, and this response was stronger if the infant's father was actively involved in caregiving.

The importance of relationship continues into the preschool years. Levendosky et al[88] suggest that in the preschool years, children's behavioral difficulties are more pronounced in their interactions with their mothers than in their general functioning. Exposure negatively affected children's observed interactions with their mothers, but not maternal reports of problem behaviors. The authors interpret this finding as suggesting that early effects of domestic violence might originate in the realm of relationships rather than the realm of children's mental health. This study also examined observed parenting variables and found that the quality of parenting in mothers who were victimized by domestic violence was tied to their mental health. Women who had elevated symptoms of depression and PTSD also had parenting problems. Women who did not have these mental health challenges seemed to compensate for the effects of violence by being more effective and responsive in their relationships with their children.

Two studies by Lieberman and colleagues[89,90] examined different sets of relationship variables in a group of preschool age children exposed to domestic violence and their mothers. One study found that the quality of the mother–child relationship as rated by clinicians, mothers' attunement to their children's sad and angry emotions, and the severity of domestic violence reported by the mother each made an independent contribution to children's externalizing behavior problems; together, these three variables explained 55% of the variance in externalizing behavior. Similar relationships did not exist, however, in relation to children's internalizing problems because there was no significant link between mothers' attunement to children's sad and angry feelings and children's internalizing behavior. In the second study, children's total behavior problems were significantly related to maternal life stress, a relationship that was completely mediated by mothers' symptoms of PTSD and the quality of the mother–child relationship.

Exposure to domestic violence also has negative effects on children's cognitive development. In a study of exposed preschoolers and their mothers compared with nonexposed child–mother pairs matched for child's age, gender, and ethnicity; mother's age and education; and annual family income, the exposed children scored significantly lower than the nonexposed ones on a measure of verbal intelligence.[91] The nonexposed children had been exposed to equivalent community violence, however, indicating that domestic violence exposure has a unique role in explaining negative cognitive outcomes over and above other stressors. A large twin study that controlled for genetic factors found an 8-point IQ loss associated with childhood exposure to domestic violence.[92] There is some indication in the literature that even these cognitive deficits may have their roots

in the quality of children's caregiving relationships. One study found that domestic violence was negatively correlated with preschool children's performance on explicit memory tasks, with children who were exposed to higher levels of violence performing more poorly. This relationship was moderated, however, by the children's mothers' positive parenting practices.[93]

Finally, there is some evidence that preschool children exposed to violence have more difficulty than their nonexposed peers in their relationships outside their families. In one study that included observations of group play and assessment of children's relationships with their preschool teachers, children exposed to domestic violence were more likely to exhibit negative affect, respond less appropriately to situations, be more aggressive with peers, and have more ambivalent relationships with their caregivers.[94] The most significant predictors of children's adjustment were psychological violence against the mother and the mother's self-esteem.

The complexity of these findings indicates that there are still many questions to be answered about the links between young children's exposure to domestic violence and emotional and behavior problems. It does appear certain, however, that children's relationships with their caregivers, and the emotional well-being of the caregivers are essential pieces of the puzzle and should be considered when assessing young children exposed to domestic violence.

Exposure to Domestic Violence in Middle Childhood

School-age children face the developmental challenge of adapting to environments and relationships outside the immediate family. In meeting this challenge, school-age children must be able to regulate emotions, to show empathy, and to accomplish increasingly complex cognitive material. As children move to these broader environments, children's development may be derailed if they are preoccupied with issues of security or if their heightened sensitivity to risk and danger causes them to process social information with a bias toward seeing ambiguous actions as hostile.[76] The most overwhelming anxiety faced by children in this age group is the fear of reemergence of longings and urges that belong to a younger age and now are be felt to be too babyish or dependent, undermining the child's emerging sense of competence and autonomy.[75] The research on school-age children's approach to domestic violence is in part responsive to these developmental issues, as researchers examine some child characteristics that may mediate or moderate the impact of children's exposure. In the main, however, studies have compared outcomes of exposed *vs.* nonexposed children, often considering the impact of family variables such as quality of parenting and parental mental health.

Although child behavior problems continue to be the outcome of interest in many studies of school-age children, researchers also investigate the level of PTSD symptoms in this population. When compared with nonexposed children, school-age children exposed to domestic violence have both higher levels of internalizing and externalizing behavior problems[95-98] and higher levels of PTSD symptoms.[99-103]

McCloskey et al[98] examined the relationship between maternal mental health, family environment, and children's outcomes. The researchers found that although women who sustained domestic violence had more mental health problems than did nonvictimized women, these problems did not mediate children's response to family violence. Further, they found that although violent families had lower levels of both sibling and parental warmth than nonviolent ones, even when these social supports were present, they did not buffer exposed children from behavior problems. These results may be something of an anomaly, however, as other studies have found family-related variables to be more impactful.

Margolin and colleagues[104] have done extensive research on how parenting variables mediate and moderate children's outcomes in families with domestic violence. Margolin's research has notable strengths: she relies on community samples that include both violent and nonviolent families and she obtains her data on parents' and children's behavior through coded observations rather than self-report. The observational data are obtained from dyadic conversations between the child and one parent and from triadic conversations among the child and both parents.

In a study that involved both dyadic and triadic interactions Margolin and colleagues[104] found that fathers' physical aggression against marital partners was associated with the fathers exhibiting more authoritarian behaviors, fewer authoritative behaviors, and more negative affect in dyadic interaction with their sons. These fathers also exhibited more controlling behaviors in triadic interactions that included sons. This pattern of findings was not evidenced in interactions with daughters. Two other findings emerged from this study: father-to-mother aggression was not associated with any negative parenting behaviors by mothers, and mothers' physical aggression in the marital relationship was not associated with any hostile, controlling, or angry behavior toward the children. Two other studies also found that violence between parents was associated with specific parenting behaviors and, in one case, with child functioning. In the first study,[105] parent-to-child hostility in triadic interactions was related to boys' increased anxiety and distracting behavior. In the second study,[106] aggression between parents was associated with lower levels of father-to-child empathy and higher levels of mother-to-child negative affect in dyadic interactions. Taken together, these findings illustrate that in homes with interparental violence, parents seem to be less emotionally available to their children, and children's repeated exposure to parents' negative affect might influence the children's own emotional reactions and behaviors. These findings appear to be stronger for boys than girls.

A study by Margolin and John[107] is unique in the literature on children's exposure to domestic violence because it relies entirely on children's own reports of the violence to which they were exposed, their parents' behaviors toward them, and their own emotional well-being. The study involved 108 children between 8 and 11 years of age recruited in the community. There were three major findings. First, aggression between parents directly influenced parenting, although the influences are different for boys and girls. Both boys and girls reported that interparental aggression was associated with parenting behaviors that were negativistic, controlling, and punitive, although this association was stronger for boys than it was for girls. Girls also reported a strong association between aggression between parents and positive parenting. Second, both boys and girls in

aggressive families reported high levels of hostility (girls', but not boys', hostility was linked to negative parenting as well as to aggression between their parents), and high levels of anxiety and depression. For both boys and girls, difficulties in functioning were nearly entirely mediated by negative parenting, meaning that once negative parenting practices were taken into account, the effects of domestic violence on children's behavior were much less pronounced. Third, violence between parents and negative parenting explained considerably more variance in boys' behavior than it did in girls'.

Maternal warmth has been found to protect children from the effects of domestic violence. One study[108] of children between ages 7 and 9 found that both boys and girls from domestically violent homes reported high levels of externalizing problems only in homes that were low in maternal warmth. The children from high-warmth homes did not have externalizing behavior problems. On the other hand, in this sample fathers' warmth interacted with children's behavior problems in the opposite way. Children whose violent fathers were warm had more behavior problems. The researchers used social learning theory[109] to explain this latter finding, asserting that when warmer bonds exist between a child and a violent parent, the child might view aggression in a more positive light, leading them to behave aggressively themselves.

Researchers have also investigated parenting variables using shelter samples. One such study[110] investigated whether women's self-reported parenting stress was associated with children's behavior problems. In this study, sheltered women and their 7- to 12-year-old children were compared with nonsheltered women and children from the same community. Physical and psychological violence against the mothers and parenting stress were measured in both samples. Interestingly, one third of the families in the nonsheltered comparison group reported domestic violence. In this study, domestic violence had a significant effect on both parenting stress and on children's behavior. Parenting stress did not differ between the sheltered and nonsheltered women, but when violence was used as a continuous variable it was significant in predicting higher levels of parenting stress. Two categories of domestic violence, physical and psychological, were examined to determine the relative effects of both on children's functioning. Although both types of violence significantly and negatively affected parenting stress, psychological violence was the stronger predictor of children's functioning. Parenting stress predicted children's functioning, over and above the effects of domestic violence. Children whose mothers suffered higher levels of parenting stress exhibited more internalizing, externalizing, and total behavior problems.

Similar findings emerged in another sample of sheltered women compared with community women in which parenting stress and violence were the variables of interest.[111] The children in this study were between 2 and 8, spanning the preschool to middle childhood stage; older children in the study, however, had more behavior problems than younger ones and girls had more problems than boys. Among both the battered women and the comparison women, parenting stress predicted children's behavior problems. Among battered women, the amount of violence in the home in the last year also predicted children's behavior problems, but even in this group, mother's parenting stress was the more robust predictor of children's functioning.

Although most of the literature on school-age children looks at the effect of adult behavior and well-being on children's functioning, there is evidence from one study of sheltered women and their children that supports the assertion of the ecological-transactional model of development that parents and children affect one another.[112] The researchers examined the relationships among the following variables: extent of interparental physical violence; children's PTSD symptoms, behavior problems, and intervention in violence between parents; and mothers' depression, anxiety, and anger. Children's PTSD symptoms were associated with the amount of physical violence that occurred; their behavioral problems, however, were related to maternal anxiety and anger. Mother's depression was associated with child intervention in episodes of violence and the quality of the mother–child relationship; anxiety was related to witnessing child abuse, child age, and child internalizing behaviors; and anger was associated with violence-related injuries, violence frequency, and children's internalizing behaviors. Although the sample for this study was small, and the resulting findings should be interpreted with caution, this study provides valuable preliminary information about the interconnected emotional functioning of battered women and their children that should be validated through further research.

A few researchers have examined child characteristics to determine their relationship with functioning after exposure to violence. The child's ability to regulate emotional response has been found to mediate the relationship between children's exposure to domestic violence at age 5 and positive play at age 9,[113] as well as negative peer group interactions, social problems, and internalizing and externalizing behavior problems at age 11.[114] Children's appraisals of violence also influence their outcomes. Children who feel more threatened by the violence, or who blame themselves for it, experience more adjustment problems.[115] In a separate study,[116] perceived threat and self-blame were found to mediate the relationship between interparental conflict (including but not limited to physical assault) for internalizing problems.

The Effect of Exposure on Adolescents

Adolescence is marked by profound changes in biological, psychological, and social functioning. Much of the internal tension experienced by adolescents is evidenced in increasingly conflicted relationships with parents as adolescents strive to achieve independence and cement important new relationships.[75] Researchers interested in the effect of domestic violence on children have studied adolescents less frequently than younger children; because adolescents are forging new relationships and becoming ever more involved in a world wider than the family. The research concerning adolescents has often examined different outcomes, including dating as well as other forms of violence committed by adolescents.

In one study of dating violence, exposure to domestic violence, destructive communication, gender stereotyping, and attitudes accepting of domestic violence mediated the observed relationship between ethnic minority status, low levels of parent education, and expressed dating violence in

13- to 19-year-olds.[117] When domestic violence and community violence are combined for analysis, violence exposure and PTSD symptoms account for as much as 50% of the variance in adolescents' violent behaviors.[118] In one large sample of African-American males living in or near public housing projects, violence exposure was strongly associated with expressed violence, but the effects were moderated when youth were less depressed and had a stronger sense of purpose in life.[119]

Researchers who separated the effects of domestic and community violence found that only domestic violence affected the functioning of a group of high-risk adolescents and that the impact was moderated by the adolescents' self-reported social support.[120] These results have limited generalizability, however. Participants were 65 inpatients between the ages of 13 and 17. Two thirds were hospitalized for suicidal ideation or behavior. The remaining third were hospitalized for homicidal ideation, combined suicidal and homicidal ideation, and assaultive behavior. Prior to hospitalization, 12 of the 65 participants lived in a residential treatment facility. Adolescents whose emotional problems are less extreme might respond differently both to community violence as a stressor and social support as a buffer. In another high-risk population of adolescents (13-18 years of age) drawn from residential treatment agencies and shelters,[121] youth exposed to violence between their parents were more likely to be depressed, run away, and be violent with parents than nonexposed youth. Exposed youth were also more likely to approve of and use violence toward dating partners, but all findings were modest and moderated by gender. The impact of witnessing violence was significant only for males and had no impact on the well-being or behavior of females.

A number of studies have looked exclusively at adolescent's internalizing, externalizing, and PTSD symptoms, with a range of findings. In a child welfare population, psychological maltreatment, as opposed to experiencing or witnessing physical or sexual assault, had the most profound effect on youth's internalizing and externalizing behaviors; witnessing family violence had a modest effect only for boys.[122] A study of a community sample of young adolescents (age 11-15) found that fathers' self-reported physical and verbal violence against mothers' significantly affected internalizing, externalizing, prosocial behavior, and cognitive functioning as reported by teachers for both boys and girls.[123] Mothers' self-reported physical and verbal violence did not affect any of the dimensions for either boys or girls in spite of the fact that mothers and fathers reported similar rates of violence.[123] In young adolescents, the use of social supports buffered the negative effects of witnessing domestic violence on participants' self-reported sense of self-worth, externalizing, and depression.[124] Witnessing violence was associated with symptoms of PTSD in both boys and girls in one study,[125] and to higher internalizing and externalizing problems for only girls in another.[126]

INTERVENTIONS FOR CHILDREN EXPOSED TO VIOLENCE

Several intervention models have demonstrated efficacy for children exposed to domestic violence across developmental levels. In this section, we discuss those models as well as some basic principles of intervention with exposed children and their nonoffending parents.

Child–Parent Psychotherapy

Child–Parent Psychotherapy (CPP) for preschoolers (age 3-5) exposed to domestic violence is a relationship-based intervention grounded in psychoanalytic, attachment, and trauma theory that also includes interventions based in social learning and cognitive behavioral theories.[127,128] Because young children organize their responses to stress and danger around their caregiving relationships, CPP promotes repair of the parent–child relationship after the trauma of domestic violence. Weekly treatment sessions involve play to promote parent understanding of the child's internal world, unstructured reflective developmental guidance, emotional support, concrete assistance with problems of living, and interpretation of behavior and feelings. CPP helps young children and their parents regulate affect, co-construct a narrative of their experiences of violence that have meaning for both of them, and restore a relationship in which both parent and child have confidence in the parent's capacity to protect the child from harm. In a randomized controlled trial comparing CPP to case management plus community intervention as usual, CPP was more effective than individual treatment in the control group in reducing children's behavior problems and PTSD symptoms as well as mother's symptoms of avoidance,[52] with improvements in behavior problems sustained at a follow-up conducted 6 months after the end of treatment.[128] PTSD symptoms were not measured on follow-up for either mother or child, but general functioning continued to improve in mothers who received CPP after the conclusion of treatment, whereas comparison group mothers' functioning did not.[128] It is noteworthy that while all of the children in this study had been exposed to at least one incident of physical violence perpetrated against their mothers by an intimate partner, they and their mothers had all suffered multiple other traumatic events as well, such as physical or sexual abuse.[52]

Project SUPPORT

Project SUPPORT is designed for children ages 4 to 9 and their mothers as they leave domestic violence shelters. Children with conduct disorders and oppositional defiant disorders and their mothers were included in a randomized controlled trial comparing the intervention to existing services. Children meet with a supportive mentor; mothers meet weekly with a therapist for parent coaching. On average, the intervention lasted 8 months with a mean number of 23 home visits per family. Trained paraprofessionals also provided advocacy and role modeling for the mothers. Children in both the intervention and comparison groups improved in their externalizing behaviors, but the children in the intervention group improved at a faster rate. Participating mothers' child management skills were enhanced,[129] and treatment gains persisted 24 months after treatment when compared with children in the control group. In addition, at follow-up intervention children showed fewer internalizing problems. There had been no significant improvements in internalizing in either group at the conclusion of treatment.[130]

Kids' Club and Kids' Club Preschool

These are group interventions designed for children age 5 to 13. The intervention is offered in both shelter and community settings. These psycho-educational groups for children, with separate groups for mothers, meet weekly for 10 weeks. Children's groups help children recover from the traumatic effects of exposure to domestic violence, and aim to prevent future problems by discussing feelings and concerns related to violence, increasing coping skills, and addressing distorted thoughts and assumptions about violence. Mothers' groups provide empowerment, parenting support, and information about the impact of violence on children.[131] An efficacy study sequentially assigned families to child only, mother and child, and wait list conditions. Children in both treatment groups had fewer PTSD diagnoses after treatment than did control children.[132] Only the mother and child group showed significant improvement in externalizing behaviors and violence attitudes compared to wait list controls.[133]

The Learning Club

This 16-week program was developed to provide advocacy services for mothers as they leave shelter and a mentoring experience plus a 10-week educational group for children ages 7 to 11. Contact with families is intense, with an average of 9 hours per family per week. Children's mentors transport the children to the educational groups and attend the groups with them. When compared with control group children, children in the intervention group improved their feelings of self-confidence. Mothers experienced increased social support. In addition, child abuse was less likely in the intervention group. These changes were maintained at 6-month follow-up.[134]

Youth Relationships Project

This group intervention, originally designed for adolescents with a history of violence exposure and risk factors for abuse, has been used in general school populations as well. Its goal is to prevent intimate partner violence and victimization and to promote healthy relationships. The group activities include psycho-education, skills training, and community involvement; youth are taught that aggression is a choice and are helped to examine the attitudes and power dynamics that foster and sustain relationship violence.[135] In a randomized controlled trial, 14- to 16-year-olds with maltreatment histories including exposure to domestic violence showed a greater decline in PTSD symptoms than did controls.[136]

Other Interventions

Although the previously mentioned interventions are the only ones demonstrated in randomized controlled trials to be efficacious with children exposed to domestic violence, other trauma-focused interventions might also be effective for these children, given the traumatic nature of domestic violence for many children and the high rates of PTSD found in some samples. The authors of two recent reviews of interventions for exposed children[137,138] suggest several features that should be included in interventions with this population: (1) a thorough assessment that takes the circumstances of exposure, family members' individual needs, co-occurring risk factors, and protective factors into consideration, (2) a focus on reexposure or similar interventions shown to be effective to treat the symptoms of PTSD, (3) education about violence and normative responses to violence, (4) a focus on processing emotional cues and affect regulation, (5) a focus on social problem-solving and interaction skills, (6) a focus on safety planning and coping with violence, and (7) inclusion of parents in the interventions. Each of the empirically validated intervention models described above includes some or all of these intervention characteristics.

IMPLICATIONS FOR HEALTH CARE PROVIDERS

Although it is clear that witnessing violence between parents has a negative effect on some children, it is impossible to predict from the current literature for whom the effect will be greatest, what conditions may contribute to or even mediate the child's distress after witnessing violence, and what conditions buffer the effect of violence on the child. What does emerge from the literature is the complex nature of exposure on developing children. How an individual child will be affected depends on the nature of the violent incident and the child's sensory exposure to it; the child's gender, individual characteristics, past experiences, relationships both inside and outside the family, and other current stressors; the stressors and protective factors that exist for the family as a whole and for the community in which it is embedded; and on what the child, family, and larger culture think about who is responsible for the violence and whether the violence is justified. Understanding all of these factors is a daunting task for an individual clinician facing an individual child and family.

HCPs do not need to complete such a nuanced picture in order to make effective interventions for the children in their care. The evidence is sufficiently strong to justify screening for domestic violence during well-child check-ups at all stages of a child's development. Internalizing and externalizing behavior problems and symptoms of PTSD are indicators of distress for children exposed to violence. There are a number of concrete things clinicians can do to help.

Ask about changes in children's moods and behavior at every well-child visit. When you hear that children are distressed, ask about stressors in the child's life at school, at home, and in the community. Tell parents how important they are to their children's recovery. Specific parenting behaviors that help are warmth, ability to listen to children's concerns and answer their questions, and ability to help children find ways to calm and soothe themselves. Become familiar with interventions for exposed children that are available in your community and take the time to make referrals.

When a child has been exposed to violence or trauma, explain to parents that when their children have been frightened, parents are their most important source of security. Children, especially young ones, feel safer when they are close to their parents. Explain that children may be more anxious than usual about separations. Tell parents that when children have been frightened, they can help by speaking with children about what happened and explaining what will happen next. Predictability and consistency help children feel secure. Parents' willingness to speak with their children about what happens in their lives gives the child a sense of being cared for and increases their feeling that the world is predictable.

Parents can enhance their children's sense of control by giving them choices that are consistent with their age and developmental stage. Remember that parents or foster parents might not understand the effect of violence or other forms of trauma on children's behavior. Their annoyance when their children misbehave or act immature and clingy does not make them bad parents. Parents need information and reassurance from their HCPs so that they can help their children.

When dealing with traumatized toddlers and school-age children, explain to parents and foster parents that their own well-being is important to their children. Help parents find intervention if they need it. Encourage parents to tell their children that the violence is not the child's fault and that the parent is trying to find ways to be safe. Encourage parents to engage in safety planning with their children so that children know where to go and what to do if they are frightened. Encourage parents to monitor their children's moods and behavior and obtain help for them if they need it. Explain to parents and foster parents that young children need predictable routines as well as physical closeness and comforting. Encourage them to spend time with their toddlers and preschoolers engaging in joint activities such as reading aloud, singing, and playing that will help restore feelings of togetherness and safety.

For adolescents, social supports are especially important. Group interventions can help tie violence-exposed adolescents to others who can understand their dilemma. Tell parents of violence-exposed adolescents that there are increased risks for self-endangering behaviors and that it is critical that they monitor changes in their adolescents' mood and behavior.

STRENGTH OF EVIDENCE AND FUTURE DIRECTIONS FOR RESEARCH

Although there is substantial evidence that exposure to domestic violence has a detrimental effect on most children, the evidence is not entirely consistent on the pattern of outcomes that children suffer. One major concern about the evidence of impact is that it may be overstated because researchers do not measure co-occurring risks and adversities that may explain more of the variance in children's outcomes than does exposure to domestic violence. The three metaanalyses of this literature[9-11] all showed that effect sizes for children's exposure ranged from small to moderate. One study that did examine co-occurring stressors found that the effect of domestic violence on children's functioning was reduced to zero for boys when the effects of other stressors were taken into account.[139] On the other hand, this finding is inconsistent with another study that found unique affects when comparing exposed children with a matched group of children who were not exposed but who had equivalent risks for poverty, ethnic minority status, living in a single mother household, and exposure to community violence.[91] Researchers would do well to recall Rutter's finding that although children can tolerate the effect of one severe stressor without declines in functioning, the experience of two stressors increases their risk fourfold.[140] This is consistent with the findings of Felitti and colleagues,[51] that children who suffered four or more adverse childhood experiences were at greatly increased risk for negative physical and mental health outcomes that extended into adulthood. In studies controlled for co-occurring adversities, researchers and clinicians would be in a better position to assert that experiencing domestic violence affects children's development.

We have pointed out some additional problems in the research earlier in the chapter. Researchers are not consistent about the way in which they define domestic violence or children's exposure to violence. Future studies should state clearly the type or types of violence to which child victims have been exposed and describe the range of participant children's sensory exposure to the violence. The two taxonomies suggested by Holden[8] are exemplary in this regard. Understanding the nature of children's exposure would help make meaning of the literature. Further, researchers in this field have greatly relied on maternal report. Observational data, and data from a variety of reporters, would enhance the validity of the findings and strengthen the evidence that witnessing violence has a genuine impact on children. Finally, the evidence would be clearer if a wider variety of outcomes were explored. In spite of the fact that trauma response symptoms are widespread among exposed children, relatively few researchers measure either symptom level or presence/absence of PTSD diagnosis. In addition, a variety of outcomes beyond behavior problems and symptoms would shed light on the effects of exposure. It is becoming easier to collect the kind of psychophysiological data that could shed light on the way exposure to domestic violence effects children's stress response systems (see Chapter 54, "Effects of Abuse and Neglect on Brain Development"). Relatively few studies have examined the effect of violence exposure on children's peer relationships. In short, we will not truly understand the phenomenological impacts of children's exposure until large enough samples of children are recruited to allow researchers to examine the effects of co-occurring stressors, to assess risk and resilience factors, and to evaluate multiple outcomes.

In addition to addressing the weaknesses in the evidence set forth above, future research might focus on four areas that have heretofore been ignored or given short shrift. First, we need longitudinal studies of children's functioning after exposure to domestic violence. With the exception of treatment outcome studies that conduct follow-ups, the literature on children's exposure to domestic violence is cross-sectional and provides only a snapshot of the child's functioning at the time. This leaves unanswered the question of whether the passage of time or developmental changes will ameliorate or exacerbate the effect of violence exposure on children.

Second, given the complexity of children's experience, intervention research is needed that can establish the extent to which interventions that are effective with populations of children exposed to domestic violence are equally effective for children with the single stressor of violence exposure and children with multiple traumatic stressors in their lives.

Third, mixed design research that captures qualitative as well as quantitative data would give a richer picture of children's responses to domestic violence. And finally, given the evidence that psychological violence between parents can have a greater effect on some children than physical violence, research is needed to examine the impact of psychological assault on large, heterogeneous groups of children, and to examine the mediators and moderators of this impact.

References

1. Jaffe PG, Wolfe DA, Wilson SK: *Children of Battered Women.* Sage Publications, Newbury Park, Calif, 1990.
2. Geffner RA, Jaffe PG, Sudermann M (eds): *Children Exposed to Domestic Violence: Current Issues In Research, Intervention, Prevention, and Policy Development.* Haworth, New York, 2000.
3. Graham-Bermann SA, Edleson JL (eds): *Domestic Violence in the Lives of Children.* American Psychological Association, Washington, DC, 2001.
4. Holden GW, Geffner R., Jouriles EN (eds): *Children Exposed to Marital Violence: Theory, Research, and Applied Issues.* American Psychological Association, Washington, DC, 1998.
5. Rossman BBR, Hughes HM, Rosenberg MS: *Children and Interparental Violence: The Impact of Exposure.* Brunner/Mazel, Philadelphia, 2000.
6. Jaffee PG, Baker LL, Cunningham AJ: *Protecting Children from Domestic Violence: Strategies for Community Intervention.* Guilford, New York, 2004.
7. Fantuzzo JW, Lindquist CU: The effects of observing conjugal violence on children: A review and analysis of research methodology. *J Fam Violence* 1989;4:77-94.
8. Holden GW: Children exposed to domestic violence and child abuse: terminology and taxonomy. *Clin Child Fam Psych* 2003;6:151-160.
9. Kitzmann KM, Gaylord NK, Holt AR, et al: Child witnesses to domestic violence: a meta-analytic review. *J Consult Clin Psychol* 2003;71:339-352.
10. Wolfe DA, Crooks CV, Lee V, et al: The effects of children's exposure to domestic violence: a meta-analysis and critique. *Clin Child Fam Psych Rev* 2003;6:171-187.
11. Evans SE, Davies C, DiLillo, D: Exposure to domestic violence: a meta-analysis of child and adolescent outcomes. *Aggress Viol Behav* 2008;13:131-140.
12. Mohr WK, Noone Lutz MJ, Fantuzzo JW, et al: Children exposed to family violence: a review of empirical research from a developmental-ecological perspective. *Trauma Violence Abuse* 2000;1:264-283.
13. Shepard M, Campbell JA: The Abusive Behavior Inventory: a measure of physical and psychological and physical abuse. *J Interpers Violence* 1992;7:291-305.
14. Straus MA: Measuring intrafamily conflict and violence: the Conflict Tactics (CT) Scales. *J Marriage Fam* 1979;41:75-88.
15. Johnson MP, Ferraro KJ: Research on domestic violence in the 1990s: making distinctions. *J Marriage Fam* 2000:62:948-963.
16. Rossman BRR: Time heals all: how much and for whom? *J Em Abuse* 2000;2:31-50.
17. Holtzworth-Munroe A, Stuart GL: Typologies of male batterers: three subtypes and the differences among them. *Psych Bull* 1994;116:476-497.
18. Field CA, Caetano R: Intimate partner violence in the U.S. general population: progress and future directions. *J Interpers Violence* 2005;20:463-469.
19. Tjaden P, Thoennes N: Prevalence and consequences of male-to-female and female-to-male intimate partner violence as measured by the National Violence Against Women Survey. *Violence Against Women* 2000;6:141-162.
20. Carlson BE: Children's observations of interpersonal violence. *In*: Roberts A (ed): *Battered Women and Their Families.* Springer, New York, 1984, pp 147-167.
21. Straus MA, Gelles RJ, Steinmetz SK: *Behind Closed Doors: Violence in the American Family.* Doubleday Press, Garden City, NY, 1980.
22. Caetano R, Schafer J, Field C, et al: Agreements on reports of intimate partner violence among White, Black, and Hispanic couples in the United States. *J Interpers Violence* 2002;17:1308-1322.
23. Fantuzzo JW, Boruch R, Beriama A, et al: Domestic violence and children: prevalence and risk in five major U.S. cities. *J Am Acad Child Adolesc Psych* 1997;36:116-122.

24. Fantuzzo JW, Fusco RA: Children's direct exposure to types of domestic violence crime: a population-based investigation. *J Fam Viol* 2007;22:543-552.

25. Fantuzzo JW, DePaola LM, Lambert L: Effects of interparental violence on the psychological adjustment and competencies of young children. *J Consult Clin Psychol* 1991;59:258-265.

26. McDonald R, Jouriles EN, Ramisetty-Mikler S, et al: Estimating the number of American children living in partner-violent families. *J Fam Psychol* 2006;20:137-142.

27. Finkelhor D, Ormrod R, Turner H, et al: The victimization of children and youth: a comprehensive, national survey. *Child Maltreat* 2005;10:5-25.

28. Bronfenbrenner U: *The Ecology of Human Development: Experiments by Nature and Design.* Harvard University Press, Cambridge, 1979.

29. Bronfenbrenner U: Ecology of the family as a context for human development: resarch perspectives. *Dev Psychol* 1986;22:723-742.

30. Cicchetti D, Lynch A: Toward an ecological/transactional model of community violence and child maltreatment: Consequences for children's development. *Psychiatry* 1993;56:96-118.

31. Schore AN: The effects of early relational trauma on right brain development, affect regulation, and infant mental health. *Infant Ment Health J* 2001;22:201-269.

32. Pynoos RS, Steinberg AM, Piacentini JC: A developmental psychopathology model of childhood traumatic stress and intersection with anxiety disorders. *Biol Psychiatry* 1999;46:1542-1554.

33. Greenspan SI: *The Growth of the Mind and the Endangered Origins of Intelligence.* Perseus Books, Reading, Mass, 1997.

34. Belsky J: The determinants of parenting: A process model. *Child Dev* 1984;55:83-96.

35. McCloskey LA, Aurelio JF, Koss MP: The effects of systemic family violence on children's mental health. *Child Dev* 1995;66:1239-1261.

36. Straus MA, Gelles RJ (eds): *Physical Violence in American Families: Risk Factors and Adaptions to Violence in 8,145 families.* Transaction Press, Brunswick, NJ, 2000.

37. Doumas D, Margolin G, John RS: The intergenerational transmission of aggression across three generations. *J Family Violence* 1994;9:157-175.

38. Lieberman AF, Van Horn P: Attachment, trauma, and domestic violence: implications for child custody. *Child Adoles Psychiatri Clin North Am* 1998;7:423-443.

39. Rutter M: Intergenerational continuities and discontinuities in serious parenting difficulties. *In:* Cicchetti D, Carlson V (eds): *Child Maltreatment: Theory and Research on the Causes and Consequences of Child Abuse and Neglect.* Cambridge University Press, New York, 1989, pp 317-348.

40. Dix T: The affective organization of parenting: adaptive and maladaptive processes. *Psychol Bull* 1991;110:3-25.

41. Maccoby EE: The role of parents in the socialization of children: an historical overview. *Dev Psychol* 1992;28:1006-1017.

42. Garbarino J: *Raising Children in a Socially Toxic Environment.* Jossey-Bass, San Francisco, 1995.

43. Mental Health: Culture, Race, and Ethnicity. A Supplement to Mental Health: A Report of the Surgeon General. U.S. Dept Health Hum Serv, SAMHSA, Rockville, Md, 2001. Available at http://www.surgeongeneral.gov/library/mentalhealth/cre/. Accessed April 5, 2009.

44. Greenfeld LA, Rand MR, Craven D, et al: Violence by Intimates: Analysis of Data on Crimes by Current or Former Spouses, Boyfriends, and Girlfriends. U.S. Dept Justice, Washington DC, 1998. Available at http://www.ojp.usdoj.gov/bjs/pub/pdf/vi.pdf. Accessed April 5, 2009.

45. Harris WW, Lieberman, AF, Marans S: In the best interests of society. *J Child Psychol Psychiatry* 2007;43:392-411.

46. Lewis ML, Ghosh Ippen C: Rainbows of tears, souls full of hope: cultural issues related to young children and trauma. *In:* Osofsky JD (ed): *Young Children and Trauma: Intervention and Treatment.* Guilford, New York, 2004, pp 11-46.

47. Osofsky JD: Prevalence of children's exposure to domestic violence and child maltreatment: implications for prevention and intervention. *Clin Child Fam Psych Rev* 2003;6:161-170.

48. Knickerbocker L, Heyman RE, Smith Slep AM, et al: Co-occurrence of child and partner maltreatment: definitions, prevalence, theory, and implications for assessment. *Euro Psychol* 2007;12:36-44.

49. Rutter M: Resilience reconsidered: conceptual considerations, empirical findings, and policy implications. *In:* Shonkoff JP, Meisels SJ (eds): *Handbook of Early Childhood Intervention.* Cambridge University Press, New York, 2000, pp 651-682.

50. Turner HA, Finkelhor D, Ormond, R: The effect of lifetime victimization on the mental health of children and adolescents. *Soc Sci Med* 2006;62:13-27.

51. Felitti VJ, Anda RF, Nordenberg D, et al: Relationship of childhood abuse and household dysfunction to many of the leading causes of death in adults: the adverse childhood experiences (ACE) study. *Am J Prev Med* 1998;14:245-258.

52. Lieberman AF, Van Horn P, Ghosh Ippen C: Towards evidence-based treatment: child-parent psychotherapy with preschoolers exposed to marital violence. *J Am Acad Child Adolesc Psychiatry* 2005;44:1241-1248.

53. McCloskey LA, Walker M: Posttraumatic stress in children exposed to family violence and single-event trauma. *J Am Acad Child Adolesc Psychiatry* 2000;39:108-115.

54. Kilpatrick KL, Williams LM: Post-traumatic stress disorder in child witnesses to domestic violence. *Am J Orthopsychiatry* 1997;67:639-644.

55. Jarvis KL, Gordon EE, Novaco RW: Psychological distress of children and mothers in domestic violence emergency shelters. *J Fam Violence* 2005;20:389-402.

56. Scheeringa MS, Zeanah C: Symptom expression and trauma variables in children under 48 months of age. *Infant Ment Health J* 1995;16:259-270.

57. American Psychiatric Association: *Diagnostic and statistical manual of mental disorders (ed 4, text rev).* American Psychiatric Association, Washington, DC, 2000.

58. Freud S: Inhibitions, symptoms and anxiety. *In:* Strachey J (ed and trans): *The Standard Edition of the Complete Psychological Works of Sigmund Freud.* Hogarth Press, London, 1926/1959 (vol 4, pp 87-156).

59. Bowlby J: *Attachment and Loss. Vol 1: Attachment.* Basic Books, New York, 1969/1982.

60. Lieberman AF: Traumatic stress and quality of attachment: reality and internalization in disorders of infant mental health. *Infant Ment Health J* 2004;25:336-351.

61. Lieberman AF, Amaya-Jackson L: Reciprocal influences of attachment and trauma: using a dual lense in the assessment and treatment of infants, toddlers, and preschoolers. *In:* Berlin LJ, Ziv Y, Amaya-Jackson L, et al (eds): *Enhancing Early Attachments: Theory, Research, Intervention, and Policy.* Guilford, NY, 2005, pp 100-124.

62. Lieberman AF, Van Horn P: *Psychotherapy with Infants and Young Children: Repairing the Effects of Stress and Trauma on Early Attachment.* Guilford, New York, 2008.

63. Gunnar MR, Quevedo K: The neurobiology of stress and trauma. *Annu Rev Psychol* 2007;58:145-173.

64. Bowlby J: *Attachment and loss. Vol 2: Separation.* Basic Books, New York, 1973.

65. Bowlby J: *Attachment and loss: Vol 3: Loss.* Basic Books, New York, 1980.

66. Lieberman AF, Van Horn P: Attachment, trauma, and domestic violence: implications for child custody. *Child Adolesc Clin N Am* 1998;7:423-444.

67. Ainsworth MD, Blehar M, Waters E, et al: *Patterns of Attachment: A Psychological Study of the Strange Situation.* Erlbaum, Hillsdale, NJ, 1978.

68. Main M: Metacognitive knowledge, metacognitive monitoring, and single (coherent) versus multiple (incoherent) models of attachment: findings and directions for future research. *In:* Parkes CM, Stevenson-Hinde J, Marris P (eds): *Attachment Across the Life Cycle.* Tavistock/Routledge, London, 1991, pp 127-160.

69. Main M, Hesse E: Parents' unresolved traumatic experiences are related to infant disorganized attachment status: Is frightened and/or parental behavior the linking mechanisms? *In:* Greenberg M, Cicchetti D, Cummings EM (eds): *Attachment in the Preschool Years: Theory, Research, and Intervention.* University of Chicago Press, Chicago, 1990, pp 161-184.

70. Lyons-Ruth K, Bronfman E, Atwood G: A relational diathesis model of hostile-helpless states of mind. *In:* Solomon J, George C (eds): *Attachment and Disorganization.* Guilford, NY, 1999, pp 35-69.

71. Pynoos RS: *The transgenerational repercussions of traumatic expectations.* Paper presented at the Southern Florida Psychiatric Society/University of Miami School of Medicine, Miami, Fla, February 1997.

72. Hughes HM, Luke DA: Heterogeneity in adjustment among children of battered women. *In:* Holden GW, Geffner R, Jouriles EN (eds): *Children Exposed to Marital Violence: Theory, Research, and Applied Issues.* American Psychological Association, Washington, DC, 1998, pp 289-334.

73. Grych JH, Jouriles EN, Swank PR, et al: Patterns of adjustment among children of battered women. *J Consult Clin Psychol* 2000; 68:84-94.

74. Cicchetti D: Developmental psychopathology: reactions, reflections, and projections. *Dev Rev* 1994;6:1-3.

75. Marans S, Adelman A: Experiencing violence in a developmental context. *In:* Osofsky JD (ed): *Children in a Violent Society.* Guilford, New York, 1997, pp 202-222.

76. Margolin G, Gordis EB: The effects of family and community violence on children. *Ann Rev Psychol* 2000;51:445-479.

77. Janoff-Bulman R: *Shattered Assumptions: Toward a New Psychology of Trauma.* Free Press, New York, 1992.

78. Osofsky JD: The effects of exposure to violence on young children. *Am Psychol* 1995;50:782-788.

79. Osofsky JD, Scheeringa MS: Community and domestic violence exposure: effects of development and psychopathology. *In:* Cicchetti D, Toth SL (eds): *Rochester Symposium on Developmental Psychopathology, Vol. 8. Developmental Perspectives on Trauma: Theory and Research.* University of Rochester Press, Rochester, NY, 1997, pp 155-180.

80. Zeanah CH, Scheeringa MS: The experience and effects of violence in infancy. *In:* Osofsky JD (ed): *Children in a Violent Society.* Guilford, New York, 1997, pp 97-123.

81. Zeitlin D, Djanjal T, Colmsee M: Maternal-foetal bonding: the impact of domestic violence on the bonding process between a mother and child. *Arch Womens Ment Health* 1999;2:183-189.

82. Casanueva CE, Martin SL: Intimate partner violence during pregnancy and mothers' child abuse potential. *J Interpers Violence* 2007; 22:603-622.

83. Jasinski JL: Pregnancy and domestic violence: a review of the literature. *Trauma Viol Abuse* 2004;5:47-64.

84. Roberts D: *Shattered Bonds: The Color of Child Welfare.* Basic Civitas Books, New York, 2002.

85. Levendosky AA, Leahy KL, Bogat GA, et al: Domestic violence, maternal parenting, maternal mental health, and infant internalizing behavior. *J Fam Psychol* 2006;20:544-552.

86. Blackburn ST, Loper DL: *Maternal, Fetal, and Neonatal Physiology: A Clinical Perspective.* WB Saunders, Philadelphia, 1992.

87. Crockenberg S, Leerkes EM, Lekka SK: Pathways from marital aggression to infant emotion regulation: the development of withdrawal in infancy. *Infant Behav Dev* 2006;30:97-113.

88. Levendosky AA, Huth-Bocks AC, Shapiro DL, et al: The impact of domestic violence on the maternal-child relationship and preschool-age children's functioning. *J Fam Psychol* 2003;17:275-287.

89. Johnson VK, Lieberman AF: Variations in behavior problems of preschoolers exposed to domestic violence: the role of mothers' attunement to children's emotional experiences. *J Fam Violence* 2007;22:297-308.

90. Lieberman AF, Van Horn P, Ozer EJ: Preschooler witnesses of marital violence: predictors and mediators of child behavior problems. *Dev Psychopathol* 2005;17:385-396.

91. Ybarra GJ, Wilkens SL, Lieberman AF: The influence of domestic violence on preschooler behavior and functioning. *J Fam Violence* 2007;22:33-42.

92. Koenen KC, Moffitt TE, Caspi A, et al: Domestic violence is associated with environmental suppression of IQ in young children. *Dev Psychopathol* 2003;15:297-311.

93. Jouriles EN, Brown AS, McDonald R, et al: Intimate partner violence and preschooler's explicit memory functioning. *J Fam Psychol* 2008;22:420-428.

94. Graham-Bermann SA, Levendosky AA: The social functioning of preschool-age children whose mothers are emotionally and physically abused. *J Em Abuse* 1998;1:59-84.

95. Jouriles EN, McDonald R, Norwood, WD, et al: Knives, guns, and interparent violence: relations with child behavior problems. *J Fam Psychol* 1998;12:178-194.

96. Jouriles EN, Norwood WD, McDonald R, et al: Physical vilence and other forms of marital aggression: links with children's behavior problems. *J Fam Psychol* 1996;10:223-234.

97. Fantuzzo JW, Lindquist CU: The effects of observing conjugal violence on children: a review and analysis of research methodology. *J Fam Viol* 1989;4:77-94.

98. McCloskey LA, Figueredo AJ, Koss MP: The effects of systemic family violence on children's mental health. *Child Dev* 1995;66: 1239-1261.

99. Rossman BRR: Descartes's error and posttraumatic stress disorder: cognition and emotion in children who are exposed to parental violence. *In:* Holden GW, Geffner R, Jouriles EN (eds): *Children Exposed to Marital Violence: Theory, Research and Applied Issues.* American Psychological Association, Washington, DC, 1998, pp 223-256.

100. Graham-Berman SA, Levendosky AA: Traumatic stress symptoms in children of battered women. *J Interpers Viol* 1998;13:111-128.

101. Lehmann P: The development of post-traumatic stress disorder (PTSD) in a sample of child witnesses to mother assault. *J Fam Violence* 1997;12:241-257.

102. Kilpatrick KL, Litt M, Williams LM: Post-traumatic stress disorder in child witnesses to domestic violence. *Am J Orthopsychiatry* 1997;67:639-644.

103. Kilpatrick KL, Williams LM: Potential mediators of post-traumatic stress disorders in child witnesses to domestic violence. *Child Abuse Negl* 1998;22:319-330.

104. Margolin G, John RS, Ghosh C, et al: Family interaction process: an essential tool for exploring abusive relations. *In:* Cahn DD, Lloyd SA (eds): *Family Abuse: A Communication Perspective.* Sage Publications, Thousand Oaks, Calif, 1997, pp 37-58.

105. Gordis EG, Margolin G, John RS: Marital aggression, observed parental hostility, and child behavior during dryadic family interaction. *J Fam Psychol* 1997;11:76-89.

106. Margolin G, Gordis EB, Oliver PH: Links between marital and parent-child interactions: moderating role of husband-to-wife aggression. *Dev Psychopathol* 2004;16:753-771.

107. Margolin G, John RS: Children's exposure to marital aggression: direct and mediated effects. *In:* Kantor GK, Jasinski JL (eds): *Out of the Darkness: Perspectives on Family Violence.* Sage Publications, Thousand Oaks, Calif, 1997, pp 90-104.

108. Skopp NA, McDonald R, Jouriles EN, et al: Partner aggression and children's externalizing problems: maternal and partner warmth as protective factors. *J Fam Psychol* 2007;21:459-567.

109. Bandura A: *Social Learning Theory.* Prentice-Hall, Englewood Cliffs, NJ, 1977.

110. Levendosky AA, Graham-Bermann SA: The moderating effects of parenting stress on children's adjustment in woman-abusing families. *J Interpers Violence* 1998;13:383-397.

111. Holden GW, Ritchie KL: Linking extreme marital discord, child rearing, and child behavior problems: evidence from battered women. *Child Dev* 1991;62:311-327.

112. Jarvis KL, Gordon EE, Novaco RW: Psychological distress of children and mothers in domestic violence emergency shelters. *J Fam Violence* 2005;20:389-402.

113. Leary A, Katz LF: Coparenting, family-level processes, and peer outcomes: the moderating role of vagal tone. *Dev Psychopathol* 2004;16:593-608.

114. Katz LF, Hessler DM, Annest A: Domestic violence, emotional competence, and child adjustment. *Soc Dev* 2007;16:513-538.

115. Skopp NA, McDonald R, Manke B: Siblings in domestically violent families: experience of interparent conflict and adjustment problems. *J Fam Psychol* 2005;19:324-333.

116. Grych JH, Fincham FD, Jouriles EN, et al: Interparental conflict and child adjustment: testing the mediational role of appraisals in the cognitive-contextual framework. *Child Dev* 2000;71:1648-1661.

117. Foshee VA, Karriker-Jaffe KJ, Reyes HLM, et al: What accounts for demographic differences in trajectories of adolescent dating violence? An examination of intrapersonal and contextual mediators. *J Adolesc Health* 2008;42:596-604.

118. Song L, Singer MI, Anglin TM: Violence exposure and emotional trauma as contributors to adolescents' violent behaviors. *Arch Pediatr Adolesc Med* 1998;152:531-536.

119. DuRant RH, Cadenhead C, Pendergrast RA, et al: Factors associated with the use of violence among urban black adolescents. *Am J Pub Health* 1994;84:612-617.

120. Muller RT, Goebel-Fabbri AE, Diamond T, et al: Social support and the relationship between family and community violence exposure and psychopathology among high risk adolescents. *Child Abuse Negl* 2000;24:449-464.

121. Carlson BE: Adolescent observers of marital violence. *J Fam Violence* 1990;5:285-299.

122. McGee RA, Wolfe DA, Wilson SK: Multiple maltreatment experiences and adolescent behavior problems: adolescents' perspectives. *Dev Psychopathol* 1997;9:131-149.

123. Kempton T, Thomas AM, Forehand R: Dimensions of interparental conflict and adolescent functioning. *J Fam Violence* 1989;4:297-307.

124. Rogers MJ, Holmbeck GN: Effects of interparental aggression on children's adjustment: the moderating role of cognitive appraisal and coping. *J Fam Psychol* 1997;11:125-130.

125. Howard DE, Feigelman S, Li X, et al: The relationship among violence victimization, witnessing violence, and youth distress. *J Adolesc Health* 2002;31:455-462.

126. Sternberg KJ, Lamb ME, Greenbaum C, et al: Effects of domestic violence on children's behavior problems and depression. *Dev Psychopathol* 1993;29:44-52.

127. Lieberman AF, Van Horn P: *Don't Hit My Mommy!: A Manual for Child-Parent Psychotherapy with Young Witnesses of Family Violence.* Zero to Three, Washington, DC, 2005.

128. Lieberman AF, Ghosh Ippen C, Van Horn P: Child-Parent Psychotherapy: six month follow-up of a randomized control trial. *J Am Acad Child Adolesc Psychiatry* 2006;45:913-918.

129. Jouriles EN, McDonald R, Spiller LC, et al: Reducing conduct problems among children of battered women. *J Consult Clin Psychol* 2001 69:774-785.

130. McDonald R, Jouriles EN, Skopp N: Reducing conduct problems among children brought to women's shelters: intervention effects 24 months following termination of services. *J Fam Psychol* 2006;20:127-136.

131. Graham-Bermann SA: *The Kids' Club: A Preventive Intervention Program for Children of Battered Women.* University of Michigan Press, Ann Arbor, 1992.

132. Graham-Bermann SA, Hughes H: Intervention for children exposed to interparental violence (IPV): Assessment of needs and research priorities. *Clin Child Fam Psychol Rev* 2003;6:189-204.

133. Graham-Bermann SA, Lynch S, Banyard V, et al: Community-based intervention for children exposed to intimate partner violence: an efficacy trial. *J Consult Clin Psychol* 2007;75:199-209.

134. Sullivan CM, Campbell R, Angelique H, et al: An advocacy intervention program for women with abusive partners: six-month follow-up. *Am J Comm Psychol* 1994;22:101-122.

135. Wolfe DA, Wekerle C, Gough R, et al: *The Youth Relationships Manual: A Group Approach with Adolescents for the Prevention of Woman Abuse and the Promotion of Healthy Relationships.* Sage Publications, Thousand Oaks, Calif, 1996.

136. Wolfe DA, Wekerle C, Scott K, et al: Dating violence prevention with at-risk youth: a controlled outcome evaluation. *J Consult Clin Psychol* 2003;71:279-291.

137. Graham-Bermann SA, Hughes HM: Interventions for children exposed to interparental violence (IPV): assessment of needs and research priorities. *Clin Child Fam Psychol Rev* 2003;6:189-204.

138. Vickerman KA, Margolin G: Posttraumatic stress in children and adolescents exposed to family violence: II. Treatment. *Prof Psychol Res Pr* 2007;6:620-628.

139. Spaccarelli S, Sandler IN, Roosa M: History of spouse violence against mother: correlated risks and unique effects in child mental health. *J Fam Violence* 1994;9:79-98

140. Rutter M: Psychosocial resilience and protective mechanisms. *In:* Rolf J, Masten AS, Cicchetti D, et al *(eds): Risk and Protective Factors in the Development of Psychopathology.* Cambridge University Press, New York, 1990, pp 181-214.

53

Effects of Abuse and Neglect on Brain Development

Joseph C. Crozier, MD, PhD, Elizabeth E. Van Voorhees, PhD, Stephen R. Hooper, PhD, and Michael D. De Bellis, MD, MPH

INTRODUCTION

Child abuse and neglect are forms of interpersonal violence that can have lasting impacts on a child's socioemotional development. Maltreated children are at increased risk for a host of behavioral and emotional difficulties including posttraumatic stress disorder (PTSD), mood disorders, and disruptive behavioral disorders, particularly attention deficit hyperactivity disorder (ADHD)[1] and substance use disorders.[2] It is thought that child maltreatment could be the single most preventable and intervenable contributor to child and adult mental and medical illness.[3] Although it is clear that child maltreatment increases the risk for the development of psychopathology, the neurobiological substrates that mediate the relation between maltreatment and psychopathology are not well understood. Given that child abuse and neglect tend to be chronic and co-morbid, the array of adverse psychological outcomes that are associated with child maltreatment can be regarded as an environmentally induced complex developmental disorder with identifiable neurobiological substrates.[4]

The main goal of this chapter is to synthesize and summarize the available literature on these neurobiological substrates using the framework of developmental traumatology. The chapter starts with a brief discussion of the field of developmental traumatology to be followed by a discussion of the relevant biological stress response systems. The focus then shifts to comparing biological stress systems and brain development in healthy and maltreated children with PTSD symptoms. The final sections of the chapter examines strength of the evidence, resilience among maltreated children, and treatment implications.

DEVELOPMENTAL TRAUMATOLOGY

Developmental traumatology is the systematic investigation of the neurobiological impact of chronic interpersonal violence on the developing child. It is a new field of study that synthesizes knowledge from developmental psychopathology, developmental neuroscience, and stress and trauma research. In this area of research, measureable aspects of traumatic experiences (e.g., type, age of onset, and duration of child maltreatment) and other biopsychosocial factors (e.g., child temperament, social support for the child and family) are regarded as independent variables, whereas behavioral, cognitive, emotional, and neurobiological measures are considered dependent variables.[5]

Abuse and neglect are extreme forms of dysfunctional family and interpersonal functioning, which often occur in the context of multiple adversities. It is therefore difficult to disentangle the effects of socioeconomic disadvantage, parental mental illness, parental alcohol and substance use disorders, and lack of social support from the effects of chronic maltreatment-related stress on brain maturation and the development of biological stress systems. An important mission for the field of developmental traumatology is to unravel the complex developmental transactions among an individual's genetic constitution, neurophysiology, and unique psychosocial environment taking into consideration experience-dependent critical periods of neurobiological and psychological development. In addition, research should be directed at discovering those processes that contribute to resilience as well as risk given that there is great variability in outcome following child maltreatment.[6-8] Ultimately, it is hoped that research in the field of developmental traumatology will contribute to an improved understanding of risk and resiliency in maltreated children, and thus lead to improved interventions for this population.

THE BIOLOGICAL STRESS RESPONSE SYSTEMS

Traumatic experiences within the context of child maltreatment include chronic neglect or maternal deprivation, physical and sexual abuse, emotional abuse, medical abuse, and exposure to domestic violence. (Domestic violence creates an environment of terror within the family.) Traumatic experiences affect an individual's development through activation of the body's biological stress systems. Stress responses are activated when external stimuli perceived via the senses are processed through the brain's thalamus, activating the amygdala fear detection circuit; projections from the amygdale then transmit signals to intermediary connections in the basal forebrain, paraventricular nucleus (PVN) of the hypothalamus, and brainstem.[9,10] In contrast to the mainly activating role of the amygdala, the hippocampus and medial prefrontal cortex (mPFC) both exert largely inhibitory control over activation of the stress response.[11] The biological stress response itself is primarily mediated by four interacting systems: the hypothalamic-pituitary-adrenal (HPA) axis, the locus coeruleus noradrenergic neurotransmitter

Supported by NIMH grants K24 MH071434 (PI: Dr. De Bellis) and R01 MH063407 (PI: Dr. De Bellis).

(LC/NA) system, the autonomic nervous system (ANS), and the immune system.[12] The purpose of the stress response is twofold: (1) to direct attention to threats in the environment, and (2) to direct metabolic resources away from homeostatic functions such as thinking and digestion to prepare for responding to environmental contingency (i.e., "fight, flight, or freezing").[13-15]

The HPA axis plays a critical role in adjusting physiological functioning in response to stressors. Activation of the stress response causes the hypothalamus to secrete corticotrophin-releasing hormone (CRH) or factor (CRF). CRH functions as both a neurotransmitter and a neuroendocrine factor. In addition to producing anxiogenic effects by binding to receptors throughout the brain,[16] CRH binds specifically to receptors in the anterior pituitary to stimulate the release of adrenocorticotropic hormone (ACTH). ACTH, in turn, binds to receptors in the adrenal cortex, resulting in cortisol secretion.

Cortisol is a glucocorticoid hormone that binds to receptors throughout the body, notably in the central nervous system (CNS). The main effects of increased cortisol secretion are suppression of the immune system, gluconeogenesis, and regulation of the stress response system.[12] In the mPFC, cortisol acts primarily to attenuate the stress response, whereas in the amygdala it has the opposite effect, promoting the stress response.[11] Cortisol exerts negative feedback control over its own secretion by inhibiting the release of both CRH by the hypothalamus and ACTH by the pituitary.

Activation of the stress response and release of CRH by the hypothalamus also activates the LC/NA system. The LC innervates a wide range of regions in the brain and is responsible for the increased release of norepinephrine. This results in elevated arousal, vigilance, and anxiety.[15,17,18] The LC/NA system and HPA axis are mutually excitatory and act together in a positive feedback loop to sustain and enhance the stress response.[13] The LC noradrenergic system also activates the sympathetic nervous system (SNS), the branch of the ANS that is classically associated with the "fight or flight" response. In addition, the SNS innervates the adrenal medulla and causes it to secrete epinephrine and norepinephrine. Increased SNS activity along with increased plasma epinephrine and norepinephrine act together to increase heart rate, blood pressure, sweating, and muscle tone; decrease renal sodium excretion; and generally prepare an individual for action by redistributing blood away from the skin, intestines, and kidney and to the brain, heart, and skeletal muscle. In addition, LC/NA system activity also acts to promote hypervigilance and to focus attention on threat-related cues in the environment.[18] For a complete review, refer to De Bellis.[18]

THE BIOLOGICAL STRESS RESPONSE SYSTEMS IN MALTREATED CHILDREN

The HPA Axis in Maltreated Children

Preclinical studies in animals have shown that early life stress results in elevated HPA reactivity in adulthood,[19] and elevated levels of CRH have been consistently reported in traumatized adults.[20] The findings regarding HPA axis regulation in maltreated children suggest a complex pattern of alterations. Most studies have found that baseline or resting

levels of cortisol are higher in maltreated children with symptoms of anxiety and depression than nonmaltreated children. Increased 24-hour urinary-free cortisol levels were found in maltreated boys and girls with PTSD[21] and in sexually abused girls,[22] and elevated mean, morning, and afternoon salivary cortisol were found in maltreated children with significant internalizing symptoms.[23] In addition, elevated mean salivary cortisol levels were found in maltreated children with impairing threshold and subthreshold PTSD symptoms.[24] Similarly, elevated salivary cortisol levels were seen in 6- to 12-year-old children raised in Romanian orphanages for more than the first 8 months of their lives, as compared with early adopted children.[25]

Studies that challenge the HPA axis show that a chronic compensatory adaptation of the HPA axis is seen in children with past abuse. Attenuated plasma ACTH responses to ovine CRH in sexually abused girls were found several years after abuse disclosure.[26] When compared with controls, the abused girls exhibited reduced evening basal, ovine CRH-stimulated, and time-integrated total plasma ACTH concentrations. Plasma total and free cortisol responses to ovine CRH stimulation did not differ between the two groups. Thus, sexually abused girls manifested a dysregulatory disorder of the LHPA axis associated with hyporesponsiveness of the pituitary to exogenous CRH, but normal overall cortisol secretion to CRH challenge. CRH hypersecretion might have led to an adaptive down-regulation of CRH receptors in the anterior pituitary, which is similar to the mechanism suggested in adults with combat-related PTSD.[27]

Priming can occur as a reflection of chronic compensatory adaptation of the HPA axis after trauma exposure. HPA axis regulation is affected by other stress biochemicals, such as arginine vasopressin and the catecholamines, both of which act synergistically with CRH.[28] A so-called primed system "hyperresponds" during acute stress. Thus, when a new emotional stressor is experienced, HPA axis functioning is enhanced (i.e., higher ACTH and higher 24-hour cortisol concentrations in response to stress). This "hyperresponse" was seen in depressed abused children, currently experiencing psychosocial adversity, during CFH challenge[29] and was seen as well in women who experienced sexual abuse and suffered from current adverse events and major depression.[30] Episodes of neglect affect the HPA axis in similar ways as child abuse. Brief maternal separations or brief neglect during infancy affect the functioning of the HPA axis and glucocorticoid receptor gene expression in the hippocampus and frontal cortex in rats.[31] Thus, the data show that in children developing some forms of internalizing psychopathology following maltreatment, cortisol levels are elevated at rest and during stress challenges. It remains to be investigated whether the dysregulation of the HPA axis contributes to the brain and cognition changes observed in maltreated children.[21]

The Locus Coeruleus Noradrenergic Neurotransmitter System and the Autonomic Nervous System in Maltreated Children

A limited number of studies in maltreated children have found evidence of increased LC/NA tone in maltreated children including elevated heart rate and decreased platelet

α_2-adrenergic receptors,[32] as well as elevated 24-hour excretion of catecholamine metabolites in sexually abused girls[22] and 24-hour catecholamine excretion in children with maltreatment-related PTSD.[21] In the latter study, levels of catecholamine positively correlated with PTSD symptoms. These findings are consistent with studies of combat-related PTSD in adults.[18-20]

The Immune System in Maltreated Children

Prolonged activation of HPA axis and the LC/NA systems can have deleterious effects on homeostatic functioning, including hypertension, accelerated atherosclerosis, metabolic syndrome, impaired growth, and immune system suppression.[15,33] Adverse childhood experiences are associated with multiple and serious health problems in adulthood.[3] For example, a significantly higher incidence of plasma antinuclear antibody titers was seen in sexually abused girls when compared with the frequency of positive antinuclear antibody titers in a sample of healthy adult women.[34] One may hypothesize that the severe stress of sexual abuse may lead to suppression of the mechanisms (T suppressor cells) that actively suppress the autoantibody-producing lymphocytes (B lymphocytes) and thus increase the incidence of positive antinuclear antibody titers in the sexually abused girls studied.[34] The influences of abuse and neglect on physical health warrant further study in maltreated children.

A REVIEW OF HEALTHY BRAIN DEVELOPMENT

Birth to adulthood is marked by progressive physical, behavioral, cognitive, and emotional development. Paralleling these stages are changes in brain maturation. Intracranial volume increases steadily until age 10, with near completion of adult intracranial volume by age 5.[35] Brain development takes place by an overproduction of neurons in utero, increases in synaptic neuropil (neuron size and synapses) during childhood, and then selective elimination of many of these neurons (apoptosis) with corresponding increases in myelination during adolescence and young adulthood.[36]

There are regionally specific nonlinear preadolescent increases followed by postadolescent decreases in cortical grey matter.[37] Neurons enlarge with age and axons become thicker as they myelinate and form neural networks, which are presumably involved in learning mechanisms. From ages 5 to 18 years, myelination by oligodendrocytes is most influential in determining brain size and function.[38] The most dramatic increase in myelination, reflected by the corpus callosum, which connects major subdivisions of the cerebral cortex, occurs from the ages of 6 months to 3 years and continues into the third decade.[39] Subcortical grey matter and limbic system structures (e.g., hippocampus and amygdala), which are involved in the regulation of emotions and memory, increase in volume nonlinearly and peak at age 16.6 years.[40] The prefrontal cortex, which subserves executive cognitive functions and regulates the stress responses, continues its development into the third decade.[41]

Interestingly, sex steroids influence neurodevelopment throughout the life span (for a review, see McEwen.[42]) However, in humans, brain maturational sex differences are an understudied area. In one pediatric neuroimaging study of healthy children and adolescents, boys showed significantly greater loss of grey matter volume and an increase in both white matter volume and corpus callosum area as compared with girls, over a similar age range, suggesting sex differences in both cerebral grey and white matter maturational processes in childhood.[43] In summary, many factors influence brain development, including early life experiences, genetics, hormones, growth factors, nutrients, and degree of environmental stimulation.

BRAIN DEVELOPMENT IN MALTREATED CHILDREN

The Brain and the Corpus Callosum in Maltreated Children

In the developing brain, elevated levels of catecholamines and cortisol can lead to adverse brain development through the mechanisms of "premature aging" or accelerated loss (or metabolism) of neurons,[44-47] delays in myelination,[48] abnormalities in developmentally appropriate pruning,[49] and/or the inhibition of neurogenesis.[50] Furthermore, stress decreases brain-derived neurotrophic factor expression.[51] Thus, the stress of child maltreatment can have adverse influences on children's brain maturation.

Myelinated areas of the brain appear particularly susceptible to the effects of early exposure to significantly elevated levels of stress biochemicals. Magnetic resonance imaging (MRI) methods are noninvasive, safe methods of observing and measuring grey and white matter brain structure, brain development, and brain function in children. MRI procedures have allowed comparison of the brain structures of healthy children to those exposed to maltreatment. This field of study is new and is limited to the study of maltreated children with PTSD symptoms. A handful of published studies indicate that adverse brain development might be a consequence of maltreatment resulting in PTSD or subthreshold symptoms of PTSD (i.e., nonspecific symptoms of anxiety and depression).[52]

Teicher et al[53] provided the initial data that suggested early childhood trauma had a deleterious effect on the development of the corpus callosum, a brain structure that anatomically and functionally connects the cerebral hemispheres. The size of the corpus callosum was affected by early adverse experience, and this effect appeared to be gender dependent. These researchers found a reduction in the middle portion of the corpus callosum in children who were hospitalized at psychiatric facilities with documented histories of abuse or neglect, as compared with psychiatric controls. These findings were more significant in males. Sanchez and colleagues[54] used structural brain MRI to study global brain differences in maternally deprived rhesus monkeys. These monkeys had a reduction in the midsagittal size of the corpus callosum, in parallel to a decrease in white (but not grey) matter volume, in the prefrontal and parietal cortices. These decreases occurred in parallel with cognitive impairments.

Imaging methods were used to examine structural differences in 44 maltreated children and adolescents with PTSD as compared with 61 age- and sex-matched controls. Many of the maltreated subjects in this study suffered from sexual abuse, and witnessing domestic violence was a common secondary form of abuse. Decreased total midsagittal area of the corpus callosum and enlarged right, left, and total lateral ventricles were seen in PTSD-diagnosed subjects compared with controls.[21] Male children with PTSD had smaller measurements of the corpus callosum, and a trend for smaller total brain volume than female children with PTSD. These findings suggested that males may be more vulnerable to the effects of severe stress on brain structures than females, although adverse effects were found in both genders. In addition, it was noted that the intracranial volume was decreased by 7%, and total brain volume by 8%, in PTSD subjects compared with controls. Earlier onset of abuse and longer duration of abuse correlated with smaller intracranial volume. Furthermore, smaller intracranial volumes and smaller total corpus callosum area were associated with elevated PTSD symptoms of reexperiencing, avoidance, and hyperarousal, as well as with elevated dissociative symptoms. These findings not only suggested adverse brain development in patients with maltreatment-related PTSD, but also indicated that adverse effects might be greater with abuse exposure in early childhood. The correlation of lower intracranial volume with longer duration of abuse also suggested that recurrent and chronic abuse might have a cumulative, harmful effect on brain development.

Another study reported that children with PTSD or subthreshold PTSD showed smaller total brain and cerebral volumes when compared with healthy age- and gender-matched archival controls.[24] In addition, attenuation of frontal lobe asymmetry in maltreated children with PTSD symptoms was observed. These findings were consistent with the earlier work.[21]

De Bellis[55] replicated this work in another study of 28 psychotropic-naïve children and adolescents with maltreatment-related PTSD. The PTSD subjects showed smaller intracranial, cerebral cortex, prefrontal cortex, prefrontal cortical white matter, and right temporal lobe volumes in comparison with 66 sociodemographically matched healthy controls. Compared with these carefully matched controls, subjects with PTSD had decreased areas of the corpus callosum and in subregions 2, 4, 5, 6, and 7, and larger frontal lobe cerebrospinal fluid volumes than controls, even after adjustment for total cerebral volume. Midsagittal divisions of the corpus callosum for quantitative MRI measurements include: Region 1 (rostrum), which reflects the orbital prefrontal and inferior premotor cortical brain structures; Region 2 (genu), which reflects the prefrontal cortical brain structures; Region 3 (rostral body), which reflects the premotor and supplementary motor cortical regions; Region 4 (anterior midbody), which reflects the cortical motor regions; Region 5 (posterior midbody), which reflects the somatesthetic and association posterior parietal regions; Region 5 (isthmus), which reflects the superior temporal and association posterior parietal regions; and Region 6 (splenium), which reflects the occipital, inferior temporal cortical regions and subcorticol limbic system.[21] Total brain volume positively correlated with age of onset of the trauma that caused PTSD (i.e., smaller volumes with earlier onset of trauma) and negatively correlated with duration of abuse (i.e., longer duration of abuse with smaller volumes). A significant gender-by-group interaction was found, with maltreated males with PTSD having larger ventricular volumes than maltreated females with PTSD (Figure 53-1).

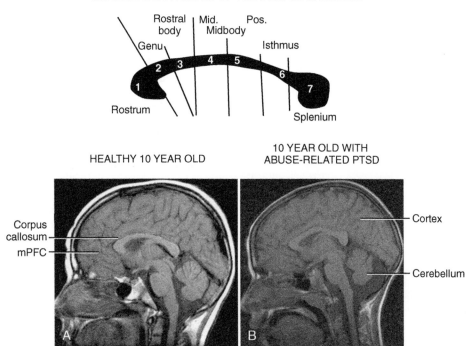

FIGURE 53-1 The midsagittal divisions of the corpus callosum, and **(A)** a midsagittal MRI of a healthy nonmaltreated 10-year-old boy compared with **(B)** a medically healthy maltreated 10-year-old boy with PTSD. Smaller cerebral area, corpus callosum, and cerebellar vermis can be seen in these comparisons. *mPFC*, Medial prefrontal cortex.

In a secondary analyses of sex differences in the published data of De Bellis et al,[52] findings of larger prefrontal lobe cerebrospinal fluid volumes and smaller midsagittal area of the corpus callosum subregion 7 (splenium) were seen in both boys and girls with maltreatment-related PTSD compared with their gender-matched comparison subjects. This finding suggests prefrontal deficits in maltreated children with PTSD, a finding similar to the data in adult PTSD.[56] Child subjects with PTSD did not show the normal age-related increases in the area of the total corpus callosum and its region 7 (splenium) compared with nonmaltreated subjects, indicating deficits in myelination in these maltreated children. This latter finding is similar to the work in nonhuman primates.

Interestingly, results of this study indicated that the absence of normal age-related increases in the area of the corpus callosum was more prominent in males with PTSD.[52] Significant sex-by-group effects demonstrated more adverse effects in brain maturation of boys compared with girls with maltreatment-related PTSD. These sex differences were seen despite the fact that boys and girls experienced similar types and durations of maltreatments.[52] Similarly, in a sociological prospective study of neglected children, maltreated males were also found to be more vulnerable than maltreated females as adults.[6] In both of these studies, maltreated males were more likely to show antisocial behaviors on follow-up.

On the other hand, 58 psychotropic-naïve maltreated boys and girls had smaller cerebellar volumes when compared with two groups of pediatric subjects who had no DSM-IV criteria A trauma histories: (1) 13 with pediatric generalized anxiety disorder, and (2) 98 healthy nonabused children and adolescents.[57] The cerebellum is involved in motor activity and in emotional and cognitive development, particularly executive functions.[58] In this study, cerebellar volumes positively correlated with age of onset of the trauma that lead to maltreatment related PTSD and negatively correlated with the duration of the abuse that led to PTSD.[57] Since there were no significant findings of sex by group interactions, the examination of sex differences in abused and neglect children is complex but an important aid to our understanding of this field. (See Figure 53-1.)

The Limbic System of Maltreated Individuals

The term *limbic system* is commonly used to designate a collection of subcortical and cortical brain regions that serve critical roles in emotion and memory. Brain regions commonly included in the limbic system include the amygdala, hippocampus, anterior thalamus, and anterior cingulate gyrus. As noted previously, the amygdala plays a key role in activating the stress response. Amygdala volumes are smaller in maltreated children compared with healthy nonmaltreated children, but this difference was not significant when controlling for brain size.[21,55]

To date, there are no published studies of amygdala function in maltreated children. Findings in traumatized adults, however, are consistent with behavioral findings in studies using tasks that depend on amygdala function, including the findings of exaggerated startle responses[59-62] and enhanced fear conditioning[63,64] in individuals with PTSD. Adults with PTSD resulting from childhood sexual abuse compared with healthy nonabused controls exhibit exaggerated amygdala activation during the acquisition of classically conditioned fear responses.[65] In addition to group differences associated with the PTSD diagnosis, amygdala activation was positively correlated with PTSD symptom severity. In a functional MRI (fMRI) study of adults with PTSD subsequent to physical/sexual assault, PTSD symptom severity was positively correlated with activation in the left amygdala for the contrast of brain activation to trauma-related vs. nonrelated words.[66] Given the amygdala's role in processing novelty, fear, and emotional memory, this is an area of developmental neuroscience that needs to be examined in maltreated children.

The hippocampus contains abundant cortisol receptors.[33] Normative levels of cortisol are necessary for the health and proper functioning of the hippocampus.[67] However, preclinical studies with animals have shown that both excess exposure to endogenous (via stressors) and exogenous corticosteroids lead to hippocampal damage including atrophy of dendritic processes, impaired neurogenesis, decreased resilience of neurons to insult, and neuronal death if exposure is high enough.[33,68] Several structural neuroimaging studies have found that male and female adults with chronic PTSD from various traumas including combat, childhood sexual abuse, and other traumas show smaller hippocampal volumes than healthy controls,[69-76] although not all studies have found this effect.[77] Consistent with the structural MRI findings, magnetic resonance spectroscopy (MRS) studies, a brain imaging technique that allows examination of biochemical markers of neuronal health, also found that chronic PTSD is associated with impaired neural integrity in the hippocampus as indexed by lower N-acetylaspartate/creatine ratios (NAA/Cr) in adults with PTSD compared with controls.[78-82]

In contrast to the findings in adults, several studies found that children and adolescents with PTSD resulting from maltreatment do not show decreased hippocampal volumes compared with healthy, nonabused control children.[5,21,24,55] A 2-year pilot study of nine children with PTSD and nine carefully matched healthy controls found that hippocampal volumes did not differ at baseline nor at 2-year follow-up.[5] In a follow-up study that combined data across several previous studies,[83] the authors found that in contrast to findings with adults, children and adolescents with PTSD compared with healthy nonabused controls exhibited larger hippocampal volumes after controlling for total cerebral volumes. Interestingly, hippocampal volumes were also positively correlated both with age of onset of trauma and with parent-rated behavior problems, although one would predict that age of onset of trauma and parent-rated behavior problems would show opposite correlations with behavior problems.

Findings of increased hippocampal volume after controlling for cerebral volumes might reflect that the developing brain of the maltreated child is more globally sensitive to stress compared with the mature adult brain. Larger hippocampal volumes in the immediate aftermath of trauma may reflect a "scarring" process reflecting a relative gain of glial processes compared with dendritic processes and that, over the course of maturation, this may actually result in decreased hippocampal volumes as these additional glial processes are pruned. The hippocampus is important for the proper functioning of biological stress systems and memory, particularly contextual memory. Given the discrepancy between the child and adult literature, additional research, particularly longitudinal work, is needed to clarify the relation between hippocampal development during childhood and PTSD.

The Medial Prefrontal Cortex of Maltreated Individuals

The mPFC exerts inhibitory control over activation of the amygdala and the stress response. The evidence from functional and structural neuroimaging suggests that child maltreatment and combat-related PTSD are associated with impaired functioning of the mPFC, particularly the anterior cingulate region.

PTSD symptoms, particularly reexperiencing symptoms of the trauma, are hypothesized to stem from conditioned fear learning.[16] The maintenance of these symptoms over time has been ascribed to a failure of extinction learning. Research in animals and humans has shown that extinction learning is associated with activity in the mPFC,[84,85] a region that includes the anterior cingulate cortex (ACC) and medial frontal gyrus. Functional neuroimaging studies using positron emission tomography (PET), single photon emission computed tomography (SPECT), and fMRI of mPFC functioning in adults with PTSD have found that symptom provocation via audiotaped trauma scripts,[86-91] cues for traumatic memories,[92] and aversive stimuli[93,94] are all associated with relative decreases in mPFC activity in adults with PTSD compared with healthy controls. In addition, women with PTSD from childhood sexual abuse exhibit relatively less mPFC activity during extinction learning of conditioned fear responses than nonabused healthy women.[65] Similarly, functional neuroimaging studies using the emotional Stroop task—a test that is sensitive to functioning of the ACC[95] and examines how emotional stimuli interfere with simple cognitive tasks—have found evidence for decreased ACC activity in adults with PTSD resulting from childhood sexual abuse.[96] Along with group differences between traumatized individuals with and without PTSD, several studies have found a negative correlation between mPFC activation and PTSD symptom severity.[90]

One potential mechanism for the relative hyporesponsivity of the anterior cingulate in PTSD is stress-related impairments in neural integrity of this region. In a study using MRS, children and adolescents with PTSD resulting from child maltreatment compared with demographically matched controls exhibited lower NAA/Cr in the ACC, which suggests neuronal loss in this region.[97] Compromised integrity of anterior cingulate was shown in adults with PTSD both in an MRS study that found decreased NAA/Cr ratios,[80] and in three structural MRI studies that found decreased volume in pregenual anterior cingulate,[98] right anterior cingulate,[99] and left anterior cingulate.[100] Given these findings, it is reasonable to speculate that maltreated children may show dysfunction of the mPFC, a large brain area important for executive functions such as problem-solving and future planning, emotional and behavioral control, and inhibition of the stress response.

THE COGNITIVE FUNCTION OF MALTREATED CHILDREN

A growing body of literature has documented the adverse effects of maltreatment on children's neurocognitive development including intellectual impairment, verbal deficiencies, and poor school performance. A literature review suggests that low intellectual ability, as reflected by low IQ scores, can be a consequence of child abuse. Poor school performance is consistently reported in abused children not evaluated for PTSD, including negative correlation between Verbal IQ score and severity of abuse. (For a review of this topic, see De Bellis et al[4]) In a well-controlled prospective study of early onset abuse or neglect (before age 11 years), lower IQ and reading ability were reported in a large sample of adult survivors of child maltreatment.[101] In a pilot study of children with maltreatment-related PTSD, more deficits in attention and abstract reasoning/executive functions were seen than in a group of socio-demographically matched controls.[102] These children demonstrated deficits on measures designed to assess frontal executive functioning (e.g., Wisconsin Card Sorting Test, Controlled Oral Word Association Test), and they were more susceptible to distraction, showed higher rates of impulsivity, and exhibited greater problems with sustained attention. In a brain imaging study, Verbal IQ, Performance IQ, and Full Scale IQ negatively correlated with duration of child abuse that led to PTSD in maltreated children.[21]

Koenen et al[103] extended these findings by focusing specifically on the relationship between exposure to domestic violence and cognitive/intellectual ability as measured by IQ. This large-scale twin study, which used 1116 monozygotic and dizygotic 5-year-old twin pairs, was aimed at assessing whether domestic violence had environmentally mediated effects on young children's intelligence. Domestic violence was associated with a negative effect on IQ in a dose-dependent fashion. Children exposed to high levels of domestic violence had IQ scores eight points lower than children who were not exposed, as measured by an abbreviated version of the Wechsler Preschool and Primary Scale of Intelligence-Revised. This effect did not differ by gender. This study revealed that domestic violence is linked to an environmental effect on suppression of children's IQ that is independent of possible confounding genetic effects on IQ. Moreover, this environmental effect was specific to domestic violence as it persisted after controlling for other maltreatment. It is critical to characterize the cognitive functioning of maltreated children, so that specialized therapeutic interventions (e.g., educational) can be designed for maltreated children.

GENETIC CONTRIBUTIONS TO OUTCOMES IN MALTREATED CHILDREN: GENE AND ENVIRONMENT INTERACTIONS

Recently, researchers have examined the interaction of genetic variables with early life stress to understand why some children experience adverse emotional and behavioral outcomes associated with child maltreatment whereas others do not. Two genes have been of particular interest in this regard over the past decade: the monoamine oxidase A (MAOA) gene and the serotonin transporter (5-HTT) gene. Two variants of these genes—a short, less active allele and a long, more active allele—have been the focus of research examining gene-by-environment interactions (G × E) with respect to depression and antisocial behavior.[104]

Serotonin is a critical element of the stress response system in that it plays important roles in the regulation of emotions (e.g., mood) and behavior (e.g., aggression, impulsivity).[18] The serotonin transporter protein is involved in the reuptake of serotonin from the synapse and is therefore critical to serotonin regulation in the brain.[4] The short allele of the serotonin transporter gene promoter polymorphism (5-HTTLPR) has been found to interact with maltreatment in the development of depression. Kaufman et al[105] found that children who were homozygous for the short allele of 5-HTTPR demonstrated a significantly elevated vulnerability to depression, but only in the presence of maltreatment.[105] Early use of alcohol was predicted by an interaction of the short alleles of 5-HTTLPR and maltreatment.[106]

The MAOA gene codes for an enzyme that selectively degrades the biogenic amines dopamine, serotonin, and norepinephrine after reuptake from the synaptic cleft, and through this mechanism influences behavioral regulation.[107] A recent metaanalysis of five published studies revealed that the association between early family adversity (particularly between neglect or physical abuse) and antisocial behavior was significantly stronger in boys with the short version of the MAOA gene, suggesting that this variant of the MAOA genotype confers greater vulnerability.[108] An extension of these findings in 7-year-old boys found an association between physical abuse and the short MAOA allele with a more general index of mental health problems, and particularly with a specific index of attentional problems and hyperactivity.[108] In addition, adolescent boys with the short MAOA allele who were exposed to maltreatment or poor-quality family relations were found to exhibit more alcohol-related problems than maltreated boys with the longer MAOA allele.[109] Further, women with a history of sexual abuse and the short MAOA allele were more likely to demonstrate alcoholism and antisocial personality disorder than were women with a history of sexual abuse and the long allele.[110]

In summary, individuals who are homozygous for the short allele of the 5-HTTLPR or the MAOA gene may be more vulnerable to mental health problems when exposed to child abuse and neglect. Early prevention and interventions for at-risk children with these genetic vulnerabilities are important ethical issues in the field of developmental traumatology and public health policy.

MALTREATMENT IS A TRAUMATIC STRESSOR: THE STRENGTH OF THE EVIDENCE

Research has clearly demonstrated that childhood maltreatment is associated with psychopathology in both childhood and adulthood. Given that the corpus of the literature indicates that age of onset and duration of maltreatment has repeatedly been shown to be associated in a dose-related fashion to a variety of poor psychological outcomes, elevated biological stress measures, and adverse brain and cognitive function, the strength of the evidence is formidable. Although genetic vulnerability exists, this vulnerability is moderated by child abuse and neglect experiences and is not predetermined.[103,105]

THE NEUROBIOLOGY OF HOPE FOR MALTREATED CHILDREN

We have outlined the effects of maltreatment on biological stress systems and brain development that have the potential to contribute to a life of depression, dissociation, numbing, substance-use disorders, and a lack of empathy, which can, in turn, lead to the continuation of the intergenerational cycle of maltreatment. Social supports and interventions, however, can free a victim to heal from their traumas and to lead a life characterized by resilience. Evidence-based treatments for PTSD symptoms attenuate depressive and externalizing symptoms, and PTSD screenings can easily be performed by health care providers.[111] Alternative mind–body medical treatments[112] might also reverse the effects of biological stress system dysregulation and lessen the potential harmful effects of trauma symptoms to an individual and society.

Particularly hopeful is evidence that the presence of strong social supports in genetically vulnerable children with maltreatment (i.e., those with two short 5-HTTLPR alleles) might reduce depression scores to levels only slightly above those of nonmaltreated children with the same genotype.[105] The researchers reporting these findings later extended them to demonstrate that the met allele of the brain-derived neurotrophic factor (BDNF) interacted with the short alleles of 5-HTTLPR to confer the highest vulnerability to depression in maltreated children, but that again the availability of social support moderated this risk.[113] Thus, there is growing evidence to suggest that early interventions can decrease the intergenerational transmission of PTSD and violence.

RESEARCH: FUTURE DIRECTIONS

Approximately one third of maltreated children grow up to repeat the cycle of abuse and neglect.[114] This is further buttressed by the findings that the majority of parents whose children are maltreated also have their own personal history of abuse and/or neglect.[115] Consequently, more research needs to be done to understand the neurobiology of risk and resilience in children of parents with histories of maltreatment. It would be cost-effective to develop and target specific interventions to at-risk children (i.e., those with parents with histories of maltreatment who have current psychopathlogy). Future research should not only focus on genetics and imaging techniques, but also on appropriate screening and engagement techniques and effective interventions for prospective parents who are at risk of maltreating their child.

References

1. Kaplan SJ, Pelcovitz D, Labruna V: Child and adolescent abuse and neglect research: a review of the past 10 years. Part I: physical and emotional abuse and neglect. *J Am Acad Child Adolesc Psychiatry* 1999;38:1214-1222.
2. De Bellis MD: Developmental traumatology: a contributory mechanism for alcohol and substance use disorders. *Psychoneuroendocrinology* 2002;27:155-170.

3. Felitti VJ, Anda RF, Nordenberg D, et al: Relationship of childhood abuse and household dysfunction to many of the leading causes of death in adults—the adverse childhood experiences (ACE) study. *Am J Prev Med* 1998;14:245-258.

4. De Bellis MD: Developmental traumatology: the psychobiological development of maltreated children and its implications for research, treatment, and policy. *Dev Psychopathol* 2001;13:539-564.

5. De Bellis MD, Hall J, Boring AM, et al: A pilot longitudinal study of hippocampal volumes in pediatric maltreatment-related posttraumatic stress disorder. *Biol Psychiatry* 2001;50:305-309.

6. McGloin JM, Widom CS: Resilience among abused and neglected children grown up. *Dev Psychopathol* 2001;13:1021-1038.

7. Flores E, Cicchetti D, Rogosch FA: Predictors of resilience in maltreated and nonmaltreated Latino children. *Dev Psychol* 2005; 41:338-351.

8. Masten AS, Wright MOD: Cumulative risk and protection models of child maltreatment. *J Aggress Maltreat Trauma* 1998;2:7-30.

9. De Bellis MD, Van Dillen T: Childhood post-traumatic stress disorder: an overview. *Child Adolesc Psychiatry Clin North Am* 2005; 14:745-772.

10. LeDoux J: Fear and the brain: where have we been, and where are we going? *Biol Psychiatry* 1998;44:1229-1238.

11. Herman JP, Ostrander MM, Mueller NK, et al: Limbic system mechanisms of stress regulation: hypothalamo-pituitary-adrenocortical axis. *Prog Neuropsychopharmacol Biol Psychiatry* 2005;29:1201-1213.

12. Glaser D: Child abuse and neglect and the brain—a review. *J Child Psychol Psychiatry* 2000;41:97-116.

13. Chrousos GP, Gold PW: The concepts of stress and stress system disorders—overview of physical and behavioral homeostasis. *JAMA* 1992;267:1244-1252.

14. Porges SW, Doussard-Roosevelt JA, Maita AK: Vagal tone and the physiological regulation of emotion. *Monogr Soc Res Child Dev* 1994;59:167-186, 250-283.

15. Tsigos C, Chrousos GP: Hypothalamic-pituitary-adrenal axis, neuroendocrine factors and stress. *J Psychosom Res* 2002;53:865-871.

16. Charney DS, Deutch AY, Krystal JH, et al: Psychobiologic mechanisms of posttraumatic-stress-disorder. *Arch Gen Psychiatry* 1993; 50:294-306.

17. Lang PJ, Davis M, Ohman A: Fear and anxiety: animal models and human cognitive psychophysiology. *J Affect Disord* 2000; 61:137-159.

18. De Bellis MD: The neurobiology of PTSD across the life cycle. *In:* Soares JC, Gershon S (eds): *The Handbook of Medical Psychiatry.* Marcel Dekker, New York, 2003, pp 449-466.

19. Sanchez MM, Ladd CO, Plotsky PM: Early adverse experience as a developmental risk factor for later psychopathology: evidence from rodent and primate models. *Dev Psychopathol* 2001;13:419-449.

20. Bremner JD, Licinio J, Darnell A, et al: Elevated CSF corticotropin-releasing factor concentrations in posttraumatic stress disorder. *Am J Psychiatry* 1997;154:624-629.

21. De Bellis MD, Keshavan MS, Clark DB, et al: A.E. Bennett Research Award. Developmental traumatology: II. Brain development. *Biol Psychiatry* 1999;45:1271-1284.

22. De Bellis MD, Lefter L, Trickett PK, et al: Urinary catecholamine excretion in sexually abused girls. *J Am Acad Child Adolesc Psychiatry* 1994;33:320-327.

23. Cicchetti D, Rogosch FA: The impact of child maltreatment and psychopathology on neuroendocrine functioning. *Devel Psychopathol* 2001;13:783-804.

24. Carrion VG, Weems CF, Eliez S, et al: Attenuation of frontal asymmetry in pediatric posttraumatic stress disorder. *Biol Psychiatry* 2001; 50:943-951.

25. Gunnar MR, Morison SJ, Chisholm K, et al: Salivary cortisol levels in children adopted from Romanian orphanages. *Devel Psychopathol* 2001;13:611-628.

26. De Bellis MD, Chrousos GP, Dorn LD, et al: Hypothalamic-pituitary-adrenal axis dysregulation in sexually abused girls. *J Clin Endocrinol Metab* 1994;78:249-255.

27. Baker DG, West SA, Nicholson WE, et al: Serial CSF corticotropin-releasing hormone levels and adrenocortical activity in combat veterans with posttraumatic stress disorder. *Am J Psychiatry* 1999; 156:585-588.

28. Chrousos GP, Gold PW: The concepts of stress and stress system disorders: overview of physical and behavioral homeostasis. *JAMA* 1992;267:1244-1252.

29. Kaufman J, Birmaher B, Perel J, et al: The corticotropin-releasing hormone challenge in depressed abused, depressed nonabused, and normal control children. *Biol Psychiatry* 1997;42:669-679.

30. Heim C, Newport DJ, Wagner D, et al: The role of early adverse experience and adulthood stress in the prediction of neuroendocrine stress reactivity in women: a multiple regression analysis. *Depress Anxiety* 2002;15:117-125.

31. Francis DD, Meaney MJ: Maternal care and the development of stress responses. *Curr Opin Neurobiol* 1999;9:128-134.

32. Perry BD, Giller EL, Southwick SM: Altered platelet alpha-2-adrenergic binding-sites in posttraumatic-stress-disorder. *Am J Psychiatry* 1987;144:1511-1512.

33. McEwen BS: The neurobiology and neuroendocrinology of stress. Implications for post-traumatic stress disorder from a basic science perspective. *Psychiatr Clin North Am* 2002;25:469-694.

34. De Bellis MD, Burke L, Trickett PK, et al: Antinuclear antibodies and thyroid function in sexually abused girls. *J Trauma Stress* 1996;9:369-378.

35. Pfefferbaum A, Mathalon DH, Sullivan EV, et al: A quantitative magnetic resonance imaging study of changes in brain morphology from infancy to late adulthood. *Arch Neurol* 1994;34:71-75.

36. Jernigan TL, Sowell ER (eds): *Magnetic Resonance Imaging Studies of the Developing Brain.* Cambridge University Press, Cambridge, UK, 1997.

37. Thompson PM, Giedd JN, Woods RP, et al: Growth patterns in the developing brain detected by using continuum mechanical tensor maps. *Nature* 2000;404:190-193.

38. Giedd JN, Snell JW, Lange N, et al: Quantitative magnetic resonance imaging of human brain development: ages 4-18. *Cereb Cortex* 1996;6: 551-560.

39. Paus T, Collins DL, Evans AC, et al: Maturation of white matter in the human brain: a review of magnetic resonance studies. *Brain Res Bull* 2001;54:255-266.

40. Giedd JN, Vaituzis AC, Hamburger SD, et al: Quantitative MRI of the temporal lobe, amygdala, and hippocampus in normal human development: ages 4-18. *J Comp Neurol* 1996;366:223-230.

41. Alexander GE, Goldman PS: Functional development of the dorsolateral prefrontal cortex: an analysis utilizing reversible cryogenic depression. *Brain Res* 1978;143:233-249.

42. McEwen BS: Neural gonadal steroid actions. *Science* 1981; 211:1303-1311.

43. De Bellis MD, Keshavan MS, Beers SR, et al: Sex differences in brain maturation during childhood and adolescence. *Cereb Cortex* 2001;11:552-557.

44. Edwards E, Harkins K, Wright G, et al: Effects of bilateral adrenalectomy on the induction of learned helplessness. *Behav Neuropsychopharm* 1990;3:109-114.

45. Sapolsky RM: Glucocorticoids and hippocampal atrophy in neuropsychiatric disorders. *Arch Gen Psychiatry* 2000;57:925-935.

46. Simantov R, Blinder E, Ratovitski T, et al: Dopamine induced apoptosis in human neuronal cells: inhibition by nucleic acids antisense to the dopamine transporter. *Neuroscience* 1996;74:39-50.

47. Smythies JR: Oxidative reactions and schizophrenia: a review-discussion. *Schizophrenia Res* 1997;24:357-364.

48. Dunlop SA, Archer MA, Quinlivan JA, et al: Repeated prenatal corticosteroids delay myelination in the ovine central nervous system. *J Matern Fetal Med* 1997;6:309-313.

49. Todd RD. Neural development is regulated by classical neurotransmitters: dopamine D_2 receptor stimulation enhances neurite outgrowth. *Biol Psychiatry* 1992;31:794-807.

50. Tanapat P, Galea LA, Gould E. Stress inhibits the proliferation of granule cell precursors in the developing dentate gyrus. *Int J Dev Neurosci* 1998;16:235-239.

51. Smith MA, Makino S, Kvetnansky R, et al: Effects of stress on neurotrophic factor expression in the rat brain. *Ann NY Acad Sci* 1995;771:234-239.

52. De Bellis MD, Keshavan MS: Sex differences in brain maturation in maltreatment related pediatric posttraumatic stress disorder. *Neurosci Biobehav Rev* 2003;27:103-117.

53. Teicher MH, Ito Y, Glod CA, et al: Preliminary evidence for abnormal cortical development in physically and sexually abused children using EEG coherence and MRI. *Ann A Y Acad Sci* 1997; 821:160-175.

54. Sanchez MM, Hearn EF, Do D, et al: Differential rearing affects corpus callosum size and cognitive function of rhesus monkeys. *Brain Res* 1998;812:38-49.

55. De Bellis MD, Keshavan MS, Shifflett H, et al: Brain structures in pediatric maltreatment-related posttraumatic stress disorder: a sociodemographically matched study. *Biol Psychiatry* 2002;52(11):1066-1078.

56. Rauch SL, Shin LM, Segal E, et al: Selectively reduced regional cortical volumes in post-traumatic stress disorder. *Neuroreport* 2003;14:913-916.

57. De Bellis MD, Kuchibhatla M: Cerebellar volumes in pediatric maltreatment-related posttraumatic stress disorder. *Biol Psychiatry* 2006;60:697-703.

58. Schmahmann JD: Disorders of the cerebellum: ataxia, dysmetria of thought, and the cerebellar cognitive affective syndrome. *J Neuropsychiatry Clin Neurosci* 2004;16:367-378.

59. Orr SP, Roth WT: Psychophysiological assessment: clinical applications for PTSD. *J Affect Disord* 2000;61:225-240.

60. Orr SP, Lasko NB, Metzger LJ, et al: Psychophysiologic assessment of women with posttraumatic stress disorder resulting from childhood sexual abuse. *J Consul Clin Psychol* 1998;66:906-913.

61. Keane TM, Kolb LC, Kaloupek DG, et al: Utility of psychophysiological measurement in the diagnosis of posttraumatic stress disorder: results from a Department of Veterans Affairs cooperative study. *J Consult Clin Psychol* 1998;66:914-923.

62. Orr SP, Pitman RK, Lasko NB, et al: Psychophysiological assessment of posttraumatic-stress-disorder imagery in World-War-II And Korean combat veterans. *J Abnorm Psychol* 1993;102:152-159.

63. Orr SP, Metzger LJ, Lasko NB, et al: De novo conditioning in trauma-exposed individuals with and without posttraumatic stress disorder. *J Abnorm Psychol* 2000;109:290-298.

64. Peri T, Ben-Shakhar G, Orr SP, et al: Psychophysiologic assessment of aversive conditioning in posttraumatic stress disorder. *Biol Psychiatry* 2000;47:512-519.

65. Bremner JD, Vermetten E, Schmahl C, et al: Positron emission tomographic imaging of neural correlates of a fear acquisition and extinction paradigm in women with childhood sexual-abuse-related post-traumatic stress disorder. *Psychol Med* 2005;35:791-806.

66. Protopopescu X, Pan H, Tuescher O, et al: Differential time courses and specificity of amygdala activity in posttraumatic stress disorder subjects and normal control subjects. *Biol Psychiatry* 2005;57:464-473.

67. Diamond DM, Bennett MC, Fleshner M, et al: Inverted-U relationship between the level of peripheral corticosterone and the magnitude of hippocampal primed burst potentiation. *Hippocampus* 1992;2:421-430.

68. Sapolsky RM: Atrophy of the hippocampus in posttraumatic stress disorder: How and when? *Hippocampus* 2001;11:90-91.

69. Stein MB, Koverola C, Hanna C, et al: Hippocampal volume in women victimized by childhood sexual abuse. *Psychol Med* 1997;27:951-959.

70. Bremner JD, Vythilingam M, Vermetten E, et al: MRI and PET study of deficits in hippocampal structure and function in women with childhood sexual abuse and posttraumatic stress disorder. *Am J Psychiatry* 2003;160:924-932.

71. Bremner JD, Randall P, Scott TM, et al: MRI-based measurement of hippocampal volume in patients with combat-related posttraumatic-stress-disorder. *Am J Psychiatry* 1995;152:973-981.

72. Gurvits TV, Shenton ME, Hokama H, et al: Magnetic resonance imaging study of hippocampal volume in chronic, combat-related posttraumatic stress disorder. *Biol Psychiatry* 1996;40:1091-1099.

73. Schuff N, Marmar CR, Weiss DS, et al: Reduced hippocampal volume and *N*-acetyl aspartate in posttraumatic stress disorder. In: Yehuda R (ed): *Psychobiology of Posttraumatic Stress Disorder*. New York Academy of Sciences, New York, 1997, pp 516-520.

74. Bremner JD, Randall P, Vermetten E, et al: Magnetic resonance imaging-based measurement of hippocampal volume in posttraumatic stress disorder related to childhood physical and sexual abuse—a preliminary report. *Biol Psychiatry* 1997;41:23-32.

75. Lindauer RJL, Vlieger EJ, Jalink M, et al. Smaller hippocampal volume in Dutch police officers with posttraumatic stress disorder. *Biol Psychiatry* 2004;56:356-363.

76. Lindauer RJL, Olff M, van Meijel EPM, et al: Cortisol, learning, memory, and attention in relation to smaller hippocampal volume in police officers with posttraumatic stress disorder. *Biol Psychiatry* 2006;59:171-177.

77. Fennema-Notestine C, Stein MB, Kennedy CM, et al: Brain morphometry in female victims of intimate partner violence with and without posttraumatic stress disorder. *Biol Psychiatry* 2002;52:1089-1101.

78. Brown S, Freeman T, Kimbrell T, et al. In vivo proton magnetic resonance spectroscopy of the medial temporal lobes of former prisoners of war with and without posttraumatic stress disorder. *J Neuropsychiatry Clin Neurosci* 2003;15:367-370.

79. Freeman T, Cardwell D, Karson CN, et al: In vivo proton magnetic resonance spectroscopy of the medial temporal lobes of subjects with combat-related posttraumatic stress disorder. *Magn Reson Med* 1998;40:66-71.

80. Mahmutyazicioglu K, Konuk N, Ozdemir H, et al: Evaluation of the hippocampus and the anterior cingulate gyrus by proton MR spectroscopy in patients with post-traumatic stress disorder. *Diagn Interv Radiol* 2005;11:125-129.

81. Menon PM, Nashrallah HA, Lyons JA, et al: Single-voxel proton MR spectroscopy of right versus left hippocampi in PTSD. *Psychiatry Res Neuroimaging* 2003;123:101-108.

82. Schuff N, Neylan TC, Lenoci MA, et al: Decreased hippocampal *N*-acetylaspartate in the absence of atrophy in posttraumatic stress disorder. *Biol Psychiatry* 2001;50:952-959.

83. Tupler LA, De Bellis MD: Segmented hippocampal volume in children and adolescents with posttraumatic stress disorder. *Biol Psychiatry* 2006;59:523-529.

84. Milad MR, Quirk GJ: Neurons in medial prefrontal cortex signal memory for fear extinction. *Nature* 2002;420:70-74.

85. Phelps EA, Delgado MR, Nearing KI, et al: Extinction learning in humans: role of the amygdala and vmPFC. *Neuron* 2004;43:897-905.

86. Britton JC, Phan KL, Taylor SF, et al: Corticolimbic blood flow in posttraumatic stress disorder during script-driven imagery. *Biol Psychiatry* 2005;57:832-840.

87. Lanius RA, Williamson PC, Densmore M, et al: Neural correlates of traumatic memories in posttraumatic stress disorder: a functional MRI investigation. *Am J Psychiatry* 2001;158:1920-1922.

88. Lanius RA, Williamson PC, Hopper J, et al: Recall of emotional states in posttraumatic stress disorder: an fMRI investigation. *Biol Psychiatry* 2003;53:204-210.

89. Shin LM, McNally RJ, Kosslyn SM, et al: Regional cerebral blood flow during script-driven imagery in childhood sexual abuse-related PTSD: a PET investigation. *Am J Psychiatry* 1999;156:575-584.

90. Shin LM, Orr SP, Carson MA, et al: Regional cerebral blood flow in the amygdala and medial prefrontal cortex during traumatic imagery in male and female Vietnam veterans with PTSD. *Arch Gen Psychiatry* 2004;61:168-176.

91. Lindauer RJL, Booij J, Habraken JBA, et al: Cerebral blood flow changes during script-driven imagery in police officers with posttraumatic stress disorder. *Biol Psychiatry* 2004;56:853-861.

92. Bremner JD, Narayan M, Staib LH, et al: Neural correlates of memories of childhood sexual abuse in women with and without posttraumatic stress disorder. *Am J Psychiatry* 1999;156:1787-1795.

93. Bremner JD, Vythilingam M, Vermetten E, et al: Neural correlates of declarative memory for emotionally valenced words in women with posttraumatic stress disorder related to early childhood sexual abuse. *Biol Psychiatry* 2003;53:879-889.

94. Shin LM, Wright CI, Cannistraro PA, et al: A functional magnetic resonance imaging study of amygdala and medial prefrontal cortex responses to overtly presented fearful faces in posttraumatic stress disorder. *Arch Gen Psychiatry* 2005;62:273-281.

95. Hamner MB, Lorberbaum JP, George MS: Potential role of the anterior cingulate cortex in PTSD: review and hypothesis. *Depress Anxiety* 1999;9:1-14.

96. Bremner JD, Vermetten E, Vythilingam M, et al: Neural correlates of the classic color and emotional stroop in women with abuse-related posttraumatic stress disorder. *Biol Psychiatry* 2004;55:612-620.

97. De Bellis MD, Keshavan MS, Spencer S, et al: *N*-acetylaspartate concentration in the anterior cingulate of maltreated children and adolescents with PTSD. *Am J Psychiatry* 2000;157:1175-1177.

98. Rauch SL, Shin LM, Segal E, et al: Selectively reduced regional cortical volumes in post-traumatic stress disorder. *Neuroreport* 2003;14:913-916.

99. Kitayama N, Quinn S, Bremner JD: Smaller volume of anterior cingulate cortex in abuse-related posttraumatic stress disorder. *J Affect Disord* 2006;90:171-174.

100. Yamasue H, Kasai K, Iwanami A, et al: Voxel-based analysis of MRI reveals anterior cingulate gray-matter volume reduction in post-

traumatic stress disorder due to terrorism. *Proc Natl Acad Sci U S A* 2003;100:9039-9043.

101. Perez C, Widom CS: Childhood victimization and long-term intellectual and academic outcomes. *Child Abuse Negl* 1994;18:617-633.

102. Beers SR, De Bellis MD: Neuropsychological function in children with maltreatment-related posttraumatic stress disorder. *Am J Psychiatry* 2002;159:483-486.

103. Koenen KC, Moffitt TE, Caspi A, et al: Domestic violence is associated with environmental suppression of IQ in young children. *Devel Psychopathol* 2003;15:297-311.

104. Cicchetti D, Rogosch FA, Sturge-Apple ML: Interactions of child maltreatment and serotonin transporter and monoamine oxidase A polymorphisms: depressive symptomatology among adolescents from low socioeconomic status backgrounds. *Devel Psychopathol* 2007; 19:1161-1180.

105. Kaufman J, Yang BZ, Douglas-Palumberi H, et al: Social supports and serotonin transporter gene moderate depression in maltreated children. *Proc Natl Acad Sci U S A* 2004;101:17316–17321.

106. Kaufman J, Yang BZ, Douglas-Palumberi H, et al: Genetic and environmental predictors of early alcohol use. *Biol Psychiatry* 2007;61:1228-1234.

107. Shih JC, Chen K, Ridd MJ: Monoamine oxidase: from genes to behavior. *Ann Rev Neurosci* 1999;22:197-217.

108. Kim-Cohen J, Caspi A, Taylor A, et al: MAOA, maltreatment, and gene–environment interaction predicting children's mental health: new evidence and a meta-analysis. *Mol Psychiatry* 2006;11:903-913.

109. Nilsson KW, Sjoberg RL, Wargelius HL, et al: The monoamine oxidase A (MAO-A) gene, family function and maltreatment as predictors of destructive behaviour during male adolescent alcohol consumption. *Addiction* 2007;102:389-398.

110. Ducci F, Enoch MA, Hodgkinson C, et al: Interaction between a functional MAOA locus and childhood sexual abuse predicts alcoholism and antisocial personality disorder in adult women. *Mol Psychiatry* 2008;13:334-347.

111. Cohen JA, Kelleher KK, Mannarino AP: Identifying, treating, and referring traumatized children: the role of pediatric providers. *Arch Pediatr Adoles Med* 2008;162:447-452.

112. Osuch E, Engel CC: Research on the treatment of trauma spectrum responses: the role of the optimal healing environment and neurobiology. *J Altern Complement Med* 2004;10(Suppl 1):S211-S221.

113. Kaufman J, Yang BZ, Douglas-Palumberi H, et al: Brain-derived neurotrophic factor-5-HTTLPR gene interactions and environmental modifiers of depression in children. *Biol Psychiatry* 2006;59:673-680.

114. Widom CS: The cycle of violence. *Science* 1989;244:160-166.

115. Kaufman J, Zigler E: Do abused children become abusive parents? *Am J Orthopsychiatry* 1987;57:186-192.

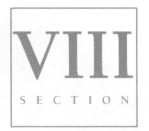

SECTION VIII

SPECIAL TOPICS

Christine E. Barron, MD,
and Carole Jenny, MD, MBA

54

SUBSTANCE ABUSE AND CHILD ABUSE

Rizwan Z. Shah, MD, and Kenneth McCann, MD, FAAP

HISTORICAL BACKGROUND

Association of child abuse and parental substance abuse is glimpsed in the works of William Shakespeare and in lithographic works of the early eighteenth century, well before Henry Kempe's article on battered child syndrome[1] brought attention to a problem that affects millions of children today. Reviews of the literature reveals a vast literature on psychosocial problems of children of alcoholics[2,3] and drug abusers.[4-7] Association of opiate addiction with parenting dysfunction and significant incident of abuse and neglect of children is reported in early child abuse journal publications.[5] Loretta Finnegan's work with infants of opiate-dependant mothers predates child abuse legislation in many states.[8] In the last 20 years, research has led to increased understanding of the relationship between child maltreatment and addiction. Substance abuse has increased in young adults of child-bearing age. In a 1999 report to Congress, the U.S. Department of Health and Human Services stated that between one third to two thirds of children in child welfare services were affected by parental substance abuse.[9]

During the last 5 years, federal legislative mandates have increased the involvement of the child protection system with addiction treatment services.[10] Similarly the Drug Endangered Children initiative[11] through the Office of National Drug Control Policy has increased the number of families involved in the child protection system.

SCOPE OF THE PROBLEM

Substance Abuse Among the Child-Rearing Population

In 2006, an estimated 20.4 million Americans over 11 years old were illicit substance users, with the highest rate among 18 to 20 year olds,[12] or over 8% of this population. Almost 20% of young adults ages 18 to 25 report illicit drug use, 16.3% using marijuana, 6.4% prescription drugs, 2.2% cocaine, and 1.7% hallucinogens. In all people over 11 years of age, males were more likely to use illicit drugs than females (10.5% vs. 6.2%). In youth ages 12 to 17, rates were similar for males and females (9.8% and 9.7%). Education was a factor in illicit substance use as well. Full-time college students used less than others in the same age group (19.2% vs. 22.6%).[12]

Illicit Substance Use and Pregnancy

According to the National Survey on Drug Use and Health (NSDUH) 2006 report,[12] 4% of pregnant women used illicit drugs and 9% used alcohol in the month prior to the survey. In addition, among pregnant women 15 to 44 years old, 11.8% reported current alcohol use, 2.9% binge drinking, and 0.7% heavy drinking. Chasnoff et al[13] studied more than 7800 pregnant women and found approximately one third had a positive drug or alcohol screen. Of pregnant women with a positive screen, 15% continued to use substances after learning of their pregnancy. NSDUH has estimated that past-month substance use is similar between new mothers and nonpregnant women. This report is concerning, since it implies new mothers are dealing with both the responsibilities and stresses of caring for a newborn while experiencing the impairments and negative effects of substance abuse.

Limitations of Available Data

Substance abuse prevalence data carry limitations, since it often relies on self-reports that are typically the "tip of the iceberg." Substance abuse carries both social stigma and the potential for negative legal consequences for the addict. Thus, substance abuse is often underreported.[14] For example, in a prospective study of more than 3000 children,[15] 43% of infants were positive for illicit substances, and of these, only 11% of their mothers reported illicit substance use. Another limitation in prevalence data on in utero exposure is that screening of newborns lacks standardized criteria. Currently, newborns are screened for illicit substance exposure at the discretion of hospital staff. This creates great variability in screening practices among hospitals.[14] Inconsistent screening practices could unfairly target minority women and women in poverty.[13]

COMMON ILLEGAL SUBSTANCES OF ABUSE

Marijuana

Marijuana is derived from the leaves of the hemp plant *Cannabis sativa*. It is a shredded green and brown mix of the plant's flowers, stems, seeds, and leaves.[16] The active chemical in marijuana is delta-9-tetrahydrocannabinol (THC). THC is passed from the lungs into the bloodstream. From the bloodstream, THC travels to the brain and other organs throughout the body. Marijuana is the most commonly abused illicit substance in the United States.[12,16] In 2006 marijuana was used by 72.8% of current illicit substance users, and exclusively used by 52.8% of these.[12]

Marijuana works on specific receptors in the brain that cause a cascade of reactions, resulting in the "high" that users experience. These receptors are located in the parts of the brain that influence pleasure, memory, thoughts, concentration, sensory and time perception, and coordinated movement. According to the National Institute on Drug Abuse (NIDA), "… marijuana intoxication can cause distorted perceptions, impaired coordination, difficulty in thinking and problem solving, and problems with learning and memory."[16]

Chronic marijuana use can cause problems in daily life and exacerbate other problems. Research has shown that chronic marijuana use impairs several important measures of life achievement including physical and mental health, cognitive abilities, social life, and career status. One way marijuana does this is by negatively affecting learning and memory.[16] According to the NIDA, these effects can last for days or weeks after the acute effects have worn off. Consequently, someone who uses marijuana daily can be constantly functioning at a suboptimal intellectual level.[16]

Many studies have shown chronic marijuana use to be associated with increased anxiety, depression, and suicidal ideation. Current evidence suggests a link between marijuana use and schizophrenia, especially when an acute psychotic reaction is precipitated in a vulnerable person after high doses of marijuana. The relationship between chronic marijuana use and mental illness blurs when considering cause and effect. One question is, does marijuana cause mental illness, or do mentally ill people use marijuana as a form of self-medication?[16]

Withdrawal symptoms following chronic marijuana use have reportedly included irritability, sleeplessness, decreased appetite, anxiety, and drug craving. These symptoms can begin 1 day after last marijuana use, peak symptoms occur at 2 to 3 days, and subside within 1 to 2 weeks of abstinence.[16]

Cocaine and Methamphetamine

Cocaine is a powerful stimulant derived from the leaves of the Coca plant. Cocaine can come in two forms: the powdered hydrochloride salt form, or a rock crystal called "crack."[17] "Crack" cocaine gets its name from the crackling sound it makes when heated. According to NSDUH,[12] in 2006 there were 977,000 people ages 12 and older who tried cocaine for the first time (about 2700 initiates per day). The average age of first use was 20.3 years. In 2006, there were 2.4 million current cocaine users.[12]

Cocaine is a strong central nervous system (CNS) stimulant. It works by blocking the reuptake of the chemical messenger dopamine. Dopamine is associated with pleasure and movement.[17] The euphoria reported by cocaine abusers is due to the nonstop stimulation of dopamine-receiving neurons. The "high" is affected by the rate of drug absorption, although rapid absorption also shortens the drug's duration of action. The high from snorting cocaine can last 15 to 30 minutes, whereas that from smoking lasts 5 to 10 minutes.[17] Other acute effects of cocaine use include reduced

hunger with resultant weight loss and reduced perceived need for sleep.

Cocaine binging, in which cocaine is used repeatedly in increasingly higher doses, can lead to irritability, restlessness, and paranoia. If continued, cocaine binging can lead to full-blown paranoid psychosis. Physical symptoms of chronic cocaine abuse can include malnourishment from chronic appetite suppression, cardiac disease, and destruction of the nasal septum for those who "snort" the drug.[17]

Cocaine use in conjunction with other substances poses additional hazards, especially when combined with alcohol. Research has shown that the human liver combines cocaine and alcohol to create a third substance, cocaethylene. Cocaethylene is postulated to increase the euphoria of the cocaine high, while potentially increasing the user's risk of sudden death.

Like cocaine, methamphetamine is a powerful CNS stimulant. Methamphetamine's effects are similar to cocaine, but the effects last longer and it costs less. Consequently, methamphetamine has been labeled the "poor man's cocaine." Methamphetamine is typically a white, odorless powder, but its appearance changes depending on how it is used. Methamphetamine can be "snorted," smoked, injected, or taken orally.

Methamphetamine can be manufactured using commonly obtained materials. The term "meth lab" is used for clandestine facilities that produce methamphetamine. In 2006, approximately 731,000 people in the United States aged 12 or older were users of methamphetamine, about 0.3% of the population.[12] Methamphetamine appears to be a substance commonly used by females. In one study, 45% of people admitted for methamphetamine abuse treatment were female.[19] In 2005 an estimated 1.3 million people aged 12 or older had used methamphetamine in the past year, and an estimated 556,000 (42%) were female.[19] The Iowa Case Management Project's analysis of 1095 clients in drug treatment showed females reported amphetamine as their substance of choice at a rate of 14%, twice the rate for male clients.[20] The study found that methamphetamine was favored by white females in their 20s.

Methamphetamine is similar to cocaine in that it blocks dopamine reuptake in the brain and produces a sense of increased alertness and euphoria. In addition, methamphetamine promotes the release of dopamine into the synaptic cleft.[21] Similar to cocaine, methamphetamine decreases fatigue and appetite. The reduced hunger can lead to weight loss, and the reduced perceived need for sleep can lead to difficulty sleeping and rapid onset of fatigue as the drug wears off. Methamphetamine users can sleep for extended periods when the drug's effects wear off, potentially leaving their children unattended or in the care of potential abusers for days. Methamphetamine also reduces thirst, which can lead to dehydration.

Methamphetamine also increases the user's sexual drive, which can lead to unsafe sex practices.[20] According to the U.S. Office for Victims of Crime, children who live with methamphetamine users often are exposed to pornographic materials or overt sexual activity.[22] Methamphetamine abuse is associated with poly-drug use, since users often use other sedating drugs such as marijuana to diminish the negative effects of the methamphetamine. This poly-drug concoction does not typically include alcohol, since users have reported that simultaneous methamphetamine and alcohol use causes an unpleasant taste.[20]

The users and the producers of methamphetamine are often the same people. As a result, the addict is subjected to the effects of the drug as well as the harmful effects of the "meth lab" environment.[23] Methamphetamine toxicity (from the drug itself as well as from by-products of its manufacture) can lead to myocardial infarction and stroke. The physical damage of chronic methamphetamine use is difficult to conceal. Skin lesions, such as excoriations and abrasions, can be seen in users picking off "meth bugs." These "bugs" are the result of methamphetamine-induced delusional parasitosis.[21,23] In addition, oral disease and dental decay ("meth mouth") is commonly seen among chronic users of the drug.[21] Dental lesions are the result of several different mechanisms, including chronic dry mouth, heavy sugar intake, and bruxism (teeth grinding) from sympathetic nervous system overstimulation.

According to the Department of Justice, parents and caregivers who are dependent on methamphetamine often become careless, irritable, and violent, and can lose their capacity to nurture their children.[22] While under the influence of methamphetamine, speech can become disorganized and difficult to understand, with abrupt shifts in thought.[20] When used chronically, the user can suffer from memory and learning impairment.[20,21] This cognitive impairment is especially obvious in areas of decision making. Chronic methamphetamine use disrupts normal sleep patterns and can cause paranoia, which can contribute to violent episodes while under the influence. Chronic use can lead to mood lability ranging from extreme depression to euphoria.[20] These negative effects intensify as the methamphetamine addict progresses through their binge-crash cycles, which last from 1 to 3 weeks.

Srisurapanont et al[24] examined 168 inpatients with methamphetamine psychosis in the United Kingdom, Australia, Japan, the Philippines, and Thailand. Their most common psychotic symptom (found in over 77% of patients) was persecutory delusions. This was followed by auditory hallucinations (over 44%), strange or unusual beliefs, and "thought reading." Negative symptoms were found in over 21% of patients. These findings are consistent with other findings in the literature.[21]

Methamphetamine withdrawal can be described in two phases: acute and subacute.[21] The acute effects of methamphetamine include increased sleeping and appetite and depression-related symptoms and sometimes anxiety, irritability, and craving of methamphetamine. The subacute phase includes marked sleepiness ("the crash") followed by insomnia.[21] Paradoxical withdrawal symptoms can include anxiety, irritability, and craving of methamphetamine. A "crash period," which involves oversleeping, begins after about 3 days of the acute withdrawal phase. Beginning on about the sixth day, a phase of insomnia follows withdrawal until about the twentieth day of methamphetamine abstinence. The symptoms of methamphetamine withdrawal are not conducive to good parenting.[21]

Heroin

Heroin is processed from morphine, which is extracted from the seedpod of the poppy plant that can be found in Asia,

Mexico, and Colombia.[25] Heroin is a brown or white powder, which is typically injected, although it can be "snorted" as well. In 2006, heroin was used by an estimated 338,000 Americans, which is more than double the 2005 estimated use by 136,000.[12] The corresponding prevalence rate increased from 0.006% to 0.14% during this period.

The effects of heroin begin shortly after a single dose and can disappear after a few hours.[25] After injecting heroin, the user feels a surge of euphoria (a "rush") accompanied by flushing of the skin, a dry mouth, and a feeling of heaviness in the extremities. The initial euphoria is followed by alternating wakeful and drowsy ("going on the nod") states.[25]

Chronic injection of heroin can lead to collapsed veins.[25] In addition, chronic intravenous heroin abuse places the user at increased risk of endocarditis, abscesses, cellulitis, and liver disease. Street heroin can include impurities and additives that do not readily dissolve. These additives can clog circulation to the lungs, liver, kidneys or brain.[25] Heroin is a CNS depressant, and chronic depression of the CNS can obscure proper mental functioning.

Heroin withdrawal can begin as quickly as a few hours after the last use. Withdrawal symptoms peak at 2 to 3 days into abstinence and subside after about 1 week. Withdrawal symptoms can include drug craving, restlessness, muscle and bone pain, insomnia, diarrhea, and vomiting. Some commonly seen withdrawal symptoms are cold flashes with goose bumps ("cold turkey") and kicking movements ("kicking the habit").[25]

COMMON LEGAL SUBSTANCES OF ABUSE

Alcohol

More than half of Americans (159 million people) over 12-years-old reported drinking alcohol in 2006.[12] More than one fifth (23%) were binge drinking at least once in the 30 days prior to the NSDUH 2006 survey. The 2006 rates of alcohol use were 29.7% among 16- to 17-year-olds, 51.6% among 18- to 20-year-olds, 68.6% among 21- to 25-year-olds, and 63.5% among 26- to 29-year-olds.[12] The rate of binge drinking peaks among 21- to 23-year-olds; 57.9% of females and 65.9% of males (age 18- to 25-years-old) reported drinking in 2006.

Alcohol's effects on behavior are complex. It works in many different ways on many different neurotransmitters and networks. Like cocaine and methamphetamine, alcohol increases the neurotransmitter dopamine, which plays a role in the motivating and rewarding effects of alcohol.[26] The sedating effect of alcohol is due to its potentiating effects on gamma-aminobutyric acid (GABA), the major inhibitory neurotransmitter in the brain. Acute alcohol use can release previously inhibited behaviors and cause the user to act impulsively and inappropriately by disrupting the normal inhibitory functions in the prefrontal networks of the brain. Many neurotransmitters are involved including serotonin, which is essential to emotional expression, and the endorphins, which can be responsible for both the "high" of alcohol intoxication and the craving to drink.[26] "Blackout," or alcohol-induced amnesia, is thought to be caused by its interference of several brain functions including memory.

Chronic alcohol abuse has a wide range of effects,[26] depending on the amount of alcohol consumed, the age at which the person began drinking, malnutrition, and psychiatric conditions such as depression and anxiety. Alcohol is considered toxic to the brain, and alcohol's neurotoxic effects are hypothesized to cause shrinkage of areas of the brain.[26] Strikingly, approximately half of the nearly 20 million alcoholics in the United States have some form of neuropsychological difficulties, which can range from mild to severe. Examples of diminished cognitive effects include alcohol-induced persisting amnesic disorder (also known as Wernicke-Korsakoff syndrome) and dementia. Compounding these problems is poor dietary habits in some alcoholics, which can lead to thiamine deficiency (vitamin B_1), contributing to damage to the brain and severe cognitive deficits.[26]

Chronic alcohol abuse can affect behavior as well as cognition. The addict can become less reactive emotionally, thus appearing "flat." In addition, alcoholics can have impaired emotional processing, including interpreting nonverbal emotional cues and recognizing facial expressions.[26]

Prolonged abuse of alcohol reduces the number of GABA (inhibitory neurotransmitter) receptors. When the alcoholic stops drinking, decreased inhibition, along with a deficiency of GABA receptors, can contribute to overexcitation throughout the brain, thus leading to withdrawal seizures within a day or two.[26]

Prescription Substances for Nonmedical Use

The National Institute on Drug Abuse (NIDA) reports that the inappropriate use of prescription medications is a serious public health concern.[27] In 2006, over 5 million people were users of nonprescribed prescription pain relievers. The three most commonly abused classes of drugs are opioids, central nervous system (CNS) depressants, and CNS stimulants.[27] Examples of opioids include morphine, codeine, oxycodone, methadone, and fentanyl. In addition to treating pain, these drugs affect regions of the brain that control the perception of pleasure, resulting in a sense of euphoria. Examples of CNS depressants include tranquilizers and sedatives. They act by decreasing brain activity, thus causing a drowsy or calming effect. The two main groups of CNS depressants are barbiturates and benzodiazepines. Barbiturates include mephobarbital and pentobarbital sodium. Examples of benzodiazepines are diazepam, chlordiazepoxide, and alprazolam.[27]

Prescription stimulants increase the user's energy, alertness, and attention. These stimulants are also associated with a sense of euphoria. Paradoxically, unpleasant feelings of paranoia or hostility can occur if these stimulants are taken at high doses repeatedly over a shorter period than prescribed.[27] If the user repeatedly takes high doses of some prescription stimulants over a short period, feelings of hostility or paranoia can occur.

IMPACT OF PARENTAL SUBSTANCE ABUSE ON CHILDREN

In 2001, more than 6 million children (approximately 10% of children aged 5 or younger) lived with at least one parent who abused or was dependent on alcohol, prescription drugs, or an illicit substance.[28] Fathers were more likely than mothers (62 % *vs.* 38 %, respectively) to abuse substances.[28,29] In 2002, nearly 5 million adults with at least one child less than 18 years of age living with them were alcohol dependent or alcohol abusing.[29] Alcohol abuse, however, does not preclude other substance abuse; in fact, it makes other substance abuse more likely.[29]

Substance Abuse and Pregnancy

As mentioned previously, of 7800 pregnant women studied, one third had a positive drug screen; of those with a positive drug test, 15% continued to use substances after learning of the pregnancy.[13] Only 25% of substance abusers register for prenatal care prior to labor, mostly in the last trimester.[30] Fewer methamphetamine users, relative to nonusers, get prenatal care (89% *vs.* 99%). They have fewer prenatal visits (11 *vs.* 14) and later first prenatal visits (15 *vs.* 9 weeks' gestational age).[31] Methamphetamine and cocaine reduces hunger and thirst and the need for sleep, resulting in malnutrition, weight loss, and dehydration in the pregnant addict. Heroin use disrupts normal menstrual cycles, therefore delaying the female addict's awareness of her pregnancy and her seeking of medical care.[30]

The pregnant heroin addict can have repeated episodes of withdrawal and overdose that are potentially fatal for the fetus.[30] Maternal opioid withdrawal is associated with increased muscular activity, metabolic rate, and oxygen consumption. Fetal activity, in turn, increases, raising oxygen demands for the fetus that might be unmet, especially in the third trimester of gestation. Unmet oxygen requirements can be dangerous for the fetus and lead to fetal demise.[30]

Early childhood is a time of close bonding of the child with the parent. Important developmental tasks including secure attachment depend on a "good fit" between the child and the parent. Children need good parenting from conception through adolescence. A substance-using pregnant woman will expose her unborn fetus to medical and psychosocial complications associated with her substance abuse, including lack of prenatal care, poor nutrition, use of drugs and/or alcohol, and existing diseases. Substance-using women often do not seek adequate prenatal care, neglect their fetuses' nutritional needs, use multiple legal and illegal substances, and suffer from coexisting chronic illnesses such as HIV infections or hepatitis. Women using heroin or other opiates during pregnancy will cause their newborn to experience drug withdrawal symptoms,[8] including feeding difficulties, irritability, sleep problems, and prolonged high-pitched crying. These infants can be challenging to nurture, especially for a mother who is struggling with her own addiction and depression.

Prenatal alcohol exposure leading to recognizable patterns of malformations and developmental disability or fetal alcohol effect is a well-defined entity.[32] Children with alcohol-related neurodevelopmental disorders, alcohol-related birth defects, fetal alcohol syndrome, or fetal alcohol effect require special care, patience, and understanding from adult caregivers, along with complex medical and rehabilitation needs.[33] Failure to provide for such essential services can result in significant secondary disabilities for the affected child.[34]

Polydrug use is a common occurrence among drug-abusing women, exposing their unborn children to multiple drugs, making it difficult to isolate effects of exposure to an individual drug. Cocaine and methamphetamine are drugs commonly used by drug abusing women during pregnancy. Early literature on infants exposed to cocaine in utero reported alarming developmental outcomes for the infants, with predictions of irrevocable brain damage requiring life-long institutional care. These opinions, which lacked a sound scientific basis, resulted in misguided policies and a tendency toward a punitive approach to pregnant women who used cocaine. The Maternal Lifestyle Study (MLS), a longitudinal, NIH-funded national prospective study, began in the 1990s.[35] This study provided more accurate data about the development of drug-exposed children, disproving many of the myths associated with "crack babies."

The MLS researchers studied 1388 mother–infants dyads (658 exposed and 730 unexposed) and reported effects of small magnitude in 5% of drug-exposed children. These effects include lower birth weight and decreased head circumference relative to birth weight,[36] lower arousal, poor quality of movement and self regulation, higher excitability, increased tone, and poorer reflexes.[35] An infant and maternal feeding study at 1 month of the infants 1 month after birth found cocaine-using mothers to be less engaged and less flexible in response to their infant's cues, whereas opiate-using mothers show higher level of activity, independent of the feeding problems shown by their infants.[37] Mothers using both cocaine and opiates along with tobacco are most likely to be at risk of insensitive, inflexible parenting during feeding.[37]

Maternal behaviors that overstimulate, control, and potentially limit feeding opportunity have been shown to compromise energy intake and future weight gain and lead to mother–infant conflict.[38]

Methamphetamine use has reached epidemic levels in the last 10 years. According to the 1999 NSDUH survey,[39] methamphetamine use was equal among pregnant and non-pregnant women. A study funded by the National Institutes of Health (the Infant Development Environment and Life-style Study [IDEAL]) examined the effects of methamphetamine use during pregnancy.[40] Subjects were recruited from seven hospitals from four clinical sites across the United States. Based on the self report of 1632 eligible mothers, the 6% of participating mothers used methamphetamine during pregnancy. Methamphetamine-exposed infants were 3.5 times more likely to be small for gestational age than non-exposed infants.[41] Methamphetamine use during the third trimester is associated with poor quality of movement. The exposed newborns were less arousable, with an apparent dose-related effect on CNS.[42]

These and other subtle but identifiable neurobehavioral characteristics of infants exposed to drugs could contribute to increased parental stress in substance-using women. Infants exposed to drugs prenatally often continue to live in environments with the compounding risks of parental depression, antisocial behavior, paranoia, family violence, lack of family support, and parents' unresolved child abuse issues. All of these factors have been associated with both poor parenting skills and poor attachment,[43] which puts the children at risk for neglect and abuse. The Keeping Children and Families Safe Act of 2003 (Public Law 108-36)[10] requires states to have policies and procedures in place ensuring that child protective services are notified of substance-exposed newborns, and to establish safety plans for newborns with symptoms resulting from prenatal drug exposure.

The Home Environment in Substance-Abusing Families

Characteristics of the home environment of substance-using families that put their children at increased risk include poverty, dangerous living conditions, environmental stress, social isolation, and overcrowding.[44] Other grave risks face children living in homes where methamphetamine is used and manufactured. The 2006 National Drug Threat Survey by the National Drug Intelligence Center[45] found that in 2004, 2474 children were found to be affected by living in homes where methamphetamine was manufactured, and 3 children were killed. The ease with which methamphetamine can be manufactured at home, using easily available ingredients, has resulted in an epidemic of clandestine "meth labs" across the Midwest and Western United States. Children from these homes require removal to a safe environment, resulting in increased demand for foster placements. Although the developmental impact of living in a home with "meth lab" toxins present has not been determined, many cases of severe neglect are reported from such homes. In addition, multiple case reports of "accidental" methamphetamine poisoning have been published.[46] Children have also suffered severe burns in household fires related to cooking methamphetamine in homes and are exposed to toxic chemicals.[47] Often "meth lab" homes have stockpiles of weapons, guard dogs, and rigged "booby traps" to protect against unwanted entry of law enforcement officials. In addition, children are exposed to criminal behavior, such as the recruitment of adolescents into the drug manufacture and delivery process. Children can be exposed to violence related to the sales and distribution of methamphetamine, or by acts of retribution and efforts to eliminate competition, which are often part of the methamphetamine trade.[20]

Many states have expanded their child abuse and neglect statutes to cover household drug use and activity, States have included the following types of conditions as actionable causes for intervening to protect children[48]:

- Manufacturing a controlled substance in the presence of a child or in a home where a child resides.
- Allowing a child to be present where the chemicals or equipment for the manufacture of controlled substance are used or stored.
- Selling, distributing, or giving drugs to a child.
- The use of controlled substance by a caregiver that impairs the caregiver's ability to adequately care for the child.
- Exposure of child to drug paraphernalia.
- The exposure to criminal sale or distribution of drugs.
- The exposure to other drug-related activity.

Substance Abuse and Social Stressors

Studies of parents whose children are abused or neglected show parental depression and substance abuse as underlying problems in many cases. Families affected by substance abuse frequently have issues around boundaries, communication, problem-solving styles, and role assignments.[49] In addition, drug and alcohol abuse can disrupt family rituals (holidays, meals, etc.), which affect children's social development and well-being.

Stress can deplete a parent's coping reserve and with a preexisting substance abuse disorder, this insult can sometimes be enough to tip the balance toward abusive responses aimed at the child. Trying to balance addictive lifestyle with demands of parenting can produce high levels of stress in women with inadequate social support and limited economic resources. Factors that challenge a parent's ability to provide for the needs of their children include lack of education, unemployment, and homelessness.

Unemployment appears to correspond with illicit substance abuse.[12] The NSDUH showed that current illicit drug use was higher among the unemployed (18.5%) than in those employed full-time (8.8%) or part time (9.4%). Conners et al[44] studied mothers entering 50 publicly funded substance abuse recovery programs. Most of the women were unemployed (88.9%), lacked a high school degree or GED (51.7%), and relied on public assistance for financial support (70.6%). In addition, 32% had been homeless in the 2 years before beginning treatment. Only 13% of mothers in this study reported receiving child support from their children's fathers.

Fathers are noticeably absent from the lives of children growing up in substance-abusing homes. In the above study, 30% of children never saw their father in the year prior to treatment entry. An additional 15% saw their fathers only once or twice in this period. The mothers in this study reported that over half (51%) of their children's fathers used illegal drugs.[44]

Substance Abuse and Parental Mental Health

The Conners study[44] reported the following historical factors in women in substance abuse treatment: depression (40.1%), psychological trauma (10.7%), bipolar disorder (6.7%), and attempted suicide (29.8%). The NSDUH showed adults with serious psychological problems were more likely to use illicit drug (27.2% *vs.* 12.3%) and to be binge drinkers (28.8% *vs.* 23.9%) compared with adults without psychological problems.[12] In addition, adults experiencing major depressive episode were more likely to use illicit substances (27.7% *vs.* 12.9%) and to drink heavily (8.6% *vs.* 7.3%) compared with nondepressed adults.

To examine the association of childhood physical and sexual abuse and parental histories of drugs or alcohol use, Walsh and colleagues[50] conducted a population-based survey of 8472 adults in Ontario, Canada. Nineteen percent of respondents were ages 15 to 24. Males reporting parental substance abuse were 1.5 times more likely to be physically abused and three times more likely to be sexually abused than those reporting no parental history of substance abuse. For girls, physical abuse was doubled, and sexual abuse was 2.5 times higher.

Addiction and Parenting

Addiction can overwhelm parents and leave them preoccupied with acquiring drugs (and other illegal behaviors), leaving little time to spend on parenting, leading to serious child neglect.[18] For example, methamphetamine users can fall into a deep sleep, sometimes for days, during which time their children are left defenseless to physical dangers in their environment as well as to abuse by other substance-abusing adults in the household.[22] Coyer[51] asked 11 women in recovery what parenting was like while using cocaine. From the mothers' responses, five themes emerged:

Lack of structure—although some of the "structure" mothers provided was physical punishment and striking out at the children.

Abandonment—Mothers knew they would not be dependable while on drugs, so they would leave children with other people indiscriminately. Similarly, adult methamphetamine addicts have reportedly drugged their children with antihistamines or benzodiazepines to keep them asleep and "safe," while their parents "crash" from their high.

Impatience and anger—Some women reported that while taking drugs, this would lead to violence against their children.

Lack of parenting knowledge—Mothers reported needing help recognizing problems in their children's growth and development that were caused by exposure to cocaine.

Repeating family of origin dysfunctional practices—It is not unusual for substance abuse to occur in an intergenerational context.

According to the NSDUH,[12] alcohol-dependent or alcohol-abusing parents were more likely to report that people in their households often insulted or yelled at each other and had more serious arguments than parents who were not abusing drugs or alcohol. Miller et al[52] examined 170 mothers with and without current alcohol and drug problems to determine discipline styles for each group. Their findings suggest that women with alcohol and drug problems are more likely to be punitive toward their children. Other factors such as mothers' histories of partner or parental violence seemed to contribute as well.

Parental Substance Abuse and Children's Behavior

The effects of parental substance abuse can be seen in the behavior of their children. Infants who are exposed to cocaine in utero can be irritable and tremulous and can show state lability on the Brazelton Neonatal Behavioral Assessment Scale.[30] These neurobehavioral effects are postulated to be due to increased catecholamine activity. When parents or caretakers are preoccupied with their addictions, they often fail to respond to infants' basic needs or to do so unpredictably. This can cause children who live in a substance-abusing environment to exhibit attachment disorders.[22]

Older children are not blind to their parent's substance abuse; by age 7 or 8, most children have developed accurate perceptions of the role of substance abuse in their family.[49] In addition, older children in substance abusing homes may often assume the roles of caretakers, causing additional stress.[22]

Scannapieco et al[55] compared families with a history of substance abuse who did and did not abuse and neglect their children. The abusive and neglectful families had fewer parental resources, less parental capability, fewer parenting skills, and less knowledge of child development. The children in the abusive families were found to be more vulnerable and fragile. In addition, the maltreating parents provided a poorer quality of physical and emotional care, and demonstrated a lack of empathy for and attachment to their children.

SUBSTANCE ABUSE AND PARENTAL INCARCERATION

Parents' incarceration resulting from drug abuse has detrimental effects on their children left behind. The United States leads the world in the number of incarcerated adults. An estimated 63% of federal prisoners and 55% of state prisoners had a minor child in 1999. The total number of minor children of these parents was about 1,498,800, or a little over 2% of the nation's 72 million children.[54] According to the Bureau of Justice Statistics,[54] 67% of parents in federal prisons were drug offenders.

Wilbur et al[55] compared the behavior of children whose fathers were incarcerated with that of children of nonincarcerated fathers. In bivariate analyses, children whose fathers were in jail had higher total scores on the Children's Depression Inventory, indicating more depressive symptoms. Teachers' reports of behaviors of children with incarcerated fathers showed more externalizing behaviors, even after controlling for age, gender, prenatal cocaine and marijuana exposure, and school-age violence exposure.

DRUG TREATMENT AND FAMILY DISRUPTION

According to the NSDUH, 4 million persons aged 12 and older received treatment for problems related to the use of alcohol or illicit drugs in 2006.[12] In one study of over 15,000 consecutive substance abuse rehabilitation admissions in California, almost 60% were parents of minor children.[56] Of these parents, 27.1% had at least one of their children removed from their custody. Of those who lost custody, 36% had their parental rights terminated. Children were more likely to be removed from their parents custody if the parent was in inpatient treatment (53%) compared with outpatient treatment (29%). The group most likely to lose custody of their children included those in treatment for narcotic addiction (80%). Even when parents enter treatment, their children can continue to experience disruption in their lives.

In substance-abusing women aged 18 to 49, the most common reasons for *not* receiving necessary treatment were[57]:

1. They felt they were not ready to stop using.
2. Cost/insurance barriers kept them from treatment.
3. They feared the social stigma that accompanies addiction.
4. They felt they could handle the problem without treatment.

SCREENING FOR FAMILY SUBSTANCE ABUSE IN THE HEALTH CARE SETTING

Given the devastating effects of substance abuse on the family, how can health care providers (HCPs) approach this issue to help families and protect children? Intervention cannot begin until a problem has been detected; therefore, screening is essential. Between birth and the age 18, HCPs have at least 20 opportunities to screen for family substance abuse issues in well-child care. A positive screen, however, does not make a definitive diagnosis of substance abuse, but indicates a potential problem. At a minimum, screening parents for substance abuse raises important issues and establishes the willingness of the provider to discuss the issue with parents.[49] Even if addicted parents do not seek treatment, other family members can get help from support groups such as Al-Anon or Alateen.[58]

Prenatal Visits

At prenatal visits, HCPs should focus on the health of the unborn child. To make the process less threatening, ask first about substance abuse in the parents' families of origin. Lifestyle questions about issues such as nutrition and smoking can be addressed, leading to a discussion about substance abuse. The provider can focus the interview on how parents' lifestyles influence the fetus, infant, child, and adolescent.[49]

Infancy and Early Childhood

Well-child visits can provide an opportunity to screen for family substance abuse problems. During these visits, emphasis can be placed on how substance abuse influences parenting decisions, exacerbates family stress and marital problems, creates potentially unsafe homes, and models drug use behaviors to children.[49]

School-Aged Children

When children are asked from whom they learn most about their health, they first list their mothers and then their physicians.[49] Anticipatory guidance about substance abuse should begin early in childhood when family standards are being assimilated. HCPs can enhance this discussion by asking if substance abuse is being discussed at school or at home, inquiring specifically about what is being discussed and whether the child understands.

Adolescents

Adolescence is a time of transition into adulthood and the adoption of either favorable or unfavorable lifestyle choices. Early identification of substance abuse risks is important to prevent continued substance abuse in adolescence.[49] For example, people who first smoked marijuana when less that 14 years old were over four times more likely to have a substance abuse problem than those who did not smoke marijuana until at least 18 years old (12.9% vs. 2.9%, respectively).[12] A similar trend was found for age of first alcohol use and future alcoholism.

As adolescents grow older, it becomes increasingly important to identify their own substance abuse. Children from homes with addiction problems are at higher risk for becoming substance abusers. Older children and adolescents should be asked if they have concerns about their parents or other family members.[49]

SUBSTANCE ABUSE SOLUTIONS FOR PARENTS

When parental substance abuse is discovered, assessment must focus not only on the parent's problems, but also on the characteristics of the child, the parents' strengths, the home environment, the social environment, and the maltreatment patterns of the family.[53] Interventions for cocaine-using mothers should focus on both the addiction and the psychopathology.[59] It is important to remember that parenting continues after infancy, thus recovering parents need long-term support.

Treatment for Pregnant Women

Pregnant women in recovery have special needs. As stated by Huestis and Choo,[30] "Substance abuse treatment for pregnant women must be non-judgmental, non-punitive, and nurturing. ... Substance abuse treatment for pregnant women needs to address poly-drug use and to provide education on the effects of licit drugs (alcohol and nicotine), illicit drugs, sexually-transmitted diseases, family planning, parenting skills, and vocational training, as well as including treatment of these women's psychiatric co-morbidities."

Therapeutic support is a more effective intervention for substance abusing parents than punishment. One example is the Rhode Island Vulnerable Infants Program (VIP-RI).[60] This program works with different providers to bring services to mothers (and fathers as well, if amenable). VIP-RI has resulted in a reduced length of stay for drug-exposed infants in the hospital, a reduction in foster care placements, and an increased rate of permanent placement including increased placement with biological families.

Family Treatment Drug Courts

The legal system is becoming involved in parental substance abuse treatment. In many areas, family treatment drug courts (FTDCs) have been established. These specialized courts collaborate with the parents, social services, substance abuse treatment programs, and other service providers.[61] FTDCs enforce parents' compliance and continued abstinence before custody of their children can be returned.

Effective Drug Treatment

Sun[62] reviewed 35 empirical studies looking at women in substance abuse treatment, identifying five elements of effective treatment: (1) single-sex programs instead of mixed-sex programs, (2) increased treatment intensity, (3) provision for child care, (4) case management and "one stop shopping" models, and (5) supportive staff and individual counseling.

Stewart et al[63] studied 1075 drug addicts in treatment. Almost half (46%) were parents. Parents (especially mothers who cared for children) were less likely to receive residential treatment. They found that women caring for children during treatment showed less improvement in psychiatric symptoms at follow-up, and concluded that women with children face special difficulties accessing services and would benefit from programs offering childcare.

Coyer[51] studied mothers in cocaine–recovery and noted that they wanted to know the consequences of prenatal cocaine exposure on their infants, appropriate methods of discipline, and their infants' developmental needs. Parenting information should be included in treatment programs for mothers.

For many women, the road to substance dependence begins in childhood experiences, such as sexual abuse, depression, and parental substance abuse. In a sample of 105 urban, African American women who used cocaine,[64] 61% reported at least one sexual abuse experience and 44% reported more than one sexual abuse incident before age 17 years. In addition, depression was common in these women (74%). Depressive symptoms started by the age of 15 years in 31% of affected women, whereas most women in this sample started using illicit drugs around 16 years old. Substance abuse was commonly noted in their families as well. Women with more drug-using family members started their illicit drug use at an earlier age. Another study of 115 cocaine-using mothers and 105 nonusers found higher levels of childhood emotional abuse, sexual abuse, and emotional neglect among the cocaine-using mothers, as well as higher levels of PTSD symptoms, antisocial behavior, anger, and hostility.[59] It is imperative, therefore, to include treatment for childhood trauma and mental health disorders in the recovery planning for substance-abusing mothers. Failure to recognize the interconnected role of childhood sexual abuse, emotional neglect, and psychiatric co-morbidities in the development and continuation of substance abuse can impact the success of treatment and recovery for this vulnerable population.

Ineffective Approaches to Drug Treatment

When the emphasis is placed on *punishing* pregnant addicts instead of offering treatment, the women are discouraged from seeking much needed prenatal care and help in achieving drug abstinence.[30] In addition, the stigma of substance abuse in pregnancy and the fear of losing custody of their children encourage pregnant women to hide their addiction from physicians and others who can offer help and support. Even if the pregnant addict wishes to seek treatment, she might meet closed doors. Many drug treatment programs will not accept pregnant or HIV-positive women.[30]

EFFECTIVE INTERVENTIONS FOR CHILDREN OF SUBSTANCE ABUSERS

By the time addicted mothers seek long-term residential drug treatment, their children usually have experienced poverty and other risks to their health and well-being that make them vulnerable to physical, academic, and social problems.[44] By age 7 or 8, most children have developed accurate perceptions of the role of alcohol and drugs. Many of them will have attachment disorders,[22] and some will have experienced stress caused by their parent's incarceration.[55] These "high-needs" children require specific, targeted interventions to restore their physical and mental health. Programs designed to address their immediate, transitional and long-term needs should be incorporated into their parents' substance abuse treatment.[44] Little research has been done on how to best meet the needs of this population of children at risk.

References

1. Kempe EH, Silverman FN, Steele BF, et al: The battered-child syndrome. *JAMA* 1962;181:17-24.
2. Lieberman DZ: Children of alcoholics: an update. *Curr Opin Pediatr* 2000;12:336-340.
3. Leonard KE, Eiden RD: Marital and family processes in the context of alcohol use and alcohol disorders. *Annu Rev Clin Psychol* 2007;3:285-310.
4. Besinger BA, Garland AF, Litrownik AJ, et al: Caregiver substance abuse among maltreated children placed in out-of-home care. *Child Welfare* 1999;78:221-239.
5. Kelley SJ: Child maltreatment within the context of substance abuse. *In:* Meyers JEB, Berliner J, Briere JN, et al*: The APSAC Handbook on Child Maltreatment.* Sage Publications, Thousand Oaks, Calif, 2002, pp 105-117.
6. Kelley SJ: Parenting stress and child maltreatment in drug exposed children. *Child Abuse Negl* 1992;16:317-328.
7. Wasserman DR, Leventhal JM: Maltreatment of children born to cocaine-dependent mothers. *Am J Dis Child* 1993;147:1324-1328.
8. Finnegan LP, Connaughteon J, Schut J: Infants of drug dependent women*: In: Practical approaches for management. Problems of Drug Dependence.* National Academy of Sciences, Washington, DC, 1975, pp 489-517.
9. Blending Perspectives and Building Common Ground. A Report to Congress on Substance Abuse and Child Protection. U.S. Department of Health and Human Services, Washington, DC, 1999. Available at http://aspe.hhs.gov/hsp/subabuse1999/subabuse.htm. Accessed April 9, 2009.
10. Keeping Children and Families Safe Act of 2003. Public Law 108-136. Available at http://www.acf.hhs.gov/programs/cb/laws_policies/policy/im/2003/im0304a.pdf. Accessed April 9, 2009.
11. Drug Endangered Children. Office of National Drug Control Policy, Washington, DC, 2008. Available at http://www.whitehousedrugpolicy.gov/enforce/dr_endangered_child.html. Accessed April 5, 2009.
12. National Survey on Drug Use and Health Report. SAMHSA-Substance Abuse and Mental Health Service Administration. 2006. Available at http://www.oas.samhsa.gov/nsduh/2k6nsduh/2k6Results.pdf. Accessed April 10, 2009.
13. Chasnoff IJ, McGourty RF, Bailey GW, et al: The 4P's Plus screen for substance abuse in pregnancy: Clinical application and outcomes. *J Perinatol* 2005;25:368-374.
14. Sun AP, Freese MP, Fitzgerald M: An exploratory study of drug-exposed infants: case substantiation and subsequent child maltreatment. *Child Welfare* 2007;86:33-50.
15. Ostrea EM, Brady M, Gause S, et al: Drug screening of newborns by meconium analysis: A large-scale, prospective, epidemiologic study. *Pediatrics* 1992;89:107-113.
16. Marijuana. Drug InfoFacts. National Institute on Drug Abuse, Washington, DC, 2008. Available at http://www.drugabuse.gov/PDF/InfoFacts/Marijuana08.pdf. Accessed April 10, 2009.
17. Cocaine. Drug InfoFacts. National Institute on Drug Abuse, Washington, DC, 2008. Available at http://www.nida.nih.gov/pdf/infofacts/Cocaine08.pdf. Accessed April 10, 2009.
18. Altshuler SJ: Drug-endangered children need a collaborative community response. *Child Welfare* 2005;84:171-190.
19. *Methamphetamine Use.* The National Survey on Drug Use and Health Report, Substance Abuse and Mental Health Services Administrations, 2007. Available at http://www.oas.samhsa.gov/2k7/meth/meth.pdf. Accessed April 10, 2009.
20. Cretzmeyer M, Sarrazin MV, Huber DL, et al: Treatment of methamphetamine abuse: research findings and clinical directions. *J Subst Abuse Treat* 2003;24:267-277.
21. McGuinness TM, Pollack D: Parental methamphetamine abuse and children. *J Pediatr Health Care* 2008;22:152-158.
22. Swetlow K: Children at Clandestine Methamphetamine Labs: Helping Meth's Youngest Victims. Office for Victims of Crime Bulletin. U.S. Department of Justice, Washington, DC, June, 2003, pp. 1-11. Available at http://www.ojp.usdoj.gov/ovc/publications/bulletins/children/197590.pdf. Accessed April 10, 2009.
23. Lineberry TW, Bostwick JM: Methamphetamine abuse: a perfect storm of complications. *Mayo Clin Proc* 2006;81:77-84.
24. Srisurapanont M, Ali R, Marsden J, et al: Psychotic symptoms in methamphetamine psychotic in-patients. *Int J Neuropsychopharmacol* 2003;6:347-352.
25. Heroin. Drug InfoFacts. National Institute on Drug Abuse, Washington, DC, May 2006. Available at http://www.nida.nih.gov/PDF/Infofacts/Heroin08.pdf. Accessed April 10, 2009.
26. Oscar-Berman M, Marinokovic K: Alcoholism and the brain: an overview. *Alcohol Res Health* 2003;27:125-133.
27. Prescription and Over-the-Counter Medications. Drug InfoFacts. National Institute on Drug Abuse, Washington, DC, July, 2008. Available at http://www.nida.nih.gov/PDF/Infofacts/PainMed08.pdf. Accessed April 10, 2009.
28. Children Living with Substance-Abusing or Substance-Dependent Parents. The National Survey on Drug Use and Health Report, Washington, DC, June 2, 2003. Available at http://www.oas.samhsa.gov/2k3/children/children.pdf. Accessed April 10, 2009.
29. Alcohol Dependence or Abuse among Parents with Children Living in the Home. The National Survey on Drug Use and Health Report, Substance Abuse and Mental Health Services Administration, Washington, DC, February 13, 2004. Available at http://www.oas.samhsa.gov/2k4/ACOA/ACOA.htm. Accessed April 10, 2009.
30. Lester BM, Derauf C, Arria AM, et al: Methamphetamine exposure: a rural early intervention challenge. *Zero to Three* 2006;26:30-36.
31. Huestis MA, Choo RE: Drug abuse's smallest victims: In utero drug exposure. *Forensic Sci Int* 2002;128:20-30.
32. Jones KL, Smith DW, Ulleland CW, et al: Pattern of malformations in offspring of chronic alcoholic mothers. *Lancet* 1973;1:1267-1271.
33. Institute of Medicine, Committee to study Fetal Alcohol Syndrome: *Fetal Alcohol Syndrome. Diagnosis, Epidemiology, Prevention and Treatment.* National Academy Press, Washington, DC, 1996, pp 4-7.
34. Streissguth A, Kanter J (eds): *The Challenge of Fetal Alcohol Syndrome: Overcoming Secondary Disabilities.* Washington Press, Seattle, 1997.
35. Lester BM, Tronick EZ, Lagasse LL, et al: The Maternal Lifestyle Study: effects of substance exposure during pregnancy on neurodevelopmental outcome in 1-month-old infants. *Pediatrics* 2002;110:1182-1192.
36. Shankaran S, Dag A, Baur CR, et al: Association between patterns of maternal substance use and infant birth weight, length and head circumference. *Pediatrics* 2004;114:e226-234.
37. LaGasse LL, Messenger D, Lester BM, et al: Prenatal drug exposure and maternal and infant feeding behavior. *Arch Dis Child Fetal Neonatal Ed* 2003;88:F391-F399.
38. Platzman KA, Coles CC, Lynch ME, et al: Assessment of the caregiving environment and infant functioning in polydrug families: Use of a structured clinical interview. *Infant Ment Health J* 2001;22:351-373.
39. National Survey on Drug Use & Health. Substance Abuse and Mental Health Services Administration, Washington, DC, 1999. Available at http://www.oas.samhsa.gov/p0000016.htm. Accessed April 8, 2009.
40. Lester BM, LaGasse L, Smith LM, et al: Parental exposure to methamphetamine and child development. *Proceedings of the Community Epidemiology Work Group* 2005;22:1-4.
41. Smith LM, LaGasse L, Derauf C, et al: The infant development environment and lifestyle study: Effects of prenatal methamphetamine exposure, poly drug exposure and poverty on intrauterine growth. *Pediatrics* 2006;118:1149-1156.
42. Smith LM, LaGasse LL, Derauf C, et al: Prenatal methamphetamine use and neonatal neurobehavioral outcome. *Neurotoxicol Teratol* 2008:30:20-28.
43. Das Eiden R, Chavez F, Leonard KE: Parental interactions among families with alcoholic fathers. *Dev Psychopathol* 1999:11;745-762.
44. Conners NA, Bradley RH, Mansell LW, et al: Children of mothers with substance abuse problems: an accumulation of risks. *Am J Drug Alcohol Abuse* 2004;30:85-100.
45. National Drug Threat Assessment 2006. National Drug Intelligence Center, U.S. Department of Justice, Johnstown, Pa, 2006. Available at http://www.usdoj.gov/ndic/pubs11/18862/index.htm. Accessed April 10, 2009.
46. Matteucci MJ, Auten JD, Crowley B, et al: Methamphetamine exposures in young children. *Pediatr Emerg Care* 2007;23:638-640.
47. Farst K, Duncan JM, Moss M, et al: Methamphetamine exposure presenting as caustic ingestions in children. *Ann Emerg Med* 2007;49:341-343.
48. Faller KC, Ziefert M: Causes of child abuse and Neglect. *In:* Faller KC: *Social Work with Abused and Neglected Children.* Free Press, New York, 1981, pp 32-52.
49. Werner MJ, Joffe A, Graham AV: Screening, early identification, and office-based intervention with children and youth living in substance-abusing families. *Pediatrics* 1999;103:1099-1112.

50. Walsh C, MacMillan H, Jamieson E: The relationship between parental substance abuse and child maltreatment. Findings from the Ontario Health Supplement. *Child Abuse Negl* 2003;27:1409-1425.

51. Coyer S: Mothers recovering from cocaine: factors affecting parenting skills. *J Obstet Gynecol Neonatal Nurs* 2001;30:45-49.

52. Miller BA, Smyth NJ, Mudar PJ: Mother's alcohol and other drug problems and their punitiveness toward their children. *J Stud Alcohol* 1999;60:632-642.

53. Scannapieco M, Connell-Carrick K: Assessment of families who have substance abuse issues: those who maltreat their infants and toddlers and those who do not. *Subst Use Misuse* 2007;42:1545-1553.

54. Mumola C: Incarcerated Parents and Their Children. Bureau of Justice Statistics. U.S. Department of Justice, Washington, DC, 2000. Available at http://www.ojp.usdoj.gov/bjs/pub/pdf/iptc.pdf. Accessed April 10, 2009.

55. Wilbur MB, Marani JE, Appugliese D, et al: Socioemotional effects of father's incarceration on low-income, urban, school-aged children. *Pediatrics* 2007;120:e678-e685.

56. Substance Use Treatment among Women of Childbearing Age. The National Survey on Drug Use and Health Report, Washington, DC, October 4. 2007. Available at http://www.oas.samhsa.gov/2k7/womenTX/womenTX.pdf. Accessed April 13, 2009.

57. Young NK, Boles SM, Otero C: Parental substance use disorders and child maltreatment: Overlaps, gaps, and opportunities. *Child Maltreat* 2007;12:137-149.

58. Information on Al-Anon and Alateen is available at http://www.al-anon.alateen.org/. Accessed April 9, 2009.

59. Eiden RD, Foote A, Schuetze P: Maternal cocaine use and caregiver status: group differences in caregiver and infant risk variables. *Addict Behav* 2007;32:465-476.

60. Lester BM, Twomey JE: Treatment of substance abuse during pregnancy. *Womens Health (Lond Engl)* 2008;4:67-77.

61. Green BL, Furrar C, Worciel S, et al: How effective are Family Treatment Drug Courts? Outcomes from a four-site national study. *Child Maltreat* 2007;12:43-59.

62. Sun AP: Program factors related to women's substance abuse treatment retention and other outcomes: a review and critique. *J Subst Abuse Treat* 2006;30:1-20.

63. Stewart D, Gossop M, Trakada K: Drug dependent parents: childcare responsibilities, involvement with treatment services, and treatment outcomes. *Addict Behav* 2007;32:1657-1668.

64. Boyd CJ: The antecedents of women's crack cocaine abuse. Family substance abuse, sexual abuse, depression and illicit drug use. *J Subst Abuse Treat* 1993;10:433-438.

55

DEFINITIONS AND CATEGORIZATION
OF CHILD NEGLECT

Christine E. Barron, MD, and Carole Jenny, MD, MBA

INTRODUCTION

Today as we embark upon a new pediatric subspecialty, Child Abuse Pediatrics,[1] it is impressive to look back and realize that Dr. C. Henry Kempe first acknowledged the existence of child abuse as a medical problem less than five decades ago.[2] With today's worldview, it is difficult to understand that many physicians questioned the validity of child maltreatment as a diagnosis when Kempe wrote his landmark paper.[3] Since then, significant advances have been made in the field of Child Abuse Pediatrics. These advances include the definition of various types of maltreatment such as physical abuse, sexual abuse, and psychological abuse. Child neglect remains less well defined, making effective research in prevention and treatment difficult.

Neglect is the most common form of child maltreatment. Child neglect accounts for over 50% of all reported child maltreatment cases,[4] and at least half of all child maltreatment fatalities.[5-7] Despite its prevalence, there is a dearth of clear definitions of neglect and research dedicated to neglect.[8] Although there is consensus that a clear definition of neglect is necessary, the task of defining neglect is daunting.

As an example of a well-defined form of child maltreatment, *physical abuse* is defined as acts of commission that result in injuries. These injuries can be visualized, they can be related to plausible mechanisms, and physicians can describe anticipated immediate and long-term outcomes based on the injury the child sustained. On the contrary, *neglect* is defined by acts of omission that often result in no clear injury. This lack of injury occurs within a context of multiple factors, and physicians can only describe potential immediate and long-term outcomes with marginal accuracy. Creating and applying a neglect definition to clinical situations is significantly more difficult than it is in other forms of child maltreatment.

A clear definition of neglect is necessary to end inconsistencies in policies, practice, and research.[9-14] Various neglect definitions have been proposed for over a decade and each has failed to gain universal acceptance. Many of the definitions place the blame for child neglect on the child's caretakers alone. For example, the definition of *child abuse* and *neglect* in the U.S. Government's Child Abuse Prevention and Treatment Act (CAPTA) is, "The physical or mental injury, sexual abuse, negligent treatment, or maltreatment of a child under the age of eighteen by a person who is responsible for the child's welfare under circumstances which indicate that the child's health or welfare is harmed or threatened."[15] Other caretaker-blaming definitions used by states and agencies include, "An omission in care by caregivers that results in significant harm or the risk of significant harm,"[16] and, "A type of maltreatment that refers to the failure by the caregiver to provide needed, age-appropriate care although financially able to do so or offered financial or other means to do so."[17] A broader definition is that neglect occurs, "… when children's basic needs are not adequately met."[18] This definition avoids blaming parents alone, and instead attributes neglect to child, parent, family, and community factors.[19]

Despite several attempts to clearly define *neglect*, clinicians are often left saying, "We know neglect when we see it!" The failure to establish a clear operational definition of *neglect* has resulted in a self-fulfilling prophecy of "the neglect of neglect."[8,20]

Neglect is multifactorial and multidimensional, encompassing a wide range of causes and consequences.[21-23] Understandably, it is a challenge to create a universal definition that can be applied to the extremely diverse set of clinical situations in which child neglect occurs, such as infants exposed to drugs in utero, infants failing to thrive based on lack of appropriate nutrition, young children left alone without age-appropriate and developmentally appropriate supervision, and children exposed to drugs and domestic violence, all of which must fit within the definition of neglect. A universally accepted definition of neglect needs to address every possible facet of the topic.

One obstacle in defining neglect is the question of perspective. Should a neglect definition be based on the perspective of the child and focus on specific unmet needs, or should a neglect definition be based on the perspective of the parents and focus on their responsibility for failing to meet the child's needs? Perspective differences in the definition of neglect are often based on two conceptual models proposed in the 1980s. Belsky[24] described a framework for understanding the etiology of child maltreatment based on the view that child maltreatment is a social-psychological phenomenon. This model identified specific factors for the individual, the family, and the community and the culture that allow all forms of child maltreatment to occur. On the other hand, Cicchetti and Rizley[25] developed a transactional model to address the causes, consequences, and mechanisms of child maltreatment. This model describes risk factors as either potentiating (increasing the probability of maltreat-

FACTORS INFLUENCING OCCURENCE
AND OUTCOME OF CHILD NEGLECT

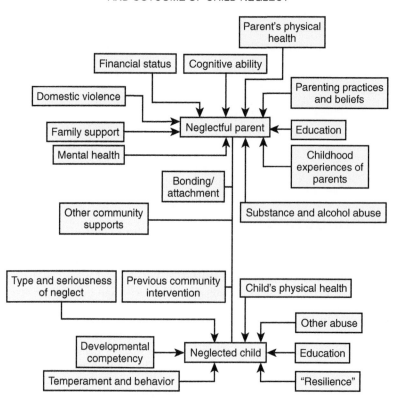

ment) or compensatory (decreasing the probability of maltreatment). Child maltreatment occurs when potentiating factors outweigh compensatory factors.[25]

Multiple factors influence the occurrence and outcome of child neglect on an individual, family, and community level (Figure 55-1). Individual factors are divided between those of the caregiver and those of the child victim. Neglectful caregivers can be influenced by inadequate parenting role models, mental health problems, physical health problems, alcohol and substance abuse, cognitive limitations, lack of education, domestic violence, impulsivity, poor anger control, unemployment, limited knowledge of the basic needs of a child, and social isolation. Factors that affect children that might lead to their neglect include age, physical and mental health, special needs, history of abuse, level of education, lack of resilience, temperament, and behavior. These intrinsic child risk factors can make child care more difficult, creating a cycle of neglect, since the failure to fulfill their needs results in increasingly difficult behaviors and inadequate bonding, which are identified as family risk factors. Other important family factors to consider include: single-parent homes, larger families, limited financial resources, inadequate food, and domestic violence. Societal influences have been identified as: poverty, unsafe neighborhoods, frequent moves, poor access to mental health and general health care, and lack of long-term community resources.[18,25-33]

There are compensatory factors to consider at each level as well. Compensatory factors include caregivers that have positive parenting role models, gainful employment, adequate support systems, and resilient children. Ideally, the balance between the potentiating and compensatory factors will identify the probability that neglect will occur.

A significant limitation of conceptual models is that although the presence of a particular factor is important to note, it does not always result in the occurrence of child maltreatment. For example, poverty has been identified as a significant risk factor for child neglect. Yet not all impoverished families neglect their children, and children that live within affluent families can be victims of neglect despite adequate available resources.

Many of the same factors influence the occurrence of other forms of child maltreatment and have not interfered with the defining of maltreatment. For example, a child that is physically abused by a caregiver within the context of poor parenting models, poverty, substance abuse, and other stressors is still diagnosed as a victim of child physical abuse. The influencing factors are taken into account to determine what intervention is most appropriate for the safety and well-being of the child. The same standard should apply for neglect. The influencing factors should be identified and used to determine the intervention necessary when neglect occurs, but these factors should not interfere with making the diagnosis of neglect.

Conceptual models allow a broader and richer understanding of the numerous complex, interwoven factors influencing the occurrence of neglect to foster a better understanding of a child's situation and to improve methods of prevention and strategies for intervention. These conceptual models, however, should not impede the establishment of a clear and consistent definition of neglect, which is needed to improve clinical assessments, research, and prevention efforts. A conceptual model cannot replace a neglect definition. Cicchetti and Lynch[34] demonstrated this by applying an ecological-transactional model to understanding the effect of community violence on the occurrence of child maltreatment. They concluded that the model provided a framework to target prevention and intervention efforts, but that violence itself needed to be defined more clearly.

The Child Protection Program at Hasbro Children's Hospital has promulgated a definition of neglect that incorporates a "multi-dimensional" approach inspired by the system used to diagnose mental illness in the DSM-IV.[35] This definitional tool looks at various aspects of neglect (the axes). The three axes are the type of neglect, the degree of neglect, and the outcome of neglect.

TYPES OF NEGLECT

The types of neglect define the unmet needs of the child. Although some children will only have one type of neglect, others experience multiple types. Types of neglect include:

- Physical neglect—inadequate food, clothing, shelter, and hygiene.
- Medical neglect—failure to provide prescribed medical care or treatment or failure to seek appropriate medical care in a timely manner.
- Dental neglect—failure to provide adequate dental care or treatment.
- Supervisional neglect—failure to provide age-appropriate supervision.
- Emotional neglect—failure to provide adequate nurturance or affection, failing to provide necessary psychological support, or allowing children to use drugs and/or alcohol.
- Educational neglect—failure to enroll a child in school or failure to provide adequate home schooling, failure to comply with recommended special education, and allowing chronic truancy.
- Other neglect—"other neglect" includes neglectful acts not covered in the above categories. It includes exposing children to domestic violence, or engaging or encouraging children to take part in illegal activities such as shoplifting or drug dealing. Another form of neglect in this category is "moral neglect" —the failure of parents to impart the values and ideals to the child needed for successful functioning in society.

Some have argued that although supervisional neglect can be grouped under physical neglect, it accounts for the most common type of neglect and should be defined as its own separate type of neglect.[36,37] In addition, within each category of neglect, further delineation of basic needs are required based on the child's age and abilities. For example, requirements for adequate supervision will vary based on a child's age and abilities. This needs to be clearly distinguished from other forms of neglect in order to research the frequency and degree to which supervisional neglect relates to childhood injuries.[38-40]

DEGREES OF NEGLECT

Child neglect is often thought of as a chronic pervasive problem. But in many cases, neglect can be a single event, sometimes resulting in disastrous consequences. For example,

a responsible, caring parent who fails to notice her 2-year-old child walking away from her into traffic could be considered supervisionally neglectful, even if she is otherwise an exemplary parent. A single act that poses serious risk to a child can also constitute neglect.[41] To define neglect, then, pattern or frequency of the neglect needs to be included as well as the type.

For our second axis, we use the term *degree of neglect*. We have defined three degrees of neglect:

- First-degree neglect—obvious, ongoing, chronic, or pervasive neglect of child.
- Second-degree neglect—a single act of negligence or inattention that puts a child at risk of harm.
- Third-degree neglect—either a single act or repetitive acts of neglect that result from a circumstance beyond the control of the caretaker. For example, if a toddler wanders away from home while his mother is responding to a health emergency of another child, that would constitute third-degree neglect. Another example is the unemployed parents of an ill child not getting timely medical care because they have to choose between taking the child to the doctor and feeding their children. A third example is the intellectually challenged mother raising a new baby without the support of friends or family who mixes formula incorrectly, resulting in poor weight gain for the baby. One caveat regarding third-degree neglect: if the parent is offered resources to make up for the deficits beyond her control and refuses those resources, third-degree neglect becomes first- or second-degree neglect. An example would be a mother of a chronically ill child who is receiving inadequate care because the mother refuses to let home care nurses into her home.

OUTCOME

Physical injury can result from neglect, but the harm to a child from many types of neglect goes beyond any immediate physical injury that might occur. Neglect has the potential to adversely affect a child's psychosocial, cognitive, and emotional development.[42-46] Neglect can result in significant emotional problems, behavioral problems and attachment disorders,[47-53] and neglect can have a greater negative affect on a child than physical or sexual abuse.[54,55] In many cases, neglect results in mental and physical health problems persisting through adolescence into adulthood.[56-65] Neglect can contribute to juvenile delinquency, adult criminal behavior, and parenting difficulties.[16]

A neglect definition needs to acknowledge that there is not a linear relationship between the types and severity of neglect and the consequences of neglect. For example, a mother who leaves her infant home alone, sleeping in his crib, every Saturday night while she goes to clubs to party is seriously neglectful of her child. But if the child never awakens and does not require any nighttime care, there will be no long-term effect of that neglect. On the other hand, the nearly perfect parent who on one occasion forgets to lock the gate to the swimming pool, allowing her child to fall in the pool has neglected the child only momentarily, but the result for her child could be lethal. All types of neglect have potential consequences along a continuum, ranging from no injuries or mental health effects to fatalities or serious mental illness. Everyone can identify the potential for any infant to sustain injuries when unsupervised, but should the first example that resulted in no harm to the child be considered less severe?

In cases of chronic neglect, separating out the specific influences of various types and combinations of neglect endured over short and prolonged periods can affect individual outcomes. Specific combinations of neglect may have cumulative effects over the long term.[66] Psychological neglect has been related to behavioral problems, and exposure to multiple types of neglect has been related to the increase of internalizing problems.[67] The currently reported worst combination of maltreatment on outcome has been the co-occurrence of physical neglect, physical abuse, emotional neglect, and verbal abuse.[68] In addition, correlating the occurrence of neglect with the child's developmental age is important. For example, experiencing child neglect in the first 2 years of life has been identified as a precursor to childhood aggression.[69]

To address the issue of the consequences of neglect, the third axis in our system of classification of neglect is referred to as *outcome*. On this axis there are four possible options:

- No current harm, and no future harm is anticipated.
- No current harm, but future harm is anticipated.
- Child experiences current harm, but no future harm is anticipated.
- Child experiences current harm, and future harm is anticipated.

The problem with using this system of categorization is that limited objective data exist to predict future harm. So putting any case into one of these categories is speculative, and different people will have different ideas of into which category the case belongs.

Applying three axes to our definition of neglect has given our multidisciplinary child protection team an effective way to communicate with each other about the cases of neglect we confront. It also offers a possible framework for future research on neglect and its effect on children.

PREVENTION

Neglect itself has been found to be a precursor to other forms of abuse.[68] Given the significant morbidity and mortality resulting from child neglect, prevention of neglect is important. Neglect prevention should include primary, secondary, and tertiary efforts because studies of child welfare systems have shown that cases of neglect have the highest risk of reoccurence.[70]

Current conceptual models of the numerous complex, interwoven factors that influence the occurrence of neglect have been used to create prevention programs.[71] Programs provided to "at-risk" families have demonstrated effectiveness,[72] but given the complexity and variation of neglect, additional individualized interventions are also necessary.[73] Federally funded projects for neglect have recognized the importance of specific strategies that include empowering families, providing in-home and out-of-home services, and using multidisciplinary teams with collaborative community partners.[74] Creating a universally accepted neglect definition

will be instrumental to creating, implementing, and evaluating the effectiveness of prevention programs.

References

1. Block RW, Palusci VJ: Child abuse pediatrics: a new pediatric subspecialty. *J Pediatr* 2006;148:711-712.
2. Kempe C, Silverman E, Steele B, et al: The battered child syndrome. *JAMA* 1962;181:17-24.
3. Jenny C: Medicine discovers child abuse. *JAMA* 2008;300:2796-2797.
4. U.S. Department of Health and Human Services, Administration for Children and Families. *Child Maltreatment 2006*. U.S. Department of Health and Human Services, Administration on Children, Youth and Families, Washington, DC, 2008. Available at http://www.acf.hhs.gov/programs/cb/stats_research/index.htm. Accessed February 22, 2009.
5. Burkowitz CD: Fatal child neglect. *Adv Pediatr* 2001;48:331-361.
6. Isaac R, Jenny C: The relation between child death and child maltreatment. *Arch Dis Child* 2006;91:265-269.
7. Crume TL, DiGuiseppi C, Byers T, et al: Underascertainment of child maltreatment fatalities by death certificates, 1990-1998. *Pediatrics* 2002;110;e18.
8. Wolock I, Horowitz B: Child maltreatment as a social problem: the neglect of neglect. *Am J Orthopsychiatry* 1984;54:530-543.
9. Dubowitz H, Black M, Starr RH, et al: A conceptual definition of child neglect. *Crim Justice Behav* 1993;20:8-26.
10. Tyler S, Allison K, Winsler: Child neglect: developmental consequences, intervention, and policy implications. *Child Youth Care Forum* 2006;35:1-20.
11. McSherry D: Understanding and addressing the 'neglect of neglect': why are we making a mole-hill out of a mountain? *Child Abuse Negl* 2007;31:607-614.
12. Zuravin SJ: Issues pertinent to defining child neglect. *In:* Mortaon TD, Salovitsz B (eds): *The CPS Response to Child Neglect: An Administrators Guide to Theory, Policy, Program Design and Case Practice*. National Resource Center on Child Maltreatment, Duluth, GA, 2001, pp 1-22.
13. Barnett D, Manly JT, Cicchetti D: Defining child maltreatment: the interface between policy and research. *In:* Cicchetti D, Toth SL (eds): *Child Abuse, Child Development, and Social Policy*. Ablex Publishing, Norwood, NJ, 1993, pp 7-73.
14. McGee RA, Wolfe DA, Yuen SA, et al: The measurement of maltreatment: a comparison of approaches. *Child Abuse Negl* 1995;19:233-249.
15. Child Abuse Prevention and Treament Act, 42 U.S.C. 5106g, §Sec. 111-2.
16. Dubowitz H: Preventing child neglect and physical abuse: a role for pediatricians. *Pediatr Rev* 2002;23:191-195.
17. Helfer RE: The neglect of our children. *Pediatr Clin North Am* 1990;37:923-942.
18. Dubowitz H, Giardino A, Gustavson E: Child neglect: guidance for pediatricians. *Pediatr Rev* 2000;21:111-116.
19. U.S. Department of Health and Human Services, Administration for Children, Youth, and Families. *Child Maltreatment 2005*. U.S. Department of Health and Human Services, Administration on Children, Youth and Families, Washington, DC, 2007. Available at http://www.acf.hhs.gov/programs/cb/pubs/cm05/cm05.pdf. Accessed February 22, 2009.
20. Dubowitz H: Neglecting the neglect of neglect. *J Interpers Violence* 1994;9:556-560.
21. Polansky B, Gaudin J, Ammonds P, et al: The psychological ecology of the neglectful mother. *Child Abuse Negl* 1985;9:265-275.
22. Brown J, Cohen P, Johnson JG, et al: A longitudinal analysis of risk factors for child maltreatment: findings of a 17-yearprospective study of officially recorded and self-reported child abuse and neglect. *Child Abuse Negl* 1998;22:1065-1078.
23. McGuigan WM, Pratt C: The predictive impact of domestic violence on three types of child maltreatment. *Child Abuse Negl* 2001;25:869-883.
24. Belsky J: Child maltreatment: an ecological integration. *Am Psychol* 1980;35:320-335.
25. Cicchetti D, Rizley R: Developmental perspectives on the etiology, intergenerational transmission, and sequelae of child maltreatment. *New Dir Child Dev* 2006;198:31-55.

26. Wise PH, Meyers A: Poverty and child health. *Pediatr Clin North Am* 1988;35:1169-1186.
27. Gaudin JM, Polansky NA, Kilpatrick AC, et al: Family functioning in neglectful families. *Child Abuse Negl* 1996;20:363-377.
28. Coohey C: Neglectful mothers, their mothers, and partners: the significance of mutual aid. *Child Abuse Negl* 1995;19:885-895.
29. Coohey C. Child maltreatment: testing the social isolation hypothesis. *Child Abuse Negl* 1996;20:241-254.
30. Ethier LS, Lacharite C, Couture G: Childhood adversity, parental stress, and depression of negligent mothers. *Child Abuse Negl* 1995;19:619-632.
31. Kotch JB, Browne DC, Ringwalt CL, et al: Stress, social support and substantiated maltreatment in the second and third years of life. *Child Abuse Negl* 1997;21:1025-1037.
32. Drake B, Pandey S: Understanding the relationship between neighborhood poverty and specific types of child maltreatment. *Child Abuse Negl* 1996;20:1003-1018.
33. Kinard EM: Social support, self-worth, and depression in offending and nonoffending mothers of maltreated children. *Child Maltreat* 1996;1:272-283.
34. Cicchetti D, Lynch M: Toward an ecological/transactional model of community violence and child maltreatment: consequences for children's development. *Psychiatry* 1993;56:96-118.
35. American Psychiatric Association: *Diagnostic and Statistical Manual of Mental Disorders DSM-IV-TR*, ed 4. American Psychiatric Publishing, Washington, DC, 2000.
36. Coohey C: Defining and classifying supervisory neglect. *Child Maltreat* 2003;8:145-156.
37. Hymel KP, Committee on Child Abuse and Neglect: When is lack of supervision neglect? *Pediatrics* 2006;118:1296-1298.
38. Garbarino J: Preventing childhood injury: developmental and mental health issues. *Am J Orthopsychiatry* 1988;58:25-45.
39. Saluja G, Brenner R, Morrongiello BA, et al: The role of supervision in child injury risk: definitions, conceptual and measurement issues. *Inj Control Saf Promot* 2004;11:17-22.
40. Peterson L, Ewigman B, Kivlahan C: Judgments regarding appropriate child supervision to prevent injury: the role of environmental risk and age. *Child Dev* 1993;64:934-950.
41. Dubowitz H, Black MM: Child Neglect. *In:* Reece RM, Christian CW (eds): *Child Abuse: Medical Diagnosis & Management*, ed 3. American Academy of Pediatrics, Elk Grove Village, IL, 2009, pp 427-463.
42. APSAC Practice Guidelines: *Challenges in the Evaluation of Child Neglect.* American Professional Society on the Abuse of Children, Chicago, 2008.
43. Campbell FA, Ramey CT: Effects of early intervention on intellectual and academic achievement: a follow-up study of children from low-income families. *Child Dev* 1994;65:684-698.
44. Greenough WT, Black JE, Wallace CS: Experience and brain development. *Child Dev* 1987;58:539-559.
45. Perry B: *Neurobiological Sequelae of Childhood Trauma: Post-Traumatic Stress Disorders in Children.* American Psychiatric Press, Washington, DC, 1994.
46. Frank DA, Klass PE, Earls F, et al: Infants and young children in orphanages: one view from pediatrics and child psychiatry. *Pediatrics* 1996;97:569-578.
47. Erickson MF, Egeland B, Pianta R: The effects of maltreatment on the development of young children. *In:* Cicchetti D, Carlson V (eds): *Child Maltreatment.* Cambridge University Press; Cambridge, 1989, pp 579-619.
48. Gaudin JM: Child neglect: short-term and long-term outcomes. *In:* Dubowitz H (ed): *Neglected Children: Research, Practice and Policy.* Sage Publications, Thousand Oaks, CA, 1999, pp 89-108.
49. Hilyard KL, Wolf DA: Child neglect: developmental issues and outcomes. *Child Abuse Negl* 2002;26:679-695.
50. Rutter M, English and Romanian Adoptees (ERA) study team: Developmental catch-up and deficits following adoption after severe global early privation. *J Child Psychol Psychiatry* 1998;39:465-476.
51. Chugani H, Behen M, Muzik O, et al: Local brain functional activity following early deprivation: a study of postinstitutionalized Romanian orphans. *Neuroimage* 2001;14:1290-1301.
52. Egeland B, Sroufe LA, Erickson M: The developmental consequences of different patters of maltreatment. *Child Abuse Negl* 1983;7:459-469.
53. Kendall-Tackett K, Eckenrode J: The effects of neglect on academic achievement and disciplinary problems: a developmental perspective. *Child Abuse Negl* 1996;20:161-169.
54. Gararino J, Collins CC: Child neglect: the family with a hole in the middle. *In:* Dubowitz H (ed): *Neglected Children: Research, Practice, and Policy.* Sage Publications, Thousand Oaks, CA, 1999, pp 1-23.
55. Erickson M, Egeland B, Pianta R: The effects of maltreatment on the development of young children. *In:* Cicchetti D, Carlson V (eds): *Child Maltreatment: Theory and Research on the Causes and Consequences of Child Abuse and Neglect.* Cambridge University Press, Cambridge, 1989, pp 203-253.
56. Clark DB, Thatcher DL, Maisto SA: Adolescent neglect and alcohol use disorders in two-parent families. *Child Maltreat* 2004;9:357-370.
57. Bolger KE, Patterson CJ, Kupersmidt JB: Peer relationships and self-esteem among children who have been maltreated. *Child Dev* 1998;69:1171-1197.
58. Kurtz PD, Gaudin JM Jr., Wodarski JS, et al: Maltreatment and the school-aged child: school performance consequences. *Child Abuse Negl* 1993;17:581-589.
59. Kaufman JG, Widom CS: Childhood victimization, running way, and delinquency. *J Res Crime Delinquency* 1999;36:347-370.
60. Widom CS, Kuhns JB: Childhood victimization and subsequent risk of promiscuity, prostitution, and teenage pregnancy: a prospective study. *Am J Pub Health* 1996;86:1607-1612.
61. Dube SR, Felitti VJ, Dong M, et al: Childhood abuse, neglect, and household dysfunction and the risk of illicit drug use: the adverse childhood experiences study. *Pediatrics* 2003;111:564-572.
62. Hussey JM, Chang JJ, Kotch JB: Child maltreatment in the United States: prevalence, risk factors, and adolescent health consequences. *Pediatrics* 2006;118:933-942.
63. Schilling E, Aseltine R, Gore S: Adverse childhood experiences and mental health in young adults: a longitudinal survey. *BMC Public Health* 2007;7:30-40.
64. Johnson JG, Smailes EM, Cohen P, et al: Associations between four types of childhood neglect and personality disorder symptoms during adolescent and early adulthood: findings of a community-based longitudinal study. *J Pers Disord* 2000;14:171-187.
65. Grogan-Kaylor A, Otis MD: The effect of childhood maltreatment on adult criminality: a tobit regression analysis. *Child Maltreat* 2003;8:129-137.
66. Dubowitz H, Pitts SC, Black MM: Measurement of three major subtypes of child neglect. *Child Maltreat* 2004;9:344-356.
67. Dubowitz H, Papas MA, Black MM, et al: Child neglect: outcomes in high-risk urban preschoolers. *Pediatrics* 2002;109:1100-1107.
68. Ney PG, Fung T, Wickett AR: The worst combinations of child abuse and neglect. *Child Abuse Negl* 1994;18:705-714.
69. Kotch JB, Lewis T, Hussey JM, et al: Importance of early neglect for childhood aggression. *Pediatrics* 2008;121:725-731.
70. DePanfilis D: Child Neglect: A Guide for Prevention, Assessment, and Intervention. U.S. Department of Health and Human Services. Administration for Children, Youth and Families, Washington, DC, 2006. Available at http://www.childwelfare.gov/pubs/usermanuals/neglect/neglect.pdf. Accessed on February 22, 2009.
71. DePanfilis D, Dubowitz H: Family connections: a program for preventing child neglect. *Child Maltreat* 2005;10:108-123.
72. Olds DL, Henderson CR Jr, Chamberlin R, et al: Preventing child abuse and neglect: a randomized trial of nurse home visitations. *Pediatrics* 1986;78:65-78.
73. Dubowitz H, Pitts SC, Litrownik AJ, et al: Defining child neglect based on child protective services data. *Child Abuse Negl* 2005;29:493-511.
74. U.S. Children's Bureau: Program Evaluation: A Synthesis of Lessons Learned by Child Neglect Demonstration Projects. U.S. Department of Health and Human Services, Administration for Children and Families, Washington, DC, 2005.

56

DENTAL NEGLECT

Rhea M. Haugseth, DMD

INTRODUCTION

According to the American Academy of Pediatric Dentistry, "Dental neglect is willful failure of a parent or guardian to seek or follow through with treatment necessary to ensure a level of oral health essential for adequate function and freedom from pain and infection."[1] Dental neglect can be further divided into three different types:

- Active neglect—intentional failure of parents or guardians to fulfill their care-giving responsibilities.
- Passive neglect—unintentional failure of parents or guardians to fulfill their care-giving responsibilities because of lack of knowledge, illness, infirmity, finances, or lack of awareness of available community support/ resources.
- Self neglect—a person's inability to provide for his or her own needs because of a physical, mental, or developmental disability or any combination of these.

Neglect can also be defined as any action or inaction by *any* person that causes harm to a vulnerable person.

RECOGNITION

Rampant dental decay or other manifestations of dental disease in a very young child should arouse suspicion of dental neglect. In the United States, health care professionals are mandated to report cases of suspected abuse and neglect of children. Each state has its own definitions of child abuse and neglect based on general standards set by Federal law. In 2006, the U.S. Department of Health and Human Services (US DHHS) reported that approximately 905,000 children were victims of maltreatment.[2] Child protective services (CPS) agencies respond to the needs of children who are alleged to have been maltreated. According to the US DHHS,[2] 64.1% of confirmed cases of child maltreatment were neglect cases. (See Chapter 5, "Epidemiology of Child Neglect.")

POSSIBLE CAUSES AND RISK FACTORS

Many factors can contribute to an increased risk of dental neglect, including family isolation, lack of finances, parental ignorance, or lack of perceived value of oral health.[3] Another contributing problem is the inability of parents to establish a *dental home* for their children, defined by the American Academy of Pediatric Dentistry as, "The ongoing relationship between the dentist and the patient, inclusive of all aspect of oral health care delivered in a comprehensive, continuously accessible, coordinated and family-centered way."[4]

DESCRIPTION

Dental neglect is often a component of overall neglect. When health care professionals recognize signs of general neglect in patients, they should look for the possibility of dental neglect. Signs of neglect include poor oral hygiene, lack of care after an injury, or poor nutrition, including inappropriate choices of food and drink for the child. The parents might also be abusing drugs and/or alcohol. Neglectful parents or caregivers commonly ignore the treatment recommendations of health care providers. This can be especially problematic in the treatment of dental disease, which is preventable in most cases.

Early childhood caries (ECC) was in the past called "nursing or baby bottle decay." It remains a common occurrence in young children who are neglected. The American Academy of Pediatric Dentistry defines ECC as, "The presence of one or more decayed, missing (due to caries), or filled surfaces in any primary tooth in a child 71 months of age or younger."[5] ECC is observed in infants and toddlers who are breastfed on demand or who are given nighttime bottles filled with highly cariogenic liquids including milk, soft drinks, juices, or sports drinks. The failure of parents to provide oral hygiene (brushing and flossing) for their children contributes to this destructive disease. The accumulation of plaque on the anterior teeth is evidence of the lack of oral hygiene care by parents or guardian (Figure 56-1).

White spot lesions (Figure 56-2) are an early indication of ECC. These are frequently initially evident on the maxillary incisors. The mandibular incisors are protected from the cariogenic liquid because of the tongue's position when sucking. Cariogenic liquids pool around the maxillary incisors when a child is put to bed with a bottle filled with a substance other than water, or when a child is breastfed on demand throughout the night. If this liquid is not removed by brushing or wiping the teeth by the caregiver, tooth decay can result.

If left untreated, ECC can worsen and progress to rampant dental caries and abscess formation (Figure 56-3). Once a health care provider has identified the dental caries and has made recommendations to the parent or guardian concerning the treatment needed, the child should be carefully followed to make sure the dental treatment is completed

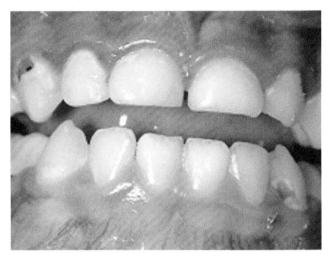

FIGURE 56-1 Visible plaque and orange algae present on unbrushed teeth.

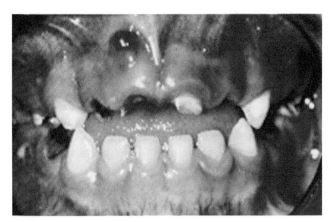

FIGURE 56-3 Early childhood caries (ECC) with rampant dental decay and dental abscesses.

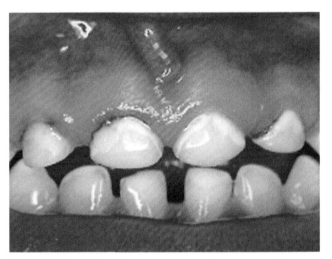

FIGURE 56-2 White spot lesions demonstrating early dental decay on maxillary incisors.

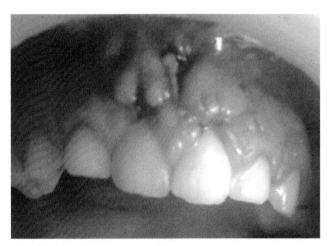

FIGURE 56-4 Unrepaired but healed torn maxillary frenum along with darkened maxillary central incisor from previous trauma.

and that the parent is providing appropriate oral health care and has established a dental home for the child. If the parent fails to comply with treatment, the health care provider should consider reporting the case to the appropriate child protective agency. Untreated rampant caries is often an indication of dental neglect.

Lack of treatment after trauma to the mouth can also be a sign of dental neglect (Figure 56-4). When evidence of a previous oral injury is noticed, care should be taken to inquire as to what happened and when.

SPECIAL NEEDS PATIENTS

In the United States, both federal and state laws deal with the neglect of the physically and/or mentally disabled. Disabled individuals are at a higher risk of being targets of neglect by caregivers than are nondisabled people. This sometimes is because parents or caregivers are simply overwhelmed by their responsibilities. Special needs individuals can be abused and/or neglected by family members, home

care attendants, or institutional health care workers, or they may even be self-neglecting.

With the current trend of mainstreaming intellectually and physically challenged people, many live in group homes. Disabled people generally have a higher incidence of dental problems because of their physical or mental limitations.[6] Those with cognitive disorders are often unaware of the need for good oral hygiene. Physical limitations can prevent some special needs individuals from performing the tasks needed to maintain their hygiene. Some people have such severe disabilities that it is difficult for even the most caring of caregivers to adequately perform the basics of hygiene, even brushing their teeth. Professionals need to be thorough in their evaluations of people with special needs.

PROFESSIONAL INTERVENTION

The first step involves taking a complete patient history, including information about the family and their home life. After analysis of this information, a thorough clinical examination should be completed. If a diagnosis of dental disease is made, appropriate recommendations for definitive treatment and referral to the proper dental care provider should be made. In addition, the family should be assisted in establishing a dental home. Monitoring of the patient should be done to determine that recommendations have been followed. Referrals to proper resources for additional education, assistance, and support should be made available to the parent or guardian. Empathy and concern for the patient should guide health care providers in their assessments.

All health professionals should be familiar with their state laws and with the mechanism for reporting suspected neglect. If a health care provider reports suspected neglect in good faith, the reporter is immune from any legal liability, even if the case is eventually unfounded. Reporting suspected neglect is a call for help for the child or disabled person.

When reporting to a local law enforcement or child protection agency, the reporter should provide a statement about his or her concerns and the reasons for suspecting neglect (including any documented evidence) and the names, addresses, and phone numbers of all involved parties. In most states, the immediate initial reports can be made by telephone, followed by written reports.

FUTURE PROGNOSIS

Dental neglect can be seen in all socioeconomic and educational levels and in all age groups. It is generally accepted that reported incidents of neglect, including dental neglect, significantly underrepresent the actual number of cases that occur. Dental neglect is often seen as a part of the more general neglect of the child. All health care providers should evaluate their patients for the presence of dental disease and assess the risk of developing dental disease in the future.

The caries disease process is multifactorial. Caries is a biofilm-mediated acid demineralization of the enamel or dentin of the teeth.[7] Dental research continues to examine the causative factors, explore genetic issues, and search for a preventive solution. Recognition and treatment of dental disease in its earliest forms is the key to preventing caries and its debilitating destruction in our most defenseless citizens.

References

1. American Academy of Pediatric Dentistry, Child Abuse Committee: Definitions, Oral Health Policies and Clinical Guidelines. Definition of Dental Neglect, 2008. Available at http://www.aapd.org/media/Policies_Guidelines/D_DentalNeglect.pdf. Access November 23, 2008.
2. U.S. Department of Health and Human Services, Administration for Children and Families. *Child Maltreatment 2006.* Available at http://www.acf.hhs.gov/programs/cb/pubs/cm06. Accessed December 27, 2008.
3. Kellogg N, Block RW, Hibbard RA, et al: Oral and dental aspects of child abuse and neglect. *Pediatrics* 2005;116:1565-1568.
4. American Academy of Pediatric Dentistry, Council on Clinical Affairs: *Definitions, Oral Health Policies and Clinical Guidelines.* Definition of Dental Home. 2008. Available at http://www.aapd.org/media/Policies_Guidelines/D_DentalHome.pdf. Accessed November 23, 2008.
5. American Academy of Pediatric Dentistry, Council on Clinical Affairs: *Definitions, Oral Health Policies and Clinical Guidelines.* Definition of Early Childhood Caries (ECC). 2008. Available at http://www.aapd.org/media/Policies_Guidelines/D_ECC.pdf. Accessed November 23, 2008.
6. Glassman P, Subar P: Improving and maintaining oral health for people with special needs. *Dent Clin North Am* 2008:52:444-461.
7. Garcia-Godoy F, Hicks MJ: Maintaining the integrity of the enamel surface: the role of dental biofilm, saliva and preventive agents in enamel demineralization and remineralization. *J Am Dent Assoc* 2008;139(Suppl):25S-34S.

57

FAILURE TO THRIVE

Deborah E. Lowen, MD

INTRODUCTION

For many clinicians, dealing with a child who is failing to thrive can invoke a complex assortment of emotions, ranging from dread to excitement. Dread arises because the evaluation and management of these children can be time-consuming, confusing, and sometimes unsatisfactory in terms of clear diagnoses, immediate results, and long-term outcomes; excitement because of the necessity to solve a possibly complex diagnostic puzzle, the potential to effect change, and the hope for a positive long-term results. This chapter discusses the history of failure to thrive (FTT) as a concept, definitions, etiology, treatment, and outcome in an attempt to move clinicians toward a clearer understanding of this often complex condition.

Early pediatric textbooks in the United States provided descriptions of malnutrition, infantile atrophy, and athrepsia that are recognizable today as FTT.[1-3] Authors speculated on etiologies, recognizing that in some cases there was no clear evidence of a medical disease causing poor growth. The terms *hospitalism* and *anaclitic depression* were used by René Spitz in the 1940s to describe both the physical and psychological effects of institutionalization and lack of a primary caregiver.[4,5] Although Spitz used these terms to describe problems more far-reaching than simple growth difficulties, he recognized the environmental effects on growth and development, the importance of a primary caregiver in the life of an infant, and the idea that psychiatric disorders can have their origins in early childhood.

Spitz's work in part led to the term *maternal deprivation syndrome*, used to describe poor growth in young children living in their own homes, but with mothers who for various reasons could not meet the children's needs.[6] This concept acknowledged the role of children's emotional and social environments in their growth and development. However, the assignment of blame to a parent, specifically a mother, could inhibit clinicians' searching for the often multifactorial etiologies of FTT and inappropriately label caregivers. Two decades ago this emphasis on parental culpability was called erroneous,[7] but "maternal deprivation syndrome" can still be found as a synonym for nonorganic FTT today.[8]

The term *nonorganic failure to thrive* has become a catchall term to describe growth failure in the absence of a major acute or chronic medical illness. With the background of Spitz's work, children with poor growth might immediately be suspected of having deficient psychosocial environments, especially as it relates to parenting. In part to avoid this rush to inappropriate diagnosis and judgment, in part to recognize the transactional nature of the disorder,[9] and in part to recognize that the main defect in these children is poor physical growth caused by lack of appropriate nutrition, several other terms have been suggested as replacements of what some feel is an obsolete description.[10] Various suggested terms include *pediatric undernutrition, inadequate growth, growth failure, growth deficiency, growth faltering*, and *failure to gain weight*. Replacement of the word *failure* is particularly desirable because of its pejorative nature[11]; others believe *faltering growth* implies something less severe or persistent than FTT.[12]

DEFINITION

Notwithstanding the concerns just mentioned, the term *failure to thrive (FTT)* will be used throughout this chapter, as well as some of the other terms mentioned. As for defining FTT, there is no accepted "gold standard" in the medical literature.[13] Although the early precursors of FTT such as anaclitic depression included both growth and developmental factors in their descriptions, FTT is almost universally defined only in terms of physical growth. At its most basic, it means postnatal physical growth that deviates from the norm. The use of anthropometric indices to define FTT is critical, but highly variable. Two commonly used criteria are weight (or weight-for-height) less than 2 standard deviations below the mean for age and sex, and/or a weight curve that has crossed more than two major percentile lines on standard growth charts after the child had achieved a previously stable pattern.[14] Even these apparently straightforward definitions are subject to interpretation, and they each evaluate a different aspect of children's growth. The first considers attained growth, a one-time measurement, whereas the second deals with growth velocity.

Different researchers and clinicians have used various definitions for growth failure when considering only the attained growth of a child as a static measure, and each method has limitations. When evaluating weight according to age and sex, varying growth charts allow clinicians to use either the fifth or the third percentiles as cutoffs. The use of Z-scores, based on standard deviations, is a similar method. However, designating as abnormal all of the lowest-weighing children for a specific age and sex is an oversimplification, since many of those children will in fact be normal but small. When a clearly undernourished child is being evaluated, however, expression of the weight as a percentage of median weight-for-age can be used to assess the severity of the malnutrition.[15] Instead of using only weight-for-age, some undernourished children are identified based on their weight-for-height being less than the fifth or third percentile. This too is not ideal as a solitary measurement, since some normal, petite children will be inappropriately labeled, whereas other children whose height growth is stunted because of chronic malnutrition will not be identified. For example, children with kwashiorkor and the edema that arises from protein malnutrition can fall within the normal range of weight-for-height percentiles. The 2000 CDC edition of growth charts includes norms for body mass index (BMI), which is now being evaluated as an assessment tool to evaluate growth failure.[16,17]

Assessing growth velocity relies on the availability of more than one measurement, providing a more dynamic view of a child's growth. When available, multiple measurements can detect a fall-off in weight-for-age by two major percentile channels, as well as changes in the child's weight-for-height. In addition, repeated measurements allow for assessment of the daily growth rate that can be compared with normative values found in incremental tables such as those developed by Guo et al.[18] Evaluating growth velocity can also allow for adjustment based upon *conditional* weight gain, consistent with the normal statistical phenomenon of regression to the mean. This tendency for weights either at the low or high end to become less extreme could lead to some children being inappropriately labeled as failing to thrive, so conditional reference charts have been developed.[19] Conditional weight gain can also be calculated using the "Thrive Index" in which changes in weight Z scores from birth to a later age are adjusted for regression to the mean.[20] This method and the conditional reference charts are predominantly used in the United Kingdom rather than the United States, just as Z scores based on standard deviations rather than percentiles are also used more commonly abroad.

Having multiple measurements to assess growth velocity is not always possible, given our highly mobile societies and the ability of caregivers to choose multiple sites for medical care, or none at all. In addition, for the most precise assessment, the anthropometric values must be obtained accurately, ideally on the same scale, by the same clinician, and with the young child in the same state of undress at each measurement.

Two reviews of the medical literature verified the problems of defining FTT using anthropometric measurements. Wilcox et al[21] and Olsen[22] performed literature reviews and found that there is no standard definition of FTT, although in Olsen's review all definitions used anthropometric indicators. In another study, Olsen used seven different anthropometric criteria for FTT to evaluate a birth cohort of 6090 children in Copenhagen. The concurrence among all seven criteria was generally poor, and none of the children identified as FTT met all the criteria. No single measurement on its own was adequate for identifying all cases of growth faltering.[23] Rather than reflecting disagreement among clinicians and researchers, this lack of a gold-standard definition represents the multiple different ways in which childhood undernutrition presents. The existing medical literature on FTT must always be evaluated in this light, especially when comparing studies using different methodologies.

Despite the varying uses of growth charts to evaluate and identify children with FTT, there is a typical progression of change on these charts when children are not gaining weight appropriately. First the weight measurement will show a drop-off from previous percentiles. If the child actually loses weight rather than simply failing to gain appropriately, the drop-off on the growth curve can be precipitous. Actual weight loss, other than that associated with an acute illness or therapeutic diet, is an indicator of pathology and is never normal in young children.[10] A malnourished child will stop normal gains in height once the inadequate weight gain continues for weeks or months, depending upon the severity. Head circumference is the last measurement to show a drop-off. If a child manifests a different pattern, a search for causes besides malnutrition, such as genetic or constitutional issues, is indicated.[14]

Acute malnutrition—when the weight-for-age has dropped to a greater degree than the height-for-age—is called wasting and is associated with a low weight-for-height. Over the longer term, as the height-for-age percentile falls, weight-for-height might normalize. This stunting is one reason that only using the weight-for-height measurement to identify poor growth is insufficient. These stunted children do not always appear malnourished at first glance, since they can seem proportionally normal. Evaluating both weight-for-age and height-for-age can make the difference in correctly identifying growth failure in these children.

Although no clear, consistent definition of FTT exists, malnutrition is the underlying defect in all cases. FTT is therefore only a descriptive term of a child's condition, rather than a diagnosis. It is the clinician's duty to determine the often multifactorial etiologies causing this malnutrition; simply identifying a child as failing to thrive is inadequate. A useful analogy is that of abdominal pain. Abdominal pain is a symptom, for which a clinician is obligated to determine the correct etiology. Simply labeling a patient as suffering from abdominal pain without searching for the cause would be inappropriate.

Even though suggestions have been made to abandon the term *failure to thrive*, there is some utility in its use of the word "thrive." To thrive generally means to have a flourishing, prosperous state.[24] In many cases, malnourished children are not only growing too slowly, but they are truly not thriving. Even descriptions of malnourished children in early pediatric textbooks discussed their loss of strength, lack of normal development, excessive crying, and later, apathy.[1-3] Children who are failing to thrive are usually affected in other ways besides growth failure, a fact that is not conveyed by terms such as *growth faltering* or *undernutrition*.

ETIOLOGY

The possible causes of FTT traditionally have been divided into two main categories: organic and nonorganic. The first referred to malnutrition caused by major illness or organ system dysfunction, whereas the latter was attributed to environmental causes such as hospitalism or the maternal deprivation syndrome.[10] In 1981, Homer and Ludwig[25] recognized that in some cases, FTT was caused by both organic problems and environmental or psychological problems. As more clinicians and researchers began studying FTT, this classification scheme has been rendered obsolete.[10] It is an oversimplification of the often multifactorial etiology of this complex problem and can result in premature, inappropriate labeling of children and/or families. Furthermore, lack of recognition of the complex interplay of different factors will make treatment more difficult, time-consuming, and possibly unsuccessful. Despite these problems with the binary categorization scheme, it continues to be taught to medical professionals[26] and to lay professionals such as child welfare workers and law enforcement personnel. Professionals should be taught that FTT is only a symptom, and that the cause or causes of malnutrition must be sought. In this chapter, the term *nonorganic FTT* is only used when the medical literature being discussed uses that term specifically.

THE BIOPSYCHOSOCIAL MODEL

In 1977 George Engel[29] presented the biopsychosocial model as a way to understand diseases and illnesses. He advocated that physicians understand not only the biomedical facts of patients' illnesses, but also the psychological and social aspects. When considering FTT, the biopsychosocial model is critically important to use. The biological, psychological, and social spheres all have the potential to greatly influence a child's growth and development.

The Biological Sphere

The most obvious problems in the biological sphere contributing to growth failure are those related to major medical illness, either acute or chronic. Even a cursory glance at Table 57-1 (categories of failure to thrive) reveals that multiple ailments can result in FTT. Medical providers sometimes focus all their attention on the search for a major medical illness. However, care must be taken to avoid attributing growth problem in an individual child entirely to a known medical cause. Growth failure can also reflect psychosocial issues. For example, an infant with unrepaired congenital heart disease might fail to thrive not only because of the increased caloric requirement inherent in the disease, but also because the caregivers are noncompliant with medications, are unable to afford special formulas, or are inadequately bonded with their special needs child. Simply treating the biomedical problem in the child will not satisfactorily resolve the growth issues.

Minor medical problems also fall within the biological realm and are capable of causing FTT. For example, even minor degrees of neurological dysfunction can interfere with a child's ability to eat and be fed appropriately.[30,31] Feeding is a complex process with three phases. Phase one involves the recognition of hunger, acquisition of food, and process of bringing food to the mouth. Phase two includes the preparation of ingested food for swallowing, with safe transfer of the food bolus to the esophagus without aspiration. Phase three is the passage of the food bolus through the esophagus into the stomach and intestines for digestion and absorption.[32] A disruption in any of these phases can result in inadequate growth. In addition to neurological dysfunction, gastrointestinal problems can also interrupt this process. Disorders that cause vomiting, such as "nervous vomiting" and rumination, can cause failure to gain weight[33] and are correctly categorized in the biomedical realm, despite their significant psychosocial components.

Certain prenatal risk factors associated with FTT are most correctly classified in the biological realm. A

Table 57-1	Categories of Failure to Thrive

Inadequate Caloric Intake

Poor Quality or Caloric Content
- Breastfeeding problems: poor latch, poor let-down, inadequate milk supply
- Formula problems: incorrect preparation, inadequate supply
- Poor nutritional content: excess juice or water, unusual diets, fixed beliefs
- Grazing
- Inadequate quantities of food given: poverty, food insecurity, neglect, purposeful withholding of food
- Medical child abuse (formerly Munchausen syndrome by proxy)

Feeding Difficulties
- Oromotor dysfunction
- Neurological impairment
- Gastroesophageal reflux ± esophagitis
- Esophageal strictures
- Vascular rings/slings
- Poor dentition
- Anorexia from various causes
- Parent–child conflict: temperament, autonomy struggles

Inadequate Absorption and/or Excess Losses

Persistent Vomiting
- Pyloric stenosis
- CNS disease
- GI obstruction
- Rumination
- Psychogenic vomiting

Gastrointestinal Disease
- Celiac disease
- Cystic fibrosis
- Protein allergies
- Lactose intolerance
- Infection: giardiasis, *Salmonella*, *Clostridium difficile*
- Liver disease
- Short gut

Increased Caloric Requirements

Cardiorespiratory Disease
- Congenital heart disease
- Acquired heart disease
- Chronic lung disease
- Cystic fibrosis
- Obstructive sleep apnea

Chronic Infection
- HIV/AIDS
- Tuberculosis
- Urinary tract infection

Other
- Malignancy
- Hyperthyroidism
- Excess activity

Defective Utilization

- Inborn errors of metabolism
- Diabetes mellitus
- Congenital adrenal hyperplasia

Adapted from Krugman SD, Dubowitz H: Failure to thrive, *Am Fam Physician* 2003;68:879-884 and Careaga MG, Kerner JA, Jr: A gastroenterologist's approach to failure to thrive, *Pediatr Ann* 2000;29:558-567.

population-based cohort study found that both parental height and higher parity were risk factors for FTT.[34] An earlier study that excluded children with "organic abnormality that could explain the lack of growth" found that medical complications of pregnancy and the perinatal period correlated significantly with later FTT. These conditions included less weight gain during pregnancy, pregnancy complications, shorter gestations, feeding difficulty in the nursery, and unresolved health questions at hospital discharge.[35]

Low birth weight itself is a risk factor for FTT, with symmetric intrauterine growth retardation carrying a worse prognosis for growth and development than asymmetric intrauterine growth retardation.[36] Low birth weight resulting from prematurity can cause confusion for clinicians. Growth curves should be corrected for prematurity up to 24 months postnatal age for weight, 40 months for height, and 18 months for head circumference.[37] Analysis of growth curves is especially important in these children to avoid either inappropriate labeling as FTT or inappropriate attribution of low weight to prematurity alone. Premature babies are often at risk for neurological, pulmonary, cardiac, and gastrointestinal problems that predispose them to growth failure. Sometimes their problems do not rise to the level of major illnesses, but even minor degrees of dysfunction can cause problems with weight gain.

Postnatally, biological risk factors for poor weight gain include weak sucking in the first 8 weeks of life, the duration of breastfeeding, and difficulty weaning.[11] An obvious postnatal risk factor is medical illness, either acute or chronic. Recurrent infections can cause FTT but can also be a secondary manifestation of immune system dysfunction associated with malnutrition. With each infection the child might lose weight or fail to grow appropriately because of a decrease in appetite, decrease in intake, higher metabolic rate, and/or increased losses caused by vomiting or diarrhea.[36] This creates a vicious cycle in which poor growth causes immune dysfunction, which causes recurrent infections, which causes poor growth.

Elevated lead levels can correlate with impaired growth. These children often have anemia and other nutritional deficits which can enhance lead absorption. They sometimes develop anorexia, causing a decrease in caloric intake. Behavioral issues can also develop, causing further difficulty for the caregivers. In children with elevated lead levels, there are often psychosocial issues at play, which themselves can contribute to their poor growth, inadequate nutrition, and exposure to lead.

The Psychological Sphere

Psychological factors in FTT usually center on the mental health issues of the caregivers, with the mother being the most often studied and evaluated. However, failure to evaluate the child's contribution is inappropriate and might lead to failure of treatment. Parents affect their children, but children also affect their parents. Each interaction influences future interactions in either a positive or negative direction. The transactional model promulgated by Sameroff and Chandler[9] considers this complex interplay and its effect on the child's ultimate development. Recognition of this transactional model in part led away from the overly simplistic idea of maternal deprivation syndrome causing FTT,[38] and

continues to lead current thinking about growth failure. It is important to consider both the child and the parent when discussing the psychological sphere of the biopsychosocial model of FTT.

A key aspect of the child's contribution to the transactional model is temperament. This behavioral style is innate in young infants but can be modified by environmental influences as they grow.[39] Components of a child's temperament include the following: activity level, adaptability, rhythmicity (the level of predictability in a child's biological functions), distractibility, initial response to stimuli, threshold of responsiveness, intensity, and persistence.[39,40] A baby who eats and sleeps on a regular schedule, responds to stimuli in a predictable manner, and is easily soothed would be described as an "easy" baby, whereas one who fusses constantly and unpredictably and does not soothe easily would be harder to parent. Some children's temperaments are not good "matches" with their parents. For instance, a young infant who sleeps a lot and must be awakened to feed might seem ideal to a depressed mother who only wants to sleep. Although this seems to be a good match for the mother, the infant might not receive appropriate feedings. In addition, as parents modify their responses to a given child's temperament, they will influence that child's future behavior.

Some studies looking at temperament in infants with growth failure found more FTT babies classified as difficult, but others provided conflicting views.[41] Darlington and Wright[41] studied 75 infants divided into three groups by their rate of weight gain: slow, average, or fast. Temperament was assessed by a validated survey completed by mothers, which assessed six domains of temperament in different settings. Infants with slow weight gain scored significantly higher than the other groups on the fear dimension, equating to rejection of new objects or persons. Infants with fast weight gain scored higher than the other groups on the distress to limitations domain, meaning they had more negative emotionality and reaction to frustrating situations. It is certainly plausible that the fast-gaining infants were more vocal with their distress, causing the mothers to respond by feeding them. Less vocal infants sometimes suffer relative undernutrition by not expressing their needs.[41] A retrospective case-control study evaluating infants with poor weight gain found that there were no significant differences in temperament between the two groups.[42] However, temperament studies done by maternal report might not be accurate, whereas studies done with observation only capture one point in time rather than the day-to-day behavior of the child.

The contribution of the child to the transactional model can be a cause or a result of growth failure. Although not specific to growth difficulties, children with feeding disorders have been shown to express more negativity and withdrawal and have been described as apathetic, or conversely, fussy and difficult.[43] Irregular sleep patterns, in addition to feeding patterns, have been described in growth deficient children, but the convenience sample was of a small size and all the children had major medical problems that could have confounded both their eating and sleeping behaviors.[44]

Parental ratings of appetite[45] as well as measurements of energy intake[46] have been found to be lower in children with FTT. Although not all children with poor appetites have difficulties with growth, the possibility exists that those children who do have growth problems have some innate differences in eating habits. Of course, children with some nutrient deficiencies develop anorexia, so once FTT is evident, a vicious cycle can ensue.

It is intuitive that parental psychological disturbance will affect the parent–child relationship, and quite possibly the child's growth and development. Recognizing this possibility is of critical importance, not for the purpose of assigning blame, but rather for offering appropriate treatment.

Evaluation of the psychological contribution of caregivers to FTT has been centered on mothers. The use of the term *maternal deprivation syndrome* clearly describes the attitudes of clinicians and researchers evaluating children who have FTT without a clear biological etiology. Early studies found a considerable degree of maternal psychopathology in these cases; however, these studies had several methodological flaws calling their conclusions into question. Boddy and Skuse[31] in 1994 published a detailed discussion of the problems with these studies. One problem was retrospective design, in which mothers were evaluated *after* their children had been identified as nonorganic FTT. The parental characteristics might have been caused in part by the identification of the growth failure. Also, study subjects were often hospitalized children with more severe FTT. The willing and truthful participation of some of these mothers could have been compromised by the labeling of their children, especially if they were under investigation.[35] In addition, some assessments of family functioning were based on parental interviews of uncertain validity[47] and might not have been appropriate for illiterate or less-educated parents.[31] In addition, observation of the mother–child relationship, especially in a hospital setting, might be subject to misinterpretation because people often act differently when their children are hospitalized.[31,48]

Families of children with FTT do not have a higher incidence of overt psychopathology than those of comparison subjects.[38] However, one study with several of the concerning methodological characteristics noted previously showed an extremely high percentage of psychopathology in parents of infants with FTT.[49] Ninety three percent of the mothers and 38% of the fathers showed Axis 1 psychopathology during the first week of their children's hospital admission. Parents were provided psychotherapy and treatment focused on the parent–infant relationship. Notably, there were significant reductions in psychopathology for both parents when reassessed 3 and 12 months later. The issue of causality is important. How much did the parental psychopathology cause or contribute to the growth failure? How much did the growth failure contribute to the psychopathology? Did the improvement in the parents result from the psychotherapeutic interventions, from the child's improvement, or both?

Perinatal depression is a common problem, with prevalence rates estimated at roughly 10% in the general population and higher among low-income and ethnic minority women.[50] A case-control study found that 21% of mothers with children falling off the growth curve were in a depressive episode compared with 11% of matched controls.[12] A selection bias in case ascertainment caused some obviously depressed mothers of growth faltering babies not to be referred for study inclusion, meaning the results could have been even more compelling. A prospective study confirmed the association of slow weight gain in infancy with postpartum depression.[51] Again, however, this association does not necessarily indicate causality, since the negative implications of their infants' growth problems might have exacerbated mood disturbances. Other studies have found that depressive symptoms and affective disorders might be more common in mothers of malnourished children.[36]

Questioning parents about their own childhoods could provide some insight. A prospective study showed a significant correlation between mothers who were physically abused or had negative perceptions of their own childhoods with the development of growth failure in their children.[35] These mothers were also more likely to reject their own mothers as role models. Perhaps this reflects a lack of adequate social or emotional support for the mothers. A case comparison study demonstrated a significantly higher percentage of mothers of children failing to thrive endorsed a history of being abused and/or neglected during childhood.[52] Despite this link between maternal childhood experiences and FTT, the association is neither direct nor inevitable.[31]

Clinicians evaluating children with poor growth often encounter very thin mothers. The possibility exists that some of these mothers are suffering from eating disorders themselves. In two case series, children of mothers with anorexia nervosa or bulimia nervosa had feeding difficulties and/or poor weight gain.[53,54] McCann et al[55] studied the eating habits and attitudes of mothers of 26 children referred for evaluation of nonorganic FTT. None of the mothers met diagnostic criteria for either anorexia nervosa or bulimia nervosa, but they did show more dietary restraint than matched controls. Even though the children all had low weight, half of the mothers were restricting the children's diet of sweets and a third restricted intake of food they felt to be fattening. Another prospective study failed to find an association with maternal dietary restraint and infant weight gain, although this study used a different scale to assess the mothers' eating attitude.[45]

Children's food intake might be purposely limited by caregivers because of other psychological issues. The disorder of medical child abuse (previously called Munchausen syndrome by proxy) can present with children failing to thrive for no reason despite extensive medical workup, often demanded by the parent.[56,57] Other parents develop a fixed belief that their children suffer from multiple food allergies requiring an extremely limited diet that can cause growth failure.[58] In some cases, double-blinded food challenges under extremely controlled medical conditions are needed to help convince parents otherwise. Some parents place children on nutritionally deficient diets because of concerns about the relationship of food to disorders such as eczema.[59] Other well-intentioned parents sometimes limit their children's diets because of a misapplication of diets for adults designed to prevent obesity or cardiovascular disease, or simply because of their own history of childhood obesity.[60]

Questions about parental competence arise in evaluation of growth-faltering children. Neglectful parenting patterns, such as poor communication and socialization at mealtimes, have been found.[61,62] The range of mothers' responses to children's poor eating can also vary greatly.[45] Although these parents' problem-solving ability needs to be high, Robinson et al's[63] study of 37 mothers found that the mothers of children with FTT performed poorer on a problem-solving evaluation than control mothers, showing a narrower repertoire of solutions and poorer quality of responses. Once again, however, the question of cause and effect arises. Were their children failing to thrive because of the mothers' skills, or were the mothers' deficits caused in part by the children's growth failure?

One other issue related to parental competence bears mentioning: maternal IQ. An older study with some of the methodological flaws mentioned above examined the homes of 58 3-year-olds who had been hospitalized as infants for FTT. Although three different interventions were applied to these cases, there were no differences in the scores evaluating the quality of the home environments. However, mean maternal IQ was quite low (80.8), and maternal IQ did account for variance in the scores.[64] Although parents of below-normal intelligence can successfully raise healthy children, in this study lower IQ was a risk factor for problems in the home environment, and quite possibly for their children's growth failure.

The Social Sphere

In this sphere of the biopsychosocial model of FTT, poverty is the most pervasive risk factor in children evaluated for growth failure.[14] Poverty can be severe enough to limit food availability.[36,65] Societal safety nets are sometimes inadequate for families to obtain enough food to avoid episodes of hunger, given the lack of appropriate funding and the nutritional needs of rapidly growing infants and young children.[36] In addition, poor families can have difficulty accessing public resources or might be concerned about their immigration status, keeping them from benefiting from governmental programs. In times of economic downturns, charitable donations to community services often dwindle, affecting the ability of nonprofit organizations to help families.

Three important points about poverty and FTT must be made. First, FTT does not occur exclusively in economically disadvantaged families, a fact recognized in early studies of the "maternal deprivation syndrome."[6,65] Second, although poverty is a risk factor for growth failure, a relative minority of poor children have FTT. Determining the exact percentage is impossible because of the inability to accurately measure the number of children living in such situations and the lack of ability to uniformly assess those children for growth failure. The sometimes restricted access to preventive medical care resulting from lack of health insurance limits the ability to detect and treat early growth failure.[36] Lack of reliable transportation, difficulty accessing primary care, and lack of adequate sources providing primary care also complicate this issue.

The third key point has arisen through recent studies questioning the long-held premise connecting poverty to FTT. Blair and colleagues[34] examined a large cohort and found that parental socioeconomic status was not related to FTT. Wright and colleagues[45] examined a prospective birth cohort and found that both the highest and lowest levels of socioeconomic deprivation were associated with faltering weight. Both of these studies took place in the United Kingdom, and the specific features of that country's benefits for families with children and the lower cost of food there could have accounted in part for these findings.[34]

In some cases, family income is associated directly with FTT, but it can also be a risk factor for other factors related to FTT. Drotar and Sturm[64] found that the quality of the home environment is related to family income. The relationship between this association and the development of FTT again leads to questions of cause and effect.

Other issues within the family that are associated with FTT include family stressors, lack of social support, social isolation, and quality of interpersonal relationships.[14,36] Regarding family stress, Altemeier et al's[35] prospective study looked specifically at sources of stress in parents of children with failure to thrive. Four maternal life stressors were significantly correlated with FTT. Of these four, three dealt with the mother's relationship with the baby's father: arguments with him, separation from him, and reconciliation with him or his family. The fourth maternal life stressor was death of a friend within the preceding year. The two paternal life stressors significantly correlating with FTT were leaving a job within the preceding year without being fired and getting arrested.

The issue of family stress is a difficult one because the identification of the child as having growth difficulties would, in most cases, be expected to cause stress in itself. Again, separating out cause and effect is difficult. In addition, the experience of stress is a personal one and depends on the parents' perceptions, which in turn is determined by individual characteristics including age and personality.[31] The role poverty plays in adding to family stress can also be significant.

Social isolation and lack of social support contribute to parents' stress and to their inability to mobilize resources in the face of other stressors. In addition, social isolation can limit the input of others outside the family to such a degree that considerable wasting is not noticed until the malnutrition is severe.

Problematic interpersonal relationships contribute to social isolation and lack of support as well as to parental stress. Drotar and colleagues[47] published results of a study of the families of children with FTT and found that they had less optimal relationships than comparison families. In addition, their scores on a standard measure of family relationships were worse both at time of diagnosis and approximately 4 years later, regardless of the type of intervention received during course of treatment. Weston and colleagues[52] found that in addition to childhood abuse, mothers of children with nonorganic FTT had experienced more abuse as adults than comparison mothers. However, the subjects were allowed to self-define abuse and no objective documentation of maltreatment, either in childhood or as adults, was provided. It is intuitive, however, that intimate partner violence would affect parental stress levels and could be associated with FTT.

Child neglect is often implicated in cases of FTT in which no clear biological etiology is detected. Yet, there are multiple other possible causes, and it is important not to assume, "… without question that poor growth in a child from a materially or emotionally deprived background adds up to neglect."[48] Although there might be elements of child neglect in many of these situations, it becomes easier to label the caregivers as negligent when there is intentional withholding of food from the child or if the family is resistant to recommended interventions[14] or is frankly noncompliant. In addition to neglect, child abuse is sometimes present in FTT cases as well. Infants in abusing families are at greater risk of FTT.[66] Severe withholding of nutrition can be classified as starvation and can result in criminal prosecution.[67]

EVALUATION

The medical evaluation of children with faltering growth should be guided by careful consideration of the many possible etiologies discussed previously. The goal is to determine the diagnosis or diagnoses causing the symptom of FTT. This section discusses the evaluation of children with FTT based on the biopsychosocial model.

Growth Charts

The medical evaluation of FTT starts with examination of the child's anthropometric data reflected in the growth chart. Accurate measurements of weight, height, and head circumference must be carefully plotted on growth charts for reliable assessments. For serial measurements, children should be weighed and measured repeatedly in the same manner to correctly assess growth over time. This can be difficult when children are taken to different medical providers, or when infants are hospitalized and different staff members weigh them each day, often on different scales.

Different growth charts are available. In the United States, the Centers for Disease Control and Prevention published new growth charts in 2000 based on data collected by the National Health and Nutrition Examination Survey (NHANES) (available at http://www.CDC.gov/GrowthCharts). These replaced charts published in 1977 by the National Center for Health Statistics (NCHS). The newer charts were an improvement because of a larger sample size, a more racially and ethnically diverse sample, the inclusion of more breastfed babies, the addition of body mass index, and statistical refinement of data analysis. In 1990, the United Kingdom also released new growth charts.[68]

The World Health Organization (WHO) had designated the 1977 NCHS growth charts as their international standard until their own charts were released in 2006. This release culminated a multiyear project that included collection of data from six countries, recruiting only nonsmoking mothers who were willing to exclusively breastfeed their infants for 4 months.[68] The goal was to create the optimum standard for growth while establishing breastfeeding as the biological norm.[69] These growth charts are meant to be used for children in all countries regardless of ethnicity, socioeconomic status, or type of feeding. Experts in pediatrics and nutrition in the United Kingdom have recommended the use of the WHO 2006 charts for UK children only after 2 weeks of age.[70]

Growth charts are available for children with specific special health issues such as Down syndrome, Turner syndrome, and velo-cardio-facial syndrome. Using typical growth charts for children with some types of health problems can lead to inaccurate labeling and unnecessary testing.

History

A thorough history will point to the correct diagnosis in the majority of cases of FTT. It is best to start chronologically in the prenatal period and proceed to the child's birth, neo-natal period, and infancy in order. Using the biopsychosocial model and remembering the different etiologies of FTT, the following tables provide examples of the type of information to be obtained. The psychological and social spheres have been combined because of the frequent overlap of issues in those categories.

Table 57-2 deals with the prenatal period. Review of the mother's obstetrical record is necessary to obtain a thorough history. No single answer is likely to indicate the etiology of a child's growth problem. For instance, if the pregnancy was unplanned and the mother considered termination, that is possibly a psychosocial issue contributing to growth failure, but it cannot be taken as a primary cause while ignoring other historical factors.

Table 57-3 refers to necessary historical information to be obtained about the baby's birth. Although having the birth records available is helpful, the parental perception might be different and must be considered. In addition, nursing or social work notes in the medical record often provide a more objective assessment of the reaction of the father or mother's partner. However, ascribing feelings to the reactions of others in such a seminal event can be difficult and should not be used to predict future behavior.

Table 57-4 discusses the time period immediately after birth, from the nursery stay until the period shortly after hospital discharge. Altemeier et al's[35] prospective study of the antecedents of FTT showed that difficulty feeding in the nursery and unresolved health questions at hospital discharge correlated with future development of FTT. Even if the medical records do not indicate a major health concern, the mother's perception might be different, either because of her own experience and knowledge or because of poor or conflicting communication from medical personnel.

Table 57-2	Historical Factors in the Prenatal Period to Be Considered in an Evaluation of Growth Failure Using a Biopsychosocial Model

Prenatal History

Biological Sphere
- Mother's medical history
- Mother's obstetric history
- Prenatal care obtained
- Infections and illnesses during pregnancy
- Medical problems with the pregnancy (e.g., preterm labor, bleeding, oligohydramnios or polyhydramnios)
- Intrauterine growth retardation
- Trauma, either intentional or accidental
- Medications used during pregnancy
- Alcohol and cigarette use/abuse during pregnancy
- Illicit substance use/abuse during pregnancy
- Maternal weight gain during pregnancy

Psychosocial Spheres
- Planned vs. unplanned pregnancy
- If unplanned, reaction of mother and father
- Timing and consistency of prenatal care
- Type and amount of social support
- Maternal mental illness before and/or during pregnancy
- Stressors during pregnancy
- Intimate partner violence
- Preparations for baby

Table 57-3	Historical Factors About the Child's Birth to Be Considered in an Evaluation of Growth Failure Using a Biopsychosocial Model

Birth

Biological Sphere
- Gestational age
- Mode of delivery
- Complications of delivery
- Weight, length, and head circumference
- Large, appropriate, or small for gestational age
- Dysmorphic appearance or congenital malformations

Psychosocial Spheres
- Maternal complications of delivery
- Maternal perception of delivery
- Father or partner's reaction to birth of baby

Table 57-4	Historical Factors About the Period Following the Child's Birth to Be Considered in an Evaluation of Growth Failure Using a Biopsychosocial Model

Neonatal Course in the Hospital Nursery and Immediately after Discharge

Biological Sphere
- Breast or bottle feeding
- Success of initial feedings
  - Trouble with latching, if breastfeeding
  - Weak or strong suck
  - Availability of lactation support
- Medical problems during initial few days
- Need for medical tests during nursery stay
- Total amount of weight loss during nursery stay
- Length of hospitalization
- Need for repeat testing after discharge
- First follow-up appointment after discharge
- Medical problems and weight at first follow-up appointment

Psychosocial Spheres
- Time for and limitations of maternal bonding
- Quality of maternal bonding
- Mother's perception of newborn's health
- Type and amount of social support during and immediately after hospitalization
- Acceptance of education while in the hospital
- Maternal length of hospitalization
- Appropriate baby supplies in the home
- Compliance with and reaction to home visitor after discharge (where available)

Table 57-5	Historical Factors About the Period After the Neonatal Period to Be Considered in an Evaluation of Growth Failure Using a Biopsychosocial Model

After the Neonatal Period, in the First Several Months of Life

Biological Sphere
- Frequency and source of routine medical care
- Growth measurements
- Immunization status
- Medical illnesses
- Hospitalizations
- Medications
- Allergies—medications, food, other
- Surgeries
- Injuries, including bruises on infants
- Feeding issues—vigorous or difficult feeder
- Breastfeeding:
  - Milk letdown
  - Sense of fullness/emptying
  - Frequency and duration of feedings
  - Maternal observation of baby swallowing
  - Maternal diet and medical problems while breastfeeding
- Formula feeding:
  - Type
  - Method of mixing (concentration)
  - Frequency and quantity of feedings
- Other intake in first few months of life, such as:
  - Water
  - Juice
  - Tea
  - Soda
  - Cereal
- Sleep schedule
- Baby's temperament
- Developmental milestones
- Use of alternative or complementary medicines

Psychosocial Spheres
- Provision of baby care, especially feeding
- Maternal sleep deprivation
- Postnatal depression or other mental illness
- Type and amount of social support
- Availability of respite for mother
- Involvement of father and/or other intimate partner
- Intimate partner violence
- Financial resources, including money for baby supplies
- Enrollment in governmental aid programs
- Parental reaction to fussing/crying
- Who lives with baby
- Reactions of others in the home to the baby
- Parental employment
- Use of daycare or babysitting
- Caregiver perception of weight gain and general appearance

Many of the issues in the biological sphere important in the first few months of life (Table 57-5) are part of a thorough pediatric medical history. Verifying some of the information via review of medical records is mandatory. Obviously there must be detailed questioning about the infant's nutritional intake. Caregivers often have difficulty answering these questions for several reasons, including poor communication between multiple caregivers about feedings, difficulty in quantifying feedings resulting from the intellectual limitations of the parent, and/or defensiveness on the parts of the caregivers caused by the detailed questioning. In addition, sometimes caregivers purposefully give false information or are knowingly feeding the baby inappropriately. Obtaining an accurate history of intake in young infants requires multiple questions phrased in different, non-judgmental ways. Parents of young infants should also be questioned about the intake of solid foods. Assuming that young infants are only receiving breast milk or formula is erroneous and will impair appropriate evaluation.

When asking about the diets of older infants and toddlers, practitioners should expand the dietary history to include the following:

- Where does the child eat (e.g., highchair, floor, table, in bed)?
- Who helps feed the child?
- Does the child feed himself or is he fed by caregivers?
- What is her eating schedule?
- How does the child's schedule coordinate with the family's eating schedule?
- What is the type and quantity of food eaten by the child?
- What is the parent's perception of the child's appetite?
- How does the parent respond to poor appetite, food refusal, or the child's desire to feed himself?
- How much liquid does she drink and how often?
- Is there a history of pica?

Although these questions will usually not provide detailed enough nutritional information for a calorie count, they help provide a sense of the family's eating/feeding style and possible disorganization around child feeding. For example, children who frequently snack or drink from a bottle or sippy cup all day might not develop enough of an appetite at mealtimes, limiting their total caloric intake. Identifying these issues helps provide an immediate starting point for remediation.

The medical history must include a detailed family history and review of systems, including the following:

Family History

- Heights and weights of parents and other children in the family
- History of parental and sibling growth problems
- Medical conditions in parents, siblings, and other family members
- Neurological disorders in the extended family
- Inborn errors of metabolism in the extended family
- Unexpected infant deaths in the family
- Consanguinity
- Mental illness in the family
- History of parental substance abuse

Review of Systems

- Constitutional: change in overall appearance, activity level, interaction, or temperament
- Respiratory: respiratory infections, wheezing, frequent cough, respiratory distress, snoring
- Cardiac: sweating with feeds, cyanosis, poor activity tolerance
- Gastrointestinal: dysphagia, vomiting, stool characteristics, diarrhea or constipation, apparent food intolerance
- Renal/urologic: polyuria, dysuria, urinary frequency

- Infection: recurrent infections including yeast infections
- Neurological: swallowing difficulties, abnormal movements, seizures, delayed development, loss of developmental milestones
- Dermatological: skin rashes, jaundice, any bruises on a young infant
- Musculoskeletal: bony fractures, deformations

Physical Examination

A thorough physical examination serves several important functions, including identification of medical disorders contributing to or causing the growth difficulties, evaluation of the severity and effects of malnutrition, and assessment for signs of neglect or abuse. An exhaustive list of physical examination findings for all the medical disorders that can cause growth difficulties is beyond the scope of this chapter. Signs of more common conditions as well as signs indicating the severity and effects of malnutrition and signs of neglect or abuse include the following:

- General—affect, interaction, absence of subcutaneous fat stores, poor muscle mass, loose skin folds
- Vital signs—hypertension or hypotension, tachycardia or bradycardia, tachypnea, hypothermia, hypoxia (by pulse oximetry)
- Head, eyes, ears, nose, throat—hair quality, hair loss, positional plagiocephaly, dysmorphic facies, cleft palate (including submucosal), poor dentition, tonsillar hypertrophy, thyroid masses
- Chest—increased work of breathing, rales or wheezes, clubbing
- Cardiac—pathological murmur, poor peripheral perfusion, cyanosis, clubbing
- Abdomen—hepatomegaly, abdominal mass, ascites
- Genitourinary and anus—anomalies, anal fistulae, signs of trauma
- Skin—skin rashes, poor hygiene, decreased turgor, scars, bruises
- Neurological—hypertonia or hypotonia, hyperreflexia, poor suck, uncoordinated swallow, developmental delay

Additional Assessment and Multidisciplinary Involvement

A complete assessment of a child with FTT is best accomplished with multidisciplinary input. Since FTT is a manifestation of malnutrition, objective assessment of caloric intake is necessary. Asking parents to recall exactly what the child ate for the prior 24 hours or longer does not always provide an accurate picture of the child's true intake. A 3-day food diary provided to parents for them to complete immediately after the initial assessment can provide more detailed information, recognizing that the evaluation itself might lead to a change in the child's diet. Parents are instructed to write down their child's entire intake, including liquids, and to estimate quantities as well as possible. Including information on the form such as timing of feeding, who fed the child, and where the child was fed can also provide valuable information about the family's feeding practices. A nutritionist can analyze the completed diet diary, not only for calorie content, but also for intake of fat, protein, and important nutrients. The diet diary cannot be used in families where the parent cannot read and write. In these families, dietary recall must be used. For children admitted to the hospital, calorie counts will be helpful but will not provide an accurate assessment of the child's intake prior to admission because of the change of environments, different people feeding the child, and different food types, preparation, and availability.

For infants failing to thrive while breastfeeding, a lactation consultant can be of invaluable assistance in identifying breastfeeding problems and helping to resolve them. This is especially true in early infancy if the mother has never successfully breastfed before. Problems in later infancy or toddlerhood often revolve around weaning issues, waning milk supply, or grazing (frequent access to small quantities of food), problems more appropriately addressed by a nutritionist or physician.

Observing feedings and parent–child interactions can occur simultaneously, although observation of the parent–child interaction not related to feeding is also helpful. Home observations of feedings and interactions can provide information that would not be readily available in the clinic or hospital setting. As Frank[36] states, these observations "… will elucidate the affective tone of the feeding process and identify dysfunctional interactions such as interrupting the feeding too often to clean the child, struggles over the child's efforts to feed independently, or inappropriate coaxing or threatening of the child." Negative reinforcement and other parental behaviors can perpetuate feeding problems[71] and might not be identified without a feeding observation. These observations will also alert clinicians to problems with clarity of the child's cues, temperament, and responsiveness to the parent, which will in turn provide a clearer portrait of their relationship.[28]

Home assessments can provide important information that parents might be unwilling to provide. Parents could be too embarrassed to admit that they have no running water, even though it affects their ability to prepare food safely. Similarly, the ability to prepare and store food depends on working utilities (electricity or natural gas) and appliances. Unusual practices such as only shopping at one location or using the refrigerator for storage of things other than food also might not be disclosed upon questioning. Other people living in the home might not come to clinic visits but nonetheless can have valuable information about the child and their own role in the family. These home observations can be conducted by social workers or nurse home visitors trained in the assessment of pediatric malnutrition.

A social worker can also do a thorough assessment of psychosocial factors affecting the child's growth and development. Sometimes medical clinicians do not have the knowledge, comfort level, or time to ask the necessary questions about the role of the psychological and social spheres in FTT. At the time of treatment, which is often multidisciplinary and multifaceted, a social worker can help with coordination of care.

A developmental evaluation is an important component in the assessment of FTT. Developmental problems are often associated with, or possibly a result of, malnutrition. Standardized assessments of a child's cognitive performance can inform caregivers about their children's strengths and weaknesses and can guide treatment plans. However, results of testing done early in the evaluation, especially if the child is poorly responsive because of malnutrition, should be interpreted cautiously and not used for prognosis; repeating the formal evaluation after nutritional rehabilitation is necessary.[36]

Three other consultants can be of great assistance in the evaluation of children with growth failure: a behavioral specialist, a psychologist, and an occupational therapist.[14] Behavioral specialists can help identify the contributions of the child's behavior to the growth failure and assist parents in dealing effectively with problematic behavior. A psychologist can assist with identification of parental psychopathology and assess its effect on the child, as well as guide treatment plans. In some cases an occupational therapist's evaluation of oral-motor functions can also be helpful.

Laboratory and Radiographic Evaluation

With a lengthy list of possible biological causes of FTT, clinicians are frequently tempted to order multiple laboratory evaluations to ferret out disease. Laboratory tests should be limited, however, and guided by findings on history and physical examination. Acute or chronic diseases causing growth failure are "rarely occult."[10] The lack of value of laboratory and radiographic testing has been clearly shown in two studies. Sills[72] reviewed the medical records of 185 children hospitalized for FTT. For the 18 children with proven organic etiologies, the history and physical examination strongly suggested the diagnosis. Only 36 of 2607 tests (1.4%) assisted in the diagnosis. Berwick's[73] review of 122 medical records of children hospitalized for FTT without apparent underlying disease showed that the infants received 4827 diagnostic tests, accounting for 24% of the total costs of hospital admission. Only 39 tests, 0.8% of all performed, were helpful in determining the etiology of the FTT.

Children undergoing evaluation for FTT are often subjected to unhelpful, expensive, and possibly harmful laboratory and radiographic evaluation, even in the absence of clues pointing to acute or chronic medical problem. Some of this might result from reliance on the old organic/nonorganic dichotomy. Some might result from the specific disciplines of the physicians evaluating FTT (e.g., gastroenterology, neurology). Certainly some is due to the litigious environment of modern medicine as well as the fact that parents sometimes demand medically unnecessary evaluations based on their own research on the Internet or discussions with friends. Some of the problem is probably related to the cognitive dissonance of the treating clinicians. Clinicians relish the idea of finding the "zebras" or unusual diagnoses, especially when the differential diagnosis is lengthy. Not only are the psychosocial causes of FTT very common, they are not perceived as being as exciting as organic causes, and are usually less readily treated. To accept common "mundane" problems such as difficulty obtaining food or postnatal depression as a cause of FTT can conflict with a clinician's self-image as a medical sleuth who solves complicated medical problems.

Since the yield of testing is so low, some experts recommend not using laboratory or radiological tests at all unless suggested by the history and physical examination.[28] Other experts advocate screening laboratory studies, with further testing based on the history, physical examination, and/or results of the screening labs. Some children with severe nutritional deficits need studies to evaluate protein status to help with clinical management.[36] Screening laboratory tests recommended by some (but not all) experts include the following:

- Complete blood count
- Serum electrolytes
- Blood urea nitrogen or creatinine
- Albumin and prealbumin
- Erythrocyte sedimentation rate or c-reactive protein
- Blood lead level
- Urinalysis
- Urine culture

In specific populations, testing for human immunodeficiency syndrome and/or tuberculosis is recommended.

There are very few medical diseases that can cause growth failure with no signs or symptoms noted on history or physical examination. Exceptions include silent urinary tract infections and renal tubular acidosis. Simultaneous testing of blood and urine pH and obtaining cultures can rule out these conditions. If a bicarbonate level obtained with serum electrolytes suggests acidosis, it should be confirmed with measurement of the pH of venous or arterial blood.[74] All other testing should result from abnormalities on history, physical examination, and/or screening labs. For instance, a history of respiratory problems and/or chronic diarrhea mandates testing for cystic fibrosis. Radiographic studies are sometimes needed to evaluate for gastroesophageal reflux, oral-motor dysfunction, or concerns about abuse.

Some laboratory tests assess the *effects* of the malnutrition. For example, serum albumin and prealbumin, zinc, and alkaline phosphatase can be affected by poor diet. A child's bone age (X-rays estimating bone maturity) can show retarded growth. Serum vitamin D levels correlated with radiographs can diagnose rickets, a disease resulting from vitamin D deficiency.

Hospitalization

The decision to admit a child to the hospital for evaluation and possible treatment of FTT is based on several factors:

- The severity of the malnutrition
- Significant dehydration
- The presence of significant medical problems, including intercurrent infections
- The safety of the child
- Concern about possible re-feeding syndrome
- The need for the involvement of multiple disciplines and/or diagnostic procedures most effectively performed in the hospital setting
- Failure of intensive outpatient management.[36,38]

Although the goal of hospitalization is often to see if normal weight gain occurs in a different setting,[48] Berwick's review of medical records of children hospitalized for FTT showed that, among children whose FTT was caused by socioenvironmental problems, many lost weight in the hospital, even though more children gained weight there. The hospital course was not a reliable indicator of the eventual

diagnosis.[73] It is not unusual for children with major medical problems causing or contributing to their growth failure to gain weight while in the hospital. Similarly, children whose FTT is primarily a result of underfeeding in the home might not easily gain weight in the hospital. A metaanalysis of the literature regarding efficacy of hospitalization specifically for children with nonorganic FTT revealed an increased probability of sustained catch-up growth in the hospital.[75]

Using severity of malnutrition as a criterion for hospitalization again depends on how FTT is defined. Determining the severity of FTT is subject to interpretation. Three commonly used systems for categorizing undernutrition include the Gomez classification, based on percentage of the median weight-for-age[15]; the Waterlow method, using the percentage of the median weight-for-height[76]; and the McLaren and Read method, based on the percentage of the median weight/height-for-age ratio.[77] Wright et al[20] compared each of these three systems for a group of 258 children referred to a multidisciplinary regional clinic specializing in FTT. There was broad variation between the number of children classified as malnourished as well as the degree of undernutrition.

TREATMENT

In light of the multiple etiologies of FTT, there is no ideal or "one-size-fits-all" treatment. Interventions must be tailored to the specific needs of the child and family,[36] although some common themes emerge. Once again, treatment is most easily addressed using the biopsychosocial model. Just like evaluation, treatment of FTT most often requires a multidisciplinary effort. In some areas specialized nutrition/growth clinics exist for management of these children. The composition of these clinics is highly variable and their ideal structure remains undefined.[78]

Treatment of Biological Issues

Depending upon severity of the malnutrition, the first step in treatment of some cases requires addressing the patient's acute medical needs. In severe cases, initial steps include stabilization of vital signs, rehydration of the child, and provision of glucose for hypoglycemia. Treatment of intercurrent infections is sometimes necessary, as well as prevention of further infections resulting from the malnutrition-related immune compromise. Infection prevention can disrupt the malnutrition-infection-malnutrition cycle and can be aided by appropriate immunization, infection-control measures (including minimizing exposure to illness), and use of appropriate antimicrobials.

If the child is failing to thrive because of a major medical illness, management of that illness is paramount to resolution of the growth failure. Involvement of various medical subspecialists is often necessary to guide additional medical evaluation and to generate a treatment plan. If the disorder is related to the gastrointestinal tract, a pediatric gastroenterologist is often consulted. In the absence of clinical indications of a gastrointestinal disorder, FTT is not necessarily a gastrointestinal problem and automatic gastroenterology consultation is not always indicated.

The pace and aggressiveness of nutritional replenishment should be dictated by the severity of malnutrition.[14] Quantification of the specific needs for nutritional repletion often requires the services of a nutritionist for calculation of caloric requirements for both catch-up growth and normal growth maintenance. A guideline for caloric requirements in infants with poor growth is based on the following equation:

$$\text{kcal per kg per day required}$$
$$= \frac{\text{RDA for age (kcal/kg)} \times \text{Ideal weight-for-height}}{\text{Actual weight}}$$

where RDA = recommended dietary allowance.

Protein requirements can also be estimated using a similar equation.[14] Depending upon the child's age, severity of malnutrition, feeding behaviors, and medical problems, a diet of routine food for age might not supply the necessary quantities of calories and protein. Methods to increase oral intake to meet the child's requirements can include concentrating formulas, provision of calorically dense supplements, removal of liquids and foods from the diet that have minimal nutritional value, and use of high-calorie additives to regular foods. Nasogastric tube feedings are also an option, especially for short-term use in infants. Nighttime drip feedings can provide nutrition, while the child is allowed and encouraged to eat during the day. If infant and young children are accustomed to "grazing" throughout the day, an intermittent daytime feeding schedule can help maintain or improve the normal hunger/satiety cycle. Nasogastric feeding tubes are only a temporary aid because of their own risks and complications. If long-term supplementation is required, placement of a gastrostomy is indicated.[29]

If the mother is having difficulty breastfeeding, modification of the timing and length of feedings, expressing breast milk, use of supplementation, and use of medication to enhance maternal milk supply are some of the available treatment options. A lactation consultant's input is likely to be valuable in this situation.

Initiation of feedings in a severely malnourished child must be undertaken with extreme caution because of a potential complication called re-feeding syndrome. Rapid re-feeding of malnourished patients can result in potentially lethal derangements of fluid and electrolytes. Hypophosphatemia can be problematic because of total body depletion and cellular uptake resulting from insulin surges related to increased glucose. Hypokalemia can result from similar mechanisms. Fluid overload, including progression to congestive heart failure and pulmonary edema, can occur with the introduction of carbohydrates to the diet followed by fluid repletion.[79] Prevention of re-feeding syndrome depends on five steps: (1) recognition of the risk in more severely malnourished children, (2) slower initiation of nutritional repletion in these children, especially in the first few days, (3) obtaining baseline laboratory tests followed by close monitoring of laboratory values as the child is nutritionally repleted, (4) frequent clinical reassessment in the early stages of nutritional repletion, and (5) early electrolyte replenishment if indicated.

All malnourished children should receive multivitamin supplements containing both iron and zinc, regardless of the presence of iron-deficiency anemia or documented zinc deficiency.[14] Serum zinc levels are not always a reliable indicator of true zinc status, and zinc supplementation results in an increase in the linear growth and weight gain of prepubertal children.[80] Appropriate additional supplementation with iron is indicated for iron-deficiency anemia, and with vitamin D in the face of vitamin D deficiency.[36]

Speech pathologists and/or occupational therapists are helpful adjuncts in the treatment of children with FTT and oral-motor problems or difficulties actually taking food into their mouths. Addressing any developmental concerns is also important. A developmental specialist, where available, can help monitor the child's developmental progress as the malnutrition and its underlying causes are treated. Early intervention services can work with the child in the home, providing necessary services such as physical, occupational, or speech therapy.

It is helpful to photograph the child to monitor his or her progress, starting at time of presentation. Depending on the child's age and the severity of the malnutrition, even weekly photographs might show drastic differences in the child's appearance. A sequence of images can provide latecomers to the treating team with a visual sense of the child's progress. It can also help parents recognize the changes in their child and encourage their active participation in the treatment plan. Finally, such photographs can be useful in court proceedings.

Close follow-up is critical in the medical management of these children. Children who are failing to thrive need frequent follow-up visits to assess their growth and other medical and developmental problems. If transportation is a problem for the family, home health nurses or aides could weigh the child at home and communicate the weights to the physician coordinating the child's care.

Treatment of Psychosocial Issues

Treatment of the psychosocial aspects of FTT is even more varied than treatment of the medical aspects. Treatment is highly dependent upon the psychosocial problems identified during the evaluation. Some issues are more easily addressed than others; again, a multidisciplinary team is often necessary. A primary care physician (the "medical home") can coordinate the various services and personnel involved, acting as a liaison among the professionals, the family, and the child.[38] Professionals helpful in the treatment of the psychosocial issues of FTT include child behavioral specialists, social workers, home visitors, nurses, parent educators, and mental health clinicians.

The psychosocial treatment should be tailored to fit the families' needs. Examples of specific treatment issues follow.

Without ensuring an adequate supply of appropriate food in the family home, a child with growth failure will not recuperate. Parents might need help in enrolling in Federal programs such as WIC (Special Supplemental Food Program for Women, Infants, and Children), SNAP (Supplemental Nutritional Assistance Program), or subsidized school lunch programs. Transportation barriers in locations with poor public transit systems might require delivery of food to the home or coordination of visits to doctors with food pick-ups. Alerting families to community service providers, or, with a family's permission, alerting community agencies about a family's needs, can help. Helping a family reconnect or maintain their utilities is sometimes necessary to ensure appropriate food storage and preparation.

Families can require financial assistance or help with other important supplies to help a child grow correctly. Cab or bus vouchers, assistance with money for gas, or referral to community services for help with transportation can ensure that the child is brought in for necessary appointments. A high chair and developmentally appropriate toys and books are beyond some families' means; again, community service agencies or even religious organizations can help with these issues.

Parental education plays a significant role in almost all cases of FTT. Families often must be taught about FTT, the difference between being "just small" and malnourished, and the reasons for concern. Treatment regimens will not succeed without parental "buy-in," which will be impaired by accusatory language, lack of clear communication from the treatment team, or the team's failure to listen to and acknowledge the parents' concerns.[36] Some parents need instruction about normal childhood nutrition, such as correct formula preparation or age-appropriate foods. Teaching families how to supplement the child's diet for catch-up growth or new methods to prepare food is usually necessary. Some families need instruction on interpreting their child's cues and responding appropriately, as well as behavioral management techniques for children with temperament issue contributing to growth failure. Educating families about developmentally appropriate stimulation and interaction can also help. Unfortunately, some parents need specific instruction for reprioritizing their spending habits, so that food for the child is purchased before nonessential items such as soda, "junk" food, or luxury items such as a new television or video game console.

Behavioral intervention is important for older children whose conduct is contributing to their poor weight gain. In some cases parents can be taught how to manage their child, but other cases require more in-depth treatment by trained professionals. An example is the child with food refusal. Providing positive reinforcement for appropriate mealtime behavior might not be enough to overcome the problem. Behavioral specialists can help add "escape extinction procedures" to prevent the child from escaping the feeding situation. When used in combination, positive reinforcement and escape extinction has helped increase food consumption in these difficult cases.[81]

As discussed previously, an assessment of the child's home is an important part of the evaluation of a child who is not growing appropriately. However, the benefits of formal home visitation programs for treatment purposes are unclear because of conflicting results of controlled studies.[82-84] Home visits can help involve other family members in the treatment plan and provide ongoing assessments of positive and negative changes in the home environment.

Treating mental health problems in the parents can be difficult but is necessary. When discussing the subject with reticent caregivers, acknowledging to the parents the strain of having a child with FTT and informing them that medical providers often recommend counseling for parents can help relieve their anxiety about the issue. Communicating the contribution of parental mental health to the child's growth must be done in a nonaccusatory, nonjudgmental way. Recognition and referral for services in situations of intimate partner violence also require judicious handling but are certainly important.

Since lack of support is a common feature in families with poorly growing children, treatment often involves becoming a de facto support team, providing guidance and positive feedback. Helping families locate sources of support is also key and can include recommending help within the community. Sometimes even simply helping find temporary daycare for the poorly growing child and/or siblings will provide some respite to a stressed caregiver. When FTT children are in daycare, quality child care situations, clear instructions on feeding, and close follow-up are all needed. In some situations, the child will do better receiving two age-appropriate meals and snacks in a daycare situation rather than in the home.

Ideally, all the contributing factors to a child's growth failure would be thoroughly addressed. However, in many situations that is not possible, but partial solutions are still worthwhile.[38] In some circumstances the child's malnutrition is too severe and/or the contributing factors either are too numerous or will take too long to resolve to provide for a safe environment for the child. In these cases, child protection services (CPS) must be notified. Other indications for involvement of CPS are signs of abuse, significant safety risks in the home caused by substance abuse or severe psychiatric or cognitive impairment, or a parent willfully withholding food with awareness of the consequences for growth.[36] Neglect is often a contributing factor to FTT, but accidental vs. intentional neglect is sometimes difficult to distinguish. Whereas intentional neglect should be referred to CPS, accidental neglect might or might not be referred, depending on whether the situation can be righted by the team's intervention.

Care must be taken to avoid assuming that neglect is the proximate cause of FTT in the absence of a clearly identifiable medical etiology.[66] Similarly, poor growth in a child from a materially or emotionally deprived background does not necessarily indicate parental negligence.[48] Neglect during treatment is also an indication for referral, but it must be accompanied by clear medical documentation that the parents were given appropriate instructions, were shown evidence of understanding the instructions and the potential adverse consequences for the child, and then failed to adhere to the interventions prescribed.[85] A referral to CPS is not a definitive statement of blame but can be a useful adjunct to help the child and family achieve stability and access services.

All children referred to CPS are not placed into protective custody. In some cases, services are provided to the family in the home. For those children removed from their parents' care, appropriate placement is paramount. Foster parents must have or must be given numerous resources including education, appropriate nutritional supplements, necessary referrals to medical providers, and a health insurance card.[36] Repeated moves to shelters or various foster homes will be detrimental to a child whose FTT is in part a result of a disorganized home environment and lack of stability. Medical providers should advocate for a stable and appropriate placement for the child. Usually, placement into foster care is not permanent, but provides a temporary period during which the parents work to correct the conditions that led to the child's growth failure. Even if the conditions are clearly correctable and the parents are already working on the issues before referral, the child's age and severity of malnutrition might be such that waiting for resolution of the family issues is not an option.

OUTCOME

Early descriptions of FTT recognized that malnourished children often have developmental delays at time of initial evaluation. The rapidity of brain growth during infancy and early childhood suggests that any biological insult during this time, including malnutrition, can affect development and cognitive outcome after nutritional repletion. Elucidating the later developmental outcomes of FTT children has been a complicated problem.

One of the earliest studies of outcome of FTT showed that children experienced delays in both physical and intellectual development.[86] Since then multiple studies performed to evaluate children's cognitive abilities after growth failure have used various methodologies and yielded conflicting results. Corbett and Drewett[87] published an excellent review and metaanalysis of 31 studies and found that "reasonably well-controlled studies" indicated FTT in infancy is associated with adverse intellectual outcomes. They estimated a loss of 4.2 IQ points, which was felt to be significant at a population level. Rudolf and Logan[88] published a systemic review of 13 studies that met their inclusion criteria and found a mean loss of approximately 3 IQ points. Also, children were lighter and shorter than comparison children, but the majority were over the third percentile for both weight and height. A more recent study by Emond et al[89] showed that weight gain between birth and 8 weeks of age had a positive linear correlation with IQ at age 8 years. Although there are not enough studies of intervention strategies to perform a systematic review, the few studies available also show conflicting results for cognitive development.[82,84,90-92]

Multiple issues cause the uncertainty regarding outcome of FTT. Many early studies were uncontrolled case studies of hospitalized children, clearly creating a problem of selection bias. Variations in other studies include case definition, exclusion criteria, loss to follow-up, time to follow-up, types of developmental testing, and types of intervention. A major issue with fully assessing development after FTT is that of confounders, including etiology of the FTT itself, parental intelligence, parental education level, parental mental health, socioeconomic status, child abuse, and other factors, all of which have individual or cumulative effects on the ultimate cognitive outcome of any child. For instance, Mackner et al[93] showed that neglect and FTT have a cumulative effect on cognitive functioning.

In summary, although the literature remains confusing, deficient growth during infancy and early childhood has potential risks for long-term growth and development.[38] Toward that end, in addition to treating the cause or causes of a child's FTT, the developmental problems accompanying FTT should also be addressed to help ameliorate deficits.[36]

STRENGTH OF THE EVIDENCE

As discussed earlier in this chapter, the definition of *failure to thrive* is ambiguous. Therefore, it is not possible to discuss the strength of the evidence in case identification when there is clear lack of consistency or uniformity on this issue. A key point is that FTT is not a diagnosis itself, but only a symptom. Assessments of strength of evidence related to case identification, treatment, and outcome are related to diagnoses, not

symptoms, and therefore the evidence base in the medical literature regarding FTT will be different than the ideal double-blinded randomized control trial. The heterogeneity of FTT is another cause of difficulty with evidence regarding case identification, treatment, and outcome studies.

Deficits in many of the earlier studies related to FTT have been discussed throughout this chapter. In addition, many of those studies evaluated nonorganic FTT only, but determining the accuracy of that now obsolete label is often not possible. Many studies over the last three decades are case studies, but some are case-control studies. None have been fully blinded, and relatively few are prospective. However, systemic reviews and metaanalyses regarding outcome of FTT were helpful and provided quite similar results.[87,88]

FUTURE DIRECTIONS FOR RESEARCH

Creating a succinct definition for FTT is a formidable goal, but one that would improve accurate case identification and allow for better uniformity of research studies. With the multifactorial etiologies, determination of a classification scheme that is more appropriate than the simplistic organic/nonorganic distinction would be immensely valuable for research into appropriate treatment and outcome. Barriers to the correct evaluation of children presenting with FTT need to be assessed and then addressed to limit unnecessary medical testing. Lastly, the development and evaluation of novel treatment programs are needed.

CONCLUSION

Despite the lack of a clear, consistent definition based on anthropometric assessments, the growth deviation from the norm seen in FTT is a sign of undernutrition. Determining the etiology—the actual diagnosis or diagnoses—requires careful consideration of the biological, psychological, and social spheres of the child and the family. The medical evaluation should focus on the history and physical examination, which in turn should guide the medical workup. Treatment needs to focus not only on nutritional repletion, but on the cause(s) of the FTT as well. Evaluation and treatment are most easily and effectively accomplished as multidisciplinary endeavors. Failure to thrive in early childhood presents potential risks to optimal growth and developmental outcome. Appropriate and timely treatment can help ameliorate those risks. Understanding this complex condition can help clinicians approach these children with eagerness, confidence, and competence.

References

1. Holt L: The derangements of nutrition. *In*: Holt L (ed): *The Diseases of Infancy and Childhood*, D. Appleton & Company, New York, 1897, pp 192-209.
2. Griffith J: Infantile atrophy. *In*: Griffith J (ed): *The Diseases of Infants and Children*, WB Saunders, Philadelphia, 1919, pp 610-615.
3. Griffith J: Malnutrition. *In*: Griffith J (ed): *The Diseases of Infants and Children*, WB Saunders, Philadelphia, 1919, pp 615-620.
4. Spitz R: Hospitalism. *Psychoanal Study Child* 1945;1:53-74.
5. Spitz R: Anaclitic depression. *Psychoanal Study Child* 1946;2:313-342.
6. Patton R, Gardner L: Influence of family environment on growth: the syndrome of "maternal deprivation." *Pediatrics* 1962;30:957-962.
7. Skuse DH: Non-organic failure to thrive: a reappraisal. *Arch Dis Child* 1985;60:173-178.

8. O'Reilly D. Maternal deprivation syndrome. Available at http://www. nlm.nih.gov/medlineplus/ency/article/001598.htm. Accessed September 1, 2008.
9. Sameroff AJ, Chandler MJ: Reproductive risk and the continuum of caretaker casualty. *In:* Horowitz F (ed): *Review of Child Development Research*, University of Chicago Press, Chicago, 1975, pp 187-243.
10. Frank DA, Zeisel SH: Failure to thrive. *Pediatr Clin North Am* 1988;35:1187-1206.
11. Emond A, Drewett R, Blair P, et al: Postnatal factors associated with failure to thrive in term infants in the Avon Longitudinal Study of Parents and Children. *Arch Dis Child* 2007;92:115-119.
12. O'Brien LM, Heycock EG, Hanna M, et al: Postnatal depression and faltering growth: a community study. *Pediatrics* 2004;113:1242-1247.
13. Argyle J: Approaches to detecting growth faltering in infancy and childhood. *Ann Hum Biol* 2003;30:499-519.
14. American Academy of Pediatrics Committee on Nutrition: Failure to thrive (pediatric undernutrition). *In:* Kleinman R (ed): *Pediatric Nutrition Handbook*, American Academy of Pediatrics, Elk Grove Village, IL, 2004, pp 443-457.
15. Gomez F, Galvan RR, Cravioto J, et al: Malnutrition in infancy and childhood, with special reference to kwashiorkor. *Adv Pediatr* 1955;7:131-169.
16. Cole TJ, Flegal KM, Nicholls D, et al: Body mass index cut offs to define thinness in children and adolescents: international survey. *Br Med J* 2007;335:194.
17. Olsen EM, Skovgaard AM, Weile B, et al: Risk factors for failure to thrive in infancy depend on the anthropometric definitions used: the Copenhagen County Child Cohort. *Paediatr Perinat Epidemiol* 2007;21:418-431.
18. Guo SM, Roche AF, Fomon SJ, et al: Reference data on gains in weight and length during the first two years of life. *J Pediatr* 1991;119:355-362.
19. Cole TJ: Conditional reference charts to assess weight gain in British infants. *Arch Dis Child* 1995;73:8-16.
20. Wright JA, Ashenburg CA, Whitaker RC: Comparison of methods to categorize undernutrition in children. *J Pediatr* 1994;124:944-946.
21. Wilcox WD, Nieburg P, Miller DS: Failure to thrive. A continuing problem of definition. *Clin Pediatr (Phila)* 1989;28:391-394.
22. Olsen EM: Failure to thrive: still a problem of definition. *Clin Pediatr (Phila)* 2006;45:1-6.
23. Olsen EM, Petersen J, Skovgaard AM, et al: Failure to thrive: the prevalence and concurrence of anthropometric criteria in a general infant population. *Arch Dis Child* 2007;92:109-114.
24. Hughes I: Confusing terminology attempts to define the undefinable. *Arch Dis Child* 2007;92:97-98.
25. Homer C, Ludwig S: Categorization of etiology of failure to thrive. *Am J Dis Child* 1981;135:848-851.
26. Pagliacelli L: Dealing with failure to thrive in children. *In: Infectious Disease in Children*, Thorofare, NJ, 2007, p 3.
27. Krugman SD, Dubowitz H: Failure to thrive. *Am Fam Physician* 2003;68:879-884.
28. Borell-Carrio F, Suchman AL, Epstein RM: The biopsychosocial model 25 years later: principles, practice, and scientific inquiry. *Ann Fam Med* 2004;2:576-582.
29. Careaga MG, Kerner JA Jr: A gastroenterologist's approach to failure to thrive. *Pediatr Ann* 2000;29:558-567.
30. Goldson E: Neurological aspects of failure to thrive. *Dev Med Child Neurol* 1989;31:821-826.
31. Boddy JM, Skuse DH: The process of parenting in failure to thrive. *J Child Psychol Psychiatry* 1994;35:401-424.
32. Rudolph CD: Feeding disorders in infants and children. *J Pediatr* 1994;125:S116-124.
33. Fleisher DR: Functional vomiting disorders in infancy: innocent vomiting, nervous vomiting, and infant rumination syndrome. *J Pediatr* 1994;125:S84-94.
34. Blair PS, Drewett RF, Emmett PM, et al: Family, socioeconomic and prenatal factors associated with failure to thrive in the Avon Longitudinal Study of Parents and Children (ALSPAC). *Int J Epidemiol* 2004;33:839-847.
35. Altemeier WA, 3rd, O'Connor SM, Sherrod KB, et al: Prospective study of antecedents for nonorganic failure to thrive. *J Pediatr* 1985;106:360-365.
36. Frank D, Drotar D, Cook J, et al: Failure to thrive. *In:* Reece RM, Ludwig S: *Child Abuse: Medical Diagnosis and Management.* Lippincott, Williams & Wilkins, Philadelphia, 2001, pp 307-337.
37. Brandt I: Growth dynamics of low birthweight infants with emphasis on the prenatal period. *In:* Falkner F, Tanner J: *Human Growth, Neurobiology and Nutrition.* Plenum Press, New York, 1979, pp 557-617.
38. Bithoney WG, Dubowitz H, Egan H: Failure to thrive/growth deficiency. *Pediatr Rev* 1992;13:453-460.
39. Turecki S: The behavioral complaint: symptom of a psychiatric disorder or a matter of temperament? *Contemp Pediatr* 2003;20:111-119.
40. Thomas A, Chess S: The role of temperament in the contributions of individuals to their development. *In:* Lerner R, Bush-Rossnagel N: *Individuals as Producers of Their Development. A Life-span Perspective.* Academic Press, New York, 1981, pp 231-255.
41. Darlington AS, Wright CM: The influence of temperament on weight gain in early infancy. *J Dev Behav Pediatr* 2006;27:329-335.
42. Wilensky DS, Ginsberg G, Altman M, et al: A community based study of failure to thrive in Israel. *Arch Dis Child* 1996;75:145-148.
43. Feldman R, Keren M, Gross-Rozval O, et al: Mother-child touch patterns in infant feeding disorders: relation to maternal, child, and environmental factors. *J Am Acad Child Adolesc Psychiatry* 2004;43:1089-1097.
44. Stewart KB, Meyer L: Parent-child interactions and everyday routines in young children with failure to thrive. *Am J Occup Ther* 2004;58:342-346.
45. Wright CM, Parkinson KN, Drewett RF: How does maternal and child feeding behavior relate to weight gain and failure to thrive? Data from a prospective birth cohort. *Pediatrics* 2006;117:1262-1269.
46. Parkinson KN, Wright CM, Drewett RF: Mealtime energy intake and feeding behaviour in children who fail to thrive: a population-based case-control study. *J Child Psychol Psychiatry* 2004;45:1030-1035.
47. Drotar D, Pallotta J, Eckerle D: A prospective study of family environments of children hospitalized for nonorganic failure-to-thrive. *J Dev Behav Pediatr* 1994;15:78-85.
48. Marcovitch H: Failure to thrive. *Br Med J* 1994;308:35-38.
49. Duniz M, Scheer PJ, Trojovsky A, et al: Changes in psychopathology of parents of NOFT (non-organic failure to thrive) infants during treatment. *Eur Child Adolesc Psychiatry* 1996;5:93-100.
50. Dossett EC: Perinatal depression. *Obstet Gynecol Clin North Am* 2008;35:419-434.
51. Wright CM, Parkinson KN, Drewett RF: The influence of maternal socioeconomic and emotional factors on infant weight gain and weight faltering (failure to thrive): data from a prospective birth cohort. *Arch Dis Child* 2006;91:312-317.
52. Weston JA, Colloton M, Halsey S, et al: A legacy of violence in nonorganic failure to thrive. *Child Abuse Negl* 1993;17:709-714.
53. van Wezel-Meijler G, Wit JM: The offspring of mothers with anorexia nervosa: a high-risk group for undernutrition and stunting? *Eur J Pediatr* 1989;149:130-135.
54. Stein A, Fairburn CG: Children of mothers with bulimia nervosa. *Br Med J* 1989;299:777-778.
55. McCann JB, Stein A, Fairburn CG, et al: Eating habits and attitudes of mothers of children with non-organic failure to thrive. *Arch Dis Child* 1994;70:234-236.
56. Moldavsky M, Stein D: Munchausen Syndrome by Proxy: two case reports and an update of the literature. *Int J Psychiatry Med* 2003;33:411-423.
57. Bools CN, Neale BA, Meadow SR: Co-morbidity associated with fabricated illness (Munchausen syndrome by proxy). *Arch Dis Child* 1992;67:77-79.
58. Roesler TA, Barry PC, Bock SA: Factitious food allergy and failure to thrive. *Arch Pediatr Adolesc Med* 1994;148:1150-1155.
59. Listernick R: Accurate feeding history key to failure to thrive. *Pediatr Ann* 2004;33:161-166.
60. Pugliese MT, Weyman-Daum M, Moses N, et al: Parental health beliefs as a cause of nonorganic failure to thrive. *Pediatrics* 1987;80:175-182.
61. Black MM, Hutcheson JJ, Dubowitz H, et al: Parenting style and developmental status among children with nonorganic failure to thrive. *J Pediatr Psychol* 1994;19:689-707.
62. Heptinstall E, Puckering C, Skuse D, et al: Nutrition and mealtime behaviour in families of growth-retarded children. *Hum Nutr Appl Nutr* 1987;41:390-402.
63. Robinson JR, Drotar D, Boutry M. Problem solving abilities among mothers of infants with failure to thrive. *J Pediatr Psychol* 2001;26:26-32.

64. Drotar D, Sturm L: Prediction of intellectual development in young children with early histories of nonorganic failure-to-thrive. *J Pediatr Psychol* 1988;13:281-296.

65. Drotar D: The family context of nonorganic failure to thrive. *Am J Orthopsychiatry* 1991;61:23-34.

66. Spencer NJ: Failure to think about failure to thrive. *Arch Dis Child* 2007;92:95-96.

67. Kellogg ND, Lukefahr JL: Criminally prosecuted cases of child starvation. *Pediatrics* 2005;116:1309-1316.

68. Wright CM: Growth charts for babies. *Br Med J* 2005;330:1399-1400.

69. World Health Organization. Nutrition Media Centre Launch of the WHO Child Growth Standards. 2008 Available from: http://www.who.int/nutrition/media_page/en/. Accessed September 1, 2008.

70. Wright C, Lakshman R, Emmett P, et al: Implications of adopting the WHO 2006 Child Growth Standard in the UK: two prospective cohort studies. *Arch Dis Child* 2008;93:566-569.

71. Piazza CC, Fisher WW, Brown KA, et al: Functional analysis of inappropriate mealtime behaviors. *J Appl Behav Anal* 2003;36:187-204.

72. Sills RH: Failure to thrive. The role of clinical and laboratory evaluation. *Am J Dis Child* 1978;132:967-969.

73. Berwick DM, Levy JC, Kleinerman R: Failure to thrive: diagnostic yield of hospitalisation. *Arch Dis Child* 1982;57:347-351.

74. Adedoyin O, Gottlieb B, Frank R, et al: Evaluation of failure to thrive: diagnostic yield of testing for renal tubular acidosis. *Pediatrics* 2003;112:e463.

75. Fryer GE Jr: The efficacy of hospitalization of nonorganic failure-to-thrive children: a meta-analysis. *Child Abuse Negl* 1988;12:375-381.

76. Waterlow JC: Classification and definition of protein-calorie malnutrition. *Br Med J* 1972;3:566-569.

77. McLaren DS, Read WW: Classification of nutritional status in early childhood. *Lancet* 1972;2:146-148.

78. Puntis JW: Specialist feeding clinics. *Arch Dis Child* 2008;93:164-167.

79. Mehanna HM, Moledina J, Travis J: Refeeding syndrome: what it is, and how to prevent and treat it. *Br Med J* 2008;336:1495-1498.

80. Brown KH, Peerson JM, Rivera J, et al: Effect of supplemental zinc on the growth and serum zinc concentrations of prepubertal children: a meta-analysis of randomized controlled trials. *Am J Clin Nutr* 2002;75:1062-1071.

81. Piazza CC, Patel MR, Gulotta CS, et al: On the relative contributions of positive reinforcement and escape extinction in the treatment of food refusal. *J Appl Behav Anal* 2003;36:309-324.

82. Wright CM, Callum J, Birks E, et al: Effect of community based management in failure to thrive: randomised controlled trial. *Br Med J* 1998;317:571-574.

83. Black MM, Dubowitz H, Hutcheson J, et al: A randomized clinical trial of home intervention for children with failure to thrive. *Pediatrics* 1995;95:807-814.

84. Raynor P, Rudolf MC, Cooper K, et al: A randomised controlled trial of specialist health visitor intervention for failure to thrive. *Arch Dis Child* 1999;80:500-506.

85. Block RW, Krebs NF: Failure to thrive as a manifestation of child neglect. *Pediatrics* 2005;116:1234-1237.

86. Glaser HH, Heagarty MC, Bullard DM Jr, et al: Physical and psychological development of children with early failure to thrive. *J Pediatr* 1968;73:690-698.

87. Corbett SS, Drewett RF: To what extent is failure to thrive in infancy associated with poorer cognitive development? A review and meta-analysis. *J Child Psychol Psychiatry* 2004;45:641-654.

88. Rudolf MC, Logan S: What is the long term outcome for children who fail to thrive? A systematic review. *Arch Dis Child* 2005;90:925-931.

89. Emond AM, Blair PS, Emmett PM, et al: Weight faltering in infancy and IQ levels at 8 years in the Avon Longitudinal Study of Parents and Children. *Pediatrics* 2007;120:e1051-1058.

90. Black MM, Dubowitz H, Krishnakumar A, et al: Early intervention and recovery among children with failure to thrive: follow-up at age 8. *Pediatrics* 2007;120:59-69.

91. Hutcheson JJ, Black MM, Talley M, et al: Risk status and home intervention among children with failure-to-thrive: follow-up at age 4. *J Pediatr Psychol* 1997;22:651-668.

92. Casey PH, Kelleher KJ, Bradley RH, et al: A multifaceted intervention for infants with failure to thrive. A prospective study. *Arch Pediatr Adolesc Med* 1994;148:1071-1077.

93. Mackner LM, Starr RH Jr, Black MM: The cumulative effect of neglect and failure to thrive on cognitive functioning. *Child Abuse Negl* 1997;21:691-700.

58

DETECTING DRUGS IN INFANTS AND CHILDREN

Kevin P. Kent, MD, and Kavita M. Babu, MD

INTRODUCTION

Drug screening facilitates the accurate assessment of the presence or absence of common xenobiotics in vivo. No drug screening methodology can or should replace the meticulous history, the physical examination, and the experience and judgment of a seasoned clinician. Still, appropriate drug screening can help answer important questions about drug exposure in the realm of child safety and can be used as an informative tool for large-scale screening to guide targeted interventions.

The term *drug screening* refers to a number of testing methods used to identify the presence or absence of medications, illicit drugs, and environmental substances in a variety of clinical situations. No single screening method can identify all substances, and each institution or facility will have its own menu of testing options and availability. It is essential for clinicians to become acquainted with the range of testing available in their clinical setting. It is equally important for clinicians to recognize that many types of new testing methods are being developed, and locally endemic drugs often necessitate acquisition of rapid testing for a particular target (e.g., methamphetamine, ketamine, or gamma-hydroxybutyrate). This can be accomplished through consultation with on-site laboratory and toxicology personnel.

The rationale for drug screening for child safety focuses on identifying drug exposure in specific populations of neonates, children, and adolescents. Often women self-report drug use during pregnancy, and many of these drugs have significant consequences for neonatal and child health and development. Concerns about stigmatization, custody issues, and forced rehabilitation may prompt pregnant women to conceal their substance abuse from medical providers. Maternal self-report has been repeatedly documented to underestimate prevalence of in utero drug exposure, with estimates of prenatal substance abuse ranging from 0.4% to 27% in various populations.[1,2] The consequences of maternal drug use during pregnancy are sometimes severe, including preterm labor, intrauterine growth restriction, congenital abnormalities, stillbirths, and neonatal abstinence syndromes.[3] Targeted drug screening protocols can help identify high risk infants and allow early intervention for possible sequelae; common criteria for targeted drug screening include a history of maternal substance abuse, prior preterm labor or placental abruption, minimal or no prenatal care, and a history of births outside of a hospital.[4]

In children, drug screening can help to identify supervisory neglect resulting in accidental exposures, the presence of illicit substances in the home, medical child abuse, or willful and unwarranted medication of children for purposes such as sedation or drug-facilitated sexual assault. (See Chapter 15, "Drug-Facilitated Sexual Assault.") These same issues can be identified in the adolescent population, as well as further elements of addiction and risk-taking behaviors.

The interpretation of drug screening results can be complex and challenging and relies on several factors, including patient history and presentation, the testing methodology, the specific target drug, and the source of the fluid tested. Knowledge about detectable toxins and turnaround times can further facilitate choosing the most appropriate test for each clinical setting.

DRUG TESTING METHODOLOGIES

There are many testing strategies that provide information on both qualitative (absence or presence) and quantitative (level of drug present in serum or blood) data for thousands of common and unusual xenobiotics. In child protection, the two most common testing methods are the immunoassay for drug screening and chromatography/spectroscopy for confirmation and quantitation of drugs of abuse.

Immunoassays and Rapid Drug Screening

Several strategies are used as initial methods in drug screening, including enzyme immunoassay, fluorescence polarization immunoassay, radioimmunoassay, and enzyme-linked immunosorbent assay.[5] Immunoassays are the most common testing methods used in the rapid drug screening found in most clinical settings and emergency departments. These antibody-based assays generally demonstrate high sensitivity and high specificity for target drugs. The ease and relative inexpense of immunoassay use (similar to home pregnancy tests) lead to rapid turnaround times and wide availability. However, problems can exist with cross-reactivity (a positive test for a substance other than the target, particularly among substances with similar structures). For example, in older assays, therapeutic use of pseudoephedrine could trigger a positive methamphetamine screen due to cross-reactivity. Newer generations of immunoassays are much more specific, with far less cross-reactivity; for the newest generation of testing, only a truly massive overdose of pseudoephedrine would interfere with the methamphetamine assay. Every laboratory will have specifications about the particular testing methodology in use, and the likelihood of cross-reaction with common drugs. Specific questions about cross-reactivity require knowledge of the exact method in use and should be answered in consultation with on-site laboratory personnel.

Chromatography

Although rapid drug screening techniques have become more specific, most laboratories still use confirmatory testing with a second method to reveal any false positives, especially given the medical, legal, and possible criminal implications of a positive drug screen. Confirmatory testing is traditionally done via chromatography and spectroscopy.[5] Chromatography and spectroscopy are highly specific processes used to physically separate individual compounds and to then identify them. In addition, these techniques can be used to obtain quantitative serum levels of many drugs. Quantitative levels can be used to help determine the time of exposure, monitor changes in concentration over time, predict toxicity, and determine treatment. Techniques like thin-layer chromatography (TLC), gas chromatography/mass spectroscopy (GC/MS) and liquid chromatography/mass spectroscopy (LC/MS) are frequently used to confirm the qualitative results obtained through immunoassays. By separating and identifying individual substances, these techniques provide reliable and accurate detection. The widespread use of chromatography is limited by its cost, as well as by the time and expertise required to perform the tests.

BIOLOGICAL MATRICES

Several sources of tissue and fluid can be used for drug screening. Urine is the most commonly-used source fluid in drug screening. The preference for urine as a testing sample stems from its ease of collection and the minimal preparation required for its analysis. Drug screening on urine, however, is generally qualitative, and little information can be obtained regarding the time of exposure beyond the window of detection in positive samples. With the exception of marijuana, few drugs of abuse are found in urine more than 72 hours after exposure (see Table 58-1 for representative intervals).[2] Considerable time and effort have been spent in finding ways to foil the standard urine drug screen, including using another individual's urine to fill the specimen cup, dilution techniques, and addition of adulterants. Although these methods are rarely successful, professional drug testing services will use indices such as specific gravity and urine temperature to prevent fraud.

Serum or blood sampling is another common source fluid. Most quantitative testing is done on serum, and certain drugs, such as alcohols, can only be accurately identified through serum sampling. One clear benefit of serum sampling is that results follow a well-defined dose response curve for many drugs, and conclusions regarding timing and intensity of exposure can be drawn in many cases, particularly with serial samples. However, obtaining blood requires expertise in phlebotomy, appropriate resources, and increased costs. In addition, the risk of needlestick and bloodborne pathogen exposure is higher for healthcare providers who draw blood.

Meconium represents a very important source fluid for drug screening in the neonatal population. Meconium is the

Table 58-1	Persistence of Selected Drugs in Urine
Drug	**Interval**
Amphetamine	2-3 days
Cocaine metabolite (benzoylecgonine)	2-3 days
Opiates	
Buprenorphine	48-56 hr
Codeine	24 hr
6-MAM (heroin metabolite)	2-4 hr
Methadone	7-9 days
Morphine	48 hr
Marijuana metabolite (tetrahydrocannabinol)	2-5 days; up to 10 days in heavy users
Methamphetamine	2 days

From Wolff K, Farrell M, Marsden J, et al: A review of biological indicators of illicit drug use, practical considerations and clinical usefulness. *Addiction* 1999;94:1279-1298.

combined debris of lanugo, desquamated alimentary tract, amniotic fluid and intestinal secretions that begins to form during the second trimester (after 16 weeks). As such, any drugs that are encountered by the mother and fetus can accumulate in meconium from the second trimester onward, and are stored until meconium is passed at or shortly after birth. Typically, 4 to 5 g of meconium is preferred for laboratory analysis, but some laboratories will be able to perform testing with as little as 2 g. The advantages of meconium as a source for testing includes greater sensitivity for illicit drug screening caused by the greater window of exposure. In one study, meconium was twice as sensitive for detecting prenatal cocaine exposure compared with neonatal urine screening; this might represent a period of maternal abstention from drug use in the days prior to delivery. In addition, meconium can be collected easily; however, it becomes increasingly mixed with stool after birth, producing a limited collection time of approximately 24 hours after delivery. Commercial laboratories are capable of performing large-scale meconium screening. Familiarity with the substances tested for, confirmatory methods, and identification of any unusual or specific testing issues requires consultation with the specific laboratory used.

Hair testing has been used to identify neonatal and childhood exposure to illicit drugs. Between 2 and 5 mg of hair are required for most assays, and frequently hair must be washed as part of the preparation for laboratory analysis to remove any external contaminants.[6] Specimens of hair are collected and subjected to mechanical disruption and extraction in various organic solvents. In contrast to meconium testing, detection of cocaine in neonatal hair identifies exposure occurring during the third trimester of pregnancy. This may have important ramifications from a child protection standpoint, since the vast majority of pregnancies would be apparent to the mother during this interval.[6] The advantages of hair testing include ease of collection and its potential to remain positive for as much as 3 months after delivery. This window can be very helpful in infants who manifest delayed symptoms suggestive of drug exposure.[6] The disadvantages of hair testing include susceptibility to external contamination and lack of standardization of testing methods among laboratories.[7] Radioimmunoassay or ELISA protocols can detect benzoylecgonine (the primary metabolite of cocaine) at very low limits (0.02 ng/g) in neonatal hair, with a sensitivity of 84%.[6]

Comparison of meconium and hair testing has shown that meconium testing is associated with superior sensitivity for identification of illicit drugs. One study demonstrated detection of cocaine metabolites in 95% of meconium samples, compared with 78% of hair samples from the same patients. Cannabis was identified in 95% of meconium samples, compared with 71% of hair, and the same frequency (87%) was found for opiates in matched specimens.[6] This difference may reflect the longer window for drug detection seen with meconium testing (second trimester onward, compared with third trimester for hair).

SPECIFIC DRUGS

Amphetamine

Because of the ease with which it can be synthesized from readily available consumer products, methamphetamine abuse in the United States saw a dramatic surge during the 1990s. The use of methamphetamine among women of child-bearing age appears to be greater than that of cocaine, with as many as 5% of U.S. pregnancies exposed to methamphetamine.[8] Other members of the phenylethylamine class, such as amphetamine, dextroamphetamine, and ephedrine, have been used clinically and/or abused for much of the twentieth century; clinical uses of methamphetamine include therapy for ADHD, obesity, and narcolepsy.

Also known as "ice," "crystal," and "speed," methamphetamine is rapidly absorbed after smoking, nasal insufflation, intravenous injection, or ingestion. The characteristic clinical effects of methamphetamine occur as a result of the widespread release of dopamine, serotonin, and norepinephrine from presynaptic neurons, as well as the inhibition of monoamine oxidase. Effects include euphoria, increased alertness, hallucinations, CNS excitation, diminished appetite, tachycardia, hypertension, and seizures.

The bulk of illegal methamphetamine used in the United States is manufactured in clandestine home laboratories, which pose added hazards to children living in the home, including burns caused by explosive reagents, exposure to lead salts, and caustic injuries from concentrated acids and organic solvents. In addition, neglect may occur during methamphetamine binges, when parents are unable to provide meals or supervise younger children. The practice of sedating children during these binges also has been reported.[9] In addition, children can be exposed to weapons, pornography, and sexual exploitation in the setting of clandestine methamphetamine laboratories.[9]

Methamphetamine readily crosses the placenta and has been linked to intrauterine growth retardation, placental abruption, and premature labor.[4] The low birth weight and other complications seen with gestational exposure to methamphetamine are likely compounded by the appetite-suppressing effects of the drug when taken regularly by pregnant women. Methamphetamine screening can be performed on meconium as well as on urine or serum.

The laboratory confirmation of exposure to methamphetamine is plagued by the problem of forensically false-positive results from licit amphetamine derivatives found in common decongestants, appetite suppressants, and CNS stimulants. The anti-parkinsonian medication selegiline is metabolized to D-methamphetamine (identical to the illegal form), and the common atypical antidepressant, bupropion, can also cause false-positive methamphetamine assays. In addition, commonly prescribed nasal inhalers (e.g., Vicks) may contain L-methamphetamine and cause false-positive methamphetamine screening results. Even gas chromatography and mass spectrometry analysis can confuse these substances, and more sophisticated methods, such as negative-ion chemical ionization mode-GC-MS testing, can be required to further differentiate these medications from illicit methamphetamine.[10]

Marijuana

Marijuana ("weed", "pot") is the most commonly abused illicit drug in the United States. It is usually smoked as cigarettes or via a water pipe ("bong"). Hashish refers to the more resinous and concentrated form of the drug.[11] Marijuana is currently a schedule I drug and is illegal to possess or cultivate according to federal law; certain state and local statutes, however, allow the use of marijuana for medical purposes. The active compound in marijuana, delta-9-tetrahydrocannabinol (THC), is responsible for its effects, including euphoria and anxiolysis. Among adolescents, marijuana use is extensive. In 2005, one study reported that 16.3% of eighth graders and 44.8% of high school seniors had used marijuana.[12]

Approximately 5% of pregnant women report smoking marijuana while pregnant.[13] Considerable controversy exists as to the effects of marijuana use during pregnancy; however, multiple studies suggest that antenatal exposure to marijuana can lead to lower birth weight regardless of gestational age and can increase the risk of preterm delivery.[14-16] Other reports suggest long-term cognitive effects after prenatal marijuana exposure and a possible increased risk of marijuana use in adolescence.[17]

Essentially any source fluid can be used for marijuana testing; screening has been conducted on urine, blood, saliva, meconium, hair, and nails. Marijuana is stored in adipose tissue and persists in urine up to 7 to 10 days in heavy users. Screening for marijuana use during pregnancy is typically conducted on meconium passed by the newborn.

Cocaine

Cocaine in its various forms is one of the most prevalent illicit substances in use in the United States. According to the 2007 National Survey on Drug Use and Health, 2.4 million Americans reported using cocaine in the previous month, with an additional 700,000 reporting use of crack cocaine.[18] Among pregnant women the prevalence of cocaine use ranges from 2.6% to 11% and appears to vary with race, socioeconomic status, and geographical setting, but is inaccurately assessed by maternal self-report.[19,20]

The use of cocaine by pregnant women can have consequences that are both unique and potentially devastating to the developing fetus. Chronic increases in vasomotor tone can impair placental perfusion and result in intrauterine growth retardation and low birth weight. Likewise, the catecholamine excess caused by cocaine can trigger placental abruption and preterm labor. Infants born after repeated exposure to cocaine can display a unique neonatal abstinence syndrome marked by poor sucking, feeding problems, irritability, hypertonia, yawning, and sneezing.

In contrast to other substances with high potential for abuse such as heroin and methamphetamine, cocaine is classified as a Schedule II substance by the U.S. Controlled Substances Act. This allows for the continued medicinal use of cocaine as a topical agent for anesthesia and vasoconstriction of mucous membranes, chiefly in otorhinolaryngologic procedures. Although used with less frequency than in decades past, its continued role in clinical medicine provide both opportunities for drug diversion as well as for positive screening test results following legitimate exposure.

Powdered cocaine represents the hydrochloride salt of the naturally occurring alkaloid benzoylmethylecgonine. The leaves of the coca plant (*Erythroxylum coca*) are harvested and extracted in a solvent such as sulfuric acid or benzene before being converted to the purified form. Crack cocaine is formed by dissolving the hydrochloride salt in a solution of sodium bicarbonate and extracting the resultant base. Cocaine can be used alone or in combination with opioids or other drugs via nasal insufflation, oral ingestion, mucosal absorption, intravenous injection, or smoking. The packaging of cocaine into well-made packets for concealment within the human body for trafficking purposes presents unique diagnostic and management challenges.[21]

Cocaine is rapidly absorbed following administration by all routes, and metabolism proceeds by three chief pathways. Approximately 5% of absorbed cocaine undergoes demethylation in the liver to produce the active metabolite norcocaine, which is capable of crossing the blood–brain barrier and producing cocaine's characteristic effects. The remainder of the absorbed dose is hydrolyzed chemically and enzymatically by plasmacholinesterase to the inactive metabolites benzoylecgonine and ecgonine methyl ester. Although these compounds have little or no clinical effect, they persist in biological fluids and tissues longer than native cocaine and thus are a more reliable target for drug testing.

Rapid drug screening methods for cocaine identify benzoylecgonine at a detection limit of 200 to 300 ng/ml, a range comparable to that of GC/MS techniques. In contrast to assays for other drugs of abuse such as opioids, cannabinoids, and amphetamines, false-positive results for cocaine are exceedingly rare. Cocaine metabolites are detectable in urine, blood, hair, nails, and meconium. Radioimmunoassay screening and GC/MS confirmation methods detect benzoylecgonine in meconium at limits of 50 ng/g with a sensitivity of approximately 96%.[6]

Ethanol

Alcohol plays a complicating role in a wide variety of child protection cases. In neonates, fetal alcohol spectrum disorder represents one of the most common preventable causes of birth defects.[22] The prevalence of fetal alcohol spectrum

disorder has been estimated as 0.5 to 2/1000 births, with an estimated cost of up to $9.7 billion per year.[23,24] Fetal alcohol syndrome refers to the more severe constellation of characteristic facial abnormalities, restricted growth, and CNS impairment seen in children exposed to heavy and chronic alcohol in utero.[25,26] Fetal alcohol spectrum disorder describes a broader range of neurodevelopmental findings seen in children exposed to prenatal alcohol, but lacking the classic facial findings. Clinicians may be alerted to prenatal alcohol exposure through maternal self-report, maternal intoxication during provider contacts or blood alcohol testing performed on the mother within hours of alcohol ingestion. Screening for maternal alcohol exposure using maternal blood or breathalyzer testing is of limited utility, given the rapid and complete elimination of alcohol in adults. In addition, many infants without the classic facies of fetal alcohol syndrome are not diagnosed for months, making testing for fetal alcohol syndrome, or the broader diagnosis of fetal alcohol spectrum disorder, challenging. Specific biomarkers can be used to assess for fetal exposure to alcohol during the prenatal period.

Fatty acid esters (FAE) are nonoxidative metabolites of ethanol that accumulate in meconium and have been used as indicators of prenatal alcohol exposure. At least one study has demonstrated a link between elevated meconium FAE levels, and limited neurodevelopmental outcomes.[27] Several FAEs are detectable using GC/MS.[28]

One unique and concerning feature of alcohol exposure in infants and small children is the potential for life-threatening hypoglycemia.[29] All infants and small children with a documented ethanol exposure require serial glucose measurements, as well as close examination of supervisory issues.

Alcohol use during adolescence has been linked to negative consequences including injury, suicide, unsafe sexual activity, and date rape.[30] In addition, early age of onset of drinking correlates with risk of alcoholism. Although screening for alcohol use among adolescents is imperative during clinical encounters, drug testing for alcohol has limited utility outside of those patients with evidence of clinical intoxication. In intoxicated adolescents, serum alcohol levels can provide a quantitative alcohol level that correlates with clinical features of intoxication (Table 58-2). This correlation is altered by chronic alcohol use and tolerance. Alcohol is generally eliminated at rates of 15-30 mg/dL/hr.[31] Minors should be observed until they have an undetectable alcohol level, or until adult supervision is available, and the patients are deemed clinically sober enough to be evaluated and are safe for discharge. All intoxicated adolescents should be referred for alcohol abuse counseling.

Opiates/Opioids

Opiate addiction is a public health problem in the United States and abroad. Myriad drugs fall into this class, ranging from hydrocodone to heroin (Table 58-3). The patient population exposed to these drugs can be widely variable, from patients receiving legitimate long-term pain management prescriptions to illicit drug abusers. The importance of accurate identification of opiate exposure is extremely important for child safety. During the antenatal period, fetuses exposed to opiates can display intrauterine growth restriction, prematurity, and low birth weight, as well as respiratory depression at birth. After birth, neonates whose mothers were addicted to opiates may suffer a neonatal abstinence syndrome, characterized by irritability, tremors, vomiting, poor feeding, and a high pitched cry.[32] Once identified, this syndrome can be effectively reversed by administration of tapered doses of opiates. In children, accidental ingestion of opiates can be lethal. The classic presentation of coma, respiratory depression, and pinpoint pupils should guide the skilled clinician to look for opiate exposure, and children exposed to longer-acting opiates (e.g., methadone and extended-release oxycodone) must be admitted for observation. In adolescents, opiate exposure can signal experimental drug use with common prescription narcotics, as well as illicit use of substances such as fentanyl, hydrocodone, oxycodone, methadone, or heroin.

Opiate screening is one of the most complex areas of drug testing. Understanding which opiates will trigger a positive screen and which will be missed requires a twofold discussion of pharmacology. The first issue relates to structure. The classic backbone of the opiate is the phenanthrene nucleus (Figure 58-1); opiates containing this structure include morphine, codeine, and 6-monoacetylmorphine (the primary metabolite of heroin). Semisynthetic and synthetic opioids, such as fentanyl, contain a markedly different backbone (see Figure 58-1). As a result, many opiate rapid drug screens cannot correctly identify the presence of these opioids, and specialized testing, such as GC/MS, is required for methadone, buprenorphine, hydromorphone, fentanyl, meperidine, tramadol, and propoxyfene. It is critically important for clinicians involved in drug screening to contact their on-site laboratory about the compounds detected on rapid drug screening and the availability of more specialized testing.

Metabolism is the second vitally important consideration since opiates are often metabolized to other commercially recognizable medications. For example, codeine is metabolized to morphine in vivo. To the unsuspecting practitioner, it may appear that the patient was exposed to two separate drugs. Examples of the metabolism of common opiates are seen in Table 58-4.

Opiates are detectable in urine, serum, and meconium. In general, opiates and opioids persist for 2 to 3 days after exposure in urine and blood, whereas meconium may reflect exposure from late second trimester to birth. Detection limits set for screening may be low enough to cause false positives from substances such as poppy seeds (liberates small amounts of codeine); however, typical confirmatory studies set limits high enough to differentiate true opiate exposure from contaminants. Given the complexities of opiate drug screening, collaboration with the clinical laboratory staff and medical toxicologists can facilitate appropriate testing and interpretation of results.

Table 58-2	Serum Blood Alcohol Levels and Correlating Clinical Symptoms
Blood Alcohol Level (mg/dL)	**Clinical Correlation**
20-50	Decreased fine motor control
50-100	Impaired coordination and judgment
100-150	Difficulty with ambulation
150-200	Difficulty maintaining posture, lethargy
300	Coma in naïve drinkers
400	Respiratory depression

From McMicken DB, Finnell JT: Alcohol-related disease. *In:* Marx JA, Hockberger RS, Walls RM, et al (eds): *Rosen's Emergency Medicine. Concepts and Clinical Practice,* ed 6, Mosby Elsevier, Philadelphia, 2006, p 2859.

Table 58-3	Commonly Encountered Opiates/Opioids

Morphine
Heroin
Codeine
Methadone
Hydromorphone
Hydrocodone
Oxycodone
Buprenorphine
Tramadol
Meperidine
Propoxyfene

Table 58-4	Examples of Opiate Metabolism

Heroin → 6-Monoacetylmorphine (6-MAM) → Morphine
 (Codeine often a contaminant)
Morphine → Codeine
Hydrocodone → Hydromorphone

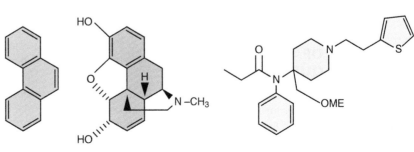

FIGURE 58-1 Structures of phenanthrene backbone, morphine, and fentanyl. *(From Gustav E: United Nations Office on Drugs and Crime. Some new analgesics and antispasmodics. Available at http://www.unodc.org/unodc/en/data-and-analysis/bulletin/bulletin_1956-01-01_1_page006.html. Published January 1, 1956. Accessed September 30, 2008.)*

Pheanthrene   Morphine   Fentanyl

MEDICAL CHILD ABUSE

Specific drug screening is sometimes indicated in cases of suspected medical child abuse, when caretakers purposely poison the children in their care. Salicylates and acetaminophen, as well as a number of opiates and benzodiazepines, can be found on the routine testing available at most hospitals. However, drugs like ipecac, sulfonylureas, insulin, warfarin and supercoumarins (a common ingredient of rat poison) are detectable only with focused testing and will not be identifiable on routine drug screens. Specialized testing can be undertaken through consultation with the laboratory staff or local toxicology resources. Comprehensive drug screening is available at some institutions, and the library of identified substances can range in the thousands; however, any drug screening method is best used when a suspected target drug or class is communicated to the laboratory personnel.

DRUG-FACILITATED SEXUAL ASSAULT

Many of the commonly used substances in drug-facilitated sexual assault are not detectable with standard rapid drug screening methodologies, and specific testing is required. For many hospitals, this testing cannot be done on-site and often requires several days for results to return. Detailed information about common "date rape" drugs and appropriate testing can be found in Chapter 15, "Drug-Facilitated Sexual Assault."

PITFALLS IN DRUG TESTING

Multiple errors can occur during the processing of laboratory samples. These errors can be described as preanalytical, analytical, and postanalytical errors depending on when they occur during specimen processing. The most common errors occur at the level of the ordering clinician (preanalytical), who either orders the wrong test or misinterprets the results.[33]

The chain-of-custody is a critical element in ensuring that results of drug screening are admissible for testimony during future legal action. Chain-of-custody requires accurate identification and association of samples to source patients during collection, transport, storage, analysis, and reporting of results.[34] Protocols for chain-of-custody should be in place for any large-scale drug or alcohol screening, and for specimens used in cases of suspected child maltreatment or in any other cases that could be of forensic importance. Critical attention should be paid to storage of specimens. By the time a screening test result is returned as positive, the original source fluid might be unavailable, and retesting the source patient might be of limited use since many drugs clear the body rapidly. Laboratories often have the ability to hold specimens for 1 week to 1 month after receipt upon request.

STRENGTH OF SCIENCE/ RESEARCH QUESTIONS

Data demonstrating the sensitivity and specificity of particular testing methodologies for individual tests have been well documented by both the medical establishment and industry. The effects of illicit drug exposure during all stages of pediatric development have also been well, if incompletely,

described. The major thrust of future research efforts could include the outcomes of large-scale drug screening and the resulting interventions in high-risk pediatric populations, since there is little in the medical literature that describes the downstream effects of drug exposure.

References

1. Lester BM, ElSohly M, Wright LL, et al: The maternal lifestyle study: drug use by meconium, toxicology and maternal self-report. *Pediatrics* 2001;107:309-317.
2. Rayburn WF: Maternal and fetal effects from substance use. *Clin Perinatol* 2007;34:559-571.
3. Ostrea EM Jr, Brady M, Gause S, et al: Drug screening of newborns by meconium analysis: a large-scale, prospective, epidemiologic study. *Pediatrics* 1992;89:107-113.
4. Smith L, Yonekura ML, Wallace T, et al: Effects of prenatal methamphetamine exposure on fetal growth and drug withdrawal symptoms in infants born at term. *J Dev Behav Pediatr* 2003;24:17-23.
5. Wolff K, Farrell M, Marsden J, et al: A review of biological indicators of illicit drug use, practical considerations and clinical usefulness. *Addiction* 1999; 94:1279-1298.
6. Bar-Oz B, Klein J, Karaskov T, et al: Comparison of meconium and neonatal hair analysis for detection of gestational exposure to drugs of abuse. *Arch Dis Child Fetal Neonatal Ed* 2003;88:F98-F100.
7. Wennig R: Potential problems with the interpretation of hair analysis results. *Forensic Sci Int* 2000;107:5-12.
8. Arria AM, Derauf C, Lagasse LL, et al: Methamphetamine and other substance use during pregnancy: preliminary estimates from the Infant Development, Environment, and Lifestyle (IDEAL) study. *Matern Child Health J* 2006;10:293-302.
9. Agnew A, Ammerman A: Methamphetamine and the pediatric patient. *Calif Pediatrician* 2006;Spring:1-3, 20.
10. Peters FT, Samyn N, Lamers CT, et al: Drug testing in blood: validated negative-ion chemical ionization gas chromatographic-mass spectrometric assay for enantioselective measurement of the designer drugs MDEA, MDMA, and MDA and its application to samples from a controlled study with MDMA. *Clin Chem* 2005;10:1811-1822.
11. U.S. Drug Enforcement Administration. Hashish. Available at http://www.usdoj.gov/dea/concern/hashish.html. Accessed September 1, 2008.
12. Johnston LD, O'Malley PM, Bachman JG, et al: *Monitoring the Future: National Results on Adolescent Drug Use: Overview of Key Findings, 2005*. National Institute on Drug Abuse, U.S. Dept of Health and Human Services, Bethesda, MD, 2005.
13. Fergusson DM, Horwood LJ, Northstone K, et al: Maternal use of cannabis and pregnancy outcome. *BJOG* 2002;109:21-27.
14. Gibson GT, Baghurst PA, Colley DP: Maternal alcohol, tobacco and cannabis consumption and the outcome of pregnancy. *Aust N Z J Obstet Gynaecol* 1983;23:15-19.
15. Zuckerman B, Frank DA, Hingson R, et al: Effects of maternal marijuana and cocaine use on fetal growth. *N Engl J Med* 1989;320:762-768.
16. Hatch EE, Bracken MB: Effect of marijuana use in pregnancy on fetal growth. *Am J Epidemiol* 1986;124:986-993.
17. Day N, Goldschmidt L, Thomas C: Prenatal marijuana exposure contributes to the prediction of marijuana use at age 14. *Addiction* 2006;101:1313-1322.
18. Results from the 2007 National Survey on Drug Use and Health: National Findings. Substance Abuse and Mental Health Services Administration Office of Applied Studies, U.S. Dept of Health and Human Services, Rockville, MD, 2007.
19. Birchfield M, Scully J, Handler A: Perinatal screening for illicit drugs: policies in hospitals in a large metropolitan area. *J Perinatol* 1995;15:208-214.
20. Bauer CR, Shankaran S, Bada HS et al: The Maternal Lifestyle Study: drug exposure during pregnancy and short-term maternal outcomes. *Am J Obstet Gynecol* 2002;186:487-495.
21. Traub SJ, Hoffman RS, Nelson LS: Body packing—the internal concealment of illicit drugs. *N Engl J Med* 2003;349:2519-2526.
22. Floyd RL, O'Connor MJ, Sokol RJ, et al: Recognition and prevention of fetal alcohol syndrome. *Obstet Gynecol* 2005;106:1059-1064.
23. May PA, Gossage JP: Estimating the prevalence of fetal alcohol syndrome. A summary. *Alcohol Res Health* 2001;25:159-167.

24. Harwood HJ, Napolitano DM: Economic implications of the fetal alcohol syndrome. *Alcohol Health Res World* 1985;10:38-43.

25. Chudley AE, Conry J, Cook JL, et al: Fetal alcohol spectrum disorder: Canadian guidelines for diagnosis. *CMAJ* 2005;172:S1-S21.

26. Sokol RJ, Delaney-Black V, Nordstrom B: Fetal alcohol spectrum disorder. *JAMA* 2003;290:2996-2999.

27. Peterson J, Kirchner HL, Xue W, et al: Fatty acid ethyl esters in meconium are associated with poorer neurodevelopmental outcomes to two years of age. *J Pediatr* 2008;152:788-792.

28. Bearer CF, Jacobson JL, Jacobson SW, et al: Validation of a new biomarker of fetal exposure to alcohol. *J Pediatr* 2003;143:463-469.

29. Vogel C, Caraccio T, Mofenson H, et al: Alcohol intoxication in young children. *J Toxicol Clin Toxicol* 1995;33:25-33.

30. Donovan JE: Adolescent alcohol initiation: a review of psychosocial risk factors. *J Adolesc Health* 2004;34:480-492.

31. Scott-Ham M, Burton FC: A study of blood and urine alcohol concentrations in cases of alleged drug-facilitated sexual assault in the United Kingdom over a 3-year period. *J Clin Forensic Med* 2006;13:107-111.

32. Johnson K, Gerada C, Greenough A: Treatment of neonatal abstinence syndrome. *Arch Dis Child Fetal Neonatal Ed* 2003;88:F2-F5.

33. Laposata M, Dighe A: "Pre-pre" and "post-post" analytical error: high-incidence patient safety hazards involving the clinical laboratory. *Clin Chem Lab Med* 2007;45:712-719.

34. Jaffee WB, Trucco E, Teter C, et al: Focus on alcohol & drug abuse: ensuring validity in urine drug testing. *Psychiatr Serv* 2008;59:140-142.

59

INJURIES RESULTING FROM FALLS

David L. Chadwick, MD, Gina Bertocci, PhD, and Elisabeth Guenther, MD, MPH

INTRODUCTION

Short falls causing minor injury occur very frequently in infants and children. Long falls causing more serious injury are not rare. Serious inflicted injuries are often falsely attributed to short falls by the persons who inflicted them.[1]

Bipedality is the quintessential characteristic of humans,[2] and the bumps and bruises from the falls of infants and young children are part of the evolutionary price paid for this advantage. Falling is universal among children who are learning to walk. In addition, young children often climb to and fall from elevated surfaces. However, if such falls were often fatal, the human race would not have survived.

In the 1960s Kravitz[3] studied infant falls by asking mothers about their children's falls. In one study, he asked the parents of infants attending a clinic to recall the falls of their children aged 10 months to 2 years some months after the falls occurred. The other focused on 336 infants under 1 year of age, asking parents to describe falls soon after they happened. Both studies were of falls from elevated surfaces rather than ground level falls. Both groups demonstrated "peaks" of fall incidence around 6 to 8 months, but both found falls at all ages including at 1 month of age. During this study, 536 infants experienced 328 falls, and about half of all infants fell at least once. Eighteen infants were hospitalized and none died. Three infants had skull fractures, two had concussion, and one had a subdural hematoma. There were no extremity fractures. Kravitz stated that child abuse was not found in any of these cases, but he did not explain how it was excluded. The most frequent circumstance leading to a fall was climbing out of a crib, and Kravitz concluded that crib design was the most important correctible factor.

Warrington and Wright[4] used the ongoing Avon Longitudinal Study of Parents and Children (ALSPAC) that had enrolled 14,000 newborn babies and their parents for prospective determination of their illnesses and injuries and associated risk factors. A questionnaire administered to all parents when the infants were 6 months of age inquired about falls and resultant injuries. Data were available for 11,466 infants; 2554 of them generated 3357 falls from "elevated places." Falls from beds or settees comprised 53% of the falls, and 10% of the infants fell from someone's arms. The rest fell from chairs, changing tables, prams, bouncers, and tables, and 5.6% "fell over" (a term not defined). An injury was sustained in 437 cases. Serious injury, defined as concussion or fracture, occurred in 21 cases (<1% of falls). Eighteen were admitted to hospital. No deaths or life-threatening injuries were reported, and the authors concluded that although falls in infants less than 6 months of age are "surprisingly common," injuries were "… infrequent, generally trivial, and almost entirely confined to the head."

Figure 59-1 captures sequential snapshots of a toddler's fall recorded in a childcare center and demonstrates why the vast majority of ground level falls in this age group are benign. Short falls have been shown to result in minor trauma such as bruising, linear parietal skull fractures, and clavicle or extremity fractures, but fatal injuries from short falls are extremely rare.[5]

A rational discussion of injury mechanisms requires the use of standard definitions. Definitions have been provided by the work of Christoffel,[6] the ICD-9,[7] ICD-10,[8] and other sources. The definitions used are found in Table 59-1.

TYPES OF FALL INJURIES

Head Injuries with Fall Histories

Most children with life-threatening head injuries present with impaired consciousness and sometimes altered breathing or full arrest. In some cases, the child is dead at the scene or on arrival at the hospital. This chapter applies to those children who survive long enough to reach a setting in which a thorough medical evaluation is possible. Many children with head injury from falls have obvious head bruising, but many do not. Certain patterns of bruising, however, would be unlikely to have been caused by a fall and should alert the clinician to the possibility of abuse. Figure 59-2 (found in Chapter 59 Supplemental Resources online at www.expertconsult.com) shows such an injury.

Complex and diastatic skull fractures (see Figure 59-3 online) have not been reported in association with short falls in observed settings such as hospitals. Their presence indicates that a major force was involved in the injury event.[9] Initial presentation with obvious severe injury and a minimal event history is typical of inflicted head injury.[10]

One type of serious cranial injury that is well known to be caused by short falls is the epidural hematoma (see Figure 59-4 online). A laceration of an artery can cause bleeding between the dura and the skull, leading to the rapid accumulation of a large, space-occupying hematoma. This can cause life-threatening increased intracranial pressure and deep coma or death. Epidural hematomas are easily recognized on CT scans and can be successfully treated if surgery is performed quickly after diagnosis.[11] In some cases,

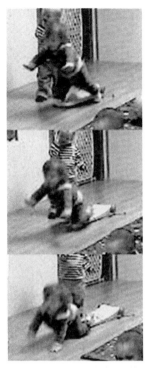

FIGURE 59-1 Illustration of a toddler's fall. These three images illustrate the use of video to study the common falls of toddlers. The toddler crumples forward, absorbing energy at multiple points on her body including her knees and hands. No damage occurs.

the epidural hematoma will communicate through a skull fracture with a subgaleal hematoma.

Abdominal Injuries with Fall Histories

Life-threatening abdominal injuries, usually present in one of two ways: (1) hypovolemic shock, which can occur shortly after injury, or (2) sepsis and peritonitis, which occur hours or days after an injury perforating a hollow viscus. There may or may not be bruising present on the abdominal skin. Sometimes bruising on the back over spinous processes provides a clue that the child was injured by deep indenting blunt trauma to the abdomen while lying on the back on a firm surface (see Figure 59-5 online).

Recognition of abdominal injury as a cause of otherwise unexplained hypovolemic shock requires experience and a high index of suspicion on the part of the physician. In these cases, shock results from blood loss into the peritoneal cavity from damaged viscera or blood vessels. Clinicians might be misled by short fall histories that do not predict life-threatening injury, and the abdomen can be soft. Children with serious intraabdominal bleeding can look fairly normal for a time and then deteriorate very quickly. Several useful articles discuss evaluating possibly inflicted abdominal injuries.[12-21] Short falls of previously healthy infants and young children are extremely unlikely to cause life-threatening abdominal injuries.[15]

Chest Injuries with Fall Histories

Unexplained healing rib fractures are sometimes found on skeletal surveys obtained in infants and toddlers who are

Table 59-1	Definitions Used in this Chapter
Elevated surface	A surface above ground or floor level
Fall	To come down by force of gravity suddenly (noun or verb).
Fall height	The change in height of the center of gravity of the falling object from the starting point to the ending point of the fall (In practice, usually the height of an elevated surface from the floor or the ground)
Ground level fall	A fall beginning and ending at ground level usually from standing to prone, supine, or sitting position
Infants	Persons at ages between birth and the first birthday
Injury	1. An event resulting in damage to a body part; 2. The damage or pathology resulting from an event
Intentional injury	Injuries that were intended to injure a person (i.e., assaults, homicides, self-inflicted injuries, and suicides)
Long fall	A fall of >1.5 meters
Nonaccidental injury	An injury inflicted by other than accidental means often without clear intent to cause injury
Outcome	The status of a case at an advanced or ultimate point
Point of recognition	The point in a case at which a health professional has a "reasonable suspicion" that the child with an injury and a fall history might be injured by "other than accidental means"
Short fall	A fall of <1.5 meters (includes falls from all household furniture items except bunk beds)
Young children	Persons between birth and the fifth birthday

being evaluated for possible child abuse (see Figure 59-6 online). Posterior and lateral rib fractures, pulmonary contusions, and hemothoraces are more likely to be caused by child abuse rather than falls, although complex falls and falls from heights can also cause these conditions.[22] Rarely, infants and children present with cardiac injuries such as hemopericardium, again a finding not likely to occur in a household fall and more often found in inflicted injuries.[23] There is a single case report of ventricular fibrillation (commotio cordis) following a fall.[24] The condition is difficult to diagnose in living children and almost impossible after death in the absence of an accurate history.[25]

Less Serious Injuries

Fractures of the extremities and linear parietal skull fractures occur infrequently (in about 1%) in the short falls that have been witnessed by multiple people in hospitals.[26-29] Other minor and moderate injuries, including concussion,[3,4] are often associated with less reliable short fall histories. Pierce et al[30] has provided an algorithm for the analysis of femur fractures occurring in association with short fall histories. It focuses the criteria suggested by Leventhal et al.[31] The algorithm points out that "… differences exist in 4 key categories: (1) history quality and detail; (2) biomechanical compatibility of the fracture morphologic features; (3) time line for seeking medical care; and, (4) presence of other injuries."[30]

The widespread use of definitions of abusive injury, which require that the injuries be severe in relationship to their explanations, has created an epidemiological anomaly. It has resulted in an apparent high case fatality rate for abusive as compared with unintentional injury. It is important to improve the recognition of minor and moderate inflicted physical injuries, because the affected children are likely to be at risk for future, more serious, injury.

Recognition and Reporting

The "point of recognition" is that point in the case at which a health professional has a reasonable suspicion that the child with an injury and a fall history might be injured by "other than accidental means." At this point a report is usually made to a child protection agency. From that point forward the process of medical assessment requires confirming or excluding that diagnosis. The point can occur as early as the first health care contact or as late as at autopsy or during an even later review by a child fatality review team. In most cases, the parents or guardians of the child should be informed that a report has been made and that an investigation will probably follow. Reporting suspected abuse is mandatory in all states, although details may vary.[32] There can be criminal sanctions and civil liability for failure to report suspected abuse.

"Points of recognition" are not unique to inflicted or abusive injuries. They occur in any medical condition, when the physician becomes aware that the facts in the case require one or more serious conditions to be diagnosed or excluded as soon as possible. However, in cases of suspected abuse when a report is made to an agency, the caretakers who are providing histories of the events leading up to the child's change of condition may adopt attitudes aimed at protecting themselves and alter the histories that they provide.

IS IT A FALL OR IS IT ABUSE? ASSESSING THE CHILD

The initial clinical assessment of the child presenting to the emergency department with the history of a fall begins by rapidly assessing the injury and medically stabilizing the child before further evaluation is undertaken. Once the child is stabilized and assessed, the process of differentiating among nonintentional trauma, abuse, or neglect begins. A complete description of the appropriate medical workup for a child presenting with the history of a fall when possible child physical abuse or neglect is being considered

can be found in Chapter 59 Supplemental Resources online at www.expertconsult.com.

Radiological Imaging

Radiological imaging, including CT, is helpful in determining the types and severity of injury and is warranted in cases in which the physical examination is unreliable because of patient age, presence of other injuries that may obfuscate the physical examination, or the presence of nonspecific signs or symptoms that could be indicative of head injury.[33,34] (See Chapter 46, "Biochemical Markers of Head Trauma in Children"; Chapter 33, "Imaging of Skeletal Trauma in Abused Children"; Chapter 34, "The Role of Cross-Sectional Imaging in Evaluating Pediatric Skeletal Trauma"; and Chapter 35, "Long Bone Fracture Biomechanics.")

CONSULTATIONS

Consultations and involvement of pediatric subspecialists in the diagnostic workup, medical management, and appropriate documentation of these cases vary significantly depending on several factors including the severity of the injury, the type of injury, the age of the child, and the examination findings. Many institutions now have multidisciplinary medical/surgical teams to efficiently manage these potentially complex cases with the associated medical, psychological, social, and legal implications.

Differential Diagnosis

When considering whether an injury is caused by a fall or by abuse, several characteristics of the injury and the event will give the clinician important information. Table 59-2 outlines these characteristics of injuries.

Biomechanical Assessment of Stated Fall Scenarios

A biomechanical assessment of a fall scenario presented as the cause of a child's injuries can provide additional objective information when attempting to distinguish abusive and nonabusive trauma. A biomechanical assessment can be best undertaken by a multidisciplinary team of clinicians and engineers; however, in the absence of an engineer, clinicians can follow some of the same basic principles in their assessment that would be used by an engineer. In particular, scene investigations and the approach outlined in the biodynamic compatibility section can be followed by clinicians when challenged to distinguish between abusive and nonabusive trauma. In contrast, biomechanical analyses must be conducted only by an engineer with the appropriate training and expertise.

Scene Investigation for Biomechanical Assessment

When conducting scene investigations, it is imperative that characteristics of the fall environment be carefully documented. Documentation should include photographs of the scene, including photographs documenting the orientation of any objects (bed, sofa, etc.) involved in the event.

Table 59-2	Differential Diagnosis of Physical Examination Findings Presenting in Cases of Alleged Falls that Can Be Associated with Abusive Injury	
Body Region/Injury Type	**Relationship to Abuse**	**Differential Diagnosis**
Head Subdural hematoma (SDH) Subarachnoid hemorrhages (SAHs) Cerebral edema Skull fractures Parietal fractures Multiple or bilateral skull fractures	20% of abused children suffer CNS trauma. It is fatal in 7-30%. 30-50% sustain permanent deficits. Injuries to the brain and spinal cord account for 75% of the deaths caused by abuse. 50% of abuse fatalities have SDH. SDH is the most common injury in shaken baby syndrome. Cerebral edema is found in 66% of abuse fatalities. Depressed, diastatic, nonparietal and complex skull fractures are more common in abuse. 80-90% of abusive skull fractures are parietal fractures.[31,35] Multiple or bilateral skull fractures are more likely caused by abuse in the absence of major accidental trauma.	Glutaric aciduria type 1 (characteristics: macrocranium, SDH, sparse intraretinal and preretinal hemorrhages, frontotemporal atrophy) and hemorrhagic disease of the newborn (risk factors: home birth, no vitamin K prophylaxis, breastfeeding). Simple linear skull fractures can result from short falls of less than 3 ft, are usually associated with scalp bruising and/or swelling. Simple linear parietal fractures can occur by toddlers falling from standing.
Skin Bruises on protected areas (neck, face, ears, trunk, buttocks, and hands)	High-velocity injuries (e.g., slap or cord mark) leave a petechial image or outline of the object.[36] Low velocity or severe forces leave a "positive" bruise image in children 0-8 months old. Bruises in protected areas are more likely caused by abuse.[36-39]	Less than 1% of bruises in infants under 6 months old have accidental bruises. Less than 3% of children who are not yet cruising have accidental bruises.[37] Other causes of bruises include accidents, coagulopathies (idiopathic thrombocytopenic purpura, vitamin K deficiency, hemophilia, von Willebrand disease), and vaculitis (Henoch-Schönlein purpura).
Head, Eyes, Ears, Nose Throat Scalp Eyes Nose Ears Mouth Neck	50% of documented abuse cases include orofacial trauma. Bald areas on the scalp can be caused by traction alopecia. Severe malnutrition causes thinning of hair. Extensive, multilayer retinal hemorrhages extending from the posterior pole to the ora serrata are often caused by acceleration/deceleration forces.[40] These types of hemorrhages are not likely to be found in impact injuries.[41] Bleeding from the nose and mouth occurring with apparent life-threatening events are associated with suffocation.[42] Pinna bruising associated with SDH, retinal hemorrhages, and cerebral edema has been called "tin ear syndrome."[43] Hemotympanum is associated with basilar or temporal bone fractures. Frenulum tears can occur with blows to the mouth or from forcing objects into the mouth. Extensive caries may indicate dental neglect. Ligature marks or finger marks can occur with strangulation.	Bald spots can be causes by tinea capitis, alopecia areata, and occipital bald spots because of the recommended supine positioning of young infants. Birth retinal hemorrhages can be extensive and multilayer, and usually clear within a few weeks. Hemotypanum can occur with leukemia. Frenulum tears of the upper lip can occur in toddler falls.
Chest Ribs	Chest injuries are more common in child abuse cases than in accidental injury cases.[44] Rib fractures in children under the age of 3 are commonly caused by abuse.[45,46]	Cardiopulmonary resuscitation was not known to cause rib fractures in the past. AP resuscitation might cause fractures.[47] More fractures are seen if the periosteum is stripped.

Continued

Table 59-2	Differential Diagnosis of Physical Examination Findings Presenting in Cases of Alleged Falls that Can Be Associated with Abusive Injury—cont'd	
Body Region/Injury Type	**Relationship to Abuse**	**Differential Diagnosis**
Abdomen Liver Duodenum Pancreas	Abdominal injury is found in 1-10% of abuse cases, but mortality in these cases is 40-50%. Bilious vomiting can be seen in abdominal injuries. Suspect liver injury if AST >450, ALT >250.[48] Liver is the most common solid organ injury in abuse. Left lobe is more commonly injured in abuse. Abused children are more likely to have a hollow viscous injury than children injured accidentally.[49] Abused children are younger and more likely to have a delayed presentation and a higher mortality rate. Pancreatic injury without a clear trauma history is suspicious for abuse.[50] Pancreatic pseudocyst can result from pancreatic injury.	Right lobe injuries are more common in accidental injuries.
Genitals/Anus	Unexplained bruises, tears, and lacerations can be caused by abuse.[51] Pregnancy and STD can be from abuse.	Straddle injuries can mimic abuse.
Extremities Classic metaphyseal lesions (CML) Diaphyseal fractures Humerus fractures Supracondylar fractures Clavicular fractures Spinous process fractures Sternal fractures Scapular fractures Vertebral body fractures and subluxations Fractures of the digits Multiple fractures of different ages	11-55% of abused children have extremity fractures. 80% of fractures caused by abuse are in children under 18 months old.[52] 2% of accidental fractures are in children under 19 months old. In immature bones, planar fractures occur through the zone of provisional calcification at the metaphysis (CML).[54] On x-ray, CML can appear as "bucket handles" or "corner fractures." Humerus fractures are suggestive of abuse in infants less than 15 months old.[55] Clavicular fractures are uncommon in abuse cases.[56] Spinous process fractures are highly specific for abuse. They can be caused by hyperflexion and hyperextension of the spine. Sternal fractures are unusual and highly specific for abuse. Scapular fractures are unusual and highly specific for abuse. Vertebral body fractures are moderately specific for abuse. They can be caused by hyperflexion and hyperextension of the spine and by vertical loading. Fractures of the digits are moderately specific for abuse. Multiple fractures of different ages are highly suspicious for abuse in the absence of bone disease.	Accidental leg fractures in infants have been associated with the use of "exersaucers."[3] Recently ambulatory toddlers can experience accidental spiral or oblique fractures of the tibia. Accidental spiral femur fractures can occur in older children who fall when running. Metabolic and genetic bone disease should be considered when abuse is suspected. Diaphyseal fractures are not specific for abuse. Supracondylar fractures can occur with falls on outstretched arms. Clavicular fractures can be caused by falls on an outstretched arm.
Other Concerning Conditions Seizures in infants Apnea or respiratory arrest Sudden infant death syndrome (SIDS)	These conditions frequently occur in abusive head trauma. Apnea/ALTE event at age > 8 months are high risk for abuse. Up to 10% of SIDS cases may actually be abuse fatalities.[57]	

Photographs should be taken from a number of vantage points or perspectives to allow for full view of the scene. Photographs of all objects that might have been involved with the injury should be obtained and movable objects should be identified as such.

A sketch of the scene, providing a plan (top) view and any necessary additional views to describe movable objects and fixed structures, along with their relative orientation to each other, should be made. Structures and objects that are a part of the scene should be measured and these measurements should be documented on a sketch. Dimensions should include height, width, and length of each object or structure. A second copy of the dimensioned sketch should be used to overlay the initial position (pre-fall) of the child as well as the resting or final position (post-fall) of the child. These positions should not only identify height of the child's feet above the impact surface, but also the child's posture (i.e., standing, sitting). Fall information should also describe final, post-fall orientation of the child (anterior, posterior, or lateral) relative to objects or structures at the scene as stated by witnesses.

In addition, samples of the impacted surfaces should be obtained when possible. For example, if the child fell onto a padded carpeted floor, samples of the carpet and padding should be obtained so that characteristics of the flooring can be determined. Similarly, if the child impacted an object during her descent, the material used to construct this object should be accurately described and documented. Information related to impact surface properties is key to a biomechanical analysis since these properties have been shown to affect biomechanical outcome measures such as resulting accelerations and force experienced by the body on impact.[58-61]

Biodynamic Compatibility of Stated Cause and Injuries

The objective of a biodynamic compatibility assessment is to determine whether the constellation of injuries is compatible with the biodynamics of the stated event.[30] In other words, as described, can the fall dynamics (how a child's body moves or falls from their initial pre-fall position to their final post-fall resting position) account for all of the presenting acute injuries? In fatal cases, *one must not only account for the underlying specific fatal injury, but also each and every acute impact injury associated with the event.* This includes all bruises, contusions, and lacerations even though they might not affect the child's overall health outcome. (Obviously, soft tissue injuries associated with medical interventions must be excluded from the biodynamic compatibility assessment.) Each of these soft tissue injuries associated with the fall will likely represent an impact or point of contact that must be accounted for in the fall dynamics. These markings provide a "roadmap" to the child's exposure. For example, a single free fall from standing on a 12-inch high chair onto a padded carpeted floor without impacting any objects during the descent cannot account for the combination of a subdural hematoma; bruising to the lateral, posterior, and anterior aspects of the head; and bruising to the buttocks and lacerations to the anterior thorax. Such a fall would lead to markings or injuries associated with impact to *one* plane of the body. If a child fell rearward from a chair, one would expect to find evidence of impact on the posterior aspect of the body, but no markings or evidence of impact on the anterior portion of the body. Using an approach that accounts for the entire "roadmap" of injuries provides an objective means of determining biodynamic compatibility of presenting injuries and their stated cause.

Biomechanical Analyses of Stated Falls

In addition to a qualitative biodynamic compatibility assessment, in some cases that proceed to litigation, a more extensive biomechanical analysis is sometimes desired. A biomechanical analysis typically strives to approximate accelerations, velocities, or forces associated with the stated impact event. These biomechanical measures, which are known to be related to injury risk, can be estimated for a particular body region or for the entire body. For example, estimated angular head acceleration can be compared with published injury thresholds to predict the risk of a subdural hemorrhage.[62-65] To estimate biomechanical measures such as acceleration or velocity, additional information must be obtained related to the child and fall event, and assumptions may need to be made. Information such as the child's mass, overall height, anthropometrics, and percentiles of growth are needed, and can influence the estimation of biomechanical measures.

In an unwitnessed fall event, assumptions regarding the fall dynamics (i.e. how the child's body moved during descent and their position upon impact with a surface), initial position and final position must be adopted for the analysis. Knowledge or assumption regarding the child's position just prior to impact is key to the analysis. For example, if a child impacts the ground head first, as opposed to feet first, this has a substantial influence on estimated head acceleration.

Biomechanical analysis is possible using a variety of methodologies, but it is critical that methods are based on the principles of physics. Such techniques can include manual calculations, use of surrogates (anthropomorphic test devices or "dummies") representing the child in fall experiments, or computer simulation modeling.[66] In each approach the goal is to determine key outcome measures associated with a given fall, which is then compared with injury thresholds to determine likelihood of injury. The advantages and disadvantages of the three methodologies are described in Table 59-3.

Manual calculations, based upon theories or laws of physics (conservation of energy, conservation of momentum, etc.), often represent the fall victim as a simplified lumped mass or rigid body with a specified mass and height (in the case of a rigid body) representative of the child. A commonly used rigid body representation is that of an inverted pendulum that consists of a rod representing the torso and lower extremities and a mass representing the pendulum or head of the fall victim. Assumptions or known facts regarding initial position, fall dynamics, and impact surface characteristics are incorporated, and physics-based computations are performed to estimated key outcome measures such as accelerations or velocities.

Surrogates have also been used in the estimation of biomechanical outcome measures associated with a fall.[67-69] These surrogates could be customized representations of the fall victim or commercially available anthropomorphic test devices. Biofidelity of surrogates (how human-like they are) relates directly to their ability to accurately predict the exposure of a child in a given circumstance. For example, when assessing head injury, the design and construction of the surrogate neck must be biofidelic in its response to exposure of force application. The surrogate must be biofidelic in all of its joint responses, as well as body segment anthropometrics and inertial properties (mass distribution). Surrogates are typically equipped with instrumentation such as accelerometers, and load cells to determine key outcome measures from various body regions. Mock fall experiments are then conducted to recreate the stated fall during which data are collected from the onboard instrumentation. Mock

Table 59-3	Some Key Advantages and Disadvantages of Various Biomechanical Analyses Methodologies	
Method	**Advantages**	**Disadvantages**
Manual physics-based calculations	Requires relatively limited time to perform Basic level engineering knowledge sufficient to perform	Greatly simplifies representation of child Greatly simplifies fall dynamics Theories or laws forming basis of calculations incorporate assumptions
Surrogate experiments	Physical device can be instrumented to assess outcomes of multiple body regions Provides visual representation of fall dynamics Ability to evaluate variations of given fall	High cost and lack of availability of surrogates Limitations in biofidelity Requires auxiliary data acquisition equipment to capture data from instrumentation
Computer simulation models	Ability to conduct parametric sensitivity (what-if) analyses Provides graphical output of fall dynamics Ability to evaluate variations of given fall	Time consuming and costly Difficult to validate Costly software needed to develop models Requires specialized expertise to develop and validate models Digitized version of child and environment Limitations in biofidelity of child surrogate

experiments again require knowledge of the initial position and fall dynamics of the child so that the surrogate can be appropriately positioned and so that the surrogate fall dynamics can be verified.

Computer simulation modeling has been used to study factors affecting injury risk associated with falls and shaken baby syndrome.[70-72] A computer simulation model of a pediatric fall consists of a discrete digital representation of the child and the fall environment. Physics-based equations of motion represented through numerical computations are used by specialized software to prescribe the child's path of motion during a fall. Outcome measures such as acceleration, velocity, and force applied to body segments can be determined by most computer simulation software programs. It is important to note that physics-based simulation software operates differently than animation software, and thus will provide different outcomes. When using animation software, the programmer has the ability to prescribe object motion of his or her choice. Therefore, when viewing visual graphics illustrating fall dynamics of a child, one must first question whether the software used to develop the graphics are physics based or animation based. *Animation-based outcomes and findings are not scientifically based and should not be considered a valid biomechanical analysis.* Although physics-based computer simulation models can provide reasonable prediction of injury risk, models must first be experimentally validated.[70-72] Experimental validation requires that the developed model be "tuned" to match data from an experiment representing the simulation. For example, to validate a computer simulation model of a pediatric bed fall, bed fall experiments using a physical surrogate that represents the model-based child surrogate must be conducted and key outcome measures from the model must match those of the experiments.[70] Only after model validation has been proved should it be used in the prediction of injury risk. Even then, one must critically assess the biofidelity of the model-based surrogate given that it is likely a representation of a commercially available surrogate that may have limited biofidelity.

It is important to note that biomechanical analyses, especially of hypothesized unwitnessed falls, inherently have assumptions incorporated into their findings. An incorrect assumption regarding fall dynamics can greatly overestimate or underestimate biomechanical measures (acceleration, velocity, etc.) leading to erroneous conclusions regarding likelihood of injury. In addition, each method described above uses a simplification of the child, the fall dynamics, and the fall environment. Engineers performing these analyses must clearly identify the limitations associated with their analysis, along with the effects that assumptions and limitations have on their findings. At a minimum, expert reports provided by engineers should provide a list of assumptions used in conducting their analysis. Although the intent of a biomechanical analysis is to provide additional objectivity, it must be cautioned that this objectivity can be compromised in the shadow of assumptions and limitations. Therefore, the findings of biomechanical analyses should be interpreted with caution and should constitute only one component of a more comprehensive assessment.

THE LIKELIHOOD OF DEATH OR SERIOUS INJURY FROM A SHORT FALL

Medicine in general, and epidemiology in particular, have used statistical analyses to assist in making quantitative probability statements comparable over time or between populations. Still, in most child abuse cases in which medical expert testimony is provided, the experts use only semi-quantitative statements such as, "Death from a short fall of a toddler is rare." Quantitative expressions of probability allow comparisons of the likelihood of different events (e.g., the comparison of deaths resulting from lightning strikes or cancer to deaths resulting from short falls).

Recently we have used an epidemiological mortality rate calculation to estimate the maximum possible likelihood of death from a short fall affecting a young child.[5] The short fall mortality rate for infants and children from birth to age 5 is less than 0.48/million young children/year. Quantitative probability expressions should be used wherever possible in litigation.

The publication of data from fall cases that lack valid observations has been a problem.[73-75] Authors have concluded that short falls resulting in fatal injuries are "possible." Some authors conclude that they are "unlikely," but they do not attempt to make quantitative or even semi-quantitative estimates. The manner in which injury events are witnessed must always be carefully described and critically analyzed. Cases of falls occurring in hospital settings can usually be considered to be valid observations.[26-28] Cases that are multiply witnessed in childcare settings are also more likely to be valid, especially if systematically and prospectively observed, recorded, and analyzed biomechanically. Such studies are badly needed and feasible with modest support.

Observations made by persons who are also suspects for possible child abuse should not be relied upon as accurate data for research purposes or for drawing general conclusions. Confessions are very useful for many purposes[76] but may not be valid in every instance. Assessing their validity can be difficult.[77]

RESPONSIBLE TESTIMONY IN CASES OF DEATH/SEVERE INJURY FROM SHORT FALLS

Responsible testimony follows the guidelines set out by the American Medical Association (AMA).[78-80] The most common form of irresponsible testimony is testimony that goes beyond the "recent and substantive experience" of the person providing the testimony, but "unique causal theory" is also common and can lead to blatant lies. Expertise requires hands-on experience as well as "book-learning" and knowledge of the literature. For child abuse cases, different types of expertise can be acquired at the bedside with patient contacts, in the laboratory, or through clinical research. Different specialists acquire expertise in different ways. Clinicians learn from patient contacts; pathologists from autopsies. Prior court appearances only confer expertise in court presentation.

The House of Delegates of the AMA has ruled that expert testimony is a part of the practice of medicine, and like any other aspect of practice, may be subject to peer review and to regulation by medical societies or governmental entities. However, review of expert testimony is a very challenging process requiring significant investments of time and knowledge. It is not generally in place at this time. A recent misguided attempt at regulation of expert testimony by the medical licensing agency of the United Kingdom has had the unintended effect of serious disruption of child protection in that country.[81]

References

1. Chadwick DL, Chin S, Salerno C, et al: Deaths from falls in children: how far is fatal? *J Trauma* 1991;31:1353-1355.
2. Kramer PA, Eck GG: Locomotor energetics and leg length in hominid bipedality. *J Hum Evol* 2000;38:651-656.
3. Kravitz H, Driessen G, Gomberg R, et al: Accidental falls from elevated surfaces in infants from birth to one year of age. *Pediatrics* 1969;44(Suppl):869-876.
4. Warrington SA, Wright CM, Team AS: Accidents and resulting injuries in premobile infants: data from the ALSPAC study. *Arch Dis Child* 2001;85:104-107.
5. Chadwick DL, Bertocci G, Castillo E, et al: Annual risk of death resulting from short falls among young children: less than 1 in 1 million. *Pediatrics* 2008;121:1213-1224.
6. Christoffel KK, Scheidt PC, Agran PF, et al: Standard definitions for childhood injury research: excerpts of a conference report. *Pediatrics* 1992;89:1027-1028.
7. International Classification of Diseases, Ninth Revision, Clinical Modification. National Center for Health Statistics, Washington, DC, 2002.
8. International Statistical Classification of Diseases and Related Health Problems, 10th Revision. World Health Organization, Geneva, 2006.
9. Hobbs CJ: Skull fracture and the diagnosis of abuse. *Arch Dis Child* 1984;59:246-252.
10. Duhaime AC, Partington MD. Overview and clinical presentation of inflicted head injury in infants. *Neurosurg Clin North Am* 2002;13:149-154, v.
11. Schutzman SA, Barnes PD, Mantello M, et al: Epidural hematomas in children. *Ann Emerg Med* 1993;22:535-541.
12. Trokel M, Discala C, Terrin NC, et al: Patient and injury characteristics in abusive abdominal injuries. *Pediatr Emerg Care* 2006;22:700-704.
13. Wood J, Rubin DM, Nance ML, et al: Distinguishing inflicted versus accidental abdominal injuries in young children. *J Trauma* 2005;59:1203-1208.
14. Cooper A, Floyd T, Barlow B, et al: Major blunt abdominal trauma due to child abuse. *J Trauma* 1988;28:1483-1487.
15. Huntimer CM, Muret-Wagstaff S, Leland NL: Can falls on stairs result in small intestine perforations? *Pediatrics* 2000;106:301-305.
16. Barnes PM, Norton CM, Dunstan FD, et al: Abdominal injury due to child abuse. *Lancet* 2005;366:234-235.
17. Gaines BA, Shultz BS, Morrison K, et al: Duodenal injuries in children: beware of child abuse. *J Pediatr Surg* 2004;39:600-602.
18. Lemburg P: [Diagnosis and clinical aspects of child abuse]. *Monatsschr Kinderheilkd* 1986;134:319-321.
19. Sibert JR, Payne EH, Kemp AM, et al: The incidence of severe physical child abuse in Wales. *Child Abuse Negl* 2002;26:267-276.
20. Sivit CJ, Taylor GA, Eichelberger MR: Visceral injury in battered children: a changing perspective. *Radiology* 1989;173:659-661.
21. Trokel M, DiScala C, Terrin NC, et al: Blunt abdominal injury in the young pediatric patient: child abuse and patient outcomes. *Child Maltreat* 2004;9:111-117.
22. Bulloch B, Schubert CJ, Brophy PD, et al: Cause and clinical characteristics of rib fractures in infants. *Pediatrics* 2000;105:E48.
23. Cohle SD, Hawley DA, Berg KK, et al: Homicidal cardiac lacerations in children. *J Forensic Sci* 1995;40:212-218.
24. Tibballs J, Thiruchelvam T: A case of commotio cordis in a young child caused by a fall. *Resuscitation* 2008;77:139-141.
25. Link MS, Wang PJ, Maron BJ, et al: What is commotio cordis? *Cardiol Rev* 1999;7:265-269.
26. Helfer RE, Slovis TL, Black M: Injuries resulting when small children fall out of bed. *Pediatrics* 1977;60:533-535.
27. Nimityongskul P, Anderson LD: The likelihood of injuries when children fall out of bed. *J Pediatr Orthop* 1987;7:184-186.
28. Levene S, Bonfield G: Accidents on hospital wards. *Arch Dis Child* 1991;66:1047-1049.
29. Lyons TJ, Oates RK: Falling out of bed: a relatively benign occurrence. *Pediatrics* 1993;92:125-127.
30. Pierce MC, Bertocci GE, Janosky JE, et al: Femur fractures resulting from stair falls among children: an injury plausibility model. *Pediatrics* 2005;115:1712-1722.
31. Leventhal JM, Thomas SA, Rosenfield NS, et al: Fractures in young children. Distinguishing child abuse from unintentional injuries. *Am J Dis Child* 1993;147:87-92.
32. Flaherty EG, Sege RD, Griffith J, et al: From suspicion of physical child abuse to reporting: primary care clinician decision-making. *Pediatrics* 2008;122:611-619.
33. Kellogg ND, American Academy of Pediatrics: Evaluation of suspected child physical abuse. *Pediatrics* 2007;119:1232-1241.
34. Campbell KA, Bogen DL, Berger RP: The other children: a survey of child abuse physicians on the medical evaluation of children living with a physically abused child. *Arch Pediatr Adolesc Med* 2006;160:1241-1246.
35. Meservy CJ, Towbin R, McLaurin RL, et al: Radiographic characteristics of skull fractures resulting from child abuse. *AJR Am J Roentgenol* 1987;149:173-175.
36. Feldman KW: Patterned abusive bruises of the buttocks and the pinnae. *Pediatrics* 1992;90:633-636.

37. Sugar NF, Taylor JA, Feldman KW: Bruises in infants and toddlers: those who don't cruise rarely bruise. Puget Sound Pediatric Research Network. *Arch Pediatr Adolesc Med* 1999;153:399-403.

38. Carpenter RF: The prevalence and distribution of bruising in babies. *Arch Dis Child* 1999;80:363-366.

39. Maguire S, Mann MK, Sibert J, et al: Are there patterns of bruising in childhood which are diagnostic or suggestive of abuse? A systematic review. *Arch Dis Child* 2005;90:182-186.

40. Levin AV: Ophthalmology of shaken baby syndrome. *Neurosurg Clin North Am* 2002;13:201-211.

41. Morad Y, Kim YM, Armstrong DC, et al: Correlation between retinal abnormalities and intracranial abnormalities in the shaken baby syndrome. *Am J Ophthalmol* 2002;134:354-359.

42. Southall DP, Plunkett MC, Banks MW, et al: Covert video recordings of life-threatening child abuse: lessons for child protection. *Pediatrics* 1997;100:735-760.

43. Hanigan WC, Peterson RA, Njus G: Tin ear syndrome: rotational acceleration in pediatric head injuries. *Pediatrics* 1987;80:618-622.

44. DiScala C, Sege R, Guohua L, et al: Child abuse and unintentional injuries. A 10-year retrospective. *Arch Pediatr Adolesc Med* 2000;154:16-22.

45. Barsness KA, Cha E, Bensard D, et al: The positive predictive value of rib fractures as an indicator of nonaccidental trauma in children. *J Trauma* 2003;54:1107-1110.

46. Bulloch B, Schubert CJ, Brophy PD, et al: Cause and clinical characteristics of rib fractures in infants. *Pediatrics* 2000;105:e48.

47. Dolinak D: Rib fractures in infants due to cardiopulmonary resuscitations efforts. *Am J Forensic Med Pathol* 2007;28:107-110.

48. Puranik SR, Hayes JS, Long J, et al: Liver enzymes as predictors of liver damage due to blunt abdominal trauma in children. *South Med J* 2002;95:203-206.

49. Ledbetter DJ, Hatch EI, Feldman KW, et al: Diagnostic and surgical implications of child abuse. *Arch Surg* 1988;123:1101-1105.

50. Servaes S, Haller JO: Characteristic pancreatic injuries secondary to child abuse. *Emerg Radiol* 2003;10:90-93.

51. McAleer IM, Kaplan GW: Pediatric genitourinary trauma. *Urol Clin North Am* 1995;22:177-188.

52. Kleinman PK: Skeletal trauma: general considerations. *In*: Kleinman PK: *Diagnostic Imaging of Child Abuse*, ed 2. Mosby, St Louis, 1998, pp 8-25.

53. Grant P, Mata MB, Tidwell M: Femur fracture in infants: a possible accidental etiology. *Pediatrics* 2001;108:1009-1011.

54. Kleinman PK, Marks SC Jr, Blackbourne B: The metaphyseal lesion in abused infants: radiologic-histopathologic study. *AJR Am J Roentgonol* 1986;146:895-905.

55. Strait RT, Siegel RM, Shapiro RA: Humeral fractures without obvious etiologies in children less than 3 years of age: when is it abuse? *Pediatrics* 1995;96:667-671.

56. Worlock P, Stower M, Barbor P: Patterns of fractures in accidental and non-accidental injury in children: a comparative study. *Br Med J (Clin Res)* 1986;293:100-102.

57. Emery JL: Child abuse, sudden infant death syndrome, and unexpected infant death. *Am J Dis Child* 1993;147:1097-1100.

58. Deemer E, Bertocci G, Pierce MC, et al: Influence of wet surfaces and fall height on pediatric injury risk in feet-first freefalls as predicted using a test dummy. *Med Engl Phys* 2005;27:31-39.

59. Lallier M, Bouchard S, St-Vil D, et al: Falls from heights among children: a retrospective review. *J Pediatr Surg* 1999;34:1060-1063.

60. Mott A, Rolfe K, James R, et al: Safety of surfaces and equipment for children in playgrounds. *Lancet* 1997;349:1874-1876.

61. Macarthur C, Hu X, Wesson DE, et al: Risk factors for severe injuries associated with falls from playground equipment. *Accid Anal Prev* 2000;32:377-382.

62. Lowenhielm P: Tolerance level for bridging vein disruption calculated with a mathematical model. *J Bioeng* 1978;2:501-507.

63. Ommaya AK: Head injury mechanisms and the concept of preventive management: a review and critical synthesis. *J Neurotrauma* 1995;12:527-546.

64. Klinich K, Hulbert G, Schneider L: Estimating infant head injury criteria and impact response using crash reconstruction and finite element modeling. In: 46th Stapp Car Crash Conference, SAE Paper 2002-22-0009; 2002.

65. Sturtz G: *Biomechanical data of children*. Proceedings of the 24th Stapp Car Crash Conference, Society of Automotive Engineers, Warrendale, PA, 1980, pp 513-559.

66. Pierce MC, Bertocci GE: Injury biomechanics and child abuse. *Annu Rev Biomed Eng* 2008;10:85-106.

67. Prange MT, Coats B, Duhaime AC, et al: Anthropomorphic simulations of falls, shakes, and inflicted impacts in infants. *J Neurosurg* 2003;99:143-150.

68. Bertocci GE, Pierce MC, Deemer E, et al: Using test dummy experiments to investigate pediatric injury risk in simulated short-distance falls. *Arch Pediatr Adolesc Med* 2003;157:480-486.

69. Bertocci GE, Pierce MC, Deemer E, et al: Influence of fall height and impact surface on biomechanics of feet-first free falls in children. *Injury* 2004;35:417-424.

70. Bialczak K, Bertocci G, Pierce MC, et al: *Pediatric bed fall computer simulation model development and validation*. ASME Summer Bioengineering Conference, June 2006, Amelia Island, FL.

71. Bertocci GE, Pierce MC, Deemer E, et al: Computer simulation of stair falls to investigate scenarios in child abuse. *Arch Pediatr Adolesc Med* 2001;155:1008-1014.

72. Wolfson DR, McNally DS, Clifford MJ, et al: Rigid-body modeling of shaken baby syndrome. *Proc Inst Mech Eng [H]* 2005;219:63-70.

73. Gardner HB: A witnessed short fall mimicking presumed shaken baby syndrome (inflicted childhood neurotrauma). *Pediatr Neurosurg* 2007;43:433-435.

74. Denton S, Mileusnic D: Delayed sudden death in an infant following an accidental fall: a case report with review of the literature. *Am J Forensic Med Pathol* 2003;24:371-376.

75. Reiber GD. Fatal falls in childhood. How far must children fall to sustain fatal head injury? Report of cases and review of the literature. *Am J Forensic Med Pathol* 1993;14:201-207.

76. Starling SP, Holden JR, Jenny C: Abusive head trauma: the relationship of perpetrators to their victims. *Pediatrics* 1995;95:259-262.

77. Kassin SM, Meissner CA, Norwick RJ: "I'd know a false confession if I saw one": a comparative study of college students and police investigators. *Law Hum Behav* 2005;29:211-227.

78. Brent RL: The irresponsible expert witness: a failure of biomedical graduate education and professional accountability. *Pediatrics* 1982;70:754-762.

79. Brent RL: Improving the quality of expert witness testimony. *Pediatrics* 1988;82:511-513.

80. Chadwick DL, Krous HF: Irresponsible expert testimony by medical experts in cases involving the physical abuse and neglect of children. *Child Maltreatment* 1997;2:315-321.

81. Chadwick DL, Krous HF, Runyan DK: Meadow, Southall, and the General Medical Council of the United Kingdom. *Pediatrics* 2006;117:2247-2251.

60

FORENSIC DENTISTRY

John P. Kenney, DDS, MS, D-ABFO

INTRODUCTION

Forensic dentistry (forensic odontology) is defined as the study of the face and oral cavity as it pertains to questions of law. Initially the focus was on use of dental evidence to identify people who were visually unidentifiable, such as victims of fire, decomposition, blast, vehicular accident, and mass disasters. The first American dental identification case of note involved Paul Revere, who in addition to his silver-smithing and midnight ride, also practiced as a barber/surgeon-dentist. He created a dental appliance for Dr. Joseph Warren, who commanded a troop of revolutionary soldiers and was killed at the Battle of Bunker Hill. Revere later identified Warren's body from the dental prosthesis he had fabricated, allowing the doctor a hero's funeral.[1]

Mass fatality identifications began in 1897 with the Bazar de la Charité fire in Paris. Dr. Oscar Amoedo, a Cuban dentist visiting Paris, suggested the use of dental records to identify the victims. His thesis on the fire and identification, "Lárt Dentaire Medecine Legale" is the seminal text on the subject.[1] The first bite mark case in Colonial America occurred during the Salem Witch Trials in 1692, where the Rev. George Burroughs was convicted and hanged for witchcraft, including biting his victims.[2]

In modern times, the first dentist member of the American Academy of Forensic Sciences (AAFS) was Dr. David Scott who joined in 1966. By 1972, 15 dentist members of the Academy came together to found the AAFS's Odontology Section. In 1970 the American Society of Forensic Odontology (ASFO) was founded,[3] and finally, in 1976, the American Board of Forensic Odontology (ABFO) was organized to provide certification examinations to ensure the highest level of competence in the field. Today there are approximately 100 active ABFO Diplomates in the United States and Canada.

Since the era of C. Henry Kempe, information on child abuse and dentistry began to appear in the dental literature.[4-7] The interest in family violence has since evolved to include work on domestic violence and elder abuse, as well as child abuse. The first edition of the Forensic Odontology Workbook, a loose leaf notebook printed by the ASFO in 1980, devoted a chapter to "Child Abuse and Neglect." These early efforts began a systematic approach to child abuse recognition and intervention by forensic odontologists and by the dental profession as a whole. This notebook evolved into the "Manual of Forensic Odontology."[8] In terms of continuing education, the Armed Forces Institute of Pathology held the first continuing education course in Forensic Odontology in 1964.[9] Child abuse and domestic violence are regular topics in their ongoing courses. The first U.S. residency in Forensic Odontology was started at the University of Texas Health Science Center, San Antonio, Texas.

Articles on the dentists' role in child abuse have been published in many journals, beginning in 1970 with an article in the New York State Dental Journal by Arthur Hazle-wood.[7] The British Journal of Oral Surgery reviewed five cases in an article the following year.[6] Bernard Sims and colleagues addressed "Bite Marks in the 'Battered Baby Syndrome'" in Medicine, Science and the Law in 1973,[10] and a number of other articles appeared in the 1970s.[11-15]

The American Academy of Pediatric Dentistry has taken a leading role for the dental profession and has an active partnership with the American Academy of Pediatrics, covering many areas of mutual interest including child abuse. Pediatric dental textbooks now routinely cover the diagnosis and management of suspected child abuse.[16-18]

Programs have been developed to educate dentists about child abuse. PANDA (Prevent Abuse and Neglect through Dental Awareness) is an educational program founded in 1992 by Dr. Lynn Mouden, in collaboration with state dental societies, the Delta Dental Plan, and state child welfare agencies (personal communication, Dr. Lynn Mouden, 2008). The program provides educational materials and training programs to participating state dental societies. It now serves 45 states, the U.S. Army Dental Command, and 10 foreign countries, providing comprehensive education for dental health professionals.[19]

OROFACIAL INJURIES IN CHILD ABUSE

Research over the past 40 years has shown that 43.5% to 65% of child abuse injuries occur in the head and neck region.[20-22] Dental professionals deal with the head and neck during the routine examination and dental health care of their patients. Child abuse injuries are not dissimilar to injuries from domestic violence or elder abuse.[23] Perioral injuries include: patterned injuries (Figure 60-1), lacerations to the lips, slap marks to the face, gag marks at the corners of the mouth, bruises, human bite marks, and burns from electrical, chemical or thermal sources.[19] Intraoral injuries include maxillary or mandibular fractures, fractured or avulsed teeth, torn frenula, other intraoral lacerations, bruising of the hard and soft palate from forced oral sex (Figure 60-2), and evidence of sexually transmitted diseases.[19]

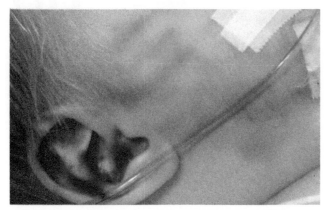

FIGURE 60-1 A "pattern mark" from a belt buckle on the face of a child.

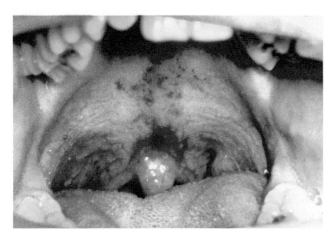

FIGURE 60-2 Palatal petechiae from forced oral sex.

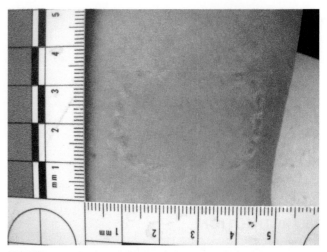

FIGURE 60-3 Bite mark of a child . The child's bite mark characteristically shows clear upper and lower arches of teeth.

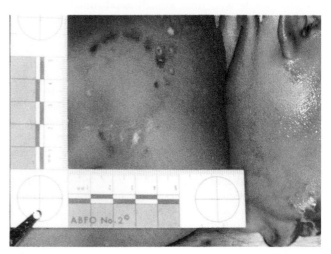

FIGURE 60-4 Bite mark of an adult. The adult bite marks are more likely to have only one distinct arch.

There are many ways forensic odontologists and PANDA-trained dentists can assist in child abuse cases. The first is assessing perioral and dental injuries as to the likely cause, treatment and outcome. Perhaps the area where the forensic odontologist plays the greatest role in child abuse is in documentation and analysis of bite marks. In some jurisdictions, forensic odontologists analyze and testify about other patterned injuries using the same techniques as in bite mark analysis.

Forensic odontologists are more familiar with the legal system and requirements for evidence collection than most hospital- or practice-based dentists. Forensic odontologists are usually actively affiliated with law enforcement agencies such as coroners/medical examiners, state police, or state forensic agencies. Odontologists have been trained to collect and handle evidence in cases of homicide, assault, and other crimes, making them valuable members of investigative teams.

BITE MARKS AND PATTERENED INJURIES

There are 4 "Rs" to consider in bite marks: Recognition, Reporting, Recording, and Referral. In addition to forensic odontologists, some specially trained allied health care professionals such as child abuse pediatricians, forensically trained pediatric nurse practitioners (PNPs), and sexual assault nurse examiners (SANE nurses) have been trained to assist hospitals in the recognition and recovery of evidence.

Recognition

A classic human bite in skin is opposing semilunar marks measuring 2 to 4 cm across, with marks along the periphery made by the individual teeth. The ABFO defines a human bite mark as "a circular or oval (doughnut or ring-shaped) patterned injury consisting of two opposing (facing) symmetrical, U-shaped arches separated at their bases by open spaces. Following the periphery of the arches is a series of individual abrasions, contusions, and/or lacerations reflecting the size, shape, arrangement, and distribution of the class characteristics of the contacting surfaces of the human dentition."[24]

Children who bite one another frequently leave fairly clear marks with both arches, whereas adult bites often only are distinct in one arch (Figures 60-3 and 60-4).[25] Specific size, class, and individual characteristics will differentiate between bite marks inflicted by human adults or children or by animals.

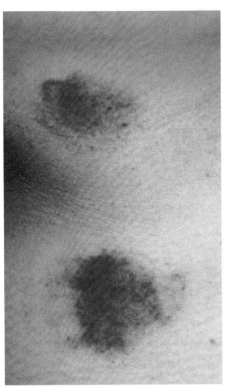

FIGURE 60-5 A "hickey" (suction mark) on the neck caused by the positive pressure of the teeth on the skin surrounding a bite mark disrupting small blood vessels.

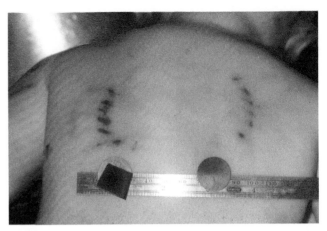

FIGURE 60-6 Bite mark from a dog bite.

Odontologists also can evaluate other skin lesions that resemble human bites and differentiate them from bite marks. In the experience of many odontologists, when one bite mark is observed by medical personnel (including forensic pathologists), a trained odontologist will often find additional, more subtle, marks. Medical practitioners trained in pattern recognition and adept at three-dimensional spatial analysis will have an advantage when recognizing and analyzing bite marks and other patterned marks.

Hickeys and Suction Marks

Bite marks can be accompanied by an area of central ecchymosis. This can be caused either by the positive pressure of the teeth on the skin surrounding the bite area, which causes disruption of the small blood vessels enclosed within the area of the bite mark (Figure 60-5), or by the negative pressure of suction or tongue thrust on the area.[23,25]

Bite Marks

The human dental arch contains two central incisors, two lateral incisors, two cuspids, four bicuspids, and six molars. Most frequently only the four or six most anterior teeth make a distinctive mark on the skin. The maxillary central incisors are wider than the laterals (approximately 8.5 *vs.* 6.5 mm) and both are linear or rectangular. The cuspids usually make the most definitive mark (triangular, or a point) because of their length and shape, and occasionally a bite mark will include the facial cusps of bicuspid teeth. The lower central and lateral incisors in the permanent dentition are about the same width (5.0 *vs.* 5.5 mm). In the deciduous or primary dentition, the maxillary central and lateral incisors are smaller, approximately 6.5 *vs.* 5.1 mm in width. The lower incisors are somewhat smaller (4.2 mm), but again, almost equal in size.[26]

A bite mark *class characteristic* identifies the group from which it originates: human, animal, fish, or other species. The teeth leave distinctive marks because of the vital response of the underlying bitten tissue, and for this reason serial photographs of living victims over several days are most useful for the odontologist to do the analysis. Generally, the upper (maxillary) arch will be larger than the lower arch, and the average maxillary intercuspid distance (cuspid to cuspid) will be approximately 33 mm. The overall width of the maxillary bite mark will be 3.5 to 4.0 cm. The mandibular mark will be on the order of 25 mm.[24] Bites by children with primary dentition (under the age of 6) will be under 3.0 cm from cuspid to cuspid. There are minor differences between the dentition of males and females, as well as between the dentition of various races, but according to research by Barsley and Lancaster,[27] age and race differences are insignificant above 12 years of age.

The *arch characteristic* is a pattern that represents the tooth arrangement within a bite mark. For example, a combination of rotated teeth, buccal or lingual version, mesio-distal drifting, and horizontal alignment contribute to differentiation between individuals. The *dental characteristic* is defined as a feature or trait within a bite mark that represents an individual tooth variation such as unusual wear patterns, notching, angulations, and fractures. The number, specificity, and accurate reproduction of these arch characteristics and dental characteristics contribute to the overall assessment of the degree of confidence that a particular suspect made the bite mark.[24]

Animal bites generally tear or avulse flesh. The dental pattern of canines and felines includes six incisors and two canine teeth in each arch. The arches are much narrower and elongated in the anterior-posterior aspect than the human dental arch (Figures 60-6 and 60-7).

Reporting

Within a hospital setting, protocols should be in place for formal reporting to the state's child protection agency as well as to the appropriate police agency. Observed or suspected

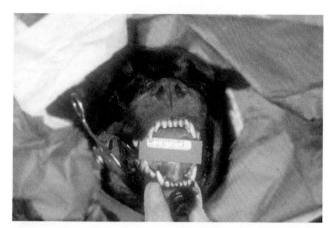

FIGURE 60-7 The teeth of the dog that bit the infant in Figure 60-7, allowing comparison of the dental arch and the bite mark.

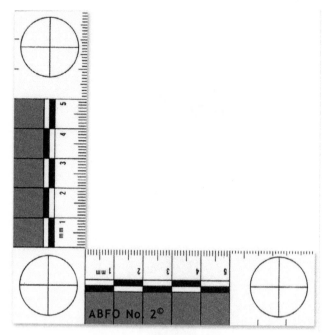

FIGURE 60-8 "L-shaped" scale developed by the American Board of Forensic Odontology for use in bite mark photography.

bite marks must be brought to the attention of law enforcement. In the case of a child who is fatally injured, the coroner or medical examiner should be advised if a bite mark is observed or suspected to be present on the child's body when the child was brought to the hospital so that evidence is collected in a timely fashion when the autopsy is done.

Recording

A body diagram should be part of the medical record, recording the initial examination and location of purported bite marks and other external injuries, as well as marks from therapeutic interventions (e.g., EKG leads, venipuncture marks, defibrillator paddles). These devices or treatment can mimic a bite mark.[28] A detailed written description of all of the injuries will be helpful when a case goes to court. In some cases, judges will not allow photos of the victim into a trial, since they might be considered overly prejudicial to the defendant. In the case of a bite mark or other patterned injury, only limited photos showing the specific area may be permitted. An accurate body diagram can be critical in laying the foundation for the expert witness testimony of a pediatrician, forensic odontologist, or forensic pathologist.

Photography

Perhaps the most significant evidence in bite mark cases is clear, accurate photographs of the injury with and without a scale in place. The ABFO initially developed the "L-shaped" evidence scale for use in bite mark photography: the ABFO #2 Photomacrographic Scale (Figure 60-8). Today it is used by police agencies and hospitals in photographs to facilitate accurate life-size depiction of lesions. It allows for life-size enlargement of photographic evidence for proper analysis. The ABFO #2 scale can be marked permanently with a Sharpie type marker and should be included in the patient record. This scale will be part of the evidence needed for analysis and courtroom testimony.

Photos should be taken by a person experienced with the particular camera/lens/flash setup used. The time for learning the camera is not at the bedside in the hectic atmosphere of an emergency department or hospital ward. A trained hospital photographer should be used to take photographs if available. Photographers will be especially helpful if they have access and knowledge of alternative light photography such as ultraviolet (UV), infrared (IR), or other alternative light sources (ALS), such as a light source in the 450-nm range. Recently, digital media has superseded the use of analog 35-mm film. Digital cameras are available with interchangeable lenses, particularly macro-focus lenses, or filtered lenses for UV, IR, and ALS photography. Higher-resolution cameras and lenses are most useful in forensic cases. While once considered "state of the art," Polaroid photography for evidentiary use is now not favored since instant images at much higher resolutions are available via digital cameras. Multiple members of the emergency department staff and/or the child protection team should also have good cameras available for evidence recording if the hospital's photographer is not available.

Salivary Swabbing

Once the area has been photographed, a sterile swab can be used to recover possible DNA evidence using the double swab technique. The first swab is moistened in sterile distilled water for approximately 10 seconds and rolled over the affected area in a circular motion. A second dry swab is immediately rolled over the same area and also placed into the same evidence box to thoroughly air dry.[29] It should be handled just as rape kit evidence is, using care not to contaminate the sample, and forwarded on to the appropriate law enforcement agency for analysis. A new test is available that presumptively identifies saliva (Rapid Stain Identification Series [RISD], Independent Forensics, Hillside, Illinois [http://www.ifi-test.com/]). If the test is positive, there will be enough cellular material present to allow for short-tandem-repeat (STR) DNA analysis for identification of the source. Swabbing the area for DNA sampling should be done prior to any washing or medical intervention of the skin to preserve necessary evidence.[29]

An important consideration for evidence collection is the activity level of the child being photographed. Good photography for bite mark analysis requires a motionless subject, and depending on where the injury occurs, it might not be possible to obtain usable photographs and/or three-dimensional impressions of the injury. If the child is to be sedated or anesthetized for other procedures, bite mark evidence collection should be coordinated to occur at the same time to allow the odontologist to collect the best evidence and to allow for ideal positioning of the subject for photographs. It might be necessary to consider sedation for the odontological examination alone in some cases. Serial photos of the injury are frequently helpful if the patient is cooperative, since the healing process will bring out more detail over a period of days, particularly of the individual tooth characteristics are present within the bite mark. If therapeutic intervention is needed to treat the bite wound or other injuries in the immediate vicinity of the bite, every effort should be made to obtain accurate and clearly scaled photographs of the bite mark *prior* to the treatment.

Impression of the Injury

Depending on the nature of the injury, it may be possible to recover a three-dimensional impression of the injury. This type of evidence will be of significant benefit to the odontologist in analysis of the bite mark or patterned injury (where a specific tool or object used could be identified). Even if not readily visible to the naked eye, discreet scratches or indentations in the skin can be recordable and reproducible. Immediate involvement of a trained odontologist by phone consultation when a bite mark is observed or suspected will assist the physician or nurse in proper handling of the patient to preserve as much evidence as possible.

Most odontologists today use either polyvinylsiloxane or polyether impression material to record surface characteristics of the area of a bite mark or patterned injury. This material is normally used within the oral cavity for dental prosthetic impressions. Because the material takes time to set, the patient must remain motionless for a period to eliminate distortion of the impression. Doing this while the victim is asleep or sedated may be necessary. A backing material of either dental stone (plaster) or Aquaplast (WFR/Aquaplast Corporation, Wyckoff NJ)(http://www.q-fix.com) for polyvinylsiloxane impressions, or 3M's Scotchcast II orthopedic casting material for polyether impressions is used.

Aquaplast, a relatively new product on the market, is a thermoplastic mesh material used for stabilization of the head for precision radiation oncology treatments. It provides a good matrix for the polyvinylsiloxane to set around so it can be rigid and undistorted when removed from the body (Figure 60-9). The Scotchcast II must be rinsed of nearly all of the fiberglass resin present on the material, or it will not adhere to the polyether. It should be noted that the Scotchcast II does not adhere well to the polyvinylsiloxane material because of the high silicone component of the impression material. Again, an experienced odontologist can select the appropriate materials for evidence recovery.

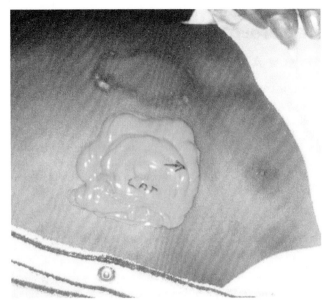

FIGURE 60-9 Polyvinylsiloxane impression of a bite mark on a victim's chest.

Invasive Analysis

If the victim dies as a result of the abuse injuries, the odontologist, with permission of the coroner or medical examiner, can actually stabilize the bite injury area with an acrylic ring "super-glued" and sutured to the body. It will be resected for additional analysis of the subcutaneous tissue. Using a technique called transillumination, teeth marks that appear as bruises or scratch marks on the subject are made much more distinct.[30]

Referral

Perhaps the most critical part in analyzing bite marks is a referral to a qualified forensic odontologist. The local coroner or medical examiner can likely identify at least one available forensic dentist. Evidence collection from bite marks and patterned injuries should be done by a qualified specialist. It is now best practice to get a second expert opinion in every bite mark case prior to trial. If an experienced forensic odontologist is not readily available, the ABFO has a website with all of the Diplomates listed geographically with contact information (www.ABFO.org). If no certified forensic odontologist is available, ABFO Diplomates are likely to be able to identify experienced dentists who will be able to assist in the analysis. It is helpful to identify local experts in advance, so that when needed, they will be available in cases of abuse or assault.

Many forensic odontologists are in private dental practice and are not government employees. They are paid on a case-by-case basis. It is sometimes necessary to get clearance from legal or child welfare authorities to authorize their work and provide for compensation. Again, making arrangements *before* the service is actually needed allows for timely consultation with expert forensic odontologists.

OTHER ASPECTS OF FORENSIC ODONTOLOGY

Dental Aging

In some cases "dental aging" of a victim is necessary to assist law enforcement. From birth through about age 21, a reasonably accurate estimation of age can be determined based on the individual's dental development. Dental aging can also be helpful to determine the age of a perpetrator, particularly if the suspect claims to be a juvenile to avoid prosecution. A panoramic dental x-ray and thorough clinical dental examination is necessary to perform this type of analysis.

Strength of Dental Evidence in Bite Mark Cases

Dental evidence in child abuse cases can be extremely compelling. The presence of bite mark is strong proof of interpersonal violence directed toward the child. Because only a limited number of individuals in a household usually have access to an infant or small child, there is a closed population of potential perpetrators to evaluate. A trained forensic odontologist can generally exclude suspected "biters," based on analysis of their dentition and of the bite mark. Arch size, class, or individual characteristics all can be used to make an initial determination. The ABFO currently uses the following terminology in describing the odontologists final determination of the evidence relating the suspected biter to the bite mark. All of these terms are used "to a reasonable degree of denial certainly": the biter, the probable biter, not excluded as the biter, excluded as the biter, and, inconclusive.[24] In recent years, there have been a few cases where DNA has contradicted the bite mark evidence. All of these have been cases of homicides of adults, where the suspect pool can be as large as the general population. To date, bite mark evidence has not been challenged in child abuse cases.

Research

A number of studies sought to show that the human dentition is unique. A small study done at UCLA School of Dentistry by Dr. Reidar Sognnaes[31] on identical twins showed adequate points of differentiation between them, even in the primary dentition. There have been studies undertaken in controlled populations,[32] and more recently in wider populations that show adequate evidence that dentition is individualized.[33] The ABFO has been involved in advancing the science of bite mark analysis since 1984.[34] A definitive and comprehensive text on this subject is *Bitemark Evidence*, edited by Robert B.J. Dorion.[35]

PARTICIPATION OF FORENSIC ODONTOLOGISTS ON HOSPITAL-BASED CHILD PROTECTION TEAMS

Child protection teams are present in many children's hospitals. Leaders of these teams have realized the value of having a dentist as a team member. Both forensic and pediatric dentists have taken part in these teams.

References

1. Barker BR: The history of forensic dentistry. *In*: Cottone JR, Standish SM (eds): *Outline of Forensic Dentistry*. Year Book Medical Publishers, Chicago, 1982, p 24.
2. Vale GL: The history of bitemark evidence. *In*: Dorion RBJ (ed): *Bitemark Evidence*. Marcel Dekker, New York, 2005, p 2.
3. Scott DB: The United States. *In*: Hill IR, Keiser-Nielsen S, Vermylen Y, et al *(eds): Forensic Odontology: Its Scope and History*. Alan Clift Associates, Solihull, UK, 1984, p 228.
4. Teuscher GT: The battered child, a social enigma (editorial). *J Dent Child* 1974;41:5-6.
5. Laskin DM: The battered-child syndrome (editorial). *J Oral Surg* 1973;31:903.
6. Tate RJ: Facial injuries associated with the battered child syndrome. *Br J Oral Surg* 1971;9:41-45.
7. Hazelwood AI. Child abuse: the dentist's role. *N Y State Dent J* 1970;36:289-291.
8. Herschaft EE, Alder ME, Ord DK, et al *(eds): Manual of Forensic Odontology*, ed 4. American Society of Forensic Odontology, Impress Printing and Graphics, Albany, NY, 2006.
9. Luntz LL: History of forensic dentistry. *Dent Clin North Am* 1977;21:7-17.
10. Sims BG, Grant JH, Cameron JM: Bite marks in the 'battered baby syndrome.' *Med Sci Law* 1973;13:207-210.
11. Grauerholz J: The role of the dentist under the child abuse and neglect reporting law. *RI Dent J* 1977;10:12-13.
12. tenBensel RW, Bastein SA: Child abuse and neglect. History, identification and reporting. *Dent Hyg* 1977;51:119-125.
13. Benusis K: Child abuse: what the dentist should know. *Northwest Dentist* 1977;26:230-263.
14. tenBensel RW, King KJ: Neglect and abuse of children: historical aspects, identification, and management. *J Dent Child* 1975;42:348-358.
15. Sopher IM: The dentist and the battered child syndrome. *Dent Clin North Am* 1977;21:113-122.
16. McDonald RE, Avery DR: Examination of the mouth and other relevant structures. *In*: McDonald RE, Avery DR (eds): *Dentistry for the Child and Adolescent*, ed 4. Mosby, St Louis, 1983, pp 19-22.
17. Braham RL, Morris ME: *Textbook of Pediatric Dentistry*. Williams & Wilkins, Baltimore, 1980, pp 80-95.
18. American Academy of Pediatrics Committee on Child Abuse and Neglect, American Academy of Pediatric Dentistry, American Academy of Pediatric Dentistry Council on Clinical Affairs: Guideline on oral and dental aspects of child abuse and neglect. *Pediatr Dent* 2008-2009;30(7 Suppl):86-89.
19. Kenny JP, Clark DH: Child abuse. *In*: Clark DH (ed): *Practical Forensic Odontology*. Wright-Butterworth-Heinemann, Boston, 1992, pp 138-148.
20. Becker DB, Needleman HL, Kotelchuck M: Child abuse and dentistry: orofacial trauma and its recognition by dentists. *J Am Dent Assoc* 1978;97:24-28.
21. Cameron JM, Johnson HR, Camps FE: The battered child syndrome. *Med Sci Law* 1966;6:2
22. Kenney JP: *The Incidence and Nature of Orofacial Injuries in Child Abuse Cases Reported by Selected Hospital in Cook County, Illinois. [Master's thesis]*. Chicago, Loyola University of Chicago, 1979.
23. Alder ME, Herschaft EE, Kenney JP, et al: Human abuse and neglect. *In*: Herschaft EE, Alder ME, Ord DK, et al *(eds): Manuel of Forensic Odontology*, ed 4. The American Society of Forensic Odontology, Albany, NY, 2006, pp 210-243.
24. ABFO bitemark terminology guidelines. In: *Diplomates Reference Manual*. The American Board of Forensic Odontology, 2009, pp 124-127. Available at www.ABFO.org/pdfs/ABFO%20manual%20revised%2010-28-09B.pdf. Accessed April 20, 2010.
25. Bernstein ML: Nature of bitemarks. *In*: Dorion RBJ (ed): *Bitemark Evidence*. Marcel Dekker, New York, 2005, pp 59-80.
26. Kraus BS, Jordan RE, Abrams L (eds): *A Study of the Masticatory System Dental Anatomy and Occlusion*. Williams & Wilkins, Baltimore, 1969.
27. Barsley RE, Lancaster DM: Measurement of arch widths in a human population: relation of anticipated bite marks. *J Forens Sci* 1987;32:975-982.
28. Dorion RBJ, Souviron RR: Patterns, lesions, and trauma mimicking bitemarks. *In*: Dorion RBJ (ed): *Bitemark Evidence*. Marcel Dekker, New York, 2005, pp 389-413.

29. Sweet D: Bitemarks as biological evidence, noninvasive analysis. *In*: Dorion RBJ (ed): *Bitemark Evidence*. Marcel Dekker, New York, 2005, pp 183-201.

30. Dorion RBJ: Tissue specimens—invasive analysis. *In*: Dorion RBJ (ed): *Bitemark Evidence*. Marcel Dekker, New York, 2005, pp 237-239.

31. Sognnaes RF, Rawson RD, Gratt BM, et al: Computer comparison of bitemark patterns in identical twins. *J Am Dent Assoc* 1985;105: 449-452.

32. Rawson RD, Ommen RK, Kinard G, et al: Statistical evidence for the individuality of the human dentition. *J Forensic Sci* 1984;29:245-253.

33. Johnson LT, Blinka DD, VanScotter-Asbach P, et al: Quantification of the individual characteristics of the human dentition: methodology. *J Forensic Sci* 2008;58:409-418.

34. Dorion RBJ: Research projects and recent developments. *In*: Dorion RBJ (ed): *Bitemark Evidence*. Marcel Dekker, New York, 2005, pp 565-591.

35. Dorion RBJ (ed): *Bitemark Evidence*. Marcel Dekker, New York, 2005.

61

MEDICAL CHILD ABUSE

Thomas A. Roesler, MD

INTRODUCTION

Medical child abuse (MCA) is defined as, "A child receiving unnecessary and harmful or potentially harmful medical care at the instigation of a caretaker."[1] MCA stands alongside physical abuse, psychological abuse, and sexual abuse within the landscape of child maltreatment. MCA shares many attributes with other forms of child maltreatment and has only a few distinguishing characteristics.[2]

Traditionally child abuse is defined as an act of commission whereas child neglect results from acts of omission. The definition of *medical neglect* is a child under the care of an adult not being provided with needed medical care, whereas *medical child abuse* is a child receiving too much medical care. Knowing why the caretaker provides either too little or too much medical care, although important, is not required to determine that the child is being harmed. The relationship between the two types of maltreatment is comparable to the relationship between physical abuse and physical neglect, or psychological abuse and psychological neglect.

SIMILARITIES AND DIFFERENCES BETWEEN MEDICAL CHILD ABUSE AND OTHER TYPES OF CHILD ABUSE

Similar to physical, sexual, or psychological abuse, children can experience medical abuse in many different ways. For example, in physical abuse, a child can be struck with an object, thrown across the room, burned, or forced to stand in an uncomfortable position for an extended period. Similarly, a child can be sexually abused in a variety of ways. A child can be medically abused by being subjected to medical interventions, including unnecessary diagnostic tests and blood draws, repeated examinations, minor or major surgeries, or unnecessary medications, when medical indications do not exist to justify these treatments.

Also, in common with other forms of child abuse, MCA ranges from mild to severe. For example, at the mild end of the sexual abuse spectrum a child can be harmed by being exposed to unnecessary parental nudity. More severe abuse consists of exposure to pornography, or even more significantly, being forced to take part in pornography. A similar continuum exists for physical and psychological abuse. It is easy to understand that being subjected to unnecessary trips to the pediatrician falls on the mild end of the spectrum of medically abusive experiences—but having part of one's pancreas removed based on false information provided by a caretaker represents a severe presentation.[3]

With all forms of child abuse, at some point along the continuum there is a threshold beyond which the child is felt to be in need of protection from his or her caretaker. The threshold is determined by society, and varies over time as well as from community to community. For example, in the United States 50 years ago, disciplining a child with a stick or a belt was considered to be within the normal range of parental behavior, even if it resulted in damage to the skin. Today in most U.S. jurisdictions the production of skin lesions constitutes behavior that rises to the level of child abuse. In much of Europe today, laws prohibit any form of corporal punishment even if no physical damage to the skin is detected. In each of these situations the threshold for protection is different.

Because the child protection community has less experience in evaluating MCA, the threshold that constitutes a need for protection has not been clearly established. A child exposed to unnecessary major surgery would meet the standard for MCA, but less severe presentations might not. Nonetheless, MCA shares this important criterion with other forms of abuse.

Continuing the comparison with other abuse experiences, MCA victims have been found to have similar long-term psychological effects from their abuse. The most common psychological effects of sexual abuse are increased risk of depression, anxiety, relationship difficulties, and higher prevalence of drug and alcohol abuse.[4] Preliminary evidence from victims of MCA shows a similar picture.

Perpetrators of the various forms of child abuse also share many characteristics. They typically disavow knowledge of how the child came to be harmed. They give many different explanations for the manifestations of the abuse in the child. For example, a caretaker of a child seen in the hospital with subdural hematomas, severe retinal hemorrhages, and encephalopathy might explain that the child rolled off a sofa onto a carpeted floor. And if that same parent had been observed by a third party violently shaking the infant, he might explain that he was afraid the child had choked and was performing the Heimlich maneuver. Perpetrators of sexual abuse notoriously deny any participation in the abuse or any ill intent if caught in the act. Similarly, parents who medically abuse their children typically deny any intent to harm their children by getting unnecessary medical care and state that their motivation was only to get their child help for a presumed illness. Another common characteristic is that perpetrators of physical, psychological, sexual, and medical abuse share is an unhappy childhood.[5,6]

The primary difference between victims of medical abuse and the other types of abuse is the type of maltreatment they received. Physical abuse victims suffer physical consequences, including cuts, bruises, burns, broken bones, or death. Victims of psychological abuse experience humiliation, threats of abandonment, or blows to self-esteem. Medical abuse victims experience medical care that is damaging or potentially damaging to their health. While the prevalence of sexual abuse seems to be fairly constant between communities and across national borders, there is at least some evidence that medical abuse is more prevalent in developed countries with more medical resources.[7]

Perpetrators of various types of abuse (physical, sexual, or medical) share many characteristics, but there is one difference. The literature notes a tendency for the perpetrator of MCA to express emotions in medical ways. They tend to have exposed themselves as well as their children to unnecessary medical care and to have multiple somatic complaints.[6] They also are almost universally female as opposed to perpetrators of sexual abuse, who are almost all male.

ISSUES OF TERMINOLOGY

This definition of MCA replaces what has been referred to as Munchausen syndrome by proxy (MSBP). Although there has been difficulty with the MSBP concept for years, it is only recently that consensus has been building that we abandon the term in favor of a straightforward definition of abuse.[1,8-14] The reason it has taken so long to clarify this question—over 30 years—is found in the involvement of the medical community in the expression of the abuse. The involvement of medical care providers as the instruments of abuse used by the parents to knowingly or unknowingly hurt the child puts the medical community in an uncomfortable position.

One of the two original case reports used to define MSBP was a child poisoned by his mother with salt.[15] At the time the paper was published, the medical community's understanding of physical abuse was quite unsophisticated. Still, there were a number of people writing about nonaccidental poisoning as a form of child abuse. For example, Dine and McGovern[16] collected a series of 48 cases from their own experiences and from examples published in the literature. It stands to reason that parents who could severely beat their children might also poison them, and in doing so expose their children to unnecessary medical care. Yet, for the early proponents of MSBP, as with physicians today, the sticking point—the obstacle that prevented them from realizing what was happening and taking the necessary steps to protect the child—was the need to deal emotionally with their involvement in the production of morbidity.

Even today when a new audience hears a description of MCA, physicians invariably ask, "So why *do* the mothers do this?" Inducing an illness in a child, such as causing seizures by obstructing the airway, is an act of physical abuse. The same is true for poisoning a child with salt. However, the subsequent medical care given to a child with an induced seizure represents MCA—the child receives medical care that would have been unnecessary if the parent had not obstructed the airway and then given a false history about what happened to the child. If a child is treated for seemingly

unexplained apnea with a bronchoscopy, that treatment is abusive. It is unnecessary and harmful or potentially harmful medical care perpetrated by the parent who induced the apnea (or gave a false history of seizure activity).

What the physicians are really asking is, "Why did this parent get me to give unnecessary medical care?" They do not ask this question about the perpetrators of sexual abuse because they are not the vectors through which the abuse is perpetrated. Being involved in bringing harm to a child is an emotionally painful experience that carries with it feelings of shame, guilt, sadness, and anger. The physician asking why the perpetrator did this is trying to understand his or her own unwitting complicity in exposing a child to potentially harmful medical care.

Unfortunately, the MSBP hypothesis has focused on the reasons why the parent put doctors in this painful position, rather than focusing on what the child is experiencing and on the need to put a halt to the unnecessary maltreatment. The other formulations offered in an attempt to deal with the shortcomings of MSBP such as pediatric condition falsification[17] or induced illness in a child by a caretaker,[18] although improvements over MSBP, suffer from the same loss of focus on the child. As some authors have written, we do not describe a child who is the victim of neglect as someone who has a parent with a syndrome known as "child neglect."[9] Physicians, rather than asking, "Why?" should be asking, "What?" or "How?" They should explore what happened to the child and how they ended up giving care that was not indicated. Although several reasons surely exist, one that seems to be frequently present is that the physician proceeded with medical treatment based on false information provided by the caretaker. In one study of victims of MCA, parents exaggerated existing symptoms in 89.7% of the cases and fabricated nonexistent symptoms in 73.6%.[1]

When false information is inserted into the medical decision-making process, the decisions that result are contaminated and potentially harmful. Numerous anecdotal accounts exist in the literature of disastrous outcomes following a caretaker providing false information. As an example, a child received an unnecessary small bowel transplant based on parent report of symptoms that in retrospect turned out not to be accurate.[19]

The discussion in the literature regarding MSBP has focused on these extreme cases.[20] As we reconceptualize a child receiving unnecessary and harmful or potentially harmful medical care as a victim of MCA, diagnosing and responding to this form of child maltreatment can be consistent with our thinking about other forms of child abuse. With this new approach, we will see examples that are not so extreme (compared with, say, a child getting an unnecessary bowel transplant) but might still be far enough along on the spectrum of clinical presentations that protection from a caretaker's behavior is indicated.

TREATMENT OF MEDICAL CHILD ABUSE

As with other forms of child abuse, management of MCA proceeds in five steps. The steps are: (1) identify the abuse, (2) stop the abuse, (3) make sure the abuse does not recur, (4) repair the physical and psychological damage experienced by the child, and (5) do all this in the least restrictive manner that ensures the safety of the child.

Identifying the Abuse

The first and most important step is to identify that abuse is occurring. Because most child abuse takes place in private, it can take considerable time for maltreatment to come to the attention of the broader community. Incest, or intrafamilial sexual abuse, can continue for many years before it comes to the attention of someone in a position to bring it to a halt. A child can be the victim of psychological, physical, or medical abuse for years as well.

With medical abuse the process of identification involves a careful examination of the medical care the child has received. Although family members or school personnel might question whether a child has been receiving inappropriate medical care, medical caregivers are in the best position to notice a child getting too much treatment. In the past when working within the framework of MSBP (or one of its other names), there was a tendency to examine the emotional makeup of the caregiver to see if she might "fit the profile." However, because receiving too much medical care constitutes MCA, the way to identify it is to determine if the medical care received was appropriate. Are there signs and symptoms of illness, independent of the possibly inaccurate history received from the parent, that supported the need for care?

In other forms of child abuse, the diagnosis is made by carefully comparing the history provided by the caretaker with the examination of the child. The same is true for MCA. A child reported to have vomited constantly over the past 24 hours would be expected to look quite ill, to be dehydrated, and would be expected to continue vomiting in the emergency department or in the hospital. If, instead, the child does not look ill, is well hydrated, and is not seen to vomit by medical personnel, a physician would be advised to question the history given and withhold aggressive treatment until objective signs and symptoms indicate a need.

This example represents a description of good medical practice. However, children who have been medically abused have caretakers who manage to persuade good physicians to give treatment in just such circumstances. Good medical practice represents primary prevention of MCA. Nevertheless, characteristics of good physicians, such as empathy, dedication to patients and their parents, and a trusting nature, can render them vulnerable to parents who, for whatever reason, insist that their child is ill and requires medical care.[21] Often the only source of information about the child's symptoms and status is from the primary caretaker and a life-or-death decision must be made based on the information the caretaker provides.

In extreme cases of MCA, a child might have been receiving unnecessary, harmful medical care for years, including receiving surgery for which there was little justification. In these situations the identification of the abuse might be the result of an intense medical record review by a child abuse pediatrician. Sanders and Bursch[22] give an excellent description of the process. There has been discussion in the literature about whether MCA can be identified by nonmedical personnel.[23] Little debate should exist about this as long as it is understood that the diagnosis is made based on the appropriateness of the medical care received. Anyone with sufficient medical knowledge to determine if the care received was indicated based on the signs and symptoms available to the treating physician is qualified to make the diagnosis of MCA.

The role of covert video surveillance (CVS) in the identification of MCA has been the subject of considerable controversy as well. In order to conduct CVS an individual or a hospital must position video cameras to observe a mother taking care of her child in a controlled setting without her knowledge. The resulting evidence, if it shows a parent smothering or otherwise physically abusing her child, can be quite convincing in a court proceeding and can aide in successful prosecution of the parent.[24] Critics have argued that subjecting a parent to video taping without knowledge or consent violates informed consent stipulations regarding research,[25-27] is tantamount to entrapment, or violates the parent's right to privacy.[28,29] Supporters of CVS say that the right of the child to be safe and healthy takes precedence over the rights of the parent, and that CVS is a tested diagnostic procedure and entirely ethical.[30] Hall[31] has suggested that every children's hospital should be capable of CVS because of its ability to prove or disprove abuse.

Although the usefulness of CVS as a diagnostic technique is clear in identifying physical abuse, and it is relatively easy to defend its ethical use, in no other form of child abuse would one expect such overwhelming evidence before proceeding to put in place protective measures. One would not send a child thought to be sexually abused to the perpetrator's apartment with a tape recorder in her pocket.

In summary, to accomplish the first step in the management of MCA (i.e., to identify that it is occurring), one must perceive that the medical care received by the child might not be indicated. This realization usually proceeds from the observation that the history given does not match the clinical picture.

Stopping the Abuse

The second step in the treatment of child abuse is to stop the caretaker's abusive behavior once it has been identified. The unique feature involved in stopping MCA is the cessation of the harmful medical care. The previous care plan for the child must be reevaluated. Unnecessary care must be eliminated and needed care reinstituted. This is easier said than done. The medical care might be the result of one physician's actions based on false information provided by the caretaker. The more common situation involves care given by a system of caregivers that might include dozens of doctors, nurses, and ancillary treatment personnel. Bringing care to a halt requires the treatment team to call a "time out" in the care, just as a surgical team might do before undertaking a procedure, to make sure that moving forward is appropriate. The medical care team then needs to review the available information, obtain whatever additional tests might inform the new course of treatment, and then institute the new care plan. Some would argue that getting all the medical care providers to reach consensus on changing the plan of care is the most difficult aspect of MCA treatment.[32]

Putting the new plan in place requires informing the caregiver and other family members of the plan, its reasons, and why the previous treatment was inappropriate. Many times this can be done expeditiously, particularly if the abuse is of the mild variety that might not even require community-based intervention. It is at this point, however, when the abuse is called to a halt, that the caregiver who has initiated the harmful medical care might act in such a way as to require legal intervention to stop the unnecessary care.

Identifying the abuse can be done without the cooperation of the abuser. Stopping it and providing for the ongoing safety of the child requires either the cooperation of the perpetrator or an intervention by community resources that ensure the abuse will not continue or be reintroduced. This is the case with MCA as it is with any other form of child maltreatment.

The motivation of the perpetrator also becomes paramount at this point. When determining if a child can remain or be returned to an environment in which he or she was previously harmed, one would like to know what the perpetrator was thinking when the harm was occurring. The motivation of the perpetrator of MCA is just as important as the motivation of someone harming their child by beating them, emotionally excoriating them, or exposing them to sexual abuse. The motivation in each case may be different, but understanding what the person was thinking is essential to making decisions about the ongoing safety of the child victim.

Making Sure the Abuse Does Not Recur

Providing for the ongoing safety of a victim of MCA requires that the child live in a family environment dedicated to the new medical treatment plan that does not allow for harmful, unnecessary treatment. This might mean excluding the parent, usually a mother, from making medical decisions, or in some cases, from even having contact with the child. However, if she can see the advantge of working with the medical team for the benefit of her child, and safeguards are in place that keep old patterns of health care abuse from reemerging, then as with other forms of abuse, one might opt for asserting family preservation as a unifying concept in ongoing family health. The determining factors include the severity of the MCA experienced by the child as well as the ability of the perpetrator to admit her contribution in the harm and her work to prevent it in the future. This may turn out to be relatively easy or completely impossible, and steps need to be taken by the child welfare community as would occur with other children when safety cannot be ensured in any other way.

Repair the Physical and Psychological Damage Experienced by the Child

Treatment of the physical effects of MCA is dependent on the types of medical care received. A child who has received intravenous immunoglobulin (IVIG) unnecessarily can simply have it stopped and the central line through which it was administered surgically removed. Similarly, children who have received a colostomy can sometimes have it surgically repaired. For some, however, the damage is permanent.[33] In general, stopping the most invasive and dangerous treatments should be done first, followed by less worrisome treatment. For example, if a child has an unnecessary implanted venous access port or gastric tube, removing these would be urgent. After this is done, less intrusive treatments and less dangerous medications can be stopped.

Psychological treatment of MCA victims parallels treatment offered to victims of other forms of child abuse. Common symptom presentations include posttraumatic stress disorder and the associated symptoms of depression and anxiety. A central feature of child abuse treatment is the need to restore trust in caregivers and others expected to keep children safe from harm. Bryk[33] gives a first-hand account about the psychological tasks facing a long-term victim of MCA.

A special feature of MCA treatment is the need to identify cognitive distortions associated with having been told for many years that one is ill and in need of medical treatment when this is not, in fact, the case. Libow[34] interviewed 10 adults victimized in childhood and described their social adaptation and attitudes to getting medical care as adults. Others have documented that being a victim of MCA might presage patterns of factitious medical utilization in adulthood as teenagers incorporate inappropriate health care–seeking behaviors into their lives.[35]

Preserve the Family if the Safety of the Child Can Be Ensured

Preserving the family is a worthwhile goal. However, as with other forms of child abuse, it is never appropriate to sacrifice the safety of a child simply to allow family members to continue to live under one roof. Having said this, Berg and Jones[36] described a series of families where children had experienced severe medical abuse and were subsequently reintegrated into their families of origin. They concluded that, in carefully selected situations, families undergoing intense treatment could experience successful family reunification.

THE MULTIDISCIPLINARY TEAM

As with other forms of child abuse, the availability of a trained child abuse pediatrician and a hospital-based multidisciplinary child protection team (MDT) is an enormous advantage. Physicians attempting to treat MCA without assistance can find themselves struggling to deal with their own emotional issues while attempting to negotiate a new treatment contract with the family. It is useful to consult with someone with prior experience with child abuse recognition and treatment in general and MCA in particular.

The MDT will find it helpful to familiarize itself with the diagnosis and treatment of MCA in the same way it diagnoses and treats other forms of child abuse. Because most jurisdictions have experience only with extreme cases and possibly not even one of these, team members should be encouraged to discuss situations that might not meet criteria for protection. Most pediatricians have a small percentage of patients and their parents where MCA is a possibility. In this way the MDT can be prepared when the situation arises in which a child might surpass the threshold of concern and need protection.

LEGAL ISSUES

The MCA formulation has been used successfully in the prosecution of several mothers in criminal court. By avoiding discussion of the motivation of the perpetrator, judges and juries are left with the facts of the case and make their decision about whether the child was harmed by the unnecessary medical care brought about by the parent. Trent[37] describes in detail the process of bringing a parent to justice for precipitating unnecessary surgery in her children.

Even though "medical neglect" carries no implication that the medical care team is neglecting the needs of the child, some have objected that "medical abuse" might refer to physicians abusing children. Having the definition of MCA include the specific stipulation that the unnecessary care is delivered "at the instigation of the caretaker" has not prevented physicians from feeling they are being singled out for criticism. There is a term for harmful medical care instigated by a physician: *malpractice*. The medical care involved in MCA is care offered in good faith, by well-meaning, competent physicians who are giving treatment that is consistent with the community standard of care. Other physicians in the community, given the same set of circumstances, would do essentially the same thing. The medical care offered that is determined to be harmful is inappropriate because the information upon which it was based is false and the person providing that false information carries the responsibility.

PREVENTION OF MEDICAL CHILD ABUSE

Physicians have a responsibility to work to minimize unnecessary medical treatment. They provide medical care in partnership with the patient and the patient's caretakers. That partnership operates with some basic assumptions that include trust between the parties. One of the responsibilities of the physician is to make a judgment about whether the trust is justified. The physician, in addition to paying attention to the nature of medical information provided by parents, and practicing good medicine, is also charged with providing only necessary care.

A number of forces promote excessive medical care use, all of which drive up the cost of medical care and decrease the availability of services. The fear of being sued for malpractice is one such force. According to one estimate, the cost of defensive medicine (ordering tests that might not otherwise be indicated, primarily to guard against future consideration that every possibility was explored) is 5% to 9% of the total health care cost in the United States.[38]

Another factor in overutilization of medical treatment is the availability of ever-increasing technical advances in diagnostic procedures and treatments. Although conventional wisdom is that more advanced medical care is better, there is growing evidence that new treatments might in some cases make things worse.[39,40] A third consideration in the growth in medical care utilization is the tendency to involve patients in choosing the course of treatment to a degree not typical several decades ago. Drug manufacturers advertise prescription medications directly to the public with an admonition to "Ask your doctor!" Doctors involve patients in more choices. Experts in medical ethics debate whether it is ethical to allow a patient to demand a medical test that has little chance in enhancing a course of treatment.[41]

Against this backdrop a small percentage of parents demand treatment for their children and provide justification for that treatment in the form of false information that can persuade a physician to prescribe unnecessary and harmful or potentially harmful medical care. It is important that physicians recognize this possibility and take steps to prevent it from occurring. No other form of child maltreatment is as preventable as MCA. As the medical care community grows more sophisticated in recognizing when children are receiving unnecessary and harmful or potentially harmful medical care, and responds to this awareness appropriately, one can only hope that fewer parents will be able to mistreat their children in the medical environment.

References

1. Roesler TA, Jenny C: *Medical Child Abuse: Beyond Munchausen by Proxy.* American Academy of Pediatrics Press, Elk Grove Village, IL, 2008.
2. Roesler TA: Defining, diagnosing and treating medical child abuse. *Brown U Child Adolesc Behav Ltr* 2007;23:1,5-6.
3. Caruso M, Bregani P, Di Natale B, et al: [Induced hypoglycemia. A unusual case of child battering]. *Minerva Pediatr* 1989;41:525-528.
4. Beitchman JH, Zucker KJ, Hood JE, et al: A review of the long-term effects of child sexual abuse. *Child Abuse Negl* 1992;16:101-118.
5. Fisher GC: Etiological speculations. *In:* Levin AV, Sheridan MS (eds): *Munchausen Syndrome by Proxy: Issues in Diagnosis and Treatment.* Lexington Books, New York, 1995, pp 39-57.
6. Bools C, Neale B, Meadow R: Munchausen syndrome by proxy: a study of psychopathology. *Child Abuse Negl* 1994;18:773-788.
7. Feldman MD, Brown RM: Munchausen by Proxy in an international context. *Child Abuse Negl* 2002;26:509-524.
8. Boros SJ, Ophoven JP, Andersen R, et al: Munchausen syndrome by proxy: a profile for medical child abuse. *Aust Fam Physician* 1995;24:768-769, 772-763.
9. Fisher GC, Mitchell I: Is Munchausen syndrome by proxy really a syndrome? *Arch Dis Child* 1995;72:530-534.
10. Morley CJ: Practical concerns about the diagnosis of Munchausen syndrome by proxy. *Arch Dis Child* 1995;72:528-529; discussion 529-530.
11. Davis PM, Sibert JR: Munchausen syndrome by proxy or factitious illness spectrum disorder of childhood. *Arch Dis Child* 1996;74:274-275.
12. Donald T, Jureidini J: Munchausen syndrome by proxy. child abuse in the medical system. *Arch Pediatr Adolesc Med* 1996;150:753-758.
13. Eminson M, Jureidini J: Concerns about research and prevention strategies in Munchausen syndrome by proxy (MSBP) abuse. *Child Abuse Negl* 2003;27:413-420.
14. Wilson RG: Fabricated or induced illness in children. Munchausen by proxy comes of age. *Br Med J* 2001;323:296-297.
15. Meadow R: Munchausen syndrome by proxy. The hinterland of child abuse. *Lancet* 1977;2:343-345.
16. Dine MS, McGovern ME: Intentional poisoning of children—an overlooked category of child abuse: report of seven cases and review of the literature. *Pediatrics* 1982;70:32-35.
17. Ayoub CC, Alexander R, Beck D, et al: Position paper: definitional issues in Munchausen by proxy. *Child Maltreat* 2002;7:105-111.
18. Bools C: *Fabricated or Induced Illness in a Child by a Carer: a Reader.* Radcliffe Publishing, Oxford, 2007.
19. Kosmach B, Tarbell S, Reyes J, et al: "Munchausen by proxy" syndrome in a small bowel transplant recipient. *Transplant Proc* 1996;28:2790-2791.
20. Rosenberg DA: Web of deceit: a literature review of Munchausen syndrome by proxy. *Child Abuse Negl* 1987;11:547-563.
21. Jenny C, Barron C, Roesler T: *Munchausen Syndrome by Proxy [Audiotape].* American Academy of Pediatrics, Elk Grove Village, IL, 2002.
22. Sanders MJ, Bursch B: Forensic assessment of illness falsification, Munchausen by proxy, and factitious disorder, NOS. *Child Maltreat* 2002;7:112-124.

23. Bursch B, Schreier HA, Ayoub CC, et al: Further thoughts on "Beyond Munchausen by proxy: identification and treatment of child abuse in a medical setting." *Pediatrics* 2008;121:444-445; author reply 445.

24. Southall DP, Plunkett MC, Banks MW, et al: Covert video recordings of life-threatening child abuse: lessons for child protection. *Pediatrics* 1997;100:735-760.

25. Evans D: Covert video surveillance in Munchausen's syndrome by proxy. *Br Med J* 1994;308:301-302.

26. Evans D: The investigation of life-threatening child abuse and Munchausen Syndrome by proxy. *J Med Ethics* 1995;21:9-13.

27. Evans D: Covert video surveillance—a response to Professor Southail and Dr. Samuels. *J Med Ethics* 1996;22:29-31.

28. Morgan B: Covert surveillance in Munchausen's Syndrome by proxy. *Br Med J* 1994;308:1715-1716.

29. Morgan B: Spying on mothers. *Lancet* 1994;344:132.

30. Yorker BC: Covert video surveillance of Munchausen syndrome by proxy: the exigent circumstances exception. *Health Matrix Clevel* 1995;325-346.

31. Hall DE, Eubanks L, Meyyazhagan LS, et al: Evaluation of covert video surveillance in the diagnosis of Munchausen syndrome by proxy: lessons from 41 cases. *Pediatrics* 2000;105:1305-1312.

32. Griffith JL, Slovik LS: Munchausen syndrome by proxy and sleep disorders medicine. *Sleep* 1989;12:178-183.

33. Bryk M, Siegel PT: My mother caused my illness: the story of a survivor of Munchausen by proxy syndrome. *Pediatrics* 1997:1001-1007.

34. Libow JA: Munchausen by proxy victims in adulthood: a first look. *Child Abuse Negl* 1995;19:1131-1142.

35. Libow JA: Beyond collusion: active illness falsification. *Child Abuse Negl* 2002;26:525-536.

36. Berg B, Jones DP: Outcome of psychiatric intervention in factitious illness by proxy (Munchausen Beyond Munchausen by proxy: identification and treatment of child abuse in a medical setting. *Prosecutor* 2008;38:1-3.

37. Trent M: A horrific case of "medical child abuse." *The Prosecutor* 2008;38:1-3.

38. Kessler D, McClellan M: Do doctors practice defensive medicine? *Q J Econ* 1996;111:353-390.

39. Fisher ES, Welch HG: Avoiding the unintended consequences of growth in medical care: how might more be worse? *JAMA* 1999;281:446-453.

40. Emanuel EJ, Fuchs VR: The perfect storm of overutilization. *JAMA* 2008;299:2789-2791.

41. Quill TE, Brody H: Physician recommendations and patient autonomy: finding a balance between physician power and patient choice. *Ann Intern Med* 1996;125:763-769.

62

CHILD DEATH REVIEW

Patricia G. Schnitzer, PhD, and Theresa M. Covington, MPH

THE PURPOSE AND SCOPE OF CHILD DEATH REVIEW IN THE USA

Child death review (CDR) is a process that works to understand how and why children die in order to take action to prevent other deaths. It involves a multidisciplinary team of professionals coming together to share case-specific information on the circumstances surrounding the death of a child. CDR team members typically include representatives from law enforcement, medical examiner/coroners' offices, public health, medicine, social services, the courts, emergency medical technicians or other first responders, mental health, and other agencies. At a review, each team member shares information available from his or her agency on the child, the family, the community, and events leading to the death. The team discussion of this information is focused on understanding and documenting the collective risk factors associated with the death and then identifying strategies to minimize these risks.[1,2]

The first CDR teams in the United States were formed in the late 1970s and early 1980s. These teams focused on evaluating the circumstances of suspicious child deaths in order to better identify deaths related to child abuse and neglect.[3] Throughout the 1990s, a number of efforts by Federal agencies and national organizations led to the growth of CDR in states and communities throughout the United States.[4-7] These efforts were greatly facilitated by the publication of the Missouri Child Fatality Study in 1993.[8] This study reviewed all injury deaths among children in Missouri under age 5 over a 4-year period. The study found that most fatal injuries of young children had been inadequately investigated, many more children died from abuse and neglect than reported, and many deaths were predictable and preventable. The authors concluded that failure to understand the circumstances of child deaths can result in misguided prevention efforts, poor policy decisions, failure to prosecute criminal conduct, and danger to surviving siblings. Based on the results of this study, Missouri passed legislation that established the Missouri Child Fatality Review Program and mandated the multidisciplinary review of all deaths of children younger than 15 years. The Missouri Child Fatality Review Program remains one of the most comprehensive CDR programs in the United States and over the years has served as a model for other state programs.

In 2002, all of the efforts of the previous decade culminated in the Federal funding of a national CDR Resource Center for Policy and Practice ("National Center"). The mission of the center is to promote, support, and enhance CDR methodology and activities at the community, state, and national levels, and to work toward standardization of death review practices throughout the United States.

In 2010, 49 states in the United States and the District of Columbia have a CDR program in place. They vary across states by the core functions they perform, the level of review (state or local), the types of deaths reviewed, agency authority for the program, availability and adequacy of funding, and the scope of state statutes that mandate or enable the review process.[9] The training and guidance provided by the National Center since 2002 has resulted in more consistency in purpose, function, and outcome across states. Details on each state's CDR program are updated annually through state surveys conducted by the National Center, available on their website (www.childdeathreview.org). Other web-based resources can be found online at www.expertconsult.com (see Chapter 62 Supplemental Resources).

ROLE OF CHILD DEATH REVIEW IN IDENTIFYING MALTREATMENT

Numerous studies have demonstrated that child maltreatment deaths are underreported in vital statistics and child welfare data.[8,10-13] These official data sources estimate that approximately 1300 children die from child maltreatment each year.[14,15] However, it is widely acknowledged that these estimates are low and that many more maltreatment deaths are likely not identified as such. CDR programs were initially created to improve the identification of deaths related to maltreatment largely by enhancing communication across agencies. It has now been demonstrated that CDR is an effective approach for better identifying fatal child maltreatment.[13]

In the past, most CDR programs focused exclusively on maltreatment deaths because of inflicted injuries (i.e., physical abuse) that were erroneously identified as accidents. Today, many programs have broadened the scope of their reviews to include all unintentional injury deaths, as well as many preventable natural-cause deaths (e.g., asthma and diabetes). Because teams have expanded the types of deaths they review, they are now more likely to discover unreported circumstances of neglect.

Unintentional or accidental injury deaths among young children most commonly occur from motor vehicle crashes, suffocation, drowning, burns, and poisoning. These deaths are routinely investigated by law enforcement and classified by coroners or medical examiners as accidents. A comprehensive review of the circumstances leading up to the injury helps to identify underlying issues of maltreatment. Some of these underlying issues include inadequate supervision of the child; substance use by caregivers; failure to appropriately use safety devices such as child restraints in motor vehicles, flotation devices, pool fencing, and smoke detectors; and failure to provide a safe sleeping environment for infants. In Michigan, the state CDR team conducted a review of unintentional injury deaths for children ages 0 to 9 from 2000 to 2001 to examine if neglect was a factor in these deaths.[13] The results were remarkable in that more than 30% of all accidental deaths of children under 10 years old had a parent or caretaker on the central registry of the state child protective services agency. After further review by the team, 82 of these accidental deaths were found to be caused at least in part by a caregiver's neglect. These deaths represented 43% of all child maltreatment deaths in the state, and a 75% increase in the number of child maltreatment deaths identified by multiple data sources over the 2-year period.[13]

In a similar retrospective case review conducted in Clark County Nevada, 47% of deaths reviewed that had not been reported to the child welfare agency were found to be related to neglect. Had these deaths been reported to child welfare, they would have merited substantiation. Reasons given in both Michigan and Nevada as to why health care providers, coroners/medical examiners, law enforcement, or other local investigators did not alert social services and/or document the neglect in death records included statements such as, "The parents did not intend harm"; "I've done the same thing with my kids—that could have been me"; and "The parents have suffered enough." These common sentiments continue to impede the classification of unintentional injury deaths as maltreatment. Some examples of injury deaths classified as accidental that were determined to be neglect when reviewed are included in Table 62-1. After conducting these special reviews in Michigan and Nevada, both states implemented changes to state and local policy to ensure that unintentional injury deaths are more closely scrutinized and that those identified as neglect-related are reported and responded to appropriately. The experiences in these two states provide compelling support to include all unintentional injury deaths in the CDR process.

Whereas the relationship of unintentional injuries to neglect has been studied, similar efforts to determine the relationship of deaths resulting from natural causes and neglect have not been undertaken. Examples where neglect might play a role in deaths from natural causes include he following:

Table 62-1	Examples of Injury Deaths that Were Considered Accidental until Child Death Review Identified Circumstances Indicating Neglect
Findings from Initial Investigation	**Additional Findings from CDR Team**
Pool drowning of 1-year-old. At 2 PM the child opens the unlocked screen door into the backyard and falls into pool.	The public health nurse providing bereavement services for family learned that the child had been left in care of 4-year-old sibling while parent took an afternoon nap.
A 5-year-old child drowns in an unfenced pond near his trailer park.	CPS review of records found that the neighbors had made numerous complaints to CPS, concerned that this child was at risk of drowning because he was frequently playing unsupervised at the pond. None of these prior reports were substantiated by CPS.
A toddler, left in a car on a hot day for 3 hours, is found dead. The child's parent was putting away groceries, then answered phone and with these distractions, forgot about child.	Case information was complete at time of investigation. CDR team discussion convinced law enforcement and district attorney to consider charges of child endangerment.
A 2-month-old infant dies while sleeping in an adult bed with both parents. The death was due to accidental suffocation/overlay by parents.	The review found that both parents had been heavily drinking alcohol and smoking marijuana before they fell asleep, contributing to their deep sleep and failure to feel the infant beneath them.
A 1-year-old child is ejected from a car during a crash. The child was in a car seat but not secured by the seatbelt and the seat was also not secured to the car. The crash was caused by another vehicle.	The review found that the father was intoxicated at the time he placed the child in the car. Even though the father was a passenger and not the driver of the car, his failure to properly restrain his child resulted in the death (child would not have been ejected if properly restrained).
A house fire kills four young children and a grandfather. The fire was started by the children who were playing with lighters. Their grandfather was babysitting them at the time, but was confined to a wheelchair and could not call for help, escape, or help the children escape.	The team found that the parents had prior CPS histories of neglect and had been told by CPS during prevention services that having the grandfather babysit was inappropriate based on grandfather's immobility and the age of the children.

CDR, Child death review; *CPS*, child protective services.

- An infant dying from prematurity and low birth weight after intrauterine drug exposure and cocaine intoxication at birth
- A child dying from asthma after the parents failed to administer his asthma medications
- A child with severe physical and developmental disabilities in whom the parents failed to provide appropriate care over time, leading to premature death.

Focusing on the link between these types of deaths and maltreatment should become a priority and will improve the identification, classification, and response to child maltreatment.

CASE REVIEW MODELS FOR IMPROVING SYSTEMS AND PREVENTING DEATHS

Many CDR programs throughout the United States have adapted strategies to adapt program models and use their review data to improve agency systems and implement prevention approaches. The following strategies are examples.

Focusing on Systems Improvements. Model focusing on systems improvements are used in both Michigan and Nevada. In Michigan, maltreatment reviews are conducted by a special state review panel. In Nevada, special reviews are conducted in response to legislative inquiries into failures of the state's child welfare system. Both states follow a process that (1) identifies potential maltreatment deaths using a variety of reporting sources, (2) obtains additional specific case information on each death, (3) conducts a comprehensive, multidisciplinary review of each death, and (4) methodically identifies systems issues, using the template in Table 62-2 to assess problems, develop recommendations, and take action on the recommendations. In both states, this process led to rapid identification of systems and problems and to the preparation of reports of the review teams' findings. Importantly, officials in both states have also issued formal responses on their plans to address the teams' recommendations, and subsequently provided updates on their progress. The template provided in Table 62-2 can be used by any CDR team to document findings and recommendations for systems changes.

Focusing on Implementing Prevention Programs. Most CDR programs have expanded their review outcomes to include action-oriented recommendations for implementing programs, services, policies, or laws to prevent future deaths. However, an analysis of over 1000 recommendations included in states' annual CDR reports found that they were often generic, nonspecific, not based on best practice, and at times not linked to actual review findings (S. Wirtz, California Department of Public Health, personal communication, July 21, 2008). Consequently, more teams are seeking training in effective methods for using CDR data to develop recommendations and strategies for implementing preventive interventions. Implementation of interventions is facilitated when local teams take responsibility for local initiatives while sharing their successes with a state advisory panel that implements policies and programs statewide.

In an effort to help review teams identify evidence-based prevention recommendations, the Harborview Injury Research Center in Seattle, Washington developed a web-based tool that offers CDR programs a variety of evidence-based prevention strategies. The tool is now maintained by the National Center. (See Chapter 62 Supplemental Resources online at www.expertconsult.com.) Examples of prevention strategies include the following:

- New or amended laws to protect children from harm such as graduated driver's licenses for teens and "safe haven" laws to prevent infant abandonment.
- New child health, safety, and protection programs, such as distribution of smoke alarms and intensive home visitation programs for new parents.
- Environmental modifications to eliminate hazards such as changing dangerous roadways.
- Widespread safety education campaigns, such as safe sleep and water safety campaigns.

THE STRENGTHS OF CHILD DEATH REVIEW

The CDR process has evolved rapidly, moving away from a punitive perspective focused on whether a child was harmed and who was responsible for harming them, to include a broader approach focused on understanding and responding to the risk factors for and circumstances leading to a child's death. A number of strengths have grounded the CDR process in states and communities:

1. *Improved interagency communication and coordination:* The heart of CDR is its power in bringing multiple disciplines together and improving communication across agencies. Effective reviews share information on the circumstances surrounding a child's death, followed by a discussion of strategies for improving systems and programs, resulting in enhanced interagency communication and coordination.[2,16]
2. *Better identification and classification of child deaths:* There is anecdotal evidence that CDR improves the quality of child death investigation and results in more accurate classification of the cause and manner of death. A recent report by the Scripps Howard News Organization found that CDR programs play an important role in detecting and accurately diagnosing infant accidental deaths.[17] They report that compared with a state with no CDR program, states with CDR programs are more likely to classify sudden unexpected infant deaths that occur in a sleep environment as resulting from accidental suffocation, rather than classifying these deaths as resulting from undetermined or unknown cause.[17]
3. *Consistent and standardized data collection:* A 2005 survey of all 50 states and the District of Columbia found that 44 states use a data collection form to document the findings from each death review, and 39 states require an annual report of their CDR findings.[18] The National Center has launched the standardized *CDR Case Reporting System*, a web-based data entry system, now in use in more than 30 states, covering more than 80% of all child deaths (ages 0-18 years) in the United States. (See Chapter 62 Supplemental Resources online at www.expertconsult.com.)

Table 62-2 A Template (with Examples) to Identify Child Protection Systems Issues in Child Maltreatment Deaths

Findings	Recommendations	Action Taken
Early or Prior Identification of Possible Harm		
No report made to CPS in suspected maltreatment deaths, because there are no surviving siblings.	Amend state law and policy to require CPS reports, regardless of sibling status.	Within 60 days, state law was introduced and policy change enacted immediately.
Delays of up to 1 week were common for reports of child abuse and neglect made by mandated reporters (e.g., law enforcement, physicians) because they could not get through on the toll-free reporting hotline.	Overhaul the 1-800 hotline reporting system, and ensure that mandated reporters have alternative methods/phone lines for reporting suspected maltreatment.	The number of phone lines was doubled, staffing increased and training for hotline workers implemented.
Investigation by CPS		
CPS did not investigate potential neglect-related deaths based on statements made by others (e.g., "the parents did not intend harm"; "there was no criminal intent"; "the death was accidental"; "parents have suffered enough"). This included failure to investigate a number of deaths with prior substantiations and/or evidence of significant neglect.	Develop a specialized unit of CPS investigators working 24/7, who are trained to respond to and investigate all potential child maltreatment deaths.	The specialized unit was created and trained and is working with other agencies (e.g., law enforcement, coroners) and conducting multidisciplinary comprehensive investigations.
Suspicious deaths reported to CPS were unsubstantiated or closed because CPS workers were unable to locate the child's parent(s)	Change policy to prohibit the closing of cases simply because parents could not be located and require intense efforts to locate parents, including working with law enforcement across state lines	A new category was added to disposition of cases to reflect that parents were not located and a new multidisciplinary team is to assume responsibility for locating parents in coordination with CPS.
Investigation by Law Enforcement		
An unexplained infant death was not investigated by law enforcement, and the criminal history of the infant's caregiver was not reviewed. Had it been checked, this caregiver's history would have revealed a prior (nonfatal) injury inflicted by this person.	Criminal background checks should become standard of practice in the investigation of all accidental or unexplained child deaths.	A multidisciplinary investigative team convened to develop plans for investigation of all child deaths. Criminal background checks are now conducted on caregivers for all accidental or unexplained child deaths
Child witnesses were not interviewed using appropriate forensic interviewing techniques.	Develop a standard of practice that all child witnesses be interviewed using accepted forensic interviewing techniques.	A series of trainings were provided to all law enforcement personnel, coroners, and CPS workers responsible for investigating child deaths.
Investigation by Coroner/Medical Examiner		
There was marked inconsistency in the determination of cause and manner of death across pathologists, even when the circumstances of the death are very similar.	Institute case conferencing on all child deaths to ensure consistency of cause and manner of death determinations.	Pathologists now hold case conferences on all child deaths. In addition, a new medical examiner position was created to help meet case load demands.
The death of a child is not referred to the coroner/medical examiner's office, despite allegations of abuse. Instead, it is signed out by a hospital physician.	Chief Medical Examiner should provide training to hospital pediatricians on the legal requirements of death certification.	The Hospital Quality Assurance Director now requires all nonnatural hospital-attended deaths be submitted immediately to the Chief Medical Examiner's Office for investigation; hospital physicians are no longer permitted to certify these deaths.

Continued

Table 62-2	A Template to Identify Child Protection Systems Issues in Child Maltreatment Deaths—cont'd	
Findings	**Recommendations**	**Action Taken**
Case Intake by CPS		
CPS investigations of child deaths were not thorough; there was little evidence that facts were verified, either through verification of available information or review of other agency records.	Create clear standards for determining which deaths must be investigated, and ensure that any death that meets these criteria is adequately investigated prior to closing the case records.	Standards were written and adopted as policy.
Services Provided by CPS		
No services are offered or ineffective services were provided for identified issues, especially in the areas of parental substance abuse and mental health needs. Service needs were not well documented in the case files.	Develop an improved tracking system to identify service needs, referrals made, and barriers to services, and ensure that these are incorporated into court petitions.	Many additional CPS service positions were created, funded, and filled to meet the need. A new computerized tracking system was implemented.
CPS investigated and closed cases when there were no surviving siblings, even if the child's mother was responsible for the death being investigated and was pregnant at the time.	CPS should keep cases open when the mother is pregnant until it can be ensured that the newborn infant will be safe.	Policy was changed to require that cases remain open when the mother is pregnant until it is ensured that the newborn infant is safe.
Response from Civil and Criminal Courts		
District Attorney's Office would not prosecute child maltreatment cases without a perpetrator confession, if there were no other witnesses.	Multidisciplinary investigative team should work with the District Attorney's Office to ensure a quality investigation that will meet evidentiary standards for successful prosecution.	A multidisciplinary team was convened (chaired by the District Attorney) to conduct case reviews on all accidental and unexplained child injury deaths.
A child died from physical abuse perpetrated by the father. Previous petitions for the removal of the child from the father had been filed by CPS but rejected by the family court judge.	Establish a feedback and peer review process for judges whose court decisions may have affected the subsequent health and safety of children.	A peer review process is under consideration.

CDR, Child death review; *CPS,* child protective services.

4. *CDRs and public health surveillance of child maltreatment:* CDR is the most promising approach for quantifying the magnitude of fatal child maltreatment in the United States. A multiyear, multistate effort to identify effective approaches for public health surveillance of child maltreatment found that CDR is the best "single source" for case identification, when compared with death certificates, child welfare case records, police uniform crime reports, and internal state child maltreatment audit systems.[13] Importantly, the *CDR Case Reporting System* developed and maintained by the National Center has the potential for becoming a system for national surveillance of fatal child maltreatment.

THE CHALLENGES OF CHILD DEATH REVIEW

The process of CDR has helped us better understand maltreatment and injury deaths, systems improvements, and prevention.[19] CDR has made significant contributions to our understanding of maltreatment. However, a number of challenges remain for practitioners using CDR to better understand maltreatment.

Establishing Uniform Definitions of Child Maltreatment

Member agencies participating in CDR have distinct definitions of child abuse and neglect, including definitions from criminal, civil, and public health perspectives. Definitions differ across states. These different definitions and perspectives make it difficult for review teams to agree on classification of maltreatment-related deaths. This in turn affects the uniform counting of maltreatment deaths.

A federal effort led by the Centers for Disease Control and Prevention (CDC) to establish uniform child maltreatment definitions for public health surveillance has been launched.[20] A pilot project to test the application of these definitions by CDR teams in three states found that the definitions were useful in reaching agreement on classifying maltreatment within a public health framework, even if the death did not meet an agency definition of maltreatment. For example, a district attorney might agree that a child who died from injuries sustained as an unrestrained passenger in a motor vehicle crash met the public health definition of neglect, even though the death might not meet his state's legal definition or standard required for prosecution.

Efforts are underway in California to create a consistent child maltreatment classification system across all of the state's local CDR teams. Using the CDC uniform definitions for child maltreatment as a starting point, the California Department of Public Health established a decision matrix to assist local CDR teams in reaching consensus on the classification of maltreatment deaths.[21] The challenge remains for widespread adoption and use of uniform definitions to classify maltreatment.

Moving Teams from Review to Action

All 49 state CDR programs now identify the prevention of future deaths as a primary purpose. Many teams, however, do not have the resources to translate their CDR findings into effective prevention strategies. A number of barriers to moving from review to action are apparent, and include the following:

- Teams frequently do not make specific, action-oriented recommendations that can be readily translated to prevention or policy interventions.
- Team members participate in reviews largely on a volunteer basis. Committing time and resources necessary to move from review to action is often prohibitive.
- Teams often do not have the expertise or financial resources to develop and implement effective prevention strategies.

For the past several years, the number one technical assistance request to the National Center has been for training on how to craft effective recommendations for preventing deaths and improving systems. Tools are now available to help teams develop action-oriented objectives. Some CDR teams are partnering with prevention-oriented organizations such as child abuse prevention coalitions, Safe Kids injury prevention coalitions, and/or local and state public health injury prevention programs.[22]

Expanding Reviews to Natural, Preventable Child Deaths

It is likely that by expanding reviews of deaths resulting from natural causes, additional maltreatment-related deaths will be identified.

Expanding Reviews to Serious Non-Fatal Injuries

Maltreatment deaths are a rare occurrence, but maltreatment-related injuries are not. The power of CDR should be expanded to review serious injuries, which provides a unique opportunity to focus on secondary prevention of additional harm to the injured children. Guidelines need to be developed to help states define and identify serious injuries for review.

STANDARDIZATION, FUNDING SUPPORT, AND A NATIONAL CDR DATABASE

Federal funding of the National Center has supported the development and implementation of a national case reporting tool and data collection system. Through these efforts, tremendous progress has been made in the standardization of CDR methodology. Continued progress will require expanded state and national funding for CDR programs.

CONCLUSION

Children are affirmations of life. When they die, their deaths present painful questions. Professional members of a CDR team must grapple with understanding the extensive array of risk factors in the deaths of our children. The answers may be complex and bewildering. Conducting quality reviews will help explain the broader questions related to risky behaviors, inadequate social systems and institutions, or dangerous environments that may have contributed to a child's death. Reviewing the circumstances of a child's death from abuse and neglect provides a way to translate these tragedies into hope, especially when the team works to translate the findings into action. The promise of effective CDR teams is that they will honor the memories of the children who have died by saving the lives of other children.

References

1. Covington TM, Foster V, Rich SK: A Program Manual for Child Death Review. National Center for Child Death Review, Washington DC, 2005. Available at www.childdeathreview.org/Finalversionprotocolmanual.pdf. Accessed April 21, 2010.
2. Covington TM, Rich SK, Gardner JD: Effective models of review that work to prevent child deaths. *In*: Alexander R (ed): *Child Fatality Review: An Interdisciplinary Guide and Photographic Reference.* GW Medical Publishing, St Louis, 2007, pp 429-457.
3. Durfee MJ, Gellert GA, Tilton-Durfee D: Origins and clinical relevance of child death review teams. *JAMA* 1992;267:3172-3175.
4. Kaplan SR: *Child Fatality Review Legislation in the United States.* American Bar Association, Chicago, 1991.
5. Maternal and Child Health Bureau: *Recommendations of the Child Fatality Review Advisory Workgroup.* Dept of Health and Human Services, Public Health Service, Washington DC, 1993.
6. Association of State and Territorial Health Officials. *State Efforts to Improve Child Death Review.* Dept of Health and Human Services, Public Health Service, Washington DC, 2004.
7. Healthy People 2000: National Health Promotion and Disease Prevention Objectives. U.S. Dept of Health and Human Services, Public Health Service, Washington DC, 1991.
8. Ewigman B, Kivlahan C, Land G: The Missouri Child Fatality Study: Underreporting of maltreatment fatalities among children younger than five years of age, 1983 through 1986. *Pediatrics* 1993;91:330-337.
9. Webster RA, Schnitzer PG, Jenny C, et al: Child death review: The state of the nation. *Am J Prev Med* 2003;25:58-64.
10. Crume TL, DiGuiseppi C, Byers T, et al: Underascertainment of child maltreatment fatalities by death certificates, 1990-1998. *Pediatrics* 2002;110:e18.
11. Herman-Giddens ME, Brown G, Verbiest S, et al: Underascertainment of child abuse mortality in the United States. *JAMA* 1999;282:463-467.
12. Overpeck MD, Brenner RA, Cosgrove C, et al: National underascertainment of sudden unexpected infant deaths associated with deaths of unknown cause. *Pediatrics* 2002;109:274-283.
13. Schnitzer PG, Covington TM, Wirtz SJ, et al: Public health surveillance of fatal child maltreatment: Analysis of 3 state programs. *Am J Public Health* 2008;98:296-303.

14. U.S. Dept. of Health and Human Services, Administration on Children, Youth and Families. *Child Maltreatment 2006.* U.S. Government Printing Office, Washington DC, 2008.

15. McClain PW, Sacks JJ, Froehlke RG, et al: Estimates of fatal child abuse and neglect, United States, 1979 through 1988. *Pediatrics* 1993; 91:338-343.

16. Sidebothom P, Fox J, Horwath J, et al: *Preventing Childhood Deaths. (Research Report DCSF-RR036)* Department for Children, Schools and Families, London, 2008.

17. Hargrove T, Bowman L: *Thousands of babies die of preventable suffocation each year.* Scripps Howard News Service, 2007.

18. National Center for Child Death Review. *2005 Survey on the Status of CDR in the United States.* National Center for Child Death Review, Washington DC, 2006 (unpublished work).

19. Hochstadt NJ: Child death review teams: A vital component of child protection. *Child Welfare* 2006;85:653-670.

20. Leeb RT, Paulozzi L, Melanson C, et al: *Child Maltreatment Surveillance: Uniform Definitions for Public Health Surveillance and Recommended Data Elements.* Centers for Disease Control and Prevention, National Center for Injury Prevention and Control, Atlanta, 2008.

21. Wirtz S, Lob S, Rose DA, et al: *Improving California's Surveillance System for Fatal Child Abuse and Neglect.* Presented at the 136th Annual Meeting of the American Public Health Association, San Diego, 2008.

22. National Center for Child Death Review. 2007 Survey on the Status of CDR in the United States. National Center for Child Death Review, Washington DC, 2008 (unpublished work).

63

RELIGION AND CHILD NEGLECT

Rita Swan, PhD

INTRODUCTION

For some sects, medicine and faith are incompatible. A study in *Pediatrics* reported on 172 U.S. children who died between 1975 and 1995 after medical care was withheld on religious grounds. It found that 140 (80%) of the children would have had at least a 90% likelihood of survival with medical care.[1]

Christian Science is the best-known religion promoting exclusive reliance on prayer for healing. It teaches that matter and spirit are opposites. The material world and its concomitant sin, sickness, poverty, war, and death are just illusions. Man is God's perfect spiritual mirror image, never born into matter and never dying.[2] Christian Science holds that disease is caused by sin, fear, or ignorance of God and that the only effective way to heal or prevent disease is to draw closer to God. Its prayer "treatments" argue that God did not make disease and therefore the disease is unreal, that the "patient" is perfect and cannot be tempted to believe he has a mortal body vulnerable to disease and death.[2]

The theology opposes medical treatment and diagnosis for both children and adults. It opposes not only drugs, but also hygiene, immunizations, health-promoting diets, chiropractic practice, vitamins, medical diagnoses, and health screenings because they are "material methods" to evaluate, treat, or prevent disease.[2] The church prohibits its healers from giving spiritual treatments to anyone who voluntarily obtains medical care unless the care is for a handful of very specific exceptions that the church founder rationalized as acceptable.[3,4]

Several small charismatic sects also oppose medical care.[5] Many are grounded in "positive confession theology," which is also known as "Name It and Claim It," the "Health and Wealth Gospel," and "Word Faith." It teaches that Jesus Christ's crucifixion was a vicarious atonement for disease as well as sin, and both are temptations from the devil. Christians must make "positive confessions" of their salvation through Jesus Christ and then the disease will disappear. The positive confession, also called "pleading the blood" by some sects, is a legalistic argument that the crucifixion has already saved them from disease. After the member makes this confession, he or she should firmly know that healing is guaranteed and ignore disease symptoms. This theology also encourages material prosperity. It teaches that God has promised Christians a right to material possessions, which they can get by ritually claiming them.[5]

Several of the charismatic faith-healing sects advocate home delivery of babies. They charge that doctors strip husbands of their God-ordained priesthood. Carol Balizet,[6] a former medical nurse, has written books promoting "Zion Births" of babies without medical attention. She praises a husband who orders his wife back into bed, although she wants to go to a hospital, and husbands who put their hands on their wives' hips and belligerently order God to enlarge them so the baby can be delivered.[6]

Many ethnic and cultural groups believe that disease has a supernatural cause and that ritual can heal it. Many have relied on shamans to enter the spirit world through trance and mediate the sick person and their community with it. They see disease as caused by imbalances among man, nature, and spirit, and by loss of spiritual power. A folk belief among the Hmongs is that disease is caused by angry spirits or by the soul leaving the body.[7]

All of these Christian and non-Christian groups believe that disease is caused by moral or spiritual factors rather than physiological and biochemical ones and is healed by ritual. For Christians, prayer for physical healing becomes a legalistic argument of affirmation and denial.

The Church of Scientology opposes some forms of medical care, but claims a biochemical basis for its beliefs, which is mixed with the science fiction written by its founder, L. Ron Hubbard. Scientology attacks psychiatry with vitriol.[8] The church claims to heal all mental health problems with its "dianetics" performed in expensive sessions by "auditors" who uncover the patient's "engrams" that are blocking health and wholeness. Then the auditors help the people to erase their "reactive mind" and reach "a state of clear."[9]

Scientologists believe babies should have a "silent birth" and not be exposed to any discomfort or language for the first week of life.[9] Words or discomfort, they believe, will be recorded by the "reptilian brain" (another term for the reactive mind). Later when one experiences the same sensory data or words, his or her reptilian brain will reenact the newborn's trauma. Hubbard claims total silence during birth is necessary to save the "sanity" of mother and baby.[9] On that basis, Scientologists refuse to have metabolic testing, immunizations, or any other injections or testing of babies until they are 1 week old.[10] Their dietary beliefs have endangered babies. Hubbard discourages breastfeeding because there are few "Guernsey-type mothers" today and recommends infants are fed "barley water" instead. Hubbard claims he "called up" the formula for barley water "from a deep past" some 2200 years ago when "Roman troops marched on barley." He calls it, "… the nearest approach to human milk that can be assembled easily."[11]

Jehovah's Witnesses are the largest denomination that stridently opposes a form of medical care. Their opposition to blood transfusions is based on Bible verses requiring abstinence "from blood" and eating meat with "lifeblood" still in it. Witness theology holds that the soul is in the blood and that Christ offered a perfect atonement for sin by shedding His blood. Accepting a blood transfusion constitutes eating blood and trampling on the sacrifice of Christ.[12] The Watchtower Bible and Tract Society, which makes policy for the denomination, prohibits transfusions of whole blood and of what they claim are its four primary components: red blood cells, white blood cells, platelets, and plasma. Because of Bible verses directing that blood be poured out on the ground, the Society prohibits storing blood for autotransfusions. As membership has grown into the millions, however, the Society has allowed several exceptions to its prohibitions against transfusions. An early one was an allowance for hemophiliacs to take clotting factors VIII and IX. The Society explained those as acceptable because they were only "minor" components of plasma. Then Witnesses were allowed to accept albumin and immunoglobulin because they too were just "fractions" of plasma and because these antibodies can pass through the placental barrier from mother to child—therefore, receiving them is a natural bodily process.[13] The Society continued to prohibit fractions derived from red blood cells, white blood cells, and platelets until 2000 when it published an anonymous statement that fractions derived from all the primary blood components were acceptable.[14] That allows Witnesses to accept interferons and interleukins from white blood cells and fibrinogen from platelets.

Blood gas analysis tests on premature infants are also allowed even though they, like autotransfusion, involve taking blood from the body and later putting it back. Witness theology, however, still prohibits the most common kind of transfusion: packed red blood cells. Jehovah's Witnesses are not faith healers. Their literature does not say that God will heal them of a need for a transfusion. Members try to persuade doctors to use blood substitutes, but if those cannot be used effectively, many claim they would rather die than accept a transfusion.

Another type of religious objection is to immunizations. Hundreds of thousands of U.S. parents refuse to immunize their children on religious or "philosophical" grounds. Often their refusal is actually based on a fear that the measles, mumps, and rubella vaccine causes autism, but their state requires them to have a religious objection to vaccines in order to get their child exempted. Some religious objectors claim that the human body is a sacred temple that should not have foreign substances injected into it.[15] Anthroposophy, an occult sect promoted at Waldorf schools in several countries, believes that children should not be vaccinated because they will have stronger immune systems if they contract infectious diseases naturally.[16]

Some conservative Catholics refuse consent for immunizations developed with aborted fetal tissue, including those for rabies, hepatitis A, varicella, and rubella. Catholic leaders, however, have encouraged members to obtain those vaccines if there is not an alternative type of a vaccine available against those diseases.[17] Some fundamentalist Catholic and Protestant groups charge that the hepatitis B and the new human papilloma virus vaccines encourage promiscuity and denigrate the morals they are teaching their children.[18] Finally, the faith-healing sects believe that one should trust God instead of vaccinations to prevent disease. Christian Science founder Mary Baker Eddy claimed that viruses and bacteria do not cause disease.[19] Her church still teaches that parents should protect children from disease not by immunizations but rather by daily "metaphysical work" to know that God is the only cause and therefore disease is unreal.[20]

Scores of vaccine-preventable disease outbreaks have occurred in groups with religious beliefs against immunizations. The largest U.S. outbreak of measles since 1992 began with a student at a Christian Science school.[21] These outbreaks are very expensive to control. Often public health departments must track exposed people through several states and even countries.

The American Academy of Pediatrics and others have suggestions for providers on how to communicate with parents who have religious objections to immunizations and other medical treatment.[22,23]

PUBLIC POLICY

With a salaried lobbyist in every state, the Christian Science church has nearly single-handedly won hundreds of religious exemptions from medical care for children. Preventive and screening measures from which many state laws provide religious exemptions include immunizations, metabolic testing, blood lead-level tests, newborn hearing screens, prophylactic eye drops at birth to prevent infections, vitamin K injections or drops, vision examinations, dental examinations, and any other health screenings. The church also works to exempt Christian Science children from having to learn about disease in school.[24]

Two states, Oregon and Pennsylvania, have religious exemptions from bicycle helmets for children. They were reportedly requested by the Sikhs.

The Jehovah's Witnesses rarely lobby legislatures. On grounds that they are actually citizens of a heavenly kingdom, the faith discourages members from holding public office or even voting. They do, however, vigorously defend their interests in court. They have won the right at the U.S. Supreme Court to proselytize door-to-door, to refuse military service, and to refuse to salute the flag or say the pledge of allegiance.[25,26]

The High Court ruled against them in the child labor case *Prince v. Massachusetts*,[27] with its famous words that "the right to practice religion freely does not include liberty to expose the community or child to communicable disease, or the latter to ill health or death. …" The case has often been cited in other rulings limiting religious freedom when a child's welfare is at stake.

Scope of Laws

The religious exemptions about medical care of sick and injured children vary widely in meaning. Several states have a religious exemption in their reporting laws or in statutory definitions of child abuse and neglect. Thirty-three states have religious defenses in their criminal codes, 19 for felony crimes against children and 14 for misdemeanors. Some of these laws are chilling in their implications. West Virginia plainly says that the statute defining the crime of murder of a child "… shall not apply to any parent … who fails or refuses … to supply a child … with necessary medical care" on religious grounds.[28] Arkansas has a religious defense to capital murder for those who cause deaths of children "under circumstances manifesting extreme indifference to human life."[29] By contrast, Rhode Island has a religious defense to a felony that "… does not exempt a parent or guardian from having committed the offense of cruelty or neglect if the child is harmed."[30] Rhode Island parents have the right to rely exclusively on prayer for healing only if the child is not harmed by the lack of medical care.

Criminal charges have been successfully pursued in several of the 33 states with religious defenses by filing charges for crimes without a religious defense or by arguing that the parent was not entitled to use the defense.[31,32] Since 1988, the U.S. Supreme Court has twice refused to review convictions of parents who withheld lifesaving medical treatment from children on religious grounds,[33,34] which suggests, although not conclusively, that the High Court regards the constitutional issues as already settled. Courts have also upheld the state's right to require immunizations and metabolic screening without a religious exemption.[35,36]

No U.S. court has held that parents have a constitutional right to abuse or neglect children. What remains unsettled, however, is whether legislatures may give parents a statutory right to withhold necessary medical care on religious grounds. A law that allows some parents to deprive their children of medical care while requiring other parents to provide it would seem to violate the constitutional rights of children to the "equal protection of the laws." Four state courts have ruled religious exemption laws unconstitutional on that basis, but only one of those rulings was at an appellate level and resulted in the voiding of an exemption statute.[37-40] Many organizations have called for repeal of these religious exemptions, including the American Medical Association, American Academy of Pediatrics, Prevent Child Abuse America, National District Attorneys Association, National Association of Medical Examiners, and Children's Healthcare Is a Legal Duty.

Issues with Adolescents

Several states give teenagers the right to consent to specific forms of medical care, such as mental health and substance abuse treatment and, most commonly, sexual health care, without their parents' permission or knowledge. Some writers argue that such laws represent an evolving concept of an adolescent's maturity and should be extended to a right to refuse any medical treatment. They want to give adolescents the free exercise, autonomy, and privacy rights that an adult has to practice his religious beliefs and control his own body.[41,42]

Minors with religious objections to medical treatment fall into at least three categories. Many minor children in faith-healing sects are not brought to medical attention when they are ill. Neither they nor their parents make decisions with the benefit of a medical diagnosis. They do not know the physical consequences of refusing medical treatment nor the

treatment options medical science has available for their illness. The children may be very devout and have a strong faith that they should rely only on God to heal them, but they certainly do not make informed decisions. There are also children such as Starchild Abraham Cherrix in Virginia.[43] He has Hodgkin's lymphoma. He completed the prescribed course of chemotherapy, but within 2 months the cancer was found again, and doctors prescribed another series of chemotherapy treatments. He refused to have more chemotherapy. He and his parents voiced nondenominational religious beliefs that a special diet would be curative. The courts allowed him to forego chemotherapy temporarily and instead have radiation and nutritional therapy from a board-certified radiation therapist and report his physical condition to the court every 3 months.

Finally, there are Jehovah's Witness children who are strongly coached to refuse blood transfusions. The Witnesses argue that they are not refusing medical treatment, but rather that they want the best medical treatment available without blood. They also argue—to providers and courts anyway—that their acceptance of most medical treatment shows that they desire to live and are not seeking martyrdom. Their internal communications, however, lavish strong praise on children who choose everlasting life in an earthly paradise over mortal life by refusing transfusions. The front cover of the May 22, 1994 issue of their magazine *Awake* has photos of 26 Witness children who died after refusing blood transfusions. The captions is, "Youth Who Put God First."

Since they are under medical care, the Jehovah's Witness children have a medical diagnosis, information about the dangers of refusing transfusions, and information about the probable success of medical treatment with transfusions. Some argue that 14- to 17-year-old Witness children should be considered "mature minors" and allowed to refuse transfusions, even at the cost of their lives.[44]

All state child protection statutes define a child as a person under 18 years of age and allow state intervention to protect unemancipated minors until their 18th birthday. Scores of court rulings have ordered medical treatment for adolescents over their and their parents' religious objections.[45-47]

The "mature minor doctrine" is said to be evolving through case law (also called common law). Some trial courts have allowed teenagers to refuse lifesaving medical treatment. Their reasoning is unknown because opinions are sealed in juvenile cases.[48] However, one finds only two U.S. appellate–level cases that allow minors to refuse necessary medical treatment on the basis of their maturity, and even then maturity must be balanced against other factors. The first is *In re E.G.* (Illinois 1989).[49] The youth was only a few months away from her 18th birthday and had acute non-lymphatic leukemia with only a 20% to 25% likelihood of 5-year survival. The appeals court gave her the right to refuse transfusions on religious freedom grounds. The Illinois Supreme Court, however, did not uphold a constitutional religious freedom right, but instead created a common law right for minors to refuse medical care if a trial court has clear and convincing evidence that the minor is "… mature enough to exercise the judgment of an adult" and to "… appreciate the consequences of her actions" and then balances the minor's right to autonomy against the state's strong interest in preserving life and special duty to protect minors, the interests of parents and other relatives, and the integrity of the medical profession, which is charged with preserving life. The Court did not rule on whether E.G. was in fact a mature minor.[49]

Oddly, the Court held that protecting the interests of parents and other third parties was more important than the state's interests. If E.G.'s parents had opposed her refusal of blood transfusions, "… this opposition would weigh heavily against the minor's right to refuse," the Court said. The ruling, therefore, can hardly be seen as giving minors autonomy. It is also revealing that the Court supported its holding with reference to criminal law allowing minors to be tried as adults, an analogy that does not show a benevolent concern for teens' welfare.

The second case also involved a 17-year-old Jehovah's Witness.[50] A hospital sought an order for a transfusion should it become necessary for treating a lacerated spleen. A trial judge granted the order. The girl was discharged without needing a transfusion, but the parents appealed. The Massachusetts Court of Appeals ruled that the trial judge should have considered the teen's maturity, among several other factors, in determining her best interests and should have taken testimony directly from her.

Factors considered by courts in determining the best interests of the minor who refuses medical care include, besides her maturity, her religious convictions, her family's attitude, the effectiveness of the proposed medical treatment, the risk of adverse side effects, the prognosis without treatment, whether treatment can safely be delayed, and the effectiveness of any proposed treatment alternatives.

As Jessica Penkower[51] notes, the "mature minor doctrine" does not really give adolescents autonomy in refusing medical treatment. The best interests of the child standard still applies. No court has given a minor the right to refuse treatment that his parents want him to have. And no reported ruling has provided an explanation of what maturity means when a child chooses to die. Penkower[51] also cites research findings that chronic or severe illness causes more anxiety and despair for adolescents than for adults. It hinders the formation of social and peer relationships, which are so important to teenagers. It may delay puberty or change their appearance in other ways. It exacerbates the feelings of self-doubt and inadequacy common to all teenagers. It increases their dependency on parents at a time when they want to pull away from parents. Those psychosocial factors might influence a teen to refuse medical treatment but be irrelevant to a chronically ill adult.

Evaluating the right of a minor to refuse medical treatment on religious grounds is problematic for many reasons. Jonathan Will[52] calls upon the courts to inquire into whether the teen has the "religious integrity" of "underlying and enduring" values and thus the "… ability to make autonomous decisions." Religion, however, is a social construct imparted to young children by parents. Furthermore, adolescence is almost by definition a time when new values are being developed.

Canadians Ian Mitchell and Juliet Guichon[53] argue that a teen's "freedom from coercion" must be established before allowing him to refuse necessary medical care. They point out that the Jehovah's Witnesses threaten members with shunning and "disfellowshipping" for accepting blood transfusions and hover over members in hospitals. Parents are enjoined to coach and role play with their children on what to say and do to resist transfusions. Children who refuse transfusions are glorified as martyrs to the faith in "Witness" magazines. Mitchell and Guichon[53] ask how a Witness child's decision to refuse a transfusion could ever be considered truly voluntary.

Furthermore, religious faith is itself generally based on assumptions that are counterintuitive to rational premises. Holding that evolution predisposes humans to have faith, anthropologist Boyer and Walker[54] argue that "… at around age seven the child acquires a conceptual ability that makes his/her religious concepts much more similar to adults', that is, based on counterintuitive assumptions *and* clearly distinguished from fiction." If courts allow minors to refuse lifesaving medical treatment based on their ability to explain their religion, they might find that 7-year-olds do as well as many adults.

A textbook case on how not to let a minor die is that of Dennis Lindberg.[55] The boy was first exposed to the Jehovah's Witness faith in 2003 when he went to live with his aunt. She became his legal guardian in 2007. On November 8, 2007, less than 2 months after his fourteenth birthday, Dennis was diagnosed with acute lymphocytic leukemia at Children's Hospital in Seattle with a 75% probability of 5-year survival. Jehovah's Witness nonrelatives were in his room around the clock. The aunt prohibited his other biological relatives from talking to him about his need for transfusions. His grandmother called several times a day; the hospital would not connect her to him, saying that grandparents had no right to talk to him against his guardian's wishes.

Although Washington law requires mandated reporters to report child abuse and neglect to Child Protective Services within 48 hours, the hospital told the aunt on November 20 that their lawyers had determined Dennis was "a mature minor" with a legal right to refuse medical treatment. On November 21, however, the hospital reported Dennis to CPS as a neglected child to, as they said, "… cover all bases and to cover the aunt." But the hospital also told CPS that their physicians thought the boy should be allowed to refuse transfusions. CPS circulated an internal memo saying they could not go to court to seek an order for transfusions because the doctors would not support it. In fact, however, CPS did have a legal right to petition the court.

On November 26, the boy's parents in Idaho were made aware that they could contact CPS and told the agency they wanted their son to have transfusions. CPS asked for a court hearing to be held the next day and flew the parents to Seattle to testify. In court the treating physician testified that Dennis still had a 70% chance of recovery with transfusions, but that he and other physicians on the team considered the boy a mature minor with the right to refuse life-saving medical treatment. He also said he had let other Jehovah's Witness children refuse transfusions and later regretted it. The judge did not see or hear from the boy since Dennis was by then comatose. The next day the judge ruled that Dennis had the right to refuse transfusions because, according to the media in attendance, the boy had religious beliefs against them and because he was mature enough to understand that he "… was basically giving himself a death sentence." Non-Witness friends and relatives attending the hearing said the judge cited no case law or statutes as the basis for his ruling. CPS did not appeal. The boy died later that day. Records of the hearing and ruling are sealed.

Redacted CPS records shown to the boy's parents indicate cursorily that Dennis was "mature, articulate, and adamantly opposed to transfusions," but also indicate that no psychological evaluation was done on the child. They show no awareness of the tremendous social pressure on him with Witnesses around the world praising his refusal on a public webpage, nor of the isolation from non-Witness relatives and friends imposed by his guardian.

Neither competence in explaining religious belief, understanding the benefits and risks of a proposed medical treatment, nor understanding the consequences of refusing treatment justify preventable deaths of children. Surely a minor's understanding that he will die without treatment is not a sufficient basis for letting him do it. Surely a higher bar should be set for a life-and-death decision than for other medical decisions that state laws allow teenagers to make on their own. The "mature minor doctrine" does not really give teens autonomy and is insidiously tied to policies that undermine our social contract to protect vulnerable children.

At the very least, no hospital should determine on its own that a child has a right to die a preventable death. All mandated reporters should promptly report a family's refusal of necessary medical care to state child welfare services, which should evaluate the psychosocial pressures upon the child. The state should promptly petition the court to order medical care, and if the court refuses to order it on the basis of a minor's maturity or religious beliefs, the state should appeal the ruling. At present we have no public records indicating how a court has evaluated a child's maturity and decided to allow a child to refuse care.

States do not allow minors to smoke, drink alcohol, play the lottery, obtain a chauffeur's license, or sign an enforceable contract. The U.S. Supreme Court recently prohibited execution of those who commit crimes as minors.[56] In those respects society acknowledges that teenagers' decision-making skills are not fully formed, and we should protect them from harmful or irreversible consequences of their decisions. Obviously the state should not impose medical treatment on children of any age if it merely prolongs dying, is only experimental, or has risks and side effects that outweigh its benefits. In this writer's view, however, the state should require that parents provide minors up to the age of 18 with the necessities of life, including medical treatment when it has a good probability of preserving life, preventing permanent harm, or significantly improving quality of life.

This should be done not only because of the state's *parens patriae* obligation to children but also because society needs these children. As the U.S. Supreme Court held in *Prince*, our "... democratic society rests, for its continuance" upon children growing "into full maturity as citizens."[27]

References

1. Asser S, Swan R: Child fatalities from religion-motivated medical neglect. *Pediatrics* 1998;101:625-629.
2. Eddy MB: *Science and Health with Key to the Scriptures.* Trustees under the Will of MBG Eddy, Boston, 1934.
3. Christian Science Board of Directors: Concerning use of drugs and medicine. *Christian Sci J* 1945;63:469.
4. Lowen M: First Church of Christ Scientist, Boston: Letter to Fellow Practitioner, April 1977.
5. Hughes R: *The Judge and the Faith Healer.* University Press of America, Lanham, MD, 1989, pp 19-22.
6. Balizet C: *Born in Zion.* Perazim Press, Grapevine, TX, 1996, pp 9-11, 25, 66, 87, 147.
7. Fadiman A: *The Spirit Catches You and You Fall Down.* Farrar, Straus & Giroux, New York, 1998.
8. Kent SA: The globalization of Scientology: influence, control, and opposition in transnational markets. *Religion* 1999;29:147-169.
9. Hubbard LR: *Dianetics: the Modern Science of Mental Health.* Bridge Publications, Los Angeles, 2007.
10. Spiering v. Heineman, 448 F.Supp.2d 1129 (Neb. 2006).
11. Hubbard LR: *The Second Dynamic.* Bridge Publications, Los Angeles, 1988.
12. Watchtower Bible and Tract Society: *How Can Blood Save Your Life?* Watchtower Bible and Tract Society, New York, 1990, pp 3-5, 24-25.
13. Franz R: *In Search of Christian Freedom.* Commentary Press, Atlanta, 1991, p 287.
14. Anon: Answer to "Do Jehovah's Witnesses accept any medical products derived from blood?" *Watchtower*, New York, June 15, 2000.
15. McCarthy v. Boozman, 212 F.Supp.2d 945 (W.D. Ark. 2002).
16. Allen A: Bucking the herd. *Atlantic Monthly* Sep. 2002:40, 42.
17. Furton EJ: Vaccines originating in abortion. *National Catholic Bioethics Center Ethics & Medics* 1999;24:3-4.
18. Lindenberger M: An STD vaccine for all girls? *Time* Jan 17, 2007.
19. Eddy MB: *First Church of Christ, Scientist, and Miscellany.* Trustees under the Will of MBG Eddy, Boston, 1925, p 344.
20. Roegge B: Safe 'in the secret place.' *Christian Science Sentinel*, Nov 14, 2005; pp 8-9.
21. MMWR: Outbreak of measles among Christian Science students—Missouri and Illinois. *MMWR* 1994;43:463-465.
22. Diekema D and AAP Committee on Bioethics: Responding to parental refusals of immunization of children. *Pediatrics* 2005;115:1428-1431.
23. Swan R: Children, medicine, religion, and the law. *Adv Pediatr* 1997;44:522-527.
24. Policy and Legal: Available at http://www.childrenshealthcare.org/. Accessed December 21, 2008.
25. West Virginia State Board of Education v. Barnette, 319 U.S. 624 (1943).
26. Watchtower Bible and Tract Society of New York, Inc. et al. v. Village of Stratton, et al., 556 U.S. 150 (2002).
27. Prince v. Massachusetts, 321 U.S. 166,167 (1944).
28. WV Code 61-8D-2(d).
29. Ark. Code 5-10-101(a)(9)(B).
30. RI General Laws 11-9-5(b).
31. People v. Rippberger, 231 Cal. App. 3d 1667 (Calif. 1991).
32. Bergmann v. State, 486 N.E.2d 653 (Ind. 1985).
33. Commonwealth v. Barnhart, 497 A.2d 616 (Penn. 1985); cert. denied, 488 U.S. 817 (1988).
34. Funkhouser v. State, 763 P.2d 695 (Okla. 1988); cert. denied, 490 U.S. 1066 (1989).
35. Douglas County v. Anaya, 694 N.W.2d 601 (Neb. 2005); Anderson v. State, 65 SE2d 848 (Ga. 1951).
36. Anderson v. State, 65 SE2d 848 (Ga. 1951).
37. Brown v. Stone, 378 So.2d 218 (Miss. 1979).
38. People v. Lybarger, No. 82-CR-205 (Colo. 1982).
39. State v. Miskimens, 490 N.E.2d 931 (Ohio 1984).
40. State v. Miller, Mercer City. Common Pleas Ct., Ohio #86-CRM30 and 31 (1986).
41. Orr R and Craig D: Old enough. *Hastings Center Report* 2007;37:15-16.
42. Derish M and VandenHeuvel K: Mature minors should have the right to refuse life-sustaining medical treatment. *J Law Med Ethics* 2007;28:109-124.
43. Bishop S: Court lets teen forego chemotherapy. *Richmond Times Dispatch*, Aug 17, 2006; A1, A10.
44. In the Matter of Berkley Ross Conner, Jr., 140 P.3d 1167 (Ore. 2006).
45. Bodnaruk ZM, Wong CJ, Thomas MY: Meeting the clinical challenge of care for Jehovah's Witnesses. *Transfus Med Rev* 2004;18:105-116.
46. E.G. v. Baum, 790 S.W.2d 839 (Texas 1990).
47. In re J.J., 582 N.E.2d 1138-1142 (Ohio 1990).
48. Driggs A: Mature minor doctrine: Do adolescents have the right to die? *Health Matrix* 2001;11:687-717.

49. In re E.G., 549 N.E.2d 322 (Illinois 1989).

50. In re Rena, 705 N.E.2d 115 (Mass. 1999).

51. Penkower J: Potential right of chronically ill adolescents to refuse life-saving medical treatment—fatal misuse of the mature minor doctrine. *DePaul Law Rev* 1996;45:1165-1213.

52. Will J: My God, my choice: the mature minor doctrine and adolescent refusal of life-saving or sustaining medical treatment based upon religious beliefs. *J Contemp Health Law Pol* 2006;22:233-300.

53. Mitchell I, Guichon J: Medical emergencies in children of orthodox Jehovah's Witness families. *Paediatr Child Health* 2006;11:655-658.

54. Boyer P, Walker S: Intuitive Ontology and Cultural Input in the Acquisition of Religious Concepts. *In:* Rosengren KS, Johnson CN, Harris PL (eds): *Imagining the Impossible: Magical, Scientific, and Religious Thinking in Children.* Cambridge University Press, Cambridge, UK, 2000, pp 130-156.

55. Swan R: Boy dies after refusing blood. Children's Healthcare Is a Legal Duty, Inc. Newsletter, Number 4, 2007; 1-12.

56. Roper *v.* Simmons, 543 U.S. 551 (2005).

64

THE PREVENTION OF CHILD ABUSE AND NEGLECT

Karyn M. Patno, MD

INTRODUCTION

The effects of abuse and neglect can be devastating. No one would disagree that to prevent abuse and neglect from ever occurring is far more preferable than to provide treatment to try and mend these broken lives. Prevention efforts can be divided into three categories. *Primary prevention* refers to those programs or interventions aimed at the general population without targeting a particular high-risk group. *Secondary prevention* refers to those programs or interventions aimed at a particular segment of the population considered at high risk for a particular condition. *Tertiary prevention* refers to those programs or interventions aimed at a segment of the population that has proved itself to be at risk because of previous experiences, and is actually an attempt to prevent recurrence or other negative consequences.[1,2]

Why has prevention of child maltreatment been so hard to achieve? One reason is that there is not, and never will be, *one* program that prevents all abuse and neglect. The problem is multifactorial and will require an armamentarium of programs. Prevention of abusive head trauma requires a much different strategy than preventing childhood sexual abuse. Likewise, preventing sexual abuse of toddlers will require a different approach from preventing abuse of middle school children.

A second consideration is that prevention does not simply deal with children. In order to prevent abuse and neglect, we must understand the *abusers* and target our intervention directly at them. There is a huge difference between the sociopath who wants to hurt a child and the parent who has no parenting skills and does not know she should not shake her baby. These two abusers require very different prevention strategies.

Another consideration is funding. Prevention is not cheap. In the past more money was available from state and Federal sources. These sources of funding are rapidly shrinking. The private sector has been able to make up for some of the loss in government funding, but in hard economic times, this source also feels the pinch. How can we get state and Federal governments to see the value of prevention? The biggest drawback with prevention is that, in most cases, the rewards are not immediate. There is a time lag between the initiation of an intervention and the resulting change in abuse/neglect statistics. Legislators are reluctant to support bills that put money into efforts that might not come to fruition during their term of office. They want to boast about big results that will bolster their chance at reelection or, at the very least, allow them to retire from office with the reputation of "having made a difference."

Another problem with prevention is that, until recently, there have not been many programs or interventions with scientific data to back up their effectiveness. Recently this has been recognized as an important aspect of prevention program development, and there are now a number of programs with good data available on their effectiveness. This will greatly aid states in their quest for effective prevention.

The goal of this chapter is to present a practical approach to effective prevention along with a resource guide highlighting specific programs. (See Chapter 64 Supplemental Resources online at www.expertconsult.com.)

VICTIM CONSIDERATIONS

Several factors must be taken into consideration when choosing a program with the best potential for effectiveness.

Age

The first factor to consider is the age of the patient. The youngest victims of abuse and neglect are unborn fetuses exposed to health hazards. The most classic example of this is fetal alcohol syndrome (FAS). Millions of children in the United States and a round the world continue to be exposed to alcohol in utero despite efforts to educate the public about the dangers of consuming alcohol during pregnancy. Why have these efforts failed? The alcohol industry is adept at creating and maintaining market share with promotions and advertising that normalizes drinking among youth, young women, and minority groups,[3] fostering the belief that there is a "safe" level of alcohol consumption, and that only those women who are "alcoholic" will damage their infants. The medical profession does not help dispel this myth when doctors tell pregnant women not to worry about having a glass of wine once in a while. If a glass of wine once in a while is acceptable, it must be acceptable to drink alcohol. Current recommendations are that no amount or type of alcohol is safe to consume during pregnancy.[4] It is essential that all medical personnel adopt this recommendation to ensure that pregnant woman understand the seriousness of this issue.

After birth, the next most vulnerable time is from immediately after birth through 12 months of age. During this time, infants and their parents are adjusting to major lifestyle shifts. Parents are often sleep deprived and many are poorly prepared for the demands of parenthood. Identifying risk factors for abuse in the newborn nursery is critical. Preterm infants, multiple gestation, and previous sibling involved with child protective services are all risk factors for abuse, as well as young parental age, lack of social support, maternal depression, and history of domestic violence. If risk factors are identified, referral to visiting nurse services or parent support programs is appropriate. Early follow-up with the primary care physician is also important. An all-too-common abusive injury during this time is abusive head trauma (AHT). Anticipatory guidance regarding infant crying should start in the newborn nursery and continue at all well-child check-ups to 6 months of age. Crying is the single most common antecedent event prior to shaking an infant, making anticipatory guidance about crying critically important.

Once the sedentary infant becomes a "mobile unit," around 10 to 13 months, new dangers await. Mobile children can now get into things and climb on things. Children who are given inadequate supervision are likely to have falls, ingestions, and other injuries, such as burns and lacerations. Toddlers are naturally active and parents who lack coping skills and patience may find themselves frustrated and exasperated by these active children. Parents may inflict injury in an effort to discipline their children and control their activities.

After children become school age, they are no longer only under the supervision of their parents. They now spend a growing portion of their day under the watchful eyes of other caregivers. With more and more children in daycare, this shift in supervisory roles has occurred at younger ages. Parents are confronted with the task of not only protecting their children from the inherent dangers in their own homes, but also from those outside the home. They must ensure that those they entrust with their children are in fact trustworthy. Those parents with poor parenting skills and poor social supports might be more likely to make poor choices in daycare providers and babysitters.

This is also the age when children need to be educated about personal safety. "Good touch-bad touch" is a confusing lesson because "not all bad touches feel bad." Rather, teaching children that they can touch their own private places but no one else should touch the child's private places—and, likewise, that they should not touch anyone else's—can be a helpful lesson. Despite our best efforts to reassure children that they will never get in trouble for telling, children are reluctant to disclose abuse.

The preadolescent presents new challenges for abuse prevention as children exercise their need for independence while lacking insight and mature judgment. Peer pressure and risk-taking behaviors begin and increase into adolescence. Prevention in this group is most effective when done in a peer setting. This may be in school with peer mentors or in group activities with peers. It is important to consider the preadolescent both as a potential victim as well as a potential perpetrator. Prevention aimed at both these aspects of abuse would be most useful in this age group. For prevention to be effective, the preadolescent must "buy in" to the message. They must identify the message as relevant to their experience.

Adolescents pose the challenge of "knowing everything" and believing that adults do not understand them or know what they are going through. The more effective prevention messages are likely to be delivered in relevant language and delivered by their peer group. Sharing real-life events and their repercussions is much more likely to be remembered by the adolescent than a discussion of the hypothetical repercussions of certain actions. Adolescents are much less likely to accept information based on "faith." They need to see and feel the wounds to believe it is real.

Developmental Level

In addition to age, developmental level is important to consider in prevention programs. Children who are developmentally disabled are thought to be at greater risk for abuse.[5,6] They also pose extra challenges to those entrusted with their care, including parents, teachers, and child care providers. These children are much more likely to trust adults and older children. They lack insight into the actions of others and often believe what they are told. Their disability may also limit their ability to report particular events or to escape frightening situations.

Estimates of the prevalence of sexual abuse among developmentally disabled children range from 25% to 83%. Some estimate that the lifelong risk of abuse among the developmentally disabled is 90%.[7] This is in contrast to the prevalence rates of 30% to 40% of girls and 13% of boys experiencing sexual abuse during childhood overall.[8]

There appears to be no clear correlation between level of disability and prevalence for abuse. However, there does appear to be some evidence suggesting that those individuals with mild mental disability are at increased risk of abuse.[7] This may be due to their higher rates of integration into society and their desire to be accepted by their nondisabled peers. Research suggests that about 80% of victims with mental disabilities were abused more then once and that 92% to 99% of the victims knew their abusers. Also, the vast majority of abuse events occurred in the victim's place of residence.[7]

A number of factors make this population of children more at risk for abuse. First is their dependence on others for assistance in activities including activities of daily living. A caregiver may engage in activities that are inappropriate but not recognized as such by the disabled child. These activities can recur on a daily basis and may become the "norm" for the abused child.[5] Also, children and adolescents with mental disabilities often lack friends and, in an attempt to be accepted, may allow themselves to be taken advantage of by other children, adolescents, and/or adults. They are more likely to regard the exploitation as love or friendship without understanding the true intent of their abusers.[6] Another very important factor that contributes to the abuse of the developmentally disabled child/adolescent is the lack of sex education.[6,9] Parents and teachers often consider them asexual and thus dismiss the need for sex education. Often the realization that their disabled child or student has sexual feelings comes too late, after pregnancy or a sexually transmitted infection has occurred. Although the mentally disabled adolescent might go through puberty at a slightly later time (depending on the cause of the disability), they all go through puberty eventually and experience the hormonal changes inherent in that process. It is important to provide education about physical development, puberty, sexuality, sexual responsibility, and safety. A child with Down syndrome will definitely need sex education. However, a mainstreamed sixth-grade classroom may not be the appropriate environment for that sex education to occur. It is important to provide the education on a level that the child can understand and incorporate into his or her life.

LOCATION OF ABUSE

When considering the choice of abuse prevention program, it is important to consider the location where the targeted abuse might occur. Abuse can occur in the home, at school, at day care, or in the community. Community locations include parks, churches, meeting of children's organizations, and at public buildings such as libraries. It is impossible for parents to have direct supervision of their child in all of these locations at all times. Effective prevention programs should consider all these locations and assess the risk of abuse for each. The risk will vary from community to community. What is assessed to be a high-risk situation in one community may be far down the list in another.

One example of location dictating prevention programs is the tragedy of the Catholic Church and its priest abusers. After many substantiated accusations came to light, the Catholic Church acknowledged a need to provide intervention. Most Catholic organizations now use a curriculum aimed at providing the students with skills and knowledge that will help them avoid victimization.

In response to the persistent occurrence of neglect and abuse among young infants, visiting nurse programs were started in an attempt to provide education and parenting training to new parents in their homes.[10] These programs allow parents to gain training in the environment where they will be using the training: in their homes with their infants.

Another example of the importance of considering location in prevention interventions is the residential care facility. Since developmentally disabled individuals face increased risk of abuse,[7] and knowing that the majority of abuse occurs in their place of residence, it is important to have interventions in place in residential facilities. Meticulous screening of employees, frequent peer review activities, video surveillance, and educational in-services on caring for and nurturing children with developmental disabilities can be helpful in ensuring a safe environment for these children.

Schools are important settings when considering child abuse prevention. There are more and more reports of bullying and sexual harassment of students by other students. Curricula are available that can be incorporated into the school academic cycle to provide students with skills and knowledge to avoid being victimized as well as to prevent them from becoming victimizers.[11]

A final example of the importance of location of abuse is the Internet. While the Internet is an amazing resource for students and young people, it has become a venue for sexual predators.[12] Teaching young users the dangers of the Internet and how to avoid exploitation is important. Prevention tools are now available aimed at electronic abuse.[13]

PERPETRATOR CONSIDERATIONS

People who *unintentionally* abuse children are particularly helped by prevention programs. They often abuse or neglect children because they do not know how to safely care for or discipline their children. There is no intent to injure although injury can occur. They are often horrified to learn that their action led to injury of their child and are quite remorseful. Education and training can often solve their problems and prevent future abuse.

Abusive head trauma is a good example in which some perpetrators might not consciously intend to injure their infants. The intent is often to quiet the infant or administer discipline for an undesired behavior. John Caffey[14] noted in his 1972 article, "On the Theory and Practice of Shaking Infants," "The most common motive for repeated whiplash-shaking of infants and young children is to correct minor misbehavior. Such shakings are generally considered innocuous by both parents and physicians." Parents, especially first-time parents, are often ill equipped to deal with the demands of a crying infant. In their efforts to comfort their child they become frustrated and angry when the infant does not respond. If they allow themselves to reach the "breaking point" of frustration, they can find themselves grabbing the infant and vigorously shaking. Again Caffey describes this as "… instinctive, almost reflex, violent actions by angry adults in the commission of willful assault. …"[14] He goes on to say that these same adults would never think of hitting their young infants but think nothing of administering a "good shake." Educational programs aimed at teaching parents the dangers of shaking have been shown to decrease occurrence of shaken baby syndrome.[2]

Parents who had poor parenting themselves are at higher risk for perpetuating abuse. C. Henry Kempe wrote in 1962, "It would appear that one of the most important factors to be found in families where parental assault occurs is 'to do unto others as you have been done by.'"[15] Choosing a prevention program that provides parenting skills and nurturing skills to high-risk parents would help break the cycle of violence.

Another group of unintentional abusers are those with mental health issues. A good example of this group is the new mother suffering from postpartum depression. When an injury occurs, she might not be capable of understanding what she is doing, even if her actions are deliberate. Depression can be so severe that mothers of newborns lose perspective on their actions and feel no emotional connection to their infants. The best intervention in this case is early recognition of postpartum depression and immediate treatment.

When child abuse is done *intentionally*, prevention becomes much more difficult. Intentional abusers are a much more diverse group, and different issues are involved when people abuse children physically, sexually, or emotionally, or when people knowingly neglect children.

Sexual Abusers

Finkelhor[16] has proposed a model consisting of four preconditions that lead to sexual abuse. Understanding these preconditions allows the targeting of interventions toward specific factors that have the potential to prevent sexual abuse. The four preconditions are (1) motivation to sexually abuse, (2) suppression of internal inhibitors, (3) lack of external inhibitors, and (4) lack of resistance by the child victim. The abuser must feel that sexually relating to the child will satisfy some emotional need and he must feel sexually aroused by the child. Sometimes there is a lack of alternative sources of sexual gratification, leaving the child as the only option.

Next the perpetrator must overcome internal inhibitors. Although he knows it is wrong to have sexual contact with the child, he finds a way to block those thoughts. This can be accomplished through the use of substances, such as alcohol or drugs. Perpetrators suffering from some types of mental illness or impulse disorders can more easily overcome internal inhibitors.

External inhibitors are those factors that usually protect the child. When a mother is not present or not emotionally connected to the child, the child is much more vulnerable to abuse. Girls from families that are socially isolated are much more vulnerable to abuse by family members as well as by family acquaintances. The girls have fewer supports and are physically available to potential perpetrators. Parents with poor parenting skills might provide poor supervision of their children, leaving them available to potential perpetrators.

The final precondition, resistance by the child, refers to the child's ability to defend herself against abuse. Children who are emotionally insecure or deprived of parental love may unknowingly allow inappropriate advances from a perpetrator. Intellectually challenged children are less able to understand that an adult is doing something bad to them and thus might allow the action. Some adults use coercion to force the child to allow the abuse to occur. The Finkelhor model is very useful when considering sexual abuse prevention strategies because an intervention can be directed at any one of the four areas described in the model.

Other Types of Abusers

Child abusers are a diverse group. For example, people with antisocial personality disorder have no consideration of others and act to meet their own aberrant needs. Prevention efforts directed toward changing their behaviors are often met with failure. The best approach with this group is to strengthen external inhibitors and/or equip the child with better avoidance skills. Another type of abuser that belongs in this group is the adult that inflicts injury on a child with the intention of hurting. They use corporal punishment or think nothing of hitting children when they misbehave. Their actions often result in minor injury but can also result in major injury or even death. Another group of intentional abusers are mothers who kill their children as acts of revenge (e.g., to get even with spouses who are "cheating on them") or as acts of mercy (e.g., killing a disabled child that will have to face a cruel and unfair world).[17]

Although this description of intentional abusers is not all inclusive, it is clear that the characteristics of the abusers vary widely, making intervention to prevent abuse very difficult. Prevention can include efforts to change the behavior of the abuser, to strengthen internal inhibitors, to strengthen external inhibitors, and to equip victims with the ability to escape and evade the perpetrators.

Reactive Child and Adolescent Abusers

Reactive abusers are a special group consisting of children who were victimized and who then become abusive to other children. Some estimates suggest that child perpetrators under age 13 account for 18% of child sexual abuse cases.[18]

If one increases the age to under age 18, the percentage of child perpetrators is as high as 40%. Children tend to perpetrate against other children younger than themselves, with the average age of child perpetrators ranging from 6 to 8 years, while their victims' average age ranges from 4 to 6 years. It is important to realize that not all child perpetrators are victims of sexual abuse, but it is definitely a risk factor. Other risk factors include high rates of familial distress (including domestic violence); sexual perpetration within the family or extended family; child physical abuse; parental arrest and incarceration; and failure to take responsibility for others' sexual abuse within the family or extended family.[18] In this group of abusers it is important to identify risk factors in the family. Prevention efforts can start with anticipatory guidance around issues such as discipline, substance abuse, and appropriate supervision. Referral to child and family counseling as well as counseling for domestic violence is essential to help break the cycle of abuse.

PREVENTION PROGRAMS WITH SCIENTIFIC DATA ON OUTCOME

Some prevention programs have good data supporting their effectiveness. There are also a few programs with little outcome data available, but the programs show promise based on program design and target. There are many programs being implemented to prevent abuse, but few have been studied carefully. Fortunately, this trend is changing. More programs are collecting data and analyzing the true effectiveness of the prevention strategies. In the future, it should be easier to identify effective evidence-based prevention programs.

CONCLUSION

When choosing a prevention program, consider several factors. First, choose the desired outcome (e.g., decrease abusive head trauma). Then identify the target population. In the above example the target population would be parents and caregivers of young infants. Next, decide on the program focus. Is the program a "primary intervention" focused at all parents and caregivers of young infants? Or will a secondary intervention be used, aimed at only high-risk parents and caregivers? Once the desired outcome and target population have been identified, the most effective intervention program can be chosen.

A description of several child abuse and neglect prevention programs can be found online at www.expertconsult.com. (See Chapter 64 Supplemental Resources.)

References

1. Barron C: Prevention of abusive head trauma in infants. *Med Health RI* 2003;86:383-384.
2. Dias MS, Smith K, deGuehery K, et al: Preventing abusive head trauma among infants and young children: a hospital-based, parent education program. *Pediatrics* 2005;115:e470-477.
3. Glik D, Prelip M, Myerson A, et al: Fetal alcohol prevention using community-based narrowcasting campaigns. *Health Promot Pract* 2008;9:93-103.
4. American Academy of Pediatrics. Committee on Substance Abuse and Committee on Children with Disabilities: Fetal alcohol syndrome and alcohol-related neurodevelopmental disorders. *Pediatrics* 2000;106:358-361.

5. Tharinger D, Horton C, Millea S: Sexual abuse and exploitation of children and adults with mental retardation and other handicaps. *Child Abuse Negl* 1990;14:301-312.

6. McCabe M, Cummins R, Reid S: An empirical study of the sexual abuse of people with intellectual disability. *Sex Disabil* 1994;12:297-306.

7. Levy H, Packman W: Sexual abuse prevention for individuals with mental retardation: considerations for genetic counselor. *J Genet Couns* 2004;13:189-205.

8. Bolen RM, Scannapieco M: Prevalence of child sexual abuse: a corrective metanalysis. *Soc Serv Rev* 1999;73:281-313.

9. Lumley V, Miltenberger R: Sexual abuse prevention for persons with mental retardation. *Am J Ment Retard* 1997;101:459-472.

10. Olds DL, Henderson CR Jr, Kitzman HJ, et al: Prenatal and infancy home visitation by nurses: recent findings. *Future Child* 1999;9:44-65, 190-191.

11. Dake JA, Price JH, Telljohann SK, et al: Teacher perceptions and practices regarding school bullying prevention. *J Sch Health* 2003;73:347-512.

12. Wolak J, Ybarra ML, Mitchell K, et al: Current research knowledge about adolescent victimization via the Internet. *Adolesc Med State Art Rev* 2007;18:325-341, xi.

13. Wolak J, Finkelhor D, Mitchell KJ, et al: Online "predators" and their victims: myths, realities, and implications for prevention and treatment. *Am Psychol* 2008;63:111-128.

14. Caffey J: On the theory and practice of shaking infants: its potential residual effect of permanent brain damage and mental retardation. *Am J Dis Child* 1972;124:161-169.

15. Kempe CH, Silverman F, Steele B, et al: The battered-child syndrome. *JAMA* 1962;181:17-24.

16. Finkelhor D: *Child Sexual Abuse: New Theory and Research.* The Free Press, New York, 1984, pp 53-61.

17. Rouge-Maillart C, Jousset N, Gaudin A, et al: Women who kill their children. *Am J Forensic Med Pathol* 2005;26:320-326.

18. Worley K, Church J: When children abuse other children. *J Ark Med Soc* 2007;103:205-208.

65

CARING FOR FOSTER CHILDREN

Kristine Fortin, MD, MPH

INTRODUCTION

UNICEF's Convention on the Rights of the Child recognizes children's right to the highest attainable standard of health and access to health care services.[1] Foster children, who numbered over half a million on a given day in the United States in 2006,[2] are susceptible to poor health. The abuse and neglect endured prior to placement, as well as the stress of being displaced from their homes, engender a high prevalence of physical, mental, and developmental health problems among foster children. Multiple barriers to health care access also impede foster children from achieving optimal health. Governments and organizations such as the American Academy of Pediatrics have set forth guidelines and policies aimed at improving the health status of foster children. Different models of foster care and health care delivery have been studied in relation to health outcomes. Older children transitioning out of foster care face many challenges and require special consideration.

PREVALENCE AND NATURE OF HEALTH PROBLEMS

Neglect, abandonment, and abuse are common reasons for foster care placement.[3] The physical and psychological consequences of physical abuse, sexual abuse, and neglect, as well as the trauma of being removed from the home, engender physical, emotional, and developmental problems. In addition, other risk factors associated with poor physical and mental health such as lack of medical care, poverty, homelessness, violence in the home, parental substance abuse, parental mental illness, and premature birth are often present.[3]

The prevalence of health problems among children in foster care has been studied using different outcome measures and timing with respect to foster care placement. Chernoff et al[4] evaluated the health status of 1407 children at the time of entry into care and found that 12% required routine follow-up only, whereas the remaining 88% required at least one referral for further medical, dental, or mental health care. Among the children referred for additional services, almost 25% required three or more referrals. The prevalence of chronic conditions among foster children has been estimated at between 30% and 80%,[5,6] and an estimated 25% of foster children have three or more chronic conditions.[5] The health problems of foster children are multiple and complex, and they affect physical, mental and developmental health.

Chernoff et al[4] found that 92% of children examined at a specialized clinic at the time of entry into foster care had at least one abnormality on physical examination. A medical problem was identified on history, physical examination, or screening tests among 60% of foster children examined at a San Francisco Child Protection Center.[7] Studies have shown that respiratory problems such as asthma and upper respiratory infections as well as allergic and infectious skin conditions were among the most common physical health problems for children entering care.[4,7] Dental caries, pediculosis, anemia, delayed immunizations, and failed vision and hearing screens are also common.[4,5,7-10] A disproportionate number of foster children are below the fifth percentile for height, weight, and head circumference.[4,5,8] Children in foster care must be evaluated for signs of inflicted injury.[8] Risk factors for vertically or sexually transmitted infections must also be assessed. Adolescents in foster care are more likely to engage in high-risk sexual behaviors compared with a group of adolescents not in care.[11]

Estimates for the prevalence of developmental problems among foster children have ranged from 20% to 60%.[5,12,13] Lack of stimulation, exposure to violence, trauma, and lack of a stable caregiver negatively affect child development. Because brain growth and development are active in infancy and childhood, children's brains are vulnerable to environmental risk factors.[14] Biological risk factors for developmental delay such as perinatal drug exposure, prematurity, and nutritional deficiencies can also be present. Neglected and abused children often fail to establish solid attachment to a caretaker. Attachment disorders can manifest with behaviors such as hiding food, self stimulation, and indiscrimination toward adults. Gross and fine motor skills as well as speech can also be compromised. Lack of stimulation makes it difficult to develop vocabulary and communication skills.[14] The effect of trauma and neglect on brain development can also lead to behavioral difficulties including hypervigilence, hyperactivity, impulsiveness, apathy, and sleep disorders.[14] School difficulties are prevalent among older children in care. In Chernoff et al's[4] cohort, 40% of school-aged children repeated a grade.

Research and practice have shown that foster children have a high prevalence of mental health and behavioral problems.[3,4,8,13,15-24] In Pilowsky's[15] review of the literature from 1974 to 1994, prevalence estimates for mental health problems among foster children ranged from 29% to 96%. Experiences prior to foster care placement including abuse, neglect, and witnessing violence place children at risk for mental health problems. The experience of being removed from the home, separation from siblings, changing schools, as well as placement changes can also be traumatic. Chernoff et al[4] found that close to 75% of their cohort of children entering care had a family history of mental illness. Traumatic experiences can result in anxiety, hypervigilence, and posttraumatic stress disorder.[3] Depression, conduct disorder, attention deficit disorder, and oppositional defiant disorder can also be present. Chernoff et al[4] found that 15% of children older than 3 years had suicidal ideation and 7% had homicidal ideation at the time of entry into care.

In addition to the physical and mental health problems experienced during childhood, children in foster care are at risk for long-term adverse outcomes. Foster children are at increased risk of unemployment, criminal conviction, substance abuse, lower educational attainment, homelessness, and poor mental health in adulthood.[25-28] In a British cohort, adults with a history of foster care were more likely to perceive their health as poor compared with controls.[26] A review of outcomes for youth leaving care showed that 18% to 42% had a history of incarceration.[28]

The prevalent physical and mental health care problems of foster children are costly. A California study of Medi-Cal claims revealed a 70% greater cost per eligible child for foster children compared with other Medi-Cal eligible children.[29] A Pennsylvania study found that expenditures for the mental health care of foster children were 11.5 times greater than those of Medicaid eligible controls,[19] and a Florida study found that behavioral health care costs for foster children were over eight times higher than for Medicaid-enrolled nonfoster children.[30] In addition to short-term direct health care costs, long-term physical and mental health problems also engender health care costs. As discussed previously, foster children are at risk for outcomes such as criminal conviction and substance abuse in adulthood, and ensuing indirect costs exist.[31] Loss of productivity and loss of tax revenues also engender costs to society.[31] The human costs of emotional and physical suffering are immeasurable.

BARRIERS TO HEALTH CARE

The prevalence of short- and long-term health problems among foster children, as well as the high human and societal costs, delineates the need for optimal health care delivery. However, multiple barriers hinder the fulfillment of foster children's health care needs. Despite their high need for quality coordinated and comprehensive services, foster children are underserved. A 1995 review of health services for children 36 months of age and younger in foster placement in New York, California, and Pennsylvania found that less than half had all of their health care needs met, and 19% and 32% had none or only some of the health care needs met, respectively.[32] In addition, 12% of children in foster placement received no routine health care and 34% received no immunizations.[32] Leslie et al[24] studied a national U.S. sample of children ages 2 to 15 in foster care and found that a quarter of children in need of mental health services had not received them after approximately 12 months in out-of-home care.[24] Furthermore, the need for services was not the only factor predicting whether services were obtained; young children and African American children were less likely to receive mental health services.[24] A national study of U.S. child welfare agencies found that 57% of the agencies

sampled did not provide comprehensive physical, mental, and developmental evaluations for all children entering foster care.[5] Recent studies highlight concerning trends in the prescription of psychotropic medications for foster children.[33,34] Among foster children receiving psychotropic medication in Texas, 41.3% were dispensed psychotropic medications from three or more drug classes at the same time.[33] Furthermore, 22.2% of foster youth with concomitant psychotropic medications were prescribed two or more drugs in the same drug class.[33] A national study of psychotropic medication use among foster youth with autism spectrum disorder found not only that foster youth were twice as likely to receive concomitant psychotropic medications compared with children on Social Security Income (SSI) but also that there was marked variation in psychotropic medication use across states.[34]

Placement instability impedes optimal health and health care. Placement changes jeopardize the continuity of care and have been associated with poor behavioral and mental health outcomes.[8,16,17,22,35] A study of foster children's use of the emergency department showed that children with multiple placements were more reliant on the emergency department for ambulatory care.[36] Rubin et al[16] categorized children according to baseline risk for placement instability and studied the relationship between actual placement stability during the first 18 months in care and behavioral outcomes. Across all levels of baseline risk for placement instability, children with unstable placement after 18 months in care were at twice the odds for behavioral problems compared with children who achieved stable placement.[16] Qualitative evidence also exists that placement instability is detrimental. Focus groups of adolescents who had at least 1 year in foster care reported that changes in foster homes had the most influence on mental health, and a participant likened foster care to "being tossed around like a little ball."[17]

Another barrier to optimal health care is a lack of information regarding children's past medical histories.[4,8,37] Fragmented health care from multiple providers can compound the difficulty of obtaining medical records.[8] Lack of information can lead to the omission or duplication of health care interventions such as immunizations and screening.[4,37] Sharing of information among social services, physicians, foster parents, biological parents, and children is an additional challenge and can lead to miscommunication.[8,9] The health care needs of foster children are complex and the resources and training necessary to meet these needs are not always available. Many health care providers do not receive training specific to foster children.[3] Providers caring for foster children require more time to address the complex needs of this population.[3,21] Foster parents often receive limited information about health care.[21] A qualitative study revealed that foster parents had difficulty accessing services and had not been adequately informed of their foster child's health care needs.[38] Lack of financial and health care resources also impede the fulfillment of foster children's health care needs.[5,8]

POLICIES AND GUIDELINES

Guidelines and policies have been established in response to the complex health care needs of foster children and the obstacles impeding the provision of optimal care. U.S.

federal policies address issues such as permanency, benefits, funding, performance tracking, and transitions out of care.[39] The first federal foster care program was established in 1961 with the Aid to Families with Dependent Children Foster care program.[39] This program, under Title IV-A of the Social Security Act, provided funds to care for children who could not safely remain with their families. However, there was little monitoring of children's care in the child welfare system, and federal laws made finding permanent homes fiscally disadvantageous.[39] The 1980 Adoption Assistance and Child Welfare Act (AACWA) under Title IV-E of the Social Security Act stipulated that "reasonable efforts" be made to prevent out of home placement and to reunify foster children with their families.[39] Another change brought about by the AACWA was that foster children were made eligible for federal adoption assistance payments and Medicaid.[39] Permanency was one of the focuses of the 1997 Adoption and Safe Families Act (ASFA). The ASFA stipulated that permanency hearings were required after no more than 12 months in care and that, with specified exceptions, termination of parental rights be initiated for children in care for 15 of the last 22 months.[39] The safety of foster children was also addressed, requiring, for example, that states develop standards for the health of children in care and that foster homes be fully licensed in order to obtain federal funding.[39] The ASFA identified kinship care as an option for permanent placement. The ASFA also required the Department of Health and Human Services to track and annually report on state performance.

Guidelines for the evaluation and treatment of the physical, developmental, and mental health care needs have been established by The Child Welfare League of America and the American Academy of Pediatrics (AAP).[9,14,21,40,41] The AAP's District II Task Force on Health Care for Children in Foster Care published a reference manual detailing guidelines for the health care of foster children.[8]

The AAP recommends that health care services for foster children be comprised of the following components: initial health screening, comprehensive health assessment, developmental and mental health evaluation, and ongoing monitoring of health status.[9] The Task Force on Health Care for Children in Foster Care recommends that the initial health screening be completed within 24 hours of removal with the goal of identifying health problems requiring immediate intervention.[8] The initial health screen should include vital signs, anthropometric measurements, examination of all body surfaces unclothed for signs of abuse, inspection of the external genitalia and anus, as well as identification of acute illness and infectious diseases such as pediculosis.[8,9] It is important to evaluate the stability of chronic illness and to ensure that necessary medications are prescribed.[8,9] The initial evaluation should also include screening for developmental and mental health problems including suicidal ideation.[8]

The comprehensive health assessment for foster children should be completed within 1 month of placement per AAP recommendations.[8,9] The goal of the comprehensive evaluation is to identify physical, developmental and mental health problems and to develop a treatment plan for the child. All available medical and social information should be reviewed. The complete review of systems should include the child's adaptation to the new living environment. A thorough physical examination should include an evaluation of the child's dentition. Clinical and laboratory screening tests should be completed as recommended by the AAP.[9] The need for sexually transmitted infection testing and pregnancy prevention counseling should be assessed. The AAP committee on Pediatric AIDS published guidelines for the identification and treatment of HIV for infants, children, and adolescents in foster care.[41] Establishing immunization status can be complicated by the unavailability of prior medical records. The Task Force on Health Care for Children in Foster Care recommends that if, despite every effort, the immunization record cannot be located after 60 days after placement, immunizations should be administered according to the AAP catch-up schedules.[8] The comprehensive evaluation should result in an individualized treatment plan and referral to the necessary health services.[8]

Comprehensive mental health and development assessments are also recommended within 30 days of placement.[8,14] Fine and gross motor skills, language, cognition, and social skills should be evaluated. Evaluation of suicidal ideation, affect, substance abuse, risky sexual behaviors, and prior history of trauma should be included in the mental health assessment. Finally, ongoing monitoring of health status is important not only to deliver routine pediatric care, but also to detect problems that were not apparent on initial evaluation and to assess adjustment to foster care.[8,9]

MODELS OF FOSTER CARE AND HEALTH CARE DELIVERY

Different models of foster care have been studied with respect to their impact on health outcomes. In light of the increasing number of foster children in kinship care,[14,18] the advantages and disadvantages of placing children with relatives or caretakers with close family ties as opposed to with nonrelative foster parents have been debated. It has been suggested that relative caretakers receive less support and follow-up from social services.[10,14,18] Kinship care has also been associated with delayed reunification[3] and fewer health care services compared with nonrelative foster placements.[10,14,18] Relative caretakers are more likely to be older, single, in poor health, and of lower socioeconomic status compared with nonrelative foster parents.[3,10] Stability has been highlighted as an advantage of kinship care. Research suggests that children placed with relatives are less likely to change placements.[10,18] Children placed with relatives experience less change in culture, religion, and family values[14,18,40,42] and are more likely to remain in the same neighborhood.[18] Studies have associated kinship care with improved behavioral outcomes.[10,18] A national study controlling for placement stability, reunification, and baseline risk and using the Child Behavioral Checklist as an outcome measure estimated that 32% of children in early kinship care had behavioral problems 3 years after initial placement compared with 46% of children in nonrelative foster care.[10]

Other models of foster care include group placements and therapeutic foster homes, which can be useful for children with significant behavioral or emotional problems.[25] Private organizations have developed foster care programs. For example, the Casey Family Programs are privately funded foster care programs offering enhanced services such as summer camps and counseling, lighter caseloads for case workers, and college scholarships for children in care.[25] When compared with youth serviced by public foster care, graduates of the Casey Family Programs had a lower prevalence of depression, anxiety, and substance abuse on interviews conducted 1 to 13 years after leaving care.[25]

Various solutions for the improvement of delivery and coordination of care for foster children have been proposed. The AAP recommends that child welfare agencies ensure transfer of medical information among health professionals and highlights the importance of communication between providers, child protection agencies, foster parents, and biological parents.[9] Medical passports and electronic records have been proposed to facilitate communication and continuity of care.[4,14,37,43] Different models of care have been used to service foster children, and their feasibility varies according to the local structure of the child protective services agency and available resources. Specialized clinics for foster children, clinics based in child protective agencies, and community-based care have been described.[6,21] A Connecticut study comparing community-based care to a specialized multidisciplinary program found that foster children serviced by the latter were more likely to be identified with mental health and developmental problems, to be referred for services, and to receive services when referred.[43]

OLDER CHILDREN IN FOSTER CARE

Youth aging out of the foster require special consideration. This population is at increased risk for homelessness, lower educational attainment, poor mental health, substance abuse, and criminal justice system involvement.[27,28,44-46] In a Midwestern U.S. study of emancipated foster youths, more than half were uninsured.[27] Policies to address the needs of this population include the Foster Care Independence Act of 1999.[39,44] This act established the John H. Chafee Foster Care Independence Program, which provides funding for independent living activities and gives states the option to extend Medicaid coverage to age 21 for emancipated foster youth.[39] Continued efforts to improve education, health care access, housing, and transition to independent living are needed for this high-risk population.

DIRECTIONS FOR FUTURE RESEARCH

A high prevalence of physical, mental, and developmental health problems among foster children has been established. New problems such as HIV have emerged since the initial studies conducted in the 1970s, underscoring the need for ongoing health status assessment for the population of foster children. Continued monitoring of health care delivery as well as of the effectiveness of policies, guidelines, and interventions aimed at improving access to care are also warranted. Further evaluation of health outcomes associated with models of foster care and health care is needed. Despite current policies and guidelines, multiple barriers to health care delivery to foster children remain, as does a need for research on the effectiveness of existing and novel solutions.

Given the growing number of children in care as well as their susceptibility to a range of health problems, many professionals will encounter the challenges and rewards of caring for foster children. The prevalence of unmet health care needs among foster children and the multiple barriers to adequate care summon advocates for individual children as well as for the foster care population as a whole.

References

1. United Nations Children's Emergency Fund: Convention on the Rights of the Child. Available at http://www.unicef.org/crc/. Accessed September 16, 2008.
2. U.S. Department of Health and Human Services Administration for Children and Families, Children's Bureau: The AFCARS Report No. 14: preliminary FY 2006 estimates as of January 2008. Available at http://www.acf.hhs.gov/programs/cb/stats_research/afcars/tar/report14.htm. Accessed September 16, 2008.
3. Simms MD, Dubowitz H, Szilagyi MA: Health care needs of children in the foster care system. *Pediatrics* 2000;106:909-918.
4. Chernoff R, Combs-Orme T, Risley-Curtiss C, et al: Assessing the health status of children entering foster care. *Pediatrics* 1994;93:594-601.
5. Leslie LK, Hurlburt MS, Landsverk J, et al: Comprehensive assessments for children entering foster care: a national perspective. *Pediatrics* 2003;112:134-142.
6. Simms MD: The foster care clinic: a community program to identify treatment needs for children in foster care. *J Dev Behav Pediatr* 1989;10:121-128.
7. Takayama JI, Wolfe E, Coulter KP: Relationship between reason for placement and medical findings among children in foster care. *Pediatrics* 1998;101:201-207.
8. AAP District II Task Force on Health Care for Children in Foster Care: *Fostering Health: Health Care for Children and Adolescents in Foster Care*, ed 2. American Academy of Pediatrics, Elk Grove Village, IL, 2005.
9. American Academy of Pediatrics Committee on Early Childhood, Adoption, and Dependant Care: Health care of children in foster care. *Pediatrics* 1994;93:335-338.
10. Rubin DM, Downes KJ, O'Reilly AL, et al: Impact of kinship care on behavioral well-being for children in out-of-home care. *Arch Pediatr Adolesc Med* 2008;162:550-556.
11. Carpenter SC, Clyman RB, Davidson AJ, et al: The association of foster care or kinship care with adolescent sexual behavior and first pregnancy. *Pediatrics* 2001;108:E46.
12. Stahmer AC, Leslie LK, Hurlburt M, et al: Developmental and behavioral needs and service use for young children in child welfare. *Pediatrics* 2005;116:891-900.
13. Leslie LK, Gordon JN, Meneken L, et al: The physical, developmental, and mental health needs of young children in child welfare by initial placement type. *J Dev Behav Pediatr* 2005;26:177-185.
14. American Academy of Pediatrics Committee on Early Childhood, Adoption and Dependent Care: Developmental issues for young children in foster care. *Pediatrics* 2000;106:1145-1150.
15. Pilowsky D: Psychopathology among children placed in family foster care. *Psychiatr Serv* 1995;46:906-910.
16. Rubin DM, O'Reilly AL, Luan X, et al: The impact of placement stability on behavioral well-being for children in foster care. *Pediatrics* 2007;119:336-344.
17. Ellermann CR: Influences on the mental health of children placed in foster care. *Fam Community Health* 2007;30:s23-s32.
18. Holtan A, Ronning JA, Helge Handegard B, et al: A comparison of mental health problems in kinship and nonkinship foster care. *Eur Child Adolesc Psychiatry* 2005;14:201-207.
19. Harman JS, Childs GE, Kelleher KJ: Mental health care utilization and expenditures by children in foster care. *Arch Pediatr Adolesc Med* 2000;154:1114-1117.
20. Zito JM, Safer DJ, Sai D, et al: Psychotropic medication patterns among youth in foster care. *Pediatrics* 2008;121:e157-163.
21. American Academy of Pediatrics Committee on Early Childhood, Adoption, and Dependant Care: Health care of young children in foster care. *Pediatrics* 2002;109:536-541.
22. James S, Landsverk J, Slymen DJ, et al: Predictors of outpatient mental health service use – the role of foster care placement changes. *Ment Health Serv Res* 2004;6:127-141.
23. Sawyer MG, Carbone JA, Searle AK, et al: The mental health and wellbeing of children and adolescents in home-based foster care. *Med J Aust* 2007;186:181-184.

24. Leslie LK, Hurlburt MS, Barth R, et al: Outpatient mental health services for children in foster care: a national perspective. *Child Abuse Negl* 2004;28:697-712.

25. Kesler RC, Pecora PJ, Willims J, et al: Effects of enhanced foster care on the long-term physical and mental health of foster care alumni. *Arch Gen Psychiatry* 2008;65:625-633.

26. Viner RM, Taylor B: Adult health and social outcomes of children who have been in public care: population-based study. *Pediatrics* 2005;115:894-899.

27. Kushel MB, Yen IH, Gee L, et al: Homelessness and health care access after emancipation: results from the Midwest evaluation of adult functioning of former foster youth. *Arch Pediatr Adolesc Med* 2007;161: 986-993.

28. Tweddle A: Youth leaving care: how do they fare? *New Dir Youth Dev* 2007;113:15-31.

29. Halfon N, Berkowitz G, Klee L: Children in foster care in California: an examination of Medicaid reimbursed health services utilization. *Pediatrics* 1992;89:1230-1237.

30. Becker M, Jordan N, Larsen R: Behavioral health service use and costs among children in foster care. *Child Welfare* 2006;85:633-647.

31. Conrad C: Measuring costs of child abuse and neglect: a mathematical model of specific cost estimations. *J Health Hum Serv Adm* 2006;29: 103-123.

32. U.S. General Accounting Office: Foster care: health care needs of many young children are unknown and unmet. Available at http://www.gao.gov/archive/1995/he95114.pdf. Accessed February 28, 2010.

33. Rubin DM, Alessandrini EA, Feudtner C, et al: Placement stability and mental health costs for children in foster care. *Pediatrics* 2004; 113:1336-1341.

34. Rubin DM, Feudtner C, Localio R, et al: State variation in psychotropic medication use by foster children with autism spectrum disorder. *Pediatrics* 2009;124:e305-e312.

35. Zito JM, Safer DJ, Sai D, et al: Psychotropic medication patterns among youth in foster care. *Pediatrics* 2008;121:e157-e163.

36. Rubin DM, Alessandrini EA, Feudtner C, et al: Placement changes and emergency department visits in the first year of foster care. *Pediatrics* 2004;114:e354-360.

37. DiGiuseppe DL, Christakis DA: Continuity of care for children in foster care. *Pediatrics* 2003;111:e208-213.

38. Lauver LS: Parenting foster children with chronic illness and complex medical needs. *J Fam Nurs* 2008;14:74-96.

39. Allen M, Bissell M: Safety and stability for foster children: the policy context. *Future Child* 2004;14:48-73.

40. Child Welfare League of America: *Standards for Health Care Services for Children in Out-of-Home Care.* Child Welfare League of America, Washington DC, 1988.

41. American Academy of Pediatrics Committee on Pediatric AIDS: Identification and care of HIV-exposed and HIV-infected infants, children and adolescents in foster care. *Pediatrics* 2000;106:149-153.

42. Barth RP: Kinship care and lessened child behavioral problems: possible meanings and implications. *Arch Pediatr Adolesc Med* 2008;162: 586-587.

43. McCue Horwitz S, Owens P, Simms MD: Specialized assessments for children in foster care. *Pediatrics* 2000;106:59-66.

44. Pecora PJ: Providing better opportunities for older children in the child welfare system. *Arch Pediatr Adolesc Med* 2007;161:1006-1008.

45. Pecora PJ, Kessler RC, O'Brien K, et al: Educational and employment outcomes of adults formerly placed in foster care: results from the Northwest Foster Care Alumni Study. *Child Youth Serv Rev* 2006;28: 1459-1481.

46. Courtney ME, Piliavin I, Grogan-Kaylor A, et al: Foster youth transitions to adulthood: a longitudinal view of youth leaving care. *Child Welfare* 2001;80:685-717.

66

THE RESPONSE OF PROFESSIONAL AND OTHER NONPROFIT ORGANIZATIONS TO CHILD MALTREATMENT

Robert W. Block, MD, FAAP, and Tammy Piazza Hurley, BA

INTRODUCTION

In the United States, the first recorded organizational response to child abuse was made by the American Society for the Prevention of Cruelty to Animals (ASPCA).[1] Responding to the now famous case of Mary Ellen in 1873, the ASPCA recognized the responsibility of organizations to prevent and intervene in cases of child abuse. However, child maltreatment was typically not an interest of health care professional organizations prior to the early 1960s. Over the last 45 years, several organizations either have added child maltreatment issues to their priorities, or have been formed primarily to respond to those issues. This has created new interest in clinical practice, scholarship, research, and advocacy to address the continuing problems of child abuse and neglect.

Many organizations deserve recognition for their important contributions to collaborative efforts to reduce and respond to the problem of violence and abuse. Those making important medically focused contributions serve as the focus of this chapter.

THE AMERICAN ACADEMY OF PEDIATRICS

The American Academy of Pediatrics (AAP) is the premier association whose mission is to improve the health and well-being of all children. The AAP was founded in 1930 in response to the need for an independent pediatric forum to address children's needs. Since its inception, the AAP has made a huge impact on advocacy, research, and practice in pediatrics in general and in the field of child abuse and neglect. The issue of child abuse and neglect was first addressed by the AAP Committee on the Infant and Preschool Child in 1962 when the AAP's Executive Board advised the Committee to address the issue of "the battered child syndrome" at the national level, working closely with the Children's Bureau, the National Council of Juvenile Court Judges and other agencies in the field.[2] In the mid-1970s, the AAP's Task Force on Child Abuse and Neglect was established to visit health-based centers to discuss child abuse and neglect under a contract with the U.S. Department of Health Education and Welfare's Health Resources Administration. The Task Force reported their findings to the government agency, which in turn passed on the report to physicians, hospitals, and state and local welfare authorities. The Task Force developed a Self-Instructional Program in Child Abuse and Neglect as an educational tool for communities. With the sun-setting on the Task Force, the Committee on the Infant and Preschool Child established a Subcommittee on Child Abuse and Neglect. The Subcommittee worked with Academy staff and the Task Force on a contract to prepare a manual on child abuse; *The Visual Diagnosis of Non-Accidental Trauma and Failure to Thrive* by Barton D. Schmitt, which was published in 1979.[3]

With a lack of dedication to child abuse and neglect by the now combined Committee on Early Childhood, Adoption and Dependent Care, the Task Force on Child Abuse and Neglect was once again established. A resolution was proposed to appoint a committee to address the widespread problem of child abuse and neglect and the dramatic increase in sexual abuse of young children. The new Task Force met for the first time on May 18-19, 1986. The Task Force became a Provisional Committee in 1988, and in 1990 it became a full standing Committee.

At the same time the Committee became official, the Section on Child Abuse and Neglect (SOCAN) was founded. The SOCAN, a special interest group of AAP members who have an interest in child abuse and neglect, provides an educational forum for the discussion of problems and treatments relating to child abuse and neglect as well as prevention. With education as its main goal, the SOCAN has developed a number of educational resources since 1990 including the current third edition of the valuable teaching resource *Visual Diagnosis of Child Abuse on CD-ROM*[4] and the now retired *Guide to References and Resources in Child Abuse and Neglect*.[5] The *Guide* provided lists of articles and selected annotations, as well as resource lists to help the pediatrician chart a path through the child advocacy system. Information on programs providing diagnostic and treatment services in the United States and Canada was also included in the manual. A revised version of this is now posted on the Section's web site: http://www.aap.org/sections/scan/medicaldiagnostic/medicaldiagnostic.htm. The SOCAN also sponsors educational sessions at the AAP National Conference and Exposition (NCE) and at the annual conference of the Pediatric Academic Societies. The SOCAN has grown to about 600 members since its creation and includes other health care professionals as affiliate members.

In 2003, members of the AAP COCAN and the SOCAN approached the AAP to support a proposal for federal funding of university-based centers of excellence, which would provide child abuse education, research, and services in a more organized manner across the United States. The Health Child Abuse Research Education and Services (Health CARES) Network proposal, based on the successful federally funded University Centers of Excellence in Developmental Disabilities, was further refined with the assistance of AAP staff and approved by the AAP Board of Directors in the spring of 2004. Shortly after, the Boards of the American Academy of Child and Adolescent Psychiatry (AACAP) and the National Association of Children's Hospitals and Related Institutions (NACHRI) endorsed the proposal. In addition, a supportive resolution was passed at the American Medical Association (AMA). Staff in the AAP Department of Federal Affairs dedicated time to advocate for support and funding of the proposal, including arranging meetings with federal agencies to gain support of the Health CARES Network. Having a long successful liaison relationship with the COCAN, the Centers for Disease Control and Prevention (CDC) Division of Violence Prevention enthusiastically expressed support of and interest in housing the Health CARES Network within their agency. Currently, AAP staff, COCAN and SOCAN members are advocating for appropriation funding of the Health CARES Network, and the CDC has provided funding for development of a report on the current status of child abuse programs providing medical services in the United States.

Over the past 18 years, AAP's support of efforts in the field of child abuse and neglect has grown tremendously. Since the creation of the COCAN and SOCAN, approximately 30 state-level committees have been organized through AAP chapters. These chapters and their respective districts have contributed greatly to advance this field through submission of resolutions in the AAP Annual Chapter Forum. These resolutions have encouraged additional research and support of child abuse prevention programs. The AAP has also been able to make great strides in child abuse research and prevention with Federal and foundation funding. Through a grant from the Agency for Healthcare Research and Quality (AHRQ), the AAP conducted a study on the child abuse recognition and reporting behaviors of pediatricians through their Pediatric Research in the Office Setting (PROS) program. The results of this study, which showed that pediatricians are not reporting 27% of the injuries they highly suspect are caused by child abuse,[6] are leading the way to additional efforts by the AAP to support pediatricians in their difficult but crucial role in protecting the child from abuse, including sponsoring a multidisciplinary conference to identify strategies to reduce or eliminate barriers to reporting and hence improve the health and well-being of these extremely vulnerable children and their families. The results were published as a supplement to *Pediatrics* in 2008.[7]

Important progress has been made in the field of child maltreatment prevention. The AAP served as an important participant in a 1999 conference sponsored by the CDC to develop a plan for CDC's work on child maltreatment prevention. The AAP and the CDC continue to have a strong relationship, and in 2005 the CDC provided a grant to the AAP through a competitive application process to enhance pediatricians' ability to prevent sexual violence. As a result of the funding, the AAP published an educational toolkit for health care professionals to assist them in incorporating sexual violence prevention messages into the health care they provide to children, adolescents, and young adults.[8]

Shortly after the CDC Child Maltreatment conference in 1999, through funding from the Doris Duke Charitable Foundation (DDCF), the AAP sponsored a conference in collaboration with Prevent Child Abuse America to determine the best approach for pediatricians to prevent child maltreatment in the office setting. Additional funding ($1.5 million) from DDCF supported the development of material to use in pediatric offices to enhance anticipatory guidance and improve screening of children ages 0 to 3, and to prevent child maltreatment. In spite of these efforts, there is much work left to be done collaboratively with other organizations and federal agencies.

The American Board of Pediatrics

The American Board of Pediatrics (ABP) was founded in 1933. As one of the 24 certifying boards of the American Board of Medical Specialties (ABMS), the ABP certifies pediatricians who meet all credentialing requirements in general pediatrics and in approved pediatric subspecialties. The ABP strives to "… continually improve the standards of its certification (and to) advance the science, education, study, and practice of pediatrics."[9]

A new pediatric subspecialty, Child Abuse Pediatrics, has been developed, with initial certificates issued in 2010.[10] Following several years of planning and preparation, representatives of the evolving subspecialty in Child Abuse Pediatrics, sponsored by the Ray E. Helfer Society and with support from the AAP, applied to the ABP for recognition as a pediatric subspecialty. After receiving approval from the ABP, the subspecialty was subsequently recognized by the ABMS, a subspecialty board was established, and work on the certifying process began. An important part of the process of establishing a new subspecialty is working with the Accreditation Council for Graduate Medical Education (ACGME) to set accreditation standards for the 3-year fellowship eventually required by all applicants for subspecialty certification. The ACGME is a private, nonprofit council established in 1981 when the academic medical community agreed about the need for an independent accrediting organization to evaluate and accredit medical residency and fellowship programs in the United States. The mission of the ACGME is to "… improve health care by assessing and advancing the quality of resident physicians' education through accreditation."[11]

The Subboard of Child Abuse and Neglect first met at the ABP headquarters on December 12, 2006. The seven subboard members and a medical editor were selected from the leadership of the AAP's COCAN and SOCAN as well as from the Helfer Society. The subboard developed requirements for certification in the new subspecialty and first offered the certification examination in November, 2009.

The purpose of the new Board certification is to create a pediatric response to child abuse and neglect by subspecialty-trained pediatricians active in research, education, and clinical service. Subspecialty recognition will encourage young physicians to continue research and scholarly activity, bring credibility to forensic testimony, and enhance multidisciplinary discourse focused on the prevention, intervention, and remediation of child abuse. By imposing standards for certification and recertification, only pediatricians who develop and maintain excellent skills and who possess the requisite cognitive knowledge base will be recognized as being certified in Child Abuse Pediatrics. In addition, certified subspecialists will be available to promote appropriate curricula in medical schools, residency programs, and continuing medical education programs. An important role will be to serve as consultants and referral sources for other physicians confronting possible child abuse or neglect cases in their practice.

The Ray Helfer Society

The Ray Helfer Society was founded in 1999 and incorporated in 2001 as an honorary society of physicians seeking to enhance the prevention, diagnosis, and treatment of child abuse and neglect. Initially, a small group of physicians with a special interest in child maltreatment met in Philadelphia to begin the discussions that led to the formation of the Society. Discussion focused on promoting education and training in the medical aspects of child abuse and neglect, and improving medical evaluation and care for children who are victims of child abuse and neglect. Other objectives of the Helfer Society are to advocate for improved resources for research in order to strengthen research and scholarly activity in the field. Society members agree it is important to promote high ethical standards for both clinical and forensic practice and research, to develop collaborative relationships with other professional organizations, and to emphasize the importance of the health consequences of child abuse and neglect. Acceptance into the Helfer Society is meant to honor an individual physician's contributions to the physical and emotional health of victims of child abuse and neglect.[12] The Society sponsors candidate members, usually younger physicians in Child Abuse Pediatrics fellowship training or in other related disciplines such as emergency medicine, public health, child psychiatry, pediatric radiology, or preventive medicine.

The Helfer Society sponsors an annual educational meeting open to regular members, candidate members, and guests. This meeting serves as a networking opportunity, a forum for state-of-the-art research presentations, and provides workshops on education, clinical guidelines, court issues, fellowship development, and other topics important to the field. Because the Society's meetings have become the principle gathering of certified subspecialists, members are working on issues related to curriculum and scholarly activities, and other important issues related to fellowship training in Child Abuse Pediatrics.

American Professional Society on the Abuse of Children

The American Professional Society on the Abuse of Children (APSAC) is a national organization whose mission is to enhance the ability of professionals to respond to children and families affected by abuse and violence.[13] APSAC

primarily fulfills this mission through providing education and other sources of information to professionals who work in the child maltreatment and related fields. Among the resources that have made a significant contribution to the field is their journal *Child Maltreatment.*

International Society for Prevention of Child Abuse and Neglect

In 1977, C. Henry Kempe, MD assembled a group of child abuse professionals from around the world to found an international organization that would support and advance their work, the International Society for Prevention of Child Abuse and Neglect (ISPCAN).[14] Today the mission of the ISPCAN remains the same. It is the only multidisciplinary international organization that brings together a worldwide cross-section of committed professionals to work toward the prevention and treatment of child abuse, neglect, and exploitation globally. ISPCAN's journal *Child Abuse and Neglect* is a preeminent publication in the field of child abuse and neglect. ISPCAN's biennial International Congress has attracted as many as 1000 professionals from 88 counties.

American Medical Association (AMA) National Advisory Council on Violence and Abuse (NACVA)

In 1991, the AMA founded the National Advisory Council on Violence and Abuse to support physicians in dealing with violence in America's communities. The Council's mission was (1) to identify, develop, and promote practices and policies that enhanced the physician's capacity to recognize and identify the presentations and consequences of violence and abuse in all their forms; (2) to ensure that physicians are capable of providing appropriate responses when these issues are identified; (3) to educate the medical community to play an appropriate role in the prevention of violence and abuse; (4) to encourage other health care organizations to identify and work toward similar goals of violence prevention; and (5) to provide leadership, advocacy, support, and guidance to other related organizations that shared their goals.[15] In the mid 1990s, the Council published a series of eight monographs on various issues of violence, abuse, and sexual violence: *Diagnostic and Treatment Guidelines on Child Sexual Abuse; Mental Health Effects of Family Violence; Domestic Violence; Child Physical Abuse and Neglect;* and *Strategies for the Treatment and Prevention of Sexual Assault.* Recently the AMA dissolved the NACVA due to financial cutbacks. The former AMA NACVA Council has formed a Transition Working Group (TWG) to develop a new organization and continue the work of the NACVA. The Family Violence Prevention Fund (FVPF) is providing an interim home and limited staff support to help the TWG determine appropriate next steps. During this transition, the organization's name is the National Health Collaborative on Violence and Abuse (NHCVA), without reference to or use of the AMA's name.

The Academy on Violence and Abuse (AVA)

Members of the American Medical Association National Advisory Council on Violence and Abuse developed the concept for the AVA when its members realized that increasing exposure to curricula focusing on violence and abuse in the core education of physicians, nurses, and other health care providers was an immediate necessity. In order to accomplish this goal, a professional membership organization was needed to give credence to this discipline. In addition, the Institute of Medicine, in its 2001 report, *Confronting Chronic Neglect: the Education and Training of Health Professionals on Family Violence*,[15] suggested such an organization was needed to improve the infrastructure necessary to support this training. The mission and vision of the AVA is to "... advance health education and research on the recognition, treatment, and prevention of the health effects of violence and abuse. By expanding health education and research, the Academy will integrate knowledge about violence and abuse into the training of all health professionals, promote the health of all people, protect the most vulnerable, and advance health and social policy that promotes safe families, safe workplaces and safe communities."[16] In 2008, the AVA released its first comprehensive report, "Building Academic Capacity and Expertise in the Health Effects of Violence and Abuse: A Blueprint for Advancing Professional Health Education."[17] The report is available from the AVA through its web site http://avahealth.org/.

Family Violence Prevention Fund

Although technically not a membership organization for professionals, the Family Violence Prevention Fund (FVPF) has made significant contributions to the health care field in an effort to prevent child maltreatment. The FVPF, whose mission is to work to prevent violence in the home and the community and to help those who have been devastated by violence, has a number of initiatives to protect children including programs aimed at improving father's roles in their child's lives. Of most significance to the health care field is their National Consensus Guidelines on Identifying and Responding to Domestic Violence Victimization in Health Care Settings,[18] which is recommended by the AAP to prevent child maltreatment.

ADVOCACY AND RESEARCH

Organizations play an important role by advocating for children, especially those that have been abused. For nearly four decades, the legislative staff in the AAP Department of Federal Affairs (DOFA) has worked to place and sustain children's health on the national agenda. Through lobbying, coalition building, and raising public awareness, DOFA has cemented the Academy's credibility and visibility on national child health issues. On issues related to child abuse, the AAP has played an instrumental role urging Congress to reauthorize the Child Abuse Prevention and Treatment Act (CAPTA) and to pass bills such as the Safe and Stable Families Act. The AAP has played an even larger role at the state level with the advocacy efforts of their Chapters. For example, because of the advocacy of the Oklahoma Chapter, physicians and child advocacy centers are able to receive compensation from the state for child abuse investigations through a special state fund created by raising the fee for filing a law suit. The Illinois Chapter worked with others in the state to get reimbursement from Medicaid for pediatricians who screen for maternal depression.

Organizations can play an increasingly important role in developing research in the field of child maltreatment. With the subspecialty of Child Abuse Pediatrics sponsored by the Helfer Society with the support of the AAP, and accepted by the ABP and the ABMS, a new generation of scholars will be created through accredited fellowships. Many studies in child abuse and neglect will benefit from collaborative, multisite projects. Organizations focused on the health consequences of violence and abuse, like the AVA and the AAP, will work to affect political policy decisions leading to funding for research. The organizations mentioned in this chapter, along with the many others focused on child maltreatment issues, can assist in the movement to recognize the critical public health consequences of all forms of violence and abuse, including child maltreatment.

SUMMARY

Education of health professions, public awareness of the health consequences of maltreatment, and influencing of political processes can all be accomplished by dedicated professionals and staff through national organizations. When addressing the issue of child maltreatment, organizations lend credence to the magnitude of the problem and the need for intervention. Groups of individuals organized around specific issues can have a greater effect. In addition to those mentioned here, organizations such as Prevent Child Abuse America,[19] the National Center for Shaken Baby Syndrome,[20] Children's Healthcare is a Legal Duty,[21] and others help create forums for the advancement of knowledge, policies, and advocacy, all important to the eventual curtailment of child maltreatment.

References

1. Lazoritz S: Whatever happened to Mary Ellen? *Child Abuse Negl* 1990;14:143-149.
2. American Academy of Pediatrics Committee on Infant and Preschool Child: Maltreatment of children. The physically abused child. *Pediatrics* 1966;37:377-382.
3. Schmitt BD: *The Visual Diagnosis of Non-Accidental Trauma and Failure to Thrive.* American Academy of Pediatrics, Chicago, IL, 1979.
4. Lowen D, Reece RM: *Visual Diagnosis of Child Abuse on CD-ROM*, ed 3. American Academy of Pediatrics, Elk Grove Village, IL, 2008.
5. American Academy of Pediatrics Section on Child Abuse and Neglect: *A Guide to References and Resources in Child Abuse and Neglect.* American Academy of Pediatrics, Elk Grove Village, IL, 1998.
6. Flaherty EG, Sege RD, Griffith J, et al: From suspicion of physical child abuse to reporting: primary care clinician decisions-making. *Pediatrics* 2008;122:611-619.
7. Flaherty EG, Sege RD, Hurley TP: Translating child abuse research into action: Improving primary care recognition and collaboration. *Pediatrics* 2008;122:S1-24.
8. American Academy of Pediatrics: Preventing Sexual Violence. An Educational Toolkit for Health Care Professions (Web Version). American Academy of Pediatrics, Elk Grove Village, IL, 2009. Available at http://www.aap.org/pubserv/PSVpreview/start.html. Accessed on March 3, 2010.
9. American Board of Pediatrics: Mission Statement. Available at https://www.abp.org/ABPWebSite/. Accessed on March 3, 2010.
10. Block RW, Palusci VJ: Child abuse pediatrics: a new pediatric subspecialty. *J Pediatr* 2006;148:711-712.
11. Accreditation Council for Graduate Medical Education: Mission Statement. Available at http://www.acgme.org/acWebsite/about/ab_mission.asp. Accessed on March 3, 2010.

12. The Ray Helfer Society: Mission Statement. Available at http://www. helfersociety.org/. Accessed on March 3, 2010.

13. Available at http://www.apsac.org/mc/page.do. Accessed on March 3, 2010.

14. Available at http://www.ispcan.org/. Accessed on March 3, 2010.

15. Cohn F, Salmon MEW, Stobo JD: *Confronting Chronic Neglect: The Education and Training of Health Professionals on Family Violence.* National Academy Press, Washington, DC, 2002.

16. Available at http://www.avahealth.org/index.asp?Type=B_ BASIC&SEC={C4499D70-5F92-4FB2-A5D8- 9F115E894507}&DE=. Accessed on March 3, 2010.

17. Mitchell C (ed): *Building Academic Capacity and Expertise in the Health Effects of Violence and Abuse. A Blueprint for Advancing Professional Health Education.* Academy of Violence and Abuse, Eden Prarie, MN, 2008. Available

at http://avahealth.org/vertical/Sites/%7B75FA0828-D713-4580- A29D-257F315BB94F%7D/uploads/%7B52050EC8-C0F9-4417- B9C1-0A6143D4466A%7D.PDF. Accessed on March 3, 2010.

18. National Consensus Guidelines on Identifying and Responding to Domestic Violence in Health Care Settings. The Family Violence Prevention Fund, San Francisco, 2002. Available at http://endabuse. org/programs/healthcare/files/Consensus.pdf. Accessed on March 3, 2010.

19. Available at http://www.preventchildabuse.org/index.shtml. Accessed on March 3, 2010.

20. Available at http://www.dontshake.org/index.php. Accessed on March 3, 2010.

21. Available at http://www.childrenshealthcare.org/. Accessed on March 3, 2010.

67

INTERNATIONAL ISSUES IN CHILD MALTREATMENT

Desmond K. Runyan, MD, DrPH, and Adam J. Zolotor, MD, MPH

INTRODUCTION

Child abuse and neglect are frequent, perhaps even ordinary, occurrences in most of the world.[1] The World Health Organization estimates that 40 million children under age 15 years around the world suffer from abuse or neglect each year requiring health and social care.[2] Using a broader behavioral definition of parental acts, the UN Secretary-General's Study of Children and Violence estimated that between 80% and 98% of children are physically punished each year and that one third or more of all children experiencing physical punishment are subjected to severe punishment with an implement.[1] Despite large numbers of children being maltreated, the recognition of child abuse and neglect as a problem is a recent phenomenon in human history, and children might be safer now than in the past.[3] Investigations, both in high and low or in middle-income countries, have demonstrated significant initial and long-term harm.[2,4-12] Clinical skills in the recognition of child abuse, even among medical professionals in countries with a history of awareness, are far from ideal, and there are few hours devoted to child abuse in medical curricula even in the United States, which has among the largest clinical literatures on the problem.[13] Among physicians in low- and middle-income countries, there is even less recognition of the problem.[14,15]

DEFINITIONS AND CULTURE

The international comparison of child abuse rates in different countries requires understanding cultural norms for parenting behavior. Definitions of what constitutes abusive or neglectful child rearing vary between countries, between professionals, and between communities in the same country. Culture is, in part, a society's shared understanding of beliefs and behaviors about child rearing and parenting. Culture includes the values, rules, and prohibitions that define acceptable parenting. Different cultures can have and have evolved different rules about acceptable practices (e.g., 24 countries have banned corporal punishment by parents).[16] However, a surprising amount of data are emerging suggesting that persons in many cultures share common working definitions of abuse and that ethnicity might not be among the important determinants of different conceptualizations of abuse.[17]

Korbin et al[18] reviewed studies in which authors presented vignettes of parental discipline to parents in different cultural groups. They noted that there was substantial agreement among community groups in a number of countries about what circumstances were harmful for children. However, there were some notable differences in perspective across societies. In one study they reviewed, the authors reported that Vietnamese parents did not perceive bruising from discipline as abusive, whereas white parents made more of an effort to distinguish spanking from other forms of hitting. Korbin[19] also noted that Asian and Pacific Islander parents were surprised to learn that U.S. law limits parental rights to physically discipline children. This review noted wide variation in parental supervision standards; some groups were less concerned about young children left unattended or left with other young children. The authors did find that there were differences in emphasis in defining abuse in different ethnic groups; African Americans were more likely to think of neglectful acts whereas European Americans were more likely to worry about physical acts.[19]

Some investigators have suggested that different cultures may have such widely divergent views on child rearing that it may not be easy to find cross-cultural agreement on what parenting practices are abusive or neglectful.[13,20] There is widespread agreement, however, that child abuse should end and considerable agreement that very harsh discipline practices and sexual abuse are abusive.[17,21] The World Health Organization's (WHO) 1999 Consultation on Child Abuse Prevention produced a definition that was acceptable to the attending group of international delegates: "Child abuse or maltreatment constitutes all forms of physical and/or emotional ill-treatment, sexual abuse, neglect or negligent treatment or commercial or other exploitation, resulting in actual or potential harm to the child's health, survival, development or dignity in the context of a relationship of responsibility, trust or power."[17]

In addition to potential variations in defining child abuse among cultures, there are other disagreements on how abuse should be defined that have a conceptual basis. Some might focus on the behaviors or acts of adults in defining abuse whereas others define abuse by the occurrence of harm or the threat of harm to the child.[22] The distinction between behavior and impact or harm becomes even more complicated if the intent of the parent is part of the definition. Some include in the definition of abuse those children inadvertently harmed through actions of a parent regardless of intent whereas others would require that harm be intended. To complicate cross-national comparisons even further, some international literature explicitly includes violence against children in institutional or school settings as child abuse.[7,23,24]

TYPES OF CHILD MALTREATMENT

This chapter attends only to parental or caregiver acts and omissions that result in harm to the child and does not address commercial exploitation or the abuse of children in institutional settings such as schools or in communities. Specifically, we examine the data, causes, and consequences for four subtypes of child abuse and neglect:

Physical abuse: An act or acts committed by a caregiver, toward a child, which produce either physical harm or have the potential for producing harm.

Sexual abuse: Acts in which a caregiver uses a child for sexual gratification.

Emotional abuse: The failure of a caregiver to provide a developmentally appropriate and supportive environment or acts that themselves have an adverse effect on the emotional health and development of a child. Restrictions of movement, belittling, denigrating, scapegoating, threatening, scaring, discriminating, ridiculing, or other nonphysical forms of hostile or rejecting treatment are all examples of emotional abuse.

Neglect and negligent treatment: Neglect is the failure of a caregiver to provide for the child in health, education, emotional development, nutrition, shelter, or safe living conditions when the caregiver is in a position to provide for the child. Neglect is usually distinguished from poverty in that neglect can occur only when there are resources reasonably available to the family or caretakers that are not offered to the child.

Fatal Abuse

Young children are at greatest risk for child abuse homicide. Rates for children 0 to 4 years of age are more than twice the rates for children ages 5 to 14 years around the world. WHO estimated 85,000 child abuse homicides among children less than 15 years of age in 1998.[17] Children under 4 from Eastern Mediterranean low- and middle-income countries have the highest rates at 14.8 per 100,000 for boys and 16.4 per 100,000 for girls. India is the next highest region with rates of 10.1 and 13.6 per 100,000 for boys and girls, respectively. Girls tend to be at higher risk of child abuse homicide. The contrast is most stark in China with rates for girls ages 0 to 4 of 15.7 per 100,000, nearly double that of boys (7.9 per 100,000). Although it seems that gender would be among the most significant risk factors for infant homicide internationally, published research indicates a surprising uniformity of risk factors for infant homicide around the world, in countries as disparate as Fiji, Cameroon, and the United States. Most child abuse homicides are to the infants of young, poor, unmarried mothers.[5,25]

Many infant deaths around the world are not routinely investigated, so it is difficult to determine child abuse homicide rates with precision in many countries. Infant deaths can be incorrectly attributed to infectious disease or malnutrition by caregivers and by health workers in countries that have limited diagnostic test access and little access to routine autopsies. A recent study in one U.S. state reported 5 fatalities in 100,000 children in the first year of life from abusive head trauma.[26] In contrast, 2.6% of parents of young children in that region reported shaking as a form of discipline.[27]

In several low- and middle-income countries, rates of shaking have been reported above 25% in the first 2 years of life.[28] Shaking is postulated to account for a significant portion of unexplained infant mortality, mental retardation, and learning disabilities in low- and middle-income countries. Child abuse fatalities are far more numerous than stated in official estimates from vital records in countries where studies of infant death have been more closely examined.[5,29,30] The leading causes of death from child abuse are, in order, abusive head trauma, blunt abdominal trauma, and suffocation.[30-33]

Nonfatal Abuse

The recent UN study on children and violence demonstrated that child abuse and neglect are global phenomena.[1] They occur in every country and civilization that has been studied. The majority of systematic studies have focused on physical and sexual abuse; less is known about neglect, emotional abuse, and other forms of maltreatment in low- and middle-income countries. At least 26 countries collect official statistics on reported abuse.[21]

The majority of countries have no legal or social systems with responsibility for responding or monitoring child abuse and neglect.[21] Case reports or case series of child abuse have been published in many countries, indicating increased professional or public awareness to this problem.[5,25,34-39] Recent population-based surveys have been completed in a number of countries including Australia, Brazil, Canada, Chile, China, Costa Rica, Egypt, El Salvador, Ethiopia, Guatemala, Honduras, India, Israel, Kenya, Mexico, New Zealand, Nicaragua, Norway, Philippines, Portugal, South Africa, South Korea, Spain, Uganda, the United States, and Zimbabwe.[4,7,8,22,24,34,38,40-57]

Physical Abuse

An estimated 40 million children around the world suffer from abuse or neglect and need health and social intervention.[2] In the United States, for 2006, 777,000 children were confirmed to be victims of either abuse or neglect and, of these, 142,000 were victims of physical abuse. The physical abuse rate was 1.9 in 100,000 children that year. Despite over 30 years of mandatory reporting of child abuse, it is almost certain that these statistics underestimate actual abuse in the United States. A 1995 Gallup poll asked a national sample of U.S. parents about disciplining their own children in the previous year. The study authors reported an abuse rate of 49 per 1000 children when defining abuse as hitting the child with an object someplace other than on the buttocks, kicking the child, beating the child up, and threatening the child with a knife or a gun. This and a similar study from a two-state probability sample in 2002 found a more than twentyfold difference in substantiated abuse and parent reports of abuse.[22,27]

International research suggests that the rates for physical abuse may be higher in low- and middle-income countries. A study from Egypt described high rates of beating and fractures. In a cross-sectional survey of children in Egypt, 37% were beaten or tied up and 26% of children reported physical injuries such as fractures, loss of consciousness or permanent disability from a beating.[24] In South Korea, severe violence (defined by the authors as kicking, beating, biting, throwing, or threatening with a knife or a gun more than two times a month) was reported by 69 of 1000 fourth and fifth graders.[34] As high as these child-reported rates appear, parent reports indicate even higher rates: South Korean parents reveal whipping children at a rate of 67%, or hitting, kicking, or beating their children at a rate of 45%.[34]

Eastern European reports of physical discipline and abuse yield similar estimates for rates of child victimization. Romanian children reported a rate of 4.6% for severe and frequent physical abuse including being hit with an object, being burned, or being deprived of food.[2] Nearly half of Romanian parents (47%) admitted to beating their children "regularly" and almost 16% reported beating their children with objects. A recent national study of parents in Georgia reported nearly 50% of children were spanked, shaken, or had their hair pulled or ears twisted in the last year.[41]

Sexual Abuse

The prevalence and incidence of sexual abuse and other forms of maltreatment have been difficult to study and compare across national samples. Definitions, methods, and measures vary widely. Most of the research into sexual abuse comes from countries in North America and Western Europe. In most cases, incidence is determined by report to social services or criminal justice authorities.[58] Victims of sexual abuse can also be counted when they present to a health care setting. However, the fundamental flaw in these approaches is that most cases of sexual abuse are only known to the perpetrator and the victim. A population-based survey of parents in the United States found that they acknowledged sexual abuse of their children 15 times more than official reports indicated.[27] One nationally representative survey of parents in the United States indicated that 1.9% of boys and girls were sexually abused in the last year and 5.7% ever.[22] The discrepancy between official reports and survey estimates might be due to unreported sexual abuse, sexual abuse reclassified as other types of abuse or neglect, or sexual abuse that is unsubstantiated or deemed not to be under the purview of child protective services. Even parent-report data are limited. It only reveals the cases of sexual abuse known to the parent being interviewed. Adolescent and adult retrospective data suggest that real rates are far higher still. Comparisons between studies are further constrained as some studies attempt to gather lifetime prevalence data whereas others attempt to ascertain incidence in the past year.

A number of studies have been done around the world surveying adolescent and adult populations about history of sexual abuse. A large study of middle-aged adults in the United States ($n = 17,337$) pooling people with private health insurance found that 24.7% of women and 16.0% of men reported sexual abuse (defined with a series of four questions pertaining to [1] touching and fondling the respondent; [2] forcing the respondent to touch or fondle the perpetrator; [3] attempt at any type of intercourse (oral, anal, or vaginal); and [4] actual completion of any type of intercourse).[59] These results are similar to estimates from studies in Europe, South America, and Africa, although national population-based survey estimates of child sexual abuse victimization on

these continents are rare.[2] A recent three-country survey in Africa, using a systematic sample of urban young adults, reported far higher rates of sexual abuse. The study reported rates of 53% in Uganda, 44% in Kenya, and 42% in Ethiopia, defined as unwanted sexual touch. Alarming rates of rape were noted, including 43% in Uganda, 30% in Ethiopia, and 26% in Kenya.[57]

Adolescents have been surveyed in several studies regarding their history of sexual abuse. There are several advantages to this approach. Adolescents can be surveyed in school settings with appropriate permission and collaboration, thus are a relatively captive audience resulting in a lower cost and a higher response rate. Furthermore, since adolescents are required to be in school in many countries up to a specific age, sampling through school systems facilitates easy access to a generalizable sample. Perhaps even more important, adolescents are closer to the events of childhood and may be more accurate in their memory of abusive trauma and less subject to recall bias. A final reason that adolescents make such an important target is that their sexual abuse history is much closer to the current reality in any national setting. That is to say, if middle-aged women report sexual abuse that occurred 20 to 40 years ago, the impact of changes in public policy and prevention cannot hope to be ascertained for many decades. However, sexual abuse peaks in adolescence,[60] so studies of adolescents can best be used to measure the current population experience with sexual abuse.

Two recent examples of surveying adolescence for history of sexual abuse come from China and Sweden. In Henan province, 21.9% of girl adolescents in a professional school program reported at least one type of sexual abuse prior to the age of 16 using a 12-item questionnaire. Sexual abuse was defined as an unwanted sexual experience for the child. This study did not include boys.[47] In Sweden, a large representative national sample of boys and girls was surveyed about sexual behavior using an instrument including 10 questions on sexual abuse. In this study, the authors inquired about only those acts that were forced; the estimates of sexual abuse were 11.2% among girls and 3.2% among boys. The study successfully recruited a population of out-of-school adolescents, a modification that is essential for national estimates because out-of-school adolescents in Sweden report nearly twice the lifetime prevalence of sexual abuse.[61] A survey of children in Ukraine reported that nearly 20% of teenagers have been sexually abused.[20] A study of adolescents from Geneva reported lifetime sexual abuse rates at 34% for girls and 11% for boys.[62] Emphasizing the importance of how the wording of questions alters estimates, another Swiss survey of adolescent girls using fewer questions and a more restrictive definition noted a somewhat lower rate (18%) for reported sexual abuse.[63] These studies are difficult to compare because of divergent definitions, varying measures, varying contexts, and sampling frames.[64]

Some studies have attempted to compare adult and child responses to surveys about sexual abuse. A survey of 1500 Romanian families obtained data from both children and adults.[2] In this study 0.1% of parents admitted to sexually abusing their children while 9.1% of children report having been sexually abused. One of the great challenges in comparing children and parents' survey response is the referent time period and possible perpetrators. The question asked of children included sexual victimization by anyone.

Men report a history of sexual abuse ranging from 1%[65] to 19%[50] among published studies of adults giving retrospective histories. International lifetime prevalence rates for child sexual victimization using adult reports range from 0.8%,[6] using rape as the definition, to 45%[50] using a much wider definition lifetime history of sexual abuse. In international journals in the 1990s the mean lifetime prevalence rate of childhood sexual victimization of women as girls was 19% and men as boys was 7%. This variation in published prevalence estimates could mask real differences in risk in different cultures or result from differences in the conduct of the studies.[64,66]

Neglect

The cross-cultural study of neglect is challenged by issues related to blame or locus of control. Some authors deem failure to meet basic needs of childhood as neglect, without placing blame on parents, government, or conditions of a local community. Others have focused on parental omissions in providing care.[67] In the United States, laws generally define a child as being neglected only when the child has been harmed by an omission in care.[67] Other authors include harm from parental omissions in care as part of the definition of abuse.[9,25,68,69]

Many societal conditions such as exposure to toxic chemicals or war can be more dangerous for children than parental omissions in care.[69] Because definitions are varied and research in neglect is far less common, it is difficult to estimate the global dimensions of the problem. In Kenya, adults asked to define child abuse most commonly cite abandonment and neglect.[68] In the United States, 60% of reports for child maltreatment are for neglect and the rate of neglect is 7 in 1000 children.[70]

Psychological Abuse

Cultural factors influence the use of parental discipline techniques and the frequency with which discipline includes psychological or emotional harms or threats. Psychological abuse itself is difficult to define, since the consequences are likely to be very different by context and by the age of the child. Surveys about child discipline demonstrate that yelling or screaming at children is common (over 80%) across many countries.[41,56] Cursing children and calling them names is also common, with 15% being the lowest rate reported by parents in a single country among a recent multinational study.[56] Rates for threats of abandonment and locking a child out of the home were widely divergent among countries.[56]

Understanding and developing prevention strategies and interventions for psychological or emotional abuse remain a major international challenge. The same threat might be much more traumatic to children in a country where that threat is unusual than it would be if the child frequently hears such threats from the parents of friends.

ECOLOGICAL CONTEXT

The causes of abuse are related to social interactions in families and communities. The ecological theory is the most widely adopted explanatory model by which to understand child maltreatment.[3,17,71,72] There are four contributory spheres of influence in this model: (1) child characteristics; (2) caregiver and family characteristics; (3) community characteristics; and (4) the social, economic, and cultural characteristics of society. The interplay of these factors can lead to abuse in one circumstance and not in another. Each of the factors appearing below has been linked to child abuse or neglect in more than one study. However, the factors listed might be only statistically associated and not causally linked.[13]

Children Characteristics

Young child age is a consistent and strong risk factor for child physical abuse.[7,24,67,73] Child abuse homicide is most common among young infants.[5,29,32,36] The peak ages of abuse vary somewhat between countries and cultures. Physical abuse is most common in the United States between 6 and 12 years of age, and similarly in India between 6 and 11. In China, however, the peak of physical abuse is between 3 and 6.[55,74] Sexual abuse is consistently most common during adolescence.[22,23,66,75]

Sex of child is a risk factor for some types of abuse. Girls are generally at higher risk for infanticide, sexual abuse, educational and nutritional neglect, and prostitution worldwide. Boys, in contrast, are at higher risk for abusive head trauma in the United States and for harsh physical discipline.[13,22,26,32,52,54]

The reasons for variation between countries in the peak age of abuse and the differential rates of types of abuse by child sex have not been well studied. Some variation may be due to acceptable parenting standards, discipline strategies, available resources, and patterns of care giving such as the use of extended families for care taking. The cultural differences in the role and value of women likely affect the rates of sexual abuse and female infanticide.

Caregiver and Family Characteristics

Gender as a risk for the perpetration of abuse has been evaluated in a number of types of studies in various countries. Women more often report using harsh physical punishment,[22,51,52,55] and children more often report violence by a mother or female caretaker.[76] In most countries, women have more responsibility for raising children and therefore for discipline and care. They also have more exposure to children in terms of time. In the United States, single mothers are more likely to self-report the use of harsh physical discipline than mothers in two-parent families. In contrast, men perpetrate more abuse resulting in severe injury.[77-79] This increase in risk may not be due to men's behavior or discipline practices, but simply due to the relative importance of strength in causing severe injuries. Sexual abuse offenders are predominantly male regardless of victim gender.[6,8,13,23,25,46,48,57,66,80,81] Rates of male perpetrators for female victims range from 92.0%[48] to 99.2%.[46] For male victims the range is between 63.2%[82] and 85.7%.[46,48]

Parents with a personal history of being abused as children appear to be at higher risk of abusing their own children.[13,73,76,78,83-85] Domestic violence and child abuse appear to be very strongly linked. They share many of the same ecological risk factors. Domestic violence has been reported as a risk factor in many countries including Colombia, China, Egypt, Fiji, India, Mexico, and the United States.[5,24,52,53,78,86,87] As many as half of abuse victims have concurrent domestic violence in their homes.[37,87] There is increasing interest in the relationship between domestic violence and child abuse in the research and policy arenas in many countries. Further work is need to understand the effect on children of exposure to both child abuse and domestic violence.[88-90]

Parents with less support and more life stress have children at higher risk for abuse.[67,72,76,91-93] Maternal mental health problems, especially depression, increase a child's risk for abuse.[92-94] Substance abuse by a parent or other household member places a child at increased risk of abuse.[2,13,17,52,68,76,78,94,95] Finally, household crowding increases a child's risk for being abused.[24,53,76] The effects of risk factors such as maternal mental health problems, household substance abuse, poverty, illiteracy, and household crowding are closely related, and further work will be needed to understand the role of each of these in diverse cultural contexts.

Community Context

Poverty is a strong risk factor for all types of maltreatment across diverse cultures.[21,46,49,52,64,66-68,72,74,96-98] Two exceptions to this finding have been demonstrated in studies in which higher income urban families had higher rates of physical abuse.[7,51] In the United States, one study found that the poorest families (incomes <$10,000/year) reported rates of physical and sexual abuse three times that of middle- and high-income families (incomes >$50,000/year).[74]

High neighborhood cohesion and the closely related phenomenon of social capital have been shown to be protective factors for child maltreatment in two studies from high-income countries.[98,99] Children in neighborhoods with less social capital have more behavioral and psychological symptoms.[91] Social networks, a component of social capital, have also been shown to decrease the risk of child maltreatment.[18,19,100]

Societal Context

The society-level risk for child maltreatment is important and complex. Factors that may mediate the risk of child maltreatment include the following: education, child support, child labor, mandatory reporting laws, laws related to corporal punishment, special criminal justice systems, value and role of children (especially girls), national health systems, home visiting services, educated health providers, larger social conflicts, and war.[1] These issues have been unexamined as they relate to child abuse in most countries but fit well into an ecological model for understanding and preventing abuse.[71,100] To study these factors would require comprehensive societal level comparative research using similar measures and definitions. Some societal level factors can compromise parental abilities to care for children (e.g., poor access to health services and education) whereas others such as access to home visiting and health care may enhance parental abilities.[1] Research is needed to examine the effect of social policy changes to enhance parenting and assist families. One example is the child care allowances and tax credits offered to parents in some countries. Research is also needed regarding the impact of aggressive pregnancy prevention policies. Perinatal home visiting programs provide important support and education for parents. Some programs have shown success in randomized trials in preventing abuse and neglect in addition to other important outcomes affecting the lives of children and families.[101-103] International comparative research could be the most powerful method of exploring how societal context decreases or increases the risk of abuse.

Education of Health Professionals

Many health professionals around the world lack the skills or inclination to identify cases of abuse. The United States has a relatively longer history of recognizing the problem of child abuse, and still they are underprepared and uncomfortable confronting child abuse. A survey of American medical schools observed that while nearly all medical school (95%) include information about child abuse in their curriculum, the median amount of class time spent on child abuse was 2 hours. Only 80% of medical students reported child abuse coursework, and they agreed with the estimate of 2 hours of instruction.[104] Given the complexity of recognizing abuse, it is clear that most students will not be well prepared for this task in the United States. As further evidence of this lack of preparedness, a recent survey of pediatricians demonstrated that 50% were uncomfortable testifying in court about child abuse, and only 30% were comfortable with diagnosing and treating child abuse as part of their professional role.[105] Recent studies have demonstrated significant lack of agreement between physicians of findings indicative of child sexual abuse and a high rate of missed diagnosis on abusive head trauma in children presenting for medical care.[77,105] Similarly, two recent studies have shown wide variation in interpretation of abusive clinical scenarios among generalists and specialists.[106,107] Anecdotal reports from the faculty of 27 medical schools from low- and middle-income countries participating in the International Clinical Epidemiology Network suggest that the problem may be even greater in other regions of the world. Little or no formal instruction in child abuse has been provided at any of the schools in this group of prestigious medical schools in Asia, Africa, and South America. A study from Turkey observed, "Some pediatricians, in a national conference, resented having to spend unnecessary time to this very local, social, non-medical problem."[37]

Physicians and other health workers need to be trained to consider child abuse in cases of unexplained injury or child psychological distress. They must interpret histories in the context of the child's development, recognize the signs and symptoms of child abuse, and distinguish suspicious findings from innocent findings. The medical determination of child abuse needs to be both sensitive and specific. The consequences of missing abuse when it is present (because of low sensitivity) can be grave and even fatal to the child. The consequences of diagnosing abuse in its absence can be grave as well, resulting in severe distress for the family and child and removal of a child from his or her home, as well as great legal and social costs.[108] Social service organizations rely on medical expertise and are not in a position to question medical interpretations of physical abuse findings.

Failure to diagnose child abuse and an unwillingness to pursue the diagnosis complicate societal efforts to protect children. Available data suggest that the preparation of physicians for work in this area is inadequate.[37,104]

FUTURE RESEARCH

Although the predominance of western publications about the problem of child abuse has led some professionals to describe child abuse as a western problem, this chapter presents data documenting that the problem is of equal or even greater severity in low- and middle-income countries. We have presented data demonstrating that child abuse is more common than many of the infectious diseases for which massive eradication programs have been mounted. Instead of rates of a few cases per thousand, child abuse and neglect affect a much larger percentage of the population and result in significant societal costs. Child abuse is a pervasive and serious global health problem and the data suggest no society is immune.

Providers seeking data about specific countries should consult the United Nation's Secretary-General's Report on Children and Violence[1] and the periodic reports issued by the International Society for the Prevention of Child Abuse and Neglect (http://www.ispcan.org). In 1996, the Secretary-General called for a global study that would address violence against children in homes and schools in a manner similar to an earlier UN study of war on children. This study was delayed until 2002 when Professor Paulo Pinheiro of Brazil was appointed the Study Director and a Secretariat for the study was established in Geneva. The report was released on October of 2006[1] and is available for no cost on the Internet. One recommendation of the report was to address the need for more research and better data on the extent and nature of child maltreatment in all nations. Improvements in measurement and expanded efforts at surveillance were called for to assess the extent of the problem and to monitor the impact of changes in policies and services for children.

One way we will better understand child maltreatment around the world is by improved use of common definitions and measures. As part of this effort and in response to the UN World Report, the International Society for the Prevention of Child Abuse and Neglect collaborated with the UN Children's Emergency Fund to develop and field-test three new survey instruments to ascertain rates of child victimization from parents, young adults, and children.[109-111] These instruments have since been field-tested in national and multinational studies.[40,41,57] The report also calls upon the world's medical schools to do a better job of educating health professionals in recognizing and responding to child abuse.[1]

We concur with the UN Secretary-General's report that there appears to be little recognition of child abuse by health professionals in most countries. Governments and academics must ascertain the epidemiology. Effective intervention strategies will need to be developed and disseminated. Prevention efforts and policies must be directed at the children, the caregivers, and the environment before, during, and after occurrences of abuse or neglect. Health professionals must learn to recognize child abuse and neglect. Professional schools in medicine, psychology, education, social work, and public health around the world must include training in this field as a prelude to successful global efforts to reduce or eliminate child abuse.

References

1. Pinheiro PS: World Report on Violence Against Children. United Nations, Geneva, 2006. Available at http://www.violencestudy.org/r229. Accessed on December 23, 2008.
2. Krug EG, Dahlberg LL, Mercy JA, et al *(eds): World Report on Violence and Health.* World Health Organization, Geneva, 2002.
3. Ten Bensel RW, Radbill S: The history of child abuse. *In:* Helfer ME, Kempe RS, Krugman RD (eds): *The Battered Child.* University of Chicago Press, Chicago, 1997.
4. Bendixen M, Muus KM, Schei B: The impact of child sexual abuse—a study of a random sample of Norwegian students. *Child Abuse Negl* 1994;18:837-847.
5. Adinkrah M: Maternal infanticides in Fiji. *Child Abuse Negl* 2000;24:1543-1555.
6. Choquet M, Darves-Bornoz JM, Ledoux S, et al: Self-reported health and behavioral problems among adolescent victims of rape in France: results of a cross-sectional survey. *Child Abuse Negl* 1997;21:823-832.
7. Ketsela T, Kebede D: Physical punishment of elementary school children in urban and rural communities in Ethiopia. *Ethiop Med J* 1997;35:23-33.
8. Krugman S, Mata L, Krugman R: Sexual abuse and corporal punishment during childhood: a pilot retrospective survey of university students in Costa Rica. *Pediatrics* 1992;90:157-161.
9. Sumba RO, Bwibo NO: Child battering in Nairobi, Kenya. *East Afr Med J* 1993;70:688-692.
10. Felitti VJ, Anda RF, Nordenberg D, et al: Relationship of childhood abuse and household dysfunction to many of the leading causes of death in adults. The Adverse Childhood Experiences (ACE) Study. *Am J Prev Med* 1998;14:245-258.
11. Anda RF, Croft JB, Felitti VJ, et al: Adverse childhood experiences and smoking during adolescence and adulthood. *JAMA* 1999;282:1652-1658.
12. Dietz PM, Spitz AM, Anda RF, et al: Unintended pregnancy among adult women exposed to abuse or household dysfunction during their childhood. *JAMA* 1999;282:1359-1364.
13. National Research Council: *Understanding Child Maltreatment.* National Academy of Sciences Press, Washington, DC, 1993.
14. Acik Y, Deveci SE, Oral R: Level of knowledge and attitude of primary care physicians in Eastern Anatolian cities in relation to child abuse and neglect. *Prev Med* 2004;39:791-797.
15. Al-Moosa A, Al-Shaiji J, Al-Fadhli A, et al: Pediatricians' knowledge, attitudes and experience regarding child maltreatment in Kuwait. *Child Abuse Negl* 2003;27:1161-1178.
16. Global Initiative to End Corporal Punishment of all Children. States with full abolition. Available at: http://www.endcorporalpunishment.org/pages/frame.html. Accessed on September 1, 2008.
17. Report of the Consultation on Child Abuse Prevention. World Health Organization, Geneva, 1999.
18. Korbin JE, Coulton CJ, Lindstrom-Ufuti H, et al: Neighborhood views on the definition and etiology of child maltreatment. *Child Abuse Negl* 2000;24:1509-1527.
19. Korbin JE: Cross-cultural perspectives and research directions for the 21st century. *Child Abuse Negl* 1991;15:67-77.
20. Facchin P, Barbieri E, Boin F, et al: *European Strategies on Child Protection.* University of Padua, Padua, Italy, 1998.
21. Hiatt S, Miyoshi TJ, Fryer GE, et al: *World Perspectives on Child Abuse: the Third International Resource Book.* Kempe Children's Center, Denver, 1998.
22. Straus MA, Hamby SL, Finkelhor D, et al: Identification of child maltreatment with the Parent-Child Conflict Tactics Scales: development and psychometric data for a national sample of American parents. *Child Abuse Negl* 1998;22:249-270.
23. Madu SN, Peltzer K: Risk factors and child sexual abuse among secondary school students in the Northern Province (South Africa). *Child Abuse Negl* 2000;24:259-268.
24. Youssef RM, Attia MS, Kamel MI: Children experiencing violence. I: Parental use of corporal punishment. *Child Abuse Negl* 1998;22:959-973.
25. Menick DM: [Problems of child sexual abuse in Africa or the imbroglio of a double paradox: the example of Cameroon]. *Child Abuse Negl* 2001;25:109-121.

26. Keenan HT, Runyan DK, Marshall SW, et al: A population-based study of inflicted traumatic brain injury in young children. *JAMA* 2003;290:621-626.

27. Theodore AD, Chang JJ, Runyan DK, et al: Epidemiologic features of the physical and sexual maltreatment of children in the Carolinas. *Pediatrics* 2005;115:e331-337.

28. Runyan DK: The challenges of assessing the incidence of inflicted traumatic brain injury: a world perspective. *Am J Prev Med* 2008;34:S112-S115.

29. Kotch JB, Chalmers DJ, Fanslow JL, et al: Morbidity and death due to child abuse in New Zealand. *Child Abuse Negl* 1993;17:233-247.

30. Meadow R. Unnatural sudden infant death. *Arch Dis Child* 1999;80:7-14.

31. Alexander RC, Levitt CJ, Smith WL: Abusive head trauma. *In:* Reece RM, Ludwig S (eds): *Child Abuse: Medical Diagnosis and Management*, ed 2. Lippincott, Williams & Wilkins, Philadelphia, 2001, pp 47-80.

32. Kirschner RH, Wilson H: Pathology of fatal child abuse. *In:* Reece RM, Ludwig S (eds): *Child Abuse: Medical Diagnosis and Management*, ed 2. Lippincott, Williams & Wilkins, Philadelphia, 2001, pp 467-516.

33. Reece RM, Krous HF: Fatal child abuse and sudden infant death syndrome. *In:* Reece RM, Ludwig S (eds): *Child Abuse: Medical Diagnosis and Management*, ed 2. Lippincott, Williams & Wilkins, Philadelphia, 2001, pp 517-544.

34. Hahm HC, Guterman NB: The emerging problem of physical child abuse in South Korea. *Child Maltreat* 2001;6:169-179.

35. Larner M, Halpren B, Harkavy O: *Fair Start for Children: Lessons Learned from Seven Demonstrations*. Yale University Press, New Haven, CT, 1992.

36. Menick DM: [Psychosocial aspects of infanticide in black Africa: the case of Senegal]. *Child Abuse Negl* 2000;24:1557-1565.

37. Oral R, Can D, Kaplan S, et al: Child abuse in Turkey: an experience in overcoming denial and a description of 50 cases. *Child Abuse Negl* 2001;25:279-290.

38. Schein M, Biderman A, Baras M, et al: The prevalence of a history of child sexual abuse among adults visiting family practitioners in Israel. *Child Abuse Negl* 2000;24:667-675.

39. Shalhoub-Kevorkian N: The politics of disclosing female sexual abuse: a case study of Palestinian society. *Child Abuse Negl* 1999;23:1275-1293.

40. Zolotor AJ, Saralidze L, Goguadze N, et al: Violence to Children in Schools Perpetrated by Adults: A National Study in Georgia. *In:* Daro D (ed): *World Perspectives on Child Abuse.* International Society for the Prevention of Child Abuse and Neglect (ISPCAN) and United Nations' International Children's Emergency Fund (UNICEF), Chicago, 2008.

41. Lynch MA, Saralidze L, Goguadze N, et al: The national study on violence against children in Georgia: the nature and extent of violence experiences by children in the home. *In:* Daro D (ed): *World Perspectives on Child Abuse.* International Society for the Prevention of Child Abuse and Neglect (ISPCAN) and United Nations' International Children's Emergency Fund (UNICEF), Chicago, 2008.

42. Speizer IS, Goodwin M, Whittle L, et al: Dimensions of child sexual abuse before age 15 in three Central American countries: Honduras, El Salvador, and Guatemala. *Child Abuse Negl* 2008;32:455-462.

43. Fanslow JL, Robinson EM, Crengle S, et al: Prevalence of child sexual abuse reported by a cross-sectional sample of New Zealand women. *Child Abuse Negl* 2007;31:935-945.

44. Machado C, Goncalves M, Matos M, et al: Child and partner abuse: self-reported prevalence and attitudes in the north of Portugal. *Child Abuse Negl* 2007;31:657-670.

45. Pereda N, Forns M: [Prevalence and characteristics of child sexual abuse among spanish university students]. *Child Abuse Negl* 2007;31:417-426.

46. Barthauer LM, Leventhal JM: Prevalence and effects of child sexual abuse in a poor, rural community in El Salvador: a retrospective study of women after 12 years of civil war. *Child Abuse Negl* 1999;23:1117-1126.

47. Chen J, Dunne MP, Han P: Child sexual abuse in Henan province, China: associations with sadness, suicidality, and risk behaviors among adolescent girls. *J Adolesc Health* 2006;38:544-549.

48. Fergusson DM, Lynskey MT, Horwood LJ, et al: Childhood sexual abuse and psychiatric disorder in young adulthood: I. Prevalence of sexual abuse and factors associated with sexual abuse. *J Am Acad Child Adolesc Psychiatry* 1996;35:1355-1364.

49. Frias-Armenta M, McCloskey LA: Determinants of harsh parenting in Mexico. *J Abnorm Child Psychol* 1998;26:129-139.

50. Goldman JD, Padayachi UK: The prevalence and nature of child sexual abuse in Queensland, Australia. *Child Abuse Negl* 1997;21:489-498.

51. Hassan F, Refaat A, El-Sayed, H, et al: Disciplinary practices and child maltreatment among Egyptian families in an urban area in Ismailia. *Egypt J Psychiatry* 1999;22:177-193.

52. Hunter WM, Jain D, Sadowski LS, et al: Risk factors for severe child discipline practices in rural India. *J Pediatr Psychol* 2000;25:435-447.

53. Kim DH, Kim KI, Park YC, et al: Children's experience of violence in China and Korea: a transcultural study. *Child Abuse Negl* 2000;24:1163-1173.

54. Shumba A: Epidemiology and etiology of reported cases of child physical abuse in Zimbabwean primary schools. *Child Abuse Negl* 2001;25:265-277.

55. Tang CS: The rate of physical child abuse in Chinese families: a community survey in Hong Kong. *Child Abuse Negl* 1998;22:381-391.

56. Runyan DK, Shankara V, Hassan F, et al: International variations in harsh child discipline. Accepted for publication, *Pediatrics*.

57. Stavropoulos J: *Violence Against Girls in Africa: A Retrospective Survey in Ethiopia, Kenya and Uganda.* African Child Policy Forum, Addis Ababa, 2006.

58. World Perspectives on Child Abuse and Neglect: an International Research Book, ed 8. International Society for the Prevention of Child Abuse and Neglect, Chicago, 2008.

59. Dube SR, Anda RF, Felitti VJ, et al: Childhood abuse, household dysfunction, and the risk of attempted suicide throughout the life span: findings from the Adverse Childhood Experiences Study. *JAMA* 2001;286:3089-3096.

60. Finkelhor D, Moore D, Hamby SL, et al: Sexually abused children in a national survey of parents: methodological issues. *Child Abuse Negl* 1997;21:1-9.

61. Edgardh K, Ormstad K: Prevalence and characteristics of sexual abuse in a national sample of Swedish seventeen-year-old boys and girls. *Acta Paediatr* 2000;89:310-319.

62. Halperin DS, Bouvier P, Jaffe PD, et al: Prevalence of sexual abuse among adolescents in Geneva: results of a cross sectional survey. *Br Med J* 1996;312:1326-1329.

63. Tschumper A, Narring F, Meier C, et al: Sexual victimization in adolescent girls (age 15-20 years) enrolled in post-mandatory schools or professional training programmes in Switzerland. *Acta Paediatr* 1998;87:212-217.

64. Finkelhor D: The international epidemiology of child sexual abuse. *Child Abuse Negl* 1994;18:409-417.

65. Pedersen W, Skrondal A: Alcohol and sexual victimization: a longitudinal study of Norwegian girls. *Addiction* 1996;91:565-581.

66. Finkelhor D: *A Sourcebook on Child Sexual Abuse.* Sage, Thousand Oaks, CA, 1986.

67. Dubowitz H, Black MM: Child Neglect. *In:* Reece RM, Ludwig S (eds): *Child Abuse: Medical Diagnosis and Management*, ed 2. Lippincott, Williams & Wilkins, Philadelphia, 2001, pp 339-363.

68. African Network for the Prevention and Protection Against Child Abuse and Neglect (ANPPCAN): *Awareness and Views Regarding Child Abuse and Child Rights in Selected Communities in Kenya.* ANPPCAN, Nairobi, Kenya, 2000.

69. Wolfe DA: *Child Abuse: Implications for Child Development and Psychopathology*, ed 2. Sage, Thousand Oaks, CA, 1999.

70. Children's Bureau: *Child Maltreatment 2006.* U.S. Department of Health and Human Services, Washington, DC, 2008.

71. Belsky J: Etiology of child maltreatment: a developmental-ecological analysis. *Psychol Bull* 1993;114:413-434.

72. National Research Council: *The Future of Public Health.* National Academy of Sciences Press, Washington, DC, 1988.

73. Hunter RS, Kilstrom N, Kraybill EN, et al: Antecedents of child abuse and neglect in premature infants: a prospective study in a newborn intensive care unit. *Pediatrics* 1978;61:629-635.

74. Straus MA, Hamby SL: Measuring physical and psychological maltreatment of children with the conflict tactics scale. *In:* Kantor GK, Jasinski JL (eds): *Out of the Darkness: Contemporary Perspectives on Family Violence.* Sage Publications, Thousand Oaks, CA, 1997.

75. Olsson A, Ellsberg M, Berglund S, et al: Sexual abuse during childhood and adolescence among Nicaraguan men and women: a population-based anonymous survey. *Child Abuse Negl* 2000;24:1579-1589.

76. Tadele G, Tefera D, Nasir E: *Family Violence Against Children in Addis Ababa.* African Network for the Prevention of and Protection Against Child Abuse and Neglect, Ethiopan Chapter, Addis Ababa, 1999.

77. Jenny C, Hymel KP, Ritzen A, et al: Analysis of missed cases of abusive head trauma. *JAMA* 1999;281:621-626.

78. Klevens J, Bayon MC, Sierra M: Risk factors and context of men who physically abuse in Bogota, Colombia. *Child Abuse Negl* 2000;24: 323-332.

79. Starling SP, Holden JR: Perpetrators of abusive head trauma: a comparison of two geographic populations. *South Med J* 2000;93: 463-465.

80. MacIntyre D, Carr A: The epidemiology of child sexual abuse. *J Child Centered Pract* 1999;6:57-86.

81. Levesque RJR: *Sexual Abuse of Children: A Human Rights Perspective.* Indiana University Press, Bloomington, IN, 1999.

82. Briere JN, Elliott DM: Immediate and long-term impacts of child sexual abuse. *Future Child* 1994;4:54-69.

83. Egeland B: A history of abuse is a major risk factor for abusing the next generation. *In:* Gelles RJ, Loseke DR (eds): *Current Controversies in Family Violence.* Sage Publications, Thousand Oaks, CA, 1993.

84. Ertem IO, Leventhal JM, Dobbs S: Intergenerational continuity of child physical abuse: how good is the evidence? *Lancet* 2000;356: 814-819.

85. Gray JD, Cutler CA, Dean JG, et al: Prediction and prevention of child abuse. *Semin Perinatol* 1979;3:85-90.

86. Zolotor AJ, Theodore AD, Coyne-Beasley TC, et al: Intimate partner violence and child maltreatment: overlapping risk. *Brief Treat Crisis Interv* 2007;7:305-321.

87. Appel AE, Holdern GW: The co-occurrence of spouse and physical child abuse: a review and appraisal. *J Fam Psychol* 1998;12:413-434.

88. Casanueva C, Kotch JB, Zolotor A: Intimate partner violence and child abuse and neglect. *In:* Kendall-Tackett KA, Giacomoni SM (eds): *Intimate Partner Violence.* Civic Research Institute, Kingston, NJ, 2007.

89. Lee LC, Kotch JB, Cox CE: Child maltreatment in families experiencing domestic violence. *Violence Vict* 2004;19:573-591.

90. Johnson RM, Kotch JB, Catellier DJ, et al: Adverse behavioral and emotional outcomes from child abuse and witnessed violence. *Child Maltreat* 2002;7:179-186.

91. Runyan DK, Hunter WM, Socolar RR, et al: Children who prosper in unfavorable environments: the relationship to social capital. *Pediatrics* 1998;101:12-18.

92. Cadzow SP, Armstrong KL, Fraser JA: Stressed parents with infants: reassessing physical abuse risk factors. *Child Abuse Negl* 1999;23: 845-853.

93. Kotch JB, Browne DC, Dufort V, et al: Predicting child maltreatment in the first 4 years of life from characteristics assessed in the neonatal period. *Child Abuse Negl* 1999;23:305-319.

94. Chaffin M, Kelleher K, Hollenberg J: Onset of physical abuse and neglect: psychiatric, substance abuse, and social risk factors from prospective community data. *Child Abuse Negl* 1996;20:191-203.

95. Cicchinelli LF: *Proceedings of the Symposium on Risk Assessment in Child Protective Services.* National Center on Child Abuse and Neglect, Washington, DC, 1991.

96. de Paul J, Milner JS, Mugica P: Childhood maltreatment, childhood social support, and child abuse potential in a Basque sample. *Child Abuse Negl* 1995;19:907-920.

97. Cawson P, Wattam C, Booker S, et al: *The Prevalence of Child Maltreatment in the UK.* National Society for the Prevention of Cruelty to Children, London, 2000.

98. Zolotor AJ, Runyan DK: Social capital, family violence, and neglect. *Pediatrics* 2006;117:e1124-1131.

99. Vinson T, Baldry E: *The Spatial Clustering of Child Maltreatment: Are Micro-Social Environments Involved?* Australian Institute of Criminology, Canberra, Australia, 1999.

100. Garbarino J, Sherman D: High risk neighborhoods and high risk families: the human ecology of child maltreatment. *Child Dev* 1980;51:188-198.

101. Daro D, McCurdy K, Harding K: *The Role of Home Visiting in Preventing Child Abuse: an Evaluation of the Hawaii Healthy Start Program.* National Committee to Prevent Child Abuse, Chicago, 1998.

102. Olds DL, Eckenrode J, Henderson CR Jr, et al: Long-term effects of home visitation on maternal life course and child abuse and neglect. Fifteen-year follow-up of a randomized trial. *JAMA* 1997;278: 637-643.

103. Olds DL, Henderson CR, Jr., Chamberlin R, et al: Preventing child abuse and neglect: a randomized trial of nurse home visitation. *Pediatrics* 1986;78:65-78.

104. Alpert EJ, Tonkin AE, Seeherman AM, et al: Family violence curricula in U.S. medical schools. *Am J Prev Med* 1998;14:273-282.

105. Theodore AD, Runyan DK: A survey of pediatricians' attitudes and experiences with court in cases of child maltreatment. *Child Abuse Negl* 2006;30:1353-1363.

106. Lane WG, Dubowitz H: What factors affect the identification and reporting of child abuse-related fractures? *Clin Orthop Relat Res* 2007;461:219-225.

107. Laskey AL, Sheridan MJ, Hymel KP: Physicians' initial forensic impressions of hypothetical cases of pediatric traumatic brain injury. *Child Abuse Negl* 2007;31:329-342.

108. Runyan DK: Prevalence, risk, sensitivity, and specificity: a commentary on the epidemiology of child sexual abuse and the development of a research agenda. *Child Abuse Negl* 1998;22:493-498.

109. Runyan DK, Dunne MP, Zolotor AJ, et al: The development of the international screening tool for child abuse—the ICAST P (parent version). *Child Abuse Negl* 2009;33:826-832.

110. Dunne MP, Zolotor AJ, Runyan DK, et al: ISPCAN child abuse screening tools retrospective version (ICAST R): delphi study and field testing in seven countries. *Child Abuse Negl* 2009;33:815-825.

111. Zolotor AJ, Runyan DK, Dunne MP, et al: ISPCAN child abuse screening tool children's version: instrument development and multi-national pilot testing. *Child Abuse Negl* 2009;33:833-841.

68

The Essentials of an Effective Child Welfare System

Thomas L. Dwyer, MA

A BRIEF HISTORY OF CHILD PROTECTIVE SERVICES IN THE UNITED STATES

The historical underpinnings of child protective services in the United States can be dated to 1874. In 1866 the New York Society for the Prevention of Cruelty to Animals was founded by Henry Bergh with a view toward more humane treatment of animals in New York City. The society's main focus was on draught horses and other work animals that were so common on the streets of New York in the late nineteenth century.[1]

Just 8 years later, in 1874, a young girl named Mary Ellen Wilson was found to be living in deplorable conditions and suffering terrible abuse at the hands of her alleged stepmother, Francis Connolly. This situation came to the attention of a Methodist missionary named Etta Angell Wheeler who tried in vain to get existing authorities to intervene in the matter. Finally, in desperation, Mrs. Wheeler turned to Henry Bergh. Mr. Bergh brought the case before the New York Supreme Court and successfully argued that the child was in imminent danger and should be removed from the home. Judge Abraham Lawrence agreed and that same day Mary Ellen was removed from home and brought before the court. After Mary Ellen's chilling testimony about the abuse and neglect she had suffered at the hands of Francis Connolly, she was permanently removed from the home and was placed with the Woman's Aid Society and Home for Friendless Girls.[2] At that time, all juveniles were handled by the New York Department of Charities and Correction, and regardless of whether a girl was homeless, orphaned, or delinquent, they were all treated the same. Consequently, Mary Ellen was placed in a home with mostly delinquent adolescents.[2]

Again, Etta Wheeler intervened with Judge Lawrence. Henry Bergh was consulted and finally it was decided to turn the child over to Etta Wheeler. Wheeler, not wanting to raise the child in the slums of New York City where she carried out her missionary work, brought Mary Ellen to her mother's house outside the city. Soon after, Wheeler's mother became ill and Mary Ellen was raised by Etta Wheeler's sister, where she thrived. She grew up to be a happy, healthy adult and lived to the age of 92.

At the time of the initial hearing and removal of Mary Ellen from her home, it was widely reported that Henry Bergh argued that the child was, first and foremost, an animal, and therefore entitled to the protection of the New York Society for the Prevention of Cruelty to Animals. In truth, this was not the argument that Bergh made. He actually made a more compelling argument. He cited Section 65 of the Habeas Corpus Act, which states, "Whenever it shall appear by satisfactory proof that anyone is held in illegal confinement or custody, and that there is good reason to believe that he will ... suffer some irreparable injury, before he can be relieved by the issuing of a *habeas corpus* or *ceriorari*, any court or officer authorized to issue such writs, may issue a warrant ... and bring him before such court or officer, to be dealt with according to law."[2]

This argument had much wider application and was subsequently used to rescue many more children from abusive and neglectful homes. A newspaper reporter who was present at the hearing when Mary Ellen was brought in to testify later wrote, "I knew that I was where the first chapter of children's rights was being written."[2]

That same year, Henry Bergh founded the New York Society for the Prevention of Cruelty to Children (NYSPCC). In 1877, it was merged with the New York Society for the Prevention of Cruelty to Animals and several other animal right groups to form the American Humane Association, which is still active in efforts to protect both children and animals.[1]

From that time on there was a growing awareness of the desperate conditions of millions of children in the United States. Cities, states, and the Federal Government began to awaken to these conditions, but actual services for these children were generally left to churches and charities. This did not change significantly until the Roosevelt era, when government began to take a greater role in social services. In 1935 Congress passed the landmark Social Security Act.[3] This was the first time that Federal funds were specifically allocated to child welfare services. Congress continued to fund child welfare services through the Social Security Act, using a series of amendments aimed at expanding funding for child welfare. This included funding for foster care for children who could not safely remain with their parents.

In 1958 Congress again amended Title V to require states to provide matching funds in order to remain eligible for Federal funds. In 1967 Title V became Title IV B of the Social Security Act titled, "Child Welfare Services." In 1961 Congress expanded Title V-A, "Aid to Families with Dependent Children" (AFDC), which included funding for foster care for children. In 1969 it became mandatory for all states to participate in this program and by 1973, more than 100,000 children were in foster care placements funded by Title IV-A.[3]

MODERN CHILD WELFARE

A landmark advance in child protection came in 1961 when Dr. C. Henry Kempe convened his now famous conference on child abuse titled, "The Battered Child Syndrome." The conference called national and international attention to the reality that many "accidental" childhood injuries were in fact the result of "battering" (abuse). The conference and the ensuing article of the same title[4] generated a demand that the issue of child abuse and neglect be dealt with more openly.

The next step in the evolution of child protection came in 1974 with the creation by the Federal Government of the "Child Abuse and Neglect Prevention and Treatment Act" (CAPTA), which in turn created the National Center on Child Abuse and Neglect. The work of CAPTA and the National Center was bolstered in 1980 with the passage of further Federal child protection legislation titled, "The Foster Care and Adoption Assistance Act of 1980." This act required, among many other things, that children not languish in foster care and that every child must have a permanent home—whether his or her own home or an adoptive home.[5]

In 1994, Congress, feeling that children were still languishing in foster care and were not sufficiently protected, passed "The Adoption and Safe Families Act." This act demanded that all states ensure the safety, permanence, and well-being of every child in the child welfare system. To ensure that the states are complying with the provisions of this act, Congress also ordered the Department of Health and Human Services, Office for Children, Administration of Children and Families (ACF) to review each state's child welfare agency to measure their compliance with this mandate. If a state was found out of compliance with the Act, ACF was to order the state to put in place a "Program Improvement Plan" (PIP) to ensure future compliance with the critical elements of safety, permanence, and well-being. On March 25, 2000 a final rule was approved identifying specifically how the Department of Health and Human Services (HHS) was going to conduct the review of each state's child welfare agency. The Children's Bureau, a division of HHS, would conduct a Child and Family Service Review (CFSR). The goal of the CFSR was to help states improve their child welfare program, the quality of which would be determined by the outcomes on the following measures[6]:

Safety: (1) Children are first and foremost protected from abuse and neglect. (2) Children are safely maintained in their homes whenever possible.

Permanency: (1) Children have permanency and stability in their living situation. (2) The continuity of family relationships and connections is preserved.

Well-being: (1) Families have enhanced capacity to provide for their children's needs. (2) Children receive appropriate services to meet their educational needs. (3) Children receive adequate services to meet their physical and mental health needs.

In addition, there were seven systemic factors that had to be reviewed and judged to be either in "substantial conformity" or "area needing improvement." Armed with these criteria, the Children's Bureau began their on-site reviews in the spring of 2002. Since that time all 50 states and the District of Columbia and Puerto Rico have been reviewed and not a single entity has been found to be in full compliance with all seven measures. As a consequence, each state, Puerto Rico, and the District of Columbia were ordered to develop a PIP to address the areas in which they were found in need of improvement.[6]

In the spring of 2007, a second round of reviews began. To date, no state has been found in compliance with all measures during the second round of reviews, leading to a second round of PIP that will be required.[7]

Through these reviews the Children's Bureau has identified a number of promising practices in child welfare but has not developed a model child protection program or identified the necessary elements of an effective child protection system.[7]

EFFECTIVE CHILD WELFARE ORGANIZATIONS

In order to be an effectively functioning twenty-first–century organization, child welfare must definitively address some of the age-old problems that have frustrated both front-line staff and administrators since its inception. It must also embrace some emerging practices that show promise for more effective child welfare organizations. The problems that must be confronted and addressed are numerous, but particular emphasis must be placed on leadership, staff turnover, burnout, secondary trauma, caseloads, and compensation.

Leadership

Leadership in child welfare must begin with the state's Governor. The Governor must be committed to the goals and mission of child welfare/child protective services (CPS) and must act accordingly. He or she must ensure adequate funding for CPS and must work with the state legislature to make children a priority of state government. Many organizations and advocates are prepared to help in this effort, but it must be led by the Governor. It is not lost on politicians that children do not vote and many of the parents of children involved with the child welfare system do not vote either. It is also imperative that the Governor choose a head of child welfare/CPS who is committed to the goals and mission of child welfare and is thoroughly qualified for the position by means of extensive experience in the field and real leadership capabilities. All too often, Child Welfare Directors or Commissioners are chosen, not for their outstanding qualifications, but for political considerations. Although no unit of government benefits from underqualified leaders, this is especially true in child welfare services where the safety and well-being of children depend upon competent leadership. The fact that the welfare of children supersedes political considerations must be understood and appreciated by all elected leaders.

Another leadership issue that must be addressed is the "culture of blame" in CPS. All too frequently when a tragic event occurs in an active child welfare case, the immediate reaction of much of the media, political leaders, and the community is to find someone to blame. This culture of blame often results in the dismissal of the child welfare director, the front-line worker, the supervisor, and other staff who were involved in the decisions in the case. The net effect of this is that child protective staff often makes decisions in an atmosphere of fear. Fear, not best practice, then drives the handling of cases. Although it is absolutely correct to hold people accountable for malfeasance and/or dereliction of duty, it is not right to destroy a worker's career for a decision made with the best information available, however poor the outcome may be. Human nature is highly unpredictable and sometimes people do terrible things that could not be reasonably anticipated. After the death of a child in the custody of child welfare services, it is usual for a panel of experts to be empanelled to review the circumstances of the case. This panel, with an abundance of time to review the case and to contemplate if the correct decision or decisions were made, then completes its report with the full benefit of hindsight. It must be understood that this process in no way resembles the realities of child welfare practice in which critical decisions must be made with limited time and limited information. This is where leaders distinguish themselves. They either "pile on" or they support their staff, if a justifiable and reasonable decision was made, even if the outcome was tragic.

Staff Turnover

Public child welfare social work is among the most difficult forms of social work practice. Unlike most other social work practice, child welfare is often confrontational, adversarial, and authoritarian. Yet child welfare social workers, like other social workers, came to the profession to help ease the burden of others. As a consequence, the turnover rate among child welfare workers is among the highest in the field and far exceeds other professions. Turnover in child welfare has been estimated at 30% to 40% annually.[8] This means that an entire child welfare staff can turn over in less than 3 years, and almost every state and county reports difficulty in recruiting competent replacement staff. There are many causes for turnover in child welfare, including high caseloads and workloads, low salaries, risk to personal safety, insufficient training, administrative burdens, secondary trauma, and "burnout."

Adding additional pressure to child welfare workers and administrators is the finding of the U.S. General Accounting Office (GAO) that in one jurisdiction, 90% of child protective staff had experienced verbal threats, 30% had been physically attacked, and 13% had been threatened with weapons.[8] The GAO also found that child welfare salaries are significantly below salaries for employees in safer and more supportive environments such as teachers, school social workers, nurses, and public health social workers. Likewise, recruitment of qualified candidates is a constant challenge and is considered one of the major problems facing child welfare administrators. This results in the inability of child welfare agencies to ensure the safety, permanency, and well-being of children in their care and the inability to comply with the requirements of the Child and Family Service Reviews.[8]

Burnout

Burnout is defined as, "A breakdown of the psychological defenses that a worker uses to cope with intense job related stress."[9] It is a syndrome in which workers feel emotionally exhausted or fatigued, withdraw emotionally from their clients, and perceive a diminution of their achievement or accomplishments.[9] Burnout results from some or all of the aforementioned reasons for turnover among child welfare social workers. In many instances burnout results in turnover, as workers leave the field for less stressful, less emotionally draining careers. In those instances in which burnout does not result in the worker leaving the agency, it results in workers providing suboptimal care to the children and families they serve, which further harms the worker and the agency. In either event, burnout takes a huge toll on the worker, the agency, and its clients.

Burnout is also related to "compassion fatigue," another phenomenon noted among child welfare personnel. Compassion fatigue results in the worker no longer being able to feel empathy for the child or family to whom they are providing services.[9]

Secondary Trauma

Secondary trauma is defined as, "The natural consequent behaviors and emotions resulting from the knowledge about a traumatizing event experienced by a significant other—the stress resulting from helping or wanting to help a traumatized or suffering person."[10] In child welfare work, it is the product of regularly witnessing human beings at their worst. There are few other professions that witness human cruelty and depravity more regularly, or more personally, than child welfare workers. Secondary trauma can be triggered by any number of experiences that child welfare workers face on a daily basis. These include sexual abuse of infants and children, extreme abuse of a child, use of children in pornography, removal of children from their homes, termination of parental rights, or the death of a child, especially one for whom the worker had responsibility. Although secondary trauma and burnout have many similarities, they are not the same thing. Secondary trauma is more personal, intense, and debilitating.

Caseloads

There is near unanimous agreement that child welfare caseloads are too high in nearly every state and county. This is made abundantly clear in the GAO report on child welfare agencies[8] that links high caseloads to the inability to meet Federal standards on safety, permanency, and well-being. In addition to the GAO, the Child Welfare League of America has established standards calling for caseloads of between 12 and 15 families per worker, while at the same time acknowledging that caseloads are frequently "… two, three and even four times that number."[11]

Compensation

Salaries in child welfare cover a very broad range. According to the Child Welfare League of America's 2005 Salary Study, the starting salary for a child protective service worker with a college degree working for a public agency ranged from a low of $24,410 to a high of $42,468.[12] Another detailed review of child welfare agencies was conducted by the National Council on Crime and Delinquency (NCCD).[13] The NCCD reviewed the overall functioning of selected child welfare agencies and grouped them into one of three clusters: high functioning, moderately functioning, and low functioning. High-functioning organizations were identified as having the lowest turnover rates, the best compliance with recognized practice standards, the highest compensation, and the lowest rate of re-abuse of children. The lowest functioning organizations had the highest turnover rates, the least compliance with recognized practice standards, the lowest compensation, and the highest rates of re-abuse of children. In the highest rated clusters, minimum salaries for child welfare workers were $56,571 and $70,057 for child welfare supervisors. In the lowest functioning clusters, minimum salaries were $32,245 for child welfare workers and $38,576 for supervisors.

Ultimately child welfare leaders must address an additional reality that plays an important role in staff turnover. In most jurisdictions, because of civil service rules, union contracts, or other structures where seniority is a critical consideration, the net result is that the least-experienced, least-trained staff are charged with the greatest responsibility: the protection of children. Because child protection and child welfare are such difficult jobs, many workers transfer out to less stressful positions, leaving the least-trained and least-experienced staff on the front lines. Child welfare leaders must implement processes and procedures that limit this practice. Accepting this "reality" puts children at risk and is a real disservice to young staff. They must also recognize that front-line child welfare workers need more time off than is typically given to a new worker. Child welfare workers must be viewed differently than other civil servants and deserve more time for rest and recover from their extraordinarily stressful jobs. They must also be allowed to rotate off the front lines for periods of time without having to give up their positions in child welfare or losing seniority.

EMERGING PROMISING PRACTICES IN CHILD WELFARE

Effective organizations should redefine their practices as new information comes to light. A body of information is emerging on a number of practices that can re-define how child welfare systems operate, described below. Effective child welfare professionals recognize that the field is dynamic and fluid and they must always be ready to re-tool the system to create a more fair and functional organization.

Differential Response in Child Protective Services

In the late 1970s and 1980s, the number of child abuse reports were increasing. Some very high profile cases demonstrated that child protective services were unprepared to manage the increasing reports. In response, child protection systems were retooled to focus more on the investigation of reports of child abuse and on documenting and preserving those investigations. Many states committed huge financial and human resources to case investigations without a concomitant commitment to the subsequent service needs of families involved in the systems. Often, investigation was the only response given to a family in crisis.

In the 1990s it became apparent that investigations that focused solely on determining if abuse or neglect occurred (and who was responsible) were not the best approach to all allegations of abuse or neglect. Some states moved to a "differential response" system, which allowed for a range of responses to allegations. This practice is also known as dual track, multiple track, or alternative responses.[14]

Although terms and definitions vary from agency to agency, differential response generally provides two types of responses to reports of child abuse or neglect: investigation and assessment (also called alternative response).

Investigation: This response focuses on investigating allegation of child abuse and neglect to determine if it occurred, and if so, who the perpetrator and victims were. If a report is proven, it is considered "indicated" or "substantiated". If the case cannot be proven, it is "unfounded" or "unsubstantiated". Indicated cases and frequently unfounded cases result in entry into the state central registry, which is a federally required repository of information on perpetrators and victims in child abuse and neglect cases. Depending on state statutes and policies, the names remain in the state central registry for years, and in some instances, forever.

Assessment: The second track in a differential response structure is assessment. Assessments are generally used in low-to-moderate risk situations and focuses not on "who did what to whom," but on a comprehensive assessment of a family's strengths and needs, and on the delivery of appropriate services to address those needs. Typically in assessment, no determination of abuse or neglect is made and no perpetrators or victims are identified. Rather, the intervention focuses on services to address the family's issues that brought them to the attention of child protective services.

Both investigation and assessment, however, focus on the safety and well-being of children. There is a mechanism to switch from the "assessment" track to the "investigative" track if a case turns out to be more serious, or if the risk to the child is determined to be greater than anticipated.

In comparison to investigations, assessments tend to be less adversarial, more focused on the strengths of the family, more likely to involve a "service remedy" rather than a "legal remedy," more likely to involve the family's natural support system, and more likely to involve community services rather than government services.[15] An effective child protective system provides both responses, depending on the level of the risk to the children, the level of cooperation of the parents, and the ability of the parents to benefit from community services.

A number of states have conducted evaluations of differential response systems. In addition, one national study found that differential response leads to better outcomes for children, especially in the area of sustained child safety, and it improves family engagement, increased community involvement, and enhanced social worker satisfaction.[15]

Family Group Conferencing

"Family group conferencing" or "family group decision-making" is a system of engaging extended family members and communities in helping families in need. It is as old as civilization and as new as the twenty-first century. In 1989, New Zealand passed the Children, Young Persons and Their Families Act.[16] This act was intended to wrap extensive services and resources around families, especially the resources of extended families, to prevent the need to remove children from their homes. This effort was largely driven by the desire to maintain the identity and culture of the native Maori people and to use the extended family and the tribal community to provide the necessary support to families in crisis who are at risk of losing their children to the child welfare system. This formal system of engaging families and communities in helping family members recognizes that families have strengths and resources to assist each other and that those resources may not be known to, or appreciated by, the child welfare system. It embraces the concept of empowering families to solve their problems in a way that works for them while at the same time ensuring the safety, permanency, and well-being of the children.

The New Zealand model was so successful in maintaining family unity that the family case conferencing model was adopted as an essential child protection tool by many child welfare systems. When a family has been respectfully engaged, and when the extended family and community can bring their strengths to bear on a family member who has become involved with the child welfare system, the net result is that children can frequently be maintained at home to the benefit of families, communities, and governments.

System of Care

In an ideal environment, child welfare services would have the capacity to deliver the right services at the right time, in the right amount, in the right place, for the right duration. Although it is unlikely that such a system actually exists, it should be the goal of every service delivery system. In order to reach that goal, agencies have adopted a comprehensive "system of care" for children and families involved in child welfare. A system of care is a unified approach to the delivery of services that seeks to ensure the safety, permanence, and well-being of every child and family through the formation of working partnerships between child welfare agencies and families. This system allows for the development of the families' capacity to meet the needs of their children in a safe and secure manner.[17]

This philosophy differs quite dramatically from the traditional delivery of services in child welfare, which usually consists of a social worker unilaterally assessing the family's needs and providing or arranging for services to address those needs, without significant input from the family and without regard to the unique strengths of the family. Services are typically delivered for a set amount of time, during which the parents are expected to "get better." Services were not individualized and not designed to meet the specific needs and strengths of the family. Such "one size fits all" service delivery systems expect the family to conform to the services, rather than having the services conform to the family.

In an effective system of care model, services are highly individualized and developed in concert with the family. Services build upon the strengths of the family, not just the deficits. An effective system of care provides a comprehensive array of services and takes advantage of the natural capacity of the community to provide viable and valuable services, which might look quite different from government services. Funding for a system of care should not be constrained by rigid funding streams and eligibility requirements but should allow for the pooling of funds from a wide variety of sources in order to build a cross-divisional, cross-departmental, and cross-agency service delivery system.

FINAL THOUGHTS

This chapter has focused on the child welfare system, which intervenes after a child has been reportedly abused or neglected. The reality, however, is that this intervention comes too late. If appropriate prevention programs were available in the community, and were of sufficient scale to be available to any family in need of the services, child welfare would not have to intervene nearly as often. This would be more beneficial to the family, to the community, and to the overburdened child welfare system. The child welfare system costs American taxpayers in excess of $33 billion a year in direct costs.[18] Can we really afford not to provide prevention and early intervention services?

References

1. American Humane Society: Mary Ellen Wilson: how one girl's plight started the child protection movement. Available at http://www.americanhumane.org/about-us/who-we-are/history/mary-ellen.html. Accessed on March 28, 2008.
2. Stevens P, Eide M: The first chapter of children's rights. *American Heritage Magazine* 1990;41(5). Available at http://www.americanheritage.com/articles/magazine/ah/1990/5/1990_5_84.shtml. Accessed on March 30, 2008.
3. Child Welfare League of America: Brief history of federal child welfare legislation. Available at http://www.cwla.org/advocacy/financinghistory.htm. Accessed on April 12, 2008.
4. Kempe CH, Silverman FN, Steele BF, et al: The battered-child syndrome. *JAMA* 1962;181:17-24.
5. Administration for Children and Families, Children's Bureau: *Child and Family Services Reviews: Procedure Manual Working Draft.* U.S. Department of Health and Human Services, Washington, DC, 2006.
6. Pagano C: Recent legislation: adoption and foster care. *Harv J on Legis* 1999;36:242-249.
7. Administration for Children and Families, Children's Bureau: Child and Family Services Reviews. Fact Sheet. Available at http://www.acf.hhs.gov/programs/cb/cwmonitoring/recruit/cfsrfactsheet.htm. Accessed on November 30, 2008.
8. U.S. General Accounting Office: Child welfare. HHS could play a greater role in helping child welfare agencies recruit and retain staff. Report GAO-03-357, 2003. Available at http://www.gao.gov/new.items/d03357.pdf. Accessed on July 20, 2008.
9. Brohl K: Understanding and preventing worker burnout. *Children's Voice* 2006;15. Available at http://www.cwla.org/voice/0609management.htm. Accessed on November 30, 2008.
10. Figley CR: *Compassion Fatigue: Secondary Traumatic Stress Disorders in Those Who Treat the Traumatized.* Routledge, New York, 1995. p 7.
11. Child Welfare League of America: Guidelines for computing caseload standards. Available at http://www.cwla.org/programs/standards/caseloadstandards.htm. Accessed on November 30, 2008.
12. Drais-Parrillo A: *2005 Salary Study.* Child Welfare League of America Press, Mt Morris, IL, 2006.
13. The Human Services Workforce Initiative: Relationship Between Staff Turnover, Child Welfare Systems functioning and recurring child abuse. National Council on Crime and Delinquency, Houston, 2006. Available at http://www.cornerstones4kids.org/images/nccd_relationships_306.pdf. Accessed on November 30, 2008.
14. Child Welfare Information Gateway: Differential Response to Reports of Child Abuse and Neglect. Administration on Children, Youth and Families, Children's Bureau, Washington, DC, 2008. Available at http://www.childwelfare.gov/pubs/issue_briefs/differential_response/differential_response.pdf. Accessed on November 30, 2008.

15. McDonald WR: National Study of Child Protective Service Systems and Reform Efforts. U.S. Department of Health and Human Services, Washington, DC, 2003. Available at http://aspe.hhs.gov/HSP/cps-status03/summary/index.htm. Accessed on November 30, 2008.

16. Children, Young Persons, and Their Families Act, 1989. *Annu Rev Popul Law* 1989;16:513-515.

17. National Child Welfare Resource Center for Organizational Improvement: Systems of Care Curriculum: Stakeholder Involvement and Interagency Collaboration, 2007. Available at http://muskie.usm.maine.edu/helpkids/rcpdfs/stakeholderfacts.pdf. Accessed on November 30, 2008.

18. Wang C-T, Holton J: Total Estimated Cost of Child Abuse in the United States. Prevent Child Abuse America, Chicago, 2007. Available at http://www.preventchildabuse.org/about_us/media_releases/pcaa_pew_economic_impact_study_final.pdf. Accessed on November 30, 2008.

69

THE COSTS OF CHILD MALTREATMENT

Kristine A. Campbell, MD, MSc

"Ignoring the direct and indirect expenditures associated with attempts to resolve this social problem will not make the task less costly nor will it result in the most efficient practice choices. While no one would argue that costs should be the sole determinant of policy, neither should costs be considered an inappropriate contributor to the decision-making process."
Deborah Daro, Confronting Child Abuse, 1988[1]

INTRODUCTION

How does one determine the costs of child maltreatment? For some, calculating a dollar value to describe the impact of maltreatment seems inappropriate. For others, the life-long effect of maltreatment on children and society makes such calculations overwhelming. Yet in a society with competing economic priorities, understanding the costs of maltreatment, as well as the costs of programs designed to prevent or respond to maltreatment, is a critical step toward effective health and social policies.

Intimate partner violence research supports this contention. Studies examining data from health maintenance organizations consistently find increased health care costs and use among women reporting a history of intimate partner violence.[2-4] Total costs of intimate partner violence in 1995 were estimated at $5.8 billion, over $1300 per victim.[2] Such data can support medical and social investments in prevention and intervention programs.

Compared with intimate partner violence, however, determining the costs of child maltreatment poses unique challenges. The mandated social response to maltreatment adds costs of protective, investigative, and legal interventions often overlooked in the analysis of intimate partner violence. Associations of child maltreatment with learning disability, juvenile delinquency, and adult health problems make it difficult to draw boundaries around cost estimates for abuse. Economic analyses in pediatrics commonly reflect costs to caregivers related to diagnosis and care of an ill or injured child, an ethically challenging proposition if the caregiver is a possible perpetrator.

It is beyond the scope of this chapter to suggest solutions to the philosophical and methodological challenges underlying the economic analysis of child maltreatment. The goals of this chapter are to provide a basic overview of approaches to economic analysis, to present best evidence related to the costs of child maltreatment, and to consider directions for future research in this area.[5]

OVERVIEW OF ECONOMIC ANALYSIS

There are several approaches to economic analysis. Selecting the appropriate analytic approach depends on the question being asked and on the data available to the researcher (Figure 69-1). At the most basic level, an economic analysis provides an understanding of the costs associated with a given condition. A cost-of-illness (COI) analysis can provide critically important information about the medical and social costs associated with a health condition. COI does not differentiate costs based on medical decision-making, nor does it try to place a value on the outcomes gained by particular interventions. As such, COI alone cannot guide rational health care policy decisions.

Cost-effectiveness analyses (CEA) and cost-utility analyses (CUA) compare costs associated with competing interventions, and balance these costs against the health-related benefits of those interventions. This approach allows decision-makers to place a proposed intervention into four possible categories: (1) improves outcomes and saves money, (2) improves outcomes but costs money, (3) worsens outcomes but saves money, and (4) worsens outcomes and costs money. Clearly, interventions in the first category should be implemented, whereas those in the fourth should be set aside. Information gained in the full CEA analysis can guide policy decisions regarding interventions falling into the second and third categories based on funding realities and social priorities.

A distinct approach to economic analysis is a cost-benefit analysis (CBA), in which the costs of medical interventions are balanced against the calculated monetary value of health outcomes. CBA provides a strictly economic perspective on medical and social interventions. Although CBA has applications in regulatory decision-making, it is unusual in the healthcare literature, where monetary valuation of health outcomes is generally viewed with skepticism or distaste.[6-8] This chapter focuses on the application of COI, CEA, and CUA in improving our understanding of the costs of child maltreatment.

Cost-of-Illness Analysis

How much does it cost to provide medical care for a child with abusive head trauma? What are the costs of mental health therapy for a child recovering from chronic sexual abuse? These are the questions answered by a COI analysis.

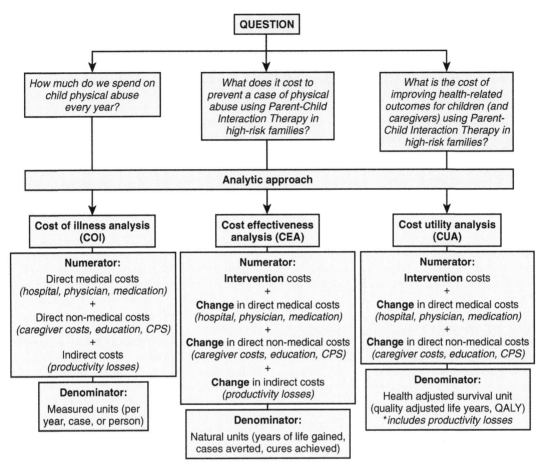

FIGURE 69-1 Visual comparison of cost-of-illness, cost-effectiveness, and cost-utility economic analyses.

As in all research, results of COI analyses are dependent on the assumptions built into the study design. Several important assumptions to consider are discussed in the following paragraphs.

Sample selection: Costs may vary widely based on the sample selected for analysis. Imagine a COI analysis for children with abusive head trauma. Substantial data exist to support the assumption that most of these children are critically ill at presentation.[9-11] It might be reasonable to assume that most of these children are admitted to intensive care units and to select a sample of PICU admissions with a diagnosis of subdural hemorrhage and child abuse for analysis. Yet this decision excludes potentially important subsets of children. As many as one tenth of children with abusive head trauma do not survive to admission (H.T. Keenan, University of Utah School of Medicine, personal communication, March 3, 2010). The proposed analysis excludes costs of children dying at home, in transport, or in the emergency room. Conversely, improvements in medical imaging and physician training may increase the numbers of mildly symptomatic children admitted to general medical or surgical services, bypassing the ICU altogether. Excluding those children never admitted to the ICU, whether because of early death or early diagnosis, could falsely inflate the medical costs associated with abusive head trauma.

Time horizon: Researchers must explicitly define the time horizon of any economic analysis. Does an accounting of the medical costs of abusive head trauma include only the costs of acute hospitalization, or extend to the lifelong costs of rehabilitation, durable medical equipment, and recurrent hospitalizations of a child with profound neurological disability?[12,13] Should the medical costs of sexual abuse be limited to the acute medical examination and specific therapies, or should there be consideration of costs of mental illness and medical complications that are increasingly linked to abusive experiences in childhood?[14-18] These decisions are driven by the objective of the analysis, but are shaped by the limitations of the data available.

Perspective: The perspective of any economic analysis defines the data used in the analysis. From a medical payer perspective, the costs of abusive head trauma are the acute care and chronic medical needs of an injured child. From a societal perspective, however, the cost burden includes child protective services and legal investigations, foster care placement, prison costs for a perpetrator, and lost wages resulting from permanent neurological disability. Both perspectives are valid, although the results of each analysis will be dramatically different.

Costs included: Estimating costs of child maltreatment raises unique questions regarding the scope of costs to be included. *Direct medical costs* are the most easily understood, encompassing the value of the health care "goods and services" needed for the proposed intervention. These can reflect the costs of a single hospitalization, or repeated encounters over time. *Direct nonmedical costs* reflect the value of resources outside of the medical system consumed by the intervention. Traditionally, these nonmedical costs account for time required of patients, family, and volunteers for the studied intervention. Nonmedical costs unique to child maltreatment can include child protection services, police investigation, legal intervention, foster care, special education, and costs of juvenile delinquency. *Indirect costs*, or productivity costs, can account for lost wages or productivity over time that can be attributed to a given health condition.

Cost adjustment: Cost data often require adjustment for economic analysis. Perhaps the most commonly recognized cost adjustment is *inflation adjustment*, which allows for comparison of cost data across many years. These calculations typically rely on the general or medical component of the Consumer Price Index (CPI).[19] A second adjustment frequently required for health care research is *profit adjustment*. In any medical system outside of a single-payer system, medical *charges* include a profit component that substantially overestimates the true medical *costs* of any intervention. There are several solutions to this dilemma. In prospectively collected data, researchers might have access to the true costs of the goods and services being used for the study. In many cases, however, researchers must rely on retrospective data that include only charge data. Under these circumstances, a cost-to-charge ratio can be applied to the economic data to better estimate true medical costs. These ratios are often available at national, regional, hospital, or departmental levels.

Cost-Effectiveness and Cost-Utility Analysis

A CEA balances costs added by a medical intervention against lives saved, cases averted, or years of life added as a result of the intervention. A CUA is a specialized subset of CEA, in which outcomes are measured with a metric that accounts for quality of life, such as the quality adjusted life year (QALY). CUA has been identified as the preferred method for economic analysis by the Panel on Cost-Effectiveness in Health and Medicine.[6] In contrast to COI analyses, which describe system costs without consideration of outcomes, CEA provides a measure of effectiveness of interventions in economic terms.

An appropriately conducted CEA can improve our understanding of the incremental improvements in health expected with new expenditures and can guide health care decision-making at a policy level. Unfortunately, CEA techniques can be challenging to conduct and interpret. A poorly conducted CEA can dramatically misrepresent cost-effectiveness estimates because of inappropriate technique, inadequate data, or investigator bias. A misinterpreted CEA might reflect a simplistic utilitarian perspective, excluding the ethical principles of nonmalfeasance, beneficence, and justice that are critically important in decision-making around child maltreatment. The following overview is in no means a comprehensive review of CEA methodology, but provides a guide to important elements to be considered in the critical review of CEA literature.

Costs: Consideration of costs for a CEA analysis includes the same element considered for COI analysis, with important additional considerations. A cost-effectiveness analysis is fundamentally a comparison of costs-to-benefit ratios between two or more interventions. Although the comparison intervention may be nothing more than "standard treatment" or "do nothing," the analysis must account for *change* in direct and indirect costs under each intervention arm. In a randomized control trial, researchers may have full access to cost data for each arm. In a one-armed observational trial, however, costs for the study population may be compared with literature-derived costs of illness to examine cost-effectiveness of the intervention. Finally, a CEA can mimic a true randomized controlled trial by relying only on literature-derived data in circumstances in which adequate data for both intervention arms already exist. Researchers must examine the strength of the cost data available for comparison when relying on literature-derived values.

Outcomes: In COI analysis, all costs are incorporated into the numerator. In CEA research, however, costs cannot simultaneously appear in the numerator, reflecting costs, and the denominator, reflecting outcomes. A CEA can include indirect costs accounting for lost work and wages in the numerator, but places years of life lost and gained in the denominator. In CUA, all indirect costs should be reflected in the health-related outcome metric used for the denominator.

The choice of outcomes in CEA research is critical and controversial. The most basic metric is years of life gained, or lives saved, by a given intervention. There is increasing recognition, however, that such measures overlook quality of life concerns. In adult medicine, the prolongation of chronic and life-threatening illness can raise health expenditures for marginal survival gains with poor quality of life. In pediatrics, similar questions are considered in analysis of health care expenditures for technologically dependent infants and children. CUA relies on "utilities" to reflect concerns of quality of life over simple survival.

The quality adjusted life years' (QALY) measure remains the most commonly used metric to express the balance between length and quality of life (Table 69-1). Although conceptually appealing, practical issues around measuring quality of life and the interpretation of these measures are subject to intense ethical debate, particularly in pediatrics.[20-22] It remains unclear how best to measure quality of life of young children. There are few—if any—validated measures of quality of life for children under 7 years of age, and researchers might rely on instruments that are

Table 69-1	**Sample Calculation of Quality Adjusted Life Years (QALYs)**		
Condition	Years (0-1)	Utility (0-1)	Total QALYs (Time × Utility)
12 months of life in perfect health	1	1	1
10 months of life in perfect health	0.8	1	0.8
12 months of life with poor health	1	0.8	0.8
6 months of life with poor health	0.5	0.8	0.4

developmentally inappropriate for a pediatric population. In children who cannot participate in quality of life studies because of age or disability, proxy responses by parents and caregivers are typical substitutes.[23,24] These issues are amplified by concerns of child maltreatment. How does one measure the impact of foster placement on the quality of life of a 15-month-old? How do we use parental proxies if we doubt the integrity of the parents? Although these considerations do not necessarily exclude quality of life metrics in the assessment of the cost-utility of an intervention, researchers must acknowledge the limitations of these measures and include analyses to account for these uncertainties.

Discounting: Many primary care health interventions are made in anticipation of future, rather than immediate, health benefits. This is particularly true for pediatrics, where the benefits of a healthy childhood can be sustained over a lifetime. It is generally assumed, however, that immediate health is valued above future health. To address this concern, most economic analyses discount both costs and benefits at about 3% to 10% per year. This practice is not without question, however, since it can lead to undervaluing of preventive or pediatric health care.[25]

Sensitivity analysis: A unique characteristic of CEA is in the reflection of uncertainty. Medical literature traditionally relies on *p*-values and confidence intervals to describe uncertainty around a result. These statistics are not helpful in CEA because of modeling techniques that allow researchers to generate sample sizes to support unrealistically tight confidence intervals. For CEA, uncertainty is reflected in sensitivity analyses, in which the analysis is repeated over a rational interval of values of costs variables and outcome probabilities. For example, CEA of a home visitation program could include the expected number of home visits or the annual salaries of the home visitors, numbers that vary by program design, by geography, and by chance. Researchers should run the model using the lowest and the highest number of

home visits as well as the lowest and the highest home visitor salaries. This type of sensitivity analysis provides the range of outcomes that can be reasonably expected under conditions of uncertainty. As almost all research in child maltreatment involves substantial uncertainty, any CEA of interventions for child abuse should reflect this uncertainty with careful sensitivity analyses.

ECONOMIC ANALYSIS IN CHILD MALTREATMENT[26]

Costs of Child Maltreatment (COI)

Several studies have attempted to describe the total costs of child maltreatment in the United States (Table 69-2). All of these studies rely on important assumptions related to the incidence of hospitalization and medical care for physical injuries, as well as the causal link between abuse and observed outcomes among children after abuse. In 1988, Daro[1] published the first estimates of the costs of child maltreatment, making informed assumptions regarding the need for inpatient treatment of abusive injury; ongoing medical, rehabilitative, and educational needs of abused children; and lifetime loss of earning potential attributed to childhood abuse. In 1996, the U.S. Department of Justice examined costs of child maltreatment.[27] The authors acknowledged the limitations of the research, commenting that "... virtually no estimates of medical costs are available for child abuse," and that "... this study's estimates for child abuse should be viewed as very rough and worthy of further study." In contrast to other studies, these authors calculated a monetary value for the quality of life costs of abuse, with estimates of $30,276 for emotional abuse, $82,506 for physical abuse, and $128,853 for sexual abuse. These intangible costs were by far the largest contributor to costs for all violent crimes in this

Table 69-2	Summary of Studies Estimating Total Annual Costs of Child Maltreatment in the United States (All Costs Adjusted to 2007 Dollars)				
Study	**Cases (n)**	**Costs Examined**	**Direct Medical Costs**	**Direct Nonmedical Costs**	**Indirect Productivity Costs**
Daro, 1988*[1] (Lifetime)	739,000 (23,648)	Costs/case	$56 ($1,761)	$3,177	$1,854-3,662
		Total costs	$41 million	$2.3 billion	$1.4-2.7 billion
Miller, 1996†[27] (Annual)	926,000 (all)	Costs/case	$3,774	$2,639	$3,157
		Total costs	$3.5 billion	$2.4 billion	$2.9 billion
	185,000 (sexual)	Costs/case	$9,025	$1,659	$3,013
		Total costs	$1.7 billion	$307 million	$557 million
	355,000 (physical)	Costs/case	$5,008	$3,079	$4,879
		Total costs	$1.8 billion	$1.1 billion	$1.7 billion
	337,000 (emotional)	Costs/case	$3,874	$3,042	$1,291
		Total costs	$1.3 billion	$1.0 billion	$435 million
Wang, 2007[28] (Annual)	1,553,800	Costs/case	$5,004	$40,520	$21,251
		Total costs	$7.8 billion	$63.0 billion	$33.0 billion

*Daro estimated medical costs based only on the acute inpatient medical care of 23,648 children with severe physical abuse and is, therefore, a substantial underestimate of the true value. Direct medical costs are provided based on the total population of abused children and the subset of those with severe physical abuse. Daro also excluded many cost categories included in subsequent analyses.
†Miller did not include child neglect in this economic analysis.

analysis. Finally, the Prevent Child Abuse America Foundation provided a recent estimate of the total national costs of child maltreatment, again relying on informed estimates for their analysis.[28] The wide range of estimates in these three studies reflects the differences in sample selected, perspective adopted, time horizon, and costs included by each of the authors.

The limitations of these studies must be recognized. There is a tendency in these analyses to suggest causation where prior epidemiological studies have only identified an association. In other words, although maltreatment is *associated* with later need for special education, it is not clear that maltreatment *causes* this educational need. It is not clear that prevention of maltreatment would eliminate all of these excess educational costs.[28] Although adult survivors of childhood maltreatment have a higher risk of illness, research identifies an additive effect of multiple childhood adversities rather than a direct correlation between child maltreatment and adult poor health.[17] It might not be reasonable to assume that prevention of child abuse will eliminate these future medical costs.

Efforts to describe acute medical costs associated with child abuse have used hospital charges for inpatient care of children diagnosed with abuse. These studies are limited by reliance on medical charges rather than medical costs, capturing medical resource utilization as well as profit margin associated with health care in the United States. By comparing medical charges in abuse-related hospitalizations to those in nonabuse-related hospitalizations, however, these studies do suggest relatively high medical resource utilization associated with child abuse (Table 69-3). These differences likely reflect the increased severity of injury, younger patient age, and increased length of stay in children with abuse-related hospitalizations.

There is increasing evidence that childhood abuse results in increased health risks sustained into adolescence and adulthood. Two authors have linked self-reports of childhood maltreatment with healthcare utilization in adult women enrolled in a health maintenance organization.[14,18] Both studies have observed moderate increases in health care costs among these women, suggesting that child abuse has a real and sustained effect on health and health care utilization among survivors.

Cost-Effectiveness of Child Maltreatment Programs

Many authors have called for improved economic analysis of child abuse prevention and intervention programs, yet few such analyses exist.[7,33-36] Population-based prevention programs tend to be resource intensive. One British study calculated that an 18-month home visiting program cost £3246 per child (2003-2004 British pounds), even accounting for costs saved in health care utilization and counseling in the intervention arm over the study period.[37] In 2007 U.S. dollars, this is $6245.* Given the early cost demands of such programs, long-term CEA provides the opportunity to weigh the initial costs against sustained benefits.

With this approach, parent training programs have been found to be cost saving in several published analyses. In an evaluation of the Nurse-Family Partnership in Elmira, New York, Olds et al[38] concluded that the program of home visitation by nurses saved $4459 per family over 48 months because of lower utilization of welfare services among families enrolled in the treatment arm of the trial. The Rand Corporation estimated cost savings of the Elmira Nurse-Family Partnership program of $24,594 per high-risk family over 15 years based on sustained reductions in welfare reliance for mother, reduced criminal justice costs for mothers and children, and increased tax revenues from maternal employment.[39] An analysis of the Family Support Center, an integrated home/school/community program for high-risk families estimated cost savings of $9564 per high-risk family over approximately 6 years.[40] Although this study relied on measured program costs over 1 year, it made broad assumptions regarding potential long-term cost savings based on literature review.

In each of these studies, the finding of overall cost savings allowed the authors to avoid the difficult calculation of lives

---

*2003–2004 UK pounds converted to 1998 U.S. dollars, then adjusted for inflation to 2007 dollars.

Table 69-3	Medical Charges Associated with Hospitalizations Related to Child Abuse (All Charges Adjusted to 2007 Dollars)			
Study	**Study Sample**	**Mean Charges Abuse Sample (n)**	**Mean Charges Nonabuse Sample (n)**	**Ratio of Charges***
Ettaro et al, 2004[29]	Children <3 yr of age with head trauma admission, 1995-1999	$49,884 (n = 89)	$19,503 (n = 288)	2.6
Irazuzta et al, 1997[30]	PICU trauma admission, 1991-1994	$42,929 (n = 13)	$41,097 (n = 34)	1.0
Libby et al, 2003[†31]	Children <3 yr with head trauma admission, 1993-2000	$33,672 (n = 283)	$14,378 (n = 814)	2.3
Rovi et al, 2004[32]	Post-neonatal pediatric hospitalization in HCUP database, 1999[‡]	$23,977 (n = 966)	$11,839 (n = 1,371,835)	2.0

*Ratio of medical charges for children hospitalized for abuse-related reasons compared with children with nonabuse-related hospitalizations.
†Charges adjusted based using 1996 (study mid-point) CPI data.
‡Healthcare Costs and Utilization Project (HCUP).

saved, cases averted, or quality of life gained. When a program saves money, and meets or exceeds the outcomes observed under current practice, there is no need to further complicate the analysis. The decision to implement these programs, if the assumptions of the analysis are accepted, should be clear. These studies identified cost savings not in violence prevention but in improved parenting, improved socioeconomic status, and improved community integration. Studies relying only on violence prevention to demonstrate cost effectiveness of a program face a much stiffer challenge.[41,42]

Although the societal costs of child abuse are substantial, few studies examine the cost effectiveness of our interventions. One study examined the cost effectiveness of rehabilitation of child sexual abuse perpetrators, concluding that treatment programs may save $124,093 compared with traditional incarceration based on decreased recidivism in the 5 years following prison release. The authors acknowledge limitations in the estimates of recidivism within this population and make appropriate sensitivity analyses, pointing out that cost savings persist as long as recidivism rates among the untreated population remained higher than 3% (compared with 25% in the treated population).[43] A more recent Australian study used a cost–benefit analysis to assess treatment programs for child sexual abuse perpetrators. Without providing specific program data, the authors conclude that the expected costs of such programs could range from a loss of $6850 to savings of $39,870 per treated prisoner (1998 Australian dollars). In 2007 U.S. dollars, this translates to savings of from $5525 to $32,160 per treated prisoner.* The estimates varied based on the interaction between the reduction in recidivism attributed to the treatment program and the range of tangible and intangible costs attributed to recidivism.[44]

Only one study has examined the cost effectiveness of a specific medical decision related to child maltreatment.[45] The dilemma over when to obtain radiographic imagining (head CT) for a well-appearing infant presenting with non-specific signs and symptoms that may reflect brain injury is common. Using literature-derived variables to model short-term cost effectiveness of CT imaging in these children, the authors found that imaging could be cost saving from a medical perspective, but only when the probability of abusive head trauma rose above 16%. From a societal perspective, identification of abuse was almost always expensive when considered over a short 1-year time frame. The authors made no attempt to identify long-term outcomes for children with earlier recognition of abuse, citing limitations in available data to address these issues.

STRENGTH OF THE EVIDENCE

It is widely accepted that violence, in its many forms, is expensive at individual and societal levels. Children can account for more than 35% of all crime victim costs.[27] Despite this, clear evidence for costs of violence against children, and the cost effectiveness of programs responding to the problem, is generally lacking. Most estimates of the costs of child maltreatment rely heavily on assumptions that fail to account

for the multiple social confounders associated with child maltreatment and with its long-term outcomes. The consistent finding of cost effectiveness of prevention programs evaluated is encouraging, yet remains limited by our poor understanding of the true costs of child maltreatment.

DIRECTIONS FOR FUTURE RESEARCH

Research in child maltreatment is rapidly accelerating. In 2007, the National Institutes of Health sought proposals for research that would move the field beyond an understanding of the epidemiology of maltreatment and toward "… large-scale, community-based, effectiveness trials" of programs to prevent and respond to child maltreatment.[46] As efforts to translate observational and behavioral science into policy and practice move forward, economic evaluation should be an integral component of emerging research. Researchers must recognize that the cost savings of many interventions might come more from secondary effects, such as reduced dependence on welfare programs or reduced need for special education, and not from primary prevention of maltreatment. Identifying the costs of abuse to victims and to society, as well as the costs of the programs proposed, will dramatically improve our understanding of the costs of child maltreatment and benefits of policies that protect children.

References

1. Daro D: The costs of prevention and intervention. *In:* Daro D (ed): *Confronting Child Abuse: Research for Effective Program Design.* The Free Press, New York, 1988.
2. National Center for Injury Prevention and Control: *Costs of Intimate Partner Violence Against Women in the United States.* Centers for Disease Control and Prevention, Atlanta, 2003.
3. Rivara FP, Anderson ML, Fishman P, et al: Healthcare utilization and costs for women with a history of intimate partner violence. *Am J Prev Med* 2007;32:89-96.
4. Wisner CL, Gilmer TP, Saltzman LE, et al: Intimate partner violence against women: do victims cost health plans more? *J Fam Pract* 1999;48:439-443.
5. Readers are referred to *Cost-Effectiveness in Health and Medicine* (Gold, 1996) and *Valuing Health for Regulatory Cost-Effectiveness Analysis* (Miller, 2006) for more detailed discussion on economic analysis and healthcare decision-making.
6. Gold MR, Siegel JE, Russell LB, et al *(eds): Cost-Effectiveness in Health and Medicine.* Oxford University Press, New York, 1996.
7. Corso PS, Lutzker JR: The need for economic analysis in research on child maltreatment. *Child Abuse Negl* 2006;30:727-738.
8. Miller W, Robinson LA, Lawrence RS (eds): *Valuing Health for Regulatory Cost-Effectiveness Analysis.* National Academy Press, Washington, 2006.
9. Hymel KP, Makoroff KL, Laskey AL, et al: Mechanisms, clinical presentations, injuries, and outcomes from inflicted versus noninflicted head trauma during infancy: results of a prospective, multicentered, comparative study. *Pediatrics* 2007;119:922-929.
10. Jayawant S, Rawlinson A, Gibbon F, et al: Subdural haemorrhages in infants: population based study. *Br Med J* 1998;317:1558-1561.
11. King WJ, MacKay M, Sirnick A, et al: Shaken baby syndrome in Canada: clinical characteristics and outcomes of hospital cases. *Can Med Assoc J* 2003;168:155-159.
12. Ewing-Cobbs L, Kramer L, Prasad M, et al: Neuroimaging, physical, and developmental findings after inflicted and noninflicted traumatic brain injury in young children. *Pediatrics* 1998;102:300-307.
13. Keenan HT, Runyan DK, Nocera M: Child outcomes and family characteristics 1 year after severe inflicted or noninflicted traumatic brain injury. *Pediatrics* 2006;117:317-324.
14. Bonomi AE, Anderson ML, Rivara FP, et al: Health care utilization and costs associated with childhood abuse. *J Gen Intern Med* 2008;23:294-299.

---

*1998 Australian dollars converted to U.S. dollars, then adjusted for inflation to 2007 U.S. dollars.

15. Chartier MJ, Walker JR, Naimark B: Childhood abuse, adult health, and health care utilization: results from a representative community sample. *Am J Epidemiol* 2007;165:1031-1038.

16. Edwards VJ, Holden GW, Felitti VJ, et al: Relationship between multiple forms of childhood maltreatment and adult mental health in community respondents: results from the adverse childhood experiences study. *Am J Psychiatry* 2003;160:1453-1460.

17. Felitti VJ, Anda RF, Nordenberg D, et al: Relationship of childhood abuse and household dysfunction to many of the leading causes of death in adults: the Adverse Childhood Experiences (ACE) study. *Am J Prev Med* 1998;14:245-258.

18. Walker EA, Unutzer J, Rutter C, et al: Costs of health care use by women HMO members with a history of childhood abuse and neglect. *Arch Gen Psychiatry* 1999;56:609-613.

19. Consumer Price Index. U.S. Department of Labor Statistics, Washington, DC, 2008. Available at ftp://ftp.bls.gov/pub/special.requests/cpi/cpiai.txt. Accessed on October 1, 2008.

20. Keren R, Pati S, Feudtner C: The generation gap: differences between children and adults pertinent to economic evaluations of health interventions. *Pharmacoeconomics* 2004;22:71-81.

21. Griebsch I, Coast J, Brown J: Quality-adjusted life-years lack quality in pediatric care: a critical review of published cost-utility studies in child health. *Pediatrics* 2005;115:e600-614.

22. Prosser LA, Corso PS: Measuring health-related quality of life for child maltreatment: a systematic literature review. *Health Qual Life Outcomes* 2007;5:42.

23. Bennett JE, Sumner W, Downs SM, et al: Parents' utilities for outcomes of occult bacteremia. *Arch Pediatr Adolesc Med* 2000;154:43-48.

24. Saigal S, Stoskopf BL, Burrows E, et al: Stability of maternal preferences for pediatric health states in the perinatal period and 1 year later. *Arch Pediatr Adolesc Med* 2003;157:261-269.

25. Brouwer WB, Niessen LW, Postma MJ, et al: Need for differential discounting of costs and health effects in cost effectiveness analyses. *Br Med J* 2005;331:446-448.

26. Except where noted, all costs have been adjusted to reflect 2007 U.S. dollars.

27. Miller TR, Cohen M, Wiersema B: Victim Costs and Consequences: A New Look. National Institute of Justice Research Report, US Department of Justice, Washington, DC, 1996. Available at http://www.ncjrs.gov/pdffiles/victcost.pdf. Accessed on November 30, 2008.

28. Wang C, Holton J: Total Estimated Costs of Child Abuse and Neglect in the United States. Prevent Child Abuse America, Chicago, 2007. Available at http://member.preventchildabuse.org/site/DocServer/cost_analysis.pdf?docID=144. Accessed on November 30, 2008.

29. Ettaro L, Berger RP, Songer T: Abusive head trauma in young children: characteristics and medical charges in a hospitalized population. *Child Abuse Negl* 2004;28:1099-1111.

30. Irazuzta JE, McJunkin JE, Danadian K, et al: Outcome and cost of child abuse. *Child Abuse Negl* 1997;21:751-757.

31. Libby AM, Sills MR, Thursston NK, et al: Costs of childhood physical abuse: comparing inflicted and unintentional traumatic brain injuries. *Pediatrics* 2003;112:58-65.

32. Rovi S, Chen PH, Johnson MS: The economic burden of hospitalizations associated with child abuse and neglect. *Am J Public Health* 2004;94:586-590.

33. Dubowitz H: Costs and effectiveness of interventions in child maltreatment. *Child Abuse Negl* 1990;14:177-186.

34. Plotnick RD, Deppman L: Using benefit-cost analysis to assess child abuse prevention and intervention programs. *Child Welfare* 1999;78:381-407.

35. Courtney ME: National call to action: working toward the elimination of child maltreatment. The economics. *Child Abuse Negl* 1999;23:975-986.

36. Weil TP: Children at risk: outcome and cost measures needed. *J Health Hum Serv Adm* 1999;21:92-108.

37. Barlow J, Davis H, McIntosh E, et al: Role of home visiting in improving parenting and health in families at risk of abuse and neglect: results of a multicentre randomised controlled trial and economic evaluation. *Arch Dis Child* 2007;92:229-233.

38. Olds DL, Henderson CR, Phelps C, et al: Effect of prenatal and infancy nurse home visitation on government spending. *Med Care* 1993;31:155-174.

39. Karoly LA, Greenwood PN, Everingham SS, et al: *Investing in our Children: What We Know and Don't Know About the Costs and Benefits of Early Childhood Interventions.* The RAND Corporation, Santa Monica, 1998, pp 73-103.

40. Armstrong KA: Economic analysis of a child abuse and neglect treatment program. *Child Welfare* 1983;62:3-13.

41. Dretzke J, Frew E, Davenport C, et al: The effectiveness and cost-effectiveness of parent training/education programmes for the treatment of conduct disorder, including oppositional defiant disorder, in children. *Health Technol Assess* 2005;9:iii,ix-x,1-233.

42. Foster EM, Jones D, Conduct Problems Prevention Research Group: Can a costly intervention be cost effective? An analysis of violence prevention. *Arch Gen Psychiatry* 2006;63:1284-1291.

43. Prentky R, Burgess AW: Rehabilitation of child molesters: a cost-benefit analysis. *Am J Orthopsychiatry* 1990;60:108-117.

44. Shanahan M, Donato R: Counting the cost: estimating the economic benefit of pedophile treatment programs. *Child Abuse Negl* 2001;25:541-555.

45. Campbell KA, Bogen DL, Berger RP: The other children: a survey of child abuse physicians on the medical evaluation of children living with a physically abused child. *Arch Pediatr Adolesc Med* 2006;160:1241-1246.

46. Available at http://grants.nih.gov/grants/guide/pa-files/PA-07-437.html. Accessed on September 29, 2008.

70

CARING FOR THE CARETAKERS

Jan Bays, MD

INTRODUCTION

After ten years of work with victims of child abuse, I found myself in a deep clinical depression. I lost interest in food, found no pleasure in gardening, dreaded going to work, and was irritable with family and friends. I thought about quitting the work I had once loved. I realized that if I (considered one of the strongest people in our program, a person whose natural state is joy, curiosity and anticipation) left the work without discovering what was wrong and how to treat it, I would be leaving my best friends and coworkers to face the same problem, but without my support and without a remedy. As a doctor, I needed to know if this disease had a name, a cause and a cure. I began to read.

Professionals who work with child maltreatment encounter aspects of human suffering that most people never experience and do not wish to acknowledge. Daily encounters with new and horrifying ways people can be cruel to children can take its mental, physical, and spiritual toll. Every job has its occupational hazards; child abuse work is no exception. Four syndromes affecting those who work closely with human suffering have been described. There is a growing body of literature and research detailing their incidence, etiology, signs, symptoms and treatment. These four are burnout, posttraumatic stress disorder (PTSD), secondary trauma, and compassion fatigue.

OCCUPATIONAL HAZARDS OF CHILD PROTECTION WORK

Burnout

When I first began this work, there were only a few physicians in the state who would evaluate abused children. Calls began pouring in. I answered these calls myself, made appointments, interviewed the families, examined and interviewed children, typed my own reports and did my own billing. Parents and caseworkers pled that every case was urgent. "You're the only one."

Burnout is "… a process in which a previously committed professional disengages from his or her work in response to stress on the job."[1] Symptoms include physical, mental, and emotional exhaustion, depersonalization, and a loss of enthusiasm and sense of mission with decreased motivation and effectiveness on the job. Signs of burnout include fatigue, irritability, anger over small issues, indifference, a decline in efficiency or overall work performance, rigidity, paranoia, and depression.[2,3] Burnout is common and, untreated, its

cost can be high. In one survey of Canadian hospital-based child protection professionals, over one third exhibited burnout on a standard burnout inventory, and two thirds had seriously considered changing their work situation.[4]

Burnout is attributed to progressive and prolonged job stress[1] related to a person's attempts to meet unrealistically high expectations. The origin of these expectations can be internal or external.[2] Burnout occurs when we set our goals too high and cannot change them when people try to give us feedback. We begin the transformation from saints into martyrs.

Azar[2] points out that unconscious assumptions held by professionals may serve as the source of unrealistic internal expectations. Here are examples:

- Family problems can always be solved and we have the tools to be helpful.
- Parents and children want my help and will be grateful for my efforts.
- Because of my role as a helper, I will be safe (e.g., I should be able to tolerate client verbal abuse and visiting unsafe neighborhoods).
- I will do no harm.
- I will approach my clients with a clear idea of my biases and have ways to keep them out of my work.
- I will always be available when someone needs my help.
- I will always be empathic, with my child and adolescent patients, their families, and even the perpetrator.
- I am on the side of truth and justice and thus the court will always agree with my point of view.
- I will be treated fairly by clients, lawyers, judges, all members of multi-disciplinary teams, and by the news media.

In describing strategies in supervision to prevent burnout in child abuse workers, Azar writes that uncovering these hidden assumptions, beliefs, and expectations is key. She also warns that they may be deeply held and that changing them requires skill and patience, since it is akin to changing a person's religion.

Unrealistic external expectations often come from the public, the media, or government officials with superficial knowledge of the difficulties inherent in attempting to intervene in the dynamics of abuse. A state legislator who angrily criticizes state agencies for failing to protect a child from abuse may also vote to cut funding for hiring and training new child protection workers or law enforcement officers.

Posttraumatic Stress Disorder

After attending an autopsy on a child who was raped and tortured I find myself sitting and staring out the window, emotionally and mentally numb. This is a blessed protection against letting the feelings of horror come up, against my mind's attempts to imagine the child's last hours. This protective effect becomes disabling when "going unconscious" renders me unable to respond to my own child's distress over a skinned knee or indifferent to a coworker complaining about a difficult client.

PTSD can occur in first responders who witness traumatic events as they unfold. Emergency response personnel rate certain events as the most stressful aspects of their occupation: death of a child, injury to a child, a personally life-threatening event, and grotesque sights and sounds, outside the usual range of human experience. Any professional evaluating and treating child victims is also likely to encounter these types of events and thus be susceptible to PTSD. Even reviewing graphic material such as autopsy pictures or videotapes of child pornography can elicit symptoms of PTSD.

Although state laws provide a measure of legal protection for mandated reporters, they do not provide protection from stressful consequences of their work. Flaherty et al[5] surveyed 56 physicians who specialize in child abuse and found that 77% had experienced at least one negative consequence of their practice. Half had been verbally or physically threatened, an average of 2.7 times, and in 5% of cases a weapon had been displayed. Half had a formal complaint filed with their employer by parents or families. One quarter had been subjected to adverse local or national media attention as a result of their work. One in six had been sued for malpractice (one to three times), and one in eight had been reported to their professional licensing agency.

Johnson[6] found that pediatricians and emergency room physicians rated court appearances as the most stressful aspect of child abuse work. Law and medicine have different rules and assumptions; law is inherently adversarial, and medicine inherently cooperative. It is acutely uncomfortable to feel pulled by both sides in what we consider an impersonal finding of facts, to be forced to reduce the complexities of human interactions and biology to yes-or-no answers, to be attacked for doing humanitarian work, or to feel that one word misspoken could set a dangerous criminal free.

Secondary Trauma

Secondary trauma (also called secondary victimization, vicarious trauma, and secondary trauma syndrome) is a group of signs and symptoms that develop through close contact with victims of "actual or threatened death, serious injury or threats to the physical integrity of self or others" and "hearing shocking material from clients."[2,3] Interviewers often describe visualizing traumatic events as they are recounted, witnessing them through the eyes of their patients and clients.

Burnout is described as a process, whereas secondary trauma can emerge after a single exposure or incident such as working with victims of a mass disaster or terrorist bombing. Burnout can occur in any occupation, but secondary trauma is specific to those who work with victims of trauma and violence. Several authors[2,3,7-9] describe symptoms attributed to secondary trauma in child abuse work. Many of these symptoms are identical to those of PTSD. The compiled list is long, but the most distinctive features are reexperiencing the traumatic event described by the patient through intrusive thoughts, dreams or visual imagery, emotional numbing, and persistent arousal, which leads to difficulty concentrating and hypervigilance.

Pearlman and Saakvitne[10] discuss six basic human psychological needs that are sensitive to disruption by actual or vicarious trauma:

Safety: Working with victims heightens the sense of personal vulnerability and the fragility of life. Symptoms include preoccupation with safety, not letting anyone babysit one's children, and hypervigilance.

Trust: Through exposure to the many cruel ways people deceive, betray, or violate the trust of others, we become overly suspicious. Symptoms include cynicism, isolation, and not trusting co-workers or one's own instincts.

Esteem: Esteem is defined as the need to perceive others as benevolent and worthy of respect. Encountering so much human cruelty can shatter our world view. Symptoms occur such as pessimism and anger at individuals or the fate of mankind in general.

Intimacy: A sense of alienation emerges from exposure to horrific imagery that cannot be shared with others, because of their distress or confidentiality requirements. This is particularly painful if your spouse cannot bear to hear what you are doing in life or what is worrying you. Symptoms are emotional numbing and withdrawal from social life and personal intimacy.

Power or control: Realizing the fragility of life and encountering clients' powerlessness, we may try to increase our sense of power in the world, by taking self-defense classes or becoming domineering. Symptoms include restricted personal freedom through fears of safety and despair about the uncontrollable forces of nature and the human world.

Frame of reference: We try to figure out the motive of the perpetrator or what the victim did wrong. How did this happen? Symptoms can be pervasive unease or loss of religious faith.

Compassion Fatigue

I believe that the most profound effect of this work is on our spiritual well being. When we remove children from abusive families and they are subjected to worse cruelty in foster homes, what have we accomplished? When people we know, ministers, police officers, protective service workers and even pediatricians abuse children, who is the enemy? It breaks through our denial. It becomes harder to hold the larger framework, the higher purpose that gives our life a sense of direction and meaning.

Compassion fatigue is the newest term. Some authors equate compassion fatigue with secondary trauma syndrome; some include both as aspects of burn out. Workers with compassion fatigue keep trying to be open-hearted and sympathetic when they feel that the inner well of empathy and kindness has run dry. They fall into cynicism ("What else can you expect from that judge?"), suspicion ("I never believe what parents tell me anymore."), despair ("The system is too broken to fix."), and depression ("Nothing I've done in all these years has changed things for the better.").[11] Compassion fatigue has also become a more general term, used, for example, to explain why people who are overexposed to media depiction of disasters and victims become cynical and cease donating to charities or why soldiers become inured to death.

PREVENTION AND TREATMENT

Preventing vicarious trauma is an active process. First, realize that anyone is susceptible to burnout, posttraumatic stress, secondary trauma and compassion fatigue. This is true no matter how many years one has been working in the field. At some point the container of human suffering may become full and begin to overflow. This is more likely to happen when stressful events in one's personal life, such as illness or death in the family, concerns over the difficulties of a parent or child, or financial or marital problems, compound the strain of working with the distress of clients.

Some tips follow:

1. Maintain a positive framework. Secondary trauma is not considered abnormal but rather a natural consequence of caring for another person and listening to them empathically, the very qualities that characterize a skilled professional who works with abused children.
2. Know your risk factors. Research indicates a higher risk of secondary trauma in those who themselves have a history of abuse or neglect, as painful emotions and memories may be re-activated.[3,9] To balance this, a history of abuse in their own childhood can provide workers with a greater sense of meaning and accomplishment in the work.[7]
3. Actively discuss and nurture what Conrad terms "compassion satisfaction,"[1] the positive benefits of meaningful work, the sense of fulfillment from helping those in distress, and involvement in supportive collegial relationships. High levels of job satisfaction seem to be protective against burnout.[4] We can create ways to celebrate our work, and, when appropriate, to honor our clients' accomplishments.
4. A combination of realism and optimism is key.[7] Acknowledge that real change is difficult and slow. An historical perspective is important, especially for young workers. The first article identifying injuries resulting from abuse appeared in the medical literature nearly 50 years ago and many doctors greeted it with disbelief.[12,13] We have come a long way—and there is still along way to go.
5. Openly acknowledge the potential side effects of sustained work with human suffering, and provide education from the start, both when hiring and training new employees, as well as part of continuing education. Actively monitor oneself and colleagues for hidden assumptions that create unrealistically high expectations or reveal negative coping strategies ("I shouldn't have lost that case in court."). Support from supervisors and colleagues is key in encouraging consultation on the job and informal, relaxed gatherings off the job. Institutional support is essential. An invaluable benefit institutions can provide is the services of lawyers and public relations staff to shield line workers from the stress of media harassment and threatened law suits.
6. Provide education about using positive coping strategies and avoiding negative ones.[9] When we ruminate over past mistakes or fall prey to anxiety and dread over future possibilities, we are incubating our own distress. Positive coping strategies focus on the present moment and restore our capacity for hope, love, intimacy, laughter, and creativity. They include exercise, time with healthy children and pets, hobbies, the arts, and travel. Activities that provide spiritual renewal are particularly important in restoring a sense of perspective. These include attending church or temple, yoga, meditation, or just being in nature. Negative strategies include complaining, isolating, blaming, or addictive behavior with drugs, alcohol, food, shopping, pornography, or gambling.

Suggested areas for routine maintenance and repair include the following:

Environmental: Balance a clinical case load with teaching and research. Limit exposure by balancing victim and nonvictim work. Set boundaries; limit weekend and night work. Make sure days off are *really* off. Find a way to work for social change.

Interpersonal: Do not work alone. Seek support from professional colleagues. Seek supervision and consultation. Develop support groups where feelings can be discussed, separate from work time.

Personal: Find healthy ways to mentally leave the past behind, remain in the present moment, and not obsess about future problems and eventualities. Understand that vicarious victimization is a normal response. Use it for growth. Use individual therapy to work on areas that are particular problems. Seek balance between personal and professional life. Make time for nonvictim-related activities that renew a sense of optimism and hope. The most common are exercise, rest, gardening, music, dance, art work, pets, time with healthy children, travel, being in nature, and doing nothing!

Spiritual: Attend to empathy. Stay anchored in the present. Develop a sense of connection to something larger than oneself. Seek spiritual renewal.

Research on the secondary effects of working with victims of trauma is relatively new and sparse. Hopefully future studies will help us understand who is relatively immune to secondary trauma and whether their immunity rests on personal differences or upon characteristics of the profession. Physicians seem to be more immune to burn out than social workers, for example.[4] Is this due to more rigorous selection of candidates, longer and more grueling training, higher pay, appreciation and status, or because their intervention is short and they have less long-term contact with troubled families? We also need to clarify what measures work, for individuals and cohorts of workers, to lessen the trauma of working with trauma.

If child abuse professionals are to remain healthy and effective in their work, they need to be aware of the potential side effects of working with victims in order to recognize and prevent these side effects, or to apply appropriate antidotes at the earliest signs of distress. It is one time that physicians *must* treat themselves. A good physician adjusts the dose of medicine to the strength of the disease. Remember, the more stress arises at work, the more time needs to be set aside as an antidote to that stress. If we take good care of ourselves, we will be able to take better care of the children we serve.

Over ten years have passed since I burned and almost crashed. I still work in child abuse, part time, and am healthier for it. I am happy that my skills and experience are still useful. The work is difficult at times, but difficult work can be done well with the help of good people, and it is continuously gratifying to find that child abuse professionals worldwide are the finest people with whom I have ever worked.

References

1. Conrad D: Compassion fatigue, burnout, and compassion satisfaction among Colorado child protection workers. *Child Abuse Negl* 2006;30: 1071-1080.
2. Azar ST: Preventing burnout in professionals and paraprofessionals who work with child abuse and neglect cases: a cognitive behavioral approach to supervision. *J Clin Psychol* 2000;56:643-663.
3. Nelson-Gardell D, Harris D: Childhood abuse history, secondary traumatic stress, and child welfare workers. *Child Welfare* 2003;82:5-26.
4. Bennett S, Plint A, Clifford TJ: Burnout, psychological morbidity, job satisfaction, and stress: a survey of Canadian hospital based child protection professionals. *Arch Dis Child* 2005;90:1112-1116.
5. Flaherty EG, Fortes DM, Sege RD: Are the protectors protected? Poster presentation at the Pediatric Academic Society Annual Meeting, Toronto, May 5, 2007.
6. Johnson CF: Child abuse as a stressor of pediatricians. *Ped Emerg Care* 1999;15:84-89.
7. Shapiro JP, Dorman RK, Burkey WM, et al: Predictors of job satisfaction and burnout in child abuse professionals: coping, cognition, and victimization history. *J Child Sex Abus* 1999;7:23-42.
8. Perron BE, Hiltz BS: Burnout and secondary trauma among forensic interviewers of abused children. *Child Adolesc Social Work J* 2006;23: 216-234.
9. VanDeusen KM, Way I: Vicarious trauma: an exploratory study of the impact of providing sexual abuse treatment on clinicians' trust and intimacy. *J Child Sex Abus* 2006;15:69-85.
10. Pearlman LA, Saakvitne KW: *Traumatic Stress: Countertransference and Vicarious Victimization in Psychotherapy with Incest Survivors.* WW Norton and Co, New York, 1995.
11. Pfifferling JH, Gilley K: Overcoming compassion fatigue. *Fam Pract Manag* 1999;6:36-42.
12. Kempe CH, Silverman FN, Steele BF, et al: The battered-child syndrome. *JAMA* 1962;181:17-24.
13. Jenny C: Medicine discovers child abuse. *JAMA* 2008;300: 2796-2797.

A

AACWA. *See* Adoption Assistance and Child Welfare Act
AAFS. *See* American Academy of Forensic Sciences
AAP. *See* American Academy of Pediatrics
Abdominal/chest injuries in abused children
  diagnostic evaluation, 329-330
    history, 329
    laboratory evaluation, 329-330
    physical examination, 329, 330f
    radiographic evaluation, 330
  directions for future research, 331
  epidemiology, 326
  introduction, 326-331
  outcomes, 331
  pathophysiology, 326-329
    associated injuries, 328-329
    intraabdominal hollow viscus injury, 327-328, 328f
    intraabdominal solid organ injury, 327, 327f
    mechanisms of injury, 326
    miscellaneous abdominal injuries, 328
    spectrum of injuries, 327
    thoracic injuries, 328
  strength of evidence, 331
Abel Assessment for Sexual Interest, 163
ABFO. *See* American Board of Forensic Odontology
ABP. *See* American Board of Pediatrics
Abrasions, 243
Abuse specific therapy, 469
Abuse-focused cognitive behavior therapy (AF-CBT), 483
Abusive burns. *See also* Skin conditions confused with child abuse
  characteristics of abuse burn perpetrators, 222-223
    classifications of burns, 222-223, 223f
  with cultural medicine practices, 230-231
  dating injuries in medical record, 233
  directions for future research, 236
  epidemiology/demographics of child abuse by burning, 222
  medical documentation, 232-233, 233f
  medical testing, 233
  neglect and, 231
  presentation of burned child for medical care, 231-232, 231t-232t
  prevention, 235-236
  psychological issues of burned child/family, 235
  scene investigation, 233-235, 234f
  strength of evidence, 236
  types/evidence of maltreatment, 223-230
    abusive thermal burn mimics, 226, 226f
    chemical burns, 228-229, 229f
    contact burns, 226-228, 227f-228f
    electrical burn injury, 229-230
    flame burns, 229, 229f
    friction/pressure burns, 230, 230f
    microwave oven burns, 230
    thermal burns, 223-226, 225f-226f, 225t, 231t
Abusive fractures, 275, 276t. *See also* Long bone fracture biomechanics; *specific fractures*
  bony injuries, 276-293
    fractures in abusive/accidental trauma, 277t, 279f-281f, 284t, 288-293, 289t, 291t-292t
    fractures in stages of healing, 276

Abusive fractures *(Continued)*
    fractures with high specificity for abuse, 277-287, 279f-280f, 285f
    incidence, 276-293, 276t, 280f
    multiple fractures, 276, 277t, 281f
    subperiosteal new bone formation, 276
  fracture assessment/injury plausibility, 275
  provided *vs.* obtained history, 275-276, 276t-278t
  summary, 293
Abusive head trauma (AHT), 6, 35, 349.
    See also Biochemical markers of AHT in children; Biomechanics of head trauma in infants/young children; Conditions confused with AHT; Epidemiology of AHT; Imaging AHT; Neuropathology of AHT; Outcome of AHT; Shaken baby syndrome; Shaking
  biomechanics role, 361
  clinical spectrum, 350
  as closed head injury, 36f
  communication, 356
  conclusion, 357
  developing brain response, 367-368, 368t
  diagnostic evaluation, 352-356
    history, 352-353, 353t-355t
    laboratory studies/consultations/secondary evaluations, 355-356, 356t
    neuroimaging, 353-355
    physical examination, 353
  diagnostic objectivity, 356
  differential diagnosis, 351, 386-387
  directions for future research, 357
  historical context, 349
  incidence/epidemiology, 349
  in infants, 36f
  injury mechanisms, 351-352
  mechanisms, 361
  missed cases, 350
  nomenclature, 349-350
  relevant forensic issues, 351
  reporting, 351
  responsibility of medical specialist, 350
  strength of evidence, 356-357
  study bias, 36t
  timing of injury, 352
Academy on Violence and Abuse (AVA), 617-618
Accidental brain injuries, 368-369
ACE. *See* Adverse Childhood Experiences
Acquaintance rape, 128-129
Acquired immunodeficiency syndrome (AIDS), 186
ACR. *See* American College of Radiology
Active/passive data collection, 6
Adams, J. A., 76, 84, 87-89, 91
Adams-Tucker, C., 471
Adelson, P. D., 360
ADHD. *See* Attention deficit hyperactivity disorder
Adolescent sexual assault/statutory rape, 127
  adolescent perceptions/attitudes, 127
  adolescent understanding sex, 131
  clinical implications, 128
  conclusions, 131-132
  IPV, 128-129
  managing response, 131
  parent requested virginity test, 131
  patient cooperation, 130-131
  patient examination, 130-131
  patient rapport/confidentiality, 130

Adolescent sexual assault/statutory rape *(Continued)*
  populations at risk, 127-128
  pregnancy, 129-130
  rape trauma syndrome, 130
  statutory rape, 129
    defined, 129
    medical/psychological consequences, 129
    pregnancy and, 129
Adoption and Safe Families Act, 629
Adoption Assistance and Child Welfare Act (AACWA), 611-612
Adverse Childhood Experiences (ACE), 26, 467
The Aetiology of Hysteria (Freud), 461
AF-CBT. *See* Abuse-focused cognitive behavior therapy
Affect expression, 470-471
Agency for Healthcare Research and Quality (AHRQ), 36-37
AHRQ. *See* Agency for Healthcare Research and Quality
AHT. *See* Abusive head trauma
AIDS. *See* Acquired immunodeficiency syndrome
Akbarnia, B., 276
Alabama Parenting Questionnaire (APQ), 480
Alcohol, 531-532. *See also* Ethanol; Ethyl alcohol
  FAS, 605
Allasio, D., 224-226
Allergic vulvar dermatitis, 96
ALS. *See* Alternate light source
Altemeier, W. A., 553
Alternate light source (ALS), 67. *See also* Bluemaxx 500; Poliray light source; Wood's lamp
  for blood detection, 113
  photodocumentation in child abuse cases, 219
  for rape kit, 109
  for screening semen/sperm, 112
American Academy of Forensic Sciences (AAFS), 579
American Academy of Pediatric Dentistry, 544, 579
American Academy of Pediatrics (AAP), 145, 364, 468, 600, 612-613. *See also* American Board of Pediatrics
  Report of Committee on Infectious Disease, 169-170
  response to child maltreatment, 615-618
American Board of Forensic Odontology (ABFO), 579
American Board of Pediatrics (ABP), 616-617
American College of Radiology (ACR), 308
American Professional Society on the Abuse of Children (APSAC), 82, 218, 617
American Society for the Prevention of Cruelty to Animals (ASPCA), 615
American Society of Forensic Odontology (ASFO), 579
AMH. *See* Anti-müllerian hormone
Amoedo, Oscar, 579
Amphetamines/methamphetamines, 121-122, 565
Anaclitic depression, 547
Anchoring, 8
Annular hymen, 70, 70f
Anogenital examination, normal/developmental variations in, 69
  directions for future research, 80
  genital embryology, 69
    cloaca, 69
    external genitalia, 69
    hymen, 69
    ovaries, 69
    primary structures, 69
    vagina, 69
  perianal variants, 78-79

Page numbers followed by f refer to figures, those followed by t refer to tables, and those followed by b refer to boxes.

Anogenital examination, normal/developmental variations in *(Continued)*
    anal dilation, 78-79
    anal skin tags, 78, 79f
    diastasis ani, 74, 78, 78f
    prominent skin folds/pectinate line, 78
    venous congestion, 79
  perineal variants, 77-78
    failure of midline fusion, 77, 78f
    infantile pyramidal protrusion, 77
    median raphe, 78
  variants in female genital anatomy, 70-77
    annular hymen, 70, 70f
    crescentic hymen, 70, 70f
    cribriform hymen, 70-72, 71f
    developmental changes to hymen, 72-74, 73f, 73t
    external ridges, 74
    factors affecting appearance, 72
    fimbriated hymen, 70, 70f
    hymenal configurations, 70-75
    hymenal tags/mounds, 74-75, 75f
    imperforate hymen, 77
    linea vestibularis, 76-77, 76f
    longitudinal intravaginal ridges, 74, 74f
    lymphoid follicles, 77
    Mayer-Rokitansky-Küster-Hauser syndrome, 72, 72f
    newborn hymen, 72, 72f
    notches/clefts, 75, 75f
    paraurethral cysts, 77, 77f
    septate hymen, 70, 71f
    sleevelike hymen, 70, 71f
    transverse hymenal diameters, 76
    vaginal septum, 70-71, 71f
    vascularity/erythema of hymen/vestibule, 76
    vestibular bands, 74, 74f
    width of inferior hymenal rim, 76
  variants in male genital anatomy, 79-80
    hydroceles, 80
    hypospadias, 80
    pearly papules, 79, 79f
    varicocele, 80
Anorectal injuries, 90
Anoxic encephalomyelopathy/infarction, 423-424, 424f. *See also* Hypoxic lesions; Ischemic lesions
Anti-müllerian hormone (AMH), 69
Aphthae, 101
Apoptosis, 368
APQ. *See* Alabama Parenting Questionnaire
APSAC. *See* American Professional Society on the Abuse of Children
AR. *See* Attributable risk
ASFO. *See* American Society of Forensic Odontology
Ashcroft v. The Free Speech Coalition, 145
ASPCA. *See* American Society for the Prevention of Cruelty to Animals
Asphyxia, 339-342. *See also* Sudden infant death syndrome
  categories, 339-340
    combinations of mechanisms that impede oxygenation, 340
    impaired oxygen transport in circulating blood, 339-340
    insufficient oxygen in surrounding atmosphere, 339
    interference with oxygen uptake at cellular level, 340
    reduced transfer of oxygen from atmosphere to blood, 339-340
  differentiation from SIDS, 342-343
  historical development, 339-342
  pathological features, 340-342
    petechiae, 341-342
    pulmonary intraalveolar siderophages, 340, 342
  pathophysiology, 339
Attention deficit hyperactivity disorder (ADHD), 472-473, 516
Attributable risk (AR), 5
Autonomic nervous system, 517-518
Autosomal dominant hypophosphatemic rickets, 263
AVA. *See* Academy on Violence and Abuse
Avulsion, 243
Azar, S. T., 641

B

Bacterial sexually transmitted infections in children
  clinical manifestations, 174-176
    diagnosis, 175
    follow-up considerations, 175-176
    forensic applications, 175
    treatment, 175-176, 176t
  directions for future research, 177
  epidemiology, 174
  STI prevalence, 174
  strength of evidence, 176-177
Balizet, Carol, 599
Bandak, F. A., 399
Bariciak, E. D., 242
Barillo, D. J., 222
Barlow, K. M., 36
Barsley, R. E., 581
Barsness, K. A., 282, 284-285
"The Battered Child Syndrome," 629
Bayley Scales of Infant Development, 453
Bays, J., 255
B-CAPI. *See* Brief Child Abuse Potential Inventory
BEAF. *See* Benign extraaxial fluid of infancy
Beals, R. K., 288
Beers, S. R., 455
Behçet syndrome, 100-101
Beijing Declaration and Platform for Action of the Fourth World Conference on Women, 139
Belfer R. A., 233
Belsky, J., 30, 503
Benedict, M. I., 31
Benign extraaxial fluid of infancy (BEAF), 386, 387f, 445-446
Benzodiazepines, 120-121
Berenson, A., 72-73, 73t, 75, 86-87, 94-95
Bergh, Henry, 628
Berliner, L., 473
Berry, Justin, 144
Bertocci, G. E., 291
Berwick, D. M., 556
Betrayal, 463
Bhat, B. V., 280-281
Bialas, Y, 242
Bias
  cognitive, 8
  confirmation, 8
  in data collection, 6
  desirability, 6
  implicit, 8
  selection, 6-7
  source in AHT studies, 36t
Big black brain, 367
Bijleveld, C. C., 159
Bilingsley, A., 31
Binkovitz, L. A., 261
Biochemical markers of AHT in children
  biomarkers in pediatrics, 430-437
    AHT *vs.* TBI, 434
    assessment/outcome, 434-435, 435t
    brain *vs.* other organs, 430-431, 431f
    candidate biomarkers of brain injury, 431-432, 432t
    development of treatment interventions, 432t, 435-436
    diagnosis of AHT, 432-434
    evaluation of treatment, 436-437
    serum brain biomarkers, 432-437
  directions for future research, 438
  introduction, 429-438
  issues in, 437
  strength of evidence, 437-438
Biomechanics of head trauma in infants/young children
  AHT mechanisms, 361
  animal models of pediatric TBI, 360-361
  computational models of pediatric head injury, 361
  introduction, 359-361
  material response of pediatric brain/skull to loads, 360
  role in AHT, 361
  TBI mechanics, 359
Biopsychosocial model, 549-553
  biological sphere, 549-550
  psychological sphere, 550-552
  social sphere, 552-553

Bird, C. R., 394-395
Birth-related head injuries, 445
Bite marks
  patterned injuries, 580-581, 581f-582f, 583
    hickeys/suction marks, 581, 581f
    impression, 583, 583f
    photography, 582, 582f
    recognition, 580-581, 580f
    recording, 582-583
    referral, 583
    reporting, 581-582
  rape kit and, 109
  saliva and, 114, 582-583
Blair, P. S., 552
Blakemore, L. C., 288
Blood
  ALS for detecting, 113
  analysis, 113
  impaired oxygen transport in circulating, 339-340
  reduced transfer of oxygen from atmosphere to, 339-340
  swab collection, 108
Blood alcohol content, 120, 120t
Blood-brain barrier, 430
Bluemaxx 500, 109
Blumbergs, P., 422-423
Bockholdt, B., 395
Bodily fluids, analysis of, 112-114
  blood, 113
  saliva, 113-114
  semen/sperm, 112-113
Bond, G. R., 102-103
Bone health/development, 260
  anatomy, 260
  anatomy/development, reproductive/endocrine disorders, 263, 267-271, 268f, 270f
  differential diagnosis, 271-272
    OI *vs.* nonaccidental trauma, 271
    TBBD, 271-272
  factors affecting bone strength, 261
  infections affecting, 268, 268f
  noninvasive measures of bone strength, 261
  physiology/disease, 261-271
    Caffey disease, 265-266
    calcium balance, 262
    calcium homeostasis, 261-267
    chronic illness, 267
    copper deficiency, 265
    hydrophosphatasia, 266
    hypomagnesemia, 262
    hypothyroidism, 262
    neuromuscular disease, 266-267
    osteoporosis, 266
    parathyroid hormone, 262
    phosphate homeostasis, 262-263
    pseudohypoparathyroidism, 262
    vitamin A intoxication, 265
    vitamin C deficiency, 265
    vitamin D, 263-265
  summary, 271t, 272-273
Bone material properties, 321-322, 321t
  anisotropy/strength, 321, 321t
  density/strength, 322, 322f
  geometric characteristics, 322
Bone scintigraphy, 296, 298f
Bonnier, C., 454-455
Bousha, D. M., 31
Boyer, Pascal, 602
Boyle, C., 82
Brain development, effects of abuse/neglect on
  biological stress response systems, 516-517
  biological stress response systems in maltreated children, 517-518
    autonomic nervous system, 517-518
    HPA axis, 517
    immune system, 518
    locus coeruleus noradrenergic neurotransmitter system, 517-518
  cognitive functioning, 521
  developmental traumatology, 516
  directions for future research, 522
  genetic contributions, 521-522
  healthy brain development, 518
  introduction, 516-522
  in maltreated children, 518-521

Brain development, effects of abuse/neglect on (*Continued*)
   corpus callosum, 518-520, 519f
   limbic system, 520-521
   mediated prefrontal cortex, 521
  neurobiology of hope, 522
  strength of evidence, 522
Brief Child Abuse Potential Inventory (B-CAPI), 479
Bronfenbrenner, U., 496
Brown, J. K., 422-423, 426
Browne, A., 462-463
Brownian motion, 374-375
Bruises/skin lesions. *See also* Skin conditions confused with child abuse
  abrasions, 243
  avulsion, 243
  bruising
   definitions, 241-243, 241t
   evolution/myths, 241t-242t, 242-243
  coagulopathies, 249-250
  complications of soft tissue injury, 250
  corticosteroid atrophy, 249-250
  directions for future research, 250
  Ehlers-Danlos syndrome, 249-250
  evaluating cutaneous injuries for child abuse, 243-248
   documentation, 244
   examination, 243-244
   history, 243, 243t
   interpretation of findings, 244-248, 245t-247t, 247f-249f, 249t
  introduction, 239-250
   anatomy of skin, 239-241, 240f
   biochemical properties of skin, 239-241
  lacerations, 243
  scratches, 243
Brunk, M., 495
Bureau of Justices, U.S., 17
Burnout, 630, 641
Burns. *See also* Abusive burns; Skin conditions confused with child abuse
  chemical, 228-229, 229f
  contact, 226-228, 227f-228f
  electrical burn injury, 229-230
  flame, 229, 229f
  friction/pressure, 230, 230f
  microwave oven, 230
  thermal, 223-226, 225f-226f, 225t, 231t
Burroughs, George, 579
Burton, D. I., 155

C

Caetano, R., 502
Caffey, John, 35, 302, 349, 364, 426, 451, 607
Caffey disease, 265-266
Cairns, A. M., 247
Calcium homeostasis, 261-267
Calder, J. D. F., 293
California Personality Inventory (CPI), 163
Camilleri, J. A., 162-163
Canadian Incidence Study (CIS), 17-18
Candida albicans, 148-149
Cannabis, 121
Canty, T. G., 331
CAP. *See* Child Abuse Potential Inventory
CAPTA. *See* Child Abuse Prevention and Treatment Act
Cardiopulmonary resuscitation (CPR), 13
Caring for caretakers
  introduction, 641-644
  occupational hazards of child protection work, 641-643
   burnout, 641
   compassion fatigue, 642-643
   PTSD, 642
   secondary trauma, 642
  prevention/treatment, 643-644
Carlson, B. E., 502
CarolinaSAFE study, 6
Carpenter, R. F., 243, 247-248
Carpentieri, U., 254
Carty, H., 394-395
Casey Family Programs, 612-613

Cassidy, L., 127
CBQ. *See* Conflict Behavior Questionnaire
CBT. *See* Cognitive behavioral therapy
CDP. *See* Centers for Disease Control and Prevention
CEA. *See* Cost-effectiveness analysis
Centers for Disease Control and Prevention (CDP), 23, 26, 36-37, 175, 186, 193, 444, 553, 596-597
Central nervous system (CNS), 517
Cerebrospinal C/Ls, 417-421
Chadwick, D. L., 445
Chaffin, 30
Chain of custody, 107
Chamberlain, D., 281-282
Chandler, M. J., 550
Charismatic sects, 599
Chemical burns, 228-229, 229f
Chernoff, R., 610-611
Cherrix, Starchild Abraham, 601
Chester, D. L., 231
Child Abuse Pediatrics, 539
Child Abuse Potential Inventory (CAP), 495
Child Abuse Prevention and Treatment Act (CAPTA), 10, 129, 490, 539, 618, 629
Child abuse surveillance pyramid, 11f
Child Behavior Checklist, 612
Child death review (CDR)
  case review models, 594
   prevention programs, 594
   systems improvement, 592, 594, 595t-596t
  challenges, 596-597
   expanding to natural, preventable deaths, 597
   expanding to serious, non-fatal injuries, 597
   moving from review to action, 597
   uniform child maltreatment definitions, 596-597
  conclusion, 597
  identifying maltreatment, 592-594, 593t
  purpose/scope, 592-597
  standardization/support/national database, 597
  strengths, 594-596
   data collection, 594
   identification/classification of child abuse, 594
   interagency communication/coordination, 594
   public health surveillance, 596
Child development/behavior, 491
Child maltreatment. *See* Epidemiological issues in child maltreatment; International issues in child maltreatment; Response to child maltreatment
Child molesters
  associated problems, 161-162
  defining, 153-154
  directions for future research, 163-164
  etiology of, 154-155
  forays, 153
  grooming by, 153
  hebephilia, 153-154
  Internet, 154
  introduction, 152-164
  obtaining evidence, 155-159
   behavioral, 156-157
   cognitive, 155-156
   victim access, 157-159
  other populations, 159-161
   females, 160-161
   juveniles, 159
   organized groups, 161
  paraphilia, 153-154
  pedophilia, 153-154, 154t
  preferential, 153
  situational, 153
  treatment, 162-163
Child neglect, definitions/categorization
  introduction, 539-542, 540f
  neglect degrees, 541
  neglect outcome, 541-542
  neglect prevention, 542
  neglect types, 541
Child physical abuse (CPA), 476. *See also* Psychological impact/treatment of CPA
Child Physical and Sexual Abuse: Guidelines for Treatment (Saunders/Berliner/Hanson), 473
Child pornography, 16, 143-145. *See also* Evaluating images in child pornography
  combating, 144-145
  ease of use, 144-145

Child pornography (*Continued*)
  predator tool, 143-144
  as profitable, 144
  victim use, 144
Child Pornography Prevention Act of 1966, 145
Child protective services (CPS), 8, 10, 16-18, 29, 32, 160, 210, 629-630
  differential response in, 631
  reporting to, 468
Child Sensuality Circle, 161
Child sexual abuse (CSA), 16
Child sexual abuse accommodation syndrome (CSAAS), 462
Child Sexual Behavior Inventory (CSBI), 463-464
Child Victim Identification Program (CVIP), 144
Child Welfare League of America, 612, 630-631
Child welfare system
  effective organizations, 629-631
   burnout, 630
   caseloads, 630
   compensations, 630-631
   leadership, 629-630
   secondary trauma, 630
   staff turnover, 630
  emerging practices, 631-632
   differential response in CPS, 631
   family group conferencing, 631-632
   system of care, 632
  final thoughts, 632
  history in U.S., 628-632
  modern, 629
Child-parent psychotherapy (CPP), 483, 510
Chlamydia trachomatis (CT), 174
  specimen collection, 198-200, 199t-200t
Choo, R. E., 536
Christian Science, 599-600
Chromatography, 564
Chronicity, 29
Church of Scientology, 599-600
Ciarallo, L., 252
Cicchetti, D., 455, 539-540
CIS. *See* Canadian Incidence Study
Clark, K. D., 231-232
Classic metaphyseal lesions (CML), 277-285, 279f-280f, 285f
  as radiographic red flags, 302, 304f
  as radiologic red flag, 302
Cloaca, 69
Closed head injury, as AHT, 36f
C/Ls. *See* Contusions/lacerations
CML. *See* Classic metaphyseal lesions
CNS. *See* Central nervous system
Coant, P. N., 326, 329-330
Coats, B., 291, 413
Cocaine, 121, 530-531, 565-566
CODIS. *See* Combined DNA Index System
Cognitive behavioral therapy (CBT), 162, 466, 470-471
  affect expression, 470-471
  cognitive coping, 471
  cognitive processing, 471
  parenting skills, 463, 471
  parenting-child sessions, 471
  psycho-education, 470
  relaxation techniques, 470
  trauma narrative, 471
Cognitive processing therapy (CPT), 470
Cohle, S. D., 394
COI. *See* Cost of illness
COI analysis, 634-638, 637t-638t
Collins, Michelle, 144
Colombo, J. L., 226
Colposcopy, 66-67
Combined DNA Index System (CODIS), 113
Compassion fatigue, 642-643
Computational models of pediatric head injury, 361
Computed tomography (CT), 308-311
  as ICI gold standard, 429
  neuroimaging examination, 373, 374f
Conditions confused with AHT
  coagulopathy/hemostasis defects, 441-444
   evaluating, 443-444
   FXIII deficiency, 442
   hemophilia (Factor VIII deficiency), 442
   PIVKA-II, 444

Conditions confused with AHT *(Continued)*
    platelet disorders, 443
    platelet functioning testing, 444
    testing for FXIII deficiency, 444
    trauma-related coagulopathy, 442-443
    vitamin K deficiency, 441-442
    vWD, 442
  conclusion, 447
  introduction, 441-447
  misdiagnosed traumatic events, 444-445
    accidents, 444-445
    birth-related head injuries, 445
  mistaken conditions, 445-447
    GA1, 446-447
    intracranial fluid collections, 445-446
    MD, 447
    scurvy, 446
Conflict Behavior Questionnaire (CBQ), 480
Connective tissue disorders, 254
Connolly, Francis, 628
Consultation on Child Abuse Prevention, 620
Consumer Product Safety Commission, 368-369, 445
Contact burns, 226-228, 227f-228f
Contact dermatitis, 96
Contributors to neglect, 30-32
  family level, 31
    chaotic families, 31
    dyadic interactions, 31
    estrangement/isolation, 31
    lack of knowledge/parenting skills, 31
    stress, 31
  individual level, 30-31
    child characteristics, 30-31
    parental characteristics, 30
  professional level, 32
  societal level, 31-32
    child welfare system, 32
    inadequate education system, 31-32
    poverty, 31-32
Controlled Substances Act, 566
Contusions/lacerations (C/Ls), 417-421. *See also*
  Cerebrospinal C/Ls; Deep C/Ls; Superficial C/Ls
Cope, O., 235
Copper deficiency, 265
Corbett, S. S., 560
Corporal punishment, 12
Corpus callosum, 518-520, 519f
Corticosteroid atrophy, 249-250
Cost of child maltreatment, 634
  directions for future research, 639
  economic analysis, 637-639
    CEA, 638-639
    COI analysis, 637-638, 637t-638t
  introduction, 634-639
  overview of economic analysis, 634-637, 635f
    CEA/CUA, 636-637
    COI analysis, 634-636
  strength of evidence, 639
Cost of illness (COI), 634
Cost-effectiveness analysis (CEA), 634, 636-639
Cost-utility analysis (CUI), 634, 636-637
Covert video surveillance (CVS), 588
Coyer, S., 536
CPA. *See* Child physical abuse
CPE. *See* Cytopathic effect
CPI. *See* California Personality Inventory
CPP. *See* Child-parent psychotherapy
CPPA. *See* Child Pornography Prevention Act of 1966
CPR. *See* Cardiopulmonary resuscitation
CPS. *See* Child protective services
CPT. *See* Cognitive processing therapy
Crescentic hymen, 70, 70f
Cribriform hymen, 70-72, 71f
Crockenberg, S., 507
Crohn disease, 95-96, 96f, 100-101
Cross-sectional imaging in evaluating pediatric skeletal
  trauma
  CT, 309-311
  introduction, 308-314
  MRI, 310f, 311-313, 312f-314f
  summary, 313-314
  ultrasonography, 308-309, 309f-310f
Crothers, B., 396
Crouter, A., 31
CSA. *See* Child sexual abuse

CSAAS. *See* Child sexual abuse accommodation
  syndrome
CSBI. *See* Child Sexual Behavior Inventory
CT. *See* Chlamydia trachomatis; Computed
  tomography
CUI. *See* Cost-utility analysis
Cultural medicine practices, 230-231
Cupping, 230-231, 255, 257
CVIP. *See* Child Victim Identification Program
CVS. *See* Covert video surveillance
Cybersex, 145-146
CyberTipline, 144
Cytopathic effect (CPE), 200

D

Daria, S., 224
Darlington, A. S., 550
Darok, M., 227
Dashti, S. R., 378-379
Date rape, 118, 125, 128-129
David, T. J., 220
De Bellis, M. D., 493, 519
De Luca, R. V., 160
Deep C/Ls, 419-421, 419f-421f. *See also* Gliding C/Ls
Degraw, M., 233
Deitch, H. R., 100-101
DeMattia, A., 175
Denton, S., 445
DePanfilis, D., 497
Department of Health and Human Services, U.S., 476,
  544
Department of Justice, U.S., 218
Depression, 466
  anaclitic, 547
  maternal, 491
Descheneaux, K. A., 327-328
Desirability bias, 6
Developmental systems theory (DST), 492-494
Developmental traumatology, 516
DFA. *See* Direct fluorescent antibody test
DFSA. *See* Drug-facilitated sexual assault
Diagnostic and Statistical Manual of the American
  Psychiatric Association (DSM-IV), 153-154, 154t
Diamond, L. J., 31
Diaper dermatitis, 93. *See also* Primary diaper
  dermatitis
Diaper Pail Friends (DPF), 161
Diastasis ani, 74, 78, 78f
Dilated hemorrhoid veins, 98
Dine, M. S., 587
Direct fluorescent antibody test (DFA), 199
Direct sampling, 6
Directions for future research
  abdominal/chest injuries in abused children, 331
  abusive burns, 236
  AHT, 357
  anogenital examination, normal/developmental
    variations in, 80
  bacterial sexually transmitted infections in children,
    177
  biochemical markers of AHT in children, 438
  brain development, effects of abuse/neglect on,
    522
  bruises/skin lesions, 250
  child molesters, 163-164
  cost of child maltreatment, 639
  documenting medical history in possible physical
    child abuse, 213
  drug screening in infants/children, 568
  ear/nose/throat injuries in abused children, 335
  epidemiological issues in child maltreatment, 9
  epidemiology of CSA, 21
  epidemiology of IPV, 26
  epidemiology of physical abuse, 14

Directions for future research *(Continued)*
  eye injuries in child abuse, 410-411
  forensic evidence kit, 110-111
  foster children, caring for, 613
  FTT, 560
  genital/anal findings conditions confused with sexual
    abuse, 103-104
  HIV/AIDS in child/adolescent victims of sexual
    abuse/assault, 190
  imaging AHT, 388-389
  imaging skeletal trauma in abused children, 306
  international issues in child maltreatment, 625
  interviewing caregivers of suspected child abuse
    victims, 58
  neck/spinal cord injuries in child abuse, 399
  outcome of AHT, 456-457
  physical findings in children/adolescents with sexual
    abuse/assault, 91-92
  psychological impact/treatment of children who
    witness domestic violence, 511-512
  psychological impact/treatment of CPA, 486
  psychological impact/treatment of neglect of
    children, 497-498
  psychological impact/treatment of sexual abuse of
    children, 473
  tests to analyze forensic evidence in child sexual
    abuse/assault, 116
  viral/parasitic sexually transmitted infections in
    children, 184
Disclosure, 49, 462. *See also* Psychological impact/
  treatment of sexual abuse of children
Dissociation, 464
DNA testing, 108
  collecting forensic evidence, 107
  legal issues, 115-116
  processing, 115
  results, 113
  role in evidence, 115
  saliva and, 114
  trace evidence, 115
  unique samples, 112-113
  valid samples, 112
Documenting medical history in possible physical child
  abuse, 209. *See also* Interviewing children/adolescents
  about suspected abuse
  directions for future research, 213
  final reports, 213
  medical record, 209-212
    developmental history, 211, 212t
    family history, 212, 213t
    HPI, 210-211, 210t
    interview circumstances, 209-210
    PMH/ROS, 211, 211t
    social history, 212, 212t
  standardized forms, 212-213
Domestic Abuse Intervention Project, 23
Domestic violence (DV), 3, 12, 23, 466. *See also*
  Psychological impact/treatment of children who
  witness domestic violence
Dorion, Robert B. J., 581
Dowd, M. D., 102-103
Downing, Steve, 349
DPF. *See* Diaper Pail Friends
Drake, J. E., 235
Drewett, R. F., 560
Drink Safe Coaster, 125
Drink spiking, 118
Drockton, P., 84
Drotar, D., 552
Drug Endangered Children, 529
Drug screening in infants/children
  biological matrices, 564-565, 564t
  DFSA, 568
  directions for future research, 568
  introduction, 563-568
  MCA, 568
  methodologies, 563-564
    chromatography, 564
    immunoassays, 563-564
  pitfalls, 568
  specific drugs, 565-567
    amphetamines/methamphetamines, 565
    cocaine, 565-566
    ethanol, 566, 567t
    marijuana, 565

Drug screening in infants/children *(Continued)*
  opiates/opioids, 564t, 566-567, 567t
  strength of evidence, 568
Drug-facilitated sexual assault (DFSA), 568
  less commonly-encountered drugs, 123t-124t
  occurrence/characteristics, 118-119, 119t
  recommendations, 122-125
  substances cited in, 119t, 120-122
    1,4-BD, 122
    amphetamines/methamphetamines, 121-122
    benzodiazepines, 120-121
    cannabis, 121
    cocaine, 121
    ethyl alcohol, 120
    flunitrazepam, 120-121
    GBL, 122
    GHB, 122
DSM-IV. *See* Diagnostic and Statistical Manual of the American Psychiatric Association
DST. *See* Developmental systems theory
Dubowitz, H., 468, 497
Duhaime, A. C., 292, 349, 360-361, 364-367
Duncan, J. M., 396
Dunstan, F. D., 247
DV. *See* Domestic violence

E

Early childhood caries (ECC), 544, 546
Ear/nose/throat injuries in abused children
  directions for future research, 335
  ear injuries, 332-333, 334f
  facial injuries, 332, 333f
  introduction, 332-335, 333t
  nasal injuries, 334
  neck/pharyngeal injuries, 335, 335f
  oral injuries, 334-335, 334f-335f
  strength of evidence, 335
Eating disorders, 466
EBT. *See* Evidence-based treatments
EBV. *See* Epstein-Barr viral infections
ECC. *See* Early childhood caries
Ecological fallacies in data collection, 7
ED. *See* Emergency department
Eddy, Mary Baker, 600
EDH. *See* Epidural hemorrhage
Edmond, A. M., 560
Edwards, C., 241
Egeland, B., 492
Ehlers-Danlos syndrome, 249-250
EIA. *See* Enzyme immunoassay
Elder abuse, 23
Electrical burn injury, 229-230
Ellingson, K. D., 36-37
E-mail, 142
Emergency department (ED), 6-8, 110
Endangerment standard, 17-18
Engel, George, 549
Enteroviruses, 171-172
Entrapment/accommodation, 462
Environmental Protection Agency (EPA), 254
Enzyme immunoassay (EIA), 199
EPA. *See* Environmental Protection Agency
Epidemiological issues in child maltreatment
  difficulties identifying child abuse/neglect, 8
    anchoring, 8
    cognitive bias, 8
    confirmation bias, 8
    implicit biases, 8
    stereotypes, 8
  directions for future research, 9
  introduction, 3-9
  problems in research in child abuse/neglect, 6-7
    data collection issues, 6-7
    ethical issues, 7
  questions answered by, 4t
  terminology, 3-5
    accuracy, 3-4
    AR, 5
    diagnostic outcomes, 4, 4f
    incidence, 3
    OR, 5
    PAR, 5
    predictive value, 4-5

Epidemiological issues in child maltreatment *(Continued)*
    prevalence, 3, 5
    RR, 5
    sensitivity, 4-5
    specificity, 4-5
Epidemiological studies in child abuse, 5-6
  CarolinaSAFE study, 6
  direct sampling, 6
  Juvenile Victimization Questionnaire, 6
  National Gallup Poll, 6
  NCANDS, 4-6, 10-11, 17-18, 17f, 476, 490
  NIS, 4-6, 8, 10-11, 17-18, 476
Epidemiology
  abdominal/chest injuries in abused children, 326
  AHR, 349
  bacterial sexually transmitted infections in children, 174
  child abuse by burning, 222
  defined, 3
  SIDS, 337
Epidemiology of AHT, 351
  introduction, 35-38
    deaths, 35
    description, 35
    quantification, 35
    unrecognized inure, 35
  male perpetrators, 37
  population at risk, 37
    adult characteristics, 37
    child characteristics, 37
    family characteristics, 37
    societal risk factors, 37
  population-based incidence studies, 36-37
  summary, 37-38
Epidemiology of child neglect
  conclusion, 32
  contributors to neglect, 30-32
    community/neighborhood level, 31
    family level, 31
    individual level: parental/child characteristics, 30-31
    professional level, 32
    societal level, 31-32
  definitional issues, 28-29
    actual *vs.* potential harm, 28-29
    adequacy of care, 28
    neglect as heterogeneous phenomenon, 29
    neglect/continuum of care, 28
    quest for evidence-based definition, 28
  incidence of child neglect, 29-30
    educational neglect, 30
    emotional neglect, 30
    fatalities, 30
    identifying, 29-30
    rates, 29
    reporting, 29
    societal neglect, 30
  introduction, 28
  protective factors, 32
    parental competence, 32
    societal capital, 32
Epidemiology of CSA
  declining CSA, 18-21
    causes, 18-19
    recurrence, 17-18
    risk/protective factors, 19-21
  directions for future research, 21
  history, 16
  strength of evidence, 21
  terminology, 16-18
    case finding, 16
    child pornography, 16
    incest, 16
    incidence, 16-18
    prevalence, 18
    rape, 16
    sexual assault, 16
    sexual exploitation, 16
Epidemiology of IPV
  dating violence, 26
  definitions, 23
    consistent, 23
    by WHO, 23
  directions for future research, 26
  effect of IPV on children, 25-26

Epidemiology of IPV *(Continued)*
  harm from research questions, 26
  introduction, 23
  risk factors, 23-24
    in sociological model, 24-25
  scope of issue, 23
    global health crisis, 23-24
  social considerations, 24-25
    assisting women, 24
    barriers to seeking help, 24-25
    motivators for victims to seek help, 25
    provider barriers, 25
  strength of evidence, 26
  women perpetrators, 26
Epidemiology of physical abuse
  active/passive surveillance, 14
  directions for future research, 14
  by injury type/body section, 12-14
    head (excluding brain/skull) and neck, 12
    skeletal injury, 13
    skin injury, 13-14
    visceral injuries, 11
  introduction, 10-14
  risk factors for physical abuse, 11-12
    caregiver characteristics, 11-14
    child characteristics, 11-14
    corporal punishment, 12
    domestic violence, 12
    neighborhood characteristics, 12
    number in household, 12
    poverty, 12
  scope of problem, 10-11
    population surveys, 10
    surveillance, 10
Epidural hemorrhage (EDH), 414-415, 415f
Epstein-Barr viral infections (EBV), 100-101, 171-172
Escherichia coli, 96
Ethanol, 566, 567t
Ethyl alcohol, 120
Evaluating images in child pornography
  introduction, 147-151
  normative studies of physical/sexual maturation, 147-148
  reviewing images/videos, 148-151
    assessing age/maturity of photographic subjects, 150-151
    physical characteristics/age ranges, 148-149
    ratings based on body size/habitus in smaller children, 150
    secondary sexual characteristics, 149-150, 149f
    supplemental secondary sexual characteristics, 150
Evidence-based treatments (EBT), 476
Ewing-Cobbs, L., 453
Examination, 243
Exline, D. L., 114
Eye injuries in child abuse
  blunt impact, 402-403, 403t
  directions for future research, 410-411
  indirect ocular/visual, 402-403
  introduction, 402-411
  ophthalmologist documentation/role, 409-410
  postmortem examination/findings, 410
  retinal hemorrhage, 403-408
    differential diagnosis, 405f, 408, 408f, 408t
    incidence, 403-404
    mechanisms, 406-408
    types/patterns, 404-406, 404f-406f
  strength of evidence, 410

F

Factor XIII (FXIII), 442
Failure to gain weight, 547
Failure to thrive (FTT), 549t
  biopsychosocial model, 549-553
    biological sphere, 549-550
    psychological sphere, 550-552
    social sphere, 552-553
  conclusions, 560
  definition, 547-548
  directions for future research, 560
  etiology, 548-549
  evaluation, 551, 553-557
    assessment/multidisciplinary involvement, 555-556

Failure to thrive (FTT) (Continued)
  family history, 555
  growth charts, 553
  history, 553t-554t, 554-555
  hospitalization, 557
  laboratory/radiographic, 556-557
  physical examination, 555-556
  review of systems, 555
  introduction, 547-560
  outcome, 560
  strength of evidence, 560
  treatment, 557-559
   biological issues, 557-558
   psychosocial issues, 558-559
Falls, 325. See also Injuries from falls
  long, 570
  short, 570, 576-577
Family Connections, 496-497
Family Environment Scale (FES-A), 480
Family resolution therapy (FRT), 472
Family therapy, 472
Family treatment drug courts (FTDCs), 536
Family Violence Prevention Fund (FVPF), 618
Fanconi syndrome, 263
Fantuzzo, J., 495, 502
Farber, F. A., 492
Farnsworth, C. L., 289-290
Farst, K., 228
FAS. See Fetal alcohol syndrome
FBI Uniform Crime Reports, 17
FDA. See Food and Drug Administration
Federal Rules of Evidence, 219
Feldman, K. W., 224, 230-231, 395-397
Felitti, V. J., 511-512
Female genital cutting (FGC), 134
Female genital mutilation (FGM)
  cultural issues, 135-136
   contributing to social stability, 136
   cultural identity preservation, 136
   health, 136
   hygiene/aesthetic reasons, 136
   marriage, 136
   religion, 136
  health complications, 137-138, 137t
  international response, 139-140
  management of, 138-139
   child protection, 138-139, 138t
   medical management, 139
  performance, 134
  prevalence/geographic distribution, 134
  terminology, 134
  types, 134-135, 135f-136f
  WHO classification, 135, 135t
Female genital mutilation/cutting (FGM/C), 134
Feminist movement, 461-462
Fenichel, G. M., 286-287
FES-A. See Family Environment Scale
Fetal alcohol syndrome (FAS), 605
Feynman, Richard, 370
FGC. See Female genital cutting
FGM. See Female genital mutilation
FGM/C. See Female genital mutilation/cutting
Field, C. A., 502
Filiano, J. J., 338
Fimbriated hymen, 70, 70f
Financial Coalition to Combat Child Pornography, 144
Finkelhor, David, 16, 18-19, 155-156, 462-463, 502
Finkelhor's precondition model, 155
Finnegan, Loretta, 529
Flame burns, 229, 229f
Flunitrazepam, 120-121
Foley, Mark, 145
Food and Drug Administration (FDA), 162
Food insecurity, 490-491
Ford, C. A., 130
Foreign bodies, 96-97, 97f
Forensic dentistry
  aspects, 584
   dental aging, 584
   research, 581, 584
  bite marks/patterned injuries, 580, 583
   bite marks, 581, 581f-582f
   hickeys/suction marks, 581, 581f

Forensic dentistry (Continued)
   impression, 583, 583f
   photography, 582, 582f
   recognition, 580-581, 580f
   recording, 582-583
   referral, 583
   reporting, 581-582
   salivary swabbing, 582-583
  hospital protection teams, 584
  introduction, 579-584
  orofacial injuries in child abuse, 579-580, 580f
  strength of evidence, 584
Forensic evidence kit, 107f. See also Rape kit; Tests to analyze forensic evidence in child sexual abuse/assault
  collecting forensic evidence, 106-107
   chain of custody, 107
   collection/handling, 106-107
   consent, 106
   DNA samples, 107
   timing, 107
  directions for future research, 110-111
  frequency of recoverable evidence, 110
   in children, 110
  introduction, 106-111
  strength of evidence, 110-111
Forensic (investigative) interviews, 41-42
  audiotaped/videotaped, 41
  factors altering disclosed information, 42t
  as grand jury evidence, 41
  interviewer training, 41
  investigative protocols, 41-42
  medical examinations and, 42
Forensic Odontology Workbook, 579
Forensic science, 112
Fossa navicularis, 90f
Fossum, R. M., 327-328
Foster Care Independence Act, 613
Foster children, caring for
  directions for future research, 613
  health care barriers, 611
  introduction, 610-613
  models, 612-613
  older children, 613
  policies/guidelines, 611-612
  prevalence/nature of health problems, 610-611
Fractures in abusive/accidental trauma, 287-293. See also Abusive fractures
  clavicle fractures, 281f, 293
  femur fractures, 279f, 287-289, 289t
  humerus fractures, 280f, 289-290
  radius/ulna fractures, 281f, 290
  skull fractures, 277t, 284t, 291-293, 291t-292t
  tibia/fibula fractures, 289
Frechette, A., 230
Freud, Sigmund, 461-462
Fridriksson, T., 434
Friction/pressure burns, 230, 230f
Friedman, S. B., 235
Friedrich, William, 463-464, 469
FRT. See Family resolution therapy
FTDCs. See Family treatment drug courts
FTT. See Failure to thrive
Fualaau, Vili, 160
Fuchs, S. M., 292
FVPF. See Family Violence Prevention Fund
FXIII. See Factor XIII
FXIII deficiency, 442
  testing for, 444

G

GA1. See Glutaric aciduria type 1
GABA. See Gamma-aminobutyric acid
Gaffney, P., 227
Galbraith, J. A., 359
Gamma-aminobutyric acid (GABA), 120
Gamma-butyrolactone (GBL), 122
Gamma-hydroxybutyric acid (GHB), 122
GAO. See General Accounting Office
Garbarino, J., 31, 503
Garcia, C. T., 229-230
Garcia, V. F., 285
Garton, H. J. L., 397-398

Garty, B. Z., 231
GAS. See Group A ß-hemolytic *streptococcus*
Gas chromatography-mass spectrometry (GCMS), 118-119
GBL. See Gamma-butyrolactone
GC. See Neisseria gonorrhea
GCMS. See Gas chromatography-mass spectrometry
GCS. See Glasgow Coma Scale
Geddes, J. F., 398-399
GEDS. See Genital Examination Distress Scale
General Accounting Office (GAO), 630
Genital embryology
  cloaca, 69
  external genitalia, 69
  hymen, 69
  ovaries, 69
  primary structures, 69
  vagina, 69
Genital Examination Distress Scale (GEDS), 468
Genital ulcers, 100-101, 100f
  aphthae, 101
  causes, 100-101
  diagnosing, 100-101
  HSV type 2 and, 100
  treatment, 101
Genital/anal conditions confused with sexual abuse, 93
  accidental anogenital injury, 101-103, 101f
   evaluating, 103, 103f
   hymen, 102-103
   nonpenetrating, 102, 102f
   from physical abuse, 103, 103f
   scrotal, 102
   straddle injury, 101, 102f
   as uncommon, 101
  anal findings
   chronic constipation, 97
   dilated hemorrhoid veins, 98
   fecal incontinence, 97
   perianal erythema, 97, 98f
   rectal prolapse, 97-98
  Crohn disease, 95-96, 96f
  directions for future research, 103-104
  foreign bodies, 96-97, 97f
  genital ulcers, 100-101, 100f
   aphthae, 101
   causes, 100-101
   diagnosing, 100-101
   HSV type 2 and, 100
   treatment, 101
  genital/anal conditions, 96, 96f
   Behçet syndrome, 100-101
  irritants/dermatitis, 93-94
   allergic vulvar dermatitis, 96
   causes, 94f, 95-96
   contact dermatitis, 96
   diaper dermatitis, 93
   Jacquet erosive diaper dermatitis, 93, 94f
   primary diaper dermatitis, 93, 94f
   resembling scald burns, 93-94, 94f
  labial adhesions, 94-95, 95f
   causes, 95
   treatment, 95
  lichen sclerosus et atrophicus, 99-100
  LS & A, 99f-100f
   diagnosis, 99
   natural history in childhood, 100
   risks with, 100
   trauma and, 99
  neoplasia, 97
  strength of medical evidence, 103-104
  ureterocele, 99, 99f
  urethral prolapse, 98-99, 98f
   medical management, 99
   resembling HPV, 98-99, 98f
   treatment, 99
   uncommon in girls, 98
  vascular problems, 97
Gennarelli, T. A., 365
Ghahreman, A., 373-374
GHB. See Gamma-hydroxybutyric acid
Gil, Eliana, 469
Giles, F. H., 424
Gilles, E. E., 454-455
Gilman, B. B., 446
Giovannoni, J. M., 31

Giradet, R. G., 63
Girvin, H., 497
Glasgow Coma Scale (GCS), 122-125, 430t, 451
  as gold standard, 429
Gliding C/Ls, 419-420
Glutaric aciduria type 1 (GA1), 446-447
Gold standard, 4
Goldstein, Paul, 349
Gomez, F., 557
Grayston, A. D., 160
Greenough, W., 493
Gresham, G. A., 242
Grooming, 153, 158
Groth, N., 153, 158
Group A ß-hemolytic *streptococcus* (GAS), 170
Group therapy, 471
Growth deficiency, 547
Growth failure, 547
Growth faltering, 547
Gruson, L. M., 255-256
Guichon, J., 602
Gully, K., 468
Gumus, K., 255
Guo, S. M., 548
Guthkelch, Norman, 35, 349

H
HAB. *See* Hepatitis B
Hammer, M. R., 397-398
Hammond, J., 222
Hangman's fracture, 396, 396f
Hankins, C. L., 226
Hanson, R., 155, 162-163, 473
Harm standard, 17-18
Harrington, W. Z., 227
Haseler, L. J., 374-375
HAV. *See* Hepatitis A
HCP. *See* Health care providers
HCUP. *See* Healthcare Cost of Utilization Project
HCV. *See* Hepatitis C
HDV. *See* Hepatitis D
Head injury, computational models of pediatric, 361.
  See also Abusive head trauma
Head Start, 495
Health care providers (HCP), 25, 476. *See also* Caring
  for caretakers
  implications in psychological impact/treatment of
    children who witness domestic violence, 511
  interviews, 479
  recognizing excessive harm, 477
  role in psychological impact/treatment of CPA,
    484-485
Health Information Portability and Accountability Act
  (HIPAA), 55-58
Healthcare Cost of Utilization Project (HCUP),
  36-37
Hearsay exception, 43
Hebephilia, 153-154
Heger, A. H., 75-76, 84, 90-91
Heider, T. R., 228
Helminths, 172
Helplessness, 462
Hemophilia (Factor VIII deficiency), 442
Hemophilus influenzae, 96
Hendriks, J., 159
Henoch-Schönlein purpura, 97
Henriques, F., 224
Hepatitis A (HAV), 180
Hepatitis B (HAB), 180-181
Hepatitis C (HCV), 179, 181
Hepatitis D (HDV), 181
Hepatitis E (HEV), 181
Hepatitis G (HGV), 181
Heppenstall-Heger, A., 83-84, 91
Heroin, 531
Herpes simplex virus (HSV), 100, 171
  diagnosis, 182
  family, 181
  recurrences, 181-182
  sexual abuse and, 182
  specimen collection, 200-201
  testing, 182

Herpes simplex virus (HSV) *(Continued)*
  transmission, 181
  treatment, 182
Herr, S., 247
HEV. *See* Hepatitis E
HGV. *See* Hepatitis G
Hicks, T. A., 233
"Hidden pediatric problem," 63
HIPAA. *See* Health Information Portability and
  Accountability Act
History of present illness (HPI), 210-211, 210t
HIV. *See* Human immunodeficiency virus
HIV/AIDS, 47, 106, 171, 174-175
  protecting against, 175
HIV/AIDS in child/adolescent victims of sexual
  abuse/assault
  directions for future research, 190
  intersection, 186-187
  introduction, 186-190
  PEP, 188-189
  risk assessment, 187-188, 188t
  strength of evidence, 190
  treatment guidelines, 189-190
Hobbs, C. J., 90, 292-293
Hoke, R. S., 281-282
Holbourn, A. H. S., 365
Holden, G. W., 501-502, 512
Holter, J. C., 235, 244
Holtzworth-Munroe, A., 501-502
Home environment in substance-abusing families, 533
Home visitation, 495-496
Home-grown porn, 161
Homer, C., 548-549
Howieson, A. J., 228-229
HPA axis, 517
HPI. *See* History of present illness
HPV. *See* Human papillomavirus
HSV. *See* Herpes simplex virus
HSV type 1, 100
HSV type 2, 100
Hubbard, L. Ron, 599-600
Huestis, M. S., 536
Hughes, L. A., 445
Human immunodeficiency virus (HIV), 186
  specimen collection, 201
Human papillomavirus (HPV), 96-97, 97f, 179-180
  active infections, 180
  diagnosis, 180
  evaluations, 180
  resembling urethral prolapse, 98f
  specimen collection, 201
  subtypes, 179
  transmission, 179
  treatment, 180
  tumors, 179
  vaccine, 180
  warts, 179
Hummel, C. S., 222
Huntimer, C. M., 329
Huppert, J. S., 100-101
Hurley, M., 119-120
Hurrell, R. M., 127
Hydroceles, 80
Hydrophosphatasia, 266
Hymel, K. P., 290, 453-454
Hymen, 67, 69
  accidental anogenital injury, 102-103
  annular hymen, 70, 70f
  crescentic hymen, 70, 70f
  cribriform hymen, 70-72, 71f
  developmental changes, 72-74, 73f, 73t
  examinations, 82
  external ridges, 74
  fimbriated hymen, 70, 70f
  hymenal tags/mounds, 74, 75f
  imperforate hymen, 77
  linea vestibularis, 76-77, 76f
  longitudinal intravaginal ridges, 74, 74f, 78
  lymphoid follicles, 77
  newborn hymen, 72, 72f
  notches/clefts, 75, 75f
  septate hymen, 70, 71f
  sleevelike hymen, 70, 71f
  transverse hymenal diameters, 76
  vascularity/erythema, 76

Hymen *(Continued)*
  vestibular bands, 74, 74f
  width of inferior hymenal rim, 76
Hymenal tags/mounds, 74-75, 75f
Hypomagnesemia, 262
Hypopharyngeal laceration, 392-393, 393f
Hypospadias, 80
Hypothyroidism, 262
Hypoxic lesions, 423-424, 424f

I
IAC. *See* International African Committee on
  Traditional Practices Affecting the Health of Women
  and Children
IBD. *See* Inflammatory bowel disease
ICAC. *See* Internet Crimes Against Children Task
  Force
ICD-9-CM. *See* International Classification of Disease
  9th Clinical Modification
ICI. *See* Intracranial injury
IET. *See* Integrated-eclectic therapy
IFPS. *See* Intensive family preservation services
Imaging AHT
  differential diagnosis, 386-388
    AHT, 386-387
    BEAF, 386, 387f
    coagulopathy, 387
    infectious/inflammatory disease, 387, 388f
    metabolic disease, 388
    parturitional head trauma, 387, 388f
  directions for future research, 388-389
  injury age determination, 376f, 382-384, 384f, 386t
  introduction, 373-389
  neuroimaging examination, 373-376
    CT, 373, 374f
    MRI, 373-375, 375f-376f
    total body MRI, 373-374
  specific injuries, 376-382
    extraaxial injury, 374f-375f, 377f, 378-382,
      382f-383f
    traumatic brain injuries, 375f, 376-378, 377f-381f
  strength of evidence, 426
Imaging skeletal trauma in abused children
  bone scintigraphy, 296, 298f
  directions for future research, 306
  introduction, 296-306
  radiographic red flags, 296-305
    characteristic fracture line, 297f, 298-299, 300f
    CMLs, 302, 304f
    multiple injuries of differing ages, 299-302,
      301f-302f
    nonambulatory children with long bone fractures,
      297-298, 299f
    rib fractures, 302-304, 304f-305f
    skull fractures, 304-305, 305f-306f
  skeletal survey, 296, 297f, 297t
  strength of evidence, 305
Immune system, 518
Immunization, 600
Immunoassays, 563-564
Imperforate hymen, 77
Implicit biases, 8
In re E.G., 601-602
Inadequate growth, 547
Incest, 16
Infantile pyramidal protrusion, 77
Inflammatory bowel disease (IBD), 95-96
Ingram, D. L., 174
Injuries from falls
  assessing abuse, 572
  consultations, 572-576
    biochemical analyses, 575-576, 576t
    biochemical assessment, 572
    biodynamic compatibility of cause/injuries, 575
    differential diagnosis, 571t, 572
    scene investigation, 572-575
  death/serious injury from short, 576-577
  introduction, 570-577, 571f, 571t
  radiological imaging, 572
  testimony when death/serious injury from short, 577
  types, 570-572
    abdominal injuries with fall histories, 571
    chest injuries with fall histories, 571

Injuries from falls *(Continued)*
head injuries with fall histories, 570-571
less serious, 572
recognition/reporting, 572
Ink/dye staining, 256
Institutional review board (IRB), 6-7
Integrated-eclectic therapy (IET), 469
Intensive family preservation services (IFPS), 472
International African Committee on Traditional
Practices Affecting the Health of Women and
Children (IAC), 139
International Centre for Missing and Exploited
Children, 135
International Classification of Disease 9th Clinical
Modification (ICD-9-CM), 36-37
International Clinical Epidemiology Network, 624
International Day of Zero Tolerance of Female Genital
Mutilation, 140
International Federation of Gynecology, 138
International issues in child maltreatment
definitions/culture, 620
directions for future research, 625
ecological context, 623-625
caregiver/family characteristics, 623-624
children characteristics, 623
community context, 624
education of professionals, 624-625
societal context, 624
introduction, 620-625
maltreatment types, 621-623
fatal abuse, 621
neglect, 623
nonfatal abuse, 621
physical abuse, 621-622, 624-625
psychological abuse, 623
sexual abuse, 622-623
International Society for Prevention of Child Abuse
and Neglect (ISPCAN), 617
Internet child molesters, 154
Internet child sexual exploitation. *See also* Evaluating
images in child pornography
case examples, 143
child pornography, 143-145
combating, 144-145
ease of use, 144-145
predator tool, 143-144
as profitable, 144
victim use, 144
children on Internet, 142-143
chat rooms, 142
dangerous behavior promoted, 142
E-mail, 142
predators and, 142
safeguards, 143
social networking sites, 142-143
solicitation, 143
text messaging, 142
cybersex, 145-146
Internet Crimes Against Children Task Force (ICAC),
143
Internet Watch Foundation, 144
Interpersonal violence, 491
Interviewing caregivers of suspected child abuse
victims, 51, 52f
contextual issues/special circumstances, 57-58
caregiver substance use/abuse/mental illness, 57
cultural factors, 57-58
MCA, 58
when caregiver is victim, 57
directions for future research, 58
documentation's role, 58
pediatric history before concern for maltreatment,
51-52
beware of bias, 52
caregiver separated from child for interview, 52
history/examination red flags, 51, 53t
interactional cues/behavioral observations, 52, 53t
pediatric interview after concern for maltreatment,
52-57
caregivers separated, 54-55
details to ask, 54, 55t
informing caregivers of concern, 55-57
questions for physical abuse, 54
rapport, 53-54
sexual abuse questions, 55, 56t-57t

Interviewing caregivers of suspected child abuse victims
(Continued)
suspected child neglect questions, 55
themes to cover, 53, 54t
strength of evidence, 58
Interviewing children/adolescents about suspected
abuse
clinical approach to medical history, 45-47
language acquisition/child development, 45, 46t
principles in interviewing children, 45-47
forensic (investigative) interviews, 41-42
introduction, 41-50
legal considerations, 43
hearsay exception, 43
outcry witness, 43
medical history components, 47-50, 48t
abusive events, 47-49
family history/response to abuse disclosure, 49
gynecological history, 49
interviews from professionals, 49
post interview information, 49-50
promises do's/don'ts, 50
questions, 49
safety issues, 49
medical history importance, 42-43
clinician interviews, 43
evidence of abuse, 42-43
parental responsibility, 42
from parent/child, 42
varies by abuse type, 42
patterns of disclosure factors, 43-45
abusers in home, 44
custody issues, 44
delayed disclosure, 43
developmental considerations, 44
gender/age, 43
nondisclosure reasons, 43
older children, 44
partial (incremental) disclosure, 44-45
protecting abusers, 44
recantation rates, 44-45
shame/embarrassment, 43
socioeconomic/cultural factors, 44
younger age, 43-44
Intimate partner violence (IPV), 23, 128-129
Intracranial fluid collections, 445-446. *See also* Benign
extraaxial fluid of infancy
Intracranial injury (ICI), 429
CT as gold standard, 429
IPV. *See* Intimate partner violence
IRB. *See* Institutional review board
Irritants/dermatitis, 93-94
allergic vulvar dermatitis, 96
causes, 94f, 95-96
contact dermatitis, 96
diaper dermatitis, 93
Jacquet erosive diaper dermatitis, 93, 94f
primary diaper dermatitis, 93, 94f
resembling scald burns, 93-94, 94f
Ischemic lesions, 424, 424f
ISPCAN. *See* International Society for Prevention of
Child Abuse and Neglect

J

Janet, Pierre, 461-462
Jaspers, Virginia, 349
Jaudes, P. K., 31
Jehovah's Witnesses, 600-602
Jenny, C., 290, 350, 433
John, R. S., 508
Johnson, C. F., 229-230, 642
Jones, J. G., 90
Jones, L. M., 18-19
Judkins, A. R., 413
Justice Appropriations Act, 143
Juvenile Victimization Questionnaire, 6

K

Kadish, H. A., 102
Kadushin, A., 31
Kashgarian, Michael, 349

Keen, J. H., 247-248
Keenan, H. T., 453-455
Keeping Children and Families Safe Act of 2003, 533
Kellogg, N. D., 54, 76-77, 82-83, 131
Kempe, C. Henry, 35, 451, 461-462, 529, 539, 579,
607, 629
KID. *See* Kids Inpatient Database
Kids Inpatient Database (KID), 36-37
King, J., 276, 289
Kinney, H. C., 338
Kirshner, R. H., 254-255
Kitzmann, K. M., 504-506
Kleinman, P. K., 278, 282, 286-287, 302, 308
Klevens, J., 484
Klinefelter syndrome, 148
Klippel-Trenanay syndrome, 252
Kochanek, P. M., 367
Koenen, K. C., 521
Korbin, J. E., 620
Krafft-Ebing, 153-154
Kravitz, H., 570
Kriewall, T. J., 360

L

Labbe, J., 244, 247-248
Labial adhesions, 94-95, 95f
causes, 95
treatment, 95
Laboratory methods for diagnosing STIs in children/
adolescents, 193, 194t-197t
serological testing, 203
reporting, 203
specimen collection
CT/GC, 193-203, 199t-200t
HPV, 201
HSV, 200-201
lice, 202-203
TV, 201-202
vaginitis/vaginosis, 201-202
strength of evidence, 203-204
Lacerations, 243
Lalumiére, M. L., 159
Lambert, M. L., 186
Lancaster, D. M., 581
Lane, W. G., 8
Langlois, N. E., 242
Language acquisition/child development, 45, 46t
Lanning, K. V., 153
Lapp, J., 31
Lawrence, Abraham, 628
Learning club, 510
Ledbetter, D. H., 327-329
Lee, Jennifer, 144
Leslie, L. K., 611
Letourneau, Mary Kay, 160
Levendosky, A. A., 507
Leventhal, J. M., 276, 290, 293, 572
Levin, A. B., 97
Lice, 172
specimen collection, 202-203
Lichen sclerosus et atrophicus (LS & A), 99-100,
99f-100f
diagnosis, 99
natural history in children, 100
risks with, 100
trauma and, 99
Lieberman, A. F., 507
Limbic system, 520-521
Lindberg, Dennis, 602-603
Lindegren, M. L., 186
Lindenberg, R., 377-378
Linea vestibularis, 76-77, 76f
Locus coeruleus noradrenergic neurotransmitter
system, 517-518
Logan, S., 560
Long, R. T., 235
Long bone fracture biomechanics
anatomy overview, 317, 318f
concepts, 317-318, 319t
force, 317, 318f
moment, 317, 320f
strain, 318, 320f
stress, 318, 319t, 320f

Long bone fracture biomechanics *(Continued)*
 factors affecting likelihood of fracture, 321-324
  bone material properties, 321-322, 321t, 322f
  combining intrinsic/extrinsic factors, 323-324, 324f
  extrinsic, 322
  intrinsic, 321-322
  intrinsic factors related to pediatric bone tissue, 322
  introduction, 317-325
  material properties, 318-321
   anisotropy, 320-321
   elasticity, 318, 320f
   ultimate strength, 320
   yield strength, 318-319
  response to rate of loading application, 323, 323f
  types/characteristics of loads, 322-323, 322f, 322t-323t
 fracture assessment, 325
 qualitative fracture assessment model, 324-325, 324f
  example: skiing incident, 325
  example: sofa fall, 325
  fracture type, 324-325
  injury causation, 324
  injury mechanism, 324
Long falls, 570
Longitudinal intravaginal ridges, 74, 74f, 78
Lowden, I. M. R., 290
Lowell, G., 230
LS & A. *See* Lichen sclerosus et atrophicus
Ludemann, J. P., 228
Ludwig, S., 548-549
Lymphoid follicles, 77
Lyons-Ruth, K., 504-505

M

Magnetic resonance imaging (MRI), 310f, 311-313, 312f-314f
 neuroimaging examination, 373-375, 375f-376f
 total body, 373-376
Maguire, S., 244
Mahabir, R. C., 287
Maibach, H. I., 240
Main, M., 504
Major outer membrane protein (MOMP), 199
Malassezia furfur, 171
Malkan, Jennifer, 349
Malnutrition, 548
Maltreatment Classification System (MCS), 479
Mann, M., 114
MAOA. *See* Monoamine oxidase A
Margolin, G., 508
Margulies, S. S., 291, 360-361, 365, 367, 413
Marijuana, 529-530, 565. *See also* Cannabis
Marks, R., 241
Marks, S. C., 286
Martin, I. M., 175
Massa, N., 228
Maternal deprivation syndrome, 551
Maternal Lifestyle Study, 529
Mature minor doctrine, 601-602
Maxeiner, H., 394-395, 416
Mayer-Rokitansky-Küster-Hauser syndrome, 72, 72f
MBP. *See* Myelin-basic protein
MCA. *See* Medical child abuse
McBride, M. T., 293
McCann, J., 74-75, 78-79, 84-85, 94-95, 551
McCloskey, L. A., 507-508
McDonald, R., 502
McGovern, M. E., 587
McGrory, B. R., 286-287
McLaren, D. S., 557
McMahon, P., 239, 248
MCMPI-III. *See* Milon Multiaxial Personality Inventory
McPherson, G. K., 360
MCS. *See* Maltreatment Classification System
MCV. *See* Molluscum contagiosum virus
MD. *See* Menkes disease
MDT. *See* Multidisciplinary team
Median raphe, 78

Mediated prefrontal cortex, 521
Medical child abuse (MCA)
 compared to other types of child abuse, 586-587
 drug screening in infants/children, 568
 interviewing caregivers of suspected child abuse victims, 58
 introduction, 586-590
 legal issues, 590
 MDT, 589
 prevention, 590
 terminology issues, 587
 treatment, 587-589
  ensuring abuse does not recur, 589
  identifying abuse, 588
  preserving family, 589
  repairing damage, 589
  stopping abuse, 588-589
Meezan, W., 495
Menkes disease (MD), 447
Mental health, 466
Mentzel, H. J., 312
Merten, D. F., 287, 293, 380
Methicillin resistant *streptococcus aureus* (MRSA), 170
Microwave oven burns, 230
Midline sparing, 76-77
Mileusnic, D., 445
Military family children, 37
Millennium Development Goals, 140
Milon Multiaxial Personality Inventory (MCMI-III), 163
Minnesota Multiphasic Personality Inventory (MMPI-2), 163
Minnesota Sex Offender Screening Tool-Revised (MnSOST-R), 163
Minns, R. A., 36, 416-417, 422-423, 426
Missouri Child Fatality Review Program, 592
Mitchell, I., 602
Mites, 172
Mitochondrial DNA (mtDNA), 113
MMPI-2. *See* Minnesota Multiphasic Personality Inventory
MnSOST-R. *See* Minnesota Sex Offender Screening Tool-Revised
Mok, J. Y. Q., 286
Mokrohisky, S. T., 256
Molluscum contagiosum virus (MCV), 96, 171, 182
MOMP. *See* Major outer membrane protein
Monoamine oxidase A (MAOA), 521-522
Moritz, A. R., 224
Morrison, C. N., 416-417
Motivators for IPV victims to seek help, 25
 addressing, 25
 consequences of IPV, 25
 increasing knowledge, 25
 understanding, 25
Mouden, Lynn, 579
MRI. *See* Magnetic resonance imaging
MRSA. *See* Methicillin resistant *streptococcus aureus*
MSBP. *See* Munchausen syndrome by proxy
MST. *See* Multisystemic therapy
mtDNA. *See* Mitochondrial DNA
Mukadam, S., 226
Multidisciplinary team (MDT), 589
Multisystemic therapy (MST), 495
Munang, L. A., 242
Munchausen syndrome by proxy (MSBP), 587-588
Murphy, S., 226
Myelin-basic protein (MBP), 431
Myhre, A. K., 78-79, 96
Myth of Classlessness (Pelton), 7

N

NAATs. *See* Nucleic acid amplification tests
NAMBLA. *See* North American Man-Boy Love Association
NAT. *See* Nonaccidental trauma
National Advisory Council on Violence and Abuse, 617
National Center for Missing and Exploited Children (NCMEC), 142, 144, 149-150
National Center for Shaken Baby Syndrome, 618
National Child Abuse and Neglect Data System (NCANDS), 4-6, 10-11, 17, 17f, 476, 490

National Child Traumatic Stress Network (NCTSN), 473, 481
National Council on Crime and Delinquency (NCCD), 630-631
National Crime Victimization Survey, 17
National Drug Threat Survey, 533
National Family Violence Survey, 502
National Gallup Poll, 6
National Incidence Studies (NIS), 4-6, 8, 10-11, 17-18, 476. *See also* Third National Incidence Study
National Institute of Child Health and Human Development (NICHD), 41-42
National Institute of Standards and Technology, 107
National Maternal and Infant Health Survey, 129
National Survey of Child and Adolescent Well-being (NSCAW), 476
National Survey on Drug Use and Health, 565
National Violence Against Women Survey, 502
Nayak, K., 244
NCANDS. *See* National Child Abuse and Neglect Data System
NCCD. *See* National Council on Crime and Delinquency
NCMEC. *See* National Center for Missing and Exploited Children
NCTSN. *See* National Child Traumatic Stress Network
Neck/spinal cord injuries in child abuse
 differentiating from nonabusive injuries, 398-399
  neck injury/shaking, 398-399
 directions for future research, 399
 indirect forces to neck, 395-396
  anatomy of neck, 395-396
 introduction, 392-399, 393t
 through mouth, 392-394
  caustic/irritating agents introduction, 393-394
  foreign body introduction, 393
  hypopharyngeal laceration, 392-393, 393f
 neck/cervical spine injuries, 396-398
  bony spine/surrounding ligaments, 396-398, 396f
  cervical structures, 397
  extraaxial hemorrhage of spine, 396-397, 397f
  presenting symptoms, 397, 398t
  recognizing cervical, 397-398
  spinal cord, 397
  vascular structures of neck, 396
 nonstrangulation blunt trauma, 395
 spine biomechanics, 396
 strangulation, 394-395, 394f
 strength of medical evidence, 399
Negative predictive value (NPV), 4-5
Neglect. *See also* Brain development, effects of abuse/neglect on; Child neglect, definitions/categorization; Dental neglect; Psychological impact/treatment of neglect of children
 abusive burns and, 231
 types of, 31
Neisseria gonorrhea (GC), 198-200, 199t
Nelson, M. D., Jr., 454-455
Neoplasia, 97
Neuropathology of AHT
 findings, 413-425
  anoxic encephalomyelopathy/infarction, 423-424, 424f
  axonal injury, 420-421, 420f-421f
  brainstem/spinal injuries, 421-422, 422f-423f
  cerebrospinal C/Ls, 417-421
  chronic lesions, 424, 425f
  deep C/Ls, 419-421, 419f-421f
  EDH, 414-415, 415f
  external examination, 413
  fractures, 413-414, 414f
  gliding C/Ls, 419-420
  hypoxic lesions, 423-424, 424f
  internal soft tissue injury, 413, 414f
  intracranial hemorrhage, 414-417
  ischemic lesions, 424, 424f
  optic nerve/retinal inure, 424-425, 425f
  parenchymal/intraventricular hemorrhage, 417
  SAH, 415f, 417
  SDH, 415-417, 415f-417f
  superficial C/Ls, 418, 418f
  TBI, 422-423, 423f
 introduction, 413-426
New York Society for the Prevention of Cruelty to Children (NYSPCC), 628

Newborn hymen, 72, 72f
NGOs. *See* Nongovernmental organizations
NHANES III. *See* Third National Health and Nutrition
Examination Survey III
NICHD. *See* National Institute of Child Health and
Human Development
Nicholson, C. E., 426
Nimkin, K., 287
NIS. *See* National Incidence Studies
Nonaccidental trauma (NAT), 308-311
Nongovernmental organizations (NGOs), 139
Nonorganic failure to thrive, 547
Nonsexually transmitted infections of genitalia/anus of
prepubertal children, 169
  normal vaginal flora/nonspecific vulvovaginitis, 169
    miscellaneous causes, 169
  specific vulvovaginitis, 169-172
    anaerobic/mixed anaerobic infections, 170-171
    fungal causes, 171
    GAS, 170
    helminths, 172
    less common bacteria, 170
    lice, 172
    miscellaneous bacteria, 171
    mites, 172
    parasites, 172
    protozoa, 172
    shigella, 170
    viral causes, 171-172
  summary, 172
Nonstrangulation blunt trauma, 395
Nork, S. E., 288
North American Man-Boy Love Association
  (NAMBLA), 156, 161
North Carolina study, 37
NPV. *See* Negative predictive value
NSCAW. *See* National Survey of Child and Adolescent
  Well-being
Nucleic acid amplification tests (NAATs), 193,
  198-200, 203-204
Nurse Home Visitation Program, 495-496
NYSPCC. *See* New York Society for the Prevention of
  Cruelty to Children

O

Odds ratios (OR), 5
Oemichen, M., 396-398
Office of Juvenile Justice and Delinquency Prevention
  (OJJDP), 143
OI. *See* Osteogenesis imperfecta
OJJDP. *See* Office of Juvenile Justice and Delinquency
  Prevention
Ojo, P., 222
O'Keefe, M., 495
Olds, D. L., 495-496, 638
Olsen, E. M., 548
Ommaya, A. K., 365
"On the Theory and Practice of Shaking Infants," 607
1,4-BD. *See* 1,4-Butanediol
1,4-Butanediol (1,4-BD), 122
O'Neill, J. A., 276
Opiates/opioids, 564t, 566-567, 567t
Oppenheim, W. L., 293
OR. *See* Odds ratios
Osteogenesis imperfecta (OI), 269-271
  diagnosis, 270-271, 270f
  laboratory findings, 270
  nonaccidental trauma *vs.*, 271
  type I, 269
  type II, 269, 270f
  type III, 269, 270f
  type IV, 263, 269-270
  type V, 270
  type VI, 270
  type VII, 270
Osteoporosis, 266
  primary, 266
  secondary, 266
Outcome of AHT
  directions for future research, 456-457
  family environment, 455
  illustrative case report, 455-456, 456f
  introduction, 451-457

Outcome of AHT *(Continued)*
  mechanisms of injury/neuroimaging findings/
    biomarkers relating to outcome, 454-455
  neurobehavioral/neuropsychological outcomes,
    451-454, 456f
    compared to noninflicted head trauma/community
      comparison groups, 453-454
    descriptive studies, 454, 456f
Outcry witness, 43
Ovaries, 69
Owings, C. L., 284

P

Palmer, W. E., 312
Palusci, V. J., 82-83, 110
PANDA. *See* Prevent Abuse and Neglect through
  Dental Awareness
PAP. *See* Prostatic acid phosphatase
PAR. *See* Population attributable risk
Paraphilia, 153-154
Parathyroid hormone, 262
Paraurethral cysts, 77, 77f
Parent training (PT), 495
Parental mental health, 534
Parent-Child Interaction Training (PCIT), 482-483
Parenting, 31, 467, 480, 482, 534. *See also* Cognitive
    behavioral therapy
  skills, 463, 471
Parenting-child sessions, 471
Parish, R. A., 231
Parks, A. G., 95-96
Parturitional head trauma, 387, 388f
Pascoe, J. M., 244
Past medical history (PMH), 211, 211t
PCIT. *See* Parent-Child Interaction Training
Pearlman, L. A., 642
Pediatric Research in the Office Setting Network
  (PROS), 147
Pedophile Information Exchange, 161
Pedophilia, 153-154, 154t
Pedophilia erotica, 153-154
Pelton, Leroy, 7
Pelvic inflammatory disease (PID), 174
Penkower, Jessica, 602
Pertussis, 402
Petechiae, 341-342, 394. *See also* Strangulation
Peters, M. L., 287, 289, 293
Photodocumentation in child abuse cases
  ALS, 219
  common errors, 219
  composition, 217-218, 217f, 218t
  conclusion, 220
  equipment, 215-217, 216f-217f
  introduction, 215-220, 218t
  legal issues, 219-220
  storage, 218
Physical examination of child with suspected sexual
  abuse
  approach, 63-64
    preparing child, 64
    timing of examination, 63-64
  debriefing child/caregivers, 67
  documentation, 67
  introduction, 63-68
  medical evaluation, 63
    document injuries, 63
    ensure child's health, 63
    establish rapport, 63
    interview child/caretaker, 63
  medical examination, 64-67
    ALS, 67
    anogenital area exam, 65, 65f
    anus/perianal area, 67
    choking injuries, 64-65, 64f
    colposcopy, 66-67
    defensive wounds, 64-65, 64f
    examination equipment, 66-67
    examination positions, 65-66, 66f
    hymen, 67
    photodocumentation, 66-67
    physician competency, 65
    self-inflicted injuries, 64-65, 65f
    specific anatomical areas, 67

Physical examination of child with suspected sexual
  abuse *(Continued)*
    speculum examination, 66-67
    vestibule, 67
  medical findings interpretations, 67-68
Physical findings in children/adolescents with sexual
  abuse/assault
  acute genital findings following sexual trauma,
    82-84
    anogenital injuries, 86f
    fossa navicularis, 90f
    injury types, 82-83, 83f
    other bodily injuries, 87f
    perihymenal injuries, 87f
    posterior fourchette, 90f
    trauma types, 82
  directions for future research, 91-92
  evaluation of serious genital injuries from sexual
    assault, 89-91
    anal injuries, 91, 91f
    under anesthesia, 90
    anorectal injuries, 90
    genital/anal injuries in males, 90-91, 90f-91f
    surgical consultation, 89-90
  healing of acute anogenital injuries, 84-85
  introduction, 82-92
  nonacute examinations of adolescents, 87-89, 87f
  nonacute examinations of prepubertal children,
    85-87
    evidence of past abuse/assault, 82, 85f-86f, 87t
    interpretation of findings, 82, 88t-89t
    long after assault, 85
  standardization of examination techniques, 82
    examination positions, 82
    multiple adjunct techniques, 82
    physical findings, 82
PID. *See* Pelvic inflammatory disease
Pierce, M. C., 244, 288-289, 324
Pigmentation disorders, 252-253
Pinheiro, Paulo, 625
PIP. *See* Program Improvement Plan
PIVKA-II. *See* Proteins induced in vitamin K absence
Plunkett, J., 368-369, 445
PMH. *See* Past medical history
POCT. *See* Point-of-care tests
Point-of-care tests (POCT), 193, 198
Poliray light source, 109
Population attributable risk (PAR), 5
Positive predictive value (PPV), 4
Posner, J. C., 77
Postacchini, F., 293
Posterior fourchette, 90f
Postexposure prophylaxis (PEP), 188-189, 188t
Posttraumatic stress disorder (PTSD), 130-131,
  464-466, 478, 516
  corpus callosum and, 518-519
  occupational hazards of child protection work, 642
Poverty, 29, 490, 552
  as contributor to neglect, 31-32
  as risk factor for physical abuse, 12
"Power and Control Wheel," 23, 24f
Powerlessness, 642
PPV. *See* Positive predictive value
Prange, M. T., 368-369
Prasad, M., 455
Predictive value, 4-5. *See also* Negative predictive value;
  Positive predictive value
Preferential child molesters, 153
Pregnancy, 129-130
Prescott, P. R., 227
Prescription substances for nonmedical use, 532
Prevent Abuse and Neglect through Dental Awareness
  (PANDA), 579
Prevention of child abuse/neglect
  conclusion, 608
  introduction, 605-608
  location of abuse, 607
  perpetrator considerations, 607-608
    abuser types, 608
    reactive child/adolescent abusers, 608
    sexual abusers, 607-608
  programs with data on outcome, 608
  victim considerations, 605-607
    age, 605-606
    developmental level, 606-607

Prevention paradox, 5
Primary diaper dermatitis, 93, 94f
Prince vs. Massachusetts, 600, 603
Principles in interviewing children, 45-47
　no prompting, 45
　patient trust, 45
　permission to share experiences, 45
　sharing information, 45-46
Program Improvement Plan (PIP), 629
Project Safe-Care, 483, 496
Project SUPPORT, 510
Prominent skin folds/pectinate line, 78
PROS. *See* Pediatric Research in the Office Setting
　Network
Prostatic acid phosphatase (PAP), 112
PROTECT Act of 2003, 145
Proteins induced in vitamin K absence (PIVKA-II),
　444
Protozoa, 172
Pseudohypoparathyroidism, 262
Psycho-education, 470
Psychological impact/treatment of children who
　witness domestic violence
　children in violent households, 502
　children's response, 505-509
　　exposure to violence by adolescents, 509
　　exposure to violence in infancy/early childhood,
　　　506-507
　　exposure to violence in middle childhood,
　　　507-509
　directions for future research, 511-512
　exposure in ecological context, 503-504
　　co-occurrence of stressors, 503-504
　　factors intrinsic to child, 503
　　power of parents, 503
　　society/culture, 503
　implications for HCPs, 511
　interventions, 509-511
　　clubs/preschool, 510
　　CPP, 510
　　learning club, 510
　　Project SUPPORT, 510
　　trauma-focused, 510-511
　　youth relationships project, 510
　introduction, 501-512
　mechanisms of action, 504-505
　　attachment, 504-505
　　dual lens – attachment/trauma, 505
　　trauma, 505
　strength of evidence, 511-512
　terminology/taxonomy, 501-502
Psychological impact/treatment of CPA
　characteristics/consequences, 477-478
　　behavior/mental health problems, 477
　　cognitive/learning attributions, 477
　　health/medical, 478
　　PTSD, 478
　　social/interpersonal competence/relationship skills,
　　　478
　　summary, 478
　continuum of force, 476-477
　　definitions, 476
　　prevalence/scope, 476-477
　directions for future research, 486
　HCP's role, 484-485
　intervention/treatment, 481-484
　　child-focused, 481-482
　　parent-child/family-focused, 482-483
　　parent-focused, 482
　　summary, 484
　introduction, 476-486
　prevention, 484
　screening/assessment/evaluation,
　　478-480
　　clinical problems/symptoms, 479-480
　　environmental context, 480
　　formal/instruments/tools, 479-480
　　functional impairment, 480
　　interviews, 478-479
　　recidivism/high-risk behaviors, 479
　　services/intervention experience, 480
　　summary, 480
　service referral/access/use, 480-481
　strength of evidence, 485-486
　summary, 486

Psychological impact/treatment of neglect of
　children
　directions for future research, 497-498
　introduction, 490-498
　long-term follow-up, 497
　predictors, 490-491
　　child development/behavior, 491
　　child temperament, 491
　　food insecurity, 490-491
　　interpersonal violence, 491
　　maternal depression, 491
　　poor maternal nutrition, 491
　　poverty, 490
　　stressful life events, 491
　programs/policies related to neglect,
　　494-497
　　family connections, 496-497
　　family interventions, 495
　　home visitation, 495-496
　　play therapy, 494-495
　psychological consequences, 491-493
　　adolescents, 492-493
　　infancy, 492
　　school-aged children, 492
　psychological functioning, 493-494
　　biological stress response, 493
　　community influences on neglect, 494
　　direct effects of neglect, 493-494
　　DST, 492-494
　　mediated effects of neglect, 494
　　moderated effects of neglect, 494
　　transactional effects of neglect, 494
Psychological impact/treatment of sexual abuse of
　children
　characterizing abuse/impacts, 462-463
　　CSAAS, 462
　　traumagenic dynamics, 462-463
　diagnosis, 465-466
　directions for future research, 473
　disclosure, 467-469
　　forensic interview *vs.*, 469
　　medical examination/interaction with child abuse
　　　team, 468
　　reporting to CPS, 468
　gender differences, 467
　history of awareness, 461-462
　introduction, 461-473
　long-term outcomes, 466-467
　　depression, 466
　　domestic violence, 466
　　eating disorders, 466
　　medical problems, 467
　　mental health, 466
　　parenting, 467
　　PTSD, 466
　　revictimization, 466
　　substance abuse/dependence, 467
　risk factors, 463
　sexual behavior, 463-464
　short-term effects, 464-465
　　adolescence/young adult (13-18), 465
　　early childhood (2-6), 464-465
　　middle childhood (7-12), 465
　strength of evidence, 473
　treatment, 469-473
　　abuse specific therapy, 469
　　affect expression, 470-471
　　CBT, 470-471
　　cognitive coping, 471
　　cognitive processing, 471
　　family therapy, 472
　　group therapy, 471
　　nonoffending parents, 471-472
　　parenting skills, 463, 471
　　parenting-child sessions, 471
　　pharmacological, 472-473
　　play therapy, 469
　　psycho-education, 470
　　relaxation techniques, 470
　　supportive therapy, 470
　　symptom-focused therapy, 469-470
　　trauma narrative, 471
PT. *See* Parent training
PTSD. *See* Posttraumatic stress disorder
Puczynski, M., 230

Purdue, G. F., 223-224, 229
Pynos, R. S., 503

Q

QALY. *See* Quality adjusted life year
Quality adjusted life year (QALY), 636-637, 636t
Quinlan, K., 230
Quinsey, V. I., 162-163

R

Raghupathi, R., 360-361
Rape, 16. *See also* Adolescent sexual assault/statutory
　rape; Date rape
　acquaintance, 128-129
Rape kit, 107-110, 107f
　ALS, 109
　bite marks, 109
　clothing collection, 108
　fingernails, 109
　hair collection, 109
　saliva collection, 109-110
　swabs, 108-109
　　blood/buccal/saliva, 108
　　collection/interpretation, 108
　　dry, 108
　　mouth, 108
　　on penis, 108
　　semen/sperm collection, 108-109
　　types/numbers to use, 108
　　vaginal/cervical, 108
　toluidine dye, 109
Rape trauma syndrome, 130
Rapid Risk Assessment for Sex Offense Recidivism
　(RRASOR), 163
Ray Helfer Society, 617
Raymond, N. C., 161-162
Reactive child/adolescent abusers, 608
Read, W. W., 557
Rectal prolapse, 97-98
Reece, R. M., 378-379, 426
Reeker, J., 471
Rees, J. L., 239
Reid, J. E., 156
Reinhart, M. A., 90
Reischle, S., 227
Relapse prevention (RP), 162
Relative risk (RR), 5
Relaxation techniques, 470
Religion/child neglect
　introduction, 599-603
　public policy, 600-603
　　issues with adolescents, 601-603
　　scope of law, 600-601
Rene Guyon Society, 161
Rennie, I., 287
Resilient peer treatment (RPT), 482
Response to child maltreatment
　AAP, 615-618
　ABP, 616-617
　advocacy/research, 618
　APSAC, 617
　AVA, 617-618
　FVPF, 618
　introduction, 615-618
　ISPCAN, 617
　National Advisory Council on Violence and Abuse,
　　617
　Ray Helfer Society, 617
　summary, 618
Revere, Paul, 579
Revictimization, 466
Review of systems (ROS), 211, 211t
Rewers, A., 289
Ricci, L. R., 242
Rimsza, M. E., 230
Rizley, R., 539-540
Robinson, J. R., 551-552
Roman Catholic Church, 600, 607
Romner, B., 434
ROS. *See* Review of systems
RP. *See* Relapse prevention

RPT. *See* Resilient peer treatment
RR. *See* Relative risk
RRASOR. *See* Rapid Risk Assessment for Sex Offense
Recidivism
Rubin, D. M., 611
Rudolf, M. C., 560
Ruppel, R. A., 367
Rutter, M., 511-512

S

Saakvitne, K. W., 642
SACA. *See* Service Assessment for Children and
Adolescents
SAH. *See* Subarachnoid hemorrhage
Salinger, Robert, 349
Saliva
analysis, 113-114
bite marks and, 114, 582-583
collection, 109-110
DNA testing and, 114
swab collection, 108
Sameroff, A. J., 550
SAMHSA. *See* Substance Abuse and Mental Health
Service Administration
Saunders, B. E., 473
Sawyer, J. R., 276
SBS. *See* Shaken baby syndrome
Scannapieco, M., 534-535
Scherl, S. A., 288-289
Schlesinger, A. E., 282
Schmidt, Barton D., 615
Schwartz, A. J., 242
SCIWORA. *See* Spinal cord injury without
radiographic abnormality
Scott, David, 579
Scottish Index of Multiple Deprivation, 37
Scratches, 243
Scrotum, accidental anogenital injury, 102
Scurvy, 446
SDH. *See* Subdural hemorrhage
Seagull, E., 31
Secondary trauma, 630, 642
Secrecy, 462
Section on Child Abuse and Neglect (SOCAN),
615-616
Seduction hypothesis, 461
Sege, R., 378-379
Selbst, S. M., 97
Selection bias, 6-7
Self-inflicted injuries, 64-65, 65f
Semen/sperm
ALS for screening, 112
analysis, 112-113
collection, 108-109
Septate hymen, 70, 71f
Serology, 113
Serotonin reuptake inhibitors (SSRIs), 162
Service Assessment for Children and Adolescents
(SACA), 480
SES. *See* Socioeconomic status
Seto, M. C., 154-155, 159
Sex hormone altering medications, 162
Sex Offender Risk Appraisal Guide (SORAG), 163
Sexual abuse, 473, 607-608. *See also* Genital/anal
conditions confused with sexual abuse; HIV/AIDS in
child/adolescent victims of sexual abuse/assault;
International issues in child maltreatment; Physical
findings in children/adolescents with sexual abuse/
assault; Psychological impact/treatment of children
who witness domestic violence; Tests to analyze
forensic evidence in child sexual abuse/assault
CSA, 16
CSAAS, 462
Sexual assault, 16, 181. *See also* Adolescent sexual
assault/statutory rape; Drug-facilitated sexual assault;
Rape; Sexual abuse
Sexual behavior, 463-464
Sexual Experience Survey, 128
Sexual maturity rating (SMR), 73-74, 147-151, 149f
Sexually transmitted infections (STIs), 47, 67, 96, 106,
130-131. *See also* Bacterial sexually transmitted
infections in children; Laboratory methods for
diagnosing STIs in children/adolescents

Sexually transmitted infections (STIs) *(Continued)*
testing, 175
treatment, 175, 176t
Shaken baby syndrome (SBS), 35, 364. *See also* Shaking
Shakespeare, William, 529
Shaking, 607. *See also* Shaken baby syndrome
accidental brain injuries, 368-369
biomechanics, 365-367
applying studies to, 365-366, 366f
brief primer, 365
infant not small adult, 366-367, 366f
developing brain response to AHT, 367-368, 368t
differentiating from nonabusive injuries, 398-399
introduction, 364-370
perpetrator confessions, 369-370
understanding TBI, 370
Shane, S. A., 292
Shaw, B. A., 289-290
Shigella, 170
Short falls, 570, 576-577
Short tandem repeats (STR loci), 112-114
"Sick Kids Child Physiology," 69
SIDS. *See* Sudden infant death syndrome
Simms, R. J., 395
Simons, M., 227
Sims, Bernard, 579
Sinclair, K. A., 179
Single nucleotide polymorphisms (SNP loci), 113
Situational child molesters, 153
Sivit, C. J., 326
Skeletal trauma. *See* Cross-sectional imaging in
evaluating pediatric skeletal trauma; Imaging skeletal
trauma in abused children
Skin conditions confused with child abuse
conclusion, 258
conditions confused with bruising, 252
congenital conditions, 252, 253f, 256f
connective tissue disorders, 254
cultural practices, 255
hematologic conditions, 254-255, 255f
hypersensitivity syndromes, 253, 253f
ink/dye staining, 256
maculae ceruleae, 256
oncological conditions, 255
photodermatitis, 255-256
topical chemical application, 256
valsalva effect, 256
vasculitic disorders, 253-254
conditions confused with burns, 256-257
accidental burns, 257, 257f
chemical burns, 257
cultural practices, 257
dermatological conditions, 256-257, 256f
infections, 256-257
dermatological conditions, 252-256
pigmentation disorders, 252-253
introduction, 252-258
Slater, S., 155
Sleevelike hymen, 70, 71f
SMR. *See* Sexual maturity rating
Smurthwaite, D., 284
SNAP. *See* Supplemental Nutritional Assistance
Program
SNP loci. *See* Single nucleotide polymorphisms
SOCAN. *See* Section on Child Abuse and Neglect
Social networking sites, 142-143
Socially disadvantaged families, 37
Socioeconomic status (SES), 7
Soft tissue injury complications, 250
Sognnaes, Reidar, 581
SORAG. *See* Sex Offender Risk Appraisal Guide
Specificity, 4-5
Speculum examination, 66-67
Spinal cord injury without radiographic abnormality
(SCIWORA), 12, 397, 399
Spine biomechanics, 396
Spitz, René, 547
Srisurapanont, M., 531
SSRIs. *See* Serotonin reuptake inhibitors
Stanley, D., 293
Staphylococcus aureus, 96
Starling, S. P., 369
Statutory rape. *See* Adolescent sexual assault/statutory
rape
Staudt, M. M., 486

STEP. *See* Systematic Training for Effective Parenting
Stephenson, T., 242
Stereotypes, 8. *See also* Implicit biases
Stevens-Johnson syndrome, 226
Stewart, D., 536
Stigmatization, 463
STIs. *See* Sexually transmitted infections
Stolfi, A., 233
Stower, M. J., 287
STR loci. *See* Short tandem repeats
Strait, R. T., 290
Strangulation, 394-395, 394f. *See also* Asphyxia
Stratified sampling strategy, 7
Strength of evidence
abdominal/chest injuries in abused children, 331
abusive burns, 236
AHT, 356-357
bacterial sexually transmitted infections in children,
176-177
biochemical markers of AHT in children, 437-438
brain development, effects of abuse/neglect on, 522
cost of child maltreatment, 639
drug screening in infants/children, 568
ear/nose/throat injuries in abused children, 335
in epidemiology of CSA, 21
in epidemiology of IPV, 26
eye injuries in child abuse, 410
forensic dentistry, 584
for forensic evidence kit, 110-111
FTT, 560
genital/anal findings conditions confused with sexual
abuse, 103-104
HIV/AIDS in child/adolescent victims of sexual
abuse/assault, 190
imaging AHT, 426
imaging skeletal trauma in abused children, 305
on impact of child abuse/neglect, 8-9
interviewing caregivers of suspected child abuse
victims, 58
laboratory methods for diagnosing STIs in children/
adolescents, 203-204
neck/spinal cord injuries in child abuse, 399
psychological impact/treatment of children who
witness domestic violence, 511-512
psychological impact/treatment of CPA, 485-486
psychological impact/treatment of sexual abuse of
children, 473
in tests to analyze forensic evidence in child sexual
abuse/assault, 116
viral/parasitic sexually transmitted infections in
children, 184
Streptococcus pneumonia, 96
Streptococcus pyogenes, 96
Stressful life events, 491
Strich, S. J., 420
Strouse, P. J., 284
Stuart, G. L., 501-502
Sturge-Weber syndrome, 252
Sturm, L., 552
Sty, J. R., 383
Subarachnoid hemorrhage (SAH), 415f, 417
Subdural hemorrhage (SDH), 364-365, 374, 380,
415-417, 415f-417f
Substance abuse, child abuse and
common illegal substances, 529-531
cocaine, 530-531
heroin, 531
marijuana, 529-530
common legal substances, 531-532
alcohol, 531-532
prescription substances for non medical use, 532
drug treatment/family disruption, 535
historical background, 529
impact of parental on children, 532-535
addiction/parenting, 534
children's behavior, 534-535
home environment in substance-abusing families,
533
parental incarceration, 535
parental mental health, 534
pregnancy, 532-533
social stressors, 533-534
interventions for children of substance abusers, 536
scope of problem, 529
among child-rearing population, 529

Substance abuse, child abuse and *(Continued)*
limitations of available data, 529
during pregnancy, 529
screening in health care setting, 535
adolescents, 535
infancy/early childhood, 535
parental visits, 535
school-aged children, 535
solutions for parents, 535-536
effective drug treatment, 536
FTDCs, 536
ineffective approaches, 536
treatment for pregnant women, 536
Substance Abuse and Mental Health Service
Administration (SAMHSA), 473, 481
Substance abuse/dependence, 467
Substances cited in DFSA, 119t, 120-122
1,4-BD, 122
amphetamines/methamphetamines, 121-122
benzodiazepines, 120-121
cannabis, 121
cocaine, 121
flunitrazepam, 120-121
GBL, 122
GHB, 122
Sudden infant death syndrome (SIDS), 337-339. *See
also* Asphyxia
autopsy findings, 338
conclusion, 343
definitions/epidemiology, 337
differentiation from asphyxia, 342-343
disorders mimicking, 338-339
introduction, 337-343
risk factors, 337-338
triple risk hypothesis, 338
Sudikoff, S., 227
Sugar, N. F., 84, 244, 247-248
Suh, D. Y., 374-375
Summit, Roland, 462, 464
Sun, A. P., 536
Superficial C/Ls, 418, 418f
Supplemental Nutritional Assistance Program (SNAP),
558
Supportive therapy, 470
Surgical castration, 162
Swischuk, L. E., 310-311
Symptom-focused therapy, 469-470
Systematic Training for Effective Parenting (STEP),
482

T

Tanzer, R. C., 446
Tardieu, Ambroise Auguste, 461
Taylor, A. S., 339
Taylor, M. T., 289
TBBD. *See* Temporary brittle bone disease
TBI. *See* Traumatic brain injury
Teicher, M. H., 518
Temporary brittle bone disease (TBBD), 271-272
Tests to analyze forensic evidence in child sexual
abuse/assault. *See also* DNA testing
analysis of bodily fluids, 112-114
blood, 113
saliva, 113-114
semen/sperm, 112-113
clinical considerations, 115
directions for future research, 116
introduction, 112-116
legal issues, 115-116
strength of medical evidence, 116
trace evidence, 114-115
analysis, 114
associations, 114
DNA testing, 115
epithelial cells, 115
locating, 114
tools, 114
transfer, 114-115
types, 114
Text messaging, 142
TF-CBT. *See* Trauma-focused CBT
Thakur, B. K., 253
Thermal burns, 223-226, 225f-226f, 225t, 231t

Thevasagayam, M. S., 392
Thibault, L. E., 365, 367
Third National Health and Nutrition Examination
Survey III (NHANES III), 65, 147, 553
Third National Incidence Study (NIS-3), 29
Thomas, S. A., 290
Thombs, B. D., 229
Titus, M. O., 224
Toluidine dye, 109
Townsend, C. W., 441
Trauma narrative, 471
Trauma Symptom Checklist for Children (TSC-C), 63,
479-480
Trauma-focused CBT (TF-CBT), 470
Trauma-related coagulopathy, 442-443
Traumatic brain injury (TBI), 349, 422-423, 423f
AHT *vs.*, 434
animal models of pediatric, 360-361
mechanics, 359
understanding, 370
Traumatic sexualization, 463
Trichomonas vaginalis (TV), 182-183
associated diseases, 183
identifying, 182
risk factors, 182
screening, 183
specimen collection, 201-202
symptoms, 183
testing, 183
transmission, 182-183
treatment, 183
Triple risk hypothesis, 338
True negative, 4, 4f
True positive, 4, 4f
TSC-C. *See* Trauma Symptom Checklist for Children
Tufts, E., 288
Turner syndrome, 148
TV. *See* Trichomonas vaginalis
Twentyman, C. T., 31

U

Udwin, O., 495
Ultrasonography, 308-309, 309f-310f
UN. *See* United Nations
UN Children's Fund (UNICEF), 134
UN Convention on the Elimination of All Forms of
Discrimination against Women, 139
UN Convention on the Rights of the Child, 139
UN Study on Violence against Children, 140
Unclassified sudden infant death (USID), 337
UNICEF. *See* UN Children's Fund
Uniformed Code of Military Justice, 163-164
United Nations (UN), 134
United Nations Population Fund (UNPF), 134
Universal Declaration of Human Rights, 139
UNPF. *See* United Nations Population Fund
Ureterocele, 99, 99f
Urethral prolapse, 98-99, 98f
medical management, 99
resembling HPV, 98-99, 98f
treatment, 99
uncommon in girls, 98
USID. *See* Unclassified sudden infant death

V

Vadivelu, R., 287
Vagina, 69
Vaginal septum, 70-71, 71f
Valsalva effect, 256
Van der Kolk, B., 465-466
Van Rijn, R. R., 398
Variable number tandem repeats (VNTR loci),
112-113
Varicocele, 80
Velangi, S. S., 239
Venereal Disease Research Laboratory, 203
Venous congestion, 79
Verma, S. K., 394
Victim access by child molesters, 157-159
choosing to interests, 157
coercion, 158

Victim access by child molesters *(Continued)*
common characteristics, 157-158
digital evidence, 159
grooming, 158
molester's home decor, 158-159
planning, 157
pressured sex, 158
secrecy, 158
targeting, 157
Vigliano, A., 235
Vinchon, M., 384, 445
Violence against women, 23
Viral transport media (VTM), 200
Viral/parasitic sexually transmitted infections in
children, 179
directions for future research, 184
hepatitis, 180-181
HAB, 180-181
HAV, 180
HCV, 179, 181
HDV, 181
HEV, 181
HGV, 181
sexual assault/abuse and, 181
HPV, 179-180, 182
HSV, 181-182
MCV, 182
pediculosis, 183
scabies, 183
strength of medical evidence, 184
summary, 183-184
TV, 182-183
Virginity test, 131
*The Visual Diagnosis of Non-Accidental Trauma and Failure to
Thrive*, 615
Vitamin A intoxication, 265
Vitamin C deficiency, 265
Vitamin D, 263-265
biochemical changes in rickets, 264
deficiency, 263-264
deficiency manifestations, 264
fractures, 264-265
metabolic cause of rickets, 264
metabolism, 263-265
rickets diagnosis, 264
sources, 263
treatment of rickets, 264
Vitamin K deficiency, 441-442
VNTR loci. *See* Variable number tandem
repeats
Vogeley, E., 219
Von Garrel, T., 286
von Willebrand disease (vWD), 442
VTM. *See* Viral transport media
vWD. *See* von Willebrand disease

W

Walsh, C., 534
Waltzman, M. L., 289-290
Warren, Joseph, 579
Warrington, S. A., 570
Waskeritz, S., 254
Waterlow, J. C., 557
Weekly Report of Abuse Indicators (WRAI), 479
Wells, R. G., 383
Wesley, N. O., 240
Weston, J. A., 552
Wheeler, Etta Angell, 628
Whiplash shaken infant syndrome, 364, 426
Whitaker, D. J., 484
Whitby, E. H., 445
White, C., 84
White, S. T., 76
WHO. *See* World Health Organization
Widom, C. S., 497
Wilbur, M. B., 535
Wilcox, W. D., 548
Will, Jonathan, 602
Willging, J. P., 392, 395
Williamson, D. M., 290
Wilson, E. F., 242
Wilson, Mary Ellen, 615, 628
Winek, C. L., 228-229

Wolak, J., 143, 154
Wood, J., 327
Wood's lamp, 109, 219, 243-244
World Fit for Children, 140
World Health Assembly, 138
World Health Organization (WHO), 23, 134, 203, 210, 553, 620
    Consultation on Child Abuse Prevention, 620
World Medical Association, 138
Worlock, P., 276, 284-285, 287, 290
WRAI. *See* Weekly Report of Abuse Indicators
Wright, C. M., 550, 570

X

X-linked hypophosphatemic rickets, 263

Y

Yordan, E. E., 73-74
Yordan, R. A., 73-74
Young, K. L., 110
Young, N. K., 529
Youth relationships project, 510

Z

Zhu, S. J., 399
Zito, J. L., 287
Ziv, N., 308-309
Zolotar, A., 35
Zubair, M., 229-230
Zubuchen, P., 256

Printed and bound by CPI Group (UK) Ltd, Croydon, CR0 4YY

08/05/2025

01864794-0004